This is the best book ever written and published on the subject of dental medicine. It encompasses the history along with a practical approach for dental implants and gives answers to many questions any doctor in private practice needs to know. It is a must for every dentist, oral surgeon, plastic surgeon, and otolaryngologist.

Dr. Borko B. Djordjevic is the editor, publisher, and translator of the original publication.
Prof. Borko B. Djordjevic, M.D. Ph.D., F.I.C.S., F.A.A.C.S.
Diplomat American Board of Cosmetic Surgery Miloja Djaka 46, 1100 Belgrade, Serbia
E-Mail: borkomd@gmail.com
Web: timelessbeauty.com
App: DrBorkoPS
Tel: (760) 880-7558

A special thanks to Roberta Kaufman, who spent countless hours assisting in the editing and translation of this book from Serbian to English.

I dedicate this book to those who have supported me the most.

First of all, I am especially indebted to my parents, because they are the founders of all that I have achieved through their great sacrifices, and because they have left me a legacy of creative spirit and perseverance to achieve the desired goals through work.

I am grateful to my beloved, patient, persevering, and devoted wife, Mary, for her understanding, for putting in a lot of effort to accompany me in my endeavors, and who is significant for a greater part of my life.

I am also grateful to my children who have supported me by rewarding me with their own successes based on true values.

I am grateful to my sister Radmila, who has always been very supportive in everything I do and encouraged me the most to leave a written trace of my creativity.

I also dedicate this book to my brother Savo, a talented dental technician who was one of the first in Yugoslavia to perform prosthetic work on implants.

Blažo Zlopaša

ORAL IMPLANTOLOGY

PRINCIPLES AND PRACTICE

BELGRADE 2025

Oral Implantology

ISBN: 978-1-967421-47-3 (Hardcover)

ISBN: 978-1-967421-48-0 (Paperback)

ISBN: 978-1-967421-49-7 (Ebook)

Contents

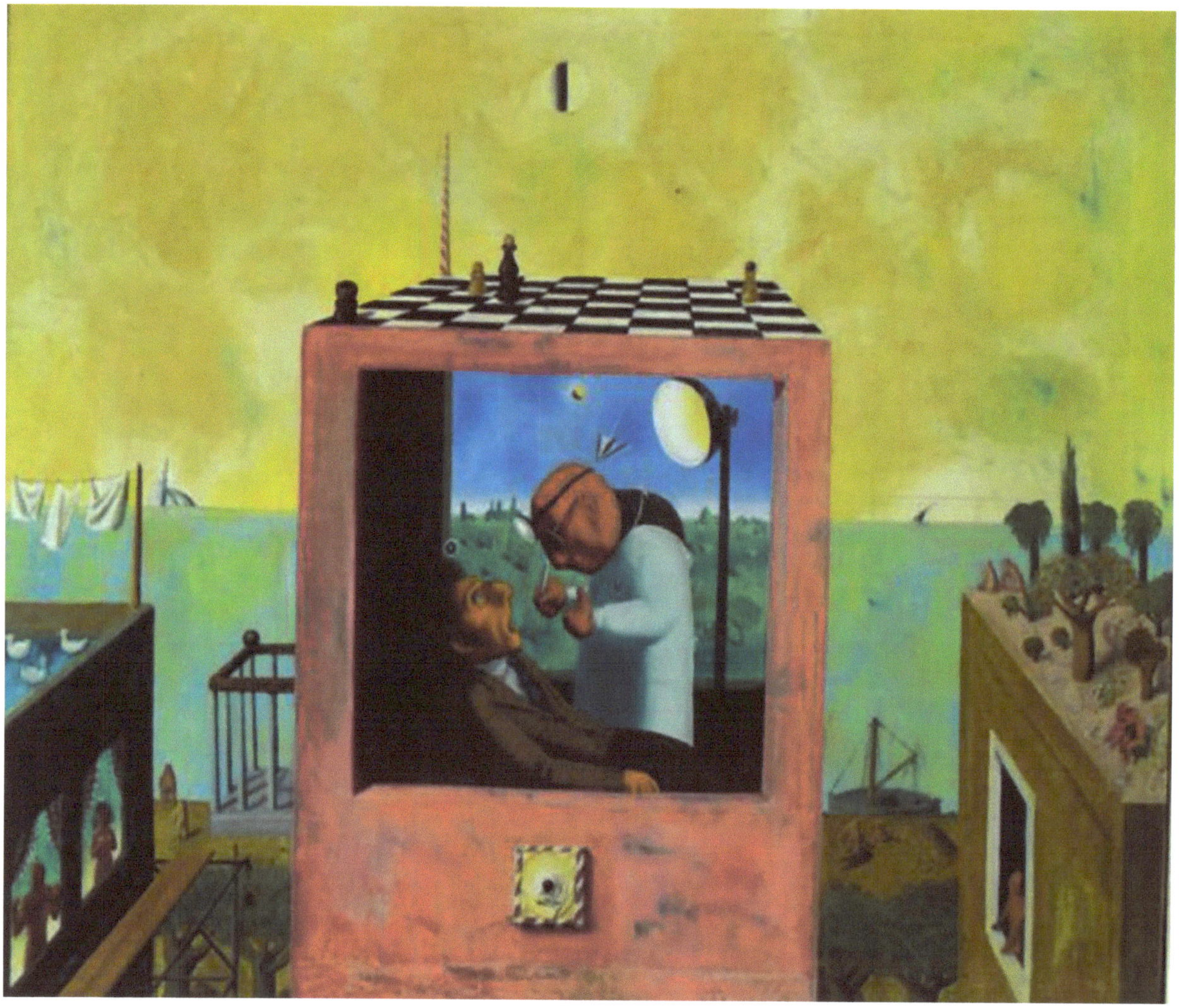

The best way not to make mistakes is to gain experience, and the best way to gain experience is to learn from your own mistakes. The purpose of life is not to live forever, but to create something that will live on after us. The best use of life is to create something that will remain after life. Experience is something that cannot be given as a gift. But it can be a valuable gift, like this one from the famous painter Voja Stanić to the author of this book. An inexhaustible source of knowledge is experience, and it only helps to notice a mistake when we repeat it. The experience was my mentor, constantly influencing the original part of me, which was enthusiastic, idealistic, and questioning.

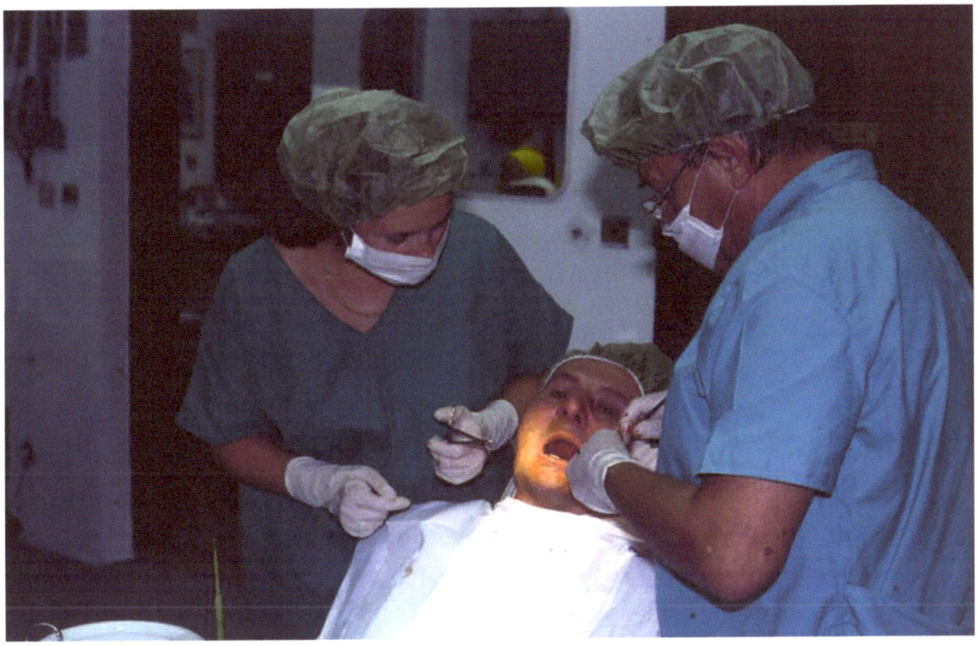

I owe the greatest gratitude to my life companion and co-worker, my wife Maria, who is the foundation of all my wishes and achievements. He who early discovers a spring with clear water, drinks healthy and clear water all his life.

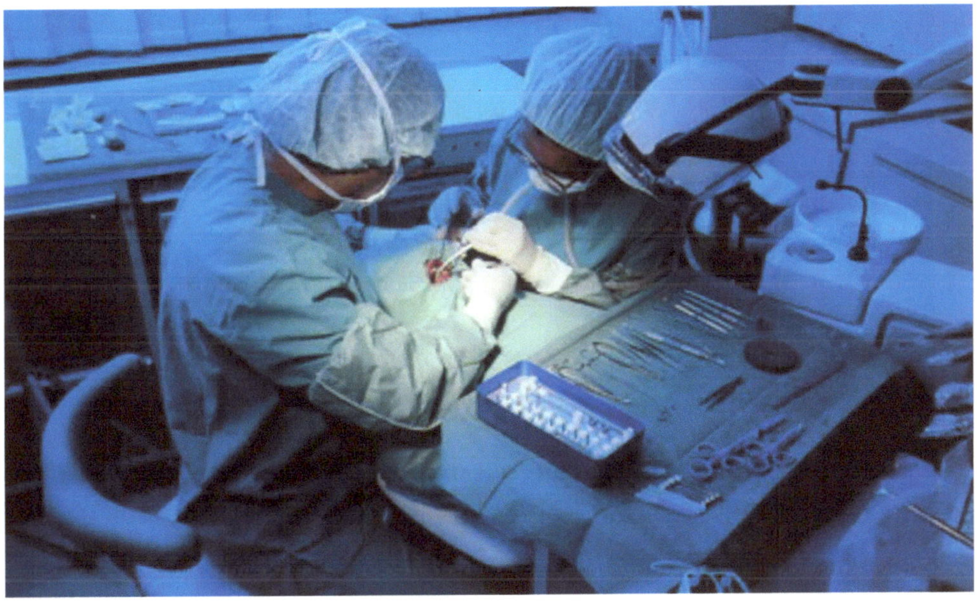

He who knows how to lay a solid foundation from the bricks that others have thrown at him is successful. Instead of aiming directly for success, focus on what you do, what you believe in, and what you love. Success will come by itself, and failure is success if we learn something from it. To succeed, one must learn from failure to know what not to do. But failure must not kill enthusiasm. Enthusiasm is the driving force that leads to success.

DR BLAŽO ZLOPAŠA AS A PROMETHEUS IN DENTAL IMPLANTOLOGY

When Dr. Blažo Zlopaša attended dental meetings in Yugoslavia sometime in the early 70s, we had a chance to learn about the European stomatology achievement firsthand. Dr. Zlopaša occasionally came from Switzerland and brought brilliant slides of his prosthetic works which caused the admiration of young colleagues, the delight of enthusiasts and, it should also be said, the envy of some distinguished experts.

After his return to Yugoslavia, Dr. Zlopaša opened a prestigious doctor's office in Cavtat near Dubrovnik, probably because private medical practice was only allowed in Croatia then.

Dr. Zlopaša, who was highly educated and experienced in the West, introduced the possibilities of modern dentistry to the Yugoslav public. This significantly encouraged dental experts across Yugoslavia to take an interest in the latest achievements in dental prosthetics and implantology.

The current generations of young dentists aren't familiar with "socialist prosthetics", which lagged behind European prosthetics by several decades. Such a situation can primarily be attributed to the population's financial resources, low health culture, and "staticity" of experts at Yugoslav dental faculties who prioritize the form in order of acquiring flattering titles. Dr. Zlopaša "chased" the essence in the profession, which brought him a great professional reputation, especially as a pioneer of implantology in Yugoslavia. The beginning of oral implantology, not only in Yugoslavia, but also in the Balkans, is related to the name of Dr. Blažo Zlopaša. It is known that the level of our profession in the socialist countries was below that of Yugoslavia. For this reason, Dr. Zlopaša's pioneering role crossed the borders of Yugoslavia.

Not even Dr. Zlopaša escaped the fate of the pioneering enterprise. Popularity and success aroused envy, so this "pioneer" of implantology and ceramic prosthetics felt a lot of bitter moments. That is why he lectured more at professional and scientific meetings on implantology abroad, where he found understanding and support. The Promethean spirit of Dr. Zlopaša did not get defensive. At numerous dental meetings, he presented his methods and the work he successfully performed. He successfully followed the achievements of his profession on the world stage. He participated in congresses abroad and brought with him the spirit of world dentistry. The devastating fact is that the "respectable" professors never invited him to lecture to the students. It is part of our mentality, and also the fate of Promethean spirits. Today's dentistry in Serbia, but also other parts of the former Yugoslavia, can also be grateful to Dr. Zlopaša for keeping up with modern European dentistry in prosthetics and oral implantology.

Even when writing this book, he remained true to himself by putting substance before form. The one who succeeds in turning essence into form is an artist. I think Dr. Zlopaša succeded in achieving that in this book.

In more than 650 pages of richly illustrated book, the author presented all aspects of this newest branch of dental medicine. In the 22 chapters of the manuscript, there is a historical overview, the anatomical foundation of the jaw region, materials and implant design, surgical techniques, indications, and contraindications for implant placement, as well as an important chapter on peri-implant infections.

The book continuously explains how to approach patients undergoing implant surgery from a psychological perspective. It is considered the best literature on implants in Serbian language.

The author talks about his pioneering venture of propagating this method on the territory of the SFRY during five decades of work, as well as about implants in dentistry, about which little was known in the Balkans at the time, and it can be said also in the world. The leaders were enthusiastic pioneers, curious people, among whom is the author of this book.

The book is written clearly with a rich lexicon both from the professional field and the literary treasury.

The systematization of the chapters introduces the cautious expert-dentist into the "secrets" of implantology, pitfalls and misconceptions, successes and possible failures.

This book can be classified as a rich medical literature, of the "PRACTICE FOR PRACTICE" type. It should be emphasized that Dr. Zlopaša is an implantologist who practiced abroad, and started in Switzerland, where the parameters of success are extremely delicate. From the book, it is documented that the beginnings of his interest in implantology are right there. It could be said that Dr. Zlopaša's book is "imported knowledge" that he selflessly, and widely offered to dental practice in Serbia and the former Yugoslavia.

The special value of the book are numerous illustrations from the author's photo library, which testify to the undoubted success of the methods and materials that the author prefers. The book certainly represents literature that every dentist should have in his library. According to all criteria of the value of professional literature, this book deserves social support for printing and publication.

Academician med. Dr. Vladimir Jokanović, member of the Croatian Academy of Medical Sciences and member of the Serbian Academy of Med. science

It is known that the human desire and the attempt to implant teeth dates back to the Incas and the Aztecs in Central and South America, as well as Ancient Egypt. The first written communication by Andrews in 1894 confirms that oral implantology is as old as dental science.

In the 70s of the last century, very little was known and written about dental implantation in our Yugoslav territories. The achieved experimental and clinical results related to the replacement of teeth by implantation of different types of implants have been presented more and more often in the developed European countries. It was during those seventies that a creative-inventive, one could say artistic and manually virtuoso nature appeared in one doctor - a dentist.

His name is Blažo Zlopaša, an oral surgeon - an implantologist, who began implementing the latest European and global achievements in oral implantology with his patients in his private practice in Cavtat, Republic of Croatia. It can be freely said that his contribution to the later increasing prevalence of tooth implantation in other parts of Yugoslavia at the time was enormous and unparalleled.

Dr. Zlopaša had many opponents in our region who went so far as to call this pioneering enterprise vivisection. He stoically and argumentatively resisted the attacks at expert meetings, because he based his work on knowledge of Bronnemark's published postulates on osseointegration. Later, in the nineties of the last century, even the biggest critics of these procedures accepted and implanted implants by consulting and carefully listening to Dr. Zlopaša's lectures at expert meetings.

The book Oral Implantology - Principles and Practice, written by our contemporary, Dr. Blažo Zlopaša, greatly contributes to the already scarce literature in these areas. The book is written in understandable language and is richly illustrated with pictures of many patients for whom Dr. Zlopaša made implants and prostheses in the most modern way. Vast clinical experience is presented in this book and it will be a good guide for young dentists - beginners in the field of oral implantology. For those with experience in this field, it will be a benchmark for their work and results. I do not see that the book is intended to be a textbook for dental students, but I am convinced that all dental graduates, specialists, and postgraduates should have this book in their professional literature. Dr. Zlopaša is the authentic creator of all chapters, written according to the highest criteria, which makes this book one of the most comprehensive manuals in this area in our region.

It is almost unimaginable that an oral surgeon-implantologist like Dr. Blažo Zlopaša would not be listed as the progenitor in this field of dental profession and science. It is necessary to emphasize that Dr. Zlopaša has an artistic and visionary spirit and a geometrical gift at the first level of ethics. That is why Dr. Blažo Zlopaša entered the gallery of the first great creative minds of oral implantology in the former Yugoslavia.

Prof. Asen Džolev, PhD,
full professor, maxillofacial surgeon

The book "Oral Implantology: Principles and Practice" is a well-designed and unique book aimed at passing on the experiences and knowledge of one of the founders of implantology to younger generations in our region and beyond. In today's dental profession, implantology is seen as an essential part, but it's important not to forget the journey this branch of dentistry has taken over the last few decades. This journey has allowed today's generations to have access to and acquire the skills and techniques needed for replacing lost teeth, including the use of dental implants.

Dr. Blažo Zlopaša is one of the pioneers of implantology in the former Yugoslavia and undoubtedly a colleague with the richest scientific and clinical experience in this field. Having decided to invest invaluable effort and write this book, he also decided to share his vast knowledge and experience with everyone who continues on this path, which is the key importance of this reading. **The book in front of you not only provides a comprehensive historical overview of the development of implantology, but also addresses many important topics and issues in contemporary implantology. The author has successfully achieved his main goal in both of these aspects. This work is well-organized and structured, covering expertly selected topics, offering an overview of all aspects of dental implantology. It starts with a historical overview and basic definitions, then moves on to different treatment options, limitations, complications, and includes a review of cases with very long follow-up times. and complications, to a review of cases with extremely long follow-up times.**

Each chapter represents a complete study dedicated to one topic or therapeutic approach. In addition, through the presentation of a large number of cases treated by the author personally, this book not only captivates with information but also with recommendations, ideas, and "tricks" for successful implant therapy. Given that it is written interestingly and understandably, without losing expertise and analyticity, the manuscript aims to enrich the reader with new ideas, encourage reflection, and invite dialogue, rather than simply aiming to please or persuade.

In Belgrade, November 5, 2016.
Prof. Zoran Aleksić, Ph.D

It is a great honor and pleasure for me that the author of this extraordinary book has entrusted me with the responsible task of objectively presenting his professional life's work.

In my professional career, I reviewed many papers published in well-known peer-reviewed journals in America and Europe. I was always very strict and demanded a precise scientific and methodological approach. This book, or the author of the book, disarmed me. I knew the author of this book before as a prominent pioneer of oral implantology in the former Yugoslavia. I listened to his lectures at several domestic and international congresses. Those lectures, in terms of content and topics, were always something new, but at the time, they were also unacceptable to most of the authorities in dentistry at that time. I knew he was writing this book and had been writing it for many years. Knowing the overall professional, scientific, intellectual, creative, artistic, and manual qualities of the author, I believed that it would be a very good, practical book. But, as I said, the author disarmed me about possible objections, the content, conception, results, illustrations, creativity, comprehensiveness, topicality, and overall quality of the book. Everything mentioned above is presented precisely, to the right extent, in an excellent style, nothing is vague. It can be said that this book has practically no flaws.

Although the material covered in the book is exclusively of a manual, artisanal nature, as it is generally thought, the author denied such an opinion and showed that oral implantology is, above all, a biological, medical specialty. Throughout the chapters, the author highlights the biological aspects of tissue and the biomechanical problems associated with implants, prosthetic superstructures, and the procedures he describes and applies. In Chapter 11, the biological aspects of living tissue and the biomechanical influences on implants and prosthetic augmentation are described in detail, with a warning of potential failure if these details are neglected. The book aims to explain the essence of oral implantology, which involves joining living tissue with inanimate foreign matter to restore lost functions of a part of the organism, using scientific knowledge from several natural sciences.

About this relatively narrow surgical field, 20 chapters have been written, in a voluminous text of 600 pages. The entire text consists of numerous theoretical and practical details, no part of the text is "empty", or redundant. Several chapters, with certain conceptual changes, could represent a separate book or a more extensive scientific work in a scientific journal. By presenting different concrete cases, the author showed how it is possible to solve many complicated and complex cases in oral implantology and major bone defects, raising the maxillary sinus, reconstruction of soft tissues, prevention, and overcoming serious complications. For such results, it is necessary to have great medical and dental knowledge, extraordinary observation, intellectual and manual dexterity, faith in oneself, faith in the almost impossible. It also presents data on the effectiveness of different bone substitutes and addresses the use of oral implants in young individuals. The chapter is a biological study and a responsible approach to an unfamiliar subject. Additionally, it delves into the risks associated with oral implantology, including risk factors, errors, consequences of risks and mistakes, iatrogenic tissue damage, prevention of errors and complications, and procedures for resolving them. Detailed attention is given to peri-implant infections, which are common yet serious complications in oral implantology. Dr. Zlopaša finds solutions even for unsolvable cases, he never gives up.

The book discusses indications, general and local contraindications for implant placement in detail. A significant part of this chapter is dedicated to "psychogenic pain" in dentistry and implantology, the causes and consequences of pain, as well as the doctor's attitude towards such patients. It is noticeable that the author, a dentist, has an excellent knowledge of medicine and basic medical sciences and strictly adheres to them in his work. An entire chapter is devoted to tooth occlusion, which is of great importance for the durability of implants. All aspects and details of dental occlusion, which are important in all dental disciplines, especially in implantology, are covered in detail through the text and numerous, original sketches. This chapter is a serious scholarly study.

Chapter 17 is titled "The Return of the Smile, Security and Self-confidence". Of all living beings only man is rewarded with a smile, as the author of this book says. The chapter features happy, smiling patients following the successful surgical and prosthetic work of Dr. Zlopaša. Chapter 18, "Conversation with a Colleague", has 150 pages, and it is something unusual, and original for a textbook. It is a virtual conversation about implantology by the author with an insufficiently knowledgeable colleague, in which the author answers essential questions related to oral implantology. It is a book within a book. Namely, this chapter goes through the entire implantology again with new text, new knowledge, new explanations, new cases, new photos, and sketches, and completes and expands the knowledge gained from the previous ones. Chapters 19 and 20 focus on conversations and contracts with patients, providing valuable insights into how a wise doctor deals with a patient. Certainly a useful guide for all doctors, especially beginners.

All chapters present important details of all aspects of oral implantology. Many different cases are presented, which, according to the stages of operation and treatment, are illustrated with numerous excellent photos and sketches. Practically, the author has connected contemporary findings from oral implantology, his decades of experience, and the results of that experience into one extraordinary book. The book by Dr. Blažo Zlopaša, a prominent figure inSerbian, Yugoslav, and European dentistry, is a unique professional and scientific work. It is at the same time an excellent scientific monograph, an outstanding atlas in the field of oral implantology, and an excellent, practical, comprehensive textbook, indispensable for those who intend to master oral implantology, a very demanding discipline of dentistry and surgery, which requires extensive knowledge of medicine and dentistry, mobility, intelligence, conscience, power of observation, manual dexterity.

Prof. Radmilo Rončević, Ph.D
maxillofacial and plastic surgeon

In my many years of work, I have conducted numerous presentations and reviews of professional and scientific studies, as well as many books, monographs, atlases, and other dental research. I am pleased to note at the outset of this review that I have never encountered anything quite like Dr. Blažo Zlopaša's book: "ORAL IMPLANTOLOGY - PRINCIPLES AND PRACTICE".

It is a great creation, which is the result of enormous effort and well-thought-out work of this pioneer of Serbian implantology. 1968 was a long time ago! Then the young dentist Blažo Zlopaša realized something that many much older, more experienced professors of the faculty did not understand, and some did not even want to accept: that dental implantology will very soon become one of the pearls of the dental profession and science. That happened in just a few decades. It must be admitted that, apart from the famous professor Leonard Linkov and a small group of enthusiasts, almost no one had this vision of the development and rapid progress of implantology. However, the Serbian visionary Dr. Blažo Zlopaša did.

Dr. Zlopaša wrote the book ORAL IMPLANTOLOGY for decades! Many colleagues, including myself, encouraged him to finish the book so it could be accessible to the professional public. However, Dr. Blažo, being the perfectionist he is, constantly added to and improved the book, causing delays in its publication. Finally, the book has been published to the satisfaction of everyone /if he did not "enrich" the book and constantly add something. Of course, this is all useful and "raises" the level of the book, but decades passed, and the book never appeared. Now she appeared and to the general satisfaction.

The book ORAL IMPLANTOLOGY is written in a rather unusual way for writing textbooks and professional books. In the book, the author presents his many decades of personal experience in the installation of implants and prosthetic care of edentulous patients. He does this thoroughly and perseveringly, looking objectively at the numerous problems that await every dentist who tries to deal with this complex branch of our profession. It is worth highlighting the huge number of examples from his office, with high-quality illustrations and displays in the form of X-rays and photographs of the condition before, during, and after the treatment of hundreds of patients. Dr. Zlopaša honestly expresses his dilemmas and problems, which he encountered and continues to during treatment. In this, he is very critical and often puts the reader on the task of how to solve some of the complex problems with implants. His critiques of professional and scientific studies by other authors, including highly respected professors in this field, are very interesting and high-quality.

All areas are covered comprehensively in this book, but the following are particularly impressive: indications and contraindications for the installation of implants, implantological treatment of young people, and especially the very instructive chapter CONVERSATION WITH A PATIENT, as well as DISCUSSION WITH A COLLEAGUE. Of the 20 chapters in the book, the mentioned areas should be highlighted, because, in many implantology textbooks, they are missing or are given only in indications. It is very impressive how Dr. Zlopaša treated the temporomandibular joint, with a series of explanations, and wonderful illustrations, with sections of the joint in various positions of the mandible, both in people without implants and in patients treated with prosthetic restorations on implants.

It is necessary to emphasize that the book by Dr. Blažo Zlopaša is written in beautiful language by a highly educated intellectual, who is also known as an excellent polemicist, and essayist, not only on professional but also on social situations. The sharpness of his observation and refined polemical spirit are therefore easily recognized in this beautiful work.

Some remarks are truly admirable. I am sure that many colleagues and patients will enjoy reading it.

I am sure that the book ORAL IMPLANTOLOGY - PRINCIPLES AND PRACTICE will be well received by the professional dental public. And not only with colleagues, who deal with implant placement but also with dental students, graduated dentists, and specialists of various disciplines of this branched medical field

Prof. Obrad B. Zelić, Ph.D
Periodontist

In the wide array of foreign and domestic literature on implantology, Dr. Blažo Zlopaša's book "Oral Implantology - Principles and Practice" is a valuable source of scientific and professional data combined with original and specific comments from the author's extensive dental and implantology experience. The special value of this book is given by its huge documentation (rarely seen in the world), which can serve for educational purposes and as an implantology atlas.

This book is important both for beginners, encouraging them and guiding them at the start of their implantology odyssey, and for experienced dentists, because it can offer them solutions to some implantology dilemmas. It is a reading that anyone dealing with implantology should have in their professional library.

The enthusiasm of Dr. Blažo Zlopaša, the progenitor and pioneer of oral implantology in this region, did not follow the known path. Instead, he chose an unknown path and left his mark in implantology practice and science.

Professor Smiljana Matić, Ph.D
oral surgeon-implantologist VMA

Today, there are many textbooks, but few books. There are many rules and many taboos.

This book is a journey through the experience of the doyen of dental implantology, which gives us the strength to reach the desired goal in our journey through implantology.

Science without practice is worthless, as well as practice without science. What unites them with a lot of moderation and honesty is given in this book, in clear language for both the beginner and the top dentist.

Professor Dr. Zoran Lazić Ph.D.
Head of the dental clinic of the VMA

Preface

Immortality exists; it is called knowledge!
Strive •to learn all your life, don't hesitate to ask, and don't be ashamed to admit your mistake!

Author

When a long journey through life has passed and the familiar autumn knocks at the door of working life, people need to take stock of their lives. When it comes to the medical profession, the question is added: How was my work, could I have done it better, differently? If a person is plagued by such questions, they will not admit that this is the end or the beginning of the end of their professional responsibility. When confronted with the end of the beginning, he has no choice but to repeatedly invoke Shakespeare's paradoxical thought that "youth comes after old age" This means never engaging in a passive strategy. Never give up.

There is another encouraging saying: "If something is not written down, it did not happen" - Verba volant, scripta manet, ars longa, vita brevis est! Perhaps in my case, personal pride required a significant effort to ensure that my work, professional experience, and life memories would not be forgotten. This compelled me to document my professional journey and the memories of my continuous efforts to pursue new knowledge in the field of oral implantology, without relying solely on clinical routine, despite its undeniable success in practice.

It was the most suitable way for me to collect the experiences of decades of work. Regardless of the passage of time, a person endures as long as they can continue to create. The decline of human creativity is associated with the end of the working age, as well as the increasing influence of the "biological clock." I believe that a person truly begins to age only when their curiosity and sense of purpose start to diminish.

This logical approach to life shows that the time for learning has always come when man wants to learn and thereby make the present better than the past. It is an attempt to correct the past. And to do so here and now to do better and best within the scope of one's own possibilities. It means being different in the present and for the sake of the future and the profession. Individual and creative strategy implies change. One should find what he missed in the past and do it better and differently in the present.

The intention to put on paper a summary of my professional activity, to record my thoughts and views on the profession is not recent. Daughter Tamara, the successor in dentistry, makes me happy and proud when I see with how much enthusiasm and love she does what her father did, and how she continues the family continuity. Here, I have crossed the fifth decade of practicing the profession to which I was devoted with great enthusiasm. It's still going on. When asked about the progress of my book, she recalls the early days of its conception with a humorous anecdote: "I remember being in Cavtat, just starting first grade. My dad was decorating a room, and when we asked what he was doing, my mom replied, 'He's starting to write a book.'" Yes, it's been a long time coming, but why the delay? I attribute it to the rapid pace of my professional growth and the demands it placed on my time. And here I am today, still in the midst of it.

The rapid development of oral implantology, it seems to me, went similarly to the development of mobile telecommunications today with new technologies. Who could write a book about all the types and models of mobile phones these days! Every time I tried to document my knowledge about implantology, I found that there were already new advancements and discoveries. It felt like trying to reach a rainbow - always just out of reach.

I didn't anticipate that creating the white paper would be more challenging than my medical work. As I reviewed, corrected, and documented my work each day, I realized that the field of oral implantology was changing faster and faster. Simply, practice and science in discovering new possibilities in oral implantology progressed faster than I could reliably follow and write down in designing and describing it all.

When God gave privileges to living creatures, He gave wings to birds and speech to man. It is all the more difficult to write words that would so fly in understanding what the man wanted to express and describe. This is what manifests itself as the complexity of life in which it is often much easier to do something than to describe what was done and how it was done in practical action. That written remains and is subject to the judgment of the majority. Describing an action takes as much time as performing it. However, the power of precise language, its clarity, and its purpose require not only theoretical education and practical knowledge, but also a broader understanding of physiology, anatomy, and psychology, which are crucial in all branches of medicine, including oral implantology.

Practice confirms both theory and science and they condition each other, but the best is the knowledge that comes from practice. Only good theory creates good practice. Good practice (practitioners) write good theory, because it is a theory of the realistically possible and achievable, not science fiction. Goethe wrote:

"Every theory, my son, is gray, the golden tree of life is green."

Any theory is just a dry word that indicates the path to follow. It is well known that many contingencies can be prevented on that road. Theory is the foundation of practice, and practice is like life. Life is usually not a journey to the desired destination, but all the unforeseen things that happen to us during the journey. A book that attempts to describe this can be a suitable read, not only for experts and students in this field, but also for other readers, e.g. for all those who want to research or think about the documentation offered or about the justification of the expressed views of the author, which, at the same time, does not prevent the right to an opposing opinion.

The right to a different opinion is always encouraging if we are freed from personal vanity. There were many opposing opinions when the author began to deal with oral implantology, showing the embedded endosseous implants, and acknowledging the opposing opinions as a challenge. The absence of different views and ideas, even if they were opposed, would slow down the progress of the profession.

When it comes to the concept of the book, certainly the author's approach to the presentation methodology could have been different. However, the realm of different approaches in presenting scientific and practical positions is unlimited, especially since practice challenges or confirms these positions. The author is deeply convinced that many of the views expressed are valid, because they are based on verification in practice, and behind this is the performance of successful work. Friedrich Nietzsche's statement: "That a gram of experience is more valuable than a load of theories", confirms the author's position that the book can be useful, as a product of practice and experience. There are also theoretical considerations to the extent that it is necessary to know to avoid risks. Albert Einstein says about the relationship between theory and practice: "Theory is when everything is known, but nothing works. Practice is when everything works, and no one knows why". The meaning of what is written is following the previously expressed thoughts.

It's important to acknowledge that there may have been mistakes in the development of ideas and the planned course of action. Failing to recognize or admit a mistake means being at risk of repeating it, which emphasizes the need for caution and provides an important lesson for future work. However, learning from these mistakes and making improvements, as demonstrated by the author's actions and descriptions, can lead to achieving better results for the patient.

A special presentation methodology has been established for writing professional books and textbooks. My goal is for the book to be different, more interesting, and thus more accessible for reading; to be different, precisely in the way that my views and attitudes about the future of the profession differed from those attitudes that fiercely challenged me.

Only when I started writing this book, did I realize that they, the authors of the textbook, also did a responsible and difficult job. I give them full recognition and gratitude.

Their skepticism and challenges to what I was saying, propagating, and doing as new in oral implantology, were the starting point and stimulus for me to persevere on the path I set out on. After all, any skepticism in science is the starting point for discovering real scientific truths. "Dubito, ergo sum!" (I doubt, therefore I exist!"

I didn't follow the required templates when writing textbooks. The content of the textbook presents facts, but lacks discussions and solutions to scientific dilemmas. I'm particularly focusing on physiology, as its explanations haven't been confirmed by practice to the extent that other fields have.

For example, it is still a big dilemma whether the installation of implants can be applied to young persons that is, to children and youth? Deepening the fundamental knowledge of anatomy and physiology, I ventured to think about it in a separate chapter.

The manner and methodology of writing the book were dictated by my experiences and practical work. I have always viewed my diploma of Doctor of Dentistry to be just an administrative entry into the professional world, and myself an eternal student devoted to the profession I chose as my life's vocation. I must admit that I was often forced to refresh my knowledge in certain areas as required by practice. For example, from anatomy, which I studied as a medical student at the University of Zagreb. However, it was necessary to renew that subject as soon as I started installing the first implants.

In the past, X-rays were not advanced enough to effectively plan oral surgeries, and the orthopantomography images were so unclear that implant installations seemed almost random. Therefore, it was necessary to update anatomical knowledge and have a detailed understanding of anatomical structures.

Probably, thanks to this attitude, I have not had any incidents in my long-term career, because risks and dangerous traps are constantly and unpredictably lurking. Dentists are exposed to those "traps" every day.

Today, many generations do not know how it used to be done and how oral implantology developed in the world and our country. I tried to describe that period with words and pictures.

I paid special attention to prosthetic care and occlusion of the temporomandibular joint due to various reasons based on my experience. The surgical procedure of installing the implant is only one part of the entire implant-prosthetic treatment. Practice has shown and confirmed that oral implantology is so interconnected with knowledge from basic biological disciplines.

To get closer to the reader and arouse his attention, but also to extract benefits and information from what was written, I came up with an "original" method that will supplement what was missed in the written chapters. Whether I managed to, through a virtual conversation "with a colleague" and "with a patient", or actually through my inner monologue, which represents the eternal unbroken questioning of an author truly dedicated to the profession, supplement what was missed, I leave it to the judgment of the reader. The reader will best answer the question of whether the book can also be useful as a textbook for supplementing the knowledge acquired and verified through practice.

In conclusion, I want to emphasize that I did not intend to write a book following the structure of textbooks and rigid consistency. Instead, I drew from my personal experiences, much like any author for whom the essence of the content takes precedence over the form. If the substance takes shape in any manner, and the form reflects the substance, then the book has achieved its purpose. When a person reaches the end of their journey, they are obligated to describe that journey, as is the motto of the book. Many doctors are unaware of what transpired on the path to oral implantology.

Hippocrates wrote: "A young doctor must know what others have discovered, examined and established before him!"

To be bold and very cautious at the same time is the art of success - Napoleon Bonaparte.

If with this book I managed to interest the readers, to help colleagues who seriously want to deal with or are already dealing with oral implantation, so that they can derive the benefit of knowledge from what is written, and especially avoid possible complications, then my invested effort has justified its goal.

AUTHOR

1

History of Oral Implantology

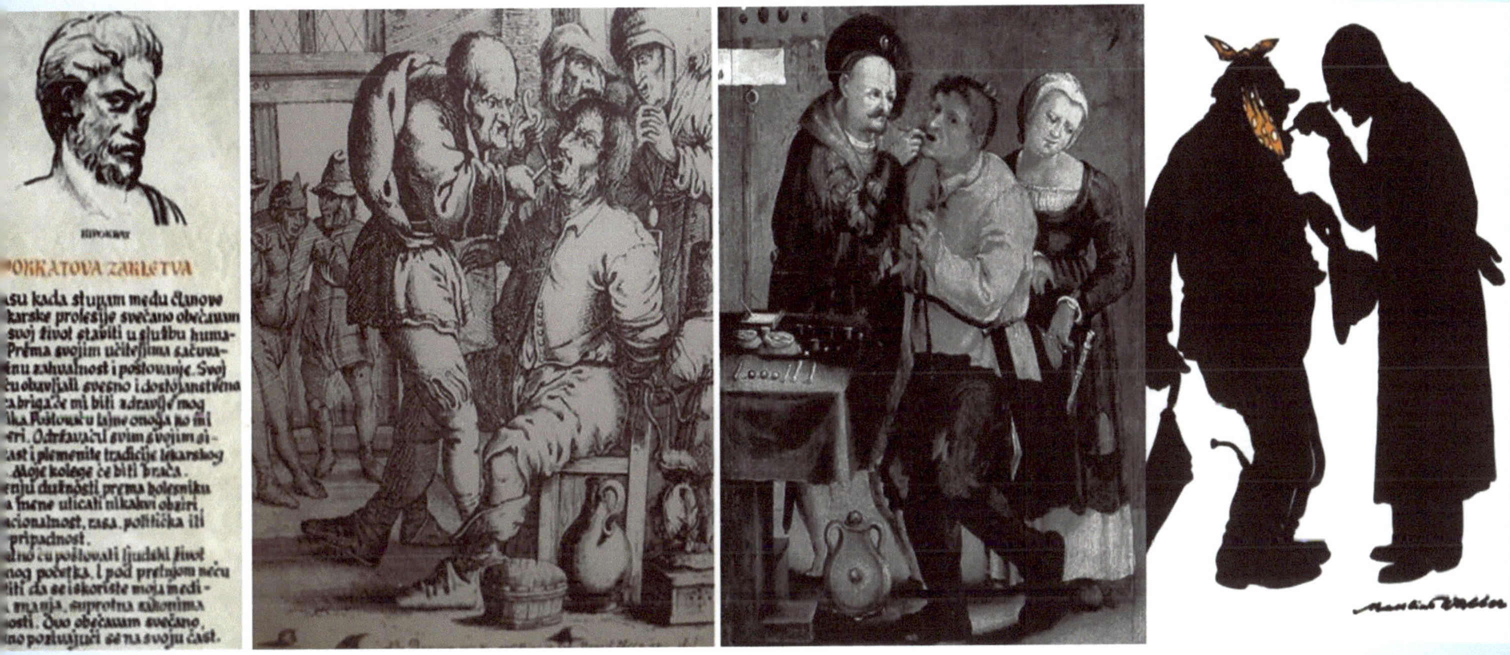

Thousands of years before Christ, people also cared about the "happenings" in their mouths. The first documented evidence says that 9,000 years ago, people used some primitive techniques, forerunners of today's, for dental procedures. In the archaeological site of Mehrgarh in Palestine, teeth with traces of a drill were found. Throughout history, people have used various ways to fill cavities in their teeth; teeth filled with precious metals, pieces of wood, shells, precious stones, etc. were found. It was not until the beginning of the 19th century that a mixture of mercury and various metals appeared to fill tooth cavities, and thus began the era of amalgam, which, despite new technologies, continues to this day. Around 500- 300 years before the Common Era, Hippocrates and Aristotle wrote about dental treatments, including the treatment of teeth and gums, tooth extraction, and the use of wires to stabilize loose teeth and mend broken jaws.

Seems that an attempt to replace a lost tooth is as old as man. According to recent findings, discovered at excavations in Honduras, it seems that implantology dates far back to the Neolithic Age. It is not known exactly when the first idea of compensating a lost tooth by inserting an object into the alveolus comes about. Some knowledge is obtained from archaeological excavations about the use of parts of some shells, bones, minerals, stones, and many objects of different materials. The development of implantology can be divided into several periods. From excavations in South America, it is known that the Inca and Mayan tribes (6000 BC) had artificial tooth roots made of quartz and bernstein and carved stone in the shape of teeth, which they inserted into the alveolus, to compensate for the loss of teeth.

The Chinese are trying to replace a lost tooth 3000 years before AD. e. The ancient Etruscans (2500 BC) are said to be the best dentists of the Old World based on the records found. They made partial dentures with gold crowns and bridges around 700 years before AD. e.The ancient Etruscans also pioneered the aesthetics of teeth, often made of ivory. Archaeological research on excavations proves that the ancient Greeks, Romans, Arabs, and members of various tribes in South America also tried to insert a foreign body ("implant") ...

It has been reported that the Indians in Central America were the first to insert stones carved in the shape of teeth directly into the wound. At Harvard University's Peabody Museum, a carved stone inserted into the lower jaw can be seen before the age of Columbus.

In addition to carved stones, various objects and materials were used to compensate for a lost tooth: by inserting ivory, gold, platinum, iridium, even lead, porcelain, and some type of acrylic. In one excavation, attempts were found to replace a lost tooth by imitating its shape made of some hardwood (most likely similar to yew or oak).

Records from medieval dentistry indicate that theories about gum disease began to emerge during this time. Dentists of that era believed that heat was the primary cause of tooth decay and deterioration. Preventive care for teeth was minimal; people accepted that their teeth would decay and eventually fall out. After losing their teeth, individuals sought various materials and objects to replace them. Initially, these replacements were primarily for cosmetic reasons, but as time progressed, there was an increasing demand for functional teeth, as these makeshift "teeth" often made it difficult to chew. Many had to remove them while eating due to their inadequate fit.

In the 16th and 17th centuries, the first prostheses were made from real natural teeth taken from another person and artificial teeth connected with silk thread. The dentists of that time inserted teeth of ivory or some larger animals into the dentures, shaping them in their own way. According to some historical records, the dehumanization of the profession for material reasons also began at that time; the "experts" of that time would acquire the "best quality" white teeth by extracting healthy teeth from the poor with a certain financial compensation and then making prostheses from those teeth for the rich.

The new owners, the rich patients, would be satisfied for a short time with such purchased teeth from the poor because the teeth fell out while eating. At every meal, the teeth would be found on the table or the plate of food. Because of this, the dentists had their hands full putting those teeth back into the prostheses.

In the Middle Ages, the first dental practice appeared - making teeth out of gold. The rich and nobles required their dentists to extract even healthy teeth and make them gold or cover healthy ones with gold crowns! In this way, they would emphasize their belonging to the upper layers of society.

Gold teeth were popular not only in the Middle Ages but also in the latter half of the 20th century. Typically, one or more healthy teeth were covered visibly in the upper jaw. In Europe, efforts to reconstruct lost teeth, including their roots, have been made for centuries.

The second period of development of implantology can be considered the period from 1809 to 1940, when enthusiastic dentists appeared whose first attempts were not successful, but were still a distant hint that something could happen in replacing lost teeth that would improve chewing.

Many emphasize today that we should remember the name of Adams from 1938, whose idea came closest to Branemark's much later idea.

The beginning of the 19th century represents the period when a small wave of a few enthusiasts started in Italy. In 1809, the Italian dentist Madolo applied the first dental implant, which was designed in the shape of a root and made of gold. Perhaps that was the first hint of the path oral implantology should take.

Eighty years later, in 1887, dentist Harris used a lead implant on which he placed a porcelain crown. At that time not enough thought was likely given, and perhaps not even known, about the toxicity of lead. The possible reason for resorting to this metal, which is toxic to the body, is most likely the ease of modeling it into the shape of a tooth root. Root molding with lead was applied in 1889 by dentists Harry and Grammy, to be "improved" by dentist Edmunds, because he did it from platinum, coated with lead in the shape of the root of the tooth.

All these attempts were unsuccessful. In explaining their failures, dentists attributed them to a lack of technique rather than the type of material used. Among the first significant advancements were the results of the Strock brothers from Boston in 1938 and 1939. In the fourth decade of the last century, Italian pioneer Formigini emerged as an influential figure in modern implantology. In 1947, he created a screw-shaped implant, which marked a notable development in the field.

Somewhat more successful use of implants began at the beginning of the fifties of the last century. In that period, subperiosteal (overbony) implants are often applied (Figures 1.1 and 1.2). Subperiosteal implants, despite the increasing use of endosseous implants, are widely used in the USA. In that period begins the application of combinations of subperiosteal and endosseous implants, especially in the lower jaw. The same combination is also used in the upper jaw, in case of strongly pronounced and lowered maxillary sinuses, where, due to insufficient available bone, the application of endosseous implants was not possible.

But none of the more "modern" implantologists base their creations on the creations of long-ago predecessors who tried to replace a lost tooth with a foreign body in the form of a root, imitating nature! In the 1950s, thoughts moved in a completely different direction.

Stefan Tramonte's implant in 1959 marked the beginning of a new era in implantology. His implant featured a screw design with wide, sharp threads. Following Tramonte's model, Italy saw the emergence of a movement where many attempted to replicate his design, each incorporating their modifications and claiming authorship of these variations. This led to a surge of new contributors in the field. Notably, the Muratori screw emerged (see Figure 1.3), and Gino Garbaggio introduced a "cortical" implant inspired by Tramonte's design, but it was much longer and thinner (see Figure 1.4).

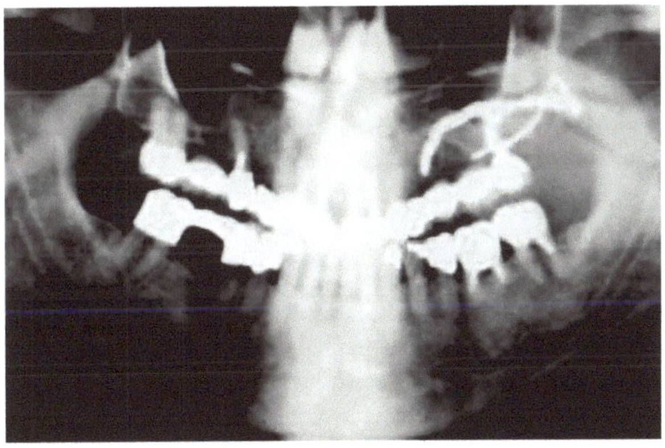

Figure 1.1. Subperiosteal implant in the lateral region of the upper jaw

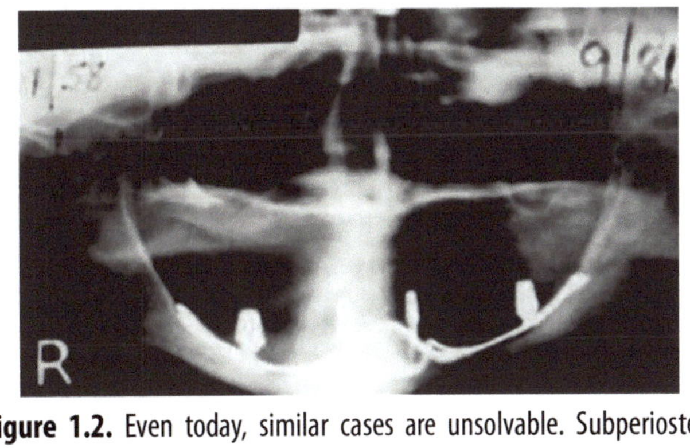

Figure 1.2. Even today, similar cases are unsolvable. Subperiosteal implant in the lateral zone

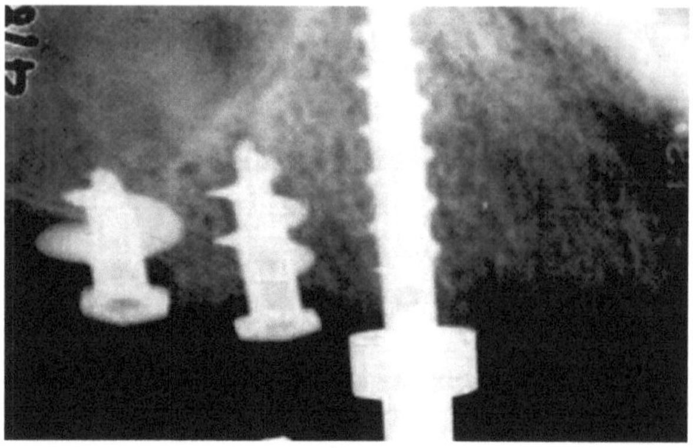

Figure 1.3. Muratorijevi zavrtanj-implantati.

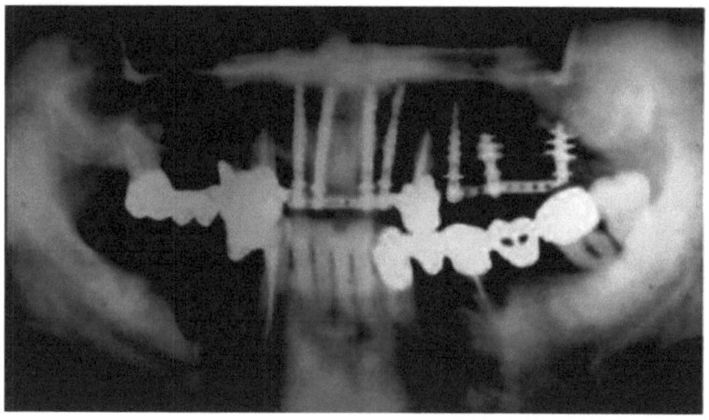

Figure 1.4. Combination of Tramonti's and Muratori's endosseous screw-implant.

All these implants are made exclusively by machine processing with a smooth surface.

It should be emphasized that Tramonte advocated immediate loading with a tantalum implant in 1961. But only after three years, in 1964, he used titanium as a material, which was not class IV. For this reason, Tramonte's first implants had a lack of bending due to low-quality titanium. Later Tramonte implants significantly improved the quality of the titanium material from which they were made. The surface of the implant was machined exclusively.

The big disadvantage of these and all similar implant forms is the vagueness in the neck area in contact with soft tissues. At the time of the launch of the implant, Tramonte once said: "Maybe my implant, although it is used a lot, has flaws, but I claim that it is an arrow and a guideline for the way to go in the creation of the implant design." It is easily accepted by the bone because it is cut into it by itself, and because of this, aggression and trauma to the bone is less than in all forms of implants today. The bone must suffer as little violence as possible during the insertion of the implant!" Tramonte's prediction was justified. During this period, Gino Garbaccio launched his bicortical implant with similar design features to Tramonte's implant. Professor Giordano Muratori from Bologna launches his implant copying Tramonte (Figure 1.7). All these implants were named after the author.

In this movement of Italian implantologists, the names Ugo and Marco Pasqualini are significant. Between the sixties and seventies of the last century, the first significant histological studies of the relationship between bone and implant were published by Professor Ugo Pasqualini. He is the first Italian implantologist who considered the problems of implantology from the aspect of implant loading, giving great importance to gnathological problems and pathological occlusion. ("Le Patologie occlusalli - principe e tecniche del riequilibrio dell occlusionsione" from 1993, published in Milan, Paris, and Barcelona).

At the end of the sixties of the last century, the right moment came that will shine a new light on implantology and accelerate its development; the works of Swede Ingvar Branemark began to be published, which will serve as an incentive for the accelerated development of oral implantology in modern prosthetics.

After those discoveries, began the rapid development of oral implantology. Thanks to a more rigorous methodology, better knowledge of indications and contraindications, as well as the development of new surgical techniques, the procedure of installing implants has been significantly facilitated. This progress was accompanied by technological innovations and the application of more modern and better prosthetic works, which all resulted in a higher percentage of success.

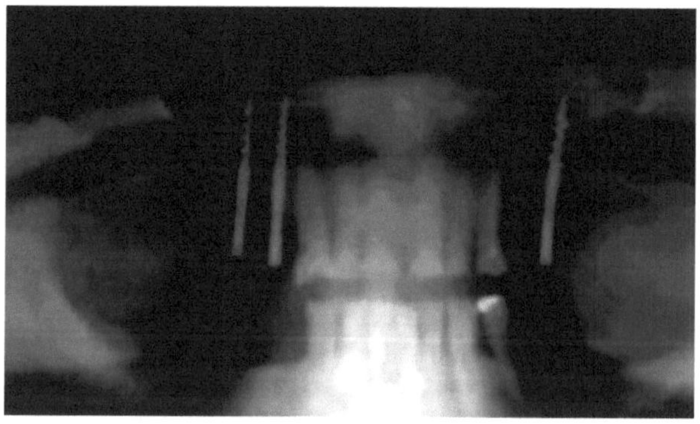

Figure 1.5. Garbaccio's endosseous cortical implant

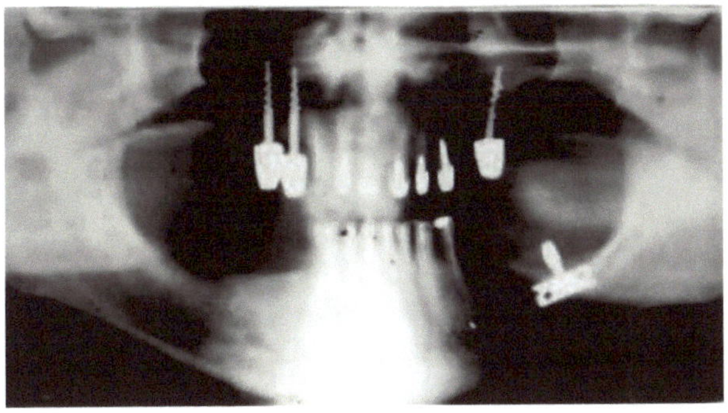

Figure 1.6. Crowns on Garbaccio's implants in the upper jaw. In the lower jaw, a one-piece leaf endosseous implant.

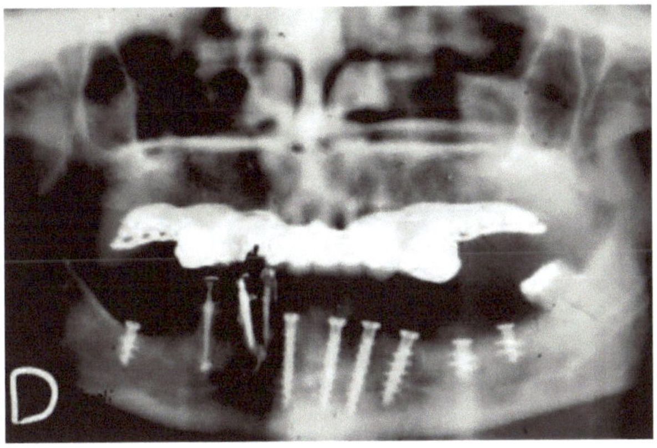

Figure 1.7. Tramonti's and Muratori's endosseous implants

In parallel with that, the study of oral implantology begins at faculties where it is given increasing importance. It was the most accepted in the French institutions for oral surgery in Paris (VII Garanciere), thanks primarily to the support of two doctors, N. Forrest and P. Giardia. Other faculties are also introducing it, putting it in graduate work and postgraduate training programs.

French oral surgeons Laure, Le Gall, and Landau, (J. F. Lauret, M. Le Gall, and C. Landeau), with their works on the analysis of occlusion and lateral movements of the lower jaw, show the mutuality of the two disciplines - implantology and prosthetics.

Thanks to such approaches and research of oral implantology and prosthetics, good planning, and precise execution of prosthetic works carried out on implants, extraordinary functional and aesthetic results are achieved.

In 1951, Leventhal was the first to point out the excellent suitability of titanium as an artificial material embedded in bone.

Since then, an entire era of implantology has been associated with the name of Leonard Linkow. For a long time, his name was mentioned as a synonym of oral implantology, and he is still being written about. The construction of his implant is the opposite of nature, the so-called two-dimensional leaf implant (blade implant). According to some data, the idea is not his (names mentioned: Leman 1959; Roberts 1965, Linkow 1968), but the fame is!

With the advent of Branemark, bony integration between titanium implants and bone was already seriously discussed.

At the clinic in Gothenburg, the group around Branemark dealt with this topic exclusively from basic research.

However, he did not go further in his investigations of the relationship between the surface of the implant and the bone. The definition of **osseous integration** completed and affirmed the Branemark implant.

More than 40 years have passed since Branemark implanted the patient Gosti Larsen. He is living proof that osseointegration exists - that the implant is fully functional and intact in the bone after the past four decades.

In the past, a low sinus floor was an insurmountable obstacle to implant-prosthetic treatment. The progress of oral implantology today can be solved using bone substitutes. The most modern approach is the fibrin clot concept based on the centrifugation of the patient's blood in test tubes without anticoagulants in the centrifuge. At the end of the centrifugation, the fibrin clot with many platelets is separated from the other formed blood elements. That fibrin clot is called **Platelet Rich Fibrin or PRF**, gradually and over a long period it releases growth factors and cytokines into the surrounding tissue - bone and soft.

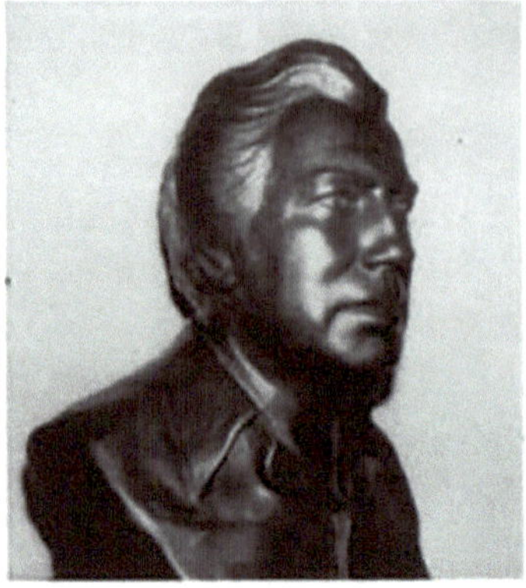

Bust of Dr. Leonard I. Linkow
Clinical Implant Society of Japan award at the 31st Annual American Academy of Implant Dentistry Convention in Las Vegas, Nevada on November 5, 1982.

To Blazo,
With my warmest personal regards to the best implantologist in Yugoslavia.
Len Linkow
10/12/83.

DENTAL IMPLANTS
CAN MAKE YOUR LIFE WONDERFUL AGAIN!!

by
Leonard I. Linkow, D.D.S.
with
Frances Minters
Drawings by Carol Morley

Robert Speller & Sons, Publishers
New York, New York 10010

The first book in the field of oral implantology was written by Leonardo Linkow (New York USA) in the early eighties of the last century.

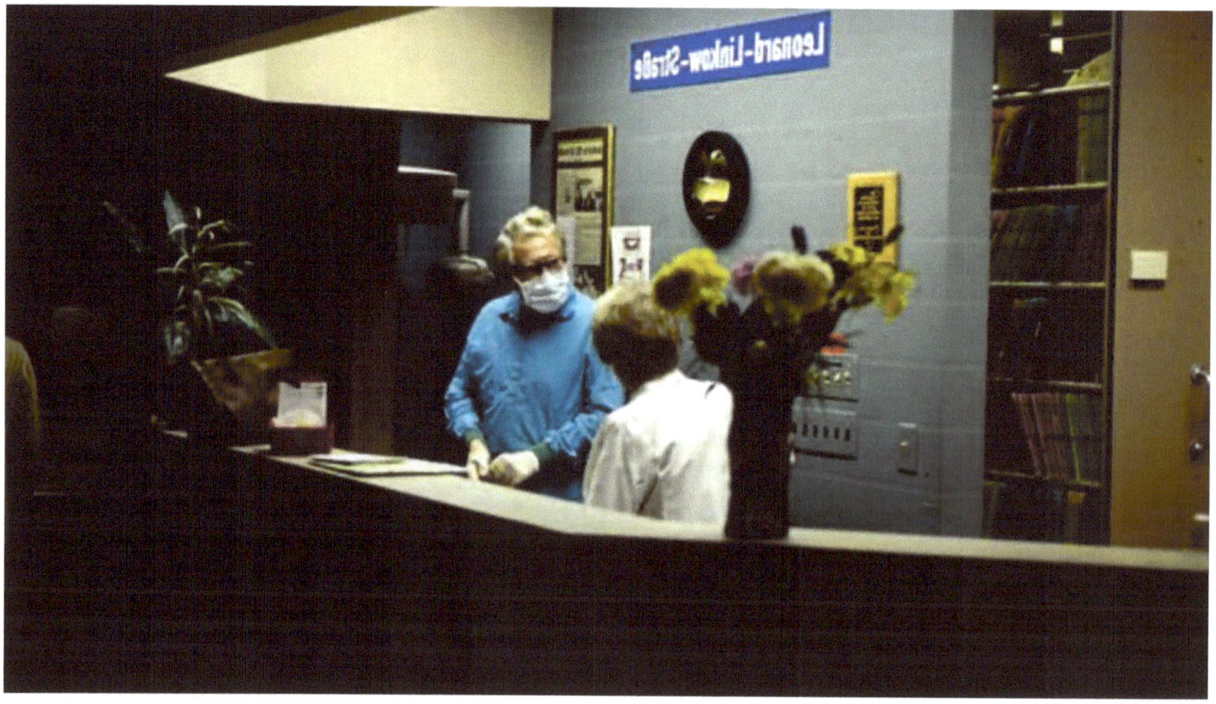

Leonard Linkow, once synonymous with oral implantology in the world - a street in the city of Bremen, Germany bears his name.

2

Anatomical Structures Important for Implantation

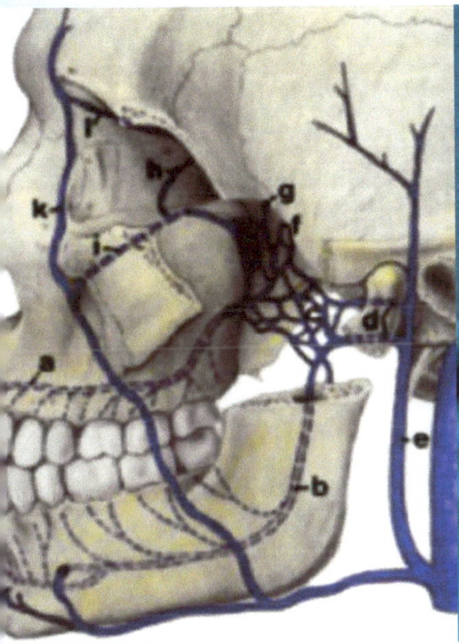

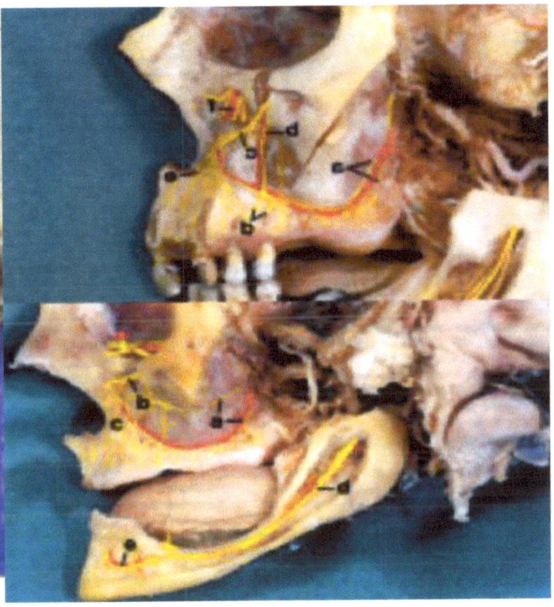

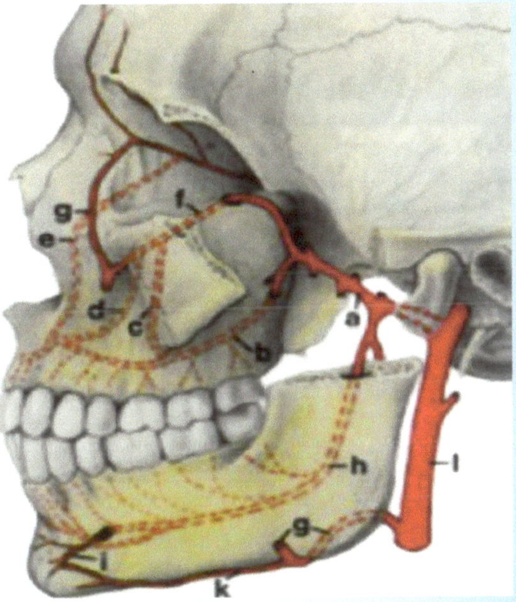

Detailed knowledge of anatomical structures and topographic relationships is extremely important for a dentist who deals with the installation of implants. Knowing these details makes it possible to see immediately, a priori, whether the installation of endosseous implants is limited by some natural limit. Knowledge of anatomy improves the assessment of the patient's condition, facilitates surgical procedures, and enables the surgeon to safely resect tissues to improve form, function, and aesthetics. Also, it must be borne in mind that certain parts of anatomical structures are exposed to changes differently during life. These changes are especially pronounced when conditions change during life due to the loss of natural teeth.

Knowing the anatomical details makes it easier for the clinician to determine the range of implant therapy in altered structures and to analyze the height and width of the alveolar ridges, which would ensure favorable conditions for implant placement.

For example, the dentist often wonders whether he can use the maxillary tubercle as a place to position the implant to avoid elevation of the sinus floor. At the same time, the shape of the tuber of the maxilla is subject to significant changes at different ages.

For this reason, the renewal of anatomical knowledge is one of the contributing factors to the success of the implant procedure. Modern implantology has expanded the field of indications for the installation of implants, which has increased caution when it comes to anatomical structures because if they are unfavorable, and especially if variations of certain anatomical structures are possible, implantation can be risky.

Zones that are of particular importance for the installation of implants in the upper jaw are its labial side and the maxillary sinus, especially its floor region, as well as the floor of the nasal cavities.

Loss of teeth reduces the width of the alveolar ridge, which differs from person to person. Bone reduction on the labial side of the maxilla is typical - the reduction in the height of the alveolar ridge in the first year is around 3 to 4 mm, especially if there are no antagonists that would maintain the height of the bone. This anatomical change on the labial side of the maxilla is extremely important during implant procedures in patients with a high smile line. The alveolar ridge in the front part of the maxilla usually consists of a thin and flexible labial cortical wall and a much thicker and thicker palatal cortical wall. Between those two parts of the cortical bone, there is a cancellous part of the bone, which is of different quality and density (Figure 2.1, a and b). The bone quality that prevails on the labial side of the maxilla is usually of medium density, in contrast to the bone density of the front side of the mandible (between two very dense cortical bones), where cortical bone is present in a higher percentage (Figure 2.1c).

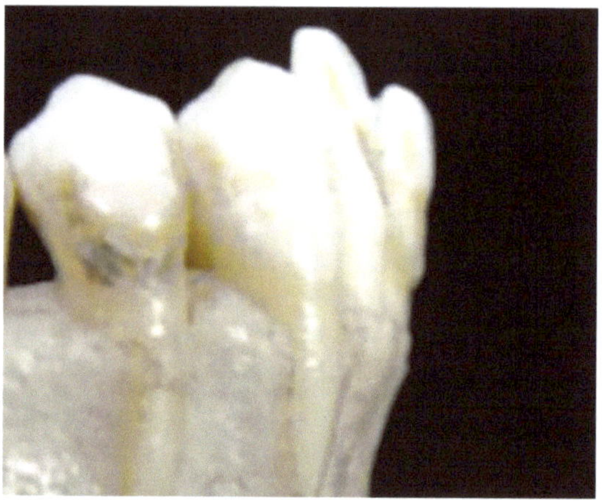

(a)

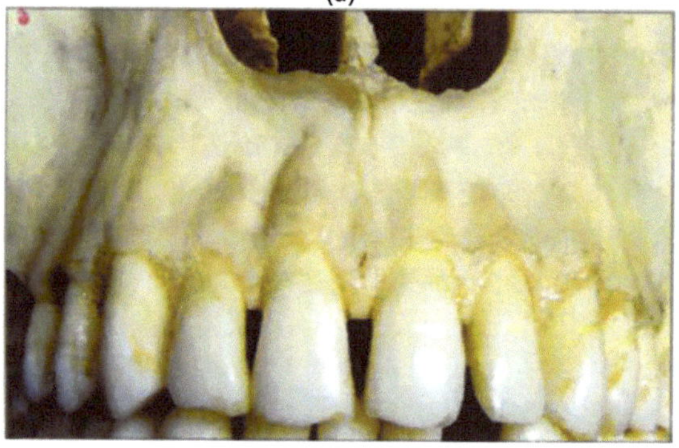

(b)

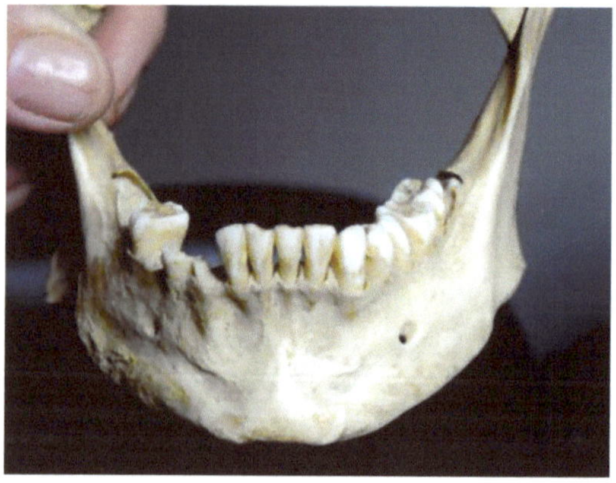

(c)

Figure 2.1. Thin labial lamellar bone in both jaws is a risk factor for implant placement, and the space between n. mentalis in case of edentulism is safe for implantation.

When it comes to the lower jaw, special attention is required to know the extension of the mandibular canal, the relationship of the chin nerve in the area of the chin opening, as well as the structures on the lingual edge of the bone. These details are of particular importance for implantation.

Among the many variants and risks that can be expected are the known maxillary sinus in the upper jaw and the existence of partitions in it, as well as the position of the sinus floor; then, the position of the opening and the course of the neurovascular structures in the region of the anterior-posterior (or buccolingual) part of the mandible and the anterior palatal part of the maxilla. Possible "traps" include anatomical variations of the chin opening (position, number, dimensions, etc.) - Figure 2.2 shows a variation with two mental openings.

Also possible are variants of the mandibular canal, unusual paths, or double canals that can be registered in people with teeth, but above all in edentulous patients. Branching of the intraosseous anterior loop of the chin nerve ("mental siphon", "front loop") is also possible, which can range from 1-7 cm, which was observed by Machado et al. in 2001. These anatomical variations are very difficult to see on conventional orthopantomographic images.

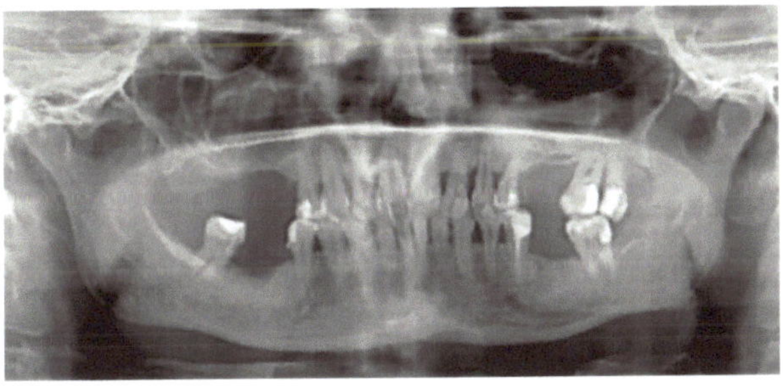

Figure 2.2. Variations of the mandibular canal on the left (from Dr. Zlopaš's office).

It is important to be aware of the potential for unwanted and unexpected injuries to specific anatomical structures during oral surgical procedures. This issue is particularly significant, as a thorough understanding of the locations of blood vessels and nerves is crucial for the safe execution of all oral surgery and periodontal treatments. This knowledge is especially vital when placing implants, making regular updates to our understanding essential for ensuring patient safety.

The floor of the oral cavity is highly vascularized and there is always a risk of injury to the blood vessels in that part of the oral cavity. Injury to larger blood vessels is especially dangerous, and the most significant is a. sublingualis, main branch of a. lingualis.

The submental artery separates from a. lingualis, and below m. myloyoideus turns forward, thus making another artery of the oral cavity that can be endangered during surgery.

During implant installation, drills may cause perforation of the lingual compact (Figure 2.3), and injury to a. sublingualis causes profuse bleeding that can threaten the life of the patient, due to bleeding and obstruction of the upper respiratory tract. The same applies to a. submentalis. That is why one should be very careful when preparing the beds for positioning the implants on the tooth sites 34, 35, 44, 45.

What to do if these blood vessels are injured?

A hemostatic suture should be placed as soon as possible and tamponed firmly!

Unlike the floor of the oral cavity, injury of a. palatine is less dangerous and does not represent a complicated therapeutic procedure (simple tamponade or thermocautery coagulation).

Anatomical structures and topographic relationships instruct the implantologist to take care of the following:

- availability of bone;
- bone structure;
- supply of different blood vessels and nerves region;
- Proximity to the nasal and paranasal cavities.

Based on this, the potential zones for implant placement can be divided as follows:

Favorable zones

- The frontal area of the lower jaw between the two mental openings.

The zone of the lateral teeth of the lower jaw if there are still natural teeth in the frontal part. In cases of total toothlessness lasting several years, the lateral area of the lower jaw is often no longer suitable for the installation of implants.

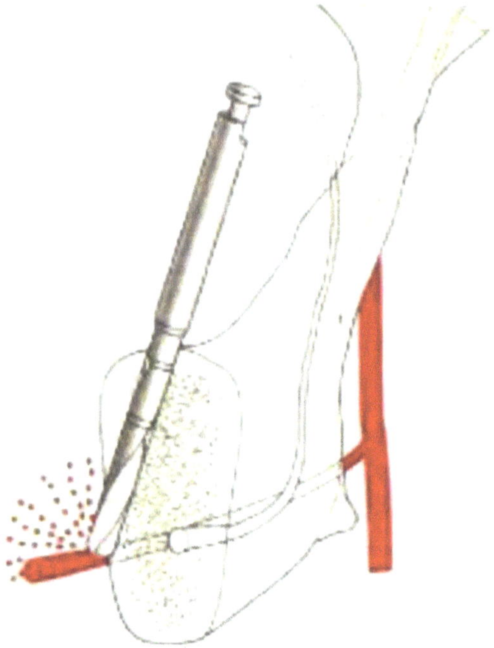

Figure 2.3. Schematic representation of perforation of the lingual compact and possible injury a. sublingual

Conditionally favorable zones:

- Upper jaw to the vicinity of the second premolars.

Unfavorable:

- The upper jaw in the lateral zone, including the tubercles of the maxilla due to the richness of the spongiosa.
- The condition of the mucous membrane that plays a significant role in implantation.

Favorable:

- Atherent tightly keratinized mucous membrane, i.e. fixed mucosa.

Unfavorable:

- Mobile mucous membrane.

Maxilla and its changes with age

The processus alveolaris of the maxilla surrounds only a small space of the roots of the teeth. For this reason, the roots of the incisors, and above all the canines, protrude, that is, emphasize the protrusions of the juga alveolaria.

The processus alveolaris of the maxilla ends behind the last molars with a tubercle, which is limited by the fissure pterygomaxillaris from the back.

The tuber undergoes incredible changes in shape during its life and also varies individually in terms of development.

Until the seventh year, the tuber exists only as an initial position and is not formed (Figure 2.4a). Around the age of twenty, the tuber is fully formed. Alveolar openings (foramina alveolaria) represent the entrance to the canals (Figure 2.4b). After the age of fifty, the tuber is increasingly subject to involution, or atrophy. The alveolar ducts turn into alveolar sulci again (Figure 2.4c). These changes explain to us why special attention must be paid to the tuber retromolaris, as a place for implant placement.

The floor of the maxillary sinus in 70% of cases is below the floor of the nasal concha. After the loss of the molar, it descends downwards, and only a thin lamella remains from the alveolar ridge. The opening of the maxillary sinus during the extraction or surgical removal of teeth in the upper jaw is not a complication in the true sense, it is mostly a consequence of anatomical circumstances or reduced attention of the dentist. Thus, one current study (M. Pasqualini) states that during extraction or surgical interventions in the upper jaw, oroantral communication is created in 24% of cases with impacted teeth and 5% if the tooth was in a normal row. Any iatrogenic opening of the sinuses requires timely and adequate treatment so that unwanted complications do not occur.

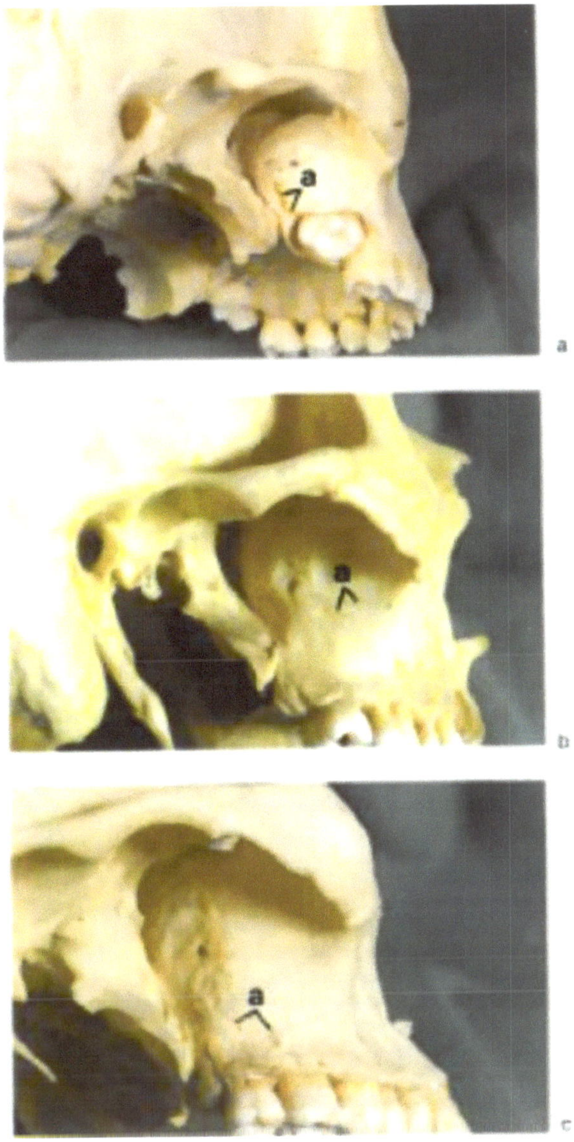

Figure 2.4.

a. Skull of a 5-6 year old child, viewed from the right side. The retromolar tubercle has not yet formed. a = alveolar sulci
b. Skull of a 30-year-old man, viewed from the right side. Strongly formed retromolar tubercle. a = alveolar foramina
c. Skull of a 62-year-old man, viewed from the right side. The retromolar tubercle is largely atrophied. a = alveolar sulci
(A. Schoreder, F. Suter and G. Krekler)

The structure of the alveolar wall

Interdental septums are 0.7-1.4 mm thick. Like the other alveolar walls, they consist of compacta and spongiosa, whereby the compacta, whose thickness is between 100 and 800 μm, due to the radial arrangement of the cementoalveolar bundles of fibers, cannot be compared with the compacta of the remaining part of the skeleton (see below).

The elastic suspension of the tooth via the alveodental ligaments loads the spongiosa, located next to the tooth root, so bone beds extend in trajectory. Due to the already mentioned removal of pressure due to chewing from the teeth of the upper jaw via the infrazygomatic ridge, the trajectory extension of the spongiosa beds in the region of the first molars is most clearly expressed (Figure 2.5). Vertically and radially distributed trabeculae are found in the compact at the height of the root tip. They are further separated from each other and inserted into the compact wall of the maxillary sinus, i.e. the floor of the nasal cavity.

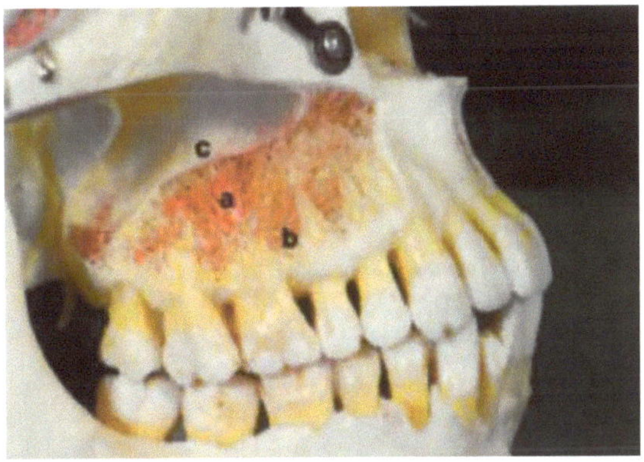

Figure 2.5. Spongiosis of premolars and molars of the upper jaw on the right side: a = vertical-radial trabeculae of the first molars (region of the infrazygomatic ridge), b = horizontal-radial trabeculae (interdental trabeculae), c = compacta of the floor of the maxillary sinus (in section). (A. Schoreder, F. Suter and G. Krekler)

This vertical-radial direction of the trabeculae likely represents the optimal biological response of the bones to the pressure force and traction force during chewing. From vertical-radial trabeculae, horizontally-radially directed bone beds formed in interdental and interradicular septums must be distinguished. In the region of the premolars and molars, they are more distinctly differentiated than those between the incisors. The horizontal-radial trabeculae probably fulfill two functions. On the one hand, they act against the pulling force through the periodontium; on the other hand, they have different loads due to the beveling of the teeth during the movement of food grinding. Whether a conceivable rotational movement of the tooth concerning the longitudinal axis in vivo theoretically occurs. In any case, this kind of movement would affect the interdental trabeculae through the traction force of the cemento-alveolar fibers.

Relationships of the teeth of the upper jaw with the maxillary sinus and the nasal cavity

For a long time, the maxillary sinus has been one of the insurmountable anatomical disadvantages when it comes to implant placement. With the development of new methods in oral surgery, implantology, and medical science in general, the maxillary sinus is no longer an insurmountable obstacle for the installation of implants. Nevertheless, despite numerous scientific achievements, when it comes to bone augmentation with some of the bone substitutes, the maxillary sinus still represents a great obstacle and a constant "trap" when installing implants. The use of bone substitutes can result in serious complications, especially when it comes to sinus lifting.

A thorough understanding of the anatomy involved in sinus lifting is becoming increasingly essential in daily practice. The spongy bone of the alveolar wall in the incisor region extends to the delicate compact bone at the floor of the nasal cavity. The frontal wall of the sinus often aligns with the canine fossa, meaning the long root of the canine sometimes reaches the height of the infraorbital foramen in the lateral wall of the nasal cavity. Nearby, there is a neurovascular structure that emerges from the infraorbital foramen. This area has the thinnest overlying bone, which is the point at which the sinus cavity is surgically accessed during the classic Caldwell-Luc operation.

The posterior wall of the sinus corresponds to the tuber of the maxilla and borders the pterygopalatine fossa, the lower wall of the alveolar process, and often coincides with the pterygoid venous plexus and numerous neurovascular structures in proximity. The lateral extension of the sinus cavity extends to the zygomatic arch and may pierce the zygomatic bone.

The spongiosis of the alveolar processes in the area of the premolars and molars borders on the thin compact of the maxillary sinus (Figure 2.5).

The mesial wall of the sinus coincides with the lateral wall of the nasal cavity and that wall is usually fragile. The sinus can have several separated chambers with septa of different heights and positions.

The beginning of the maxillary sinus is located below the floor of the nasal cavity in 70% of cases. Most often, the floor of the maxillary sinus is concave and has smooth walls. The smallest distance to the maxillary sinus is shown by the tips of the roots of the second molars, and often also the first molars. The alveolar wall of both these teeth can cause bulging of the floor of the maxillary sinus, resulting in a more or less pronounced chamberization of the maxillary sinus (Figure 2.6). These surface characteristics of the sinus floor play a significant role when it is desired to raise it by augmentation.

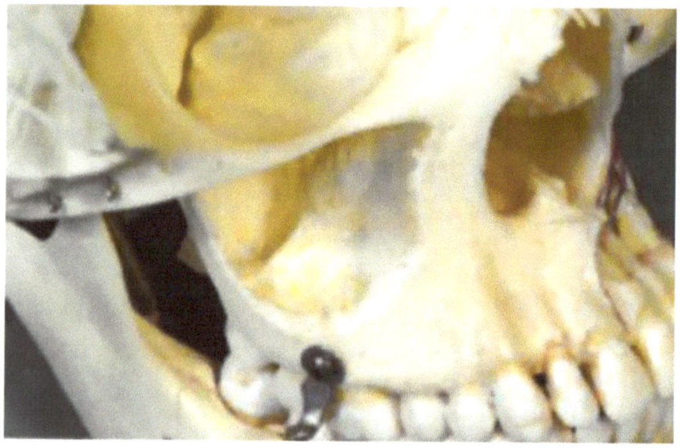

Figure 2.6. Right maxillary sinus, open. Incomplete septation of the maxillary sinus, due to the roots of the second and third molars.

The maxillary sinus is lined with a multi-layered ciliated epithelium (Schneider's membrane), and its thickness is from 0.13 to 0.5 mm.

After tooth loss, there is not only atrophy of the alveolar process of the maxilla but also a lowering of the floor of the sinus, so that after years of absence of teeth, often only one thin bone lamella separates the bone of the alveolar process from the maxillary sinus.

The role of its communication with the nasal cavity through the osteomeatal complex is important for the health of the maxillary sinus. This complex has a semilunar opening that opens into the nasal cavity below the middle turbinate. Therefore, it is usually positioned above the level to which the planned augmentation should be performed.

The mucosa of the sinus itself is poorly vascularized. However, the maxilla has an excellent blood supply of several branches of the maxillary artery: a. infraorbitalis, superior alveolar, paranasal, and palatal artery.

The blood supply is supplemented by the branches of the upper temporal artery, that is, the facial artery. Then, numerous anastomoses contribute to good collateral circulation. With sinus pneumatization, some of these arteries are suppressed and lie within grooves on the surface of the sinus walls. Detailed knowledge of the anatomy and physiology of the maxillary sinus is very important if any intervention in that region is planned, especially implantology.

The palatal root of the first molar is located at least 1.56 mm from the floor of the maxillary sinus, while the palatal root of the second molar is approximately 2.4 mm from the sinus floor. Additionally, the disto-buccal root of the second molar is about 2.79 mm away from the sinus floor. The greatest distance between the apex of a root and the floor of the sinus is found at the buccal tip of the first premolar's root, measuring 6.18 mm. The space from the tip of the palatal root to the floor of the sinus is 7.05 mm.

It is important to note that these anatomical relationships can vary from person to person. For instance, the distance from the apex of the root of the second premolar to the floor of the maxillary sinus can range from 10.12 mm to 15 mm, and in some cases, this distance may even be zero.

The sensory and secretory innervation of the maxillary sinuses is carried out via the upper posterior alveolar nerves (n.n. alveolares superiores posteriores), which enter the tuber of the maxilla through the foramina alveolaria, and then into the sinus. In the infraorbital sulcus, from the infraorbital nerves are separated n. alveolaris superior medialis. Before exiting through the foramen infraorbitalis, from n. infraorbitalis are separated n. n. alveolares superiores anteriores, which innervate the mucosa of the front wall of the maxillary sinus. Vascularization of the maxillary sinus takes place through several arteries: a. infraorbitalis, a. palatine major, a. incisive and a. alveolaris posterior superior. Blood from the maxillary sinus drains through c. facialis, v. sphenopalatine, pterygoid plexus and pharyngeal plexus. The described details are shown in Figures 2.24, 2.25 and 2.27. Knowing all these anatomical details is extremely important, as operations in this region can be extremely complicated and should not be performed without good training.

Bone structure of the lower jaw and its changes with aging

Configuration of the mandible

Spatially, the trigonum of the retromolar mandible is located opposite the tuber of the maxilla. This bony triangle forms at the transition from the ramus of the mandible to its body (see Figure 2.7). It is bounded lingually by the cristo temporalis and buccally by the linea forma. In younger individuals, the retromolar trigone may raise considerations regarding implantation, as a normal jaw angle of 120° positions the mandibular canal anteriorly, approximately 8 mm mediocaudal to the floor of the retromolar trigone.

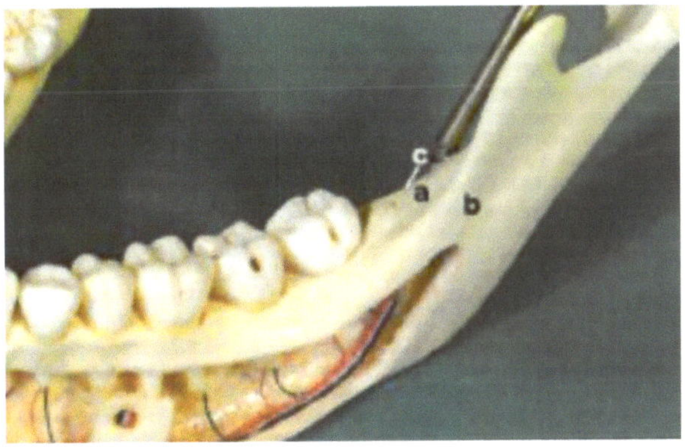

Figure 2.7. Left side of the lower jaw with the opening of the mandibular canal: a = fossa retromolaris, b = linea obliqua, c = crysta temporalis (A. Schroeder, F. Sutter, G. Krekler)

The distance between the retromolar trigonums (trigonum distance) is 60-65 mm, which is distinctly greater than the distance between the retromolar tubercles of the maxilla (tuber distance), averaging around 50 mm. This indicates that the arch of the upper jaw is significantly shorter than the basal arch of the lower jaw.

However, when measuring the distance between the distal cusps of the lower molars (molar distance) and comparing it to the midpoint of the crown surface of the upper molars, it turns out that the dental arches are approximately 55 mm in length, making them similar in size (see Figure 2.8).

Due to the oblique position of the tooth axis and the varying points of contact between teeth, different bone arches can be balanced out. When using the retromolar trigone as an implant placement site, these anatomical factors should be considered.

Tooth axis

The shafts of the teeth of the lower jaw are slanted inwards to the vertical line, so that the sides of the crowns that lie towards each other are closer than their roots, Figure 2.8. regarding the alveolar wall, this means that the lingual cortex is more strongly formed than the buccal. The bony walls of the alveolar wall of the mandible in adults, as a whole, both lingually and buccally, are more compact than the corresponding structures of the upper jaw.

Regarding the formation of trajectory-directed beds of spongiosa of the alveolar wall of the lower jaw, both the vertical-radial trabeculae, which start from the tips of the roots, and the horizontal-radial trabeculae of the interdental and interradicular septums have a similar structure. In principle, the relations are the same as for the upper jaw. However, the mandibular vertical trabeculae are, compared to the relationships at the level of the upper jaw, more evenly distributed to the teeth (Figure 2.9). The reason for this is that the supporting column in the infratemporal ridge of the upper jaw is formed as a pressure relief system for strong occlusal chewing forces, which is missing in the lower jaw.

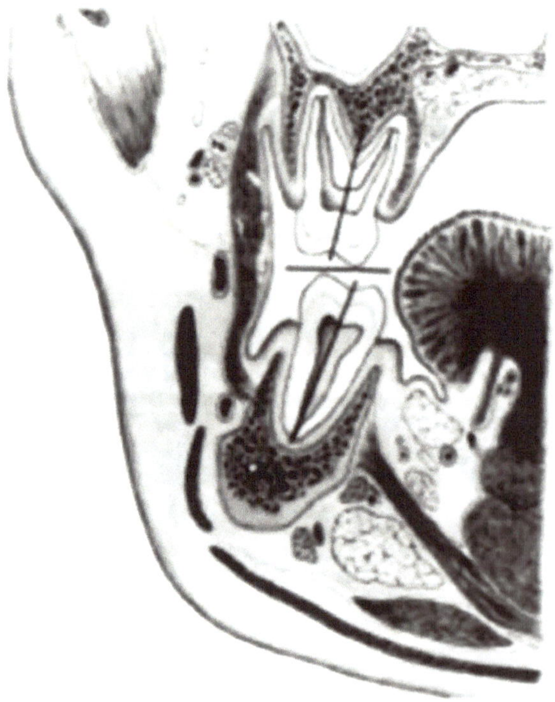

Figure 2.8. The distance between the retromolar trigones of the upper and lower jaw.

Flow of the mandibular canal

The mandibular canal begins at the mandibular foramen, located in the middle of the ramus, approximately 1 cm above and 2 cm behind the crown of the third molar. From there, the canal extends obliquely downward through the ramus, eventually reaching the cancellous body of the mandible, situated roughly midway between the lingual and buccal compacta (see Figure 2.7).

In the area of the third molars, the horizontal portion of the compact bone is about 3-4 mm above the bottom of the dental alveoli, while in the region of the first molars, this distance increases to about 8 mm. At regular intervals, the alveolar canals of the mandible extend vertically from the main canal into the dental alveoli (see Figure 2.10).

Between the first and second premolars, the canal makes a sharp turn toward the buccal side, known as the mental canal (canalis mentalis), which opens externally at the mental foramen. Just before this opening, a small arched canal branches off medially from the spongiosa.

This is the incisive canal (canalis incisivus), which houses the nerves and blood vessels supplying the canines and incisors.

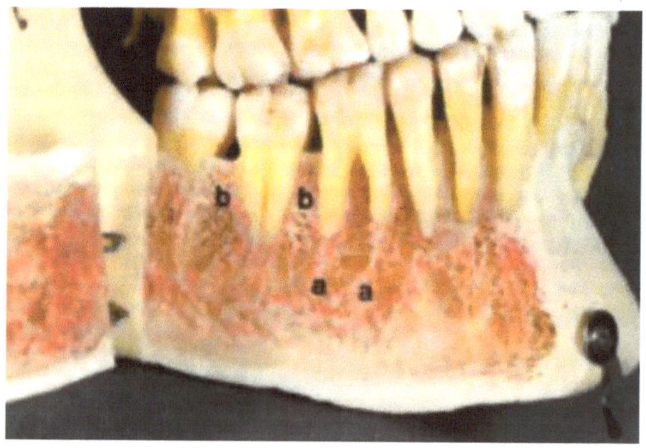

Figure 2.9. Spongiosis of premolars and molars of the right side of the lower jaw: a = vertical-radial trabeculae, b = horizontal-radial trabeculae.

Changes in the shape of the mandible during life

In newborns, the upper part of the mandible, known as the alveolar part, is twice as high as the lower part, or basal part. By adolescence, the growth of the basal part increases fourfold, while the alveolar part grows to only about twice its height at birth. After tooth loss, the alveolar part experiences significant atrophy. Additionally, in old age, severe destructive changes occur in the basal part of the mandible, primarily affecting the lingual side rather than the buccal side.

The disappearance of the compact bone on the lingual side of the mandible, possibly caused by the pressure from a poorly fitted prosthesis, may contribute to this phenomenon. In a case involving a 65-year-old individual who wore full dentures, it was observed that the mandibular canal was exposed on the lingual side over a significant area. As a result, the inferior alveolar nerve, along with its blood vessels, was positioned directly beneath the lingual mucosa (see Figure 2.11). Due to severe resorption changes, the roof of the bone canal had fenestrated, transforming into a bony groove.

In the case of a 62-year-old man, n. incisivus lay directly under the mucous membrane of the floor of the oral cavity (Figure 2.13). The presented topographical position of these sensitive nerves must have led to severe pain in the patient under the compression prosthesis, confirmed by the medical history in both this and the previous case.

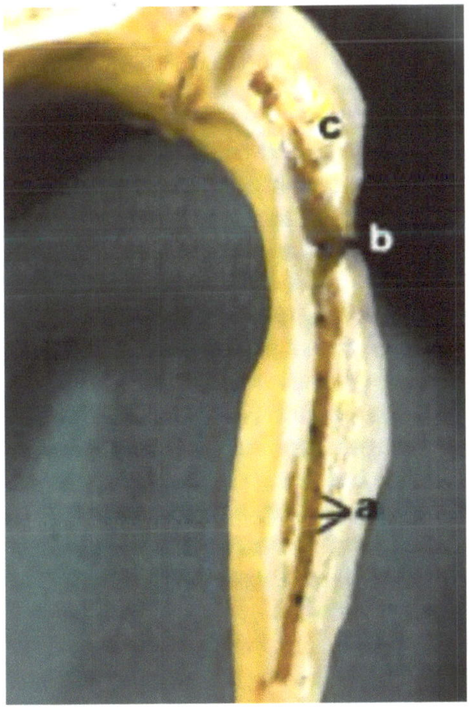

Figure 2.10. Mandibular canal of the right side of the lower jaw open caudally: a = canaliculi alveolaris, b = foramen mentale, c = canalis incisivus. (A. Schroeder, F. Sutter, G. Krekler)

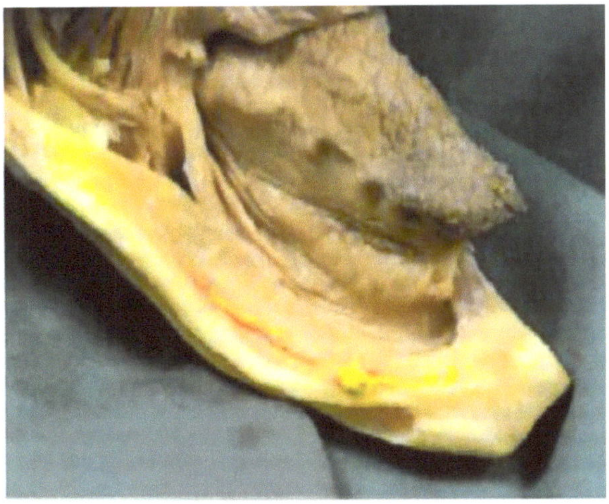

Figure 2.11. The right side of the lower jaw of a 65-year-old man, bent buccally. A view of the lingual surface. After removing the mucous membrane of the bottom of the oral cavity, n. alveolaris inferior and a. alveolaris inferior, due to atrophic decomposition of the bone with the opening of the alveolar canal towards the medial side, lie free. (A. Schroeder).

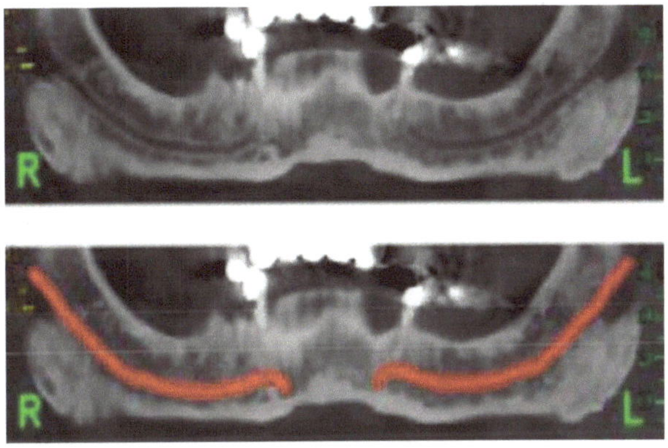

Figure 2.12. The possibility of 3D-tomography to clarify the position of the mandibular canal by staining. (from Dr. Zlopaš's office).

Senile atrophy of the alveolar body of the mandible is typically caused by tooth loss, leading to changes in the angles of both jaws. In older individuals, the angle of the lower jaw can shift to resemble the angles seen in childhood, potentially exceeding 160°. This alteration in angle also impacts the retromolar trigone, causing it to descend into the bone that is affected by senile atrophy. As a result, the retromolar trigone loses its viability as an implant site in areas of senile atrophied bone, due to its close proximity to the oblique part of the mandibular canal. With the development of the most modern three-dimensional technique, extremely precise visibility of the position of the mandibular canal is possible (Figure 2.12).

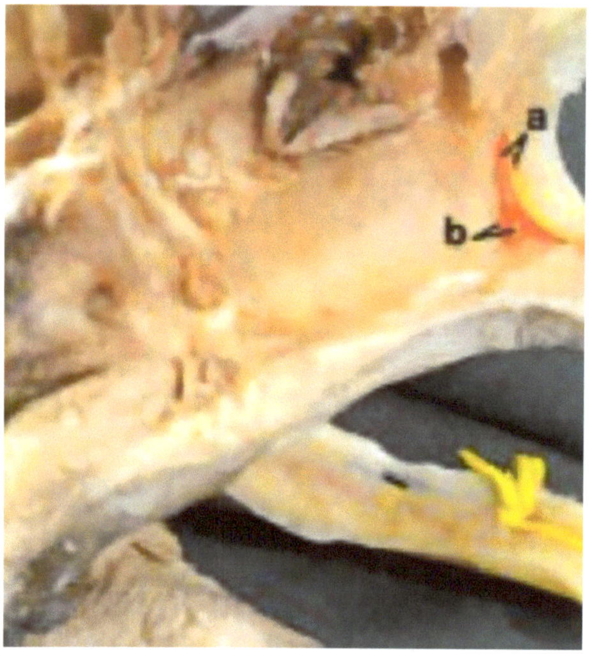

Figure 2.13. The right side of the mandible of a 62-year-old man. Atrophy of the basal part with an open incisive canal. N. incisivus lies directly under the mucous membrane of the floor of the oral cavity. a = nerve and artery nasalis lateralis, b = ramus perforans to plexus caninus. (A. Schroerder, F. Sutter and G. Krekele).

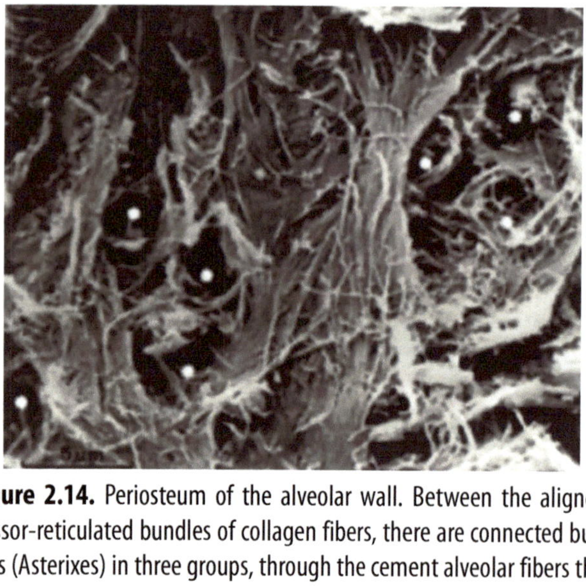

Figure 2.14. Periosteum of the alveolar wall. Between the aligned, scissor-reticulated bundles of collagen fibers, there are connected bundles (Asterixes) in three groups, through the cement alveolar fibers that extend to the edge of the alveolar wall (image magnified 1.600 times). (Orale Implantologie, Andre Schroeder, Franz Sutter und Gisbert Krekler).

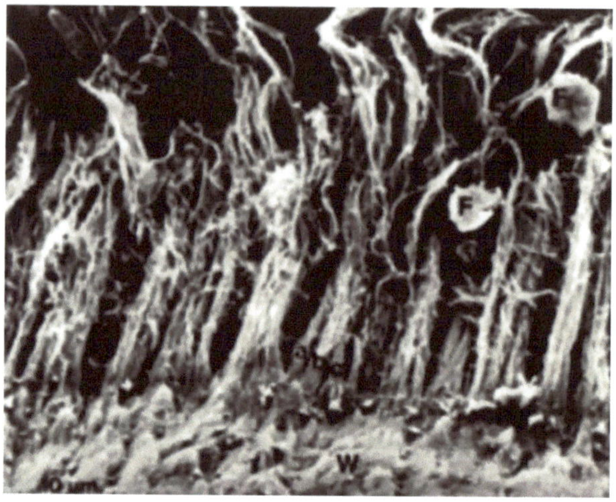

Figure 2.15. Bundles of cement alveolar fibers of one premolar in the middle third of the root. Bundles of collagen fibers leave the cementum at right angles (900). Always three bundles of fibers create one functional morphological unit (Orale implantologie, A. Schreder, F. Sutter and G. Krekeler).

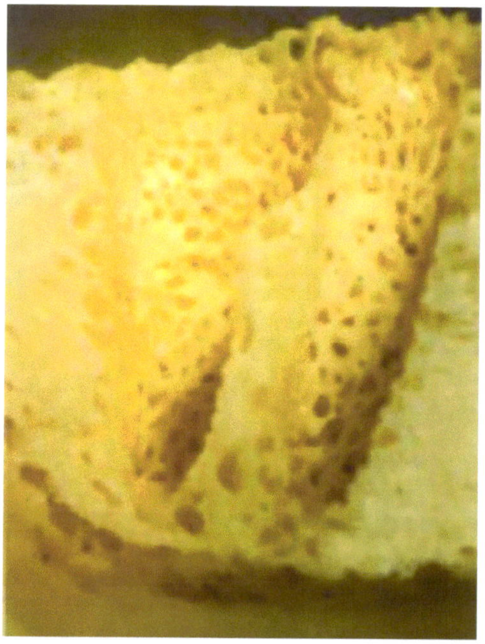

Figure 2.16. Bony lingual wall of the alveolus of the first molar (lower jaw of a 55-year-old man). Expansion of the cemento-alveolar zone of fixation until the transformation of the compact into spongiosis (magnification 1500 times).

Bone quality

Very often, even after a well-established diagnosis, when planning the location and number of implants, the doctor encounters the obstacle that the patient's bone is porous, or that there is too little high-quality bone mass, both in the vertical and horizontal levels.

K. Misch and M. Judy were the first to describe the different categories of bone quality from an implantological point of view (Fig. 2.16, 2.17, and 2.18). Lekholm and Zarb even better devised a classification system for determining bone quality. Today, we can more precisely analyze the quality of the bone with computerized tomography using histograms and the Houndsfield scale.

Wolff's rule (orthopedics call it Wolff's law) indicates the bone's need for function. Unstressed bone undergoes degenerative osteolytic changes and accelerated atrophy (Figures 2.18 and 2.19), while under physiological stress, the opposite occurs, the creation of new bone until a stable balance is reached. But, likewise, an overloaded bone is subject to even faster bone degeneration and deterioration if it is overloaded. This rule only confirms the general law of biology; function, but proper, maintains the organ, and the absence of function equals overload and destroys the organ. (discussed in more detail in the chapter on the legality of biomechanics in oral implantology.

Wolf's rule supports the justification for immediate loading of dental implants. This approach allows chewing forces to be transmitted onto the teeth and implants within physiological limits. As a result, it helps preserve and strengthen the surrounding bone. Conversely, a lack of mechanical load can lead to a decline in bone quality, causing resorption of the internal supporting structures around the implant. This process results in a loss of bone support and stability for the implant.

In conclusion, physiological loading is both functional and constructive, maintaining the volume and quality of the bone. In contrast, excessive loading can be destructive and demineralizing for the jawbone.

Divisions by bone quality groups

Misch and Judy described the quality of bones and divided them into four groups:

D1 group is characterized by: dense cortical bone with a small amount of spongiosis, which is most pronounced in the frontal part of the lower jaw, in atrophied regions.

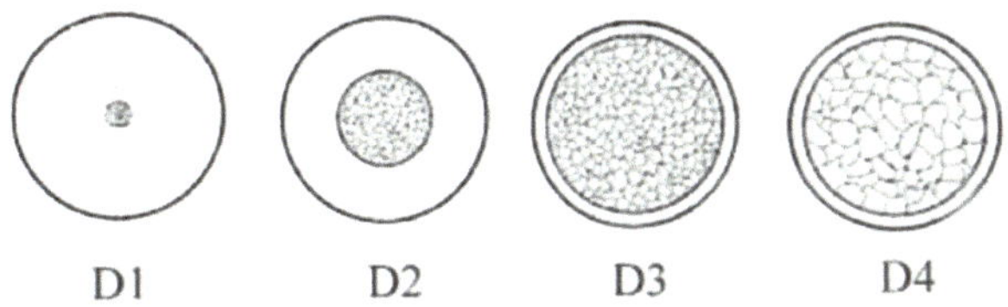

Figure 2.17. Division of bone quality according to K. E. Misch

Advantages of bone quality D1: achieving primary stability up to 90-98% and the possibility of applying shorter implants.

Disadvantages: poor vascularization, which slows healing during implant placement. Due to the compactness of the bone, there is a risk of overheating the bone during preparation. The use of long-used and dull drill bits increases the risk.

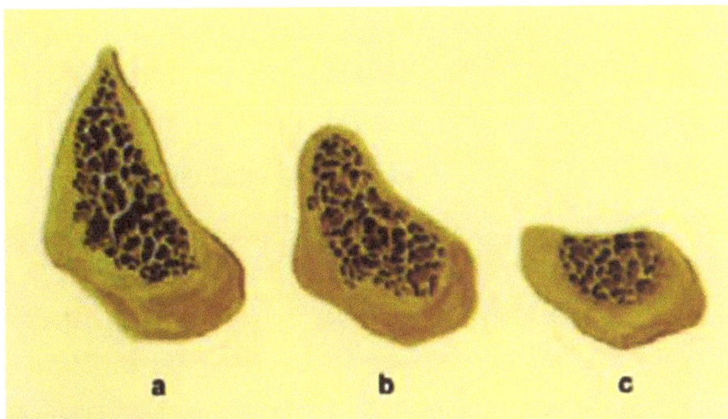

Figure 2.18. Atrophied alveolar ridges in the lower jaw (K. E. Misch).

The D2 group is characterized by dense cortical bone along with a denser region of cancellous bone, primarily found in the lateral areas of the mandible and the palatal section of the upper jaw. While the primary stability in this group is lower compared to the previous one, the vascularization of the bone is better. Advantages of D2 include faster bone healing and a simpler implantation technique.

The D3 group features thin cortical bone and low-density spongiosa, particularly in the lateral part of the upper jaw. This group presents a heightened risk of not achieving primary stability during implantation. Although D3 offers good blood supply and quicker healing, it also has disadvantages such as challenging osteotome application and difficult bicortical anchoring. To mitigate these risks, it is recommended to use a larger number of implants connected by a prosthetic superstructure.

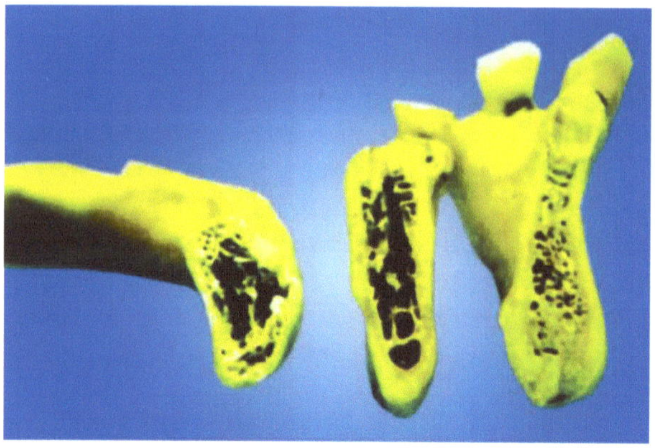

Figure 2.19. Illustration of internal bone resorption with emphasized empty spaces (Carl. E. Misch).

D4 bone quality group is the most risky for implant placement. This group is characterized by extremely thin cortical bone with widely expressed spongiosis in all parts of the upper jaw. The primary stability of the implant is reduced to a risky 25%.

The bone in the maxilla and mandible differs significantly both in quantity and quality, as well as in the shape of the formed alveolar ridges.

The alveolar ridge at the front of the upper jaw features a very thin, flexible cortical labial wall and a thicker, denser palatal cortical wall. The space between the labial and palatal cortices is filled with cancellous bone, which typically has a medium density. When the upper front teeth are lost, both the width and height of the ridge decrease. The most significant height loss occurs in the first year, averaging about 3 to 4 mm, and this loss is particularly evident in the labial portion of the bone. As a result of these anatomical changes and the greater resorption of the labial bone, dental implants are always placed toward the palatal side.

Great attention is given to the quality of the bone in the posterior part of the maxilla due to common challenges associated with implant installation. Bone loss frequently occurs on the buccal wall at the height of the ridge. The most significant bone loss in the lateral area of the upper jaw is caused by the destruction of the periodontium. Additionally, one of the major anatomical obstacles for implant placement is the enlargement of the maxillary sinuses. The degree of sinus pneumatization can vary, with the most common limitations occurring around the first molar region.

The sinus can extend from the pterygoid process to the canine area in the mesial direction. The cortical part of the floor is very thin. If the cortical bone of the sinus floor is too thin, where the occlusal loads are the highest, implant placement in this part is achieved by raising the sinus floor.

Gawood and Howell classified the shape of the alveolar ridge of the posterior part of the maxilla. They described what kind of ridge forms in the back of the maxilla after tooth loss:

a) immediately after the extraction, a small concavity is formed on the ridge;
b) after 8-10 weeks, the ridge takes on a rounded shape, of adequate width and height;
c) after a long period and delay of implantation, the ridge takes the shape of a knife, of adequate height and inadequate width;
d) flat shape of inadequate height and width;
e) and finally, there is a reduced ridge shape, with a clear basal loss.

Significant loss of alveolar bone in the posterior part of the maxilla is mostly due to long-term periodontal destruction. The main characteristic of bone quality and quantity in the posterior part of the maxilla is very thin cortical bone and very scarce trabecular spongiosa. The bone density in this region decreases distally, and may extend to the premolar region and is usually of medium density.

When considering implant placement in the back of the maxilla, keep the following points in mind:

1. Avoid proximity to the maxillary sinus.
2. The critical amount of bone must not be less than 7 mm in thickness.
3. Access from the buccal mesial side is straightforward, so the implant should be angled accordingly.
4. If conditions permit, it is beneficial to use implants with a wider diameter, ensuring that primary stability is achieved.

Adequate conditions can be established in this region for the installation of implants using autogenous bone grafts and for performing a sinus lift.

When evaluating the posterior region of the maxilla for implant placement, it's important to note that the bone quality in this area is typically weak, and the occlusal forces are high.

To meet biomechanical requirements, it's necessary to elevate the bone crest using grafts for both height and width, along with a sinus lift procedure to achieve sufficient bone volume. However, these interventions can be complex, and the success rates may vary.

Innervation zones of the upper and lower jaw

Innervation of the teeth of the upper jaw

The infraorbital nerve and its branches primarily innervate the upper jaw. The posterior superior alveolar branches emerge from it, traveling through the infraorbital nerve, which passes through the inferior orbital fissure to reach the orbit. These nerves exit the pterygopalatine fossa via the pterygomaxillary fissure and extend obliquely downward over the tubercle of the maxilla. Through the superior alveolar foramina, they ascend into the maxillary sinus, forming the superior dental plexus at its base. From there, the branches extend towards the molar roots, interdental septa, and interradicular septa (see Fig. 2.19). The cranial branches of the posterior superior alveolar nerve, after providing smaller branches to the mucous membrane of the maxillary sinus, continue forward to join the superior dental plexus, which innervates the spongy bone on the anterior aspect of the maxilla (see Figures 2.20 and 2.21).

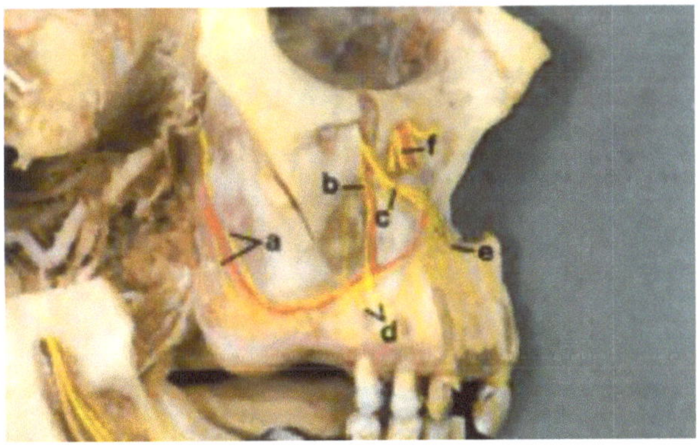

Figure 2.20. Innervation of the teeth of the upper jaw of a 70-year-old man: a =n.n. alveolares superiores posteriores, b = n. alveolaris superior medius, c = n.n. alveolares superiores anteriores, d = plexus dentalis, e = plexus caninus, f = n. infraorbitalis.

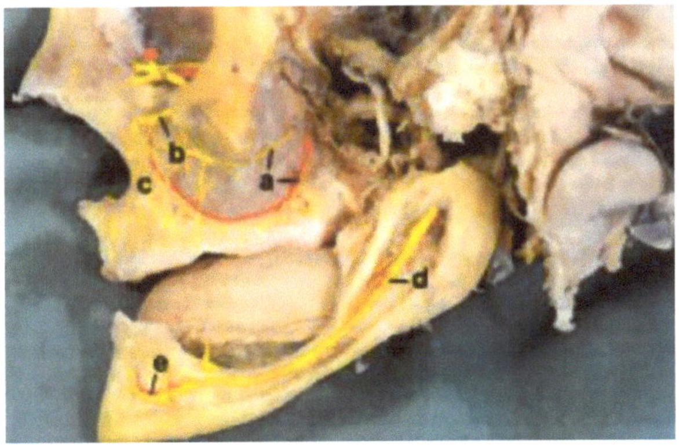

Figure 2.21. Innervation of the teeth of the upper jaw. A 92-year-old woman: a = n.n. alveolares superiores posteriores, b = n. alveolares superiores anteriores, c = plexus caninus, d = n. alveolaris inferior, e = n. incisive. (n. alveolaris inferior anterior).

This nerve plexus also includes nervus alveolaris superioris medius and n.n. alveolares superiores anteriores. All three branches at the bottom of the sinus form the plexus dentalis superior, from which the branches for bone, teeth, and gums are separated. The gum from the buccal side innervates n. bucalis from the last molar to half of the second premolar.

Plexus dentalis is in the area of the canine fossa, a shallow pit on the front wall of the maxillary body below the infraorbital foramen, of particular density. It seems justified to designate this anterior part of the plexus dentalis as the plexus caninus (Fig. 2.19). This independent designation is justified because some other nerves besides those already mentioned also participate in forming the canine plexus. It is about n. nasalis lateralis, the final branch of the anterior ethmoid nerve. N. ethmoidalis anterior represents a branch of n. nasociliaris, and belongs to the ophthalmic nerve. It seems particularly interesting that the afferent fibers from the canine and incisor teeth are carried by the ophthalmic nerve. Based on this fact, it can be explained that patients with toothaches in the area of canines or incisors complain of radiating pain in the frontal part of the forehead. The term "canine" used in the vernacular may explain the connection between that tooth and the eye area.

The lateral nasal nerve, followed by the artery of the same name, extends downward under the mucosa of the lateral nasal wall. One large branch pierces the lateral nasal wall and enters the plexus caninus (Figure 2.19).

The infraorbitalis nerve, after leaving the infraorbital foramen with its branches, no longer participates in the innervation of the teeth or gingiva.

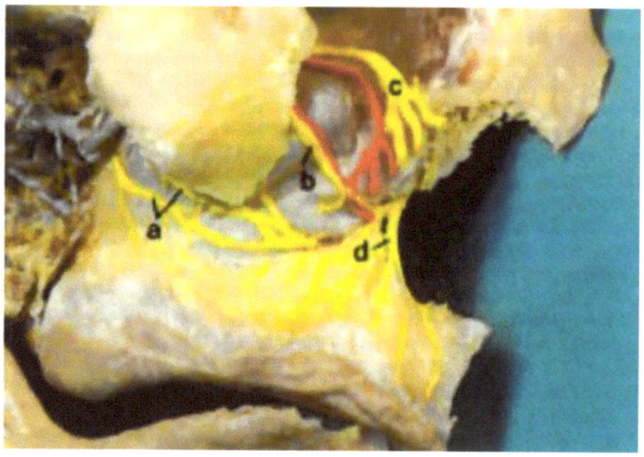

Figure 2.22. Innervation of upper jaw teeth, 47-year-old woman: a = nn. alveolares superiores posteriores, b = n. alveolaris superior medius, c = n. infraorbitalis, d = n. nasalis lateralis after preparation of the path of one part of the lateral bony wall of the nose. Take care of the formation of branches n. nasalis lateralis with plexus caninus.

Innervation of lower jaw teeth

N. mandibularis is the third branch of the trigeminal nerve. The lower jaw is innervated by the lower alveolar nerve, a branch of the mandibular nerve.

N. alveolaris inferior passes through the mandibular canal in a solid periosteal sheath (Figures 2.23-2.25), which extends from the foramen of the mandible to the foramen mentale. So, on the entire passage through the bony tunnel of the mandible. However, that periosteal sheath does not belong to the neurovascular bundle, which is mentioned, but belongs to the inner wall of the mandibular canal. The periosteal sheath, in addition to the nerve, also includes the lower alveolar artery and vein, as well as the central lymphatic vessel of the teeth of the lower jaw. At irregular distances, the said sheath is pierced by nerve branches that pass freely through the spongiosa and provide dental and interdental branches that depart almost vertically.

Due to implant procedures, it is important to emphasize that at a short distance, in the area of the mental foramen, from n. alveolaris inferiora separates n. incisivus for canine and incisors. Lateral branches of n. mentalis and n. alveolaris inferior innervate bone, teeth, and gums. As previously mentioned, n. alveolaris inferior anterior, as a rule, intersects with n. mentalis. Crossing from the upper side was never observed, as the textbooks generally state.

When opening the periosteal sheath, it can be observed that the dental-gingival branches with their accompanying vessels separate early. Another segment passes inside the periosteal sheath, before breaking through it (Figure 2.23). In a third of cases, n. alveolaris inferior already before entering the mandibular canal divides into its final branches:

1. n. mylohioideus, which as a motor branch extends through the sulcus mylohioideus on the inner side of the mandible to its area of innervation
2. as a rule, two dentogingival nerves
3. the longest branch, n. alveolaris inferior anterior (n. incisivus), i
4. the strongest branch of n. mentalis (Figure 2.23). The sensitive innervation of the palatal gingiva and the mucous membrane of the palate takes place via n. palatinus and n. nasopalatinus that anastomose with each other.

In the area of the lower jaw, the buccal nerve provides innervation of a small field, buccally in the area of the first molars. The remaining part of the gingiva is innervated buccally by n. dentogingivales of the lower alveolar nerve, labially by n. alveolaris inferior anterior (n. incisivus), and lingually by the lingual nerve (Figure 2.23).

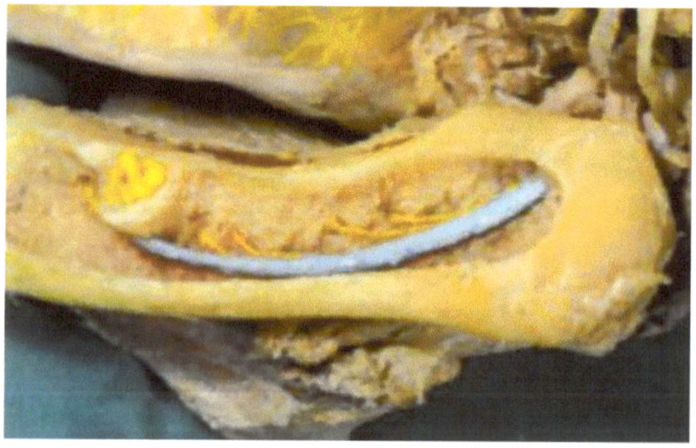

Figure 2.23. Left side of the lower jaw of a 68-year-old man: Open mandibular canal. The tough periosteal sheath extending from the mandibular foramen to the mental foramen is colored blue.

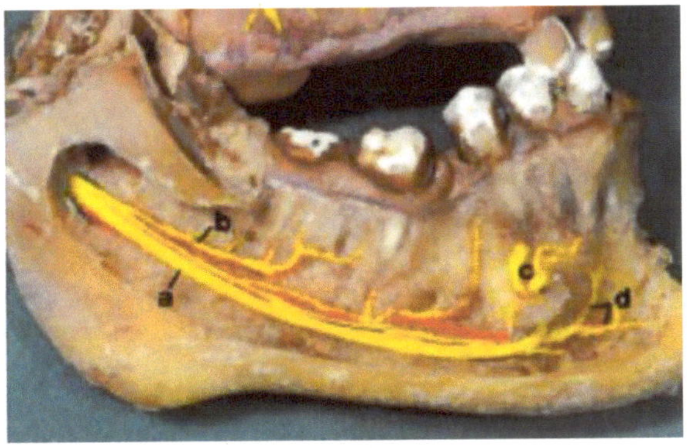

Figure 2.24. Right side of the mandible of a 57-year-old man: Open mandibular canal and elimination of the periosteal sheath; a = n. alveolaris inferior, b = n. dentogingivalis, c = n. mentalis, d = n. incisive. (n. alveolaris inferior anterior).

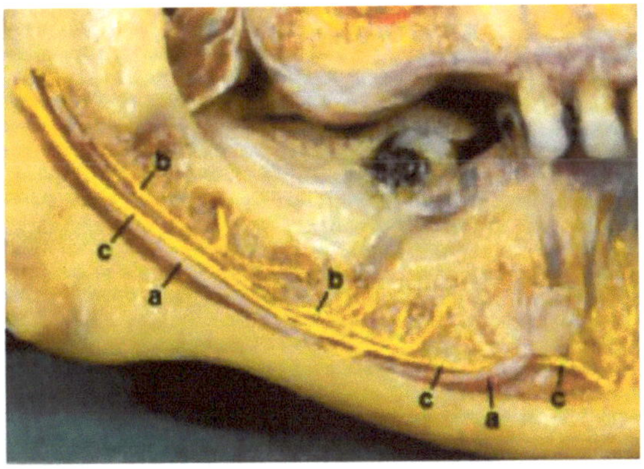

Figure 2.25. The right side of the lower jaw of a 79-year-old man. High separation n. alveolaris inferior. In the canalis of the mandible there are: a = n. mentalis (not color coded), b = n. dento-gingivalis, c = n. incisive (n. alveolaris inferior anterior).

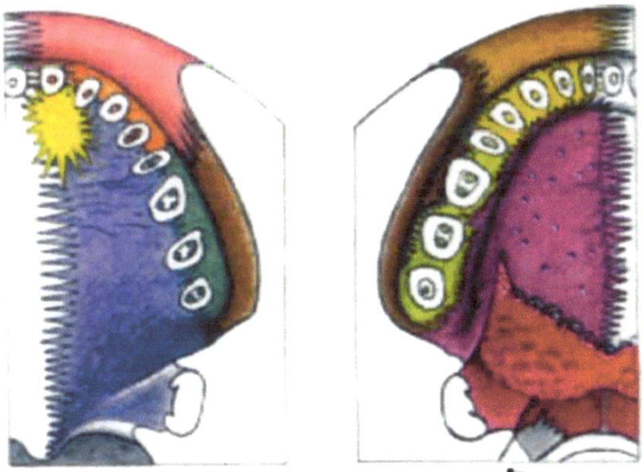

a b

Figure 2.26a and 2.26b. Sensitive innervation of the gingiva. a: upper jaws: labial vestibular: orange = plexus caninus, green = plexus dentalis (nn. alveolares superiores posteriores et medii). Palatal: blue = n. palatinus major, yellow = n. nasopalatinus. n. infraorbitalis (purple) and n. buccalis (brown) do not participate in the sensitive innervation of the gingiva of the upper jaw; b: mandibles. Labial buccal: yellow = n. incisivus (n. alveolaris inferior anterior), brown = n. bucalis, green = n. dentogingivalis; lingual: purple = n. lingual. n. mentalis (light brown) does not participate in the sensitive innervation of the gingiva (according to Pernkopf).

Arteries of the upper jaw

The upper jaw is supplied with blood from the branches of a. maxillaris, a. infraorbitalis and a. palatine descedens (Figures 23 and 24). With a. maxillaris are connected a. alveolaris superior media and a. alveolaris superior anterior that separate from a infraorbitalis, the final branch of a. maxillaris (Figures 2.27 and 2.28).

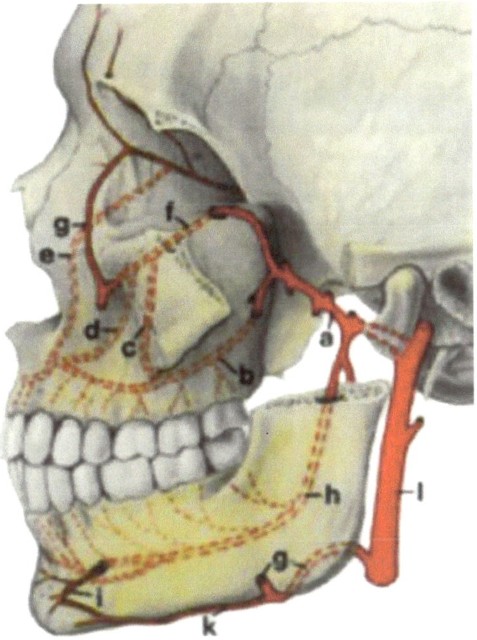

Figure 2.27. External arterial vascular ring of upper and lower jaw teeth: a =a. maxillaris, b = a. alveolaris superior posterior, c = a. alveolaris superior media, d = a. alveolaris superior anterior, e = a. nasalis lateralis, f = infraorbital artery, g = facial artery, h = inferior alveolar artery, i = a. mentalis, k = a. submentalis, l = a. carotid externa.

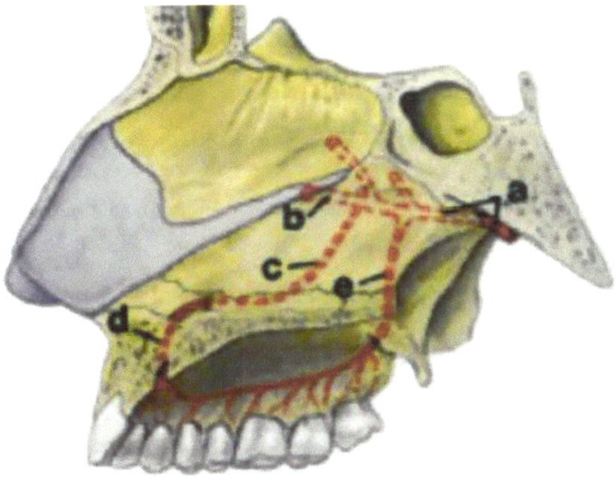

Figure 2.28. Internal arterial vascular ring for the blood supply of the gingiva of the teeth of the upper jaw: a = maxillary artery, b = spheno-

palatine artery, c = a. nasalis posterior septi, d = ramus anastomoticus, e = descending palatine artery (a. palatina major).

Arteries of lower jaw teeth

The teeth of the lower jaw are also supplied with blood through a vascular ring. The main blood vessel is the lower alveolar artery, which passes through the mandibular canal and reaches the teeth of the lower jaw via the dental branches. A. alveolaris inferior over the mental artery and the submental artery forms one external vascular arch with the facial artery (Figure 2.29). The internal vascular arch connects the lower alveolar artery with the deep lingual artery through the supragenioideus ramus, and with the sublingual artery through the interincisive branches (Figure 2.29).

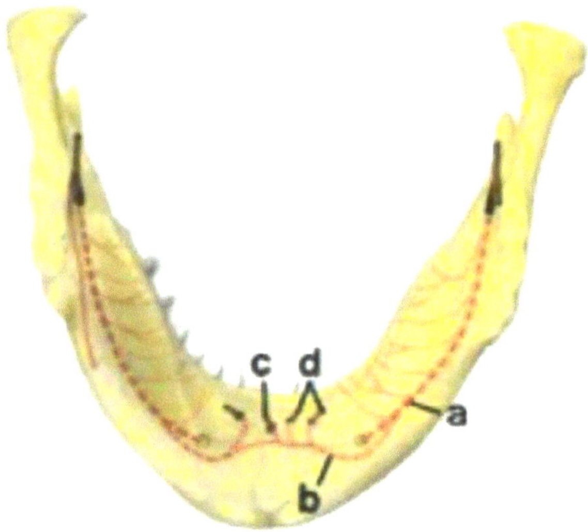

Figure 2.29. Internal anastomoses of the lower alveolar artery: a = a. alveolaris inferior, b = a. incisive (a. alveolaris inferior anterior), c = ramus supragenoideus of the deep lingual artery, d = rami interincisive of the sublingual artery.

Venous drainage of upper and lower jaw teeth

Venous blood from the pulp flows via superior alveolar veins and inferior alveolar veins into the pterygoid plexus, a venous vascular network located on the lateral surface of the medial pterygoid muscle. This venous vascular network drains blood via the maxillary veins into the vena retromandibularis (Figure 2.30). Of special importance is the fact that the plexus pterygoideus has four drainage courses that lead to the cavernous sinus: 1. through the plexus foraminis ovalis, 2. through v. meningea media, 3. via an anastomosis between the lower ophthalmic vein to the upper ophthalmic vein, and 4. via the infraorbital vein (or v. faciei profunda) to the facial vein, and from there, via the angular vein and vena dorsalis nazi, it affects the upper ophthalmic vein. These connections with the cavernous sinus are, for this reason, of special clinical importance, since infections from the area of the teeth of the upper and, much less often, the lower jaw can, through the mentioned vessels and arterio-venous anastomoses, lead to thrombosis of the cavernous sinus, with consequent, life-threatening, consequences.

For the craniomandibular relationship, see Chapter 8.

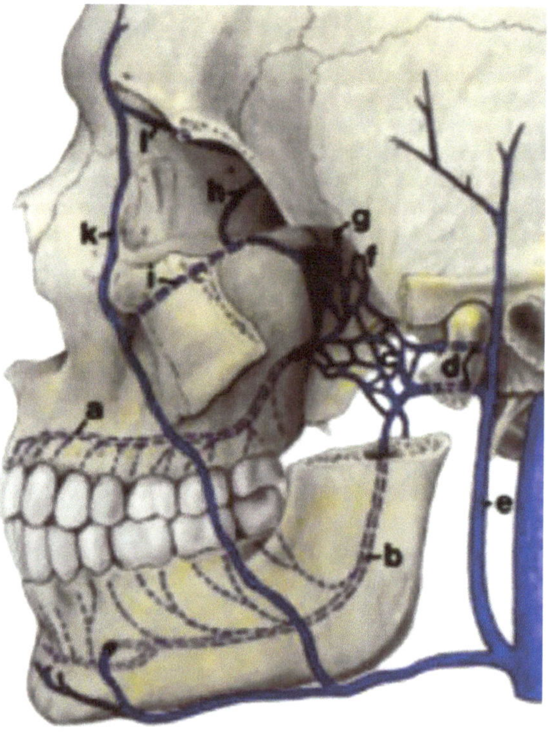

Figure 2.30. Venous Drainage in the Upper and Lower Jaw Teeth Area. Venous blood from the tooth area drains through the superior alveolar vein (a) and inferior alveolar vein (b) into the pterygoid plexus (c). From there, it flows through the maxillary veins (d) into the retromandibular vein (e). There are various connections with the cavernous sinus via the foramen ovale plexus (f), the medial meningeal vein (g), the inferior ophthalmic vein (h), and the infraorbital vein (i). The infraorbital vein has an anastomosis with the facial vein (k), which also connects with the dorsalis nasi vein (l) originating from the superior ophthalmic vein.

3
Role and Design of the Implants

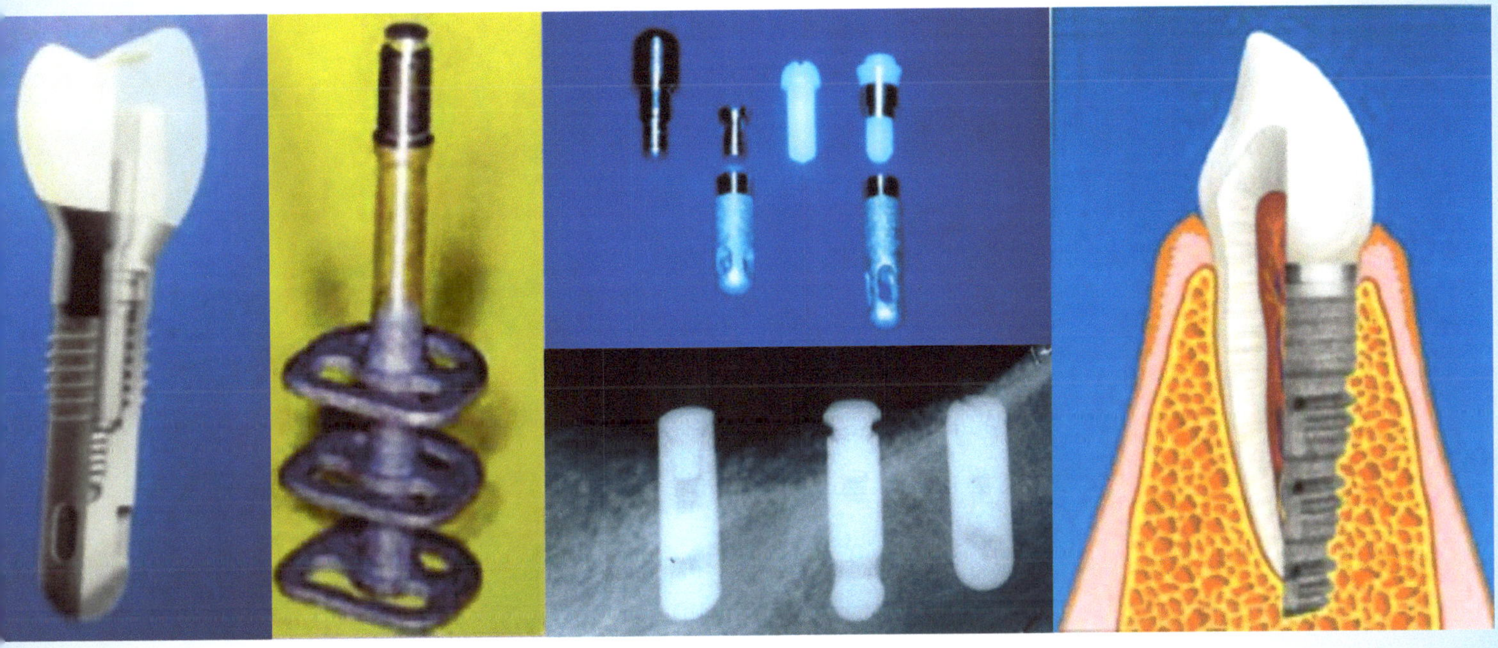

Implants have their basic role in replacing lost teeth that bother people when eating and distort their appearance. The shape of the part of the implant that lies in the bone imitates the root of the tooth by design (Figures 2.1-2.3). In the past, there was a lot of confusion when it came to the component elements of the implant, the part that lies in the bone, and the part that is in contact with the soft tissues - the implant neck and the support (abutment). In the end, a logical solution followed that it is best to make an implant the way nature did it precisely. Experience confirms that the design of the implant depends on its stability in the bone.

One or more teeth, i.e. single-rooted and multi-rooted teeth, can be compensated by implant installation in regions where there are conditions for implant installation: sufficient amount of available bone, favorable anatomical structures, and favorable position of interjaw relationships (Figures 2.4-2.16).

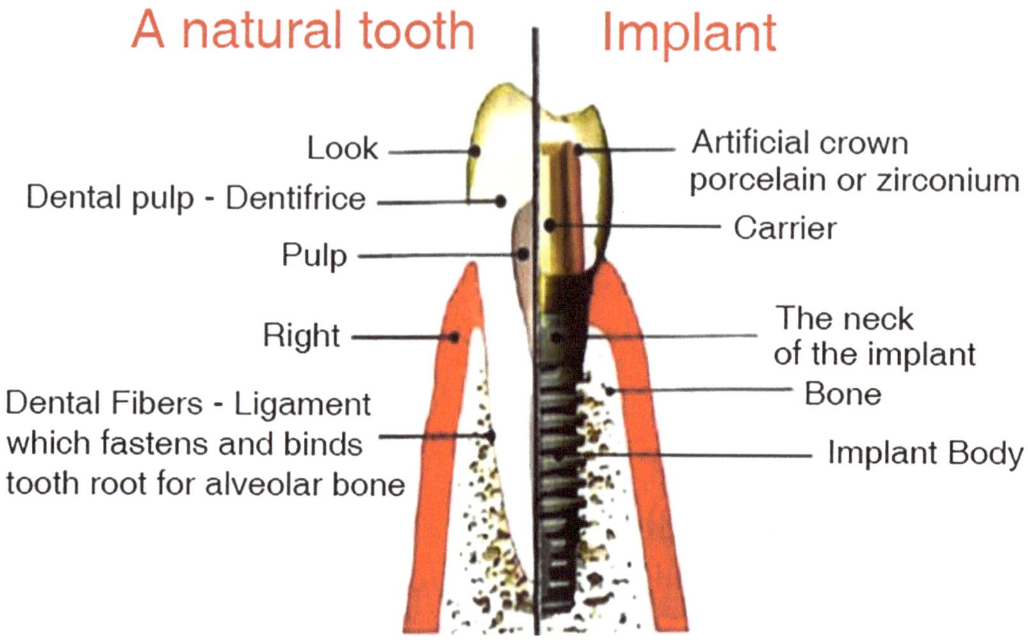

Figure 3.1. Schematic representation of the root of a natural tooth and an implant. Approaching the shape of the implant to the shape of the natural root, following this logic, the conical design of the implant for stability in the jawbone is the best.

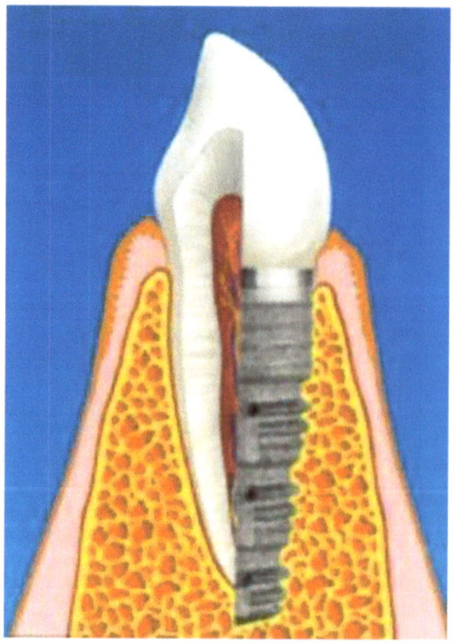

Figure 3.2. Schematic representation of the position of the implant in the bone as a substitute for a natural tooth.

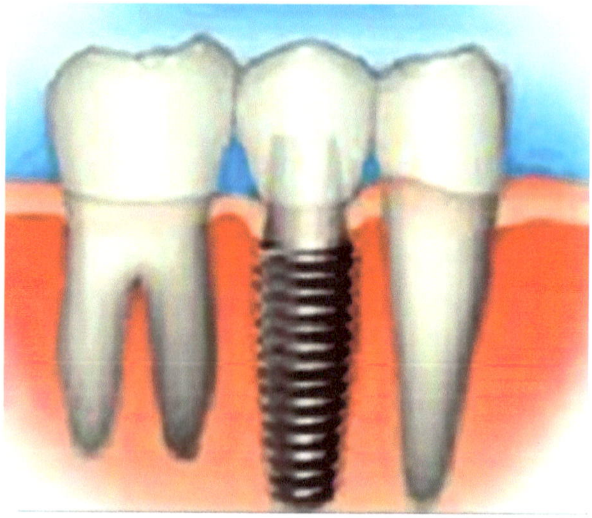

Figure 3.3. Schematic representation of premolar restoration.

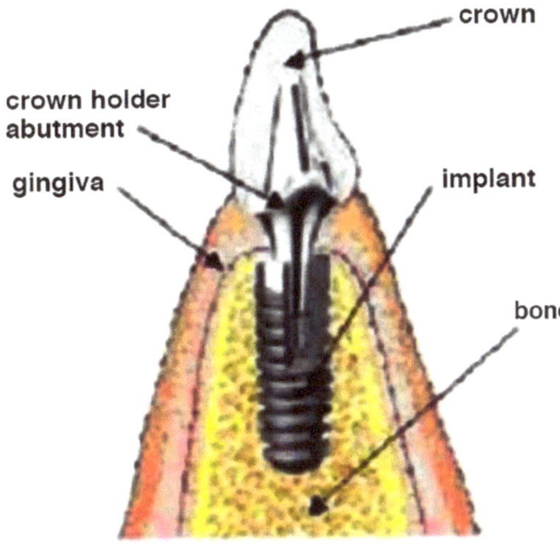

Figure 3.4. Schematic representation of the relationship between the soft tissues and the neck of the implant - the body of the implant and the bone with the support and the crown.

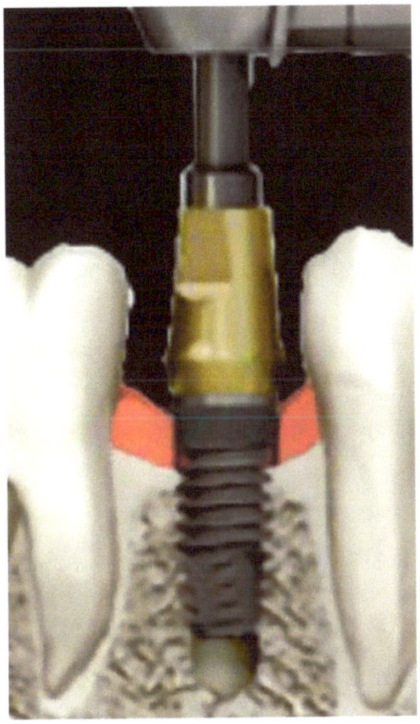

Figure 3.5. Schematic representation of the replacement of one tooth with an implant.

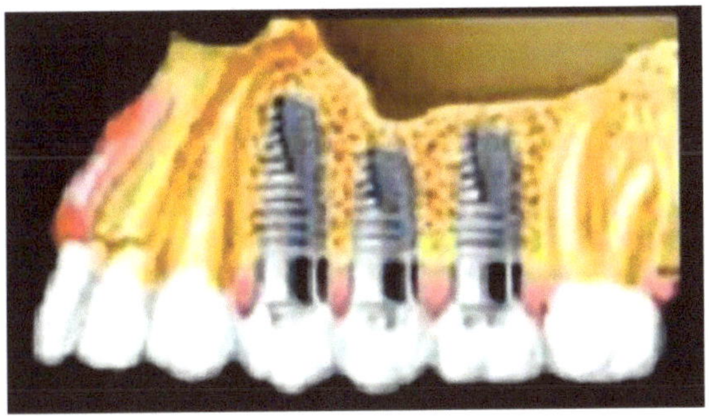

Figure 3.6. Schematic representation of implants of different lengths adapted to the anatomical configuration of the maxillary sinus.

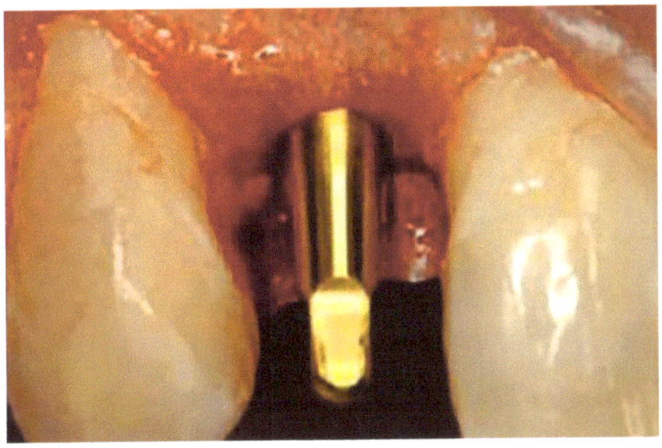

Figure 3.7. Abutment (support) of a one-piece implant with a narrow diameter.

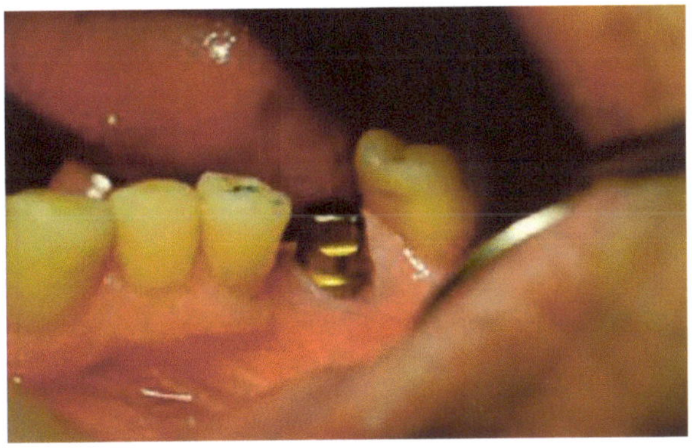

Figure 3.8. Molar replacement with a wide diameter implant.

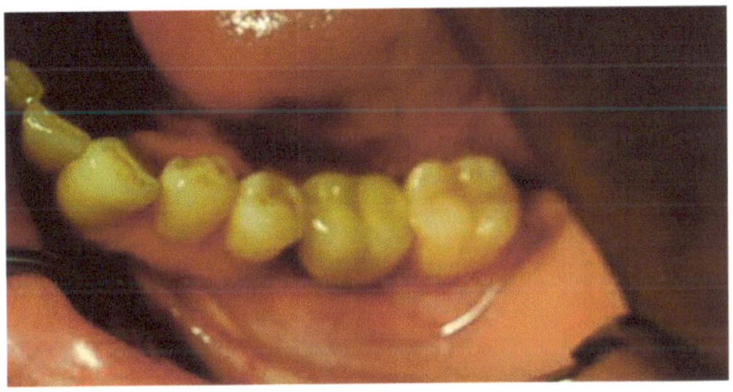

Figure 3.9. Metal-ceramic molar crown on a wide-diameter implant.

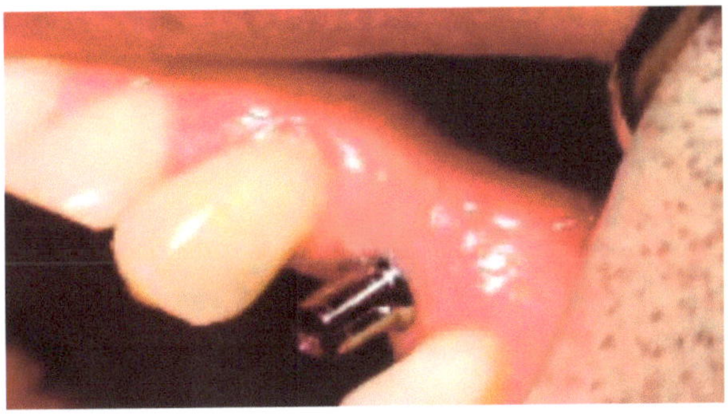

Figure 3.10. Compensation of the first premolar for installation of Nobel-Biocare implants.

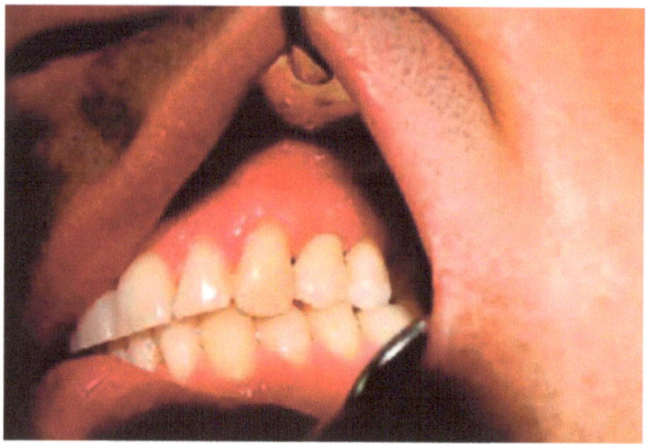

Figure 3.11. Appearance of the crown of the first premolar on the implant (Figure 3.10).

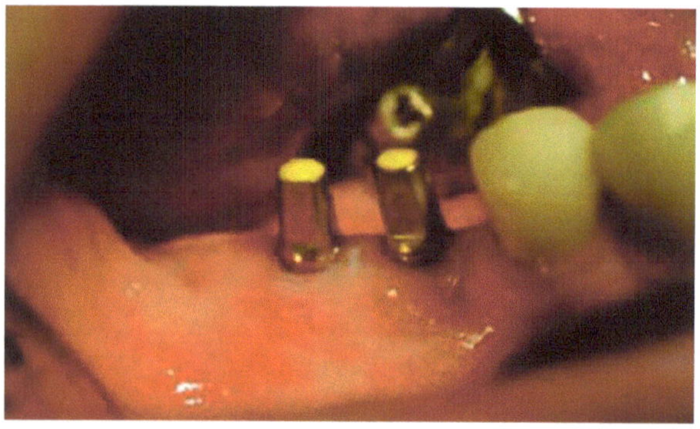

Figure 3.12. The appearance of the healed gingiva around the supports (abutments) placed immediately after the immediate installation of Nobel-Biocare implants, immediately loaded with temporary acrylic crowns.

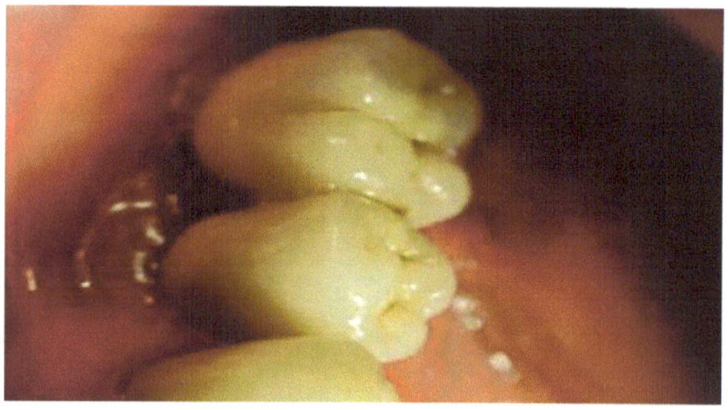

Figure 3.13. Definitive crowns on metal-ceramic abutments (Figure 3.12).

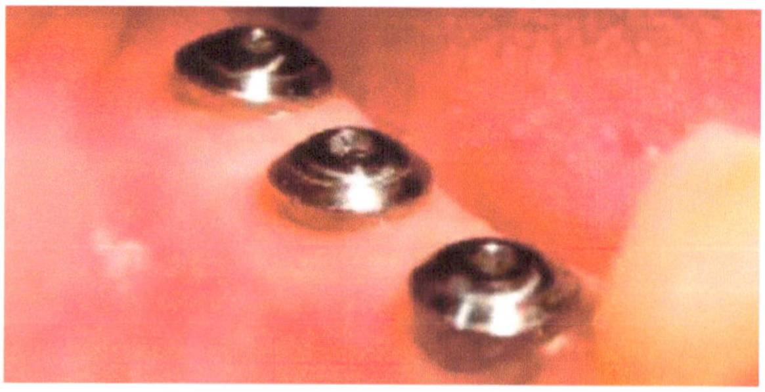

Figure 3.14. Formation of gingival sulcus with dedicated elements (screw healing).

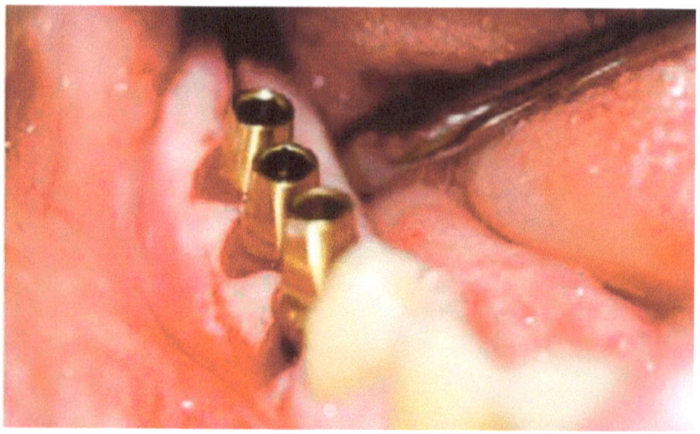

Figure 3.15. The current established procedure for the formation of the gingival sulcus with the elements of the gingival former (screw healing) is the opinion of the author of the book that the placement of a definitive abutment immediately after the installation of the implant is a more justified procedure.

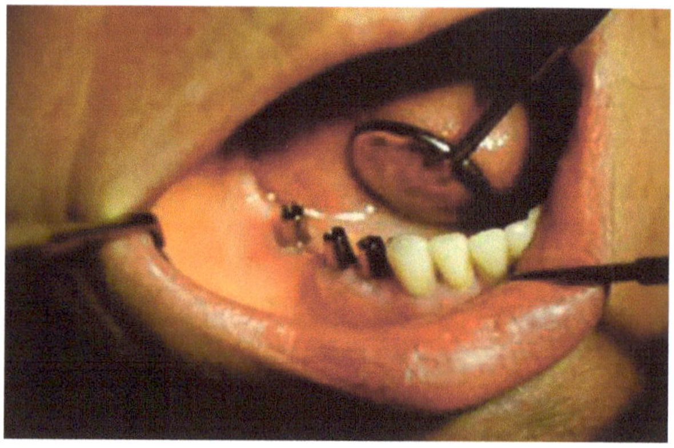

Figure 3.16. Abutments placed on a two-part implant immediately after implant placement without raising the flap.

Losing one or more teeth disrupts both the natural and aesthetic harmony of the mouth and face, affecting the overall dental structure. When a tooth is partially lost, it results in a decrease in bone mass in that area because the bone loses its natural productive function associated with the tooth root. The absence of a natural tooth leads to subtle changes in the angulation of the remaining teeth, reducing the spaces between them. This reduction can cause issues with tooth alignment, which may also affect the relationships between the upper and lower jaws. These changes can lead to discomfort or complications in the jaw joint. When a tooth is lost, the adjacent teeth can begin to shift, become misaligned, or even fall out entirely. This often leads to complications during dental procedures, such as the fitting of crowns and bridges, especially if a patient delays visiting the dentist. The situation can become more complex when it involves dental implants. As the natural teeth shift, the space between them decreases (refer to Figures 3.17-3.19). If this interdental space is less than 3 mm, placing an implant is not advisable, primarily for aesthetic reasons, since it becomes difficult to create a crown of the proper size and shape. To create the necessary space for a narrow-diameter implant, orthodontic displacement may be needed.

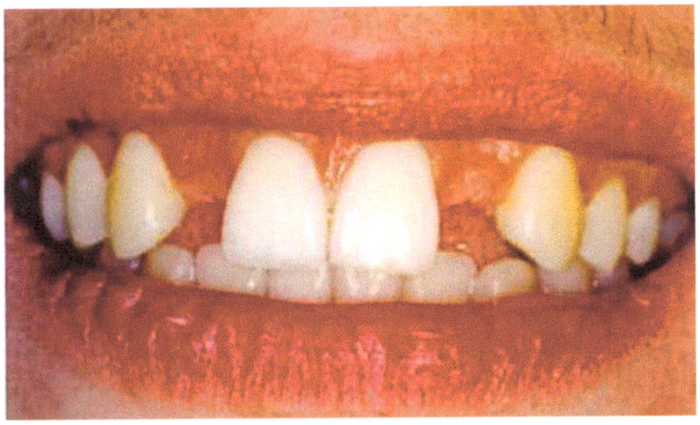

Figure 3.17. Anodontia of the lateral incisors is an indication for implant placement.

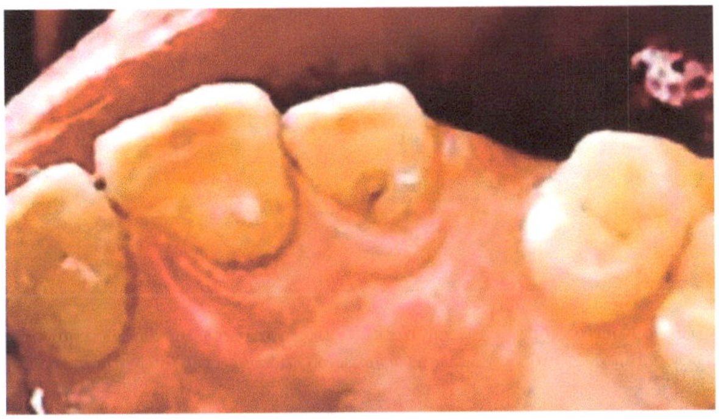

Figure 3.18. Long retention of a milk canine or premature loss of a lateral incisor leaves the result of a narrow interdental space, which makes implant placement an aesthetic risk factor.

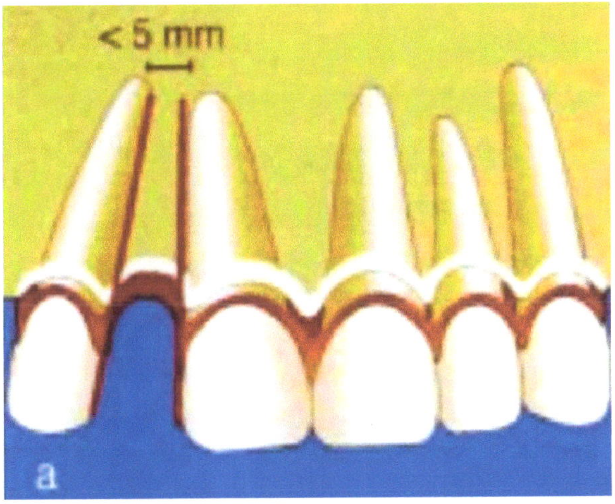

Figure 3.19. Schematic representation of a narrow interdental space caused by anodontia or loss of a natural tooth.

Nature has ensured that the forces received by the tooth with its supporting apparatus during chewing are properly absorbed and atraumatically distributed within physiological limits. For this reason, it was important to copy nature when it came to implant design to the extent possible.

Over time, periodontal disease can cause natural teeth to drift out of their sockets, leading to a condition known as "floating teeth." This phenomenon, previously termed passive tooth growth, is now more accurately referred to as pathological tooth migration. When teeth lose their proper alignment and harmony, they are subjected to the forces of chewing in an abnormal way. This additional stress can create leverage, causing teeth to loosen and eventually fall out. The longer the periodontal disease persists, the more alveolar bone is lost. Teeth with strong enamel, which resists wear on the occlusal surface, are particularly susceptible to these changes. Some individuals may experience more pronounced abrasion than others. Teeth that are prone to abrasion tend to be more resistant to periodontal changes. By reducing the clinical crown through abrasion above the maxillary ridge, the leverage effect is minimized, resulting in weaker and less favorable chewing forces. When considering implant extension, it's important to note that the material used for the crown differs from that of a natural tooth (see Figures 3.20 and 3.21). Porcelain is two to three times harder than tooth enamel, and zirconium is even harder. Therefore, using these materials for immediate loading in prosthetic work is not advisable, as the lack of abrasion can negatively impact the integration process. A significant disadvantage of prosthetic superstructures on implants is the application of materials that have a hardness similar to that of natural tooth enamel on the biting surfaces. Consequently, for immediate loading, provisional prosthetic work should be made with much softer materials than ceramics. Remember that ceramics are 2.5 times harder than natural tooth enamel, which is crucial to consider during the initial healing phase to promote successful integration.

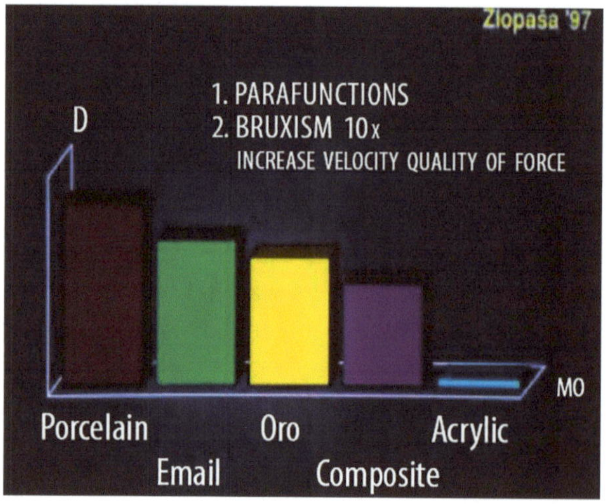

Figure 3.20. Hardness of materials used in prosthetic restorations. (From the lecture of the author of the book at the world symposium of implantologists in Bologna).

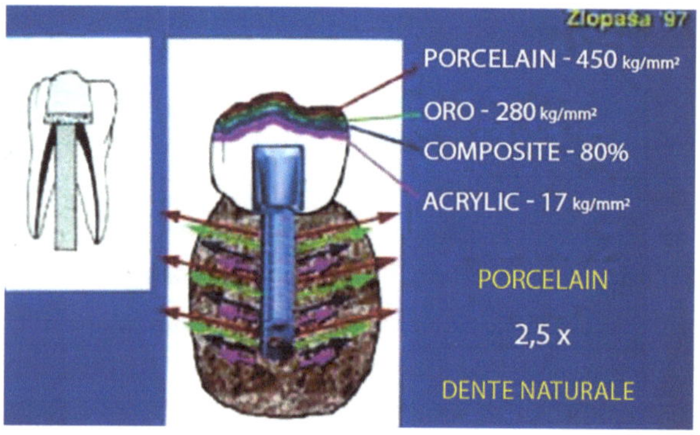

Figure 3.21. Schematic representation of differences in the hardness of different building materials. The occlusal surface made of ceramics is 2.5 times harder than the enamel of a natural tooth (from the author's lecture at the World Congress of Implantologists in Bologna).

Nature made an effort to ensure that the building material receives the action of chewing forces on the bone and distributes them within physiological limits, which is supported by the position of the teeth, and the position and number of roots. Therefore, the conical design of the implant is the most justified solution. In the natural series of teeth, there are single-rooted and multi-rooted teeth. The strongest chewing forces are expressed in the regions of the molars, which must always be kept in mind when installing implants in that region.

Natural harmony is reflected in the number, shape, and arrangement of the teeth, as well as in the number, arrangement, and shape of the roots. For the molars, where the action of chewing forces is the strongest, and due to the great difference in bone density and compactness, in the upper and lower jaw, nature determined the number, position, and shape of the roots, and adapted the hardness of the biting surfaces to physiological requirements.

The above should be kept in mind in order to understand biomechanical events on prosthetic restorations on implants, to which a separate chapter is dedicated (11).

In terms of the building material used for implant crowns and the hardness of the occlusal surfaces of natural teeth, the occlusal surfaces of artificial implant crowns are much harder. When biomechanical events are taken into account, the hardness of the occlusal surfaces of prosthetic works can adversely affect the integration processes. For this reason, the creation of prosthetic works in zirconium on implants in the lateral regions should be avoided - this is the opinion of the author.

Upper molars are three-rooted, and in the lower jaw two-rooted, and this natural law must be respected when replacing molars with implants to reduce the reception of chewing forces to physiological limits. Compensate the shape, length, position, and number of roots: position, number, diameter, and length of the implant, and harmonize the prosthetic work with biomechanical and aesthetic requirements.

Most often, when replacing four incisors in the lower jaw, the number of natural roots cannot be compensated with the same number of implants due to the disproportion between the diameter of the natural root and the diameter of the implant (Figure 3.22). The disproportion between the diameters of the roots of natural teeth in the front of the lower jaw is particularly pronounced in the mesiodistal direction. The diameter of the incisor root in the lingual-labial direction is usually around five millimeters or less, and the mesiodistal thickness of the root is around two millimeters. Placement of implants with standard or wider diameters could compromise osseous integration due to insufficient inter-implant bone space and very thin bucco-valve lamellar bone, therefore there is a risk of fenestration.

In the case of restorations in the front regions of the jaws, the positioning of the implants determines, therefore, both the functional and the aesthetic outcome.

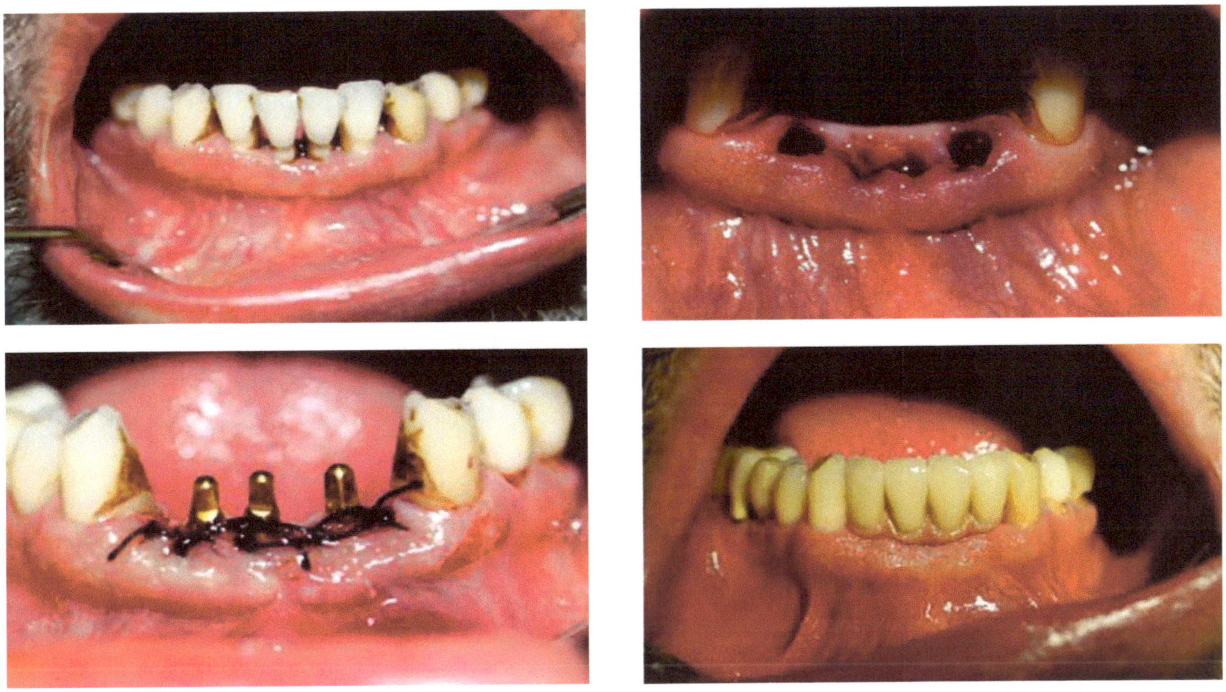

Figure 3.22. Presentation of the installation of Biohorizons implants with a diameter of 3 mm in the region 42, 41, 31, 32 of the lower jaw, which are immediately loaded. The diameter and design of the implant is not identical to the design and diameter of the natural root. For this reason, the number of extracted teeth cannot compensate for the same number of implants. Appearance of definitive prosthetic work in metal-ceramics on implants.

The molars bear the greatest pressure from chewing forces. Chewing forces that are neutralized are distributed appropriately to the length and shape of the root. Physiological biomechanical harmony is harmonized with a preserved dental row. Incisors are exclusively single-rooted and serve to cut food. When replacing front teeth with implants, in addition to functional ones, it is important to fulfill aesthetic requirements. Loss of teeth disrupts that harmony. By placing an implant, an attempt is made to restore the disturbed harmony.

For a long time, implantology has stagnated in terms of implant design, the complexity of chewing forces, their reception, and decomposition so as not to damage the bone.

Not infrequently, with the installation of implants of today's outdated designs, large bone destructions caused by traumatic aggressive implant installation and biomechanical inconsistencies followed in practice.

A long-standing question in experimentation has been how to design an implant. It was necessary to imitate nature, which gave it to the ancient divine invention, the natural tooth, in the most perfect way: the hardness and elasticity of the building material, taking into account all the anatomical disadvantages in both jaws.

Imitation of the root of the tooth (Figures 3.23 and 3.24), as previously emphasized, is considered as an optimized copy of what nature has created.

However, when it comes to this copy of nature, it can never be completely achieved, but it can be theoretically discussed how close to nature can be with creations. Science has advanced considerably when it comes to oral implantology. Implant design is important, but the main component of tissue engineering technology is the matrix of biomaterials from which the implant is made. The bioinert material titanium from which the dental implant or hip, heart valves and other partial substitutes of natural tissues are made, replacing certain tissue, provides mechanical, but not metabolic function. For this reason, in contrast to the fact that a copy of the root design of a natural tooth is optimized by an implant, it entails disadvantages that do not exist in a natural tooth. Despite the ankylosing stiffness, it is possible to have the same events that we have in natural teeth: periodontal disease, and in the case of implants, the appearance of peri-implantitis and complications of treatment.

When replacing a lost tooth with implants, the primary goal is to achieve optimal osseous integration. This term refers to how closely the bone approximates the surface of the implant (see Chapter 7 on osseous integration). While a rigid connection between the implant and the bone might be perceived as unnatural, it is considered normal with embedded implants. Although these concepts are more theoretical, they are not crucial to practical applications. The focus is primarily on the design of the implant's shape.

There are two main shapes used for implants: cylindrical and screw-shaped (see Figures 3.23-3.25). The cylindrical shape is becoming less common.

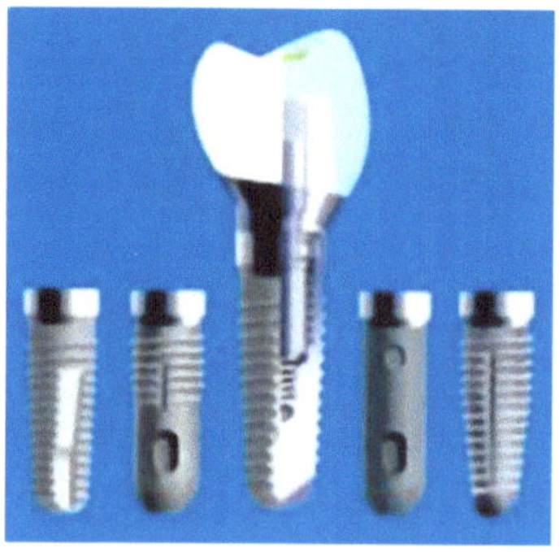

Figure 3.23. The combination of screw and cylindrical implant is no longer in use.

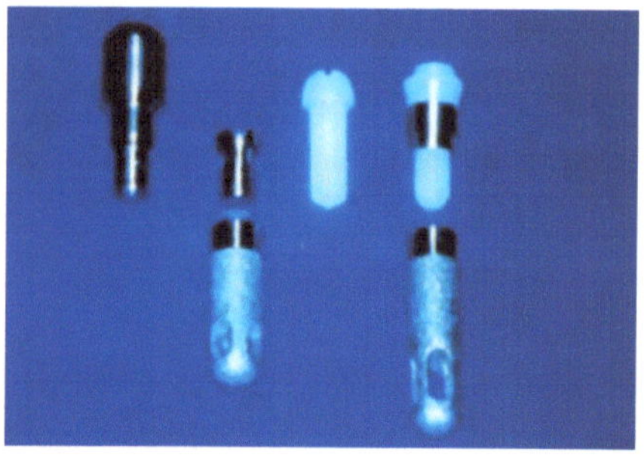

Figure 3.24. Cylindrical shape of the implant.

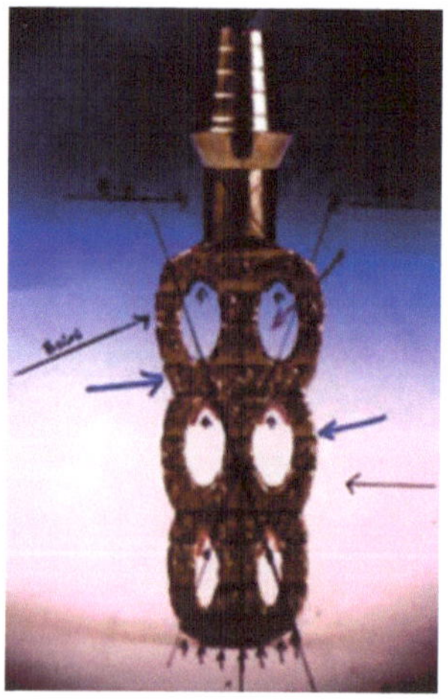

Figure 3.25. Leaf implant design intended for implant placement in the frontal regions (picture from a lecture by the author of the book "Reception and distribution of forces in leaf implants", Liege, Belgium, 1981).

When there is a lack of space in the jaw in the vertical direction, short implants can also be applied, which can be satisfactorily functional (Figures (3.29 and 3.30).

It is also possible to connect two or more implants using the so-called Dolder or Ackerman crossbars (Figures 3.31-3.33).

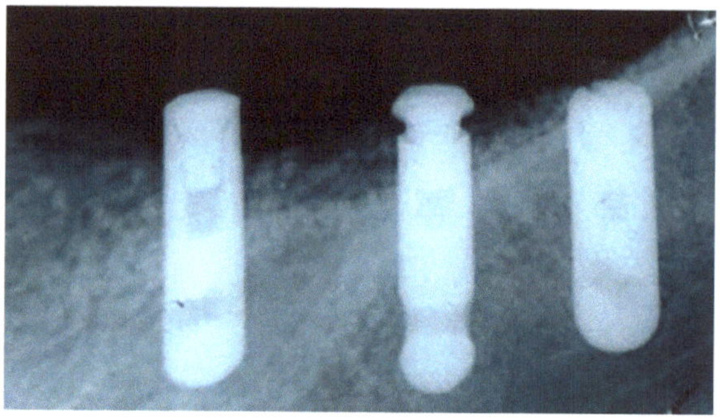

Figure 3.26. Cylindrical forms of implants

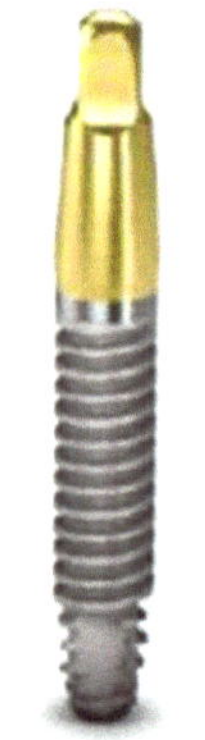

Figure 3.27. The one-piece form of the implant has a diameter of 3 mm. Implant neck coated with "laser-luck" technology.

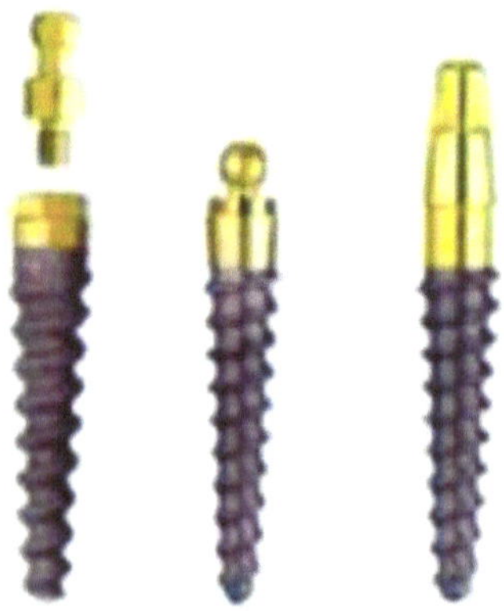

Figure 3.28. Different thread design for implants with a narrow diameter of 3 mm.

One-piece implants (3.0 mm) have different surface treatments. (pictures 3.27 and 3.28) and the possibility of adjusting the abutment without transferring heat to the implant body. The neck part of the one-piece implant, which remains above the level of the bone, is processed with "laser-luck" technology, which promotes better attachment of peri-implant soft tissues (picture 3.27) and a design that lacks this processing (picture 3.28). Recently, implants with wider diameters have been designed.

The application of one-part and two-part implants with a narrow diameter in the frontal part of the lower jaw has proven to be a good solution for the functions of uncomfortable and unstable total acrylate prostheses. It is about the so-called "mini" or standard forms (depending on the width and length of the alveolar bone). All forms of one-piece implants must be loaded immediately.

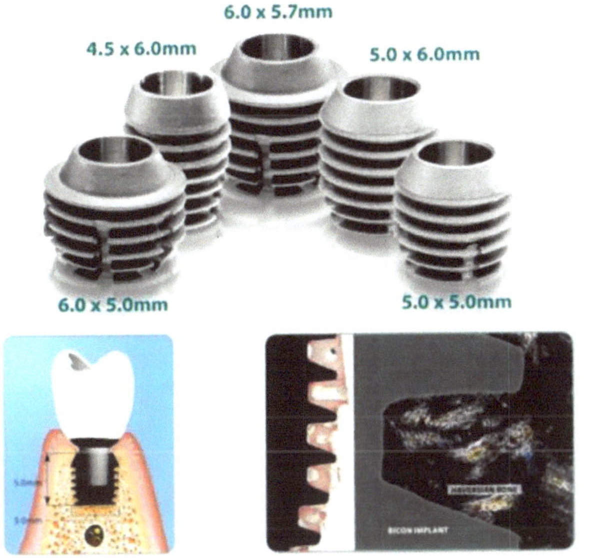

Figure 3.29. Design of short implants with wide diameters and heights between 5 and 6 mm. Microscopic view of bone growth between the threads of the implant body and histological view of bone integration on the thread.

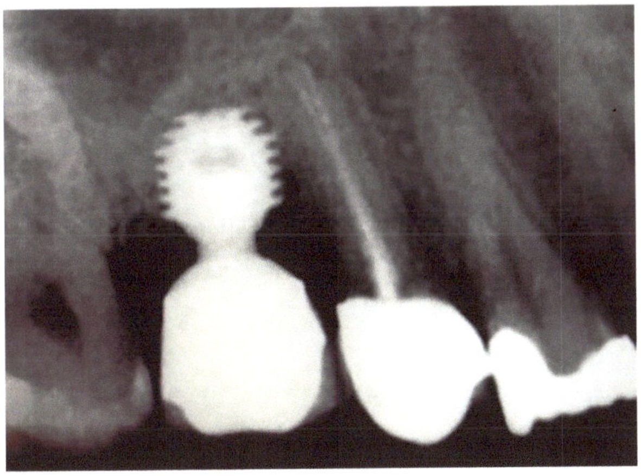

Figure 3.30. Design of short implants with a diameter of 6 mm and a height of 6 mm. Control shot after 2 years.

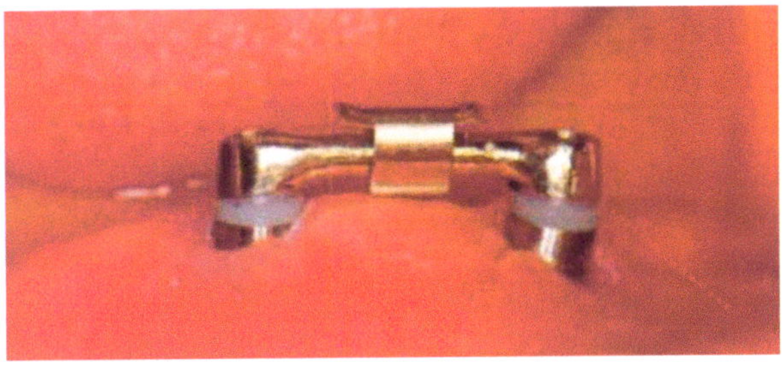

Figure 3.31. Dolder bar on two implants with retention-resilient riders and inserted Teflon rings.

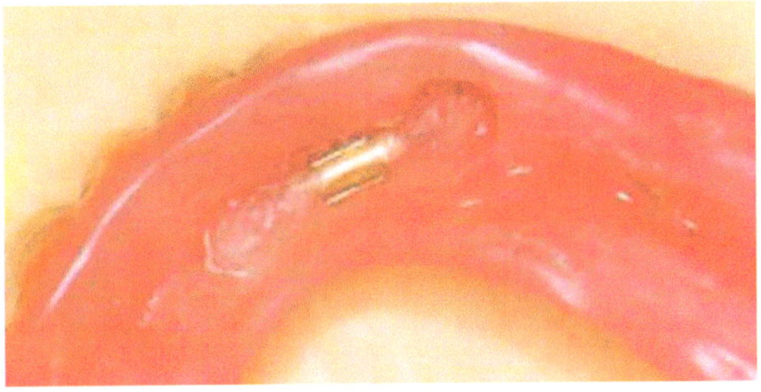

Figure 3.31a. Retention grip for Dolder's bar.

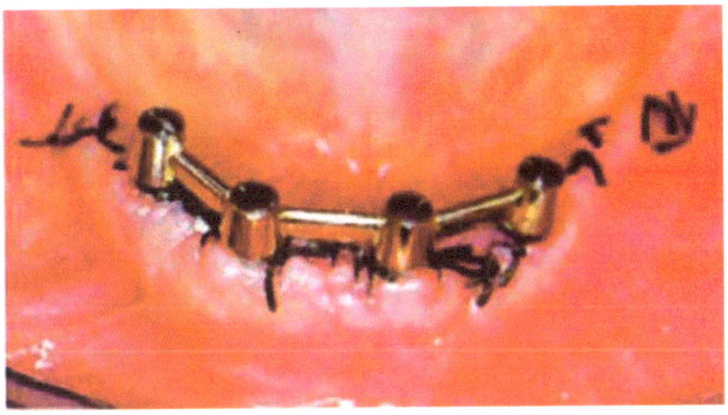

Figure 3.32. Connection of multiple implants for stabilization of the lower total prosthesis with a Dolder bar.

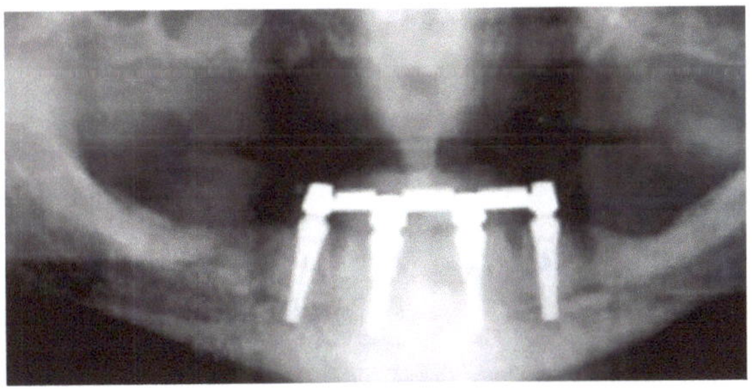

Figure 3.33. Four implants of a conical design connected by a Dolder bar. Control shot after 6 years.

The use of a crossbar, onto which specialized clips rest, significantly improves the stability of a mobile and unstable total prosthesis that previously moved around in the patient's mouth. This anchoring method allows for secure attachment, enabling the patient to perform actions like biting into an apple comfortably. The images (Figures 3.35-3.47) display various implant designs that have been utilized or are currently in use in practical implantology. Stabilization of the lower total prosthesis is demonstrated using Dolder and Ackerman retention bars along with resilient grippers in the following images: 3.31, 3.31a, 3.32, 3.33, 3.39, 3.40, 3.41, 3.45, and 3.46.

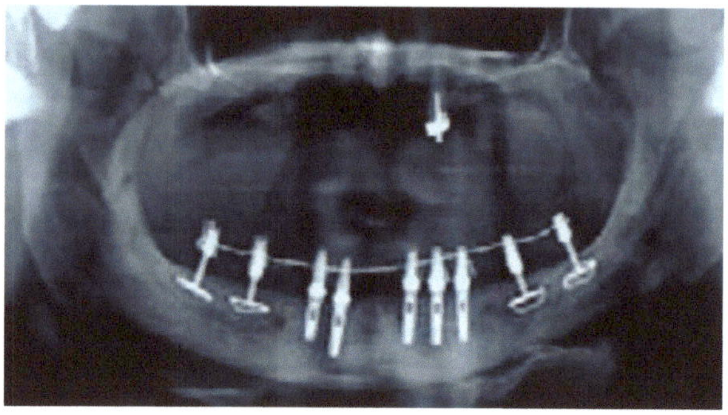

Figure 3.34. Display of "Ihdeo-disk" implants. A copy of the failed "Max Julius-Disc" implant. The author of the book abandoned the installation of these implants in the 80s.

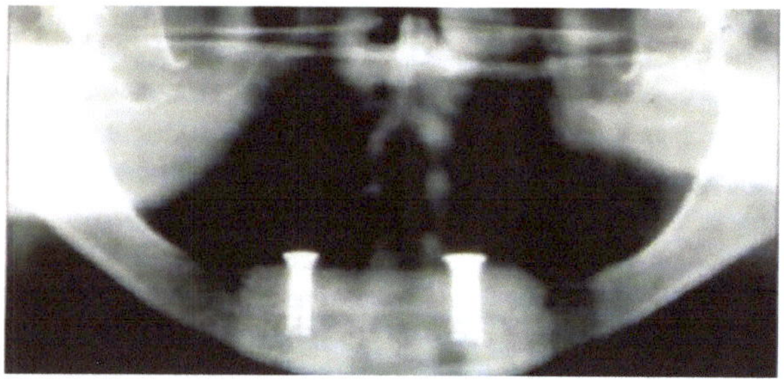

Figure 3.35. The role of natural roots after extraction, for the stabilization of the lower total prosthesis, is taken over by implants (surpassed implant design, opposite to the design of the natural root of the tooth).

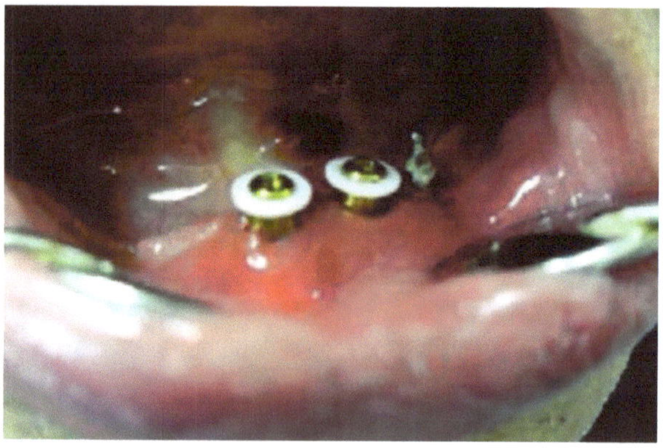

Figure 3.36. Two implants of standard diameter (sufficient amount of available bone) and one implant of narrow diameter (2.4 mm) subsequently added. Placement of cushioning rings before bonding to the acrylic part of the prosthesis.

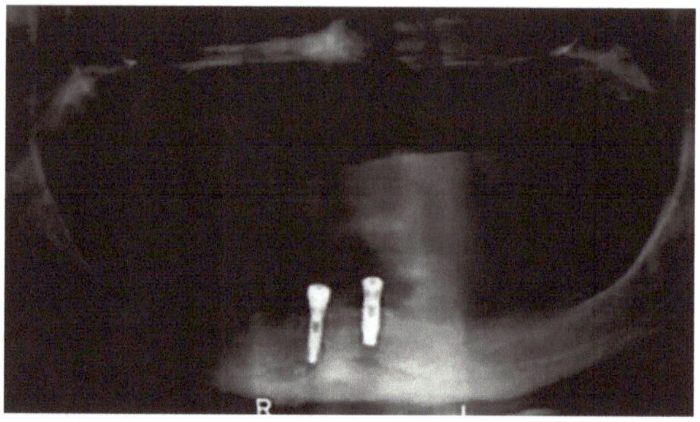

Figure 3.37. Photo after installation of 2 implants of standard diameters.

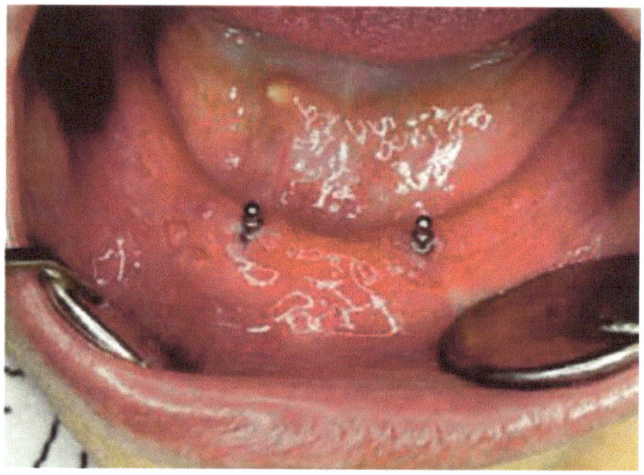

Figure 3.38. Presentation of endosseous one-piece implants with a narrow diameter of 3 mm with spherical heads ("O-ball abutments").

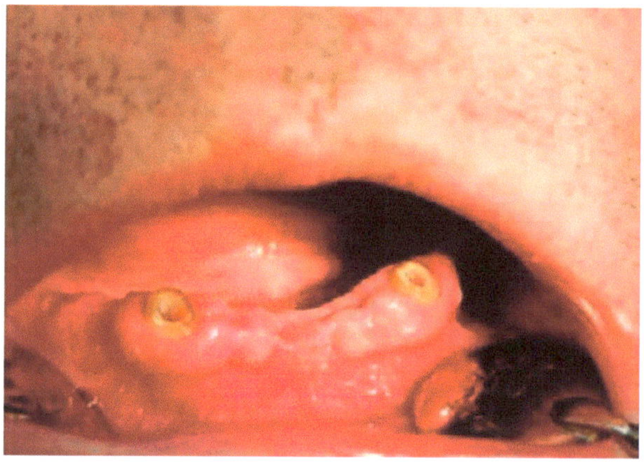

Figure 3.39. The use of natural, cured roots is still an applicable method of stabilizing lower dentures today. There are two options: by installing retention clips or by connecting a Dolder or Ackerman bar on the roots of natural teeth and not losing roots on installed implants.

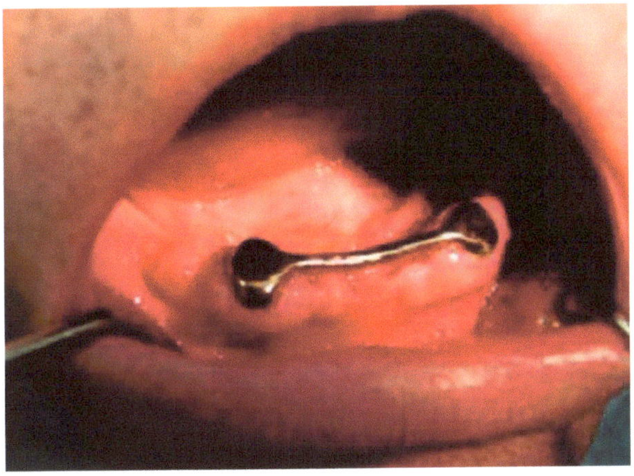

Figure 3.40. Connecting the roots with an Ackerman bar, the difference from a Dolder bar is that it can be adapted to the configuration (relief) of the lower jaw.

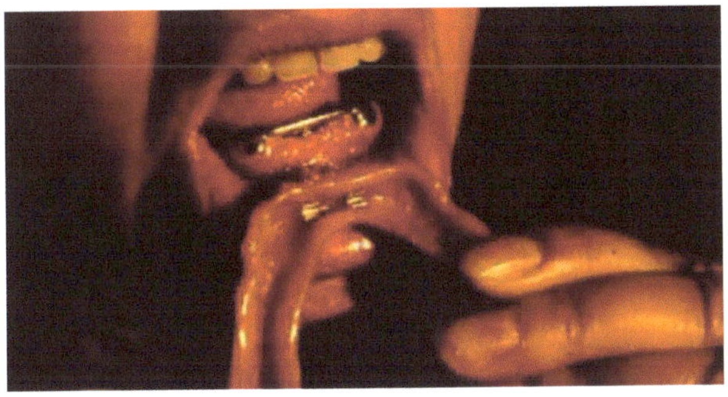

Figure 3.41. Dolder's crossbar placed on natural roots.

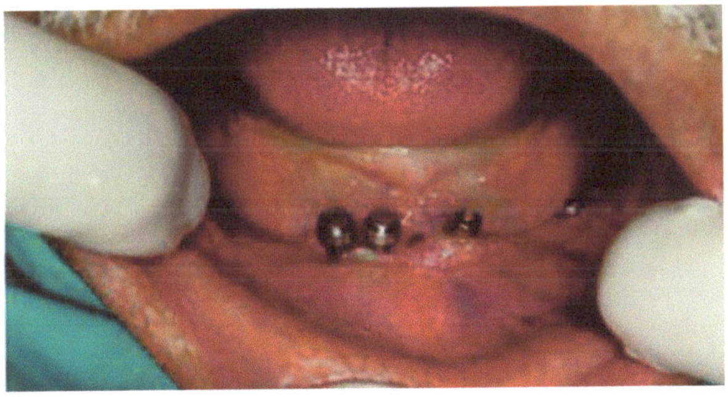

Figure 3.42. Retention clips on wide-diameter two-piece implants - added narrow-diameter implant due to insufficient horizontal amount of alveolar bone.

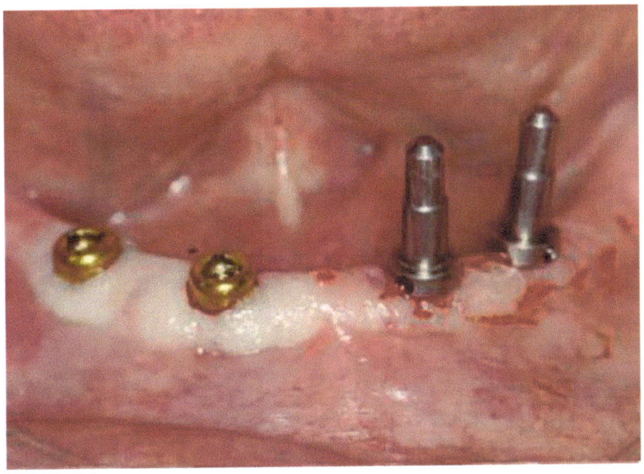

Figure 3.43. Extreme alveolar bone resorption in the lower jaw (Figure 3.47) makes it impossible to use any implant system. The available bone determines the solution: retention clips or Dolder and Ackerman cross-bars (Figures 3.40 and 3.45.).

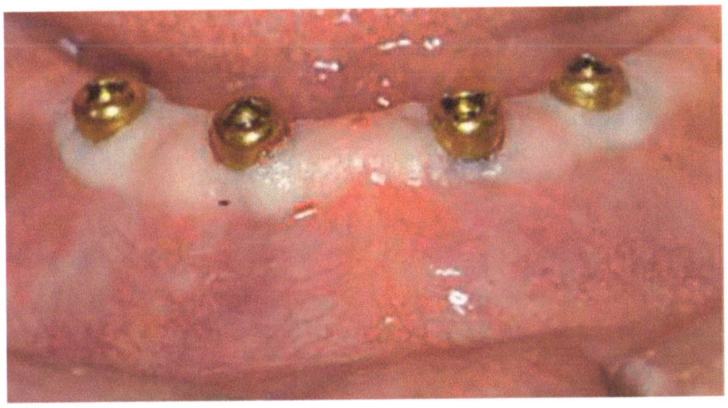

Figure 3.44. Implants of standard diameters are installed, and the available bone determines the solution: retention clips or Dolder and Ackerman bars. (pictures 3.40 and 3.45, 3.47.)

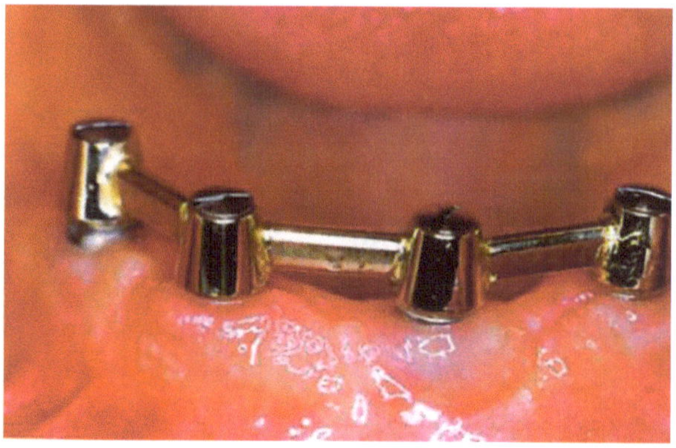

Figure 3.45. Retention clips on implants with a round head ("O-ball abutments") increase the stability of the lower total acrylic prosthesis and comfort in the mouth (picture 3.38), but the use of Dolder (pictures 3.31 to 3.33) and Ackerman bars is a better solution, depending on the amount of available bones in the frontal region.

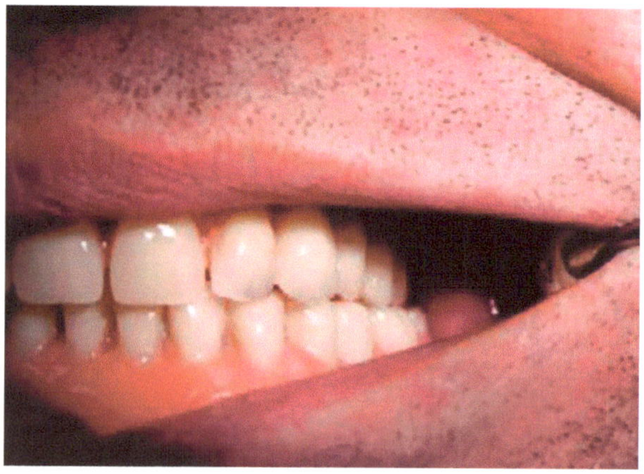

Figure 3.46. Stabilization of the lower total acrylate prosthesis with a Dolder bar anchor on the implants is the optimal solution, considering the impossibility of implantation in the lateral regions due to extreme atrophy of the alveolar bone. It is extremely important from the aspect of biomechanical laws to establish a balanced occlusion.

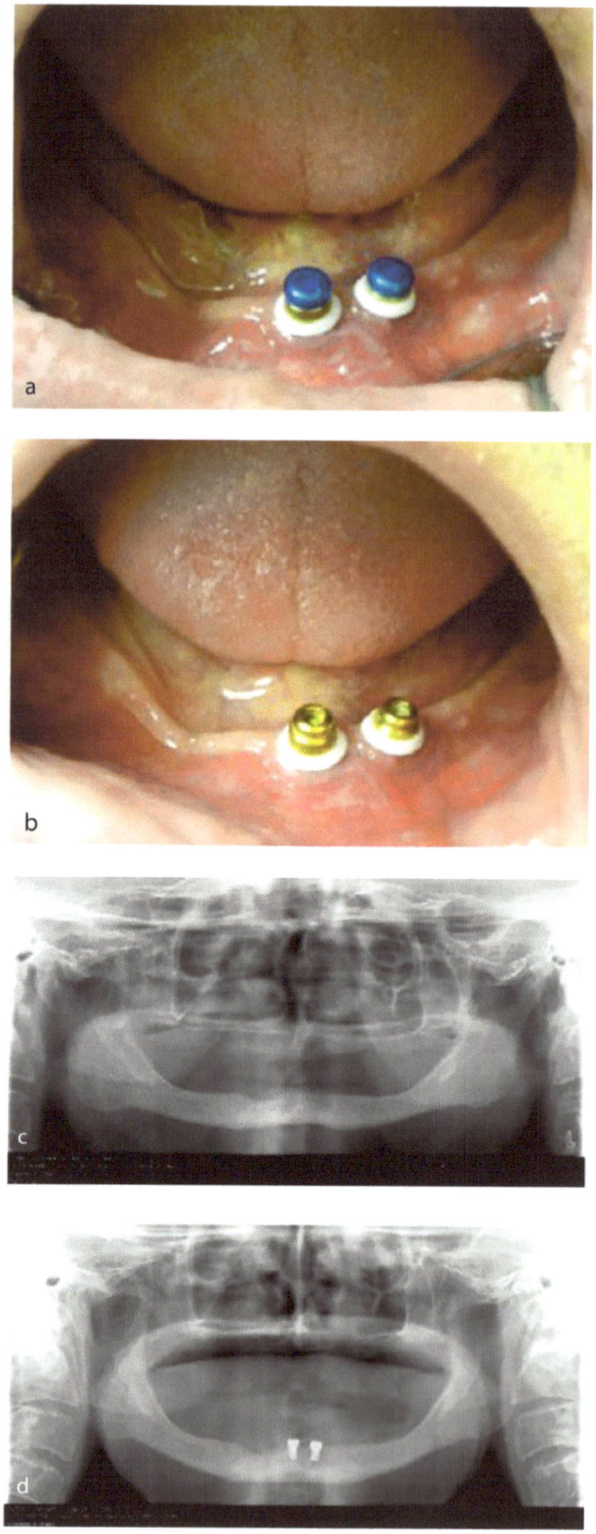

Figure 3.47. The use of two-part implants (a, b, c and d) of wider diameters with shock-absorbing rings enables resilient settlement and neutralizes the effect of forces during mastication (BioHorizonts system).

Different implant system

The manufacturing technology of various implant systems is so advanced today that over 500 implant systems are offered on the market. On this and the next page, only some of them are shown.

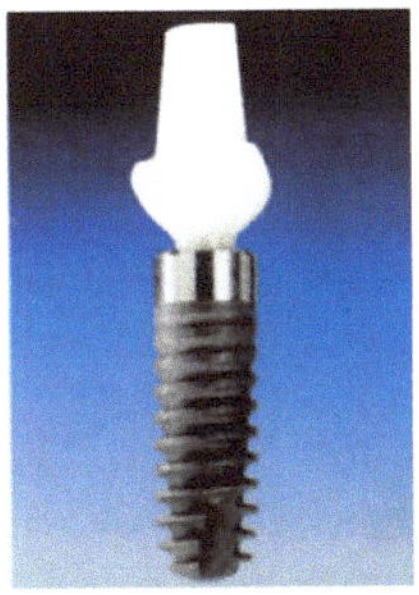
FRIADENT - DGUSSA DENTAL IMPLANT with ceramic abutment

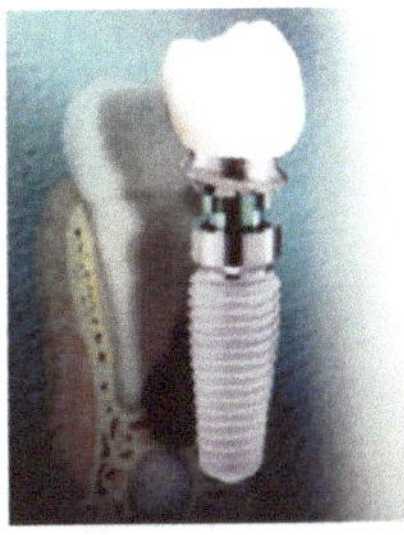
NOBEL BIOCARE IMPLANT

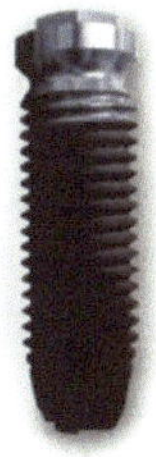
INNOVATION IMPLANT

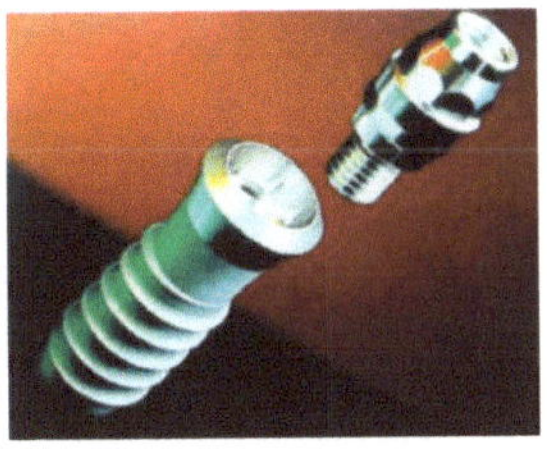
STRAUMANN IMPLANT

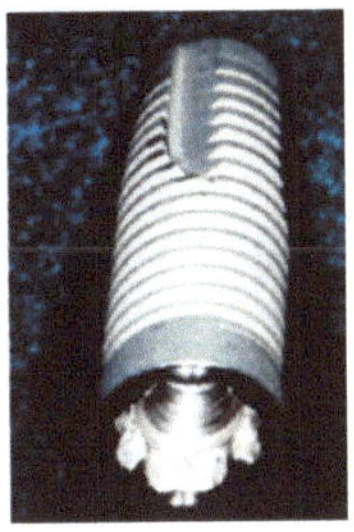
CRESCO TI SYSTEMS

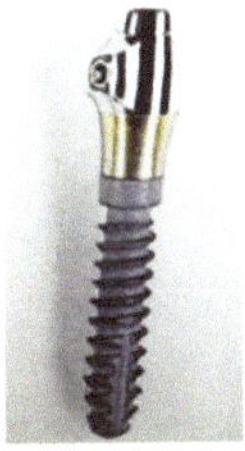
ZL MICRODENT ATTACHMENT IMPLANT

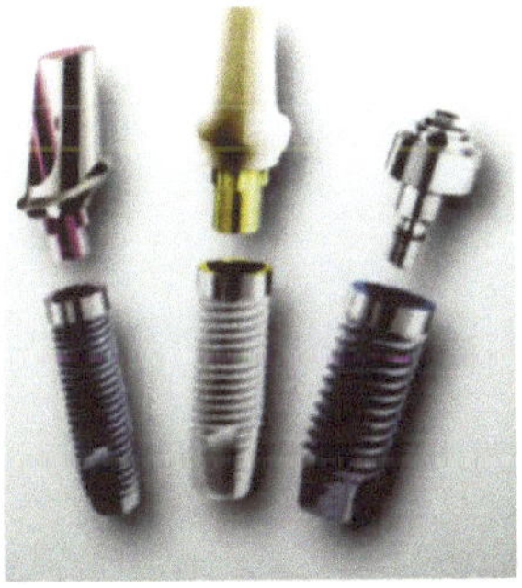
NOBEL BIOCARE IMPLANTS

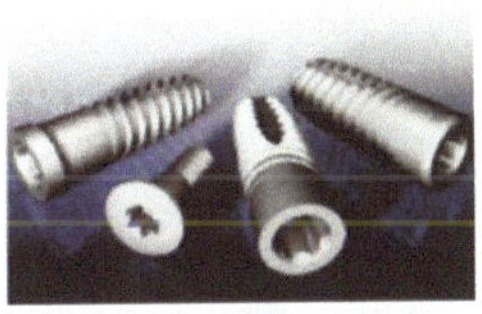
STAR-GROUP IMPLANT

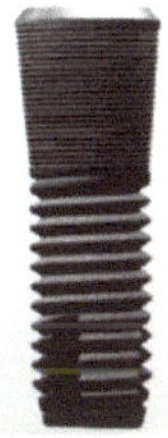
ASTRA TECH IMPLANT

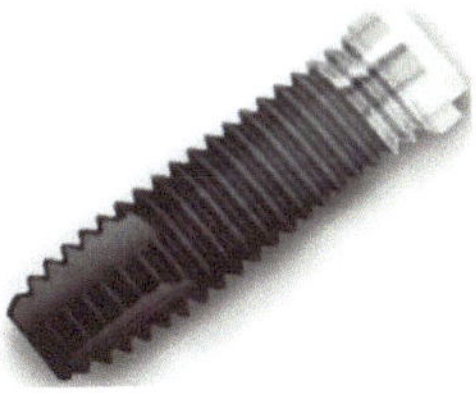
LIFECORE BIOMEDICAL IMPLANT

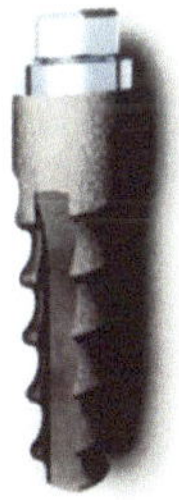
TIOLOX IMPLANT

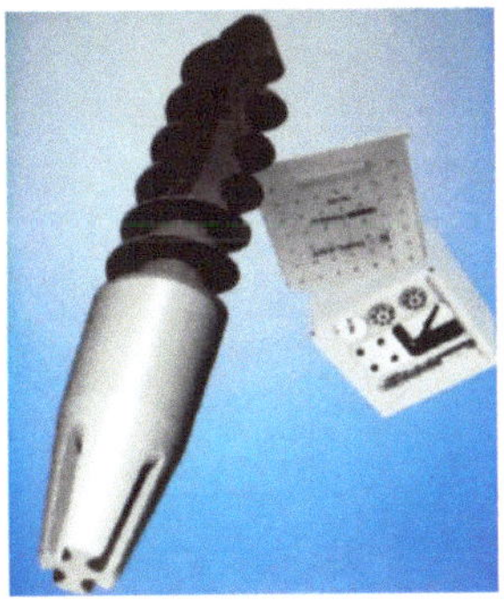
TRINON TITANIUM IMPLANT

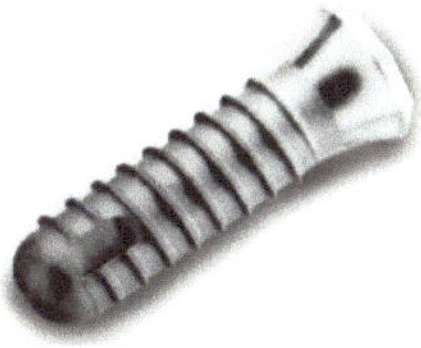
LIFECORE BIOMEDICAL IMPLANT

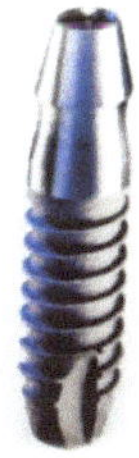
THOMMEN MEDICAL IMPLANT

Figure 3.48

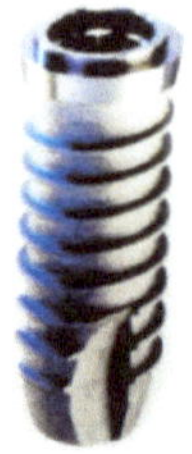
DR IHDE IMPLANT

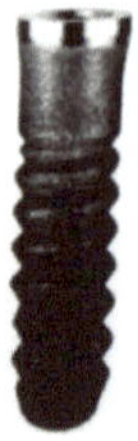
SCHUTZ DENTAL IMPLANT

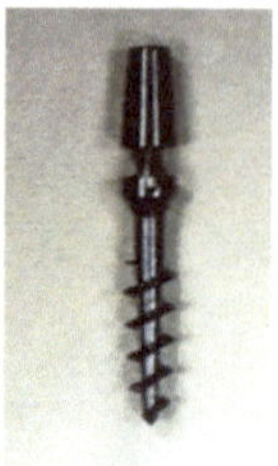
DR IHDE DENTAL IMPLANT

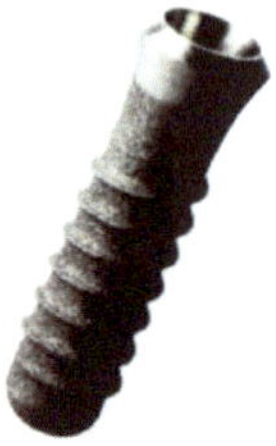
THOMMEN MEDICAL IMPLANT

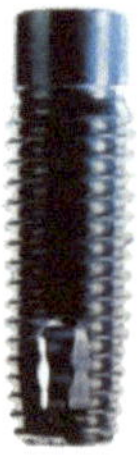
DR IHDE IMPLANT

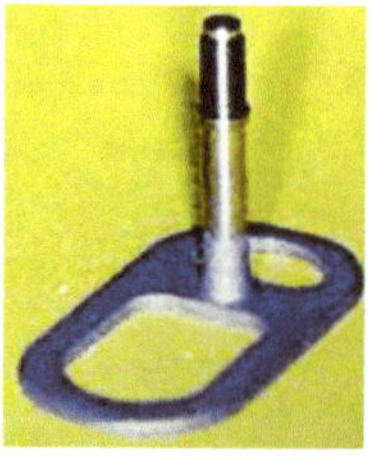
DR IHDE IMPLANT

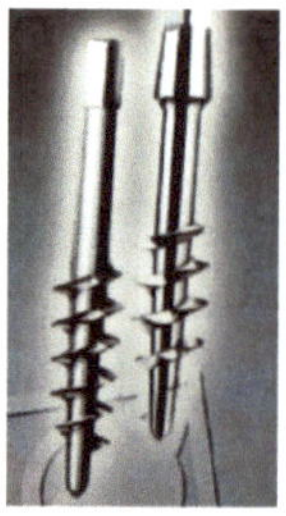
GARBAGGIO ORALTRONICH IMPLANT

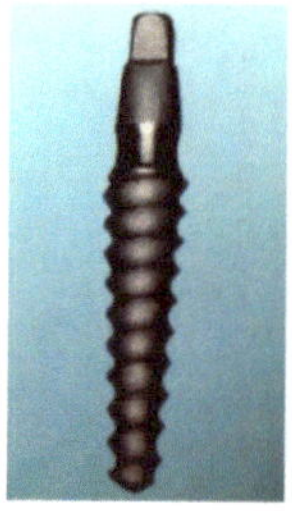
KSI-SCHRAUBE IMPLANT

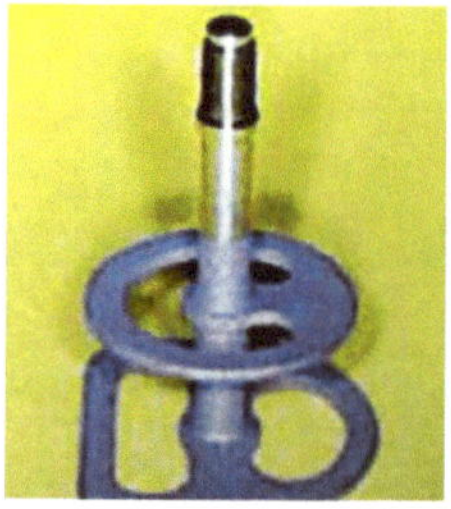
DR IHDE IMPLANT

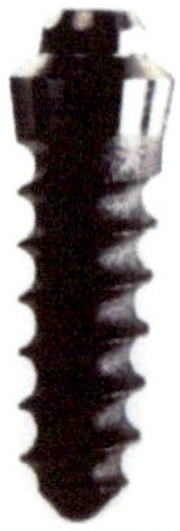
DR IHDE IMPLANT

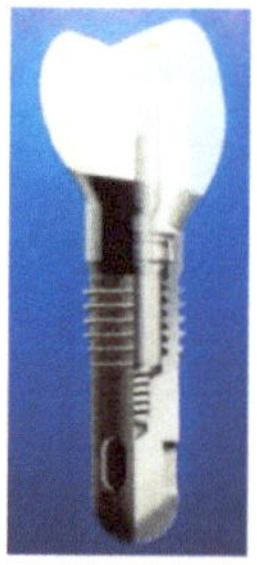
IMPLADENT IMPLANT

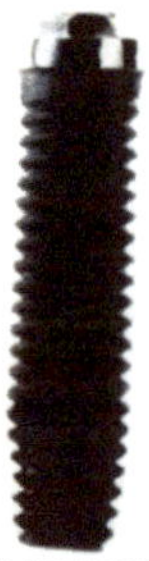
DR IHDE IMPLANT

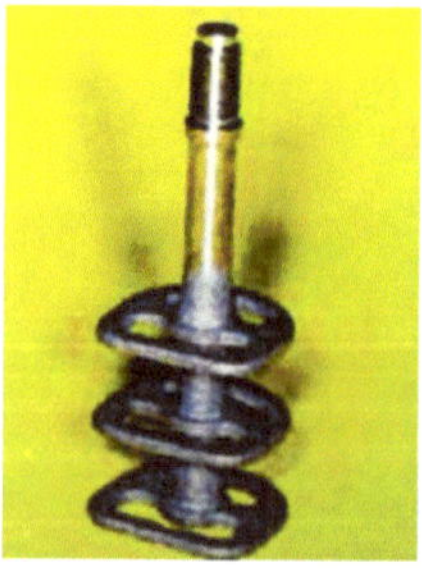
DR IHDE IMPLANT

Figure 3.48

Transforming new implant designs

Among many high-quality implant systems, Nobel Biocare and Zimmer Dental System stood out - high quality, but also high price, which increasingly prevented their wider use. It was necessary to create a system combining their qualities into one system, but also with a lower price. Direkt Implant System confirms the quality of the mentioned implant systems with a certificate.

The design of the Implant Direkt system was launched in 2006 by Dr. Gerald Niznicke, a prosthetist. The Implant Direct system is designed in several systems: RePlant, Legacy, and Swish plant systems. The advantage of these systems is that they are compatible with implant systems Nobel Biocare, Strauman, and Zimmer Dental systems, according to the "all in one" principle.

The most widely used Legacy system is designed in three different systems: Implant Legacy TM 1 which is compatible with the Zimmer Dental Tapered Screw –Vent system with the following features:

a) Internal hexagonal connection, color-coded and with an inlet chamfer.
b) The surface of the implant is treated with the technology of the soluble medium of hydroxyapatite crystals in order to improve bone integration with its rough texture.
c) The system is obtained "all in one" – implant, support, cap for healing, gingiva former (part for forming the gingival sulcus) and analogue (transmitter).

Diameters: 3.7 mm, 4.7 mm and 5.7 mm.

d) Implant lengths: 8.10, 11.5, 13 and 16 mm.
e) Microthreads with double entry standard "V" thread shape, which allows easy self-tapping into the bone, with reduced stress on the bone itself.

This system is designed to be compatible with the Zimmer Dental Tapered Screw-Vent system, with an internal hex connection, color coded and SBM (dissolving synthetic medium) surface treatment and HA sheath; it has double microthreads that enable self-tapping with reduced stress on the surrounding bone. The advantage of the Direct implant system is that the design and quality of the titanium was compatible with the most successful implant systems, such as Nobel Biocare, Straumann, Zimmer Dental Implant and Spectra System.

This system is designed to be compatible with the Zimmer Dental Tapered Screw-Vent system, with an internal hex connection, color coded and SBM (dissolving synthetic medium) surface treatment and HA sheath; it has double microthreads that enable self-tapping with reduced stress on the surrounding bone. The advantage of the Direct implant system is that the design and quality of the titanium were compatible with the most successful implant systems, such as Nobel Biocare, Straumann, Zimmer Dental Implant and Spectra System.

Characteristics of one design option from the Direct implant system, e.g. the Swish System, which is designed in two options: Swish Plus and Swish Plant. The Swish Plus option features a 2 mm semi-structured neck for placement at a gingival level for aesthetic reasons. The Swish Plant is also a 2mm neck, impregnated for placement at bone or gingival level. The microthreads of both designs provide self-tapping and stress reduction to the surrounding bone. Double-threaded grooves provide faster and easier insertion and good primary stability.

The Swish Plant implant—both surgical and prosthetic—is compatible with the Straumann system. One of the key advantages of this implant package is that, for the same price, you receive not only the implant but also a healing cap, gingiva former, transfer, and a titanium definitive superstructure. On the other hand, the Legacy TM 2 System is compatible with the Zimmer Implant System. This system shares the same hexagonal length, features a color-coded connection, and has an implant surface processed using the same technology as the Swish Plant. The contents of the implant package are similar to the previous system, with the addition of a temporary suprastructure (support). While the lengths of the implants are the same as those in the Swish Plant system, they come in different diameters: 3.7 mm, 4.2 mm, 5.7 mm, and 7.0 mm.

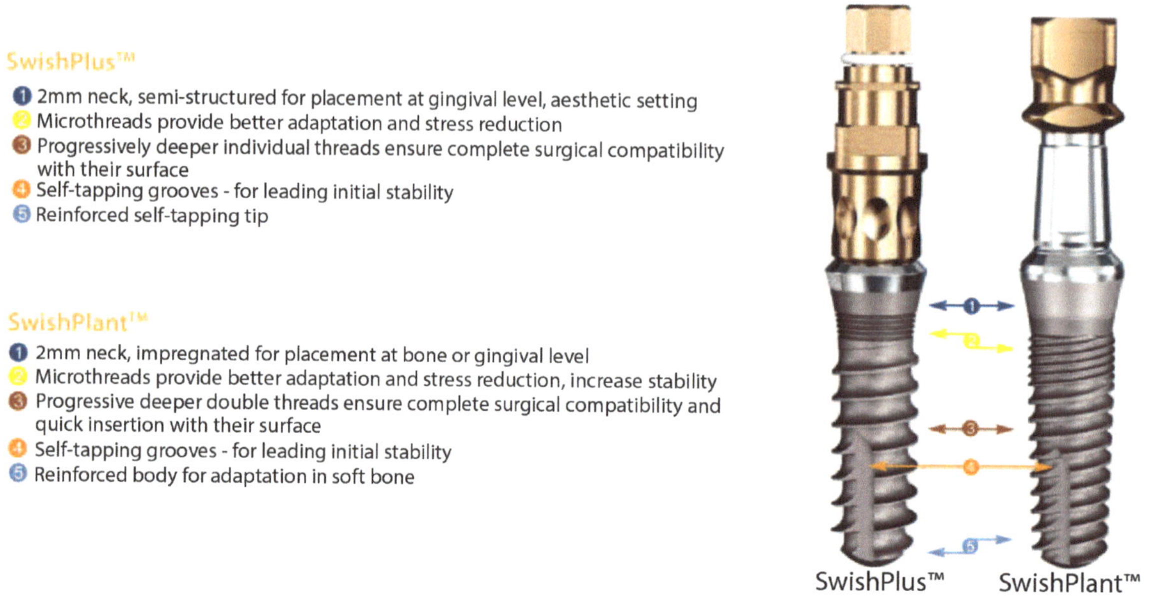

Figure 3.48

The Imlantata Legacy TM 3 is compatible with the Zimmer Implant System. Both systems share the same connection and surface treatment, and the implant package includes a definitive titanium support. While the lengths remain consistent with the previous system, there are differences in diameters, which are coded in different colors.

The Implant Direct system has made significant advancements with the introduction of short implants featuring wider diameters. A key characteristic of the short Implant Direct implants is their aggressive threading, which facilitates easier and faster achievement of primary stability.

The Legacy TM2 design incorporates microthreading with a double progressive wider spiral thread, allowing for improved self-tapping and a more conical shape.

Additionally, the direct implant system is unique in developing one-piece implants with wider diameters, making it possible to replace a single lost tooth. This particular one-piece implant design simplifies the surgical procedure while ensuring primary stability, which enables immediate prosthetic work.

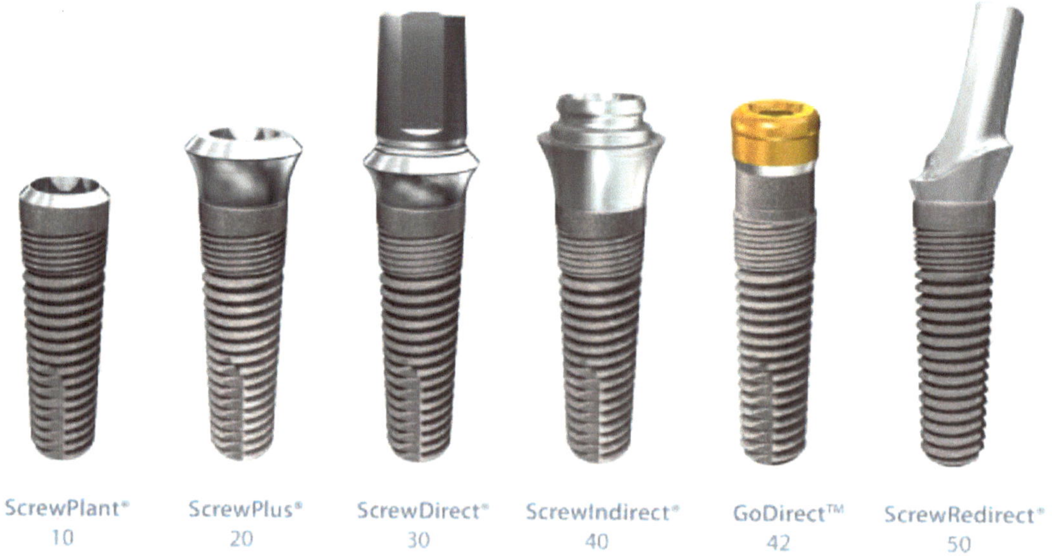

Figure 3.49

SWISCH PLUS IMPLANT

The implant is surgically and prosthetically compatible with Straumann. It features an internal octagonal connection design, which includes both a wider and a narrower diameter. Additionally, the connection has an internal hexagonal shape. The lengths and diameters are compatible with Straumann implants, available in sizes of 6, 8, 10, 12, 14, and 16 mm. The surgical protocol for this implant is the same as that used for Straumann implants.

Characteristics of this implant: surgical and prosthetic, it is compatible with Strauman:

The connection has an internal octagon, and the narrower diameter has an internal hex connection. The surface is treated with a soluble hydroxyapatite medium. The surgical set corresponds to the Straumann set. The implant includes a healing cap and gingiva former of 2 mm height with an implant length transmitter of 6, 8, 10, 12, 14, and 16 mm.

SwissPlant implants

The SwissPlant implant is compatible with Straumann systems. It features an octagonal connection for wider diameters and a hexagonal connection for narrower ones. The installation can be performed using the Straumann surgical set. This system offers various implant lengths, including short options of 6 mm and 8 mm, as well as longer lengths of 10 mm, 12 mm, 14 mm, and 16 mm. One of the key advantages of this implant system is that it allows for the secure attachment of both temporary and definitive prosthetic works using a permanent titanium support.

Design Of The El Esthetic Line Implant System

This implant system, made of quality titanium (type IV), is designed with features that enhance osseointegration and the formation of soft tissues. Its thread profiles enable self-tapping during installation, aligning with biomechanical requirements. Overall, this design places the implant system in a high class of implant technologies.

EL ESTHETIC LINE IMPLANT has outstanding characteristics and has a wide range of implant-prosthetic indications. The design of this implant is conical, and it is characteristic that in the apical third has aggressive threads that allow easier installation, with significantly reduced stress on the bone during insertion. This design detail ensures good primary stability in soft bone as well.

The prosthetic connection of the EL implant offers stability and safety through its support (abutment) for the prosthetic work. This design effectively eliminates micromovements and microcracks that can occur between the abutment and the implant body. A key feature of the implant is the beveled shoulder, which has been specially designed to enhance integration processes by allowing bone to grow over it. This design detail helps ensure the long-term survival of the implant. Since occlusal forces are strongest on the first threads of the implant, the design of these threads facilitates the distribution of these forces evenly across the cortical bone. Additionally, positioning the implant subcrestally is ideal for aesthetic regions, as it contributes to the long-term stability of the surrounding soft tissues.

Platform-switching and concave aesthetic design of the support (abutment) enables successful shaping of soft tissues, which is of primary importance for a successful aesthetic result. The surface design is characterized by three different thread profiles with double thread shaping, which ensures not only good primary stability but also a more intimate bone-implant contact.

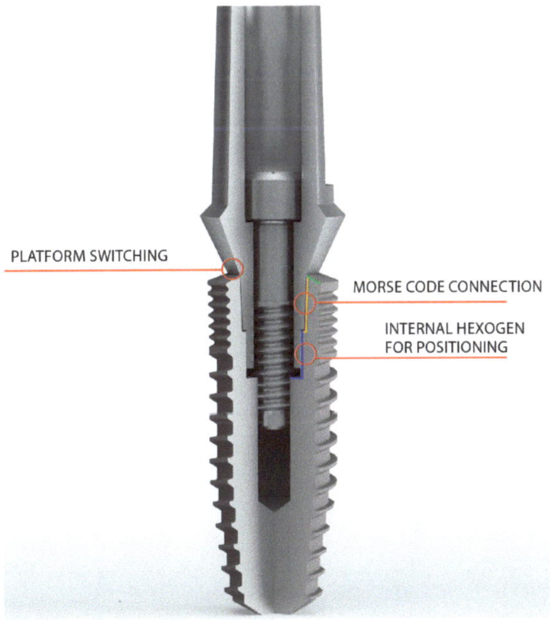

Figure 3.50. Cross-sectional view of the design of the EL ESTETIK LINE implant system with an abutment (support).

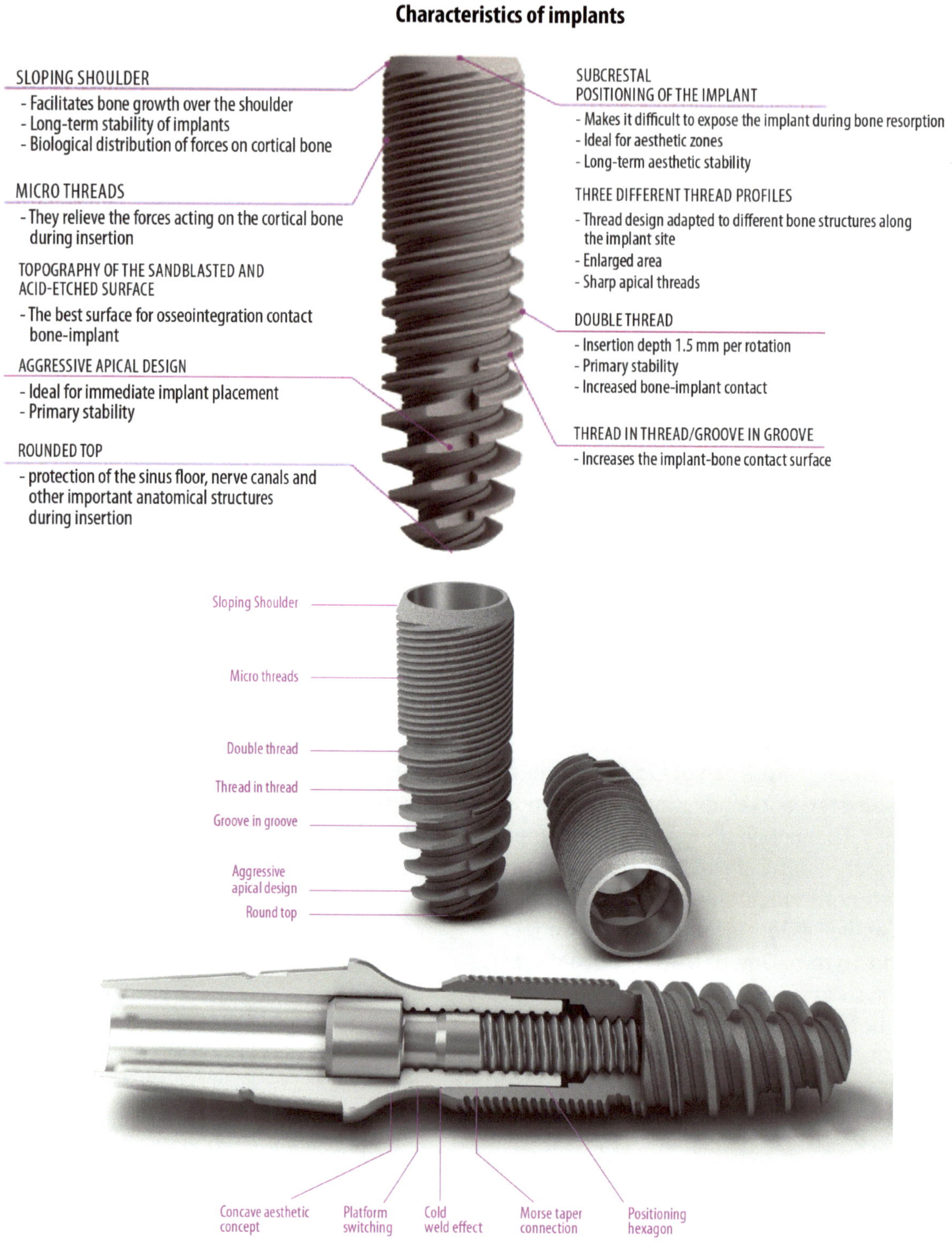

Figure 3.51. Characteristics of the EL Estethic Line implant system: the design of the implant is the fifth generation of this implant system, with double aggressive threads, especially in the apical third. The surface designed in this way allows achieving good primary stability in many indications of oral surgical treatment. Decades of experience in the application of many implant systems confirms that this system has top quality.

Characteristics of the El Esthetic Line implant system (see the application of this system in chapter 18 Conversation with a colleague).

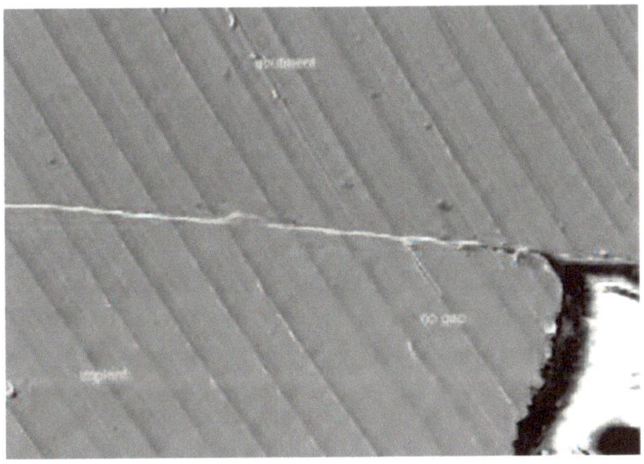

Figure 3.52a. Display of the connection of the implant and the support (abutment) of the prosthetic work. This implant system is characterized by the complete absence of microcracks, which prevents the deposition of calculus, bacterial plaque and the penetration of microorganism colonies. The characteristic of this connection is that it prevents micromovements and unscrewing of the support (abutment) from the endosseous body of the implant.

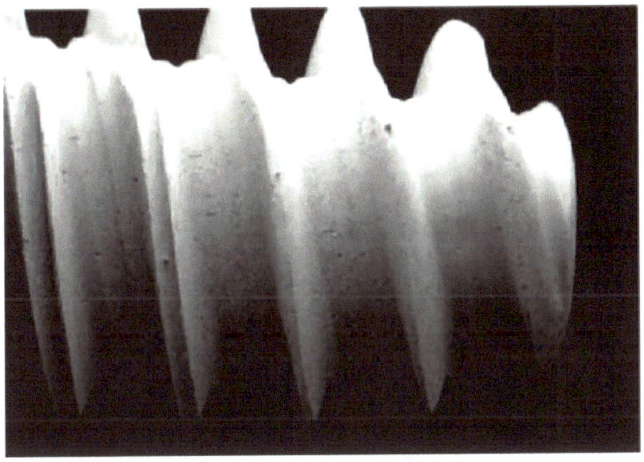

Figure 3.52b. Microscopic view of the El Esthetic Line implant surface. The design of the thread and technological treatment of the surface of the thread enables easier self-cutting into the bone, with less trauma, as well as achieving good primary stability of the embedded implant.

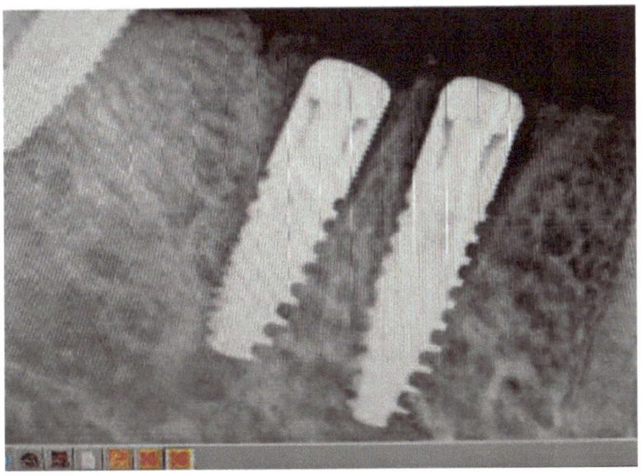

Figure 3.52c. Embedded El Esthetic Line implant (image with RVG intraoral sensor). Compare the thread design of this implant system with Nobel Biocare Replace implants (Figure d). Thread design and technological processing of the El Esthetic Line implant system facilitates the installation of self-tapping implants by reducing stress and trauma to the bone. The safety of implant installation, in addition to 3D imaging, is significantly increased by the use of the RVG intraoral sensor (work by T. Zlopaša).

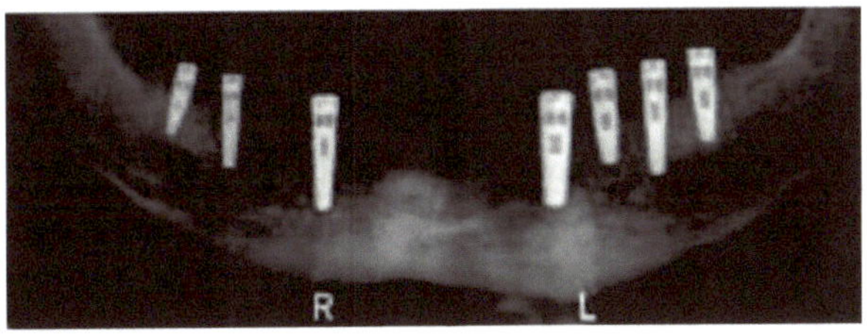

Figure 3.52d. Built-in implants of the Nobel Biocare Replace system of standard and larger diameters. After extraction of the teeth and preservation of the alveoli, the implants were immediately installed and immediately loaded 15 years ago. After the elapsed time, the implants are well integrated without peri-implant changes (see chapter 18). The degree of achieved primary stability of the implant determines the next stage of the procedure - primary or delayed loading. Compare the El Esthetic Line implant design with the Nobel Biocare Replace implant design. The progress of oral implantology and the accumulated experiences also led to the improvement of the surface design of many implant systems (work by the author of the book).

The following pictures show both Implant Systems Installed Direct Implant System and El Estethic Line Implant System

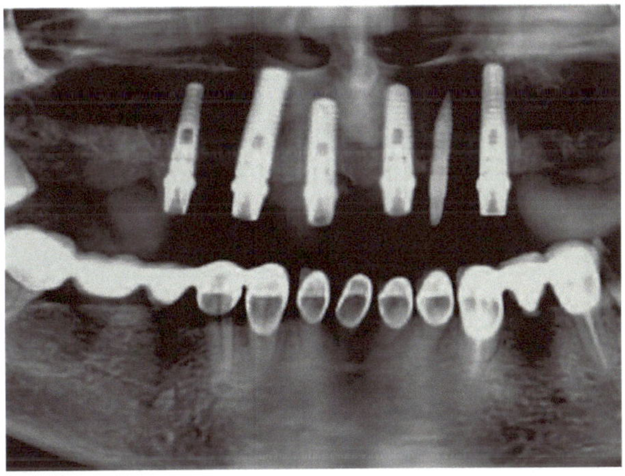

Figure 3.53. After tooth extraction, Direkt Implant System implants are immediately installed. In region 22, the horizontal dimension of the available bone, due to resorption of the lamellar bone, allowed the installation of a narrow-diameter implant. Immediately after installation, the implants are immediately loaded with fixed prosthetic work in acrylate.

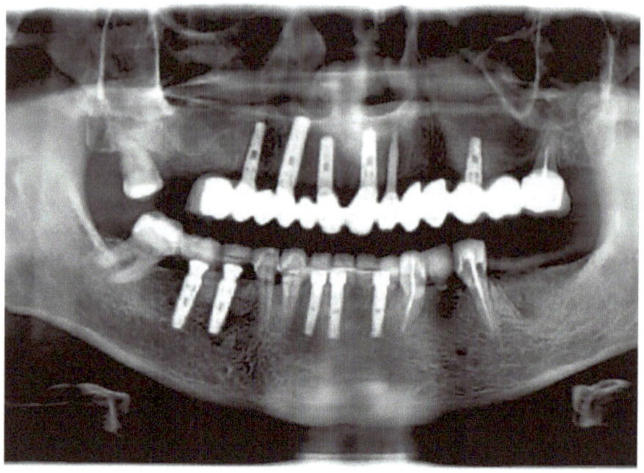

Figure 3.54. Orthopan tomographic image of the installed implants in the upper jaw of the Direkt Implant System design and in the lower jaw El Esthetik Implant System. Compare the design details of both systems. Both implant systems are immediately installed and immediately loaded with fixed prosthetic works in acrylate.

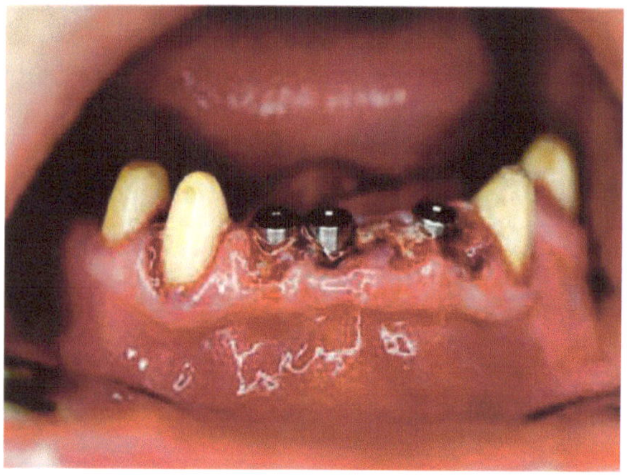

Figure 3.55. After 5 years from the installation of the Direkt implant system in the upper jaw, the patient applied for implant-prosthetic treatment in the lower jaw. After the extraction of the incisors (32,31,41,42), El Esthetic System implants were immediately inserted. Compare with the design of the Direct Implant System in the upper jaw.

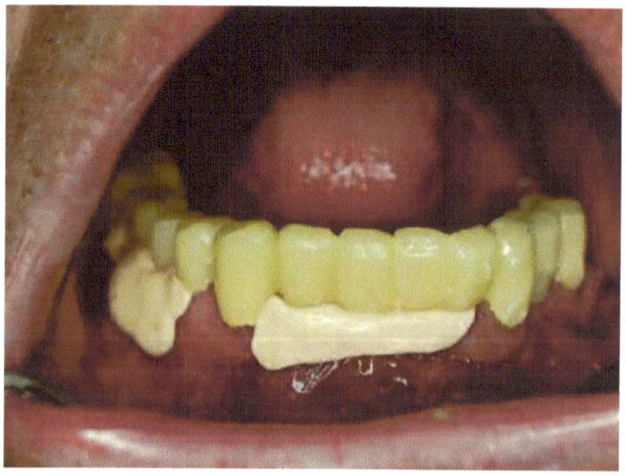

Figure 3.56. After tooth extraction and immediate installation of implants, placement of immediate provisional fixed prosthetic work, packaging with Reso-pak, which promotes healing of soft tissues, was carried out.

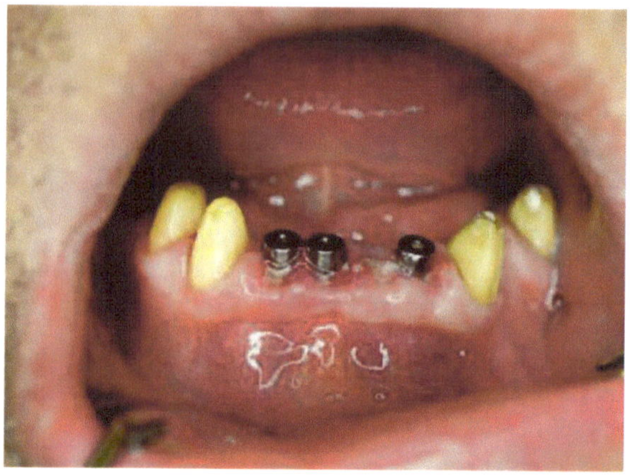

Figure 3.57. Appearance of healing 7 days after implant placement.

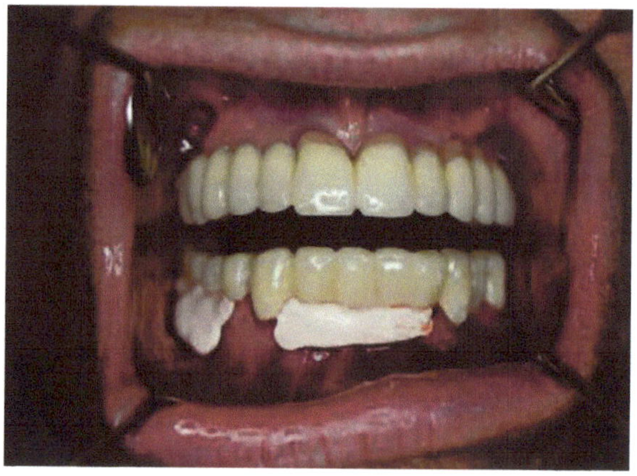

Figure 3.58. With the immediate installation of the implant and the immediate loading of the patient, the patient's comfort was not reduced during the implant-prosthetic treatment in both jaws. Appearance of definitive prosthetic work in the upper jaw, with well-integrated implants and stably formed soft tissues after 5 years.

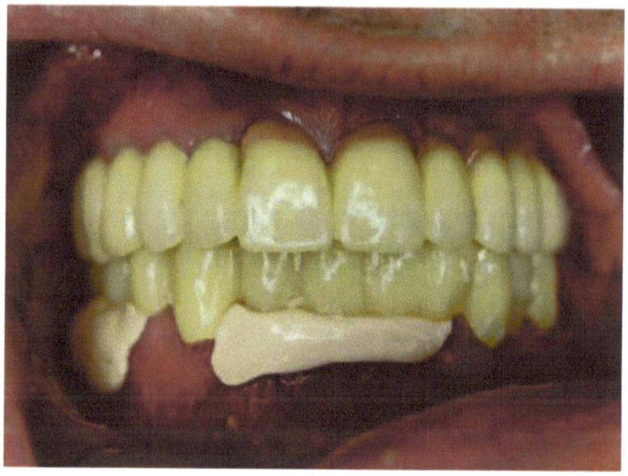

Figure 3.59. Establishing a well-balanced occlusion is of crucial importance for the promotion of osseointegration processes, whether it is definitive or temporary prosthetic work. (work by T. Zlopaša).

4

Review Of The Past, Ranges Of The Present, Look Into The Future

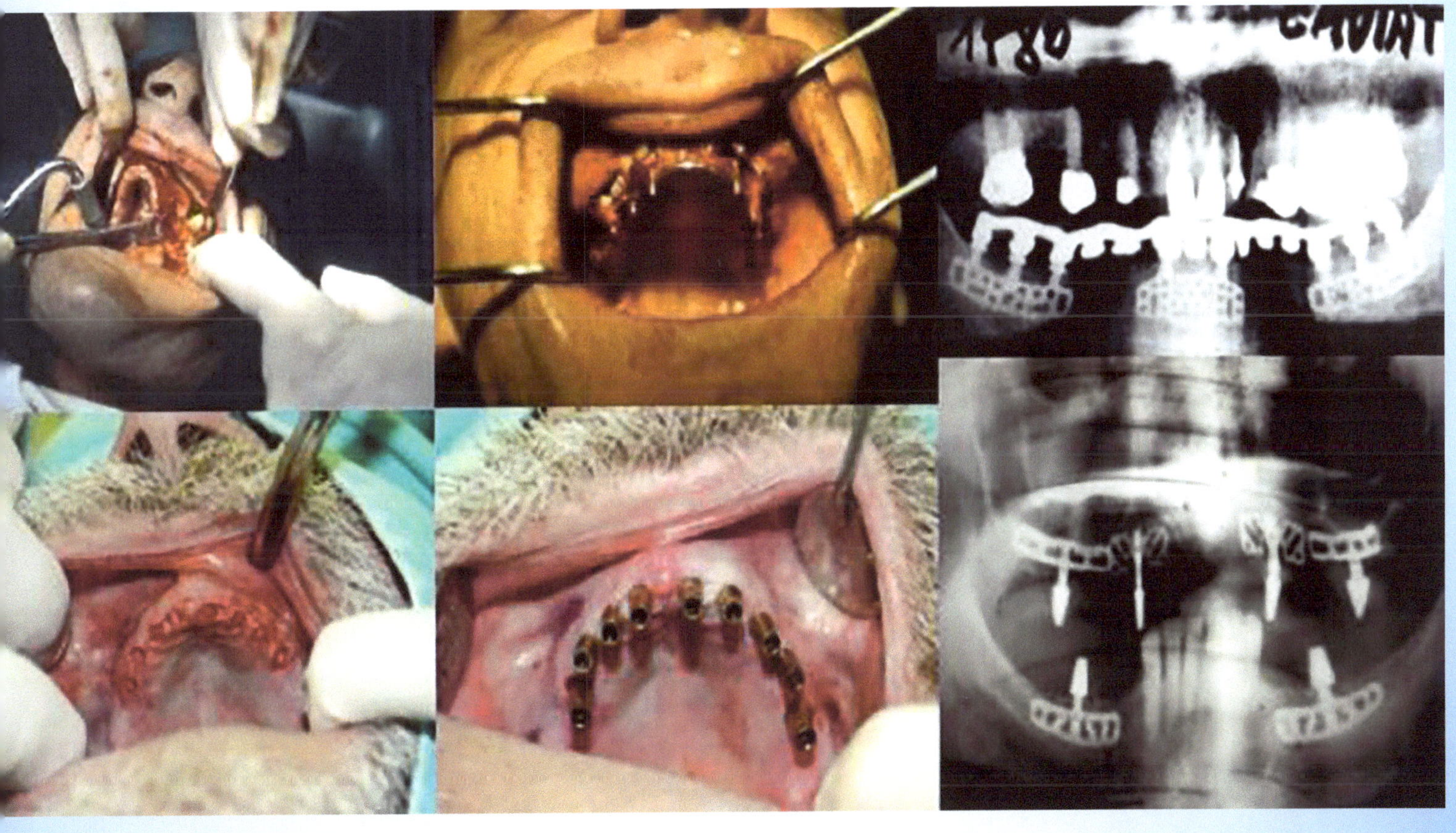

Implantology is a science, and oral implantation, the installation of implants is today a recognized therapeutic procedure, scientifically explained and practically confirmed. The past times, when numerous dentists and skeptics considered oral implantology unreliable and impractical, are behind us.

Of all branches of medicine, the era of pioneering efforts lasted the longest in oral implantology. At that time, only a few dentists used implants. Some of the pioneers developed their own implant systems, which they commercialized.

Scientific institutions, professional class associations, and universities kept them aside. However, enthusiastic pioneers, provoking criticism, unaccepted and misunderstood, assured that there would be a period when implantology would try to prove its qualities and capabilities. It should be emphasized that no training in implantology was organized at any university until 1980, due to fierce resistance. It seems that the ferocity of the resistance was nowhere as manifested as here.

Only rare individuals, enthusiasts, recognized the vision. The clinical results of enthusiasts have increasingly predicted that oral implantology will be a reliable branch of oral rehabilitation.

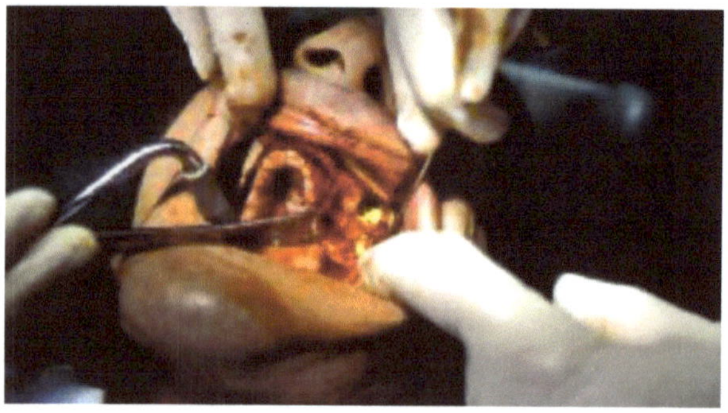

Figure 4.1. Such interventions from the past, uncovering the entire alveolar ridge and palate with a flap, are unimaginable today in oral implantology. Surgical intervention for the installation of subperiosteal implants.

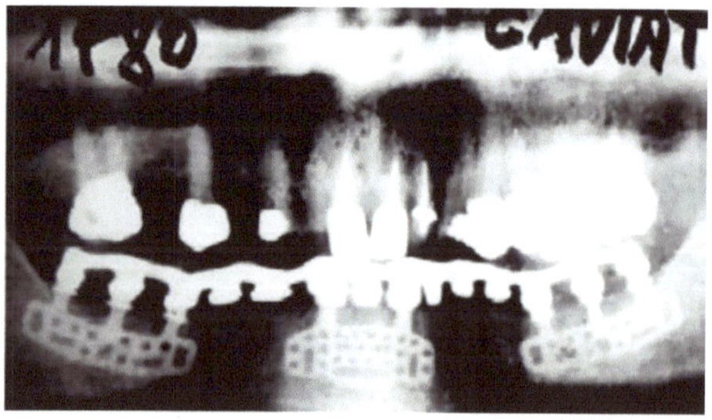

Figure 4. 2. One-piece leaf implant in the lateral regions with three supports and one arch leaf implant in the frontal region with two supports.

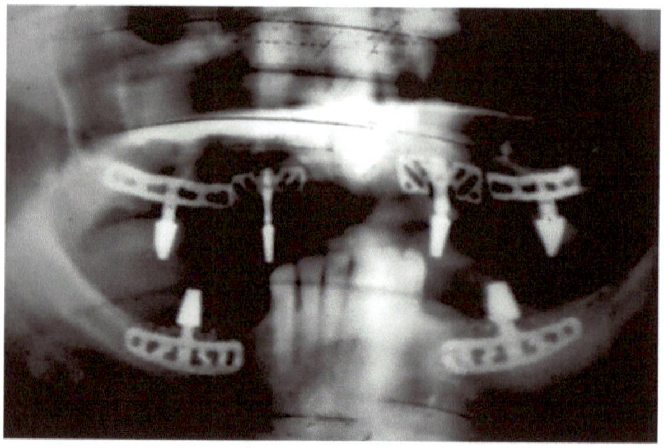

Figure 4.3. Complicated and aggressive installation of Linkov's Blades implants (author's work in 1977).

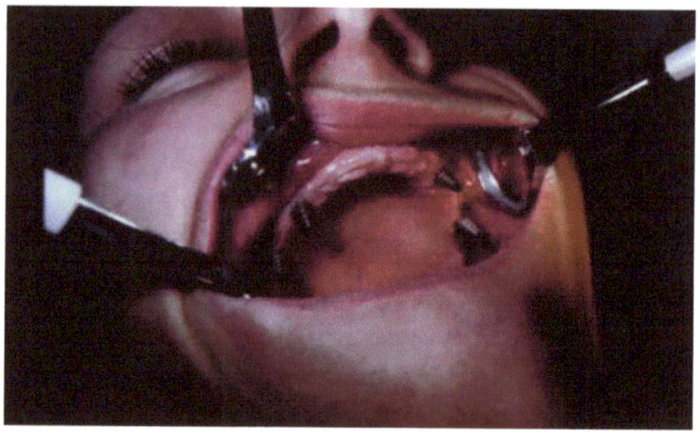

Figure 4.4. Appearance of healing after 4 weeks of insertion of one-piece Linkov leaf implants (paper by the author of the book 1976).

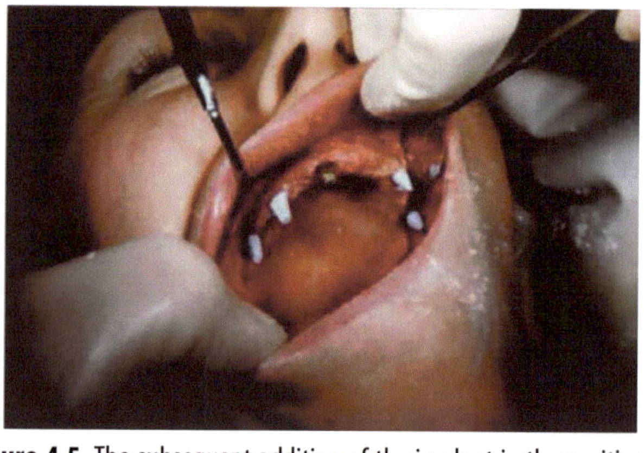

Figure 4.5. The subsequent addition of the implant in the position of the central incisor significantly improved the support of the prosthetic superstructure.

Total toothlessness, especially in the lower jaw, has been a significant challenge even for the most skilled prosthetists. For a long time, dentures, particularly complete ones, posed substantial issues for patients. Experienced dentists have explored various solutions to address these challenges. One of the first attempts to stabilize complete prostheses outside the traditional prosthetic approach involved the installation of subperiosteal implants.

Leonard Linkov, a notable figure in oral implantology, was inspired to help his mother, who struggled with a lower complete prosthesis. He became one of the first to implant an endosseous implant in her. Similarly, the author, who faced the same issue with their mother's lower prosthesis, dedicated a significant portion of their professional career to oral implantology as a result of this challenge. Since then, numerous innovations have been made to enhance prosthetic rehabilitation by integrating various implant systems.

Advanced atrophy of the alveolar ridge was a stumbling block in prosthetics at the time, especially in lower total dentures. One of the solutions to stabilize it to some extent was to increase the weight of the prosthesis. It is weighed down by gold, the part that lies on the ridge, and due to the high price of gold, many made it heavier by incorporating amalgam from the lingual sides of the prosthesis.

Many tips, in cases where it was necessary to make a total prosthesis in the lower jaw, the author learned as an intern from Dr. Vojin Petrović, professor of the Academy of Medical Sciences in Belgrade. An experienced practitioner would advise that every root that can be cured should be preserved in the lower jaw and used to stabilize the lower total prosthesis. He knew that the longer the healing roots stay in the lower jaw, ground to the level of the gums and filled with amalgam, significantly slows the atrophy of the alveolar bone. That procedure would significantly contribute to the stabilization of the lower total denture. At that time, retention clips that were installed on the roots of the teeth, significantly stabilizing the total dentures, were not known. By using residual roots in the lower jaw, by installing retention clips on them, good stability of the total prosthesis could be achieved, but only for a certain period, because such roots are exposed to decay over time.

The practice involved grinding down the remaining teeth and covering them with crowns, while the use of acrylic or metal prostheses was one solution for rehabilitation. However, this method often led to "passive growth," where coated teeth would eventually loosen and fall out over time.

The author gained valuable insights into stabilizing complete prostheses at the University of Zurich (Switzerland) under Professor Gerber. These new findings supported the views of Professor Vojin Petrović. Despite the advancements in knowledge, there was limited progress in Switzerland at that time regarding complete edentulism and the stabilization of lower complete dentures. The concept of implanting a foreign body into living bone was still largely unknown, though a few rare individual enthusiasts in the US had documented cases.

Together with our Swiss colleague Otto Buhler in Lugano (1968), the two of us drew attention to the possibility of installing tantalum needle implants, which we connected with a special apparatus with cold soldering to a gold rail, for which an acrylate prosthesis was retained.

The application of retention clips, as a frequent solution, filled the patient with satisfaction. By connecting two or more roots with a Dolder or Ackerman bar, the stability of the prostheses is increased. The benefit and satisfaction of the patient from the initial stabilization with this method was great, because the period of getting used to it compared to an unstable prosthesis was significantly shorter, and wearing the prosthesis was much more comfortable.

Modern implantology has progressed further. Instead of the impossibility of using the remaining roots in the stabilization of the lower total prosthesis, implants are a far more favorable and long-lasting solution. A special advantage is that existing prostheses can be anchored in this way, loading the installed implants immediately.

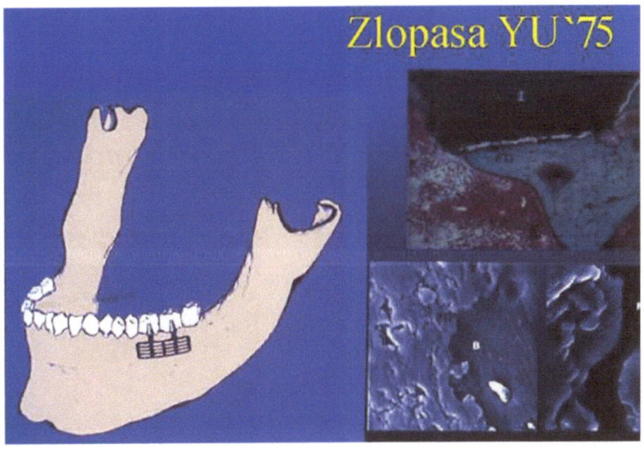

Figure 4.5a. Presentation from the lecture of the author of the book in the period of application of one-piece endosseus leaf (razor) implants (Blades Implant). Osseous integration was not much discussed in prac-

tice, because scientific research was in its infancy. The application was based on achieving a good primary fixation by driving the implant into the prepared bed with circular burs (pictures 4.69 and 4.71), and survival in the bone was based on the growth of new bone through the designed endosseous part in the form of a grid. The attitude of waiting 3 weeks to load was quickly abandoned. The action of lingual forces and their moments on the fixed supports of the prosthetic work compromised the achieved primary fixation by loosening and losing the implant.

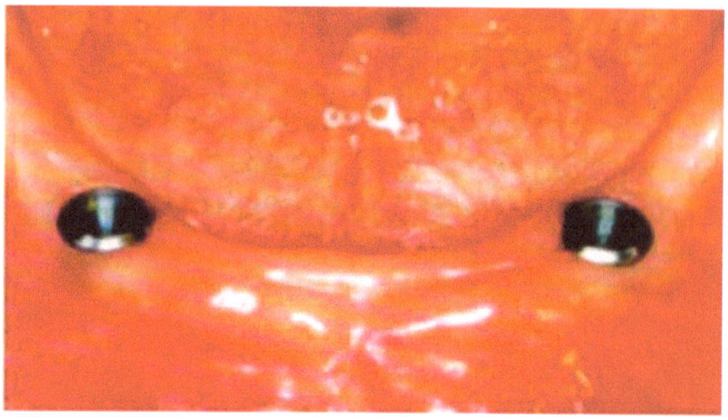

Figure 4.6. The development of oral implantology is followed by the beginning of the period of application of two-part implants.

Implants of narrow diameter MDI - mini implants

Given that the installation of implants in the USA is a very expensive process, it was necessary to innovate a more social solution for the stabilization of often poorly made and uncomfortable prostheses, which would be acceptable to millions of users.

On the implant market, one such narrow diameter implant was first launched by IMTEC Sendax MDI Implant (Mini Dental Implant). Wide application of narrow-diameter implants proved to be justified very quickly. The success of installing narrow diameter implants of 1.8 mm, 2.1 mm and 2.4 mm, aroused the interest of manufacturers and influenced the significant improvement of one-piece and two-piece narrow diameter implants. The improvement was manifested in the increase in diameter to 3.0 mm, better technological processing, as well as the two-part form of the implant with a narrow diameter. The part surrounding the soft tissues was treated with laser technology (pictures 4.7- 4.11).

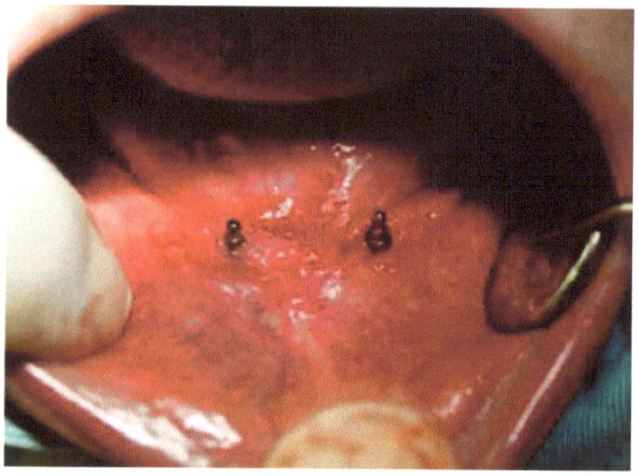

Figure 4.7. One-piece narrow-diameter implant with retention clips immediately after immediate implant installation.

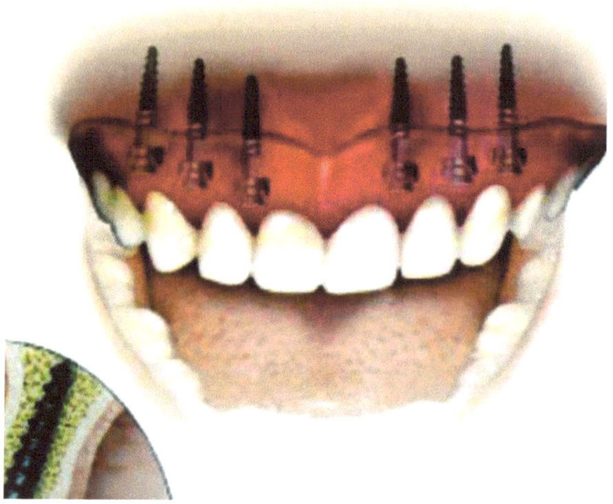

Figure 4.8. Schematic representation of six one-piece MDI implants.

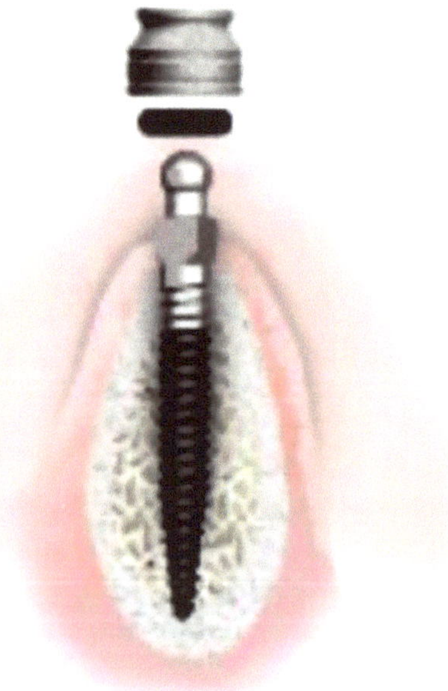

Figure 4.9. Schematic representation of a one-piece implant: with a retention clip of the part that lies in the bone, a cap with an amortizing ring that lies in the acrylic part of the prosthesis.

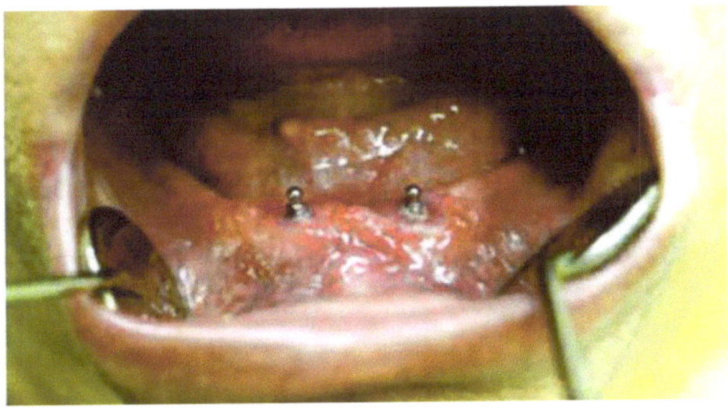

Figure 4.10. Embedded implants with a diameter of 3 mm after 3 years (see Figure 4.7).

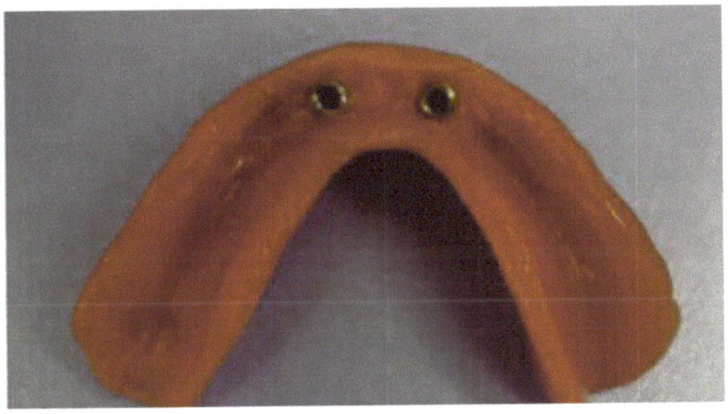

Figure 4.11. After 3 years, the base of the acrylate prosthesis was replaced with soft acrylate (Molisol, Detax, Germany).

The main features of narrow-diameter implants are:

1. minimally invasive surgery - most often there is no raising of the flap and suturing;
2. simple and painless installation under local or general anesthesia;
3. the possibility of immediate loading;
4. quick healing;
5. there is no bone destruction at the site of the lost implant;
6. simple installation of the retention part of the matrix in the already existing prosthesis;
7. low cost;
8. the entire procedure was significantly shortened in time;
9. the patient, due to the noticeably increased comfort in the mouth, leaves the office satisfied.

Due to the low price and simple application, this type of implant soon found wide use, firsst in dental practices throughout America, and today in all countries.

This type of implant is particularly suitable in cases where the narrowness of the alveolar ridges does not allow the use of implants of standard diameters. The longer the implant is inserted into the narrow alveolar ridge, if there are anatomical conditions for it, the more favorable the prognosis (Figures 4.12 and 4.13).

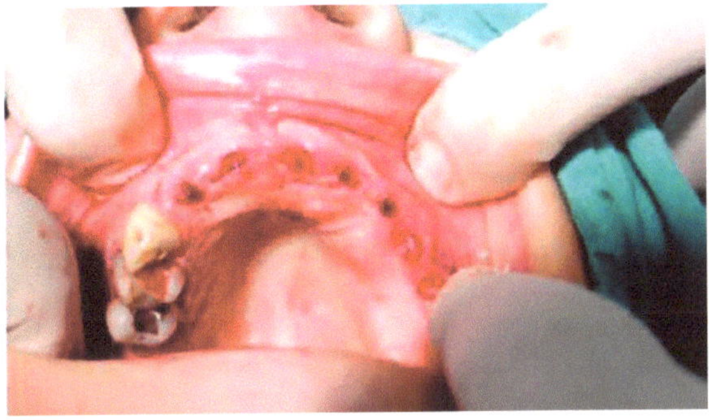

Figure 4.12. With narrow-diameter implants, quick temporary and permanent solutions are possible.

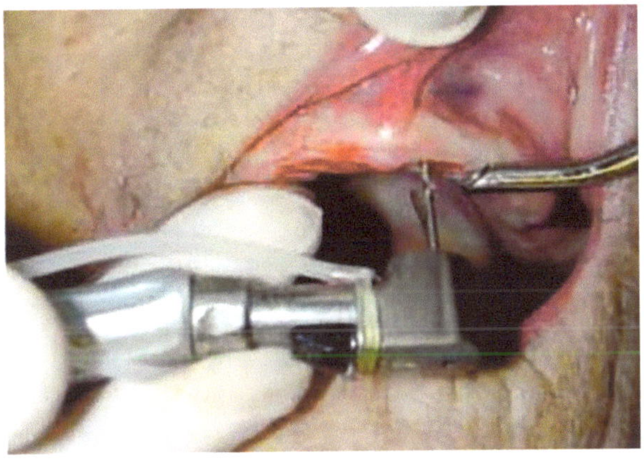

Figure 4.13. Implant placement is simplified.

The frontal part of the lower jaw is an extremely favorable region for the installation of one-piece implants either for anchoring mobile or fixed prosthetic restorations. The area between the two mental openings has no anatomical obstacles for the installation of any type of implant.

The diameters of IMTEC MINI implants are 1.8 mm, 2.1 mm and 2.4 mm, and the lengths are 12, 13, 15 and 18 mm.

The new forms of narrow implants with a diameter of 3 mm have been improved as far as the thread itself is concerned, so that they enable easier self-tapping and even easier installation in very hard bone. This enables good primary stability in the cortical part of the bone (Figure 4.14.)

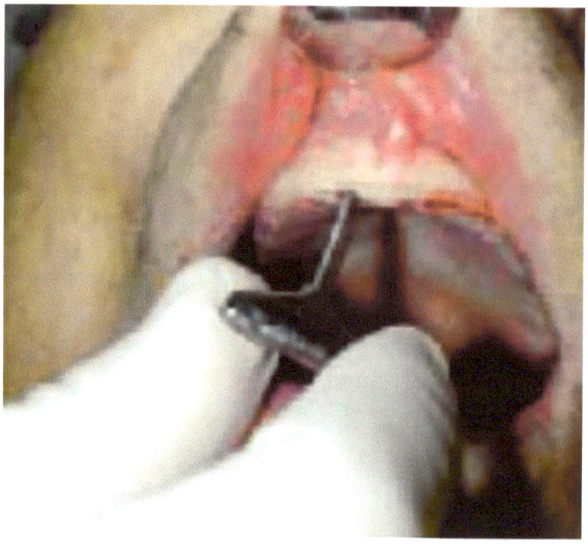

Figure 4.14. Manual insertion of the implant into the bone.

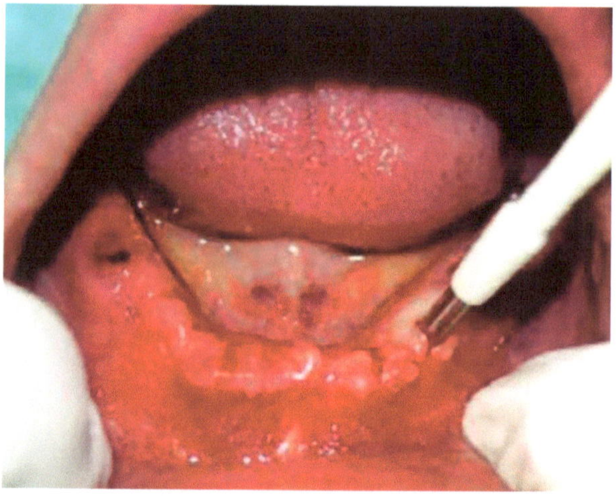

Figure 4.15. Soft tissue preparation for implant positioning.

For the installation of narrow implants from 1.8 to 2.4 mm, only one new drill bit (picture 10) is needed, which enters the bone, and at the same time a pilot drill with a diameter of 1.3 mm. This drill is recommended for very dense D1 bone.

For installing the implant, in addition to the manual adjuster, there is also an adjustable wrench that shows the tension that occurs when the implant is screwed into the bone. There are two forms of adjustable wrenches: a larger one with 10-60 Ncm of maximum force and a smaller one with an indication of tension in the range of 10-40 Ncm. The first, larger, is needed for extremely strong bone (D1), with a maximum force of 60 Ncm.

When using this key, whose arm has the power of a lever, you should always keep in mind precautions: do not cut the implant with great force quickly, (diameters 1.8 mm, 2.1, and 2.4 mm) because due to the narrow diameter, fractures of the implant itself are possible implants, which can be an undesirable complication.

The convenience of installing this type of implant in a located place is the fact that the mucoperiosteal flap is not removed, but the bone is accessed with a special tubular round scalpel intended for this purpose (tissue punch), which can also be used to reveal two-part implants after the healing phase. A special relief is provided by the drill guides.

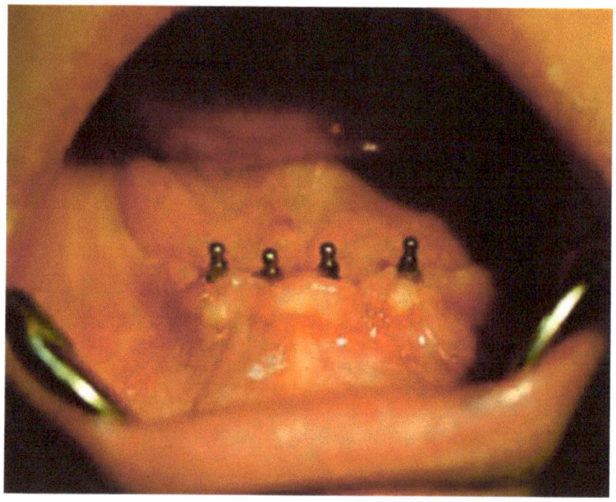

Figure 4.16. One-piece implants of 3.0 mm diameter with spherical heads ("O-ball abautmens").

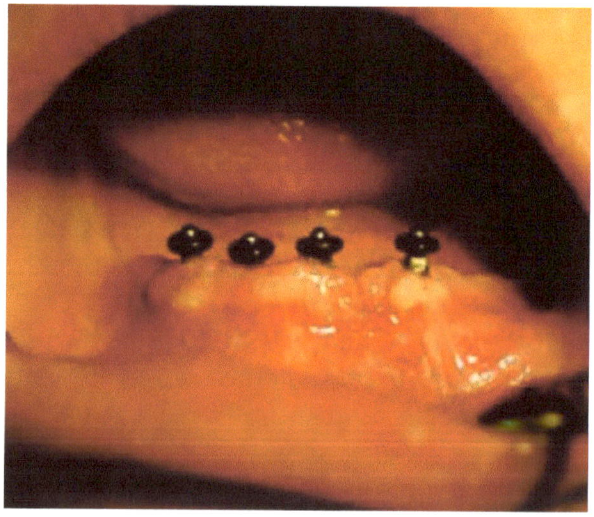

Figure 4.17. Resilient rings that fit into the retention caps that connect the acrylic prosthesis to the implants.

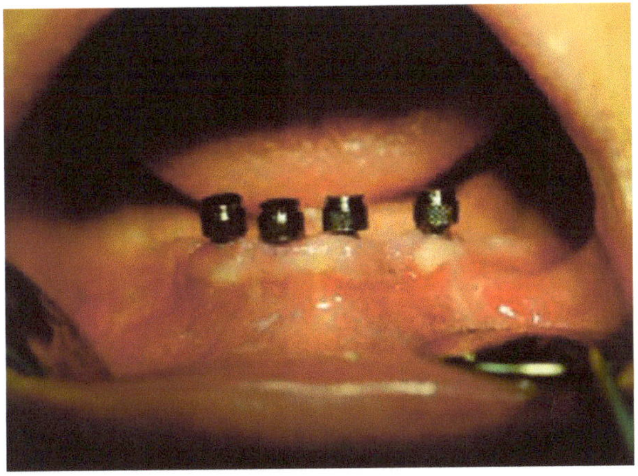

Figure 4.18. Complete cap with inner rings.

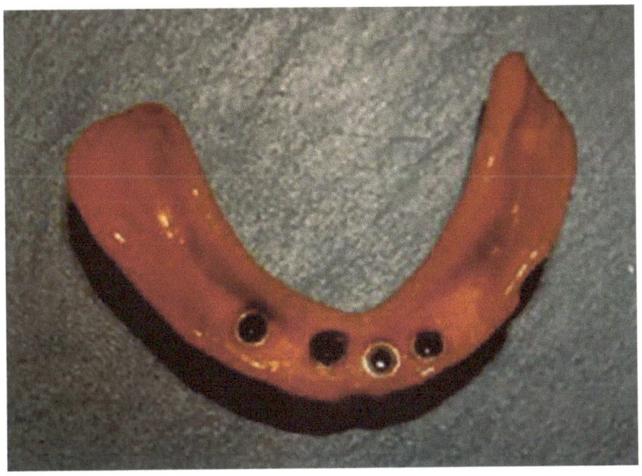

Figure 4.19. Retention caps in a total acrylate prosthesis with a soft acrylate base. A reshaped partial acrylic prosthesis that the patient had previously used for a long time.

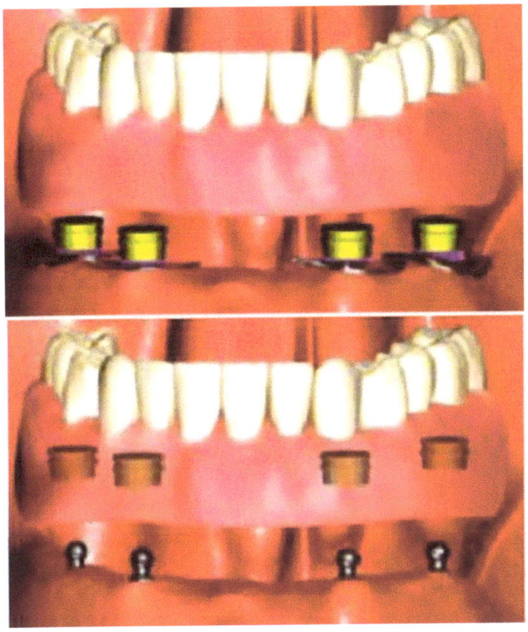

Figure 4.20. Schematic representation of MDI one-piece implants with a narrow diameter and the position of the retention clips in the acrylate part of the prosthesis.

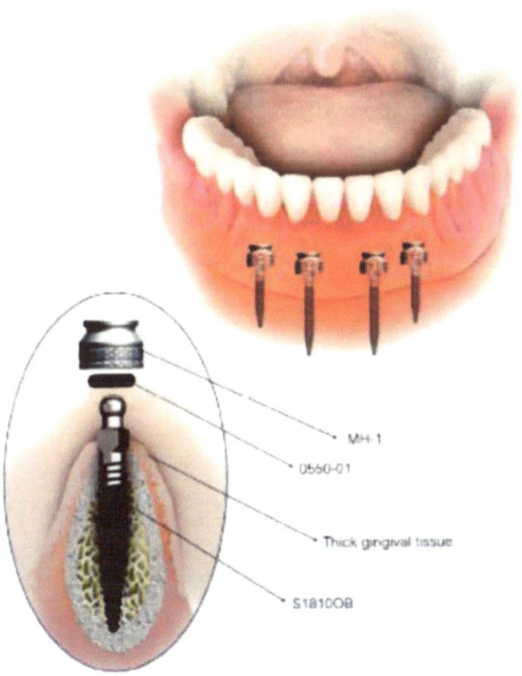

Such solutions with narrow-diameter implants can often be used as temporary, in certain cases, anchoring of temporary prosthetic works in acrylate (Figure 4.20). If failure occurs, removal of the embedded implant due to its narrow diameter does not leave any consequences on the bone where the implant was placed. The healing is complete as if nothing was done in that place.

To satisfy patients' impatience and desire to be able to chew food (and also to improve aesthetics), implants of narrow diameters (and appropriate lengths) can be used as a temporary solution for anchoring fixed temporary acrylic bridges. This procedure, regardless of whether narrow implants or implants of standard diameters are used, is most often determined by the patient's professional obligations, so that he does not end up without teeth, and also for better comfort in the mouth (pictures 4.21-4.25).

In patients, as is the case shown in the pictures of 4.22. until 4.34. to achieve a good functional and aesthetic result, after planning the implant-prosthetic rehabilitation, oral surgical procedures require a specific sequence. After the extraction of diseased teeth, preserve the alveoli. Fill the alveoli with bone substitute. To establish aesthetic and functional comfort, it is necessary to make an immediate acrylic prosthesis as a provisional solution, which promotes the formation of the alveolar arch. In the presented case, the positioning of implants in the places of extracted teeth is out of the question due to the diastema of the central incisors and the low frenulum from the middle of the alveolar ridge, it is impossible to achieve an ideal aesthetic effect. A frenulectomy is necessary. After the healing of the shaped alveolar ridge, the position of the implant and the appearance of the future fixed prosthetic work are planned, followed by modeling wax on a plaster model (fig. 4.27 and 4.28). The exact location of the implant is determined by placing the stent on the alveolar ridge. Fixed prosthetic work in metal ceramics on implants can be performed as a temporary or social solution with implants of narrow diameters. These can easily be replaced with implants of standard diameters when the alveolar bone is completely healed.

The following pictures show a complex case in the upper and lower jaw of a 27-year-old female patient. For a good aesthetic result, healing and a shaped arch of the alveolar ridge were required (pictures 4.23 and 4.26). The sequence of procedures shown in pictures (4.21 to 4.40).

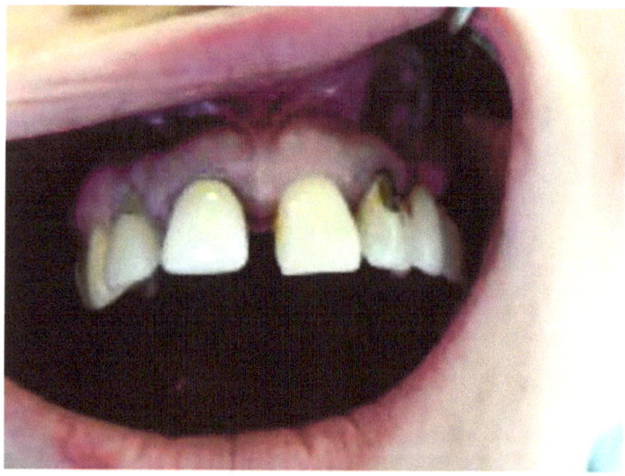

Figure 4.21. A 27-year-old patient - the only flaw in her beauty was her teeth.

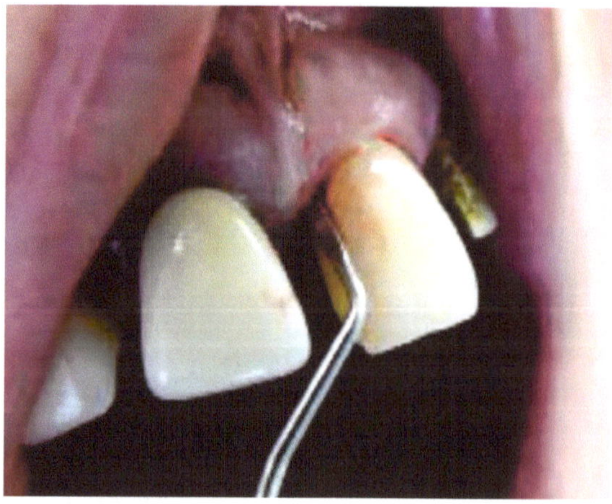

Figure 4.22. Bad prosthetics - wide crowns, followed by the terminal stage of periodontopathy.

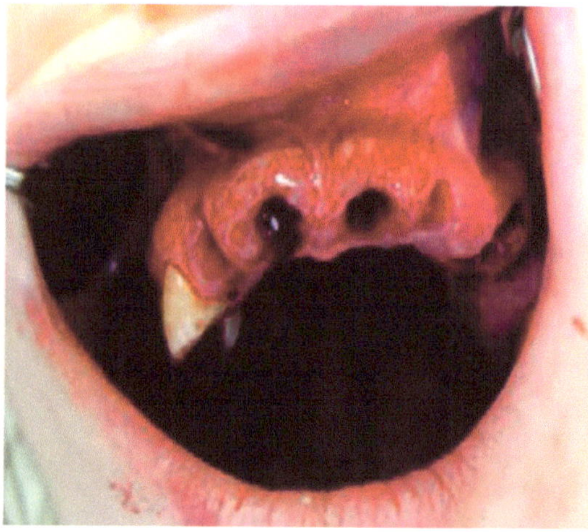

Figure 4.23. A typical case where preservation of the alveoli is indicated, and filling with a xenogeneic bone substitute, shaping of the alveolar arch, and after bone and soft tissue healing, using a stent to determine the position of the implant in order to achieve a good aesthetic result.

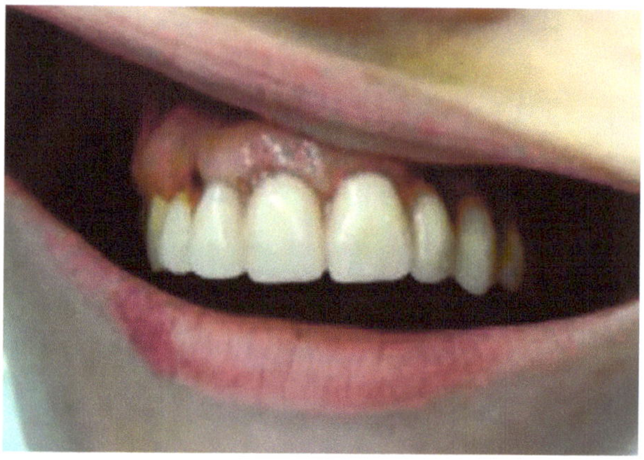

Figure 4.24. Temporary prosthetic rehabilitation immediately after the extraction of diseased teeth. Achieved aesthetic appearance of the patient and the possibility of chewing function.

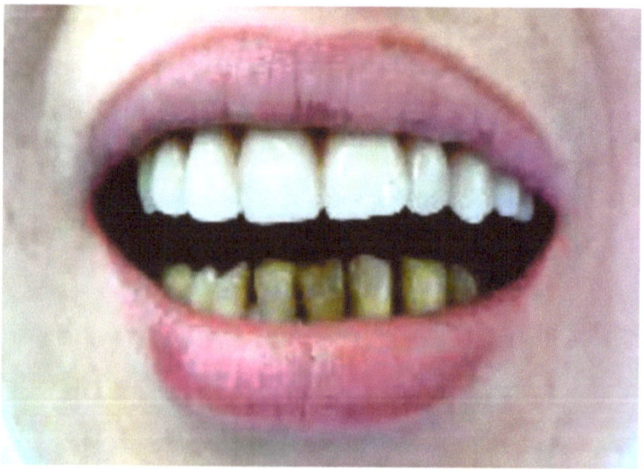

Figure 4.25. Patient satisfaction with the temporary solution, treatment in the lower jaw was also advised, but postponed at the patient's request.

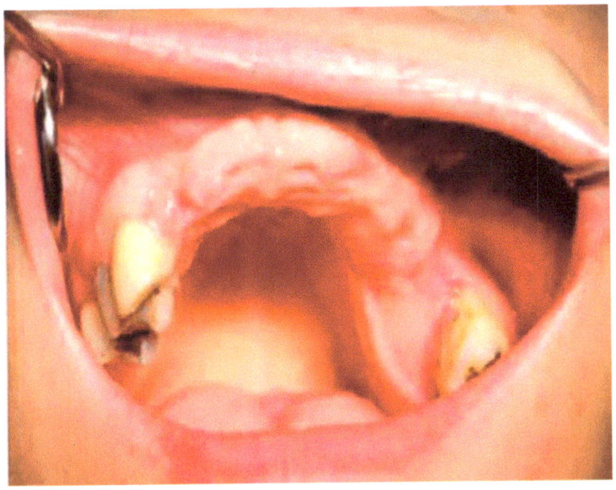

Figure 4.26. Alveolar ridge three months after tooth extraction and alveolar arch augmentation.

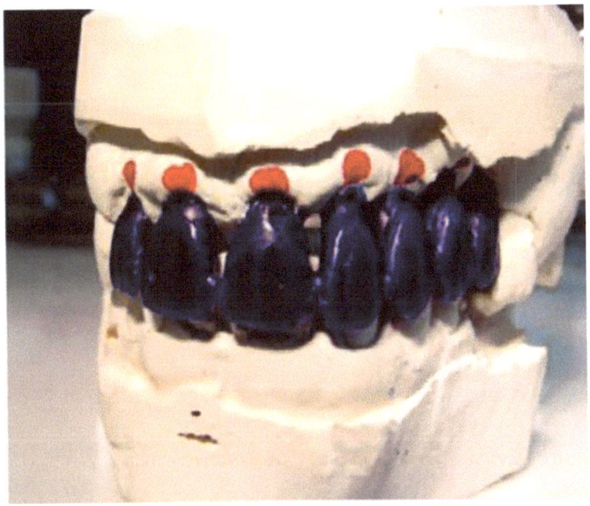

Figure 4.27. Planning the implant position of future temporary prosthetic work on mini-implants.

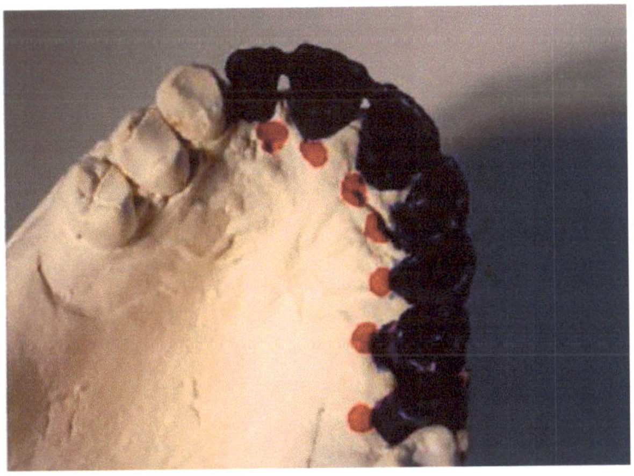

Figure 4.28. Appearance of the marked position of the implant from the palatal side on the plaster model.

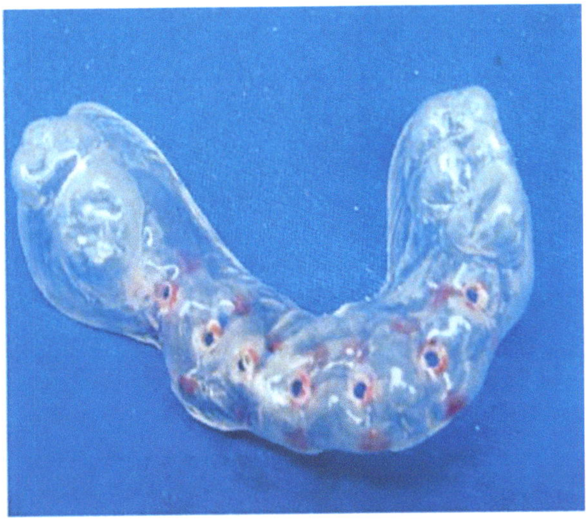

Figure 4.29. Stent for determining the number and position of the implant.

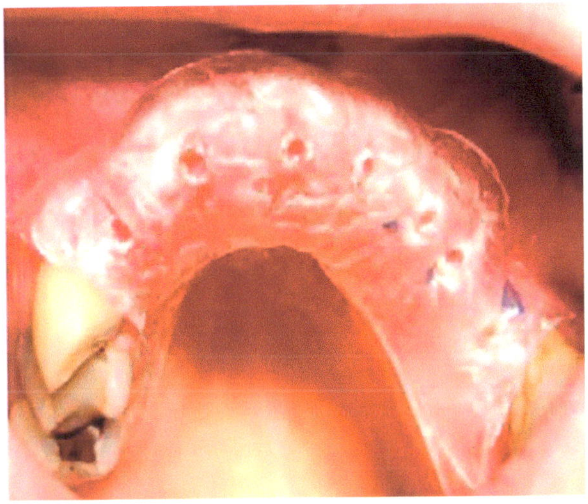

Figure 4.30. Placed stent on the alveolar ridge to locate the implant position.

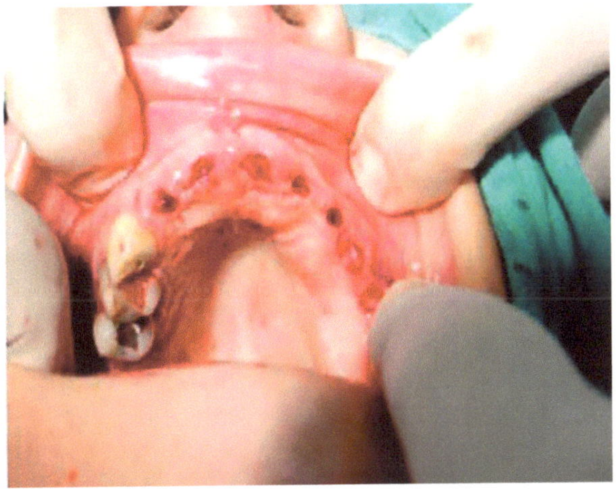

Figure 4.31. Marking with a special instrument the position of the implant for preparation of the bed without raising the flap.

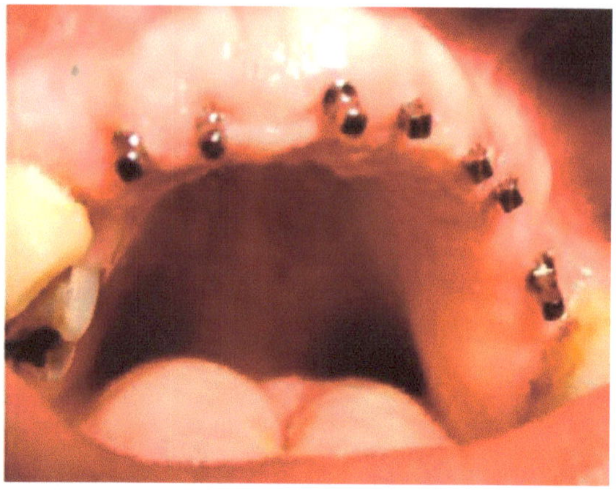

Figure 4.32. Built-in implants of a narrower diameter - a temporary (social) solution. Parallel caps made of cast metal (picture 4.33)

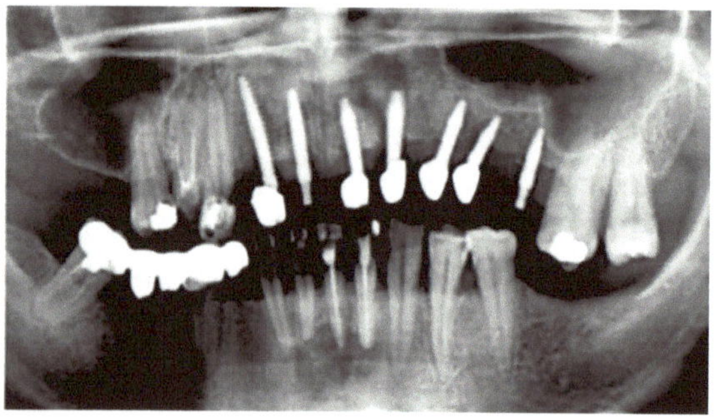

Figure 4.33. Built-in implants for temporary fixed prosthetic work. Adapted brackets cast in metal.

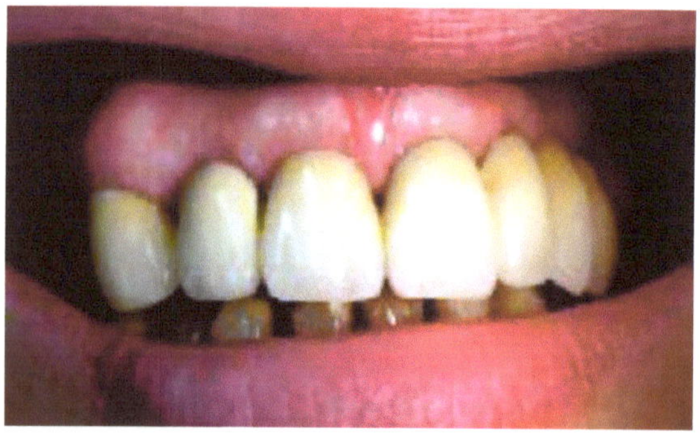

Figure 4.34. Appearance of prosthetic work after 6 months from extraction and augmentation.

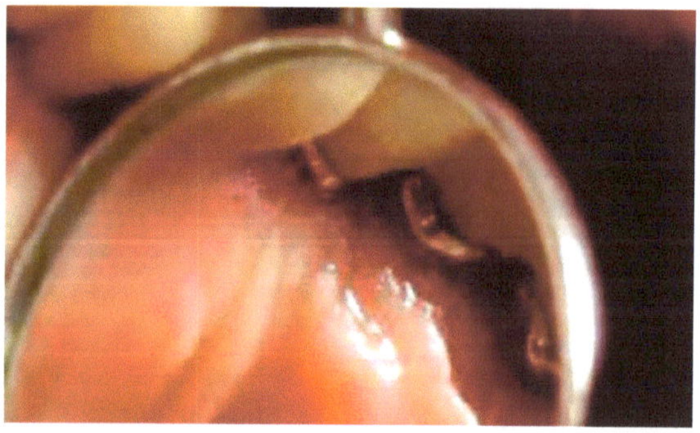

Figure 4.35. Appearance from the palatal side High collars left and the possibility of maintaining oral hygiene.

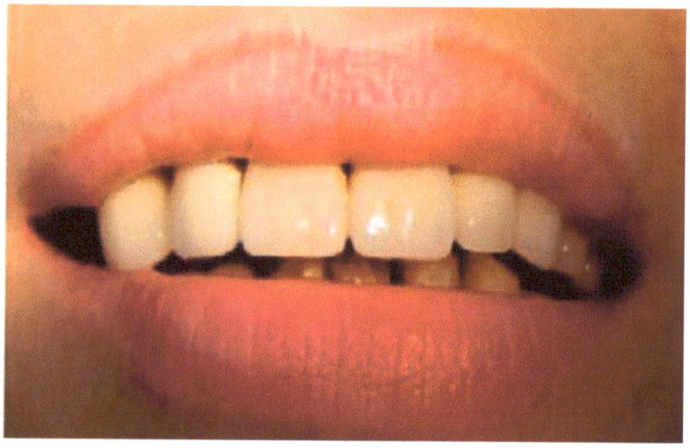

Figure 4.36. The shape of the upper lip and the favorable smile line. After 12 years, the patient does not want to fulfill the original plan, the replacement of mini implants with implants of standard diameters, diameters, because she is satisfied with aesthetics and function.

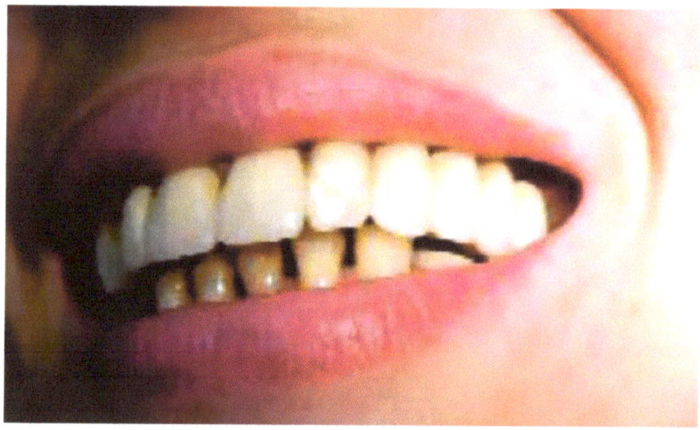

Figure 4.37. The patient was advised that he needed rehabilitation in the lower jaw as well; endodontic treatment of roots and teeth, removal of prosthetic work in the lower jaw and installation of implants in regions 36 and 37. Shortening of molars in the upper jaw; endo treatment or extraction (27 and 28). See Figure 4.33.

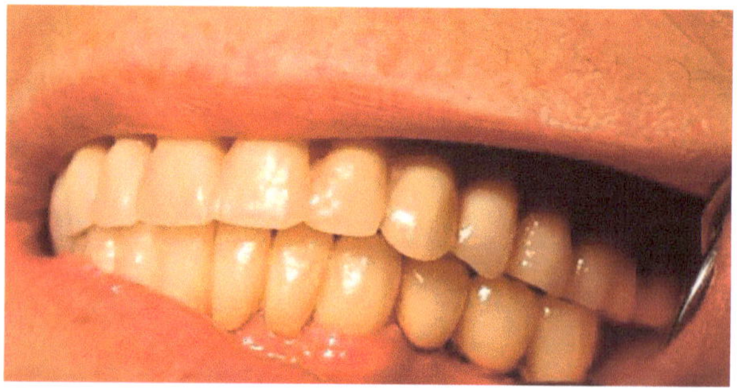

Figure 4.38. Rehabilitation in the lower jaw, endonal, prosthetic and implant-protest procedures (regions 34, 34, and 36).

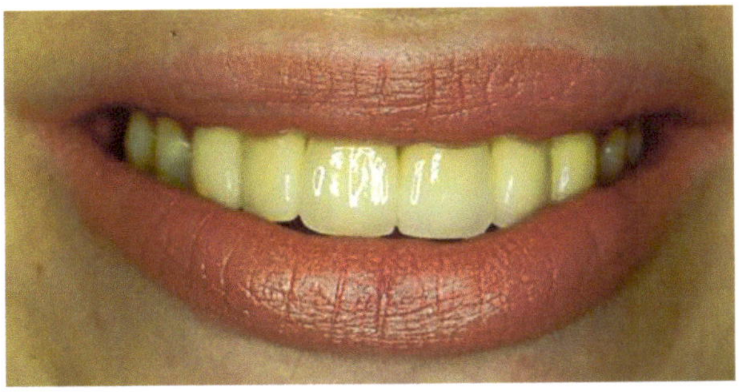

Figure 4.39. When it comes to surgical implant-prosthetic rehabilitation, patients are more and more informed about the scope of oral implantology and insist more on satisfying the aesthetic outcome of the treatment.

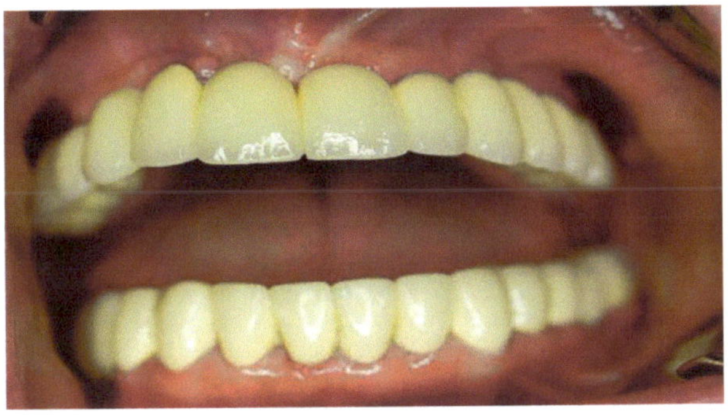

Figure 4.40. The patient's first and most important request is successful aesthetics, but they do not see what is important; establishment of physiological interjaw relationships, occlusion and articulation, which ensures long-term osseointegration of the implant into the jawbone.

The success of implant-prosthetic treatment is determined at the beginning by determining the position and number of implants. There are several ways of marking the position where the implant should be placed. In practice, the most appropriate way is to use a stent. On the toothless alveolar ridge, modeling in wax shapes the morphology of future teeth, that is, the appearance of future prosthetic work. The positions of the implants are marked on the plaster model (fig. 4.27 and 4.28), which are transferred to the alveolar ridge via the acrylic stent (fig. 4.29 and 4.30) (fig. 4.31).

The procedures described above achieve a good aesthetic and functional result (fig. 4.35- 4.40). Palatal and lingual, it is necessary to have a metal collar in case of definitive prosthetic work in the gingival area, which avoids the deposition of plaque and easier and better maintenance of oral hygiene (fig. 4.35).

Temporary bridges, made of acrylate or composite materials, can be placed on implants of standard or wider diameters, where the load is delayed for several months. Narrow-diameter implants, which are immediately loaded with temporary prosthetic works, serve to wait for the healing phase and enable better bony integration of the installed standard two-part implants.

Patients with narrow-diameter implants that are immediately loaded can chew freely, without exerting any pressure on standard and wider-diameter implants. This type of temporary fixed compensation is extremely comfortable for people whose profession requires smooth daily verbal communication.

After a year or more, the temporary prosthetic work can be removed along with the thin implants that temporarily hold it in place. Thin implants can then be replaced with implants of standard diameters. The convenience of the procedure is a well-healed bone and a formed alveolar ridge.

Science and many experiences confirm that the degree of osseous integration of unloaded implants that waited a six-month healing period was the same as that of implants that were immediately loaded. Experiences, however, show that with a properly immediately loaded implant, the bone-implant connection was even better, which is also our experience (plctures 4.41-4.48).

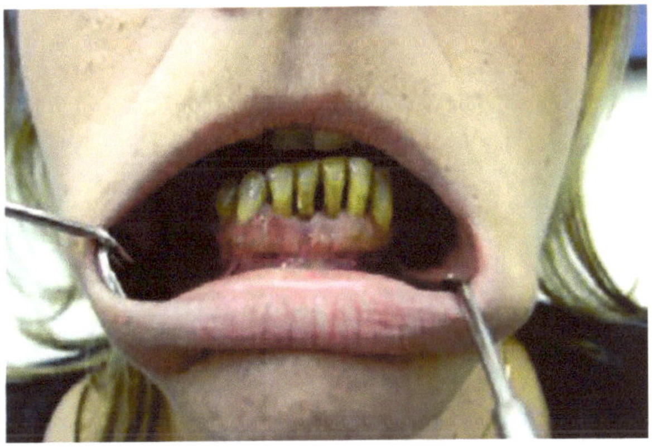

Figure 4.41. Dislocated incisors in the front of the lower jaw with periapical changes, the only correct solution is the extraction of the affected teeth.

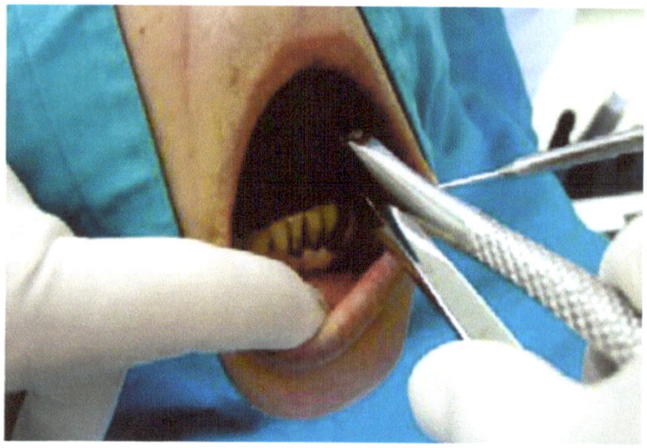

Figure 4.42. Extraction of periodontally diseased teeth. Due to professional obligations, the patient's request to receive fixed prosthetic work on the same day was fulfilled according to the set plan. Temporary prosthetic work with an acrylate mobile prosthesis would compress soft and bony tissues, promoting their resorption.

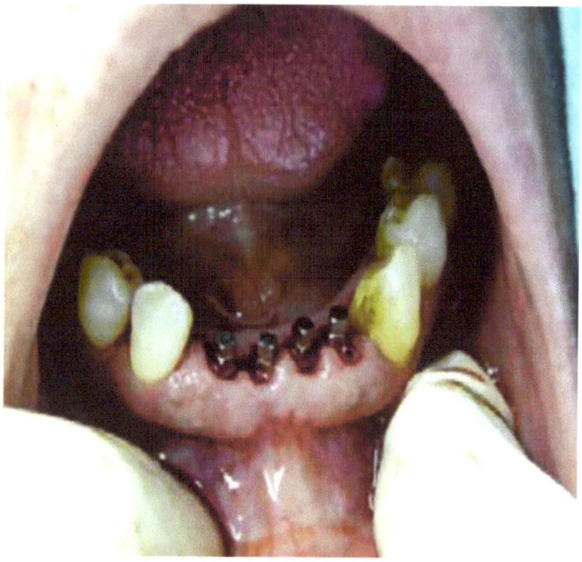

Figure 4.43. The patient's professional obligations required immediate implantation. Today there are more suitable forms of narrow gauges.

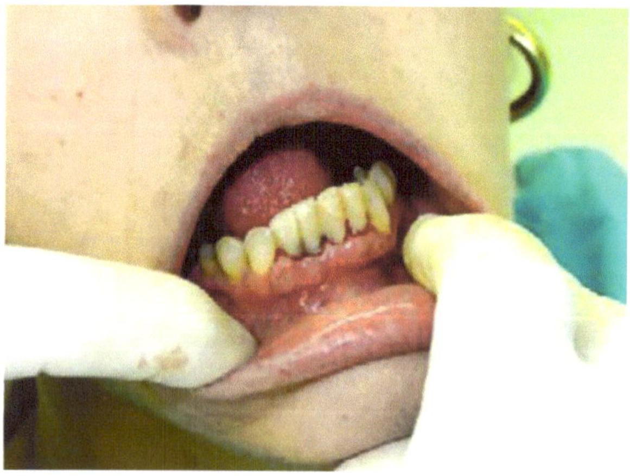

Figure 4.44. A temporary acrylic bridge installed on the same day after tooth extraction and immediate implant installation.

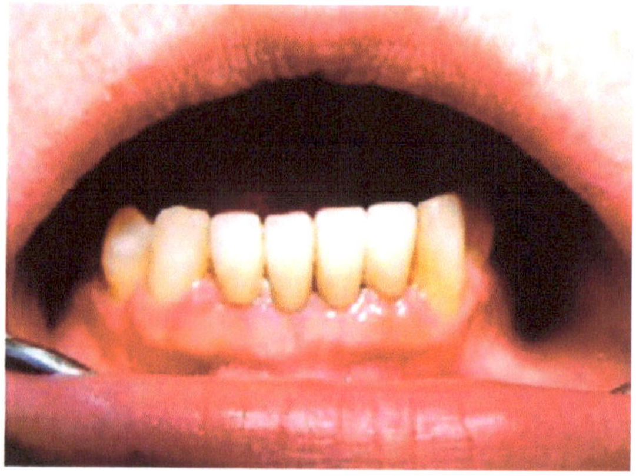

Figure 4.45. Definitive prosthetic work in metal-ceramics.

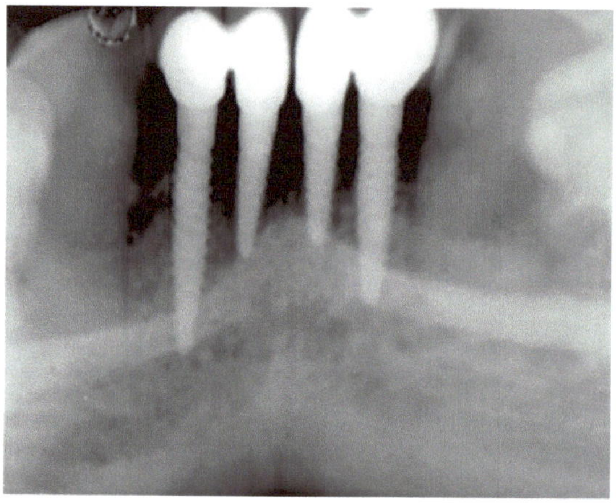

Figure 4.46. A control image after 10 years.

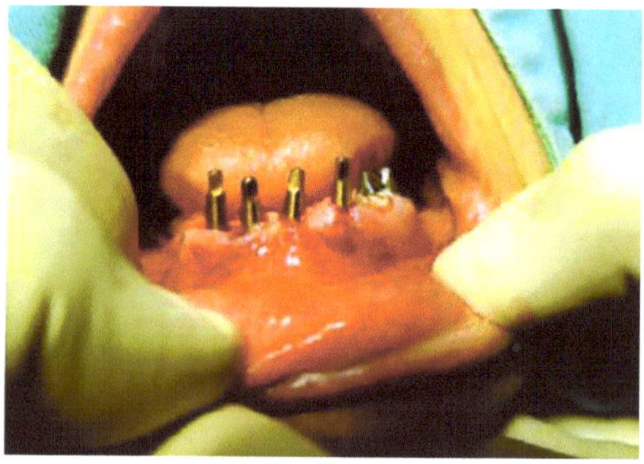

Figure 4.47. Implants with a narrow diameter of 3 mm. Immediately burdened with fixed prosthetic work.

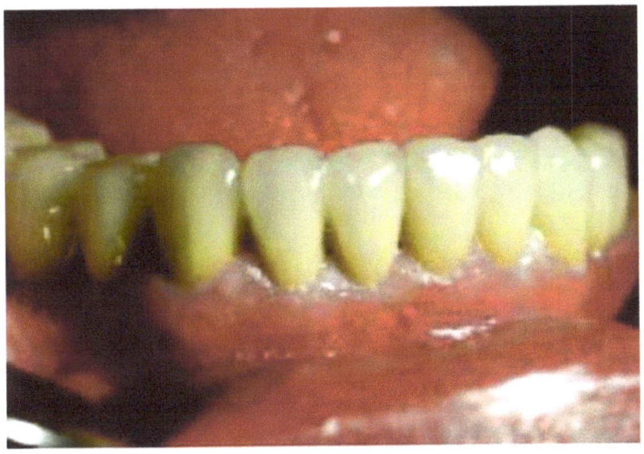

Figure 4.48. Definitive prosthetic work in metal ceramics on implants. Stable soft tissues with forimar interimplant papillae.

After the good results of immediate loading, these requirements forced the production of one-piece implants with a slightly wider diameter of 3.0 mm and 3.2 mm with a length of 12, 15 and 18 mm. Due to biomechanical requirements, the shortest length of narrow implants with a diameter of 3.0 mm was until recently 12 mm.

Thanks to the good results and successful solutions with narrow diameter implants (3 mm), shorter implants with a length of 10 mm (10, 12, 14 and 16 mm) were launched. Recently, one-piece implants with a diameter of 3.0 mm have exactly those lengths: 10, 12, 14 and 16 mm.

Based on favorable experiences with the 3.0 mm diameter one-piece implant, some implant systems have launched a 3.5 mm diameter one-piece implant, which is significantly closer to the standard 3.75 mm diameter.

One-piece implants with a diameter of 3.0 mm enable the processing of an abutment that is fixed with the part of the implant that enters the bone.

What should be emphasized?

1. One-piece implants with a narrow-diameter (1.8, 2.1, and 2.4 mm) are most successfully used in case of total edentulousness of the narrow alveolar ridge, which is of insufficient width and favorable height if immediate loading is possible.
2. Application is also possible in cases where one wants to plan a fixed prosthetic work (3 mm), and not only a combined fixed-mobile compensation.
3. Using one-piece implants significantly shortens the time to satisfy the patient's needs and wishes, because immediate loading is possible, and from the experience of the author of the book, this is both recommended and increasingly applicable (Wolf's law in orthopedics).
4. When installing one-piece implants, parallelism must be strictly taken into account, because the abutment is not at an angle. Subsequent adjustment of parallelism by grinding a fixed abutment should be avoided, despite the advantage highlighted above (softness of the abutment material). Grinding of the abutment should be reduced to the smallest possible extent and with great care to avoid even the smallest microtrauma of the implant. The manufacturers also thought of that, adding a special hard (hard) drill for single use to each package of implants.
5. When using implants with a narrow diameter, all the requirements that apply to the implantation of standard diameters and general requirements should be applied, as with all oral surgical procedures. It is necessary to adhere to all principles - from anamnesis, inspection, palpation, and radiographic analysis of anatomical limitations - paying attention to everything that can be a risk, and suggest to the patient the obligation to maintain oral hygiene.
6. By palpating the labiogingival bony ridge in the symphysis region of the mandible, we must determine the direction and angulation of the drill, using the drill guide to achieve parallelism. The procedure is the same for installing two-part implants.
7. The drills used must be sharp and should not all have the same diameter. This is important because the implants are self-tapping. The correct angle for placement is crucial, and achieving primary stability is the most critical part of the initial movement when positioning the implant. In the symphysis region of the lower jaw, the bone is often more condensed (D1). Careless insertion of drills or prolonged drilling without sufficient cooling with saline can lead to **thermal trauma due to overheating the bone**. Therefore, attention must be given to overheating during implantation. To avoid this, it's essential to take short breaks between drilling operations and to irrigate the area abundantly with a physiological

solution. Additionally, it is particularly important to pause during the screwing process to allow the bone to "rest" from the stress on its walls. This resting period prepares the bone to accept the next threads during the cutting process.

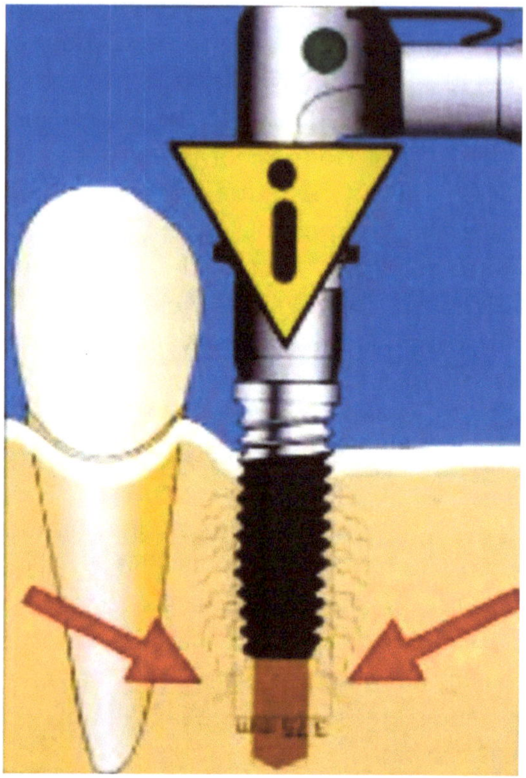

Figure 4.49. Too strong and fast tightening of the implant when screwing it into the bone can cause microfractures in the bone (M.Davarpanah, H.Martinez et al.).

Exercise maximum caution when using abutments, as they can potentially lead to significant issues. The thread of the abutment may not align with the thread of the implant, which can compromise primary stability. It is advisable to use the cutting tool exclusively at the very beginning, specifically in the cortical bone, to facilitate easier placement of the implant in the drilled area.

Using the threads of the implant as self-tapping mechanisms in the bone is the most efficient approach. The guidelines for inserting thin implants into the bone should be similarly applied to standard diameter implants, particularly when working with good-quality, narrow, and dense bone.

Bone, as a living tissue, experiences stress at the points where the implant rests on it—specifically at the contact surface of the implant (see picture 49). To manage this, it is advisable to pause the screwing process once the implant makes initial contact. Back off by one or two threads and allow the bone some time to "rest" before continuing. This approach allows the implant to proceed more smoothly to its final positioning.

What else is important to know when installing immediately loaded implants with a narrow diameter?

The patient's motivation to accept such a treatment is an extremely important factor accompanied by a detailed explanation by the doctor. The most important and most common motive of the patient is to get teeth as soon as possible.

One-piece implants with a diameter of 3.0 mm and 3.5 mm can give good results as definitive immediately loaded solutions.

Recently, two-part implants of the same diameters (3.0 and 3.5 mm) have been launched.

Before deciding on implantation, it is necessary to learn about the patient's expectations and fears by talking to them. We often encounter exaggerated fears, but also unrealistic demands and expectations.

During the patient interview, it's important to guide them to ask questions about both the operative and postoperative periods. When patients formulate their own questions, we can better understand their expectations regarding implant placement. It's essential to give them ample time to think and articulate their queries throughout the entire rehabilitation process. Additionally, we must clearly explain why narrow-diameter implants are being used and why standard or wide-diameter implants cannot be considered.

The patient should be motivated by suggesting some questions that he should ask, such as:

1. you must never hesitate to ask the selected dentist questions that will influence your decision and trust;
2. don't pay attention to many newspaper ads and advertising websites, because young, inexperienced beginners are usually prone to exaggerated ads. Five questions from the patient are inevitable:
    1. for guidance, how many implants should be installed and why?

2. Why do so many implants need to be installed?
3. which selected implant system should be implanted? Is it the best system and is there a better one?
4. Do you believe that implants are the last option or that tooth loss can be solved in another way?
5. Can you guarantee that the implants will last a long time and what is the guarantee period?

If the implantologist claims that there is a warranty period, one should doubt his experience. Today, there are doctors who guarantee everything with advertisements, and in medicine, guarantees cannot be issued, because in medicine there are biological, not mechanical laws. Implantology is a serious medical field that requires great responsibility, expertise and experience, as well as from the aspect of medical ethics.

Likewise, do not bypass questions to the patient, such as:

a) what are his expectations?
b) the patient's fears - is he afraid and why?
c) aesthetic expectations?
d) what are the expectations when eating?
e) is he already familiar and does he accept the obligation to come for regular check-ups?
f) Does he know that he should maintain perfect oral hygiene?
g) what are the patient's financial capabilities?
h) is he a heavy smoker?

and. is he aware that smoking is one of the contraindications for implantation and that smoking interferes with wound healing after surgery?

What should be done to extend the life of the implant?

With the installation of the implant, provided that everything is done correctly, the responsibility is assumed by the patient. Attendance at regular periodic check-ups is mandatory and the dentist's instructions on maintaining oral hygiene must be strictly adhered to. The progress in the development of new means for maintaining oral hygiene is also significant.

Explain to the patient (assistant's duty) that there are many brushes of various shapes and qualities on the market for maintaining oral hygiene with embedded implants. Many antiseptic, disinfectant and deodorant mouthwashes are in use, which inhibit harmful bacterial flora in the mouth.

Digital X-ray technology (digital intraoral sensor RVG) is so advanced that it is possible to see with accuracy whether there have been changes around the implant during check-ups after a few years.

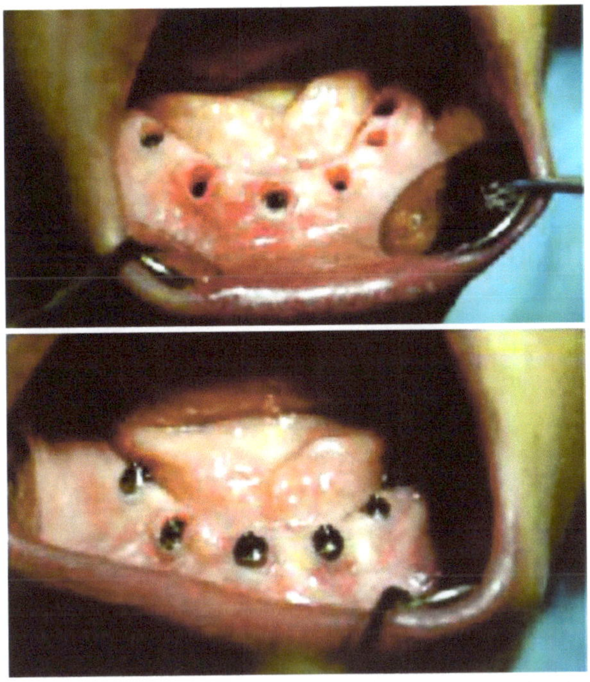

Figures 4.50 and 4.51. Strong motivation of the patient for fixed work in the lower jaw (55-year-old female patient). Branemark type implants.

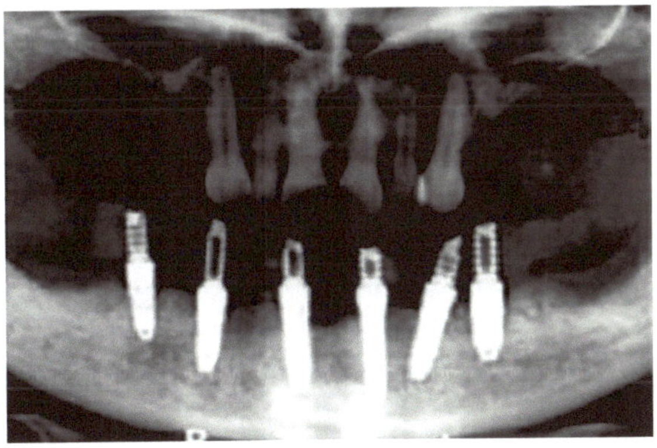

Figure 4.52. X-ray view of Branemark implants (work of the author of the book).

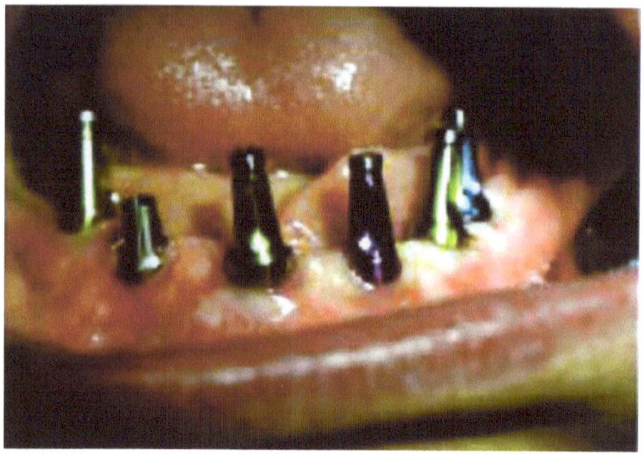

Figure 4.53. Placed supports (Brenemak implant system) for impression taking.

Control with an intraoral recording is an unavoidable procedure. It is greatly facilitated by the RVG technique. If changes around the implant are noticed in time, small interventions can eliminate the problems that have arisen and significantly extend the life of the implant. One of the bone substitutes can be placed in the place where the bone has broken down.

Another great innovation in oral implantology is the laser preparation of the implant bed as well as the laser action on the bone around the implant, so that this method can stimulate all the positive factors used in implanted implants. Laser (acronym for "Light amplification by stimulated emission of radiation") stimulates the surrounding tissues with light emissions and mild radiation.

The future of implantology is evident. This is also evidenced by the fact that a few years ago, the USA invested in the development of implantology as much as the Japanese company "Mitsubishi" in the development of the automobile industry. American implantologist Irwin Smigel said: "We are at the beginning of the XXI century - it seems that the dream of thousands of years about replacing lost teeth with third teeth, implants, has become a reality." In the conclusion of the American Dental Association, it was stated: "Uncomfortable dentures have come to an end." But it all comes at a cost."

Many understandings have also been changed. Dentists, and those who do not deal with the installation of implants, should know the possibilities that implantology offers today, so that they can advise and explain to the patient and guide him to satisfactory solutions.

It is necessary to explain to the patient that his case can be solved by avoiding uncomfortably moving prostheses (either total and partial acrylate, or metal skeletonized) by installing implants (Figures 4.50-4.57).

All possibilities and options must be presented to the patient in order to solve his case in the best way. All therapeutic possibilities must be explained to him (excerpt from the author's lecture at a scientific symposium, Munich, Germany, 1987).

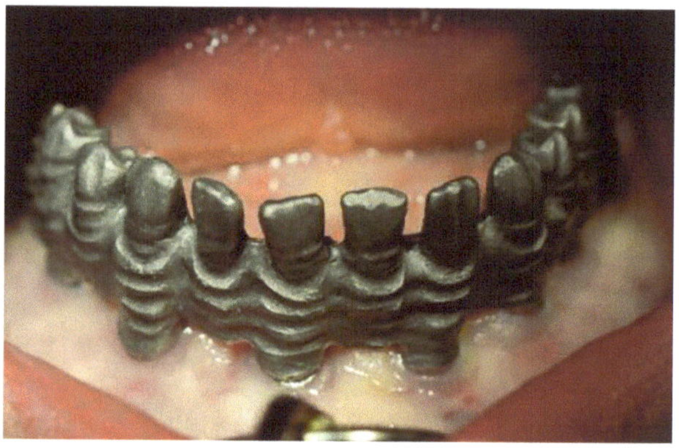

Figure 4.54. Appearance of metal construction for fixed prosthetic work on Branemark implants.

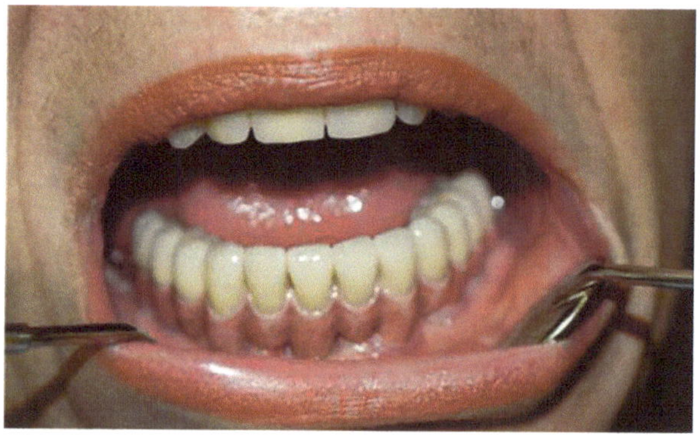

Figure 4.55. Appearance of definitive prosthetic works in both jaws.

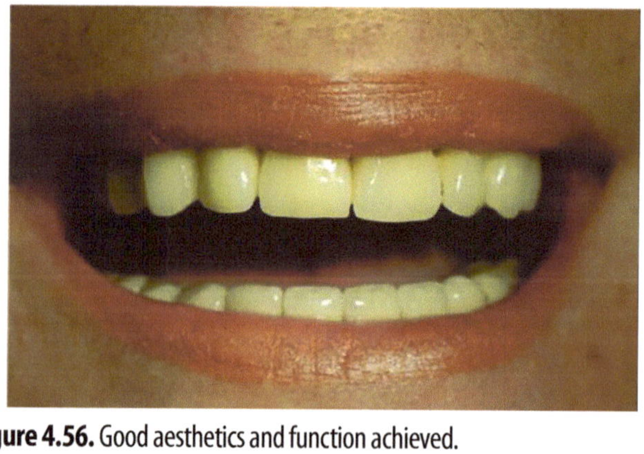

Figure 4.56. Good aesthetics and function achieved.

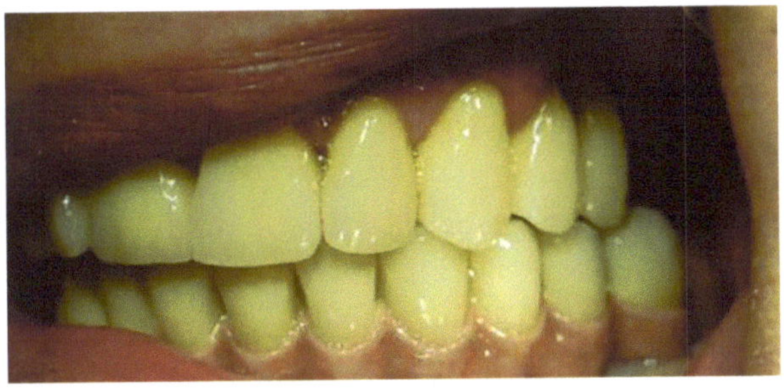

Figure 4.57. Balanced occlusion achieved.

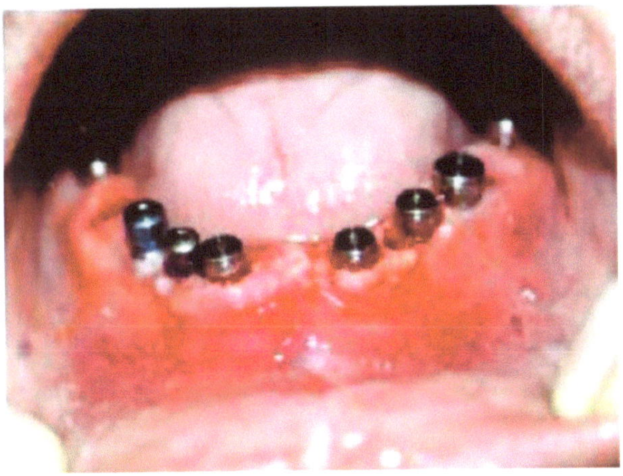

Figure 4.58. Total toothlessness in the lower jaw can be restored with comfortable fixed work instead of uncomfortable total dentures, (Work by Dr. T. Zlopaša and Dr. B. Zlopaša).

Gone are the days when only implantologists were competent to explain the possibilities of implantology. The development of the profession imposed an obligation for most dentists to be educated to explain the benefits of implant placement to patients.

How should one approach the practice of implantology, according to the quote at the end of the book "Oral implantology" by Leonard Linkov: "It is imperative that dentists who want to practice implantology must complete several well-organized courses." Never, never, should dentists dare to install implants only after reading a short article about it or listening to a lecture on implant installation".

Dentists across all specialties should explain to their patients the possibilities of realizing their wishes and clarify the role of the dentist who specializes in implant installation to ensure the best possible outcome. Among all medical fields, implantology has faced considerable resistance. The pioneers of implantology, who shared their initial results and experiences at international congresses and professional gatherings, encountered far more skepticism at dental weeks and congresses throughout the former Yugoslavia. Consequently, the author chose to deliver most of his lectures and share his experiences at foreign congresses and scientific gatherings. At these events, practitioners increasingly showcased successful outcomes, demonstrating that the justification for installing implants could no longer be challenged. Attention then shifted exclusively to the physiological processes that occur after implant placement.

Physiology serves as the foundation of medicine and can be considered a medical bible. It has increasingly influenced the development of dental implantology, enhancing our understanding of physiological events at the bone-implant interface. This relationship is known as osseointegration.

Recently, advances in physiology have made it essential for every dentist to have a basic understanding of osseointegration processes. This knowledge involves understanding what occurs between the bone and the surface of the implant.

For a long time, aesthetic results were not a major consideration in implantology. This focus primarily on functionality was reasonable for that period, as the primary goals of implant placement were based on functional needs rather than aesthetic ones. However, in the last decade, there has been a significant shift towards addressing aesthetic requirements, particularly in cases of individual tooth loss and partial toothlessness. As a result, patients' demands for satisfactory aesthetic outcomes are steadily increasing.

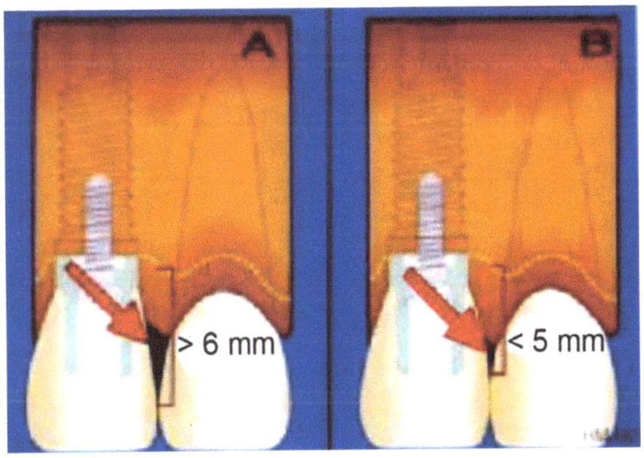

Figure 4.59. Preservation of the crestal bone during implant placement is extremely important for the regeneration of the papilla. Incomplete regeneration of the interdental papilla occurs when the distance between the top of the interdental papilla and the top of the bone crest is greater than 6 mm; (a), is reduced twice. Complete regeneration of the papilla occurs when the distance from the crestal bone is less than 5 mm, (b) (M.Davarpanah, H.Martinez).

To meet these requirements, it is essential to position the implant optimally. Before this, any necessary soft tissue procedures should be performed, and if bone mass needs to be increased, bone substitutes should be used— an aspect that received insufficient attention in the past.

Today, oral surgeons and periodontologists not only perform bone augmentation but are also able to reconstruct the lost papilla around the implant (as shown in Figure 4.59). Only after these steps can it be concluded that the desired functional and aesthetic results have been achieved. With this understanding, oral surgeons and periodontologists can create an aesthetic outcome that closely resembles the natural appearance of a tooth, with soft tissues that closely mimic healthy tissue.

There is less and less dilemma whether a lost or diseased tooth should be replaced with an implant. Such dilemmas and thoughts belong to the past. Attention is directed to the precise positioning of the implant and to the details that are important, in order to achieve good bone integration and form soft tissues, achieving a good functional and aesthetic result. Reconstruction of the papilla is an aesthetic priority.

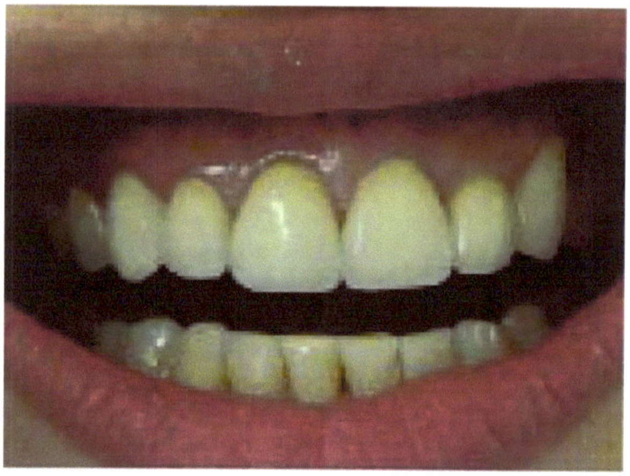

Figure 4.60. The appearance of the preserved papilla in the reconstruction of frontal teeth on implants in the upper jaw.

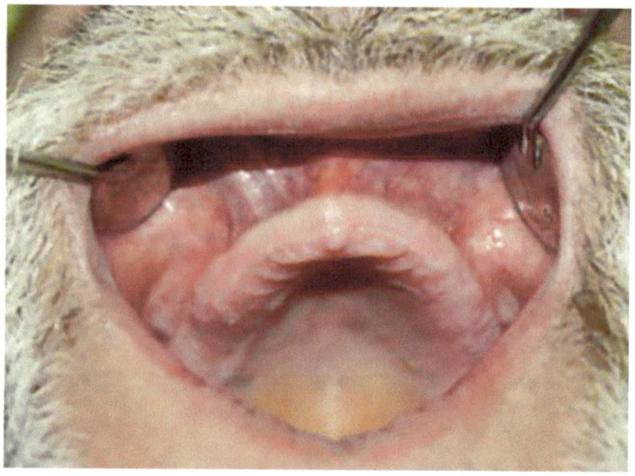

Figure 4.61. In case of total edentulism, the type and number of implants and their positioning determine the predictable success of the outcome.

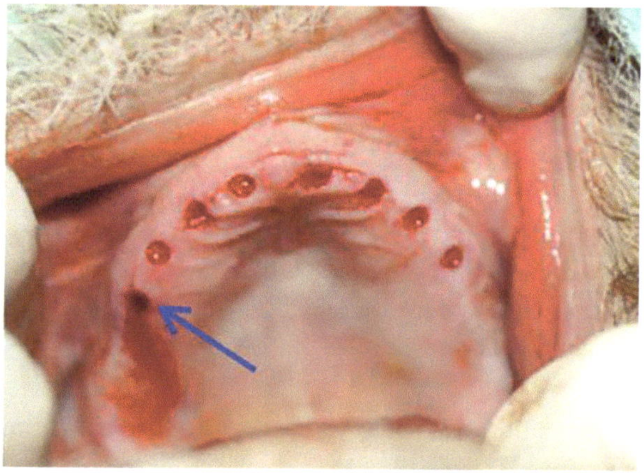

Figure 4.62. In case of long-term toothlessness, it is possible to move palatal blood vessels with minor or major iatrogenic incidents.

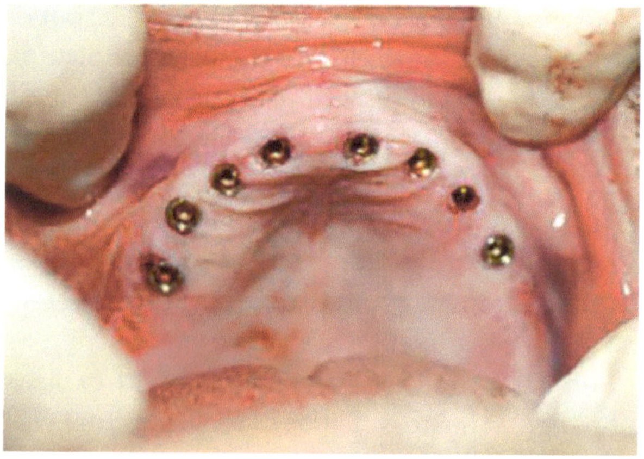

Figure 4.63. Display of the completed implantation of the implant without raising the flap.

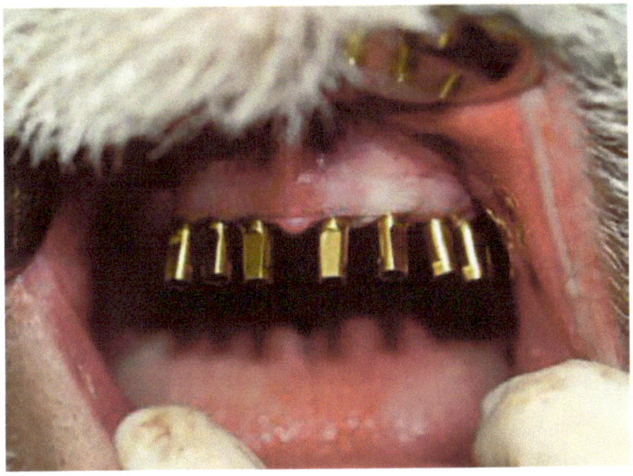

Figure 4.64. Placed definitive abutments assume the role of a "healing abutment".

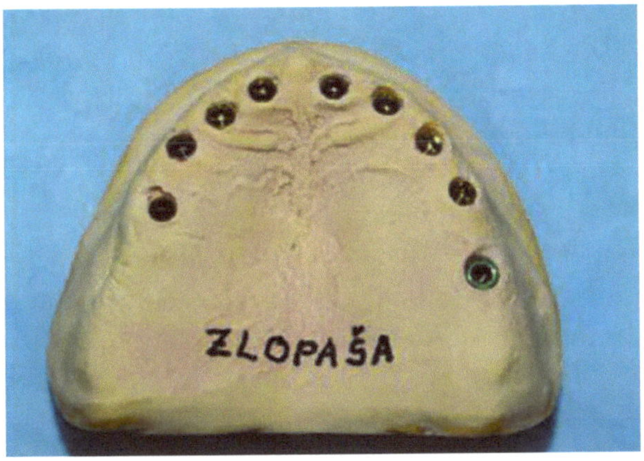

Figure 4.65. Appearance of the position and paralysis of the installed implants without raising the flap on the plaster model (see picture 64).

The alveolar ridge bone plays a crucial role in the function of the interdental papillae. After placing the implant, it is important to monitor the distance between the contact points of the crown and the bone, as this distance significantly affects the complete regeneration of the papilla. If the distance is less than 5 mm (see Figure 4.58), the regeneration of the papilla is typically complete. However, as this distance increases, the likelihood of incomplete papilla regeneration rises. For instance, if the distance exceeds 6 mm, the potential for papilla reconstruction is halved. If the distance goes above 7 mm, the chances of successful papilla reconstruction are further compromised.

Additionally, the precision and quality of temporary restorations are vital in facilitating proper papilla formation. Successful papilla reconstruction is essential for achieving the final aesthetic outcome of an implant placement and the associated prosthetic work (see Figures 4.67- 4.68). Ultimately, the position of the implant influences the reconstruction of the papilla (see Figures 4.63 and 4.64).

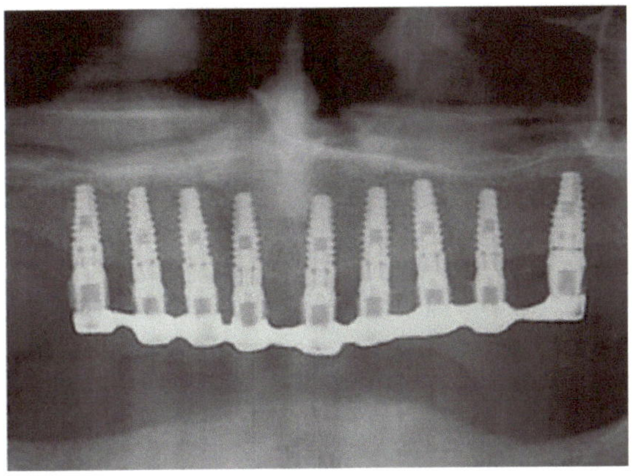

Figure 4.66. Implants immediately installed without raising the flap (reduced trauma and shortened healing time of soft tissues) immediately loaded with temporary precise fixed prosthetic work in composite on a precise metal base.

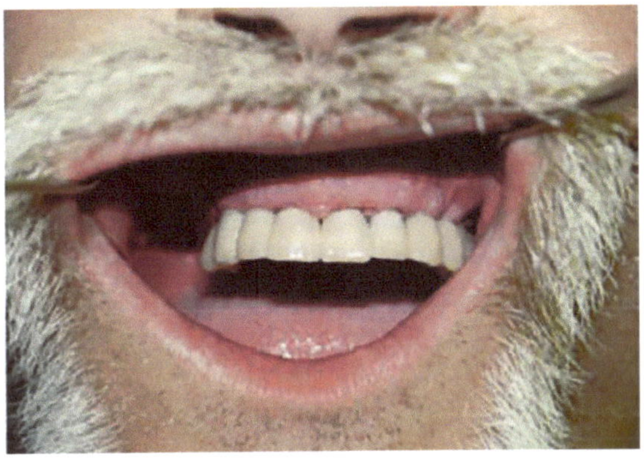

Figure 4.67. Provisional immediate prosthetic work on immediately loaded implants.

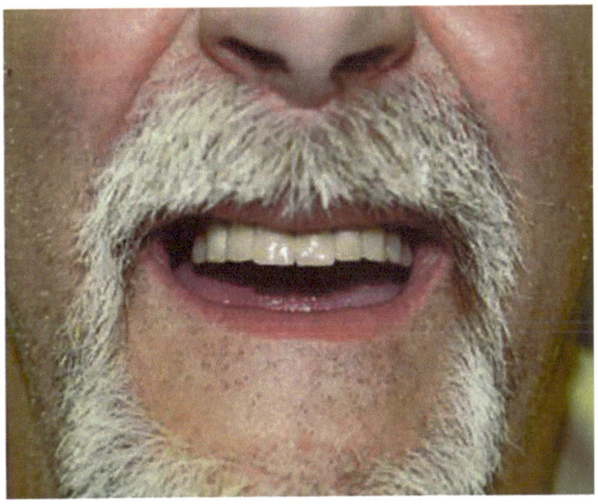

Figure 4.68. Aesthetic and functional satisfaction of the patient one week after the intervention.

Modern oral implantology has resolved many of the past debates regarding when, why, and how to use implants. However, questions still arise from dentists who do not specialize in implants, as well as from patients. The answers to these questions can vary significantly, so it's essential that they are simplified and made understandable for patients.

The role of implants in modern dentistry is crucial and offers advantages that go beyond traditional care. Even dentists who do not perform implant procedures should be aware of their importance. While traditional restoration treatments can sometimes be sufficient, in cases where more conventional options are viable, the use of implants may be unnecessary unless partial acrylic or skeletal prostheses are being considered as a solution.

The use of implants offers a promising option for preserving both hard and soft tissue. Patients who receive implants often report high levels of satisfaction, as it has been shown to enhance self-confidence and improve overall quality of life.

Choosing the appropriate solution or technique—whether surgical or purely prosthetic—depends on a careful assessment of individual needs and indications. The decision of which implant solution to use is influenced by a variety of factors. Unlike in the past, there is now a wide range of systems available on the market, with hundreds of variations. However, only about twenty major systems dominate the landscape.

The quality of an implant is determined by several factors, including the quality of the titanium used, the treatment of its surface that interfaces with the bone, and the area where soft tissues form around it. The enhancement of the surface on the endosseous part of the implant began with plasma treatment, which improves the healing surface. Current technological surface treatments include acid etching, sandblasting, and more recently, laser technology.

Different implant systems have distinct features and unique surfaces that optimize osseointegration. Osseointegration, as defined by Branemark, is based on microscopic research and refers to the structural and functional connection between living bone tissue and the implant surface that is mechanically loaded with masticatory forces.

Some implant systems are coated with hydroxyapatite. Due to the failed technological connection of the hydroxyapatite and the titanium surface, however, there was a separation of the hydroxyapatite from the metal part of the implant that lies next to the bone. This would be manifested by periimplatitis, the swelling of unhealthy granulation tissue, and eventually the loss of the implant.

Forms of overcome implant systems

In the development period, according to their purpose and surgical technique, until recently, implants were divided into suprabony (subperiosteal), intrabony (endosseus), transdental and submucosal.

The development of implantology has made the application of subperiosteal, transcendental, and submucosal (intramucosal) implants a thing of the past in surgical implantology.

Describing the details of some forms that are completely out of practical application, such as: "ramus frame" implant, which extends bilaterally from the ascending region of the ramus in the lower jaw to the region of the symphysis as one-piece, then pterygoid and zygomatic implants, do not deserve the attention of describing the details, because they are out of everyday practical application and belong to the history of oral implantology.

The black points of subperiosteal implants were, in addition to a very aggressive surgical technique, numerous complications, primarily on soft tissues (inflammation, accompanied by swelling and pain, especially when chewing), which is why, after a short stay in the mouth, they had to be removed.

And many endosseous implants, which stood the test of time and lasted for several years, even decades, also belong to the historical past. This primarily refers to leafy forms. This type of implant was created in several forms, which confused clinicians as to when and which form should be applied. The quality of leaf implants was not uniform, depending on the manufacturer. Experienced implantologists, who used multiple implant systems depending on the case, knew when to apply which system.

Podiatry in the application of implants is not desirable, and it followed that time. Everything the market offered was accepted, which resulted in failure more often than success. The choice for a certain implant system was determined by the success of certain forms, the dexterity and experience of the practitioner.

There are other ideas. Attempts are being made again with the application of implant forms that were launched thirty or more years ago, such as the so-called "disk" implant (Figures 4.69 and 4.70).

At the beginning of 1980, Mark Julie (Paris) launched a "disc" implant, which did not find wider application in practice due to:

a) aggressive surgical implantation techniques;
b) non-physiological action on the bone itself and uneven reception and distribution of chewing forces;
c) bad technological solution;
d) at the site of the extracted implant, there was a large loss of bone, and compensation with any bone substitute resulted in failure and complications, and it was usually not possible to compensate for such bone destruction with augmentation.

A distinct disadvantage of the "disk" implants of the time was that it was not cast from one piece, but a long arm with a thread for the abutment was soldered to the implant foot that rests in the bone. The black dot was also the place of soldering, and the long arm easily broke and separated from the implant foot, probably due to the unfavorable shear moments of forces during chewing. The condition of the soft tissues with the "disk" implant was not thought about at all.

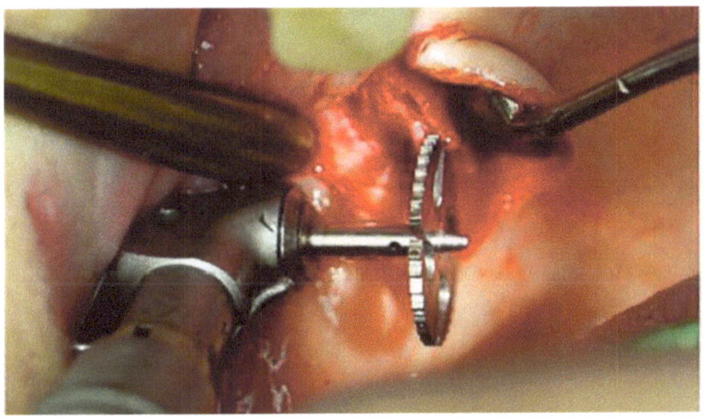

Figure 4.69. Aggressive preparation of the tray for the installation of "disk" implants. Danger of serious injuries to the surrounding tissues.

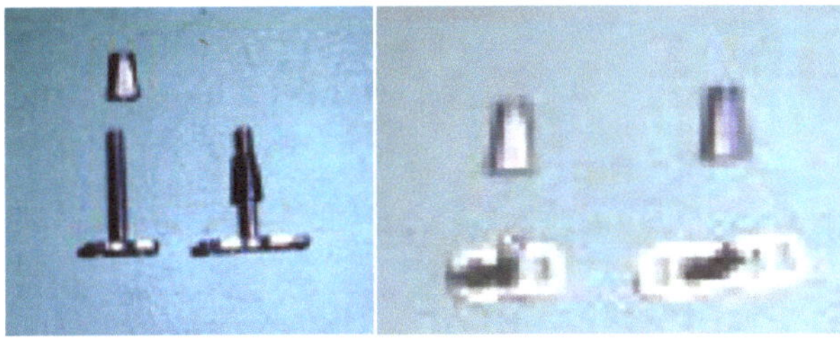

Figure 4.70. Overcome disc implant Appearance of the "disc" implant rate (Mark Julie Paris, 1980).

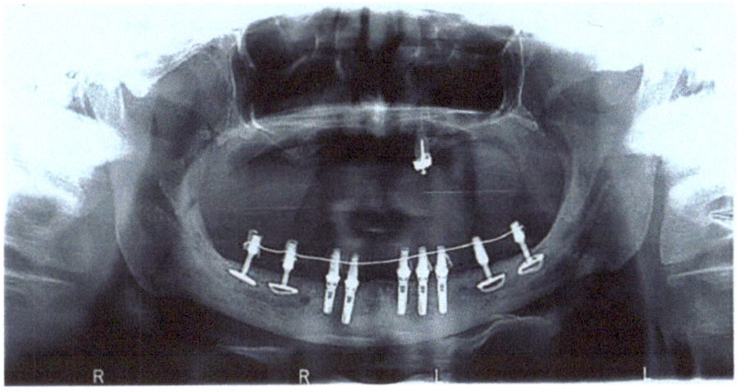

Figure 4.71. "Disc" implants have two main disadvantages: aggressive implantation (see pictures 4.69 and 4.72, marked by red arrows) and the risk of fracturing the long arm of the support for the prosthetic work (refer to picture 4.70). This fracture occurs when the support separates from the plate base of the endosseous portion of the "disk" implant, which is typically connected by soldering. The extraction of this component can lead to patient mobility issues and destruction of the surrounding bone.

Additionally, extreme bone atrophy in the upper jaw is evident in attempts to stabilize a total acrylic prosthesis using a retention clip on the residual root (indicated by the yellow arrow).

The use of these implants doubled the aggression on both the soft tissues and the bone: the first time, during the installation of the implant in the bone using rough circulatory saws (Fig. 4.71), and the second time it would be repeated with even greater aggression, during the very complicated extraction of the broken off part of the implant.

Thus, this technique, due to the aforementioned shortcomings, was abandoned as having been overcome. However, Dr. Ihde has recently launched a supposedly "improved" version, named the "basal disc implant", also calling it "plate". Unlike earlier "disk" implants, which had a single base plate, these "basal implants" consist of multiple base plates that are connected to the vertical part of the implant (shaft) with external threads to which the abutment is attached.

Ihde's "basal implants" are installed similarly to earlier models, being inserted aggressively from the outside of the jaw and anchored directly through the bone and its cortical layer (see Figure 4.72). The creator of these implants, Dr. Ihde, emphasizes that basal implants primarily transmit load through the cortical parts of the bone initially, and it is not necessary for the vertical components to integrate with the bone. Ihde has developed 24 variations of the basal plate, which bear a resemblance to the colorful design of the "Fifth Generation of Linkov Implants."

Despite these "improvements," which are intended for use in cases of very low alveolar ridge height, this implant retains all the characteristics of Marc Juli's long-abandoned "disc" implant, which has since been surpassed. The creation of these 24 implant designs appears to stem more from a profit motive rather than a scientific need.

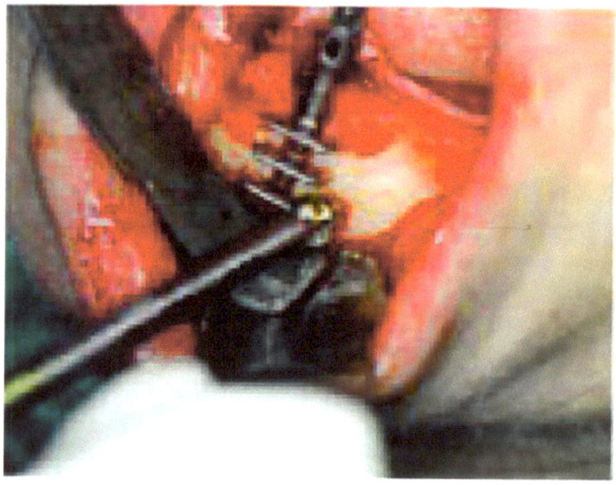

Figure 4.72. Installation of Ihde's "disk" implant - modified Mark Julius implant.

From today's perspective on the development of implantology, the idea that a specific type of implant (such as the BAC-type) can be partially used as a subperiosteal implant is unacceptable. This represents a regression in the field, not just one step backward.

Ihde's concept of "basal" and "disk" implants is based on the belief that the invasive technique of bone transplantation should never be employed to position the implant correctly for prosthetic purposes, as the outcomes are often unpredictable and unreliable.

While Ihde's stance on using bone substitutes for augmentation may have some merit, it is important to evaluate each case individually. Furthermore, literature indicates significant complications associated with such procedures, as noted by Fouad Khoury in "Augmentative Verfahren in der Implantologie," published by Quintessenz Verlag, Berlin, in 2009.

The initiative by Swiss Ihde to return to the long-abandoned implant system is particularly relevant in cases where there are anatomical disadvantages in the lower jaw due to insufficient height of the alveolar ridge.

Based on personal experience and literature data regarding the application of "disk" implants, the following points can be noted:

a) The use of rough and hazardous circular saws (see Fig. 4.71), which were previously employed for installing leaf implants, represents a step backwards.
b) There is no precise guide for the rough and dangerous circular saw used to cut bone. Engraving becomes complicated and imprecise with this implant, especially when it features multiple basal plates.
c) The variety of shapes (25) mirrors the so-called "Fifth Generation Leaf Implants," which previously confused implantologists regarding which form should be applied.
d) the indication that one of these forms of implants (BACtip) Ihdea can partly be used as a subperiosteal implant confirms the view that this is a long-overdue thinking.
e) in the case of complications and loss of such implant forms, the loss of bone is such that reconstruction with bone substitutes is unsuccessful and almost impossible.
f) the author's experience is that it is more justified to install a leaf implant, if the "new" implant systems already go back to the past, because, at least, the aggression during implant installation is much less.

The most important things to know before starting the implant installation

Implant placement requires training. In many countries, there have long been several courses organized by implant companies, dental associations, and individual practitioners who have licenses from their chambers.

Despite the progress of implantology on a scientific basis, some dentists still misinform patients when it comes to implantology. However, misinforming the patient is an ethical violation. Recently, a case like this happened: a colleague in Switzerland lost a court case with a patient who sued him in court. Even though her prosthetic work (combination of fixed and mobile) was done extremely correctly, before starting the work, the aforementioned colleague had to explain and present to her that her case could also be solved with the implant installation method, although he does not deal with implant installation. The court concluded that he was obliged to point out this possibility to the patient.

The patient's request for an implant restoration requires an exhaustive and detailed analysis of the situation.

In many cases, patients may not be suitable for implant treatment, making conventional solutions a better option. This determination is made after a thorough analysis that includes X-rays, a review of the medical history, detailed anamnesis, objective findings in the mouth, and laboratory blood tests (such as prothrombin time and bleeding time). It's essential to identify any underlying conditions like osteoporosis, osteomalacia, or diabetes. Additionally, we must assess oral hygiene, the condition of remaining teeth, periodontal health, as well as the patient's overall general and psychological well-being. Finally, the patient's preferences and financial capabilities are also important factors to consider.

Initial consultation

During the initial consultation, it is very important to determine the patient's primary motive for installing the implant. It used to be based on the basic rule that aesthetics in itself is not an indication, but primarily the establishment of the chewing function. However, with the development of implantology, these concepts have been completely changed. It should be studied in detail whether the aesthetic requirements can first be satisfied with a conventional bridge. If the proposed solution derives from the functional need and satisfaction of the patient's need, and the function is nevertheless a key requirement that must occupy the attention of the doctor. That's the right approach.

Psychological factors require our careful consideration. Patients seeking implants often have various and intriguing motivations, which can be social and psychological in nature. Many expect a boost in self-confidence, enhanced attractiveness, and a way to overcome shyness. However, some patients may have unrealistic demands and expectations, which necessitates caution on the part of the implantologist.

Particular care should be taken with women experiencing menopause, as they may be hoping to regain their youthful facial appearance and smile—something that is often unattainable. It can be challenging for these patients to achieve their wishes and expectations, and this may sometimes lead to unpleasant legal disputes.

For these reasons, many reputable implantologists require patients to read a specific information form thoroughly at home before signing an agreement.

Contraindications must be well known when installing implants, to which a separate chapter of this book is dedicated.

It is of the utmost importance that the patient gains trust in the doctor before the implant procedure, which certainly makes the surgical procedure easier.

Clinical examination

The clinical examination involves a thorough inspection of the oral cavity. After conducting a detailed medical history, a functional examination should be performed using an articulator to analyze the interjaw relations. This analysis is crucial for effective planning and achieving a successful outcome. Pre-surgical analysis on the models in the articulator is extremely important, as having sufficient available bone is not always the deciding factor for the placement of an implant and its positioning. For this reason, dedicated sections will address this topic. As Winston Churchill once said, "He who does not know how to plan, plans to fail."

Following this, a routine examination of hard and soft tissues should be conducted. Notably, high mobility of soft tissue serves as an absolute contraindication for implant placement. The condition of the alveolar ridges must be examined closely, as an atrophied or excessively sharp alveolar ridge may render it unsuitable for implantation.

The intraoral examination should check the state of the periodontium of the remaining teeth, the presence of caries on them, and the quality of oral hygiene. All these procedures are followed by high-quality digital orthopan X-ray and tomographic analysis.

Recently, radiographic technology has advanced so much that the classic orthopantomographic image can be said to have already been surpassed in comparison with three-dimensional images.

The latest three-dimensional imaging technology is additionally enriched with photographs of the condition found with the same device. This is extremely important for both the patient and the doctor, so that after the implantology treatment, one can see where it started (Figure 4.73). This detail is significant in potential court cases.

With modern technology, anatomical structures can be displayed, which allows good planning and simulation of implant position (Figures 4.73 and 4.75). The presentation of the face profile also refers to the state of interjaw relations, i.e. the vertical dimension (Figure 4.74).

Before implant installation, it is essential to rehabilitate the gums and any decayed teeth, remove remaining roots, clear dental calculus from surrounding teeth, and conduct orthodontic movements if necessary.

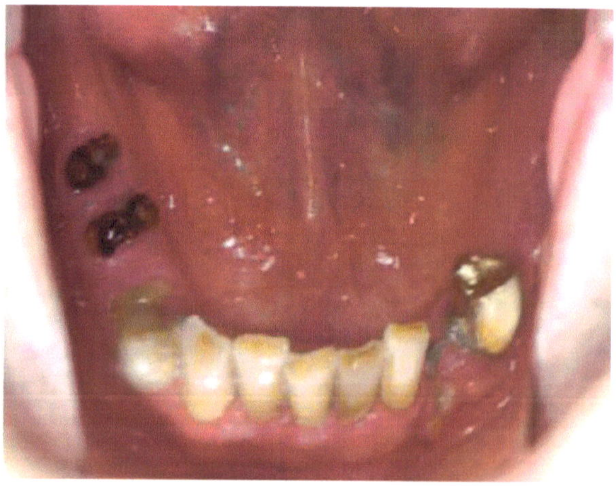

Figure 4.73. With the new technology, the same device, a photographic overview of the found condition of the oral cavity is obtained.

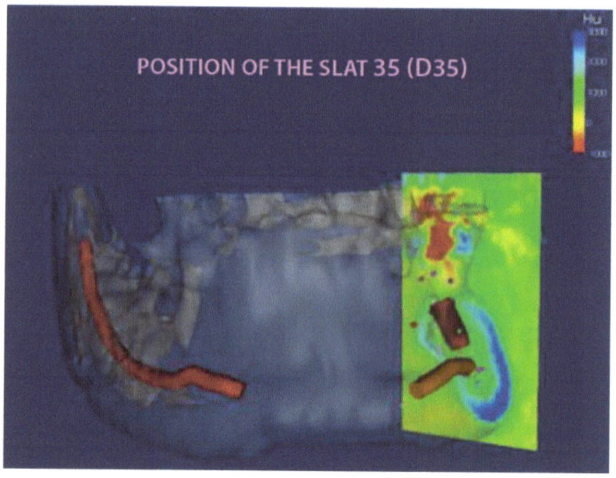

Figure 4.74. The same technology allows simulating the position of the implant, which makes implant placement safe.

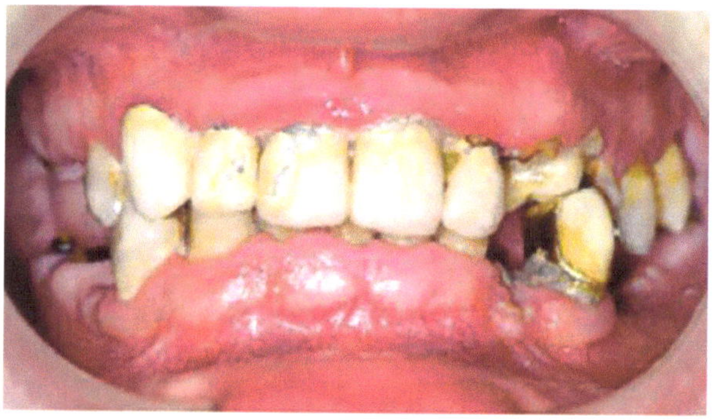

Figure 4.75. An intraoral finding made with a device that simultaneously provides computed tomography data of targeted bone sections and photographic data of the intraoral condition of the oral cavity. (see chapter 12).

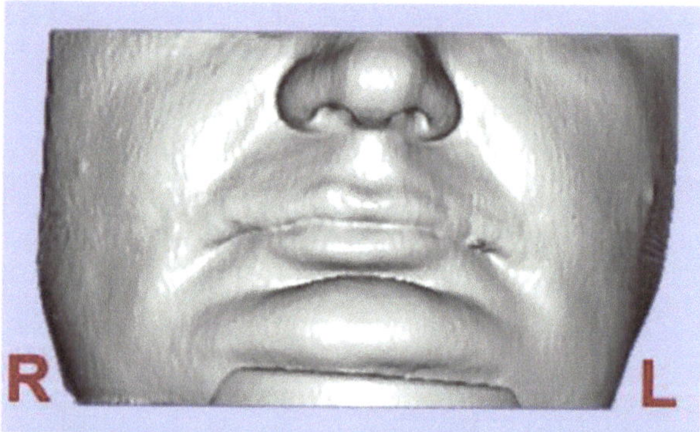

Figure 4.76. In addition to the three-dimensional display of anatomical structures, the computer device also provides profile photos of the patient's face, i.e. the vertical relationship of the upper and lower jaw.

5

Developmental Path Of Oral Implantology

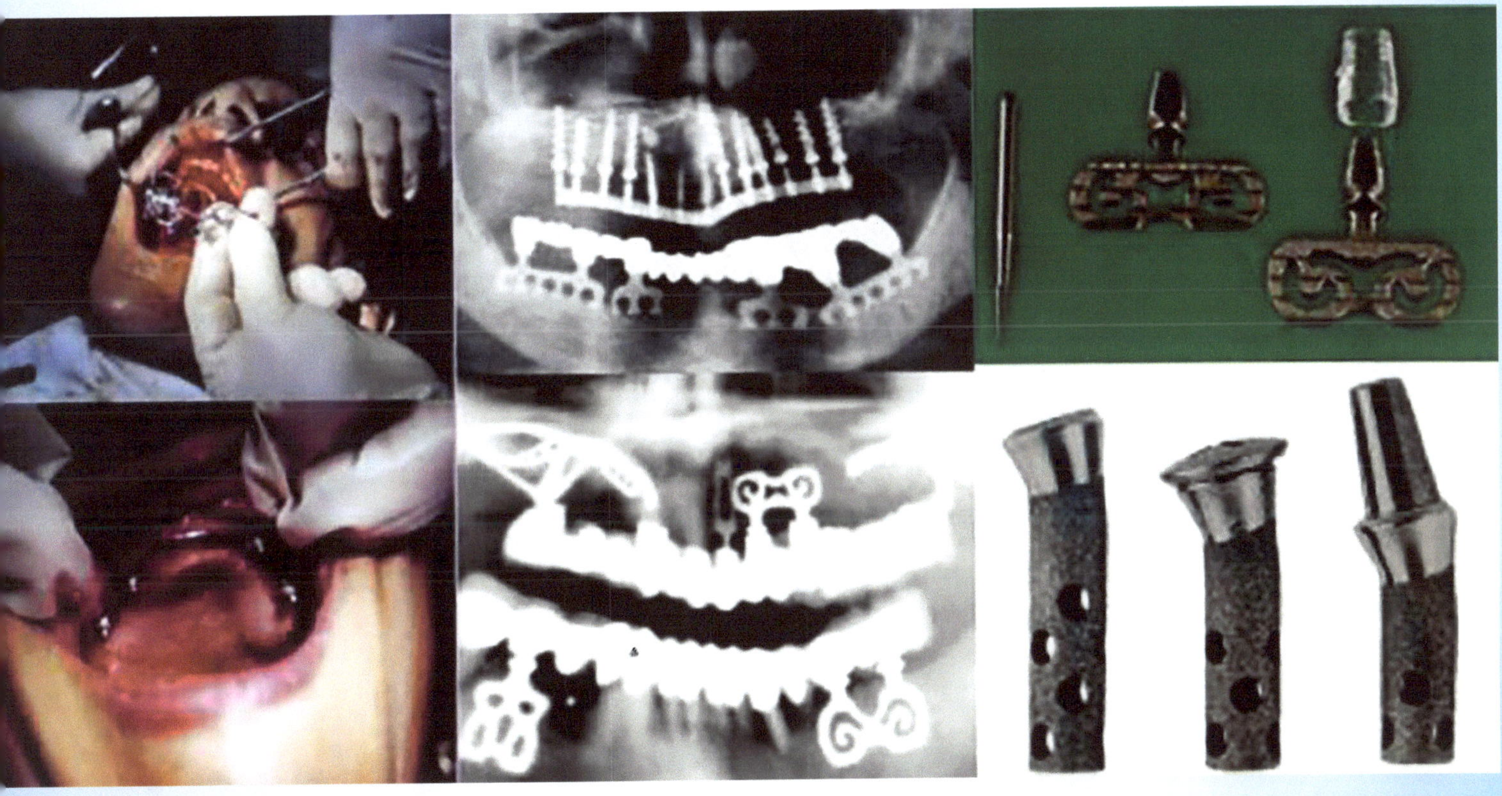

The development of oral implantology is ongoing and far from complete. Today, the forefront of this field is found in some of the largest and most prestigious universities and research institutions that have established oral implantology as a scientific discipline. The field continues to grow, and as new experiences and innovations emerge, the success rates are becoming increasingly reliable. In modern dentistry, oral implantology has become an essential component.

The fast development of oral implantology is best illustrated by the following example. Among the first serious books on oral implantology, printed at the beginning of the eighties of the last century are: "Implantationen im Kieferbereich - Indikazionen und Techniken" supplemented with an atlas for practice, by Charles A. Babbusch, published in Munich, and the other; "Les implants dentaires - Bases fondamentales", Techniques chirurgicalesi Aplicationen cliniques by Marc Burt, published in Paris in 1987. Today, these books (with over 300 pages) represent the past in everything, and everything written in those books is no longer applicable in practice. This conclusion was recently confirmed by Mark Burt himself, who wrote a new book with the same title, in which there is not a single sentence, not a single representation from the previous edition.

Despite the rapid development of oral implantology, much remains undefined, and many positions are not entirely clear and defined. We are witnessing too long wandering in the design of implants. The biggest difficulty of the long-contested enthusiasts, who endured the burden of resisting oral implantology for a long time, was the fact that, at that time, implantology practice was not encouraged by science. Anything and everything that was offered and available on the market was implanted (forms of implants from subperiosteal to endosseous, made of various materials).

The materials from which they were built also wandered: tantalum, titanium, vitalium, various alloys, such as chrome-cobalt-nickel and ceramics were used. All of that was not aligned with biological and natural laws.

The design of the implants was not by nature and did not come close to the design of the natural root. The development of science confirmed this inevitable demand, which was realized by modern oral implantology, bringing the shape of the implant closer to the shape of the root of a natural tooth.

In the future development of oral implantology, in terms of design, not much will need to be added or changed. The ratio of the bone to the surface of the implant, thanks to new technologies, the implantation success rate is 98%. The search for the most optimal conditions for the relationship between implants and soft tissues is still ongoing. For the above reasons, the division of implants used in practice today is not the same as before.

The development of oral implantology significantly changed the previous criteria and made many forms of implants belong to the implantological past.

The criteria by which the implants were classified were: position of the implant in relation to the available bone, purpose and surgical technique. According to the place where the implants were inserted, they are divided into:

- subperiosteal;
- endoseal;
- transdental and
- submucosal.

Subperiosteal implants

The installation of subperiosteal implants is quite a complicated procedure, starting from the surgical technique to the procedure of its manufacture. The implant was placed on the bone itself under the periosteum (Figure 5.1). The indication was exceptional atrophy of the alveolar bone.

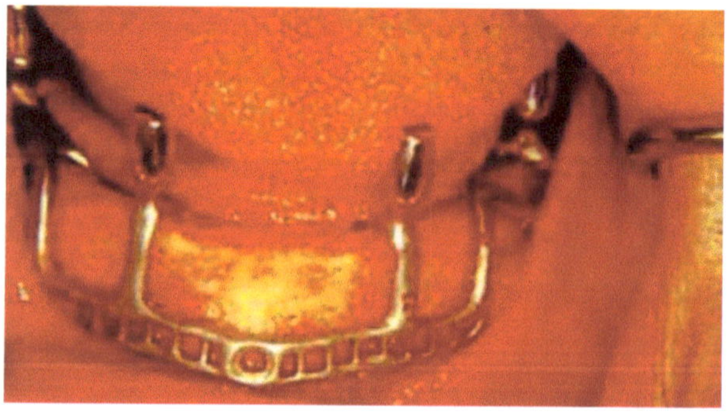

Figure 5.1. Arched subperiosteal implant in the frontal region of the lower jaw. The treatment of similar cases with implant-prosthetic treatment using a modern approach shows the enormous achievements of oral implantology.

After a short time after installation, complications arose in the form of infection, which spread along the implant, affecting soft tissues and bone. Inflammation is accompanied by swelling and pain, especially when chewing. Beneath the implants made of chromium-cobalt-molybdenum alloy, bone destruction occurred due to uneven pressure (Figure 5.2).

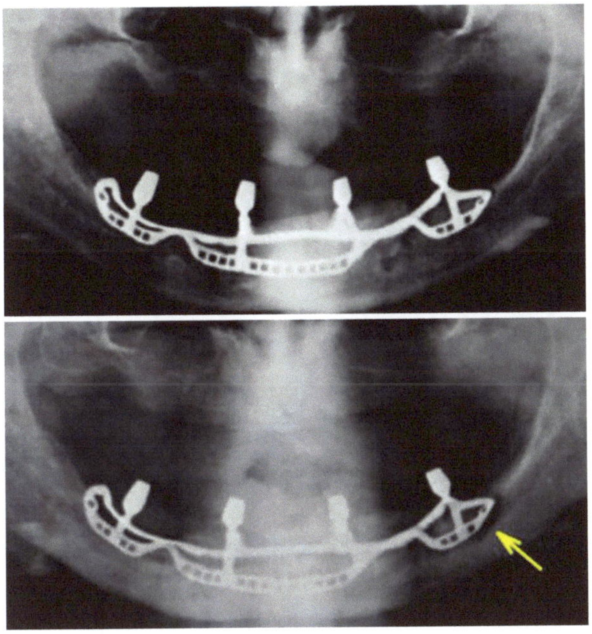

Figure 5.2. Bone destruction caused by uneven fit of the structure (indicated by an arrow).

Already at the beginning of 1937, the first subperiosteal implants were installed by Muller, by inserting under the mucous membrane - a grooved subperiosteal wire mesh with four pins that protruded into the oral cavity, perforating the mucous membrane. Gustav Dahl (G. Dahl) continued to apply these types of implants using alloys of vitalium, chromium, cobalt and molybdenum as material. The Americans Gerschkoff and Goldberg (Gerschkoff & Goldberg) stated that from 1949 - 1957, they made the constructions of these implants from the same alloy, and they justified their failures by the incorrect fit on the bone of the palate, caused by a compressive impression over the closed palatal mucosa.

For this reason, Ogus (1951) opened the palatal mucosa and took a direct impression of the exposed bone. The second procedure - the insertion of the cast implant structure (picture 5.3) had to wait until the wound had completely healed, at least four weeks because the modeling and casting of the metal lasted for several days (pictures 5.4-5.8).

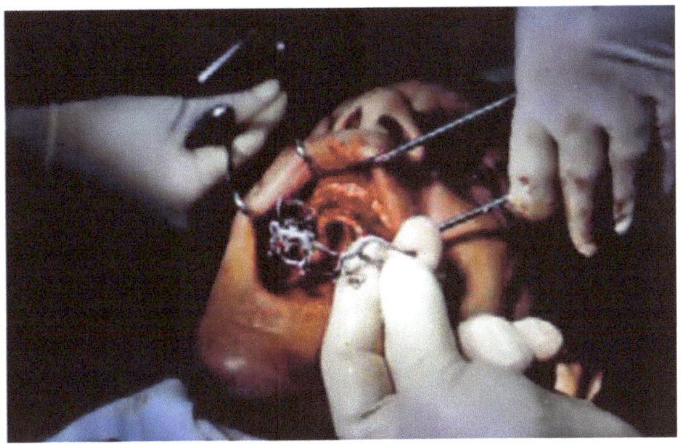

Figure 5.3. The cast construction of the subperiosteal implant is placed by raising the entire palatal flap. From the practice of the author of the book during his education in New York (1983).

The wave of making subperiosteal implants swept Germany and in 1955, Hammer and Reichenbach were the first in Germany to deal with the installation of these types of implants. In the same year, Marciani simplified the entire procedure by using holey tantalum as a working material. The skeleton is made of tantalum by forging, and it was returned to the mouth in a one-time procedure. It only took two hours to make the tantalum skeleton. This method was extremely inaccurate.

In 1955, Germany experienced a surge in the use of subperiosteal implants, with Hammer and Reichenbach being the first to perform these procedures in the country. That same year, Marciani streamlined the process by utilizing holey tantalum as the material for the implants. The tantalum skeleton was created through forging and could be inserted into the mouth in a single procedure, taking only two hours to complete. However, this method had significant inaccuracies.

From 1958 to 1962, Schwindling improved the procedure, because he needed only 6-7 hours for the implant skeleton, using the chrome-cobalt-molybdenum alloy casting method, which significantly improved the accuracy of the anatomical relief of the surface of the palatine bone. This encouraged other authors to devote themselves to subperiosteal implants with great enthusiasm. Mostly they were German names: (Schmutziger, Obwegezer (1958), Kole (1963), Wunderer (1964).

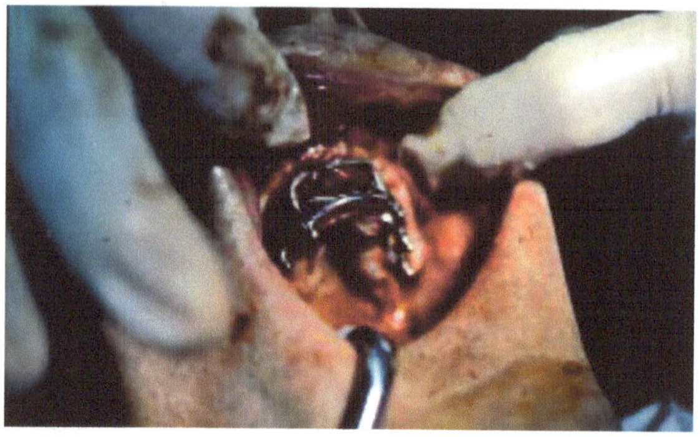

Figure 5.4. Placed subperiosteal implant.

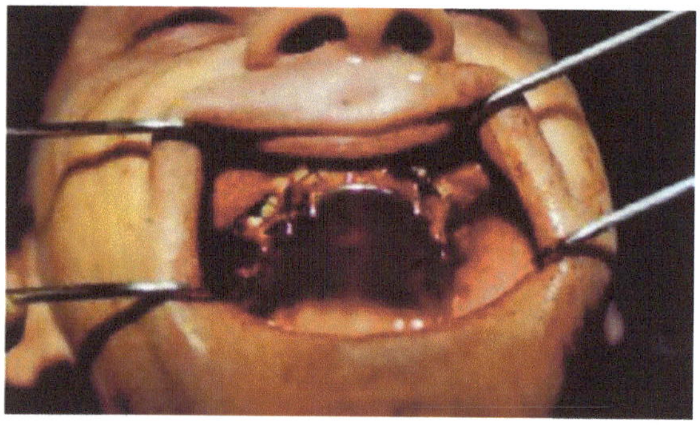

Figure 5.5. Appearance of the subperiosteal implant in the final stage.

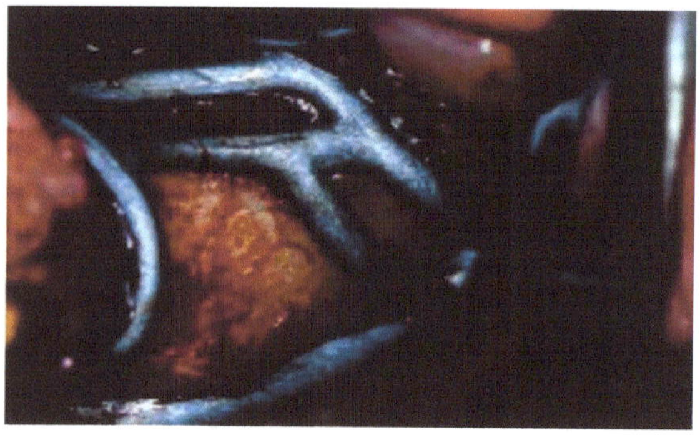

Figure 5.6. Appearance of the part of the implant that lies above the periosteum.

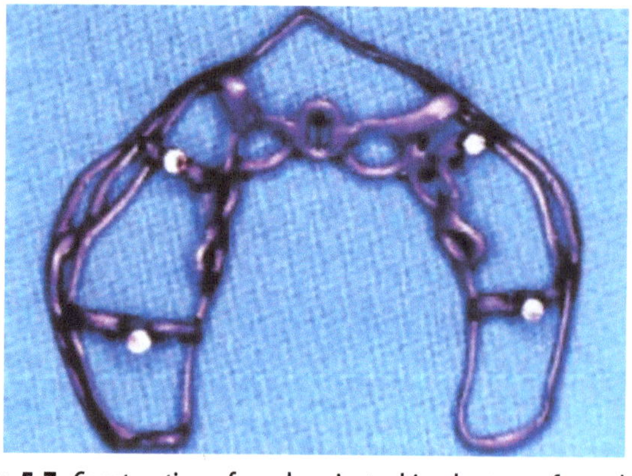

Figure 5.7. Construction of a subperiosteal implant cast from chromium-cobalt-molybdenum alloy.

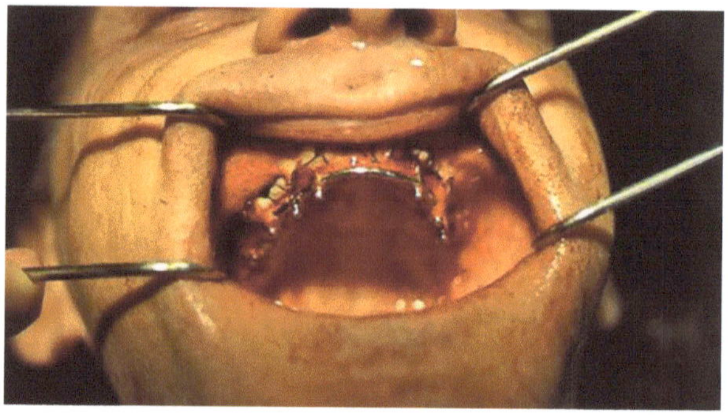

Figure 5.8. Installation of subperiosteal implants is an extremely complicated and traumatic procedure: raising the flap of the alveolar ridge and palatum (fig. 5.1) to take an impression for a metal construction in chrome-cobalt molybdenum alloy (fig. 5.7).

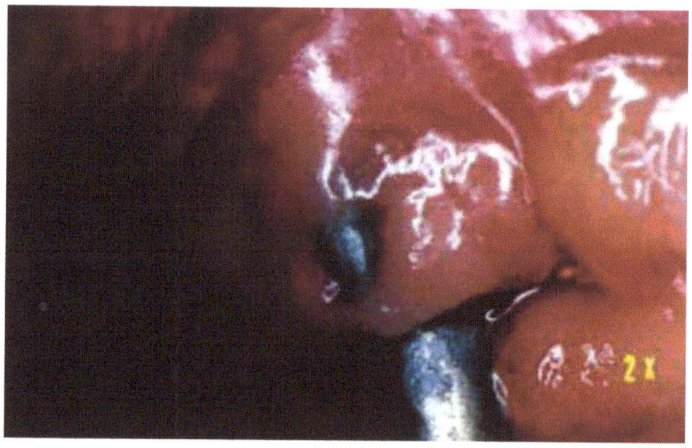

Figure 5.9. Dehiscence of part of the implant through the soft tissues followed by an inflammatory process.

In those years, A. Tavčar and A. Tašković installed several subperiosteal implants at the Academy of Medical Sciences in Belgrade. That attempt of theirs ended after a short time in failure and with numerous complications (Figure 5.9).

Large failures continue with the combination of superiostal implants in the lateral regions connected with endosseous implants or with natural teeth (Figures 5.10 and 5.11).

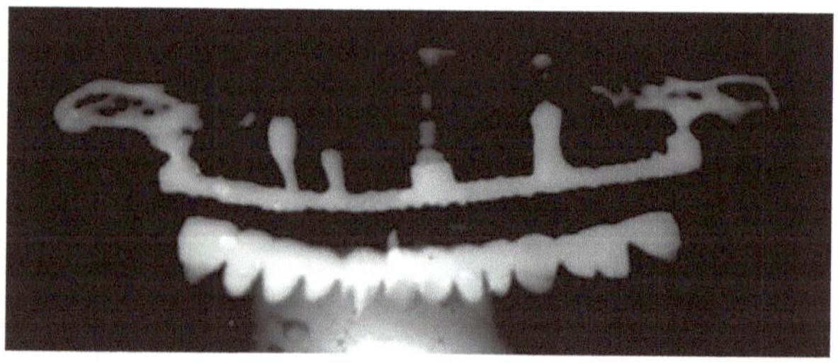

Figure 5.10. Subperiosteal implants in the lateral regions.

When evaluations of the use of subperiosteal implants began to be given based on longer-term observations, it was determined that complications arose in the largest number of patients, so that the success rate dropped to a "modest figure", as stated by Obwegeser, definitely giving up on this method. Only a few authors reported on "functional success", and only one author cited a case of ten-year success.

It's important to note that the main advocates of subperiosteal implants do not have access to accurate and detailed statistics. Although the use of these implants often led to negative outcomes, subperiosteal implantology was primarily utilized in America during the 1980s for a relatively short period. During my time with Professor Leonard Linkow in New York, many cases were successfully addressed using subperiosteal implants. Despite this familiarity, I chose not to continue using them in my practice due to their complex and aggressive soft tissue treatment procedures.

After the initial incision to lift the flap and take the impression, it was necessary to wait at least four weeks before repeating the incision to place the cast structure. This implantation method was frequently followed by complications, ranging from bone decubitus to inflammation of the soft tissues, which could lead to ulcerations. Not long after that period, the era of subperiosteal implants was considered to be over.

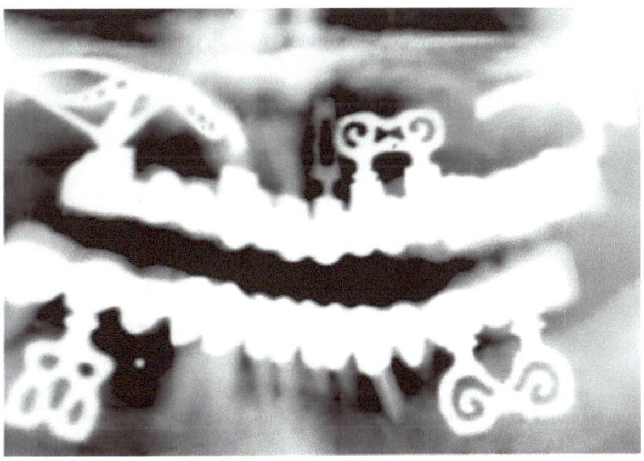

Figure 5.11. A combination of subperiosteal and sheet one-piece implants bonded to natural teeth.

In the sparse literature at the time, no valid statistical data on the success or failure of subperiosteal implants were ever published. At that time, everyone hid their failures. Such a way of "reporting" has followed endosseous implants for a long time.

It is likely that the high failure rate of subperiosteal implants directed thoughts towards the transition to endosseus implantation.

Endosseus implants applied in the past

Intraosseous implant systems are directly implanted into the bone using various surgical techniques. Endosseous implants are classified by their shape into four categories: cylindrical, leaf-shaped, needle-shaped, and screw-shaped implants. Cylindrical implants come in several forms, including threadless (inserted by tapping), threaded, hollow (available in different designs), and solid implants (see Figures 5.12-5.35).

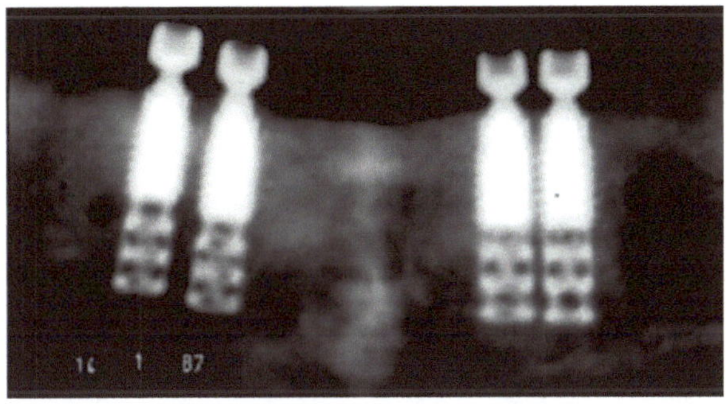

Figure 5.12. Hohlzylinder implant – Typ-F (launched 1974).

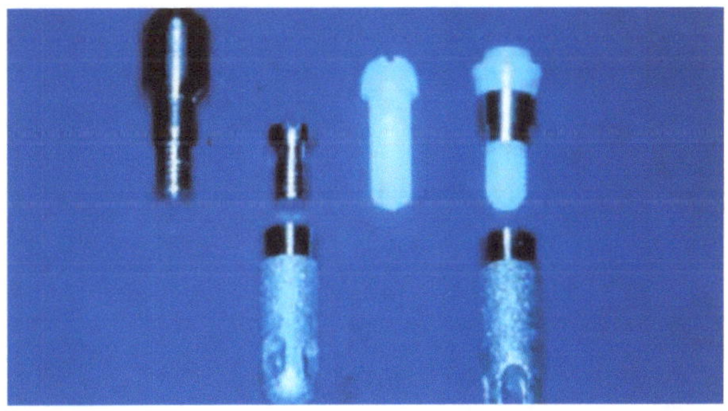

Figure 5.13. A combination of solid and hollow implants.

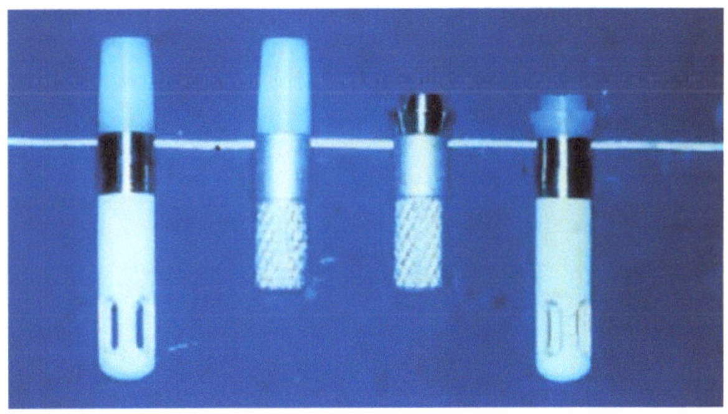

Figure 5.14. Cylindrical implants.

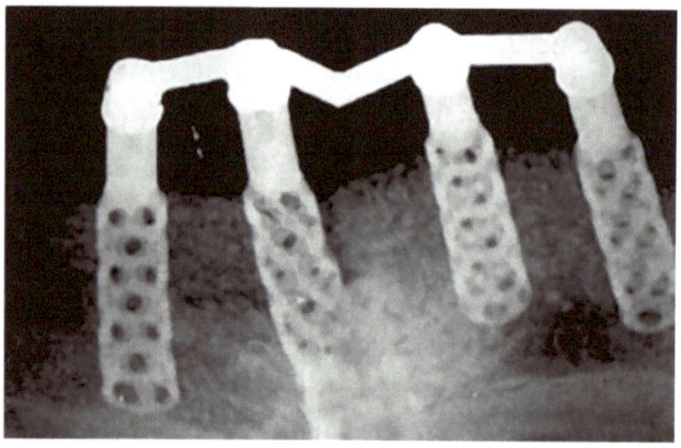

Figure 5.15. Bonding of multiple hollow cylindrical implants.

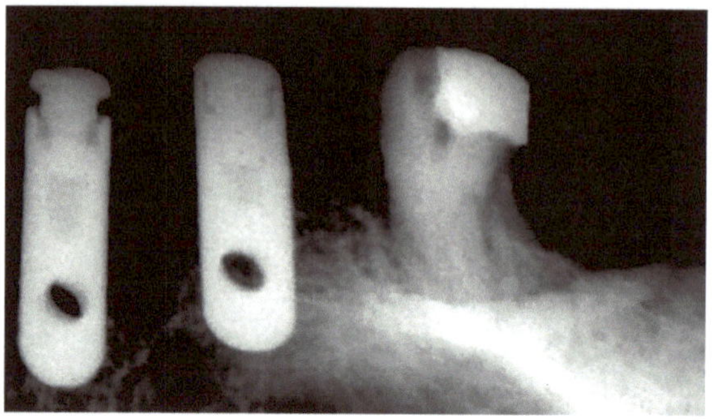

Figure 5.16. A hammered cylindrical implant with a perforation in the basal part for bone growth.

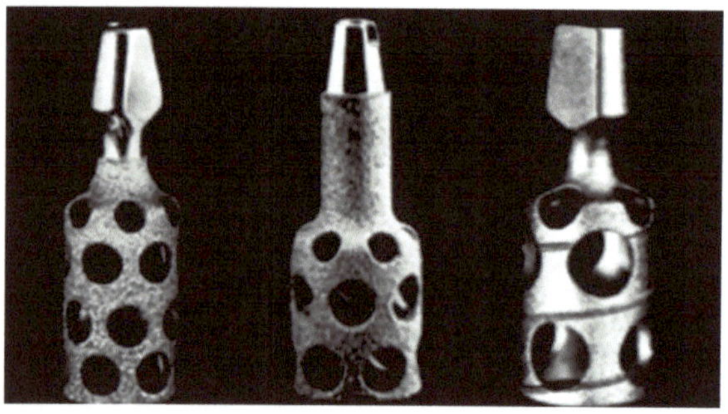

Figure 5.17. In 1974, hollow cylindrical implants (Hohlzylinder) with a fixed support and hollow cylindrical implants with a screw-on support were developed.

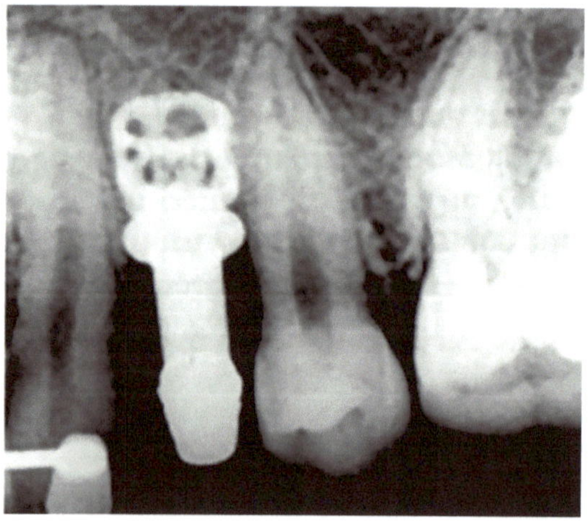

Figure 5.18. Implant shape launched in 1966. Control shot in late 1986.

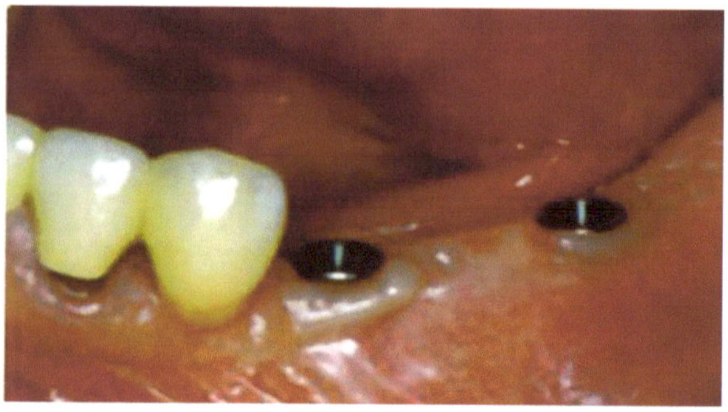

Figure 5.19. Built-in implants Type-F-HS.

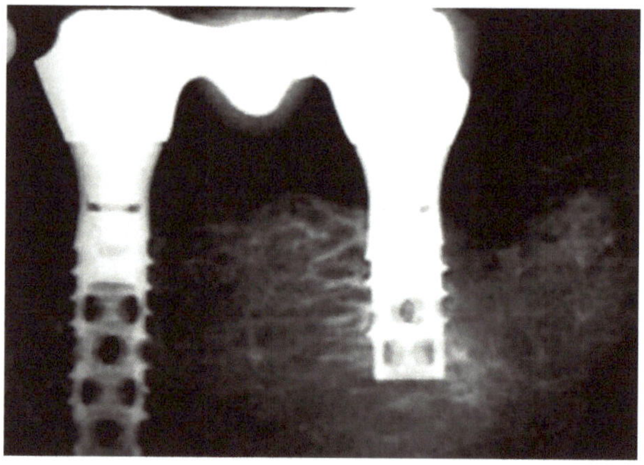

Figure 5.20. X-ray control of F-HS implants.

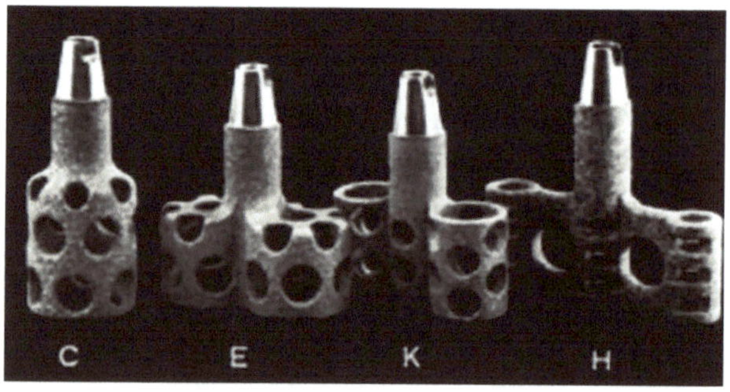

Figure 5.21. Forms of ITI implants (1976) with screw-on abutments, and the surface of the implant is covered with titanium-plasma.

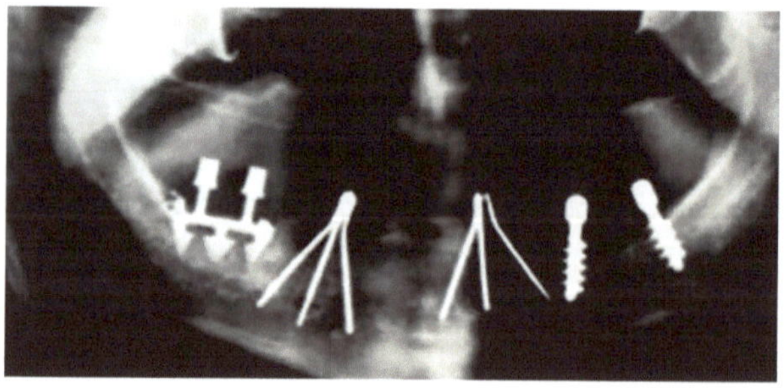

Figure 5.22. Various implant designs. Kombi (Heinrich), needle and screw implants.

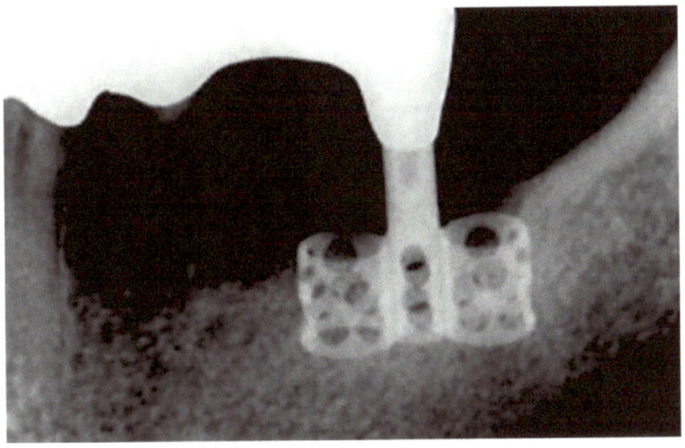

Figure 5.23. ITI implant (1976). X-ray control after one year.

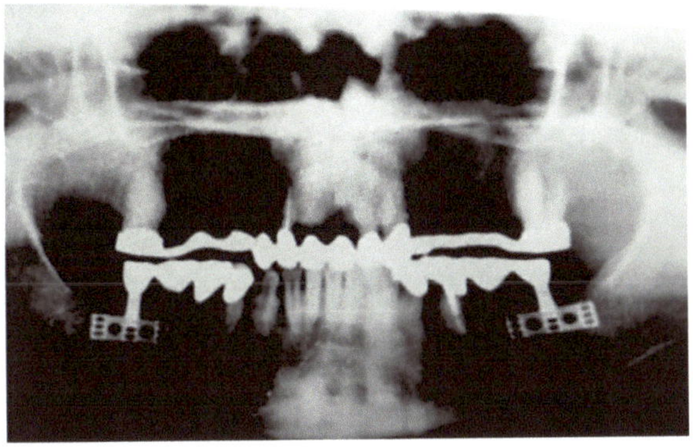

Figure 5.24. Design of Type-H implants

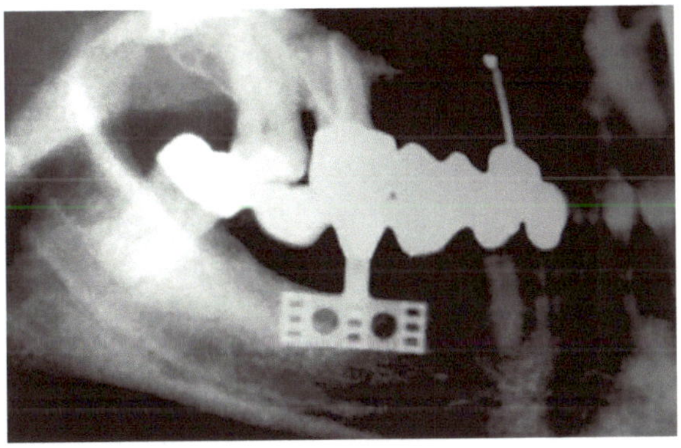

Figure 5.25. Type-H implant as a support for a long-span bridge.

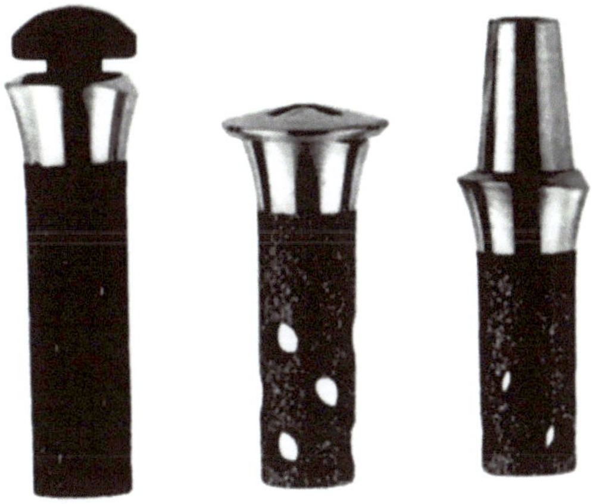

Figure 5.26. Type-F implant: with a cap for gingival formation, a covering cap in the healing phase and an implant with an abutment.

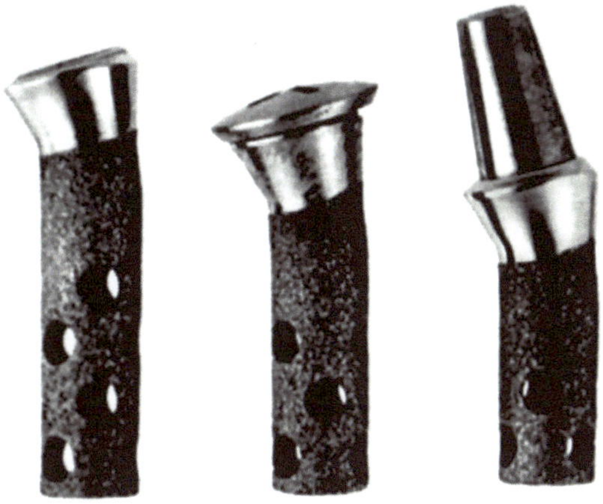

Figure 5.27. Type-F implant design with implant neck slope of five different lengths: 8mm, 10mm, 12mm, 14mm and 16mm.

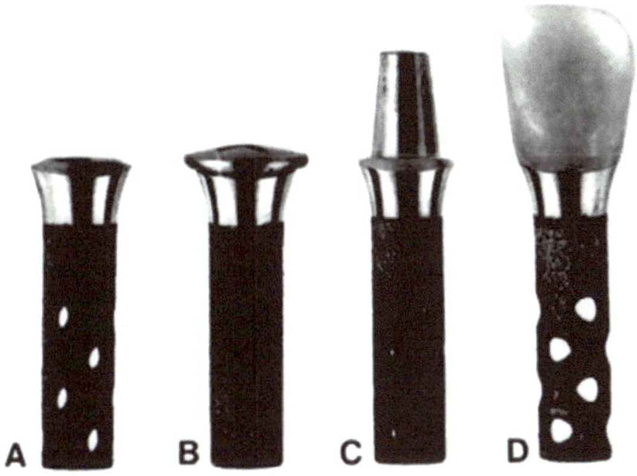

Figure 5.28. Tio-F implants length 8 mm, 10 mm and 12 mm.

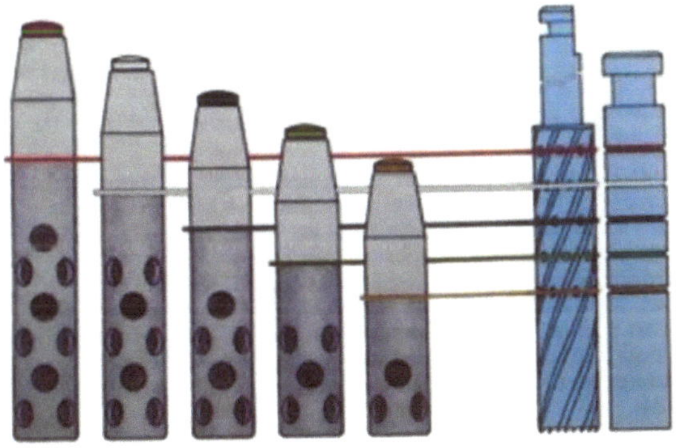

Figure 5.29. Dimensioned drill bits for bone preparation.

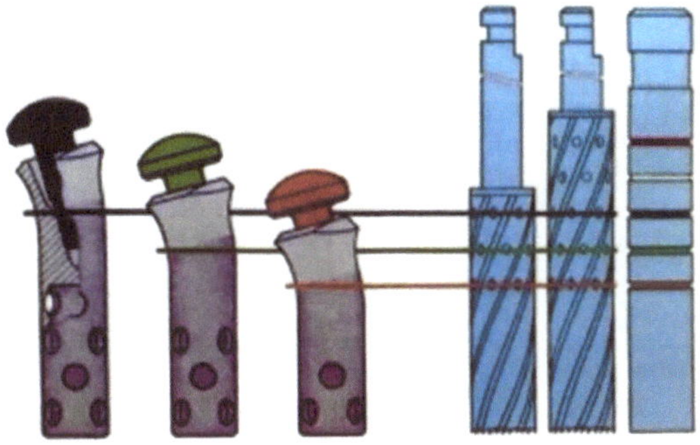

Figure 5.30. Dimensioned drill bits for bone preparation.

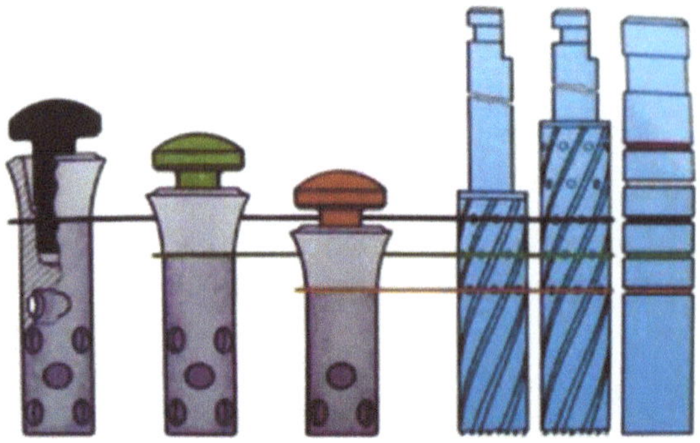

Figure 5.31. Schematic representation of the bone preparation drill and the bone preparation depth gauge.

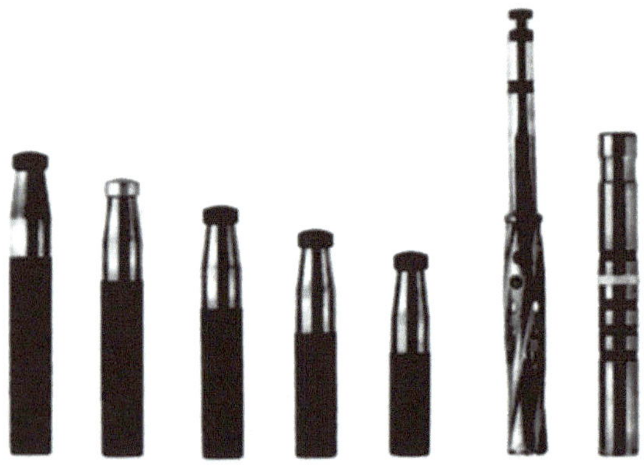

Figure 5.32. Different lengths of the part that lies in the bone.

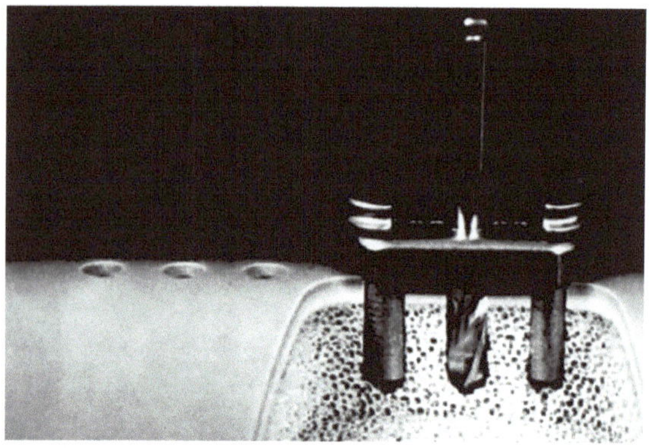

Figure 5.33. Positioning of drills for the preparation of the Holcinder implant bed.

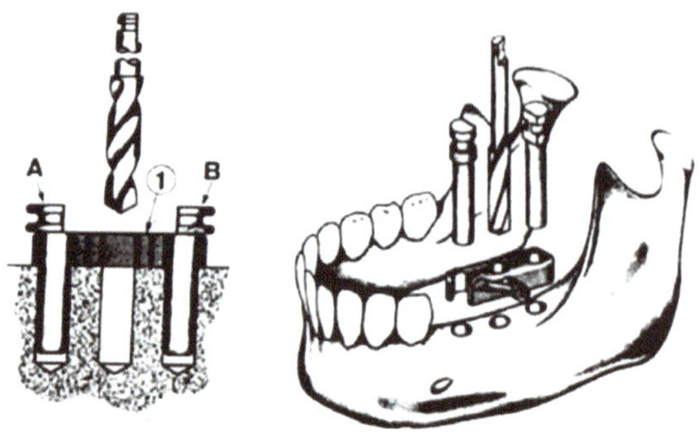

Figure 5.34. Part of the instrumentation for positioning and preparation of the socket for a hollow cylindrical implant.

Most forms of endosseous implants are no longer in use. Implants with screws have been used for the longest time due to the possibility of cutting and self-cutting into the bone. The basic function of implants, it was believed at the time, was to serve as carriers of prosthetic works, and that chewing forces, via the endosseous part, were completely transferred to the alveolar bone. Aesthetics were neglected. Today, according to the construction, one-part and two-part implants are in use, and according to the surgical technique and stages of implantation, these implants are divided into one-phase and two-phase.

One-piece implants have one part that goes into the bone, on which the abutment (carrier) continues, which carries the prosthetic work. One-piece implants are installed using a simplified one-phase surgical technique. The neck of the implant, which is connected to the abutment, in newer generations is covered with "laser-lock" technology. To better adapt the soft tissue, the abutment is placed transmucosal in the mouth above the alveolar ridge. The abutment is made of a much softer material than the endosseous part, which allows easy processing and prevents the transfer of thermal aggression to the bone. Due to reduced diameters, lengths below 12 mm did not exist until recently. Narrow one-piece implants, diameter 3 mm, with the possibility of processing abutments (shortening and establishing parallelism), lengths: 10, 12, 15, and 18 mm. These implants can be immediately loaded and are indicated for narrow alveolar ridges with sufficient height.

Two-phase endosseous implants consist of several parts: the body of the implant, which is embedded in the alveolar bone of the jaw, the healing cap, the part for the formation of soft tissues, the support, the transfer necessary to accurately transfer the position of the implant to the working model in the laboratory, and the analog of the implant. The bracket is made in several shapes, i.e. angles (15, 20, and 25 degrees), with which it is possible to correct the disparity of the implant, and the brackets meet certain aesthetic requirements.

Two-phase (multipart) endosseous implants are recommended in situations where a period of rest lasting several months is necessary, often due to weak primary stability. After the implants are installed, they are covered with a mucoperiosteal flap, and a cap may be placed to shape the gum tissue. The duration of the resting period is determined by the doctor.

Experience often suggests that the mucoperiosteal flap should not be completely covered by the caps to allow for better healing of the implants. This is important because, after the resting period, a second phase of the surgical intervention is required. During this phase, the caps of the implant body are revealed, and adjustments may be needed to properly form the gingival margin.

The length of time the implant remains in the bone before loading, as well as the specific timelines for each case, depend on the clinician's judgment. Thus, the experience and expertise of the dentist play a critical role in making an accurate assessment.

If we refer to the period after implantation as "rest time" instead of "waiting time," we can pose an important and debatable question: "Will the integration process be faster and more effective in a resting phase or a functional phase for the bone?" The most reliable answers to this question come from clinical results and success rates.

Additionally, there is ongoing debate about whether the implant should be covered, if a component for gingival formation should be placed, or if an abutment should be installed immediately after implantation for gingival formation purposes. Based on the author's experience, the best results are achieved when a definitive abutment is used, especially if the implants are loaded early.

It is also advisable to minimize the number of times definitive abutments are placed for several reasons, including the potential for trauma and infection of the soft tissues.

Today, physiological knowledge favors function, because bone in function promotes regeneration, and when it comes to an implant, this implies faster and better apposition of new bone directly on the surface of the implant.

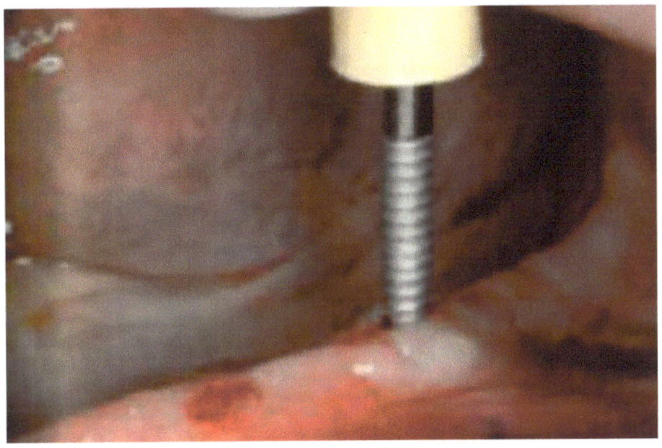

Figure 5.35. Implantation without raising the flap.

Transdental implants

These implants are needle-shaped, they are inserted through the root canal, and the length of the implant is greater than the length of the root, because the implants lie mostly in the bone. The transdental implant extends the root shaft (Figures 5.36 and 5.37). Such a system could rather be called transdental fixation (which was confirmed by G. Pruin in 1974) rather than an implant. Strock and Strosch, in 1943, report on a method by which loosened teeth, with a disturbed clinical crown-to-root length ratio, are refixed endosseusly with the help of an implant, i.e. a vitalium wedge embedded through the root canal in the jawbone. After Hammer (1955), who propagated this idea, it was accepted by Staegeman (1957-58), and continued by Orlay (1960). Pruin gave some metallurgical explanations, using tantalum wedges instead of titanium.

How did the idea of transdental fixation come about?

Proponents of this method considered endosseous implants an "open" issue, arguing that it is impossible to achieve an epithelial grip - an epithelial attachment for a part of the implant located in an open environment such as the oral cavity. By leaving the natural tooth with the root, using transdental implants, that epithelial connection was untouched as a "biological collar" (Frenkel 1973).

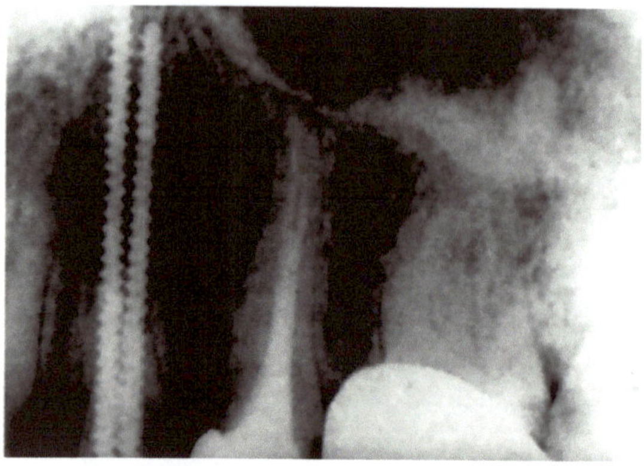

Figure 5.36. Transdental implants on the first premolar.

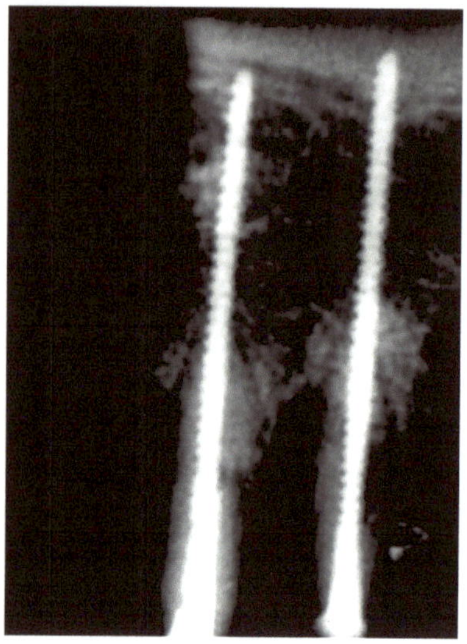

Figure 5.37. Transdental implants with resorbed roots.

Since at that time, indeed, the weak point of all endosseous implants was the impossibility of epithelial attachment with the alloplastic material - the support of the prosthetic superstructure, these thoughts had a basis, to some extent. However, all possible events surrounding the devitalized root, subject to permanent resorption, must be considered (Figure 5.38 and 5.39).

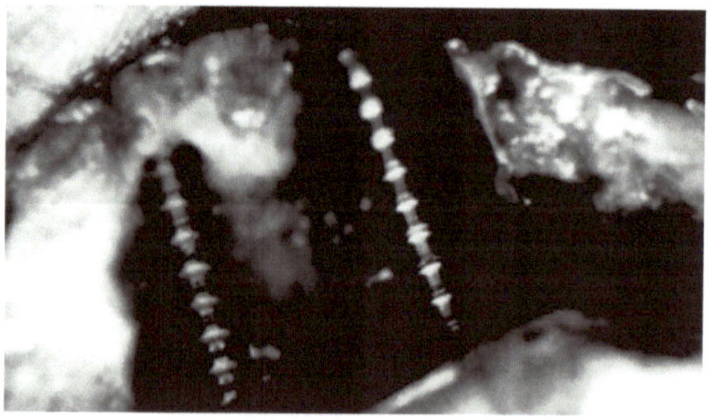

Figure 5.38. Root resorption and bone destruction around transdental implants.

After some time, root resorption occurred (Fig. 5.36 and 5.38), and the site of root resorption was not replaced by good bone. The most common consequence is the destruction of the surrounding bone. (Figures 5.36 and 5.38.) If one can talk about the justification for the use of these implants, then, according to the author of this book, the only justification for their use is in frontal tooth root fractures of children at an age where the growth of the jaw ridges has not been completed implantation is not indicated. The method of transdental fixation thus postpones tooth loss and preserves space for implantation after the age of 18.

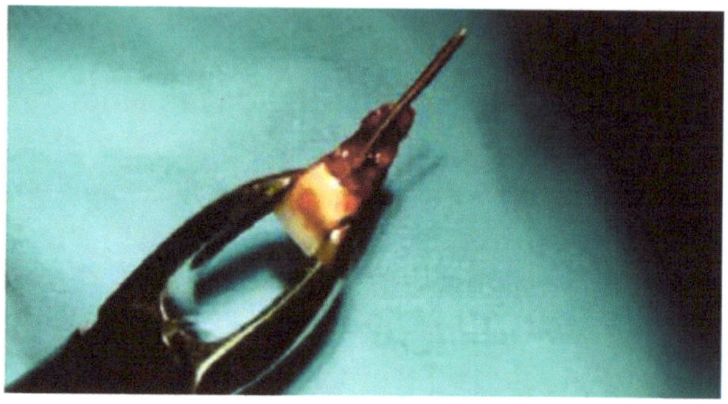

Figure 5.39. Resorbed root with transdental implant. The author of the book has never accepted transdental implant treatment, arguing that it is a total failure.

The development path continues with an attempt to cover the cylindrical implants of the hydroxylapat with titanium. Installation of these implants often resulted in failure because a solid connection between the two materials: metal and hydroxyapatite could not be achieved (Figures 5.40 and 5.41).

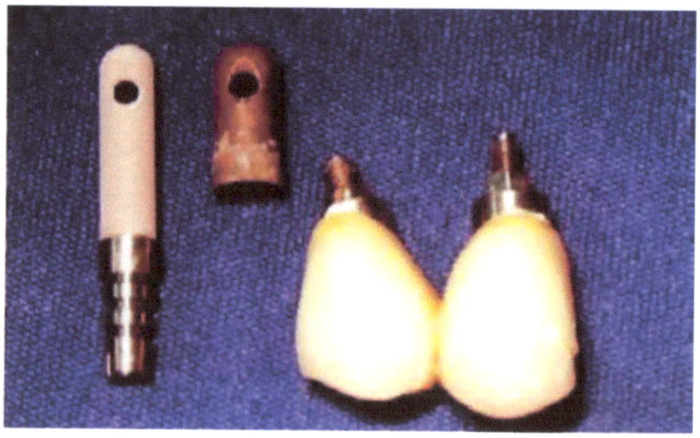

Figure 5.40. Cylindrical implant coated with hydroxyapatite (left) and extracted implant (top right). At the site of decomposed hydroxyapatite, granulation tissue was formed around the implant.

Through ionization in an electrolytic medium, a chemical reaction occurred, resulting in the separation of hydroxyapatite from the smooth titanium surface of the implant. This created a space that led to the formation of granulation tissue. The failed bond between the metallic titanium surface of the implant and the hydroxyapatite particles quickly resulted in peri-implantitis (see picture 5.41 - yellow arrow).

In several cases where I used a combination of "Pitt Eissy" implants on one side and cylindrical implants coated with hydroxyapatite on the other, I observed two different outcomes. In the first case, the "Pitt Eissy" implant showed good stability during the follow-up examination after three years, with minimal marginal bone loss of up to 1 mm. Conversely, on the other side (Figure 5.41 - red arrow), where the hydroxyapatite-coated implant was placed, peri-implantitis developed, accompanied by all the signs of inflammation.

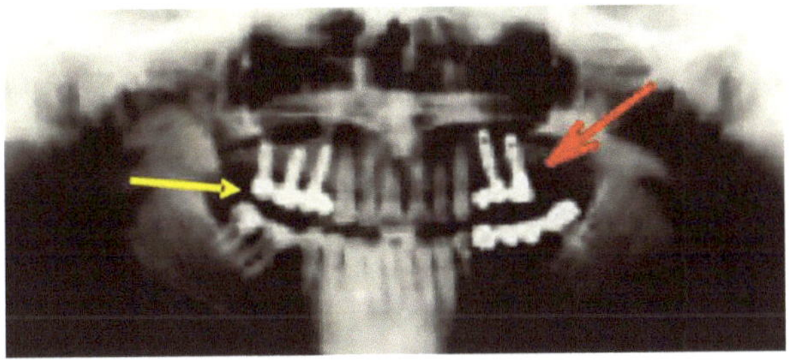

Figure 5.41. On the right, three implants coated with hydroxyapatite (yellow arrow) and on the left a "Pitt eissy" implant (red arrow).

After the symptoms of inflammation subsided, to preserve the prosthetic work, the granulation tissue was radically removed. The bone defect was compensated with a bone substitute (Bio-Oss) and mixed with autogenous bone was covered with a resorbable membrane. During the control examination, by raising the mucosal flap, it was established that the inserted graft was firmly attached to the surface of the implant and treated with a titanium brush. After 15 years, the implant is still functioning well, and all "Pitt Eissy" implants in other patients, after fifteen years, show extraordinary stability.

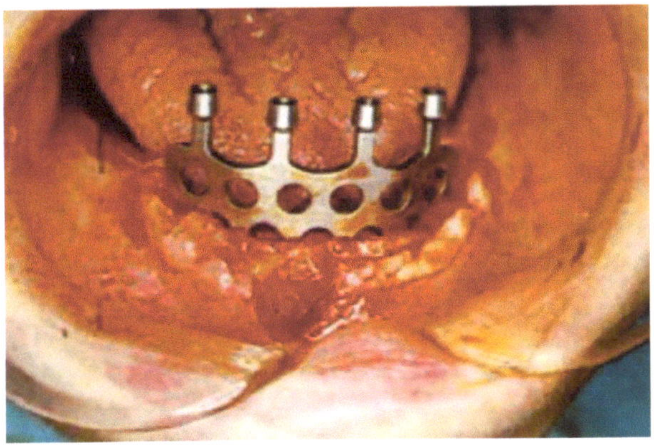

Figure 5.42. Installation of an arched one-piece Linkov implant. Complicated surgical procedure with significant patient morbidity and trauma to the alveolar bone along its entire length.

Of all the endosseous leaf implants, the most complicated, bone-aggressive and imprecise method was the installation of Linkov's leaf arch implant in the front region of the lower jaw (Figures 5.42-5.44).

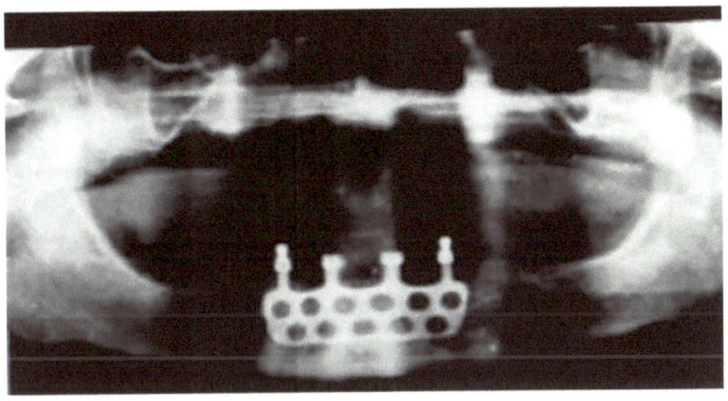

Figure 5.43. X-ray view of the arch implant.

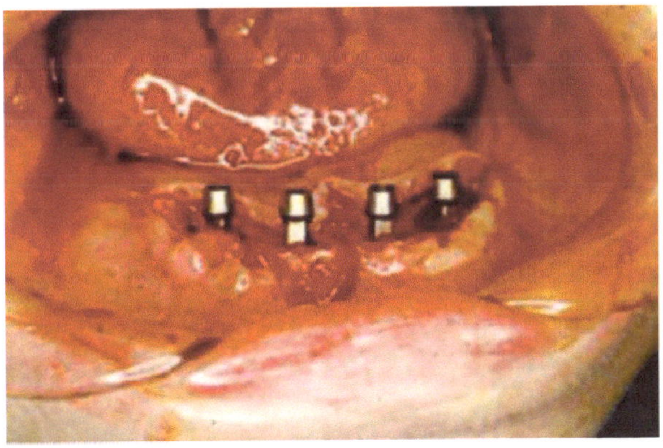

Figure 5.44. Built-in arch implant with supports.

A major disadvantage of this surgical technique was the imprecise execution of the cut with sharp cutters without a guide when forming a suitable implant bed. At one time, this was standard surgical protocol. Based on those implants, a one-piece implant cast in a chromium-cobalt-molybdenum alloy was launched at the VMA in Belgrade for installation in the entire mandible. With certain modifications, these implants were used in traumatology, especially in war injuries of the lower jaw. An absolute failure was the "Kombi implant" launched by Benedict Heinrich, launched in the mid-eighties of the last century (Figures 5.45 and 5.46).

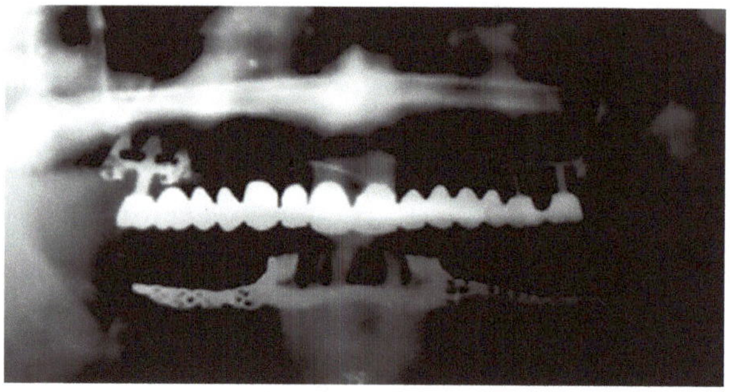

Figure 5.45. Built-in Combi implants with subperiosteal flaps.

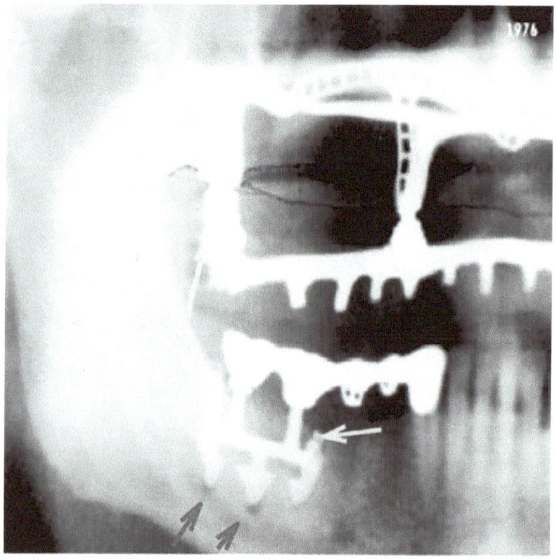

Figure 5.46. Illustration of wings resting on the periosteum (yellow arrow) and bone destruction (red arrow). The work of the author of the book is an excerpt from a lecture by Dr. Zlopaša in Munich, 1976).

The combination of endosseous and subperiosteal implants failed. In this absolute failure, everything is imperfect: from the material (tantalum) to the design. The first indicators of this imperfect implant were manifested in the destruction of the bone under the wing that rested on the periosteum, perforating the mucous membrane in the oral cavity. At the same time, I was staying at the clinic in Bremen with Prof. Heinrich, I suggested to him that the combination of endosseous and subperiosteal implant is problematic and that before installation those wings should be removed, which he accepted (Figure 5.47).

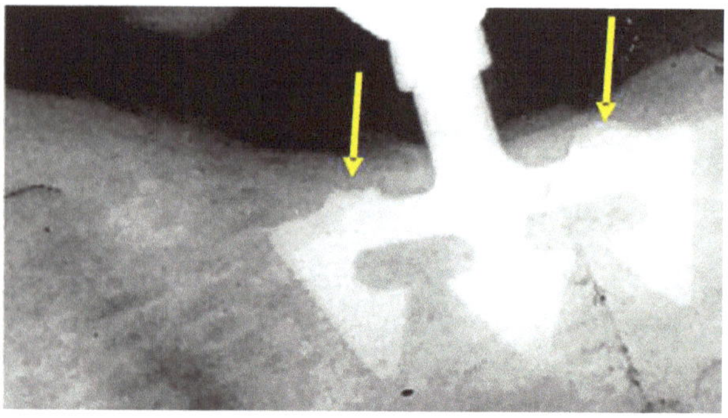

Figure 5.47. Heinrich's "Kombi" implant with reduced subperiosteal flaps that Heinrich (B. Heinrich) "reduced" at the suggestion of the author of the book at the Congress in Munich.

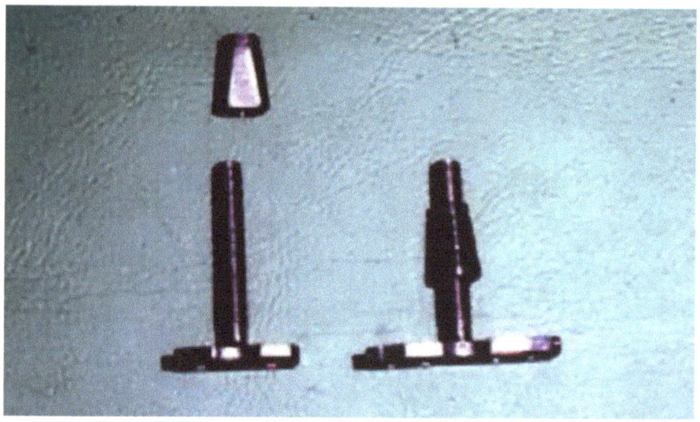

Figure 5.48. Marc-Jouli disc implant

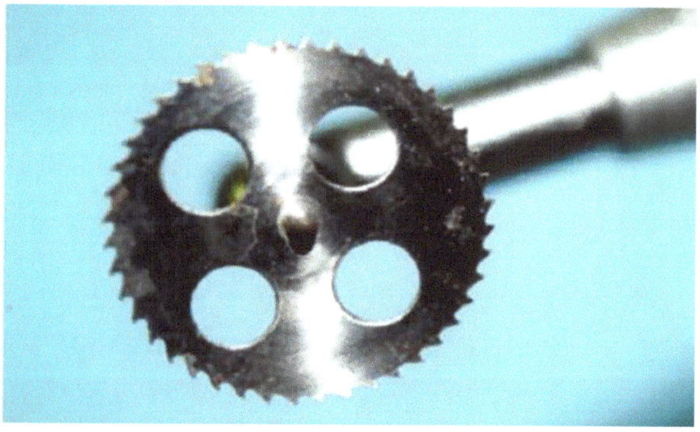

Figure 5.49. The use of circular burs was dangerous due to more severe iatrogenic injuries to the tongue and surrounding soft tissues.

The so-called "disk" implants (Figure 5.48) were not widely accepted in oral implantology due to several disadvantages. Their installation required a complicated and aggressive surgical technique, affecting both the bone and the soft tissues. A significant technological drawback was that these implants were not made from a single piece. Instead, the foot of the implant and the supporting arm for the future prosthetic work were joined by soldering. This design meant that the long arm, to which the abutment was attached, acted as a lever, resulting in stress from shearing forces at the connection point between the arm and the implant foot. This connection was prone to breakage.

Furthermore, the process of part installation was highly complicated and led to substantial bone defects. Once such a defect occurred, it became impossible to insert an endosseous implant at that location. Recently, Dr. Ihde introduced a similar implant, which will be discussed in more detail in the chapter on risks in oral implantology.

Submucosal implants

Submucosal implants involve the placement of alloplastic buttons in the mucous membrane of the palate, creating a perforation similar to a "patrice." The other component, known as the "matrix," is integrated into the acrylic portion of the prosthesis that covers the palate. This configuration forms a type of "dricker" (clip) that serves as a connection between the palate and the acrylic total prosthesis (see Figure 5.50).

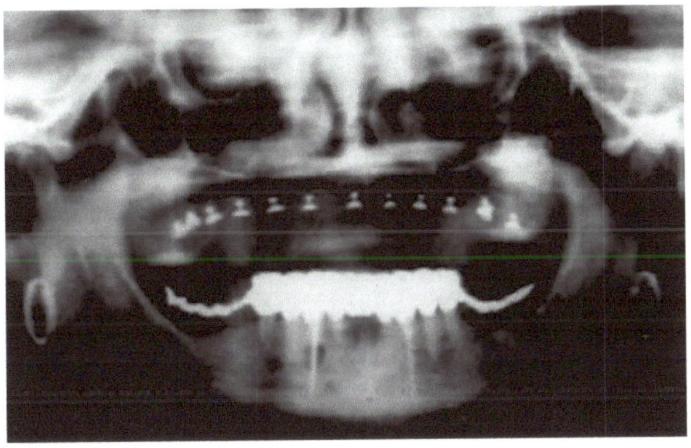

Figure 5.50. X-ray view of submucosal implants.

In 1943, Mr. Dahl was the first to implement this form of implantation for anchoring in cases of total edentulism. Dentists Lew and Kestenbaum published the earliest written works on this type of implant as early as 1953. Professor Giordano Muratori from Bologna perfected and applied this system of submucosal implants in practice. This technique began to spread in Italian dental offices under the name "sucieti submucosi."

Although this method was not considered physiological, it is surprising to note that American dentists started to adopt a modified version of this procedure, known as the "mucosal insert." This approach was widely promoted by American dentists in literature as a major advancement in the oral rehabilitation of total edentulism. However, time and practical application ultimately revealed it to be a failure.

Submucosal implants were rejected due to complications: occurrence of pain, decubitus, and ulceration on the mucous membrane; in addition, they did not significantly increase the stability of the prosthesis.

If all forms of implants that are no longer in use are considered from today's time distance, it can be concluded that endosseous leaf implants survived the longest. Such Linkov implants were applied almost until the beginning of the last decade of the last century, even though the method of augmentation and shaping of the alveolar bone began to be applied in countries and outside of America.

The Frenchman Marc Bert devotes an entire book to leaf and "disc implants" that are not used today. Linkov's implants*[1] were developed in five generations. In each generation, the design would change, from an open and finally to a closed form. Attention was mainly paid to the design. The last, V generation of Linkov leaf implants differed from the previous ones. Some forms were made of two parts, and the part lying in the bone was coated with "titanium-plasma" Increasing the roughness of the surface of the endosseus part of the implant (Fig. 5.51).

1 The first books on practical implantology were written about Linkov implants (Marc Bert "Les implants dentaires", Josef Franke "Der heutige Stand der Implantologie", (1979) Ralph V. McKinney, Jr. Jack E. Lemons "The Dental Implant" - Clinical and Biological Response of Oral Tissues. Contemporary Implant Dentistry" (1993), Charles M. Wiss - "Dental implants: physiologic and clinical comparisons of fibroosteal and osteal integration" (1988), L. Linkow - "Maxillary implants; (1977) and "Mandibular implants" (1978).

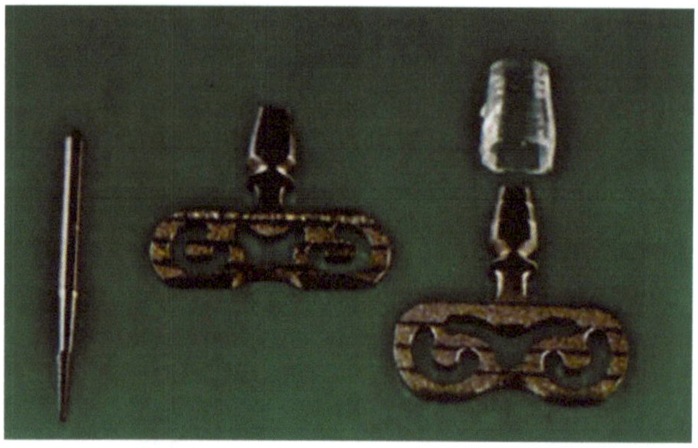

Figure 5.51. Closed plasma plated one-piece leaf Linkow implant, bone cutting bur and plastic casting cap.

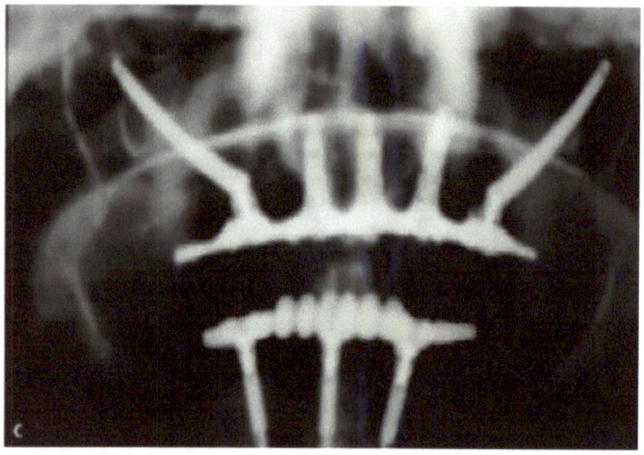

Figure 5.52. Two zygomatic implants in the upper jaw.

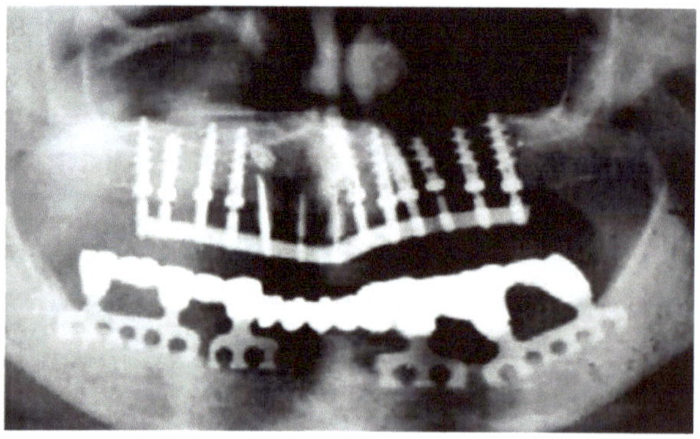

Figure 5.53. Application of screws (Tramonte's) in the upper jaw and open leaf implants (Linkov's, 1st generation) in the lower jaw.

And as for the technological processing of the implant surface, only in the so-called In the "fifth" and last generation, which was created in 63 forms, there was a technological improvement of the surface of the implant that lies in the bone and a better adhesion to it.

A large number of forms of leaf implants were explained by anatomical specificities (tubes and the position of the sinus in the upper jaw and the position of the inferior alveolar nerve and mentalis nerve in the lower jaw) and possible variations of the anatomical structures. And as for the carrier, in his neck, around which the soft tissues are formed, there have been no changes in all five generations. That was and remains the weakness of leaf implants. Marginal bone loss started from the necks of the implants, and the greatest bone loss was between the supports of the same implant, because the bone was losing its function in that place. Despite these shortcomings, many cases were solved successfully at that time.

The material from which Linkov's leaf implants were made was not even pure titanium, but a mixture of titanium, 6% aluminum and 4% vanadium: Ti Al6 V4. The success and length of stay in the bone of these implants was evaluated on the basis of clinical results, because they remained in the bone for ten or even more years. Figures 5.54-5.62 show various types of implants and their combinations, most of which were installed by the author himself, including some of the complications. Today, these implants represent history!

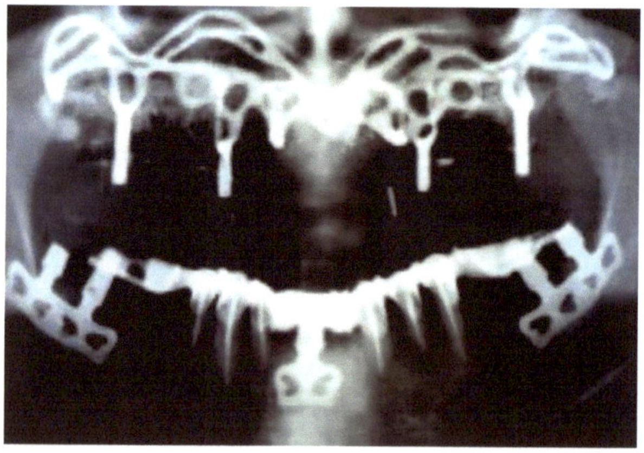

Figure 5.54. Subperiosteal implant in the upper jaw and connection of leaf Linkov implants of the V generation with natural teeth.

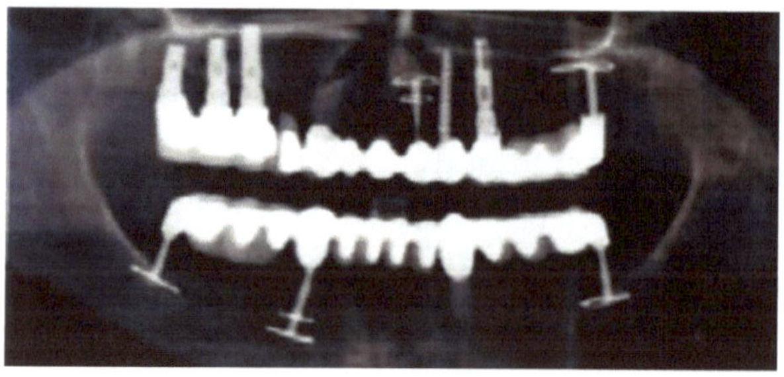

Figure 5.55. Display of the combination of Ihde's "disc-implants" two-part standard and narrow diameters. Absolute failure.

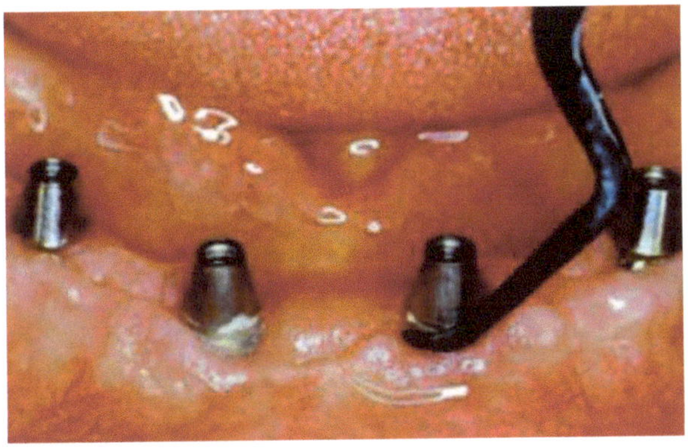

Figure 5.56. Arch Linkov implant abutments.

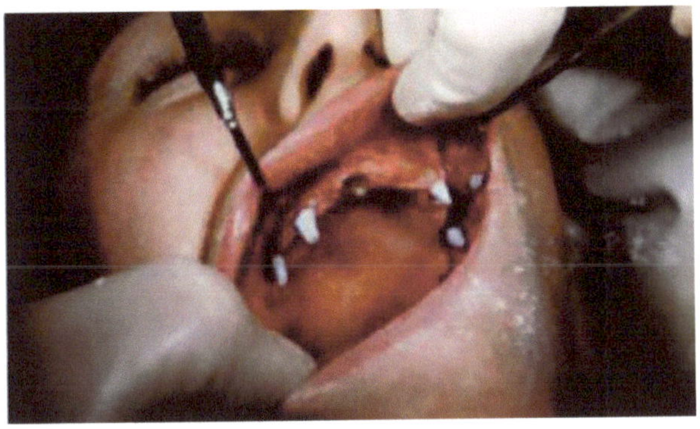

Figure 5.57. Total toothlessness of a 35-year-old patient. Embedded leaf Linkow implants. Work of the author in 1976.

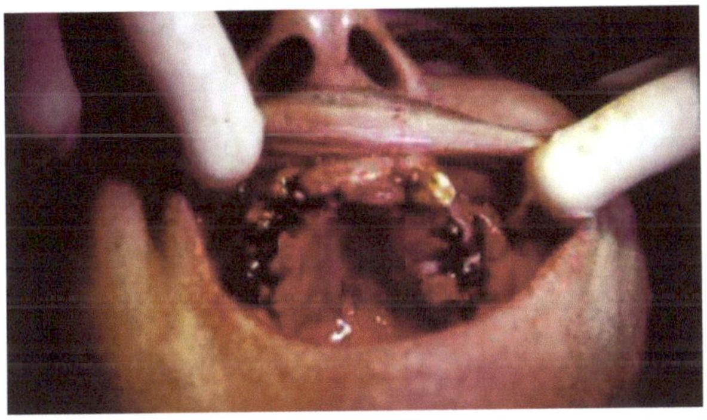

Figure 5.58. Embedded one-piece Linkov leaf implants in the edentulous upper jaw. The work of the author of the book in 1977.

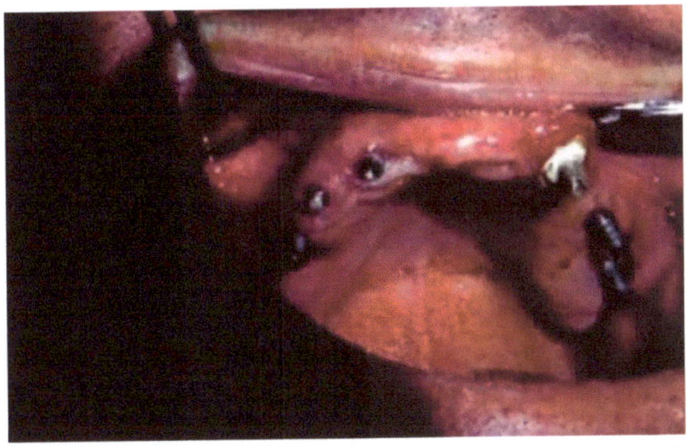

Figure 5.59. With Linkov implants, the inability to form a gingival sulcus around the abutments was their weakest feature.

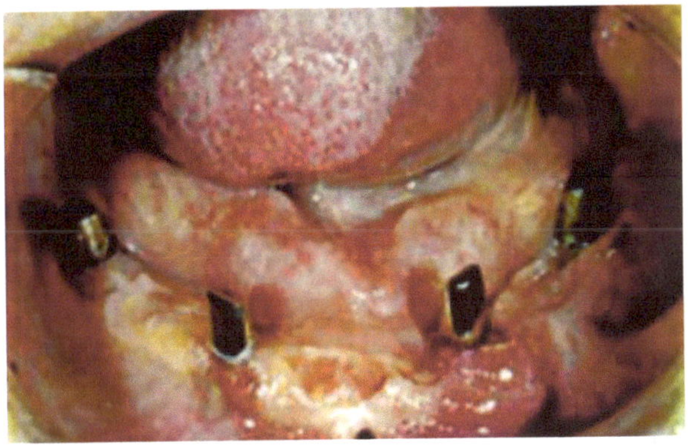

Figure 5.60. Ulceration caused by a subperiosteal implant.

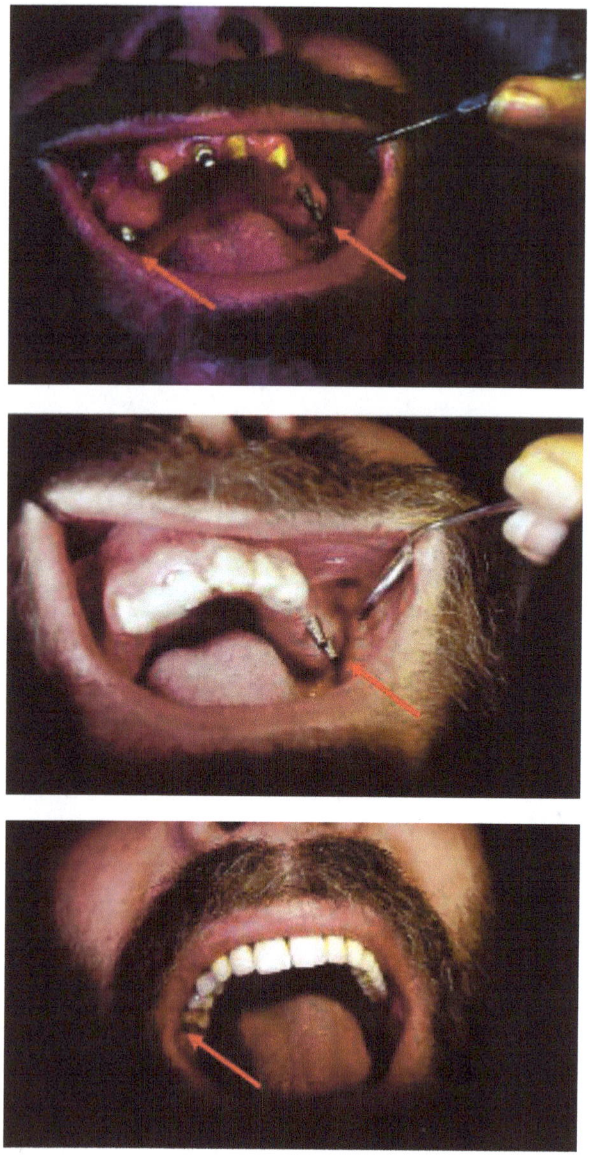

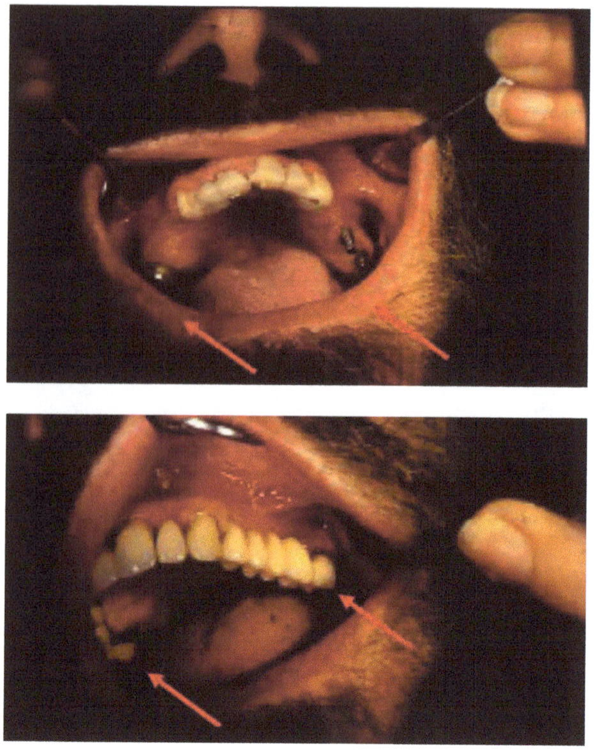

Figure 5.61. Embedded leaf implants (Linkow Blade Implant) where a functional and aesthetic result was achieved that the patient was satisfied with. The work of the author in 1977. Dental technician Savo Zlopaša.

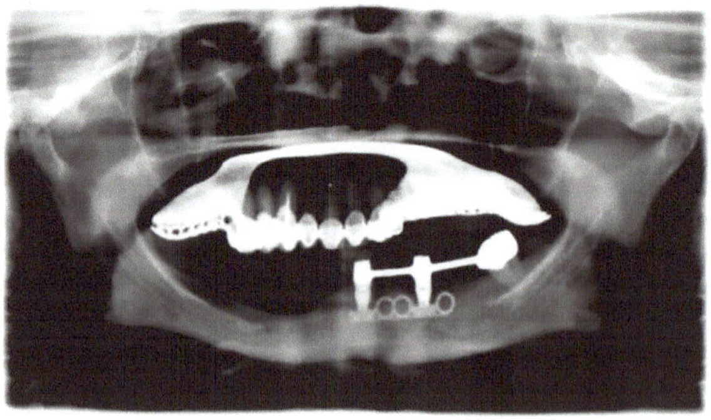

Figure 5.62. BTC endosseous implant (author A. Škundrić, VMA Belgrade), control image after 26 years.

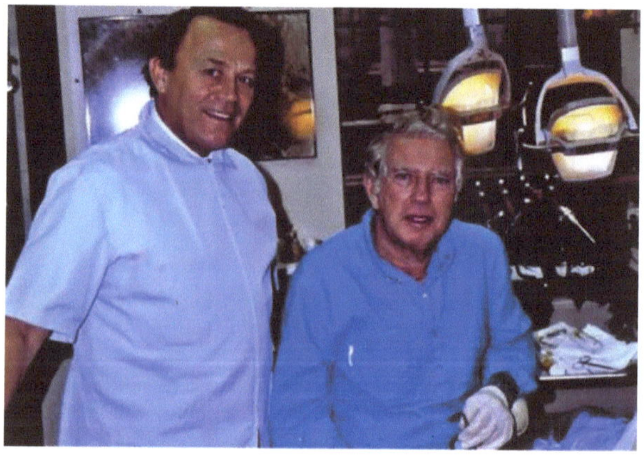

Author of a book with Leonard Linkow, the man who marked an epoch in the development of oral implantology - grateful to the teacher who gave me courage and caution (New York, 1983 to 1985).

6
When Implant Installation Is Justified

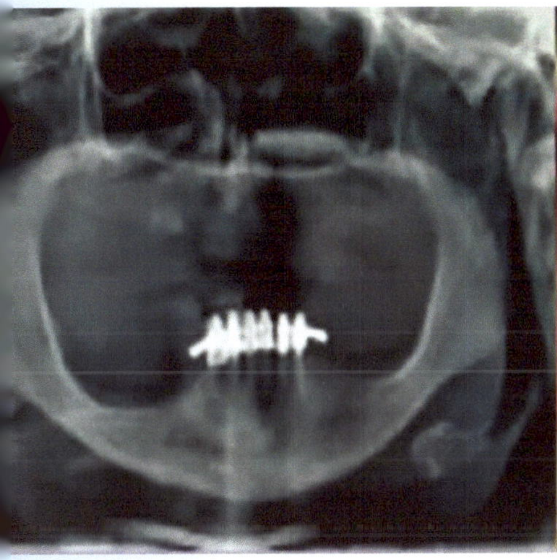

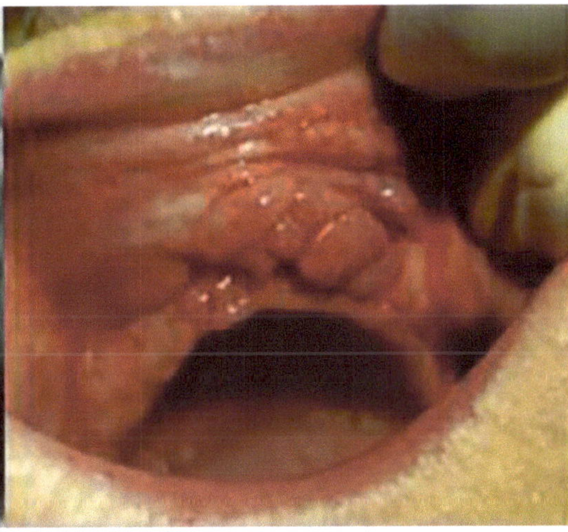

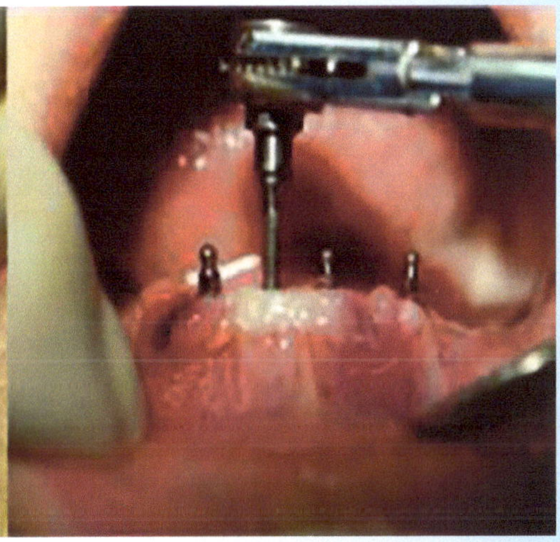

Many dentists desired to gather the courage and knowledge to start installing the first implants. It was a challenge to help patients with uncomfortable and unstable acrylate total dentures. It started with the intention to stabilize and improve chewing function with acrylic prostheses. It was easier for patients to get used to the upper total prosthesis, but for many patients it remained a continuous psychological trauma. The biggest challenge was how to stabilize the lower total prosthesis, problematic even for many experienced prosthetists.

Total toothlessness, especially in the lower jaw, brought many problems. One of the problems, in addition to the quantitative loss of alveolar bone to critical limits, which prevented the stability of the lower total prosthesis, was also macroglossia, the enlargement of the tongue. Macroglossia, as a consequence of premature tooth loss, as already emphasized, was followed by alveolar bone atrophy. The instability of the prosthesis was especially manifested when speaking and chewing food. In many patients, such lower total prostheses stayed in their pockets and purses more than in their mouths.

It all started from there. Function was primary, and aesthetics, it was considered: as much as could be achieved. With the installation of implants, at that time, not much could be achieved in terms of aesthetic creation. However, implantology, since it stopped being a routine skill of individuals, and enthusiasts, it has been transformed into a science and is developing at an unimaginable speed. Dentists dealing with implant placement for several decades can best appreciate the enormous progress of oral implantology.

A natural and healthy tooth, despite the great progress of oral implantology, cannot replace even the most modern implant. In the case of a diseased tooth, where the dentist is in a dilemma whether such a tooth should be extracted or left, replacing it with an implant is a more justified and reliable solution.

However, as the development of implantology advanced by Himalayan leaps, the indications for the installation of implants have expanded significantly, and the contraindications have significantly decreased. A few decades ago, the only indication was the restoration of chewing function. Today, with the installation of implants, functional requirements are equated with aesthetic ones.

When a single tooth is missing in either jaw, the best solution is to install an implant. This is in contrast to previous practices where two adjacent healthy teeth were ground down in order to replace one missing tooth, which is now considered completely unacceptable.

Replacing a missing tooth—referred to as an "Appendix"—is biomechanically a poor choice. Grinding down a healthy tooth results in the loss of significant structural integrity, potentially jeopardizing the vitality of that tooth. Additionally, a prosthetic tooth that is not anchored properly can create leverage on a single point of support. Such dental work will eventually weaken the periodontal tissue and may cause the supporting tooth to loosen due to unfavorable chewing forces and uneven pressure distribution.

Using movable acrylic prostheses—often called "frogs"—as a permanent solution to compensate for the loss of one tooth should be avoided whenever possible, even if they are used temporarily. Relying on such prosthetic replacements as a definitive solution is not advisable for several reasons.

Modern oral implantology has advanced significantly, allowing for remarkable functional and aesthetic results, even in challenging cases, through the installation of implants. For replacing a single missing tooth, an implant is often the most effective solution.

When the surgical procedure and protocol are followed correctly, the longevity of the implant in the bone is typically characterized by long-term survival, resulting in both functional and aesthetic benefits.

It is essential to share these insights, gained from practical experience, with students and future implantologists to help them draw informed conclusions and reap the benefits of this knowledge. Additionally, a crucial aspect of the process involves educating the patient about the advantages of implant placement, thereby fostering collaboration towards achieving a common goal.

Before the installation of the implant, it is vital to clarify various professional ambiguities to the patient. This includes explaining the function of a natural tooth and how the implant serves as its replacement.

Natural teeth are anchored in the jawbone by the periodontium, a fibrous tissue that nourishes the tooth and allows it to receive various stimuli, such as cold, warmth, sourness, and sweetness. One of the key functions of periodontal tissue is to cushion and distribute the forces generated during chewing, a function that implants do not possess.

The periodontal connective tissue secures the natural tooth within its socket, known as the alveolus, much like how a healthy tree's roots anchor it in the ground. If the roots of a tree become diseased and dry up, they must be cut; similarly, if the supporting structures of a tooth—the periodontium—deteriorate, the tooth will be lost. The extent of periodontal disease directly influences how long a natural tooth can remain in the jawbone.

Various factors can lead to the decay of the periodontium, resulting in tooth loss. When a tooth is lost, the space where the tooth once was begins to lose function, which can lead to bone loss, a condition known as jaw atrophy or resorption. Therefore, premature tooth loss accelerates the reduction of alveolar bone, which is visibly manifested by a decrease in the height of the jaw (alveolar) ridges.

The use of removable prosthetics, whether temporary or permanent, such as partial acrylic dentures, metal skeletonized dentures, or complete dentures, can accelerate the loss of jawbone, particularly due to the reduction in chewing function. It's important to note that losing a single tooth can lead to severe consequences if a "frog" (a temporary solution) is used, especially when an implant is planned for that area. This non-prosthetic approach can compress the soft tissues, and during the first four weeks, when bone loss is most significant, it can promote the atrophy of the alveolar bone in that location. This further complicates the installation of an implant and may result in unfavorable aesthetic outcomes.

What happens when the implant is placed in the jawbone?

In individuals with intact front teeth, tooth loss can occur unilaterally or bilaterally, which is typically addressed using traditional prosthetic solutions. These classic restorations often involve uncomfortable and non-functional acrylic partial dentures with unsightly wire hooks. As a more comfortable alternative, skeletal prostheses have been explored.

However, it's important to note that both types of prostheses, which rest on the jaw ridges, contribute to bone resorption and significantly accelerate the loss of bone mass. Additionally, they can damage the periodontium of the remaining teeth, particularly if they are secured with hooks, leading to tooth loosening. With these mobile prosthetic devices, achieving optimal chewing function is impossible, depriving patients of the experience they had with natural teeth.

When younger individuals are provided with such solutions, the risk of accelerated bone resorption increases, resulting in often insurmountable consequences later in life. By preserving the teeth in the frontal region, the amount of bone can be maintained. A similar effect is observed when implants are placed within the jawbone, as this approach helps slow down bone resorption.

In a computed tomographic analysis of a specific case, the ridge width measured 1 mm at a distance of 2 mm from the top to the plateau, indicating that implantation would not be feasible without prior augmentation.

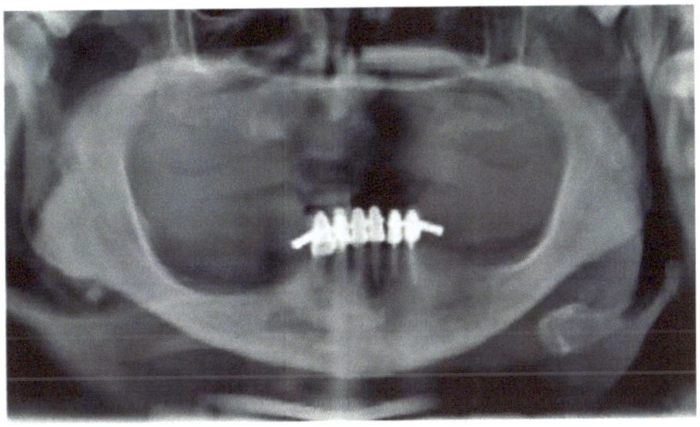

Figure 6.1. Extreme atrophy of the alveolar ridge in the lateral regions in a 45-year-old female patient.

An example of a 60-year-old patient (see Figure 6.2) shows similar issues in the upper jaw, where the alveolar ridge has atrophied and is covered with abundant, mobile soft tissue. After removing the hyperplastic soft tissue (refer to pictures 6.3 - 6.5), if it is not possible to deepen the vestibule due to significant bone loss, the only solution is to use a total acrylic prosthesis, which requires the permanent application of adhesive pastes or glues for prostheses.

What solutions are available for the lower jaw in cases of substantial bone loss due to the aforementioned causes?

The possibility of installing an implant depends on the type and extent of alveolar bone loss in both width and height. If there is sufficient height of the alveolar bone but insufficient width, the ridges may have razor-sharp edges. In such cases, augmentation with bone substitutes can create more favorable conditions for implant placement. However, this process tends to be time-consuming, complicated, and expensive.

If there is enough height, it may be possible to place a narrower diameter implant (for example, 1.8 mm) with a spherical head and retention clip.

Overall, augmentation is a long-term and often complex procedure aimed at creating optimal conditions for implant installation. The patience of the patient and their financial resources are crucial factors in this treatment. However, based on the situation shown in Figure 6.2, attempting augmentation may not be advisable.

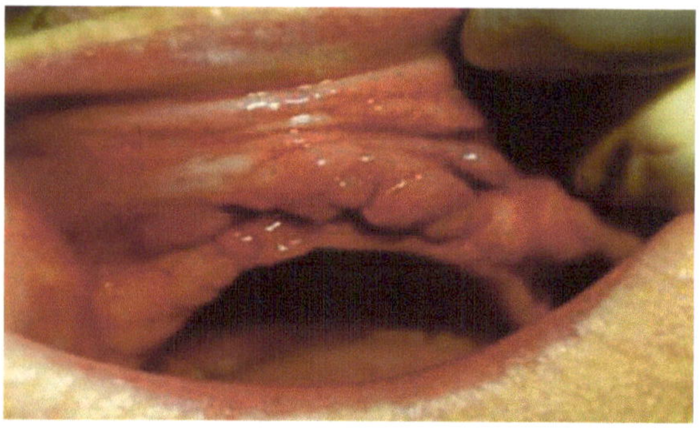

Figure 6.2. The consequences of premature loss of natural teeth, large loss of alveolar bone and wearing a bad acrylic prosthesis leave consequences that exclude the possibility of immediate installation of implants.

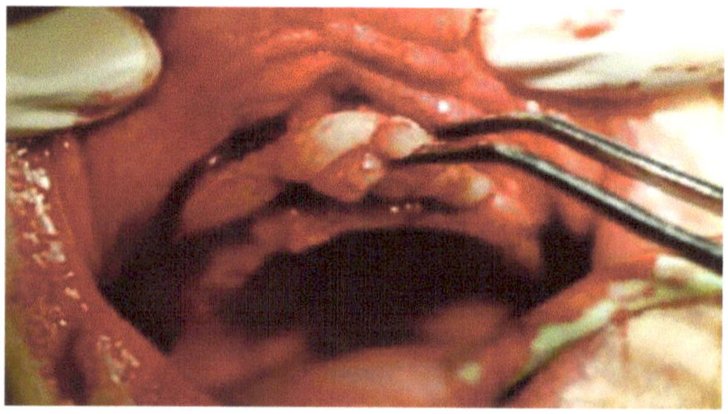

Figure 6.3. Removal of hyperplastic mucosa.

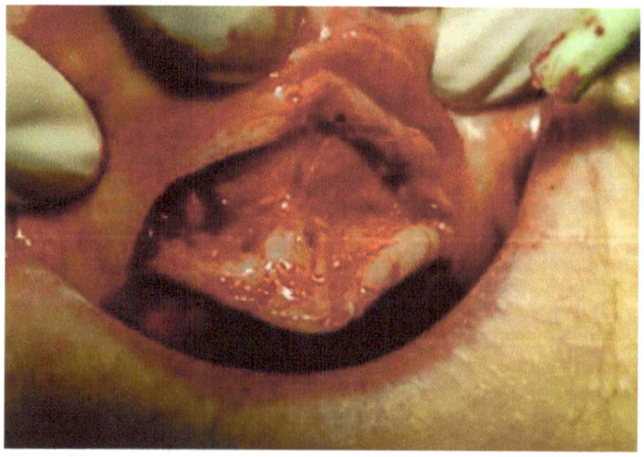

Figure 6.4. Elevation of the lobe - there is no alveolar ridge.

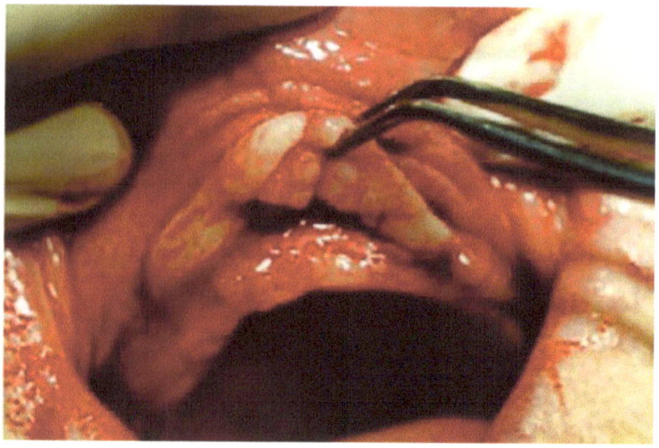

Figure 6.5. Removal of hyperplastic soft tissue, deepening and formation of the fornix for the upper total prosthesis. Extremely resorbed alveolar bone - an absolute contraindication for immediate implant placement.

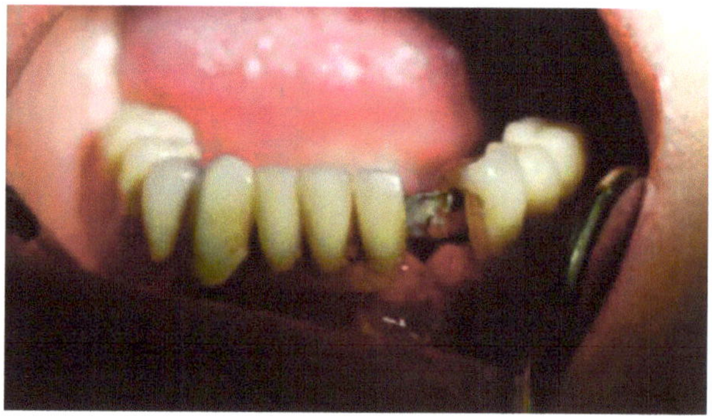

Figure 6.6. Presentation of a 48-year-old female patient where the inadequate "solution" did not consider the later consequences (see Figure 6.1).

The wishes, hopes and demands of the patient shown in Figure 6.6 were to get rid of uncomfortable prostheses. The financial situation was not posed as an obstacle to the desired requests. However, the situation in the mouth indicated the only possible solution: a mobile acrylic prosthesis and the eventual installation of an implant with retention clips. Given the extreme alveolar bone loss and unfavorable anatomical structures, this attempt may be futile. After the removal of the loosened tooth (Figure 6.7), implants with a narrow diameter (2.4 mm) were inserted due to the unfavorable width of the alveolar bone, and a maximum length of 16 mm. Amortizing rings and positioned metal caps are placed on the installed implants (pictures 6.8 6.10). An existing prosthesis that had narrow saddles and sharp edges was used. The procedure was performed in two stages: cap transfer and fixation in an acrylic plate by taking a functional impression. The acrylate part lying on the alveolar ridges was replaced by a soft acrylate mass (Figure 6.11). A satisfactory aesthetic and functional solution was achieved by all the procedures mentioned above (Figure 6.12).

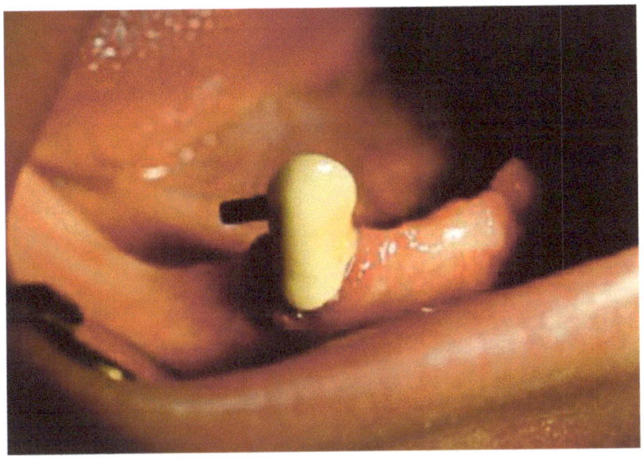

Figure 6.7. By wearing a skeletonized metal prosthesis, the central incisors and the left canine were first lost, and the remaining right canine, loosened by the inflammation process, was extracted.

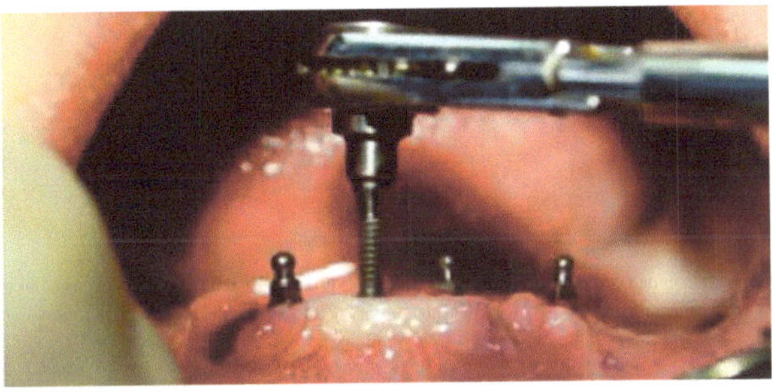

Figure 6.8. Installing a narrow diameter implant (3 mm) is the only possible solution.

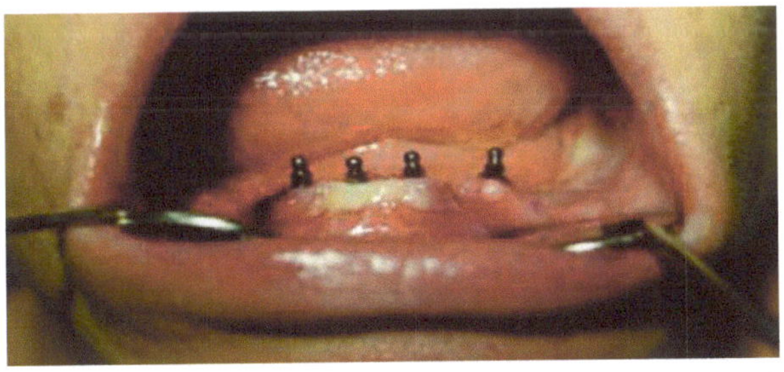

Figure 6.9. The final stage of immediately installed one-piece implants for stabilization of the lower total prosthesis.

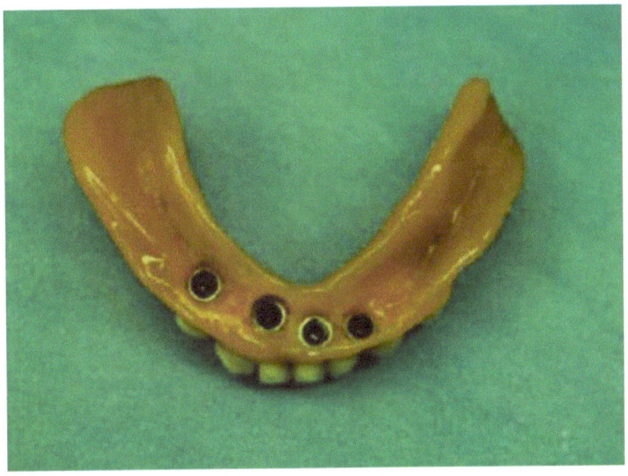

Figure 6.10. Preformed existing acrylic partial denture with added teeth and embedded retention clasps. Acrylate part of the prosthesis replaced by soft acrylate (Molisol, Detax) (picture 6.11).

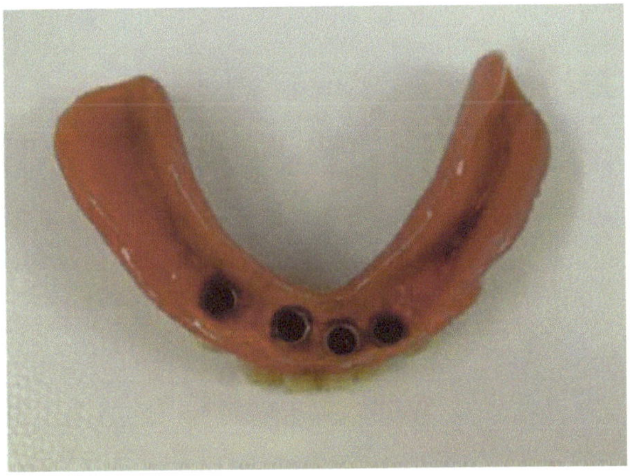

Figure 6.11. Modified acrylate base of the existing partial denture (picture 6.10) with soft acrylate more comfortable for the patient.

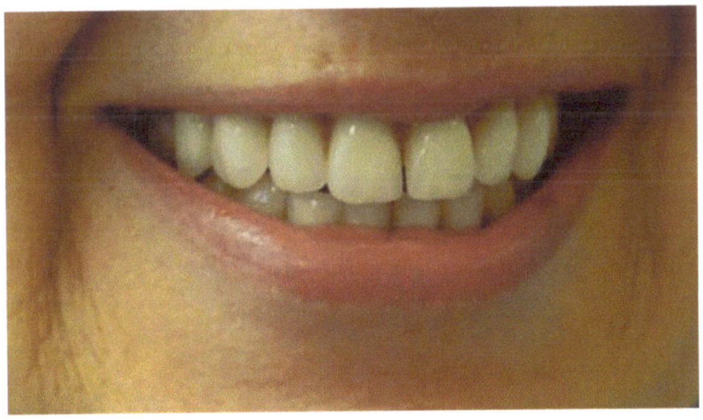

Figure 6.12. An aesthetically and functionally acceptable solution for stabilization of total acrylate prostheses with retention resilient clips.

The justification of implant placement in a specific case and convenience for the patient is fulfilled in the following:

a) treatment time is significantly shortened;
b) the implants are immediately loaded;
c) the old prosthesis to which the patient has become accustomed was used;
d) in the upper jaw, the existing prosthesis served as an individual spoon;
e) the occlusion that could not be achieved with the old prostheses due to the change in position and wobble of the frontal teeth is aligned.

In this example, the most important thing was to achieve good mastication. The aesthetic result with acrylic total dentures was easily achievable because the laugh line was favorable.

During normal mastication, the natural teeth for crushing food provoke a pressure, more or less around 16 kg per square centimeter of bone, which in extremely strong bites can reach up to 90 kg per cm2.

However, with braces, the average chewing pressure drops to 50 kg per cm, and with some lateral movements necessary to grind food down to 25 kg per square centimeter. From these data, with dentures, there is an enormous loss of chewing forces, which will cause many changes in the way of eating and choosing the type of food. Denture wearers must avoid certain types of food, which cannot be chewed well due to the reduction of chewing forces with the help of classic dentures. They are forced to change the way they chew, and thus the way they eat, and to change many habits related to the loss of natural function.

This affects the quality of food digestion, which manifests in overall health. By installing implants behind the remaining teeth, mastication is established approximately at the same level as when there were natural teeth.

Insertion of the implant into the jawbone significantly slows down the resorption of the alveolar bone. By the ingrowth of bone cells into the millimicron pores of the implant surface, an ankylosing bond, which is referred to as bone integration of the implant, is more and more firmly established. With the installation of the implant, the bone regains its function, which was lost due to the loss of the tooth, i.e. to hold, support, and feed someone, receiving forces from the external environment and dispersing them to the advantage of action.

In the area around the implant, the bone becomes dynamic again, because it sets in motion osteogenesis and remodeling with osteoblasts and osteclasts, whose activity must be physiologically balanced, which will result in the processes of osteogenesis and osteolysis. This physiological dynamic is that the bone must once again support the implant in the place where it replaced the tooth, with which it was also in a dynamic relationship. All this means that the atrophy of the alveolar ridge is significantly slowed down, although it cannot be said that it has been completely stopped. In the case of early tooth loss, along with loading the alveolar bone with an acrylate plate, the degenerative processes are accelerated.

The installation of implants in the lower jaw should take place immediately after tooth loss. This is important because the premature loss of teeth in the lower jaw can lead to macroglossia. In cases of advanced edentulism, macroglossia may become a contraindication for the successful placement of implants, as it can create unfavorable lingual forces and moments from those forces.

Given this information, it is essential for the dentist who is performing the implant installation to engage in a thorough dialogue with the patient (refer to chapter 19). This conversation is not straightforward, as it requires mutual understanding. The dentist must assess the type of patient they are dealing with and clearly explain the rationale for implant installation. Additionally, the patient should be able to derive pertinent questions from the dentist's explanation.

It is crucial for both parties to exercise patience during this discussion to prevent any misunderstandings and potential disputes in the future.

A patient cannot embark on a complicated procedure without being informed about all the details and the outcome, possible complications and the like. Of course, the price is also one of the important factors that the patient must know before installing the implant. Implantology is a serious branch of medicine and requires great responsibility, expertise and experience of the implantologist both from the aspect of ability and medical ethics.

What should be advised to the patient to make the life of the implant as long as possible?

After the implant surgery, the patient assumes significant responsibility for their own well-being, provided that everything has been performed correctly. It is crucial to strictly follow the dentist's instructions for maintaining oral hygiene. Recent advancements in hygiene products are also noteworthy. Patients should receive clear explanations about hygiene maintenance, typically provided by a trained dental assistant with experience in hygienist training courses. This assistant will demonstrate how to maintain hygiene around the implant using specialized brushes designed for this purpose. There is a wide variety of brushes available on the market, made in different shapes and qualities, specifically for cleaning around implants. Additionally, numerous antiseptic, disinfectant, and deodorizing pastes and mouth rinses are available that offer prolonged antiseptic effects to neutralize harmful bacteria. It is important for the dentist to explain these options to the patient.

Digital X-ray technology has advanced significantly, allowing us to accurately monitor changes around dental implants over time, including the degree of any potential bone resorption. If any changes are detected early, they can often be addressed with minor interventions, greatly extending the lifespan of the implant. In areas where bone breakdown has occurred, we can use bone substitutes that promote healing. Additionally, one remarkable innovation in implantology is the use of lasers to remove granulation tissue around implants, which can stimulate regeneration.

However, heavy smokers are considered a risk group for successful implant-prosthetic treatment. There are differing opinions on this matter, but the author's experience indicates that healing of soft tissues is often slower in smokers, and they tend to accumulate more plaque.

7

Bone Integration

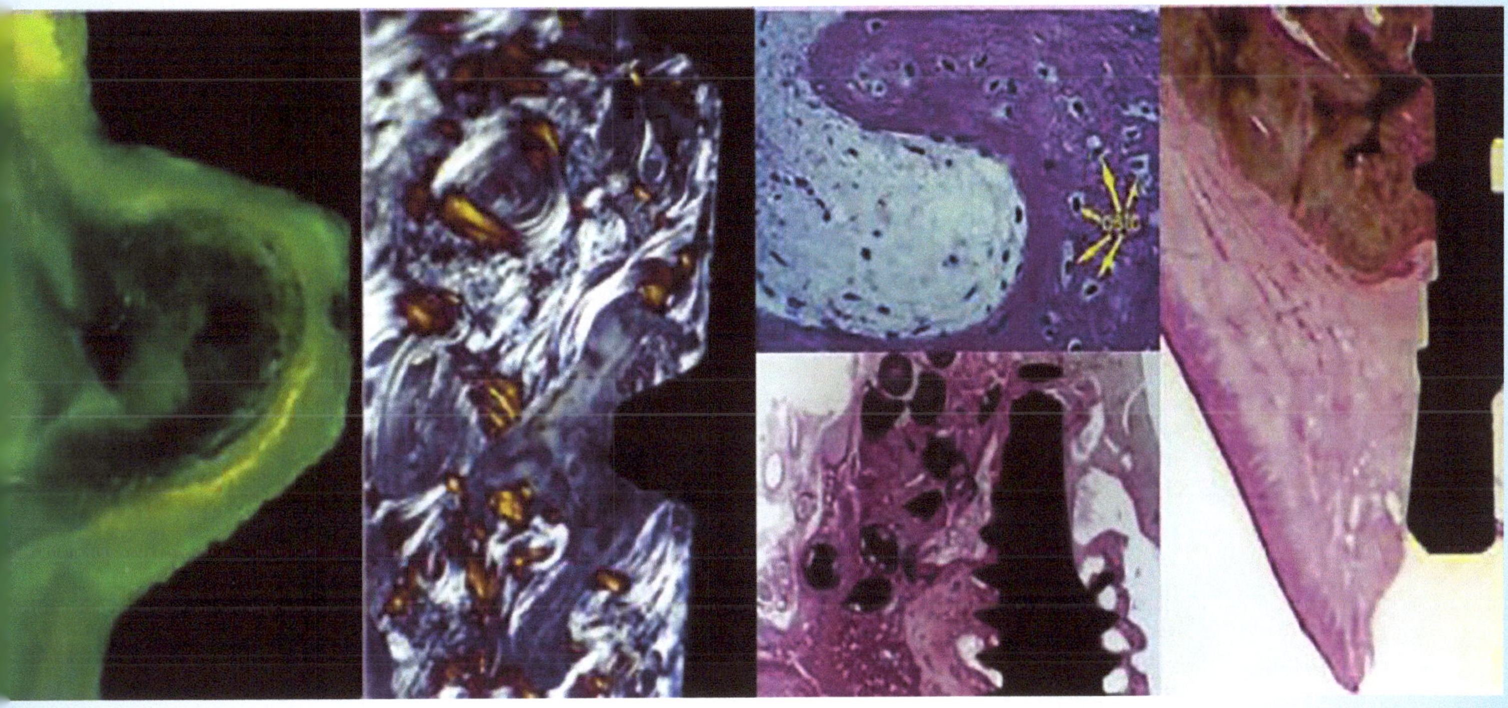

When Branemark published his work in 1965, it marked the beginning of modern oral implantology based on scientific principles. Clinically, osseointegration can be defined as a state in which a solid anchorage of the alloplastic material (the implant) is achieved in the bone and maintained during functional loading (Albrektsson and Zarb, 1993).

Today, our understanding of the relationship between the surface of an implant and the bone has advanced significantly, thanks to the scientific and clinical studies published by Branemark. He initiated systematic research into the interaction between the implant and the surrounding bone, challenging the previous belief that the formation of fibrous connective tissue in this gap was typical. Over many years, strong clinical outcomes have been documented, primarily by Swedish researchers, demonstrating that direct bone-implant contact is a more reliable connection over the long term. This direct contact between the bone and the implant surface is referred to as osseointegration.

Many dentists believed that achieving complete bone integration with titanium, an inert material, at the biological, chemical, and even cellular and molecular levels, was impossible. The interaction between the implant's surface and the bone has been a long-standing concern in dentistry and oral surgery, fueling hopes and expectations within the field. To better understand the various processes occurring in the dynamic environment of bone, it's essential to continually update our knowledge of bone structure. It is a significant mistake to consider the area used for dental implant placement as an autonomous microregion. All events should be viewed within the context of the entire complex system, including the interactions and reactions that take place.

Bone is a solid form of connective tissue that possesses unique mechanical and biological properties. Its matrix provides strength and stability to the bones.

Histologically, bone consists of two main types: cortical (compact) bone and trabecular (cancellous) bone. Trabecular bone has a distinct three-dimensional structure, which contributes to its different mechanical properties.

Cortical bone makes up about 80% of total bone mass and is characterized by densely packed lamellar sheets. This density is crucial for the placement of implants, as cortical bone is 10 to 20 times denser than cancellous bone. Because of this density, cortical bone is much more suitable for implant placement.

In orthopedics, implants have historically lacked the longevity that dental implants possess. This difference is partly because orthopedic implants are embedded in cancellous bone, whereas dental implants are placed in the denser cortical bone. Additionally, orthopedic implants tend to be heavier and are typically fixed in place using cement within the cancellous bone. This results in a complex relationship consisting of bone, cement, and implant.

If this physiological process occurs in the maxilla and mandible, the mineralized bone can be classified into two types:

- **Fibrous (primary) bone**
- **Lamellar (secondary) bone**

The classification depends on the degree of development or healing.

Fibrous bone is formed in the early stages of bone development. It consists of irregularly arranged collagen fibers that are not fixed in place, serving as a foundation for mineralization. Hydroxyapatite crystals adhere to these collagen fibers.

In comparison to lamellar bone, fibrous bone is softer and less dense due to differences in structure and mineralization. However, the mechanical properties of fibrous bone improve over time through remodeling and replacement by lamellar bone. Since fibrous bone has weaker mechanical properties than lamellar bone, it provides less mechanical support during implant installation. Therefore, experienced dentists recommend leaving the implant in fibrous bone unloaded for an extended period. It is advisable to allow at least three to six months of rest in the bone before loading the implant.

There are varying opinions regarding the timing of implant stress. Some experts argue that the implant should be subjected to physiological stress as soon as possible, accompanied by precisely crafted prosthetic work. This approach would facilitate the replacement of fibrous lamellar bone, resulting in remodeled bone that provides a solid support for the longevity of the implant.

In conclusion, remodeled lamellar bone surrounding the implant site has distinct advantages over fibrous bone, a factor to consider when selecting the implant placement location.

Additionally, the success rate for implants in the lower jaw is significantly higher than in the upper jaw. This preference for implant placement in the mandible over the maxilla is primarily due to the denser cortical bone in the lower jaw, especially noticeable on the anterior side. In contrast, while the upper jaw does have denser cortical bone, it is generally found in the lateral sections and the frontal region.

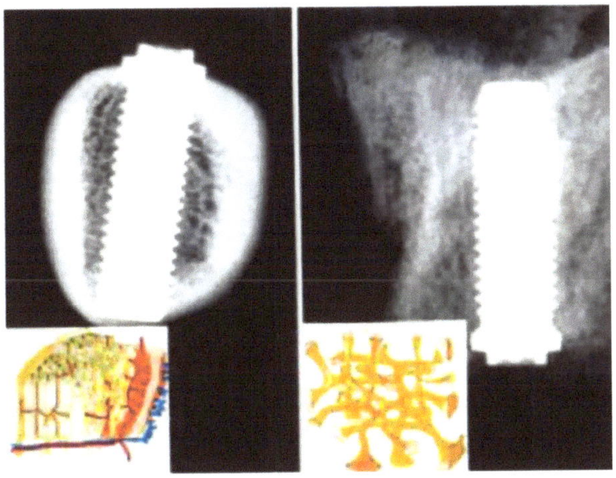

Figure 7.1. Radiographic view of dense bone in the lower jaw and cancellous bone of the upper jaw. Schematic representations of the three-dimensional architecture of cortical bone (left) and cancellous, trabecular bone (right).

The upper jaw differs from the lower jaw in its composition; it includes a thin layer of cortical bone along with spongiosa of varying density and quality. These structural differences in bone, along with unique anatomical features of the upper and lower jaws, influence the intensity of the integration processes.

The process of bone integration begins with the surgical placement of the implant and is influenced by the extent of trauma inflicted on the bone using the appropriate drills for creating the implant bed. The level of trauma is closely related to the surgeon's skill during the preparation and the force applied when screwing the implant into the bone. Additionally, the integration process depends on the degree of primary contact between the bone and the implant's surface, within the space formed by bone, bone marrow, and hematoma mixed with bone fragments created during the drilling process.

Therefore, soaking the implant in saline prior to its insertion into the bone is a significant mistake that should be avoided.

The clean, intact, and dry surface of an implant should be closely surrounded by blood within the bone to ensure that the primary coagulum forms as quickly as possible. The healing process that occurs with bone loss or fractures also takes place around the implant embedded in the bone. Inflammatory and mesenchymal cells migrate from the surrounding tissues into the space between the implant and the bone. The initial hematoma is replaced by proliferating granulation tissue and non-mineralized connective tissue. Over time, multinucleated giant cells cover the surface of the implant that faces the unmineralized tissue.

This reaction of the organism to the presence of an implant, particularly in relation to materials like titanium, is not yet fully understood and remains an area for scientific exploration. For instance, the body's response to achieving homeostasis in the environment of such bioneutral materials is still unclear.

As time progresses, the number of multinucleated giant cells decreases, leading to an increase in bone-to-implant surface contact. During the formation of new bone at the cortical region near the surface of the implant, the number of secondary osteons increases, resulting in fibrous bone developing in the space between the bone and the implant.

When considering the processes involved in cylindrical and threaded implants—commonly used today—we can conclude that the degree of bone-implant contact improves with the amount of newly formed bone on the implant threads. This correlation between the quantity and quality of bone on the implant's threads contributes to increased implant stability over time, ensuring its long term integration within the bone.

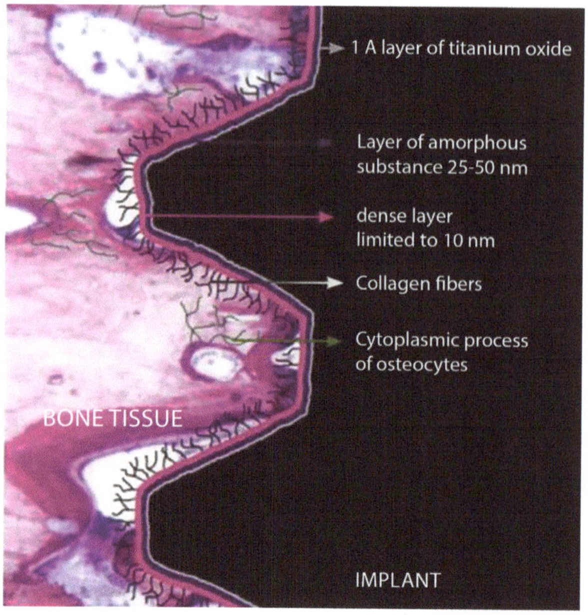

Figure 7.2a. Display of the surface of the integrated implant and bone.

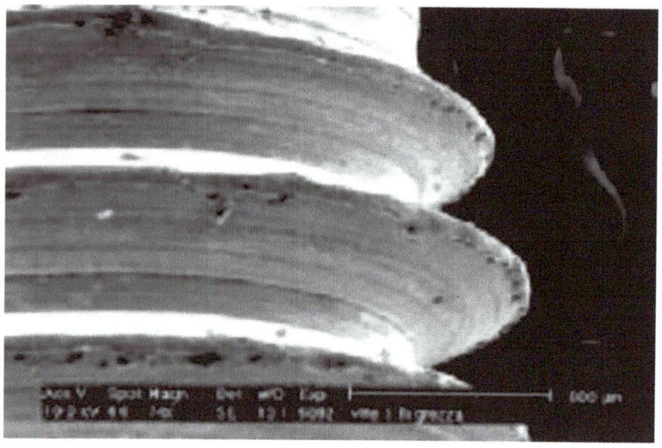

Figure 7.2b. Appearance of the microscopically enlarged endosseus surface of the implant treated with laser technology. The speed and quality of osseointegration processes depends on the quality of titanium and the treatment of the implant surface.

Clinical tests with cylindrical implants without threads showed constant marginal bone resorption (Figure 7.3), and in a larger percentage of this type of implant, there was a major failure. In the case of embedded cylindrical implants, marginal resorption was also proven in dense bone.

Threaded implants demonstrate superior primary fixation and integration compared to cylindrical implants, resulting in significantly less marginal bone loss. This advantage is largely due to the design of the threads, specifically the thread pitch. The thread pitch, defined as the vertical distance between threads, should be at least 1 mm, while the horizontal depth should range from 0.3 mm to 0.5 mm. These specifications ensure good primary stability during the immediate placement of implants, particularly following the extraction of periodontal teeth. In these scenarios, achieving good primary stability can be accomplished with 2-3 threads in healthy bone, specifically in the area above the apical region of the tooth being extracted. Experience indicates that implants placed and loaded immediately after extraction tend to integrate well with the bone and yield successful outcomes. Additionally, the use of longer implants greatly enhances the success of this procedure.

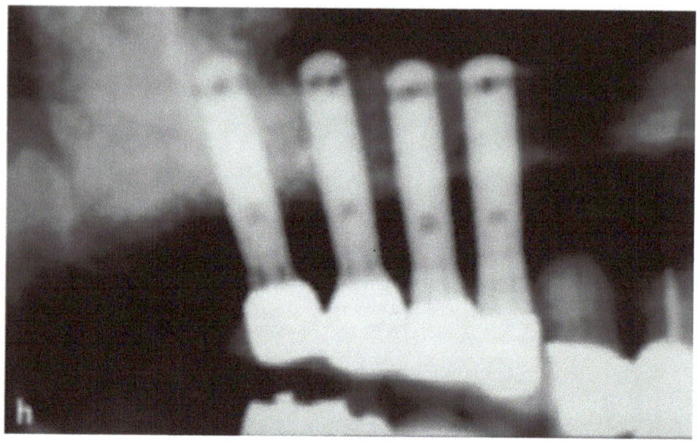

Figure 7.3. Bone resorption in cylindrical implants coated with hydroxyapatite (author's paper, 1988).

Clinical studies have shown that failures with shorter implants were higher than with longer ones. Many studies have proven that poor bone quality is a major risk for the placement of wide implants. Researchers and manufacturers focused the most attention on "soft bone", and solutions for implant stability were mainly tied to the design of the implant, its surface and the quality of pure titanium, ie titanium oxide (TiO).

The further course of osseointegration processes depends on the degree of fixation of the implant in the first phase of healing (primary stability).

In the realm of healing, differing perspectives continue to exist today. Previously, the prevailing belief was that implants should be allowed to heal and integrate with the surrounding bone before they were loaded with pressure. Immediate loading of implants was generally not recommended due to perceived higher risks and unpredictability of outcomes. This view contributed to the two approaches advocated by Branemark himself. However, numerous studies on bone-integrated implants have demonstrated that a healing period may not always be necessary, provided certain conditions are met. It is now understood that allowing the implant to heal prior to loading is not an absolute requirement for long-term success. The precise duration needed to achieve complete stability and optimal bone integration has not been thoroughly established, but it is believed to occur within a timeframe of 3 to 6 months. This period is considered sufficient for achieving lasting results in both the upper and lower jaws. Based on experience, the durability of high-quality implanted devices can typically be evaluated within six weeks at the latest.

Experienced dentists understand that implants placed in soft bone tend to exhibit less primary stability compared to implants in dense bone. However, over time, the stability of implants in soft bone increases significantly more than those in dense bone from the moment of implantation to loading. By twenty months after implantation, all implants achieve a similar level of stability, regardless of the quality of the bone or the initial primary stability.

The longer an implant remains in the bone, the more stable it becomes, although this is influenced by several factors, including the load placed on the implant, the quality of the implant itself, and its surface properties. In the later stages of healing, the surface treatment of the implant promotes the replacement of fibrous bone with lamellar bone, which is substantially stronger.

Another important aspect of the implant is the design of the neck area, which is essential for proper soft tissue formation. Clinical results, supported by radiological and histological evidence, indicate that the healing process around the implant in soft bone—characterized mainly by spongy trabecular bone—leads to changes in the quality of the bone that comes into contact with the implant surface. Dynamic changes in bone around an implant and the loading process appear to have a stimulating effect. When all parameters are appropriately adjusted to distribute chewing forces effectively, the resulting forces can place physiological stress on the bone tissue surrounding the implant. This stress likely contributes to the transformation of trabecular bone into laminar bone.

Numerous studies and clinical findings related to soft bone indicate several important points: in soft cancellous bone, implants should ideally be as long as possible to ensure adequate primary stability. In such conditions, an extended healing period is necessary to achieve satisfactory stability before the implant is subjected to loading. However, this does not imply that the implant should remain inactive for an extended period.

Many studies have shown that the same implants in a similar bone structure, which after installation showed little primary stability and different behavior, loaded immediately after installation, promote the condensation of trabecular bone around the loaded implants and a faster recovery process than with implants that lay in the bone without load. At the end of the chapter, the author of the book proves it by solving very complex cases.

Experience indicates that when good primary stability is achieved, early loading—if kept within the limits of physiological masticatory forces—can enhance the stability of the implant. The decision to load the implant immediately or to allow for a healing period to ensure adequate stability depends on the judgment and experience of the dentist.

To achieve this stability, it is essential to have satisfactory horizontal and vertical dimensions of the alveolar bone, which serves as the foundation for the implant. Preserving the alveolar bone during and after tooth extraction is particularly important because the bone associated with the periodontium is inevitably lost when teeth are removed. The loss of buccal bony walls during tooth extraction leads to a decrease in both horizontal and vertical dimensions of the bone. This resorptive process is especially pronounced on the buccal walls of the alveolar bone in the upper jaw and is most significant in the first three months following tooth extraction.

Maintaining the vestibular wall of the alveolar bone, especially in the frontal regions of both the upper and lower jaws, is crucial for meeting both functional and aesthetic requirements.

The clinician should evaluate whether the use of bone substitutes or autologous bone augmentation is necessary for successful implant placement. It is crucial to maintain the volume of the bone in all three dimensions to preserve the bone structure and facilitate complete integration around the implant.

Both function and aesthetics are important in the frontal region. Therefore, the thickness of the buccal wall of the alveolar bone should be no less than

2 mm. However, in many patients, this wall is often thinner than 1 mm. Additionally, in the first year following tooth extraction, the loss of height in the vestibular wall typically ranges between 2 and 4 mm mm, where the resorptive process takes place most strongly in the first three months. It depends on the judgment of the clinician, first of all his experience, whether the augmentation will be performed before or during the installation of the implant, by filling the space with a bone substitute and covering the tissue with a resorbable membrane.

Practice, and theory, indicate that with implants where weak primary stability has been achieved, a healing period of 3 to 6 months is sometimes required.

It is important to highlight that the most critical period for implant stability occurs during the initial healing phase, which lasts 4 to 6 weeks. During this time, the dentist's expertise and assessment skills are vital. In many cases where rapid loading is avoided, it is recommended to allow the first phase of healing to extend for at least three months, and in some instances, even up to 12 months or longer.

The surgical technique and its execution play a crucial role in establishing conditions that promote effective bone integration and implant stability. The success of this process heavily depends on the implant system used, particularly the quality of the components. Specifically, the drill bits utilized for preparing the bone must be sharp and made of high-quality, non-corroding metal. *Many manufacturers advise that a drill should only be used for a limited number of implants before needing to be replaced with a new one.*

This manufacturer's recommendation can be understood from two perspectives. First, high-quality drills designed for repeated use are made from non-corroding materials, which are more expensive. In contrast, drills intended for one-time use are often made from cheaper, corrosive materials, resulting in higher profits for the manufacturer. The quality of the surgical set also reflects the quality of the implant system.

Blunt drills that are not adequately cooled can cause the greatest trauma to bone tissue. These drills can generate excessive heat, raising the temperature of the bone beyond acceptable limits and operating at inappropriate speeds. When the bone overheats, proper contact between the bone and the implant surface is compromised, leading to a higher likelihood of implant failure within a short period. This crucial phase of implant installation is emphasized throughout the case presentations in the book.

The diameter of an implant significantly impacts its stability. Numerous studies have indicated that a weak connection between the implant and the bone may occur with wider implants if they are not surrounded by an adequate amount of bone. During surgical procedures, it's common for an implant inserted into the prepared site to exhibit little to no primary stability. In such cases, it may be necessary to consider using an implant with a larger diameter, as long as it is surrounded by sufficient amount of bone to ensure good blood supply.

Numerous experiences and clinical studies conducted by implantologists have demonstrated that this method of implant placement can lead to successful outcomes. Typically, a larger diameter implant is used during the procedure to optimize primary stability, particularly when a standard diameter implant would not suffice. This larger implant is often kept as a "spare" to ensure minimal stability is achieved during surgery.

The relationship between the diameter of the implant and the integration process

It is important to note that having a wide diameter for an implant does not guarantee its stability over time if it is not surrounded by an adequate amount of bone to ensure proper blood supply. During the installation of the implant, the torque applied can increase shear stresses, resulting in trauma to the bone. This trauma can, in turn, cause ischemia in the bone, which often has very thin surrounding walls. Based on the author's experience, this series of events frequently leads to necrosis. As a result, even if satisfactory primary stability is achieved, the implant may still be lost.

In any case, many experiences and studies have shown a weaker bond between bone and a 5 mm diameter implant than a standard implant (3.8 mm). 5 mm implants last for 3-5 years. One of the reasons for the loss of implants with a wide diameter of 5 or 6 mm is that they are usually short (6 and 9 mm) and were used in cases where primary stability could not be established with a standard implant. Even though they had all the properties of standard implants, and the installation was performed under the same conditions as with standard implants (with a diameter of 3 to 3.75 mm), the wide implants did not have long-term survival in the bone.

Immuno-histological research

The initial histological studies of leaf implants were conducted by several authors prior to the research of Branemark. In 1951, Leventhal highlighted the excellent suitability of titanium as an artificial material for implants, emphasizing its advantages over tantalum and other alloys that were primarily used at the time. A group of researchers, including Babbusch and R.D. Manderson (1972), R.A. James (1974), F. Doms (1974), and M. Meenagham et al., were among the first to investigate the ratio of the area of the leaf implants.

Scientific research works on the fibrointegration bond have shown that the results obtained after the implants are not stable in the long term, even that the failures increase over time. All the results proved that the percentage of failure is significantly higher and faster in the upper jaw than in the lower jaw.

For a long time, it was thought that the insertion of connective tissue between the implant and the bone replaces the periodontium of the natural tooth and assumes the role of a shock absorber for receiving strong chewing forces. It must be admitted that the classic idea of traditional implantology was based on this connection. It was only offered to patients as a temporary solution, something more long-term in the lower jaw with fixed and mobile prosthetic restorations.

Research on fibrointegration in dental implants has shown that the results achieved are not stable over the long term, with failure rates increasing over time. Studies indicate that the percentage of failure is significantly higher and occurs more quickly in the upper jaw compared to the lower jaw.

For many years, it was believed that the presence of connective tissue between the implant and the bone could replace the periodontium of a natural tooth, acting as a shock absorber to handle strong chewing forces. This traditional concept of implantology was based on this connection. Initially, implants were offered to patients as a temporary solution, while more durable options were considered for the lower jaw, including fixed and removable prosthetic restorations.

After Branemark's research and scientific evidence demonstrated direct contact between implants and bone, a new era began, allowing patients to receive more stable, long-term solutions for both the upper and lower jaws. In 1981, Branemark further explored the concept of direct implant-bone contact through additional scientific studies, establishing the term "bone integration." His clinical results indicated a significantly better connection between the implant and the bone compared to a fibrous connection.

One of Branemark's major contributions was his pioneering research into the biological compatibility of the materials used in implant construction. Results from his studies, along with later research by others, clearly showed that the quality of titanium is crucial to the success or failure of implant placement. Branemark determined that titanium must be of high purity, with impurities not exceeding 0.25%. Although commercially pure titanium is significantly more expensive and more challenging to process, many implant systems on the market are made from "impure" titanium, often consisting of a mixture of titanium, aluminum, and vanadium.

The biotolerance of pure titanium has been proven by many scientists in animal and human experiments. To date, no toxic reaction to titanium has been reported anywhere in the literature, and this has been confirmed by scientific research. Even high concentrations of titanium did not produce any toxic reactions. Regarding titanium, no carcinogenic or allergic reaction to titanium has ever been observed, both experimentally and clinically.

Scientific research on the behavior of cells in implant-bone contact (T.R.I.Gould 1981, M.Kasemo 1985, Mac Qveen 1987) shows that bone cells are extremely vital when they come into contact with pure titanium. Only Gould in 1981, through animal experiments, noticed, but very rarely, giant multinucleated cells (macrophages) in the vicinity of titanium.

Titanium is a highly reactive material when exposed to oxygen. This tendency towards oxidation, however, contributes to its resistance to corrosion from tissue fluids. After installation, titanium is protected by a thin but durable layer of titanium oxide, which is why it demonstrates the highest corrosion resistance among all metals.

The mechanical properties of titanium implants are influenced not only by the metal's strength but also by its biochemical characteristics. These properties arise from the titanium oxide layer, which plays a crucial role in the physiological dynamics within the peri-implant space. This physiological effect was scientifically explained by J. Lausmaa in 1984 and B. Kasemo in 1986. They demonstrated that the titanium oxide layer forms more stable titanium oxides that, from a biochemical perspective, help maintain homeostasis in the peri-implant environment.

From the extensive bibliography and works of scientists who have studied titanium as a material from which implants are made and its behavior in the body, one brief conclusion can be given about what you need to know about titanium during its application in implantology:

1. titanium and its compounds possess such mechanical properties that make them an ideal material for oral implantology and orthopedics;
2. titanium and its compounds show oxidation when exposed to air. Titanium oxide, on the surface, is extremely stable in the physiological environment of the body;
3. the stability and inertness of the oxide layer helps to protect titanium from corrosiveness when it is incorporated into the physiological milieu of the bone, i.e. the body, in dentistry as a tooth replacement, and in orthopedics as a replacement for a diseased hip or knee;
4. during the preparation of titanium for the manufacture of dental implants, it is very important to eliminate all impurities that can affect bone integration processes. Many systems are offered on the market, some of questionable quality, where titanium impurities exceed the permitted 0.25%. When choosing an implant system, an experienced dentist should choose the most reliable companies, despite the expensive price of the implant system. Higher quality implant systems have their secret in technological processing, so many competing companies that produce copies of such implants cannot enter the secrets of technological processing of the implant surface;
5. titanium, in the body, can contact metals whose passivity is close to or equal to it (such as the chromium-cobalt alloy used in the production of superstructures), because there will be no galvanic corrosion.

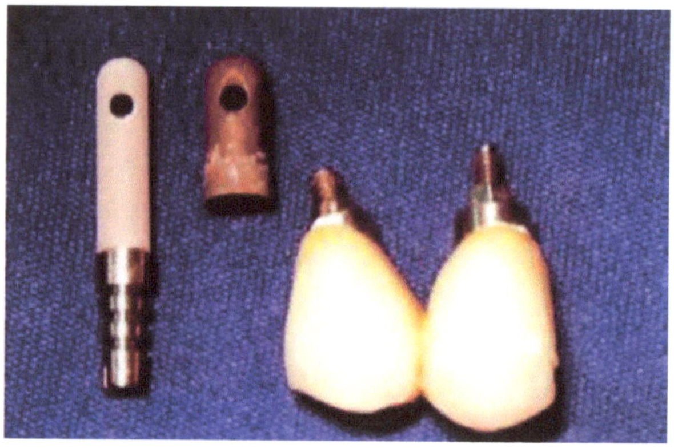

Figure 7.4. The cylindrical shape of the implant coated with hydroxyapatite (left) and the cylindrical implant after being in the bone, the layer of hydroxyapatite does not exist (author's work).

Today, commercially pure titanium can be considered a universal bioinert material in oral implantology and has exceptional properties, but based on long-term clinical results, we are still far from the ideal properties of implant materials for ideal osseointegration. In order to achieve this, an attempt was made to coat titanium with hydroxyapatite (M.Bert, 1994). With all installed hydroxyapatite-coated implants, after a few years, these two materials separated, and this led to the loss of the implant (Figure 7.4). Based on all the clinical results, the advantage is on the side of pure titanium, which has proven to be successful after decades of use.

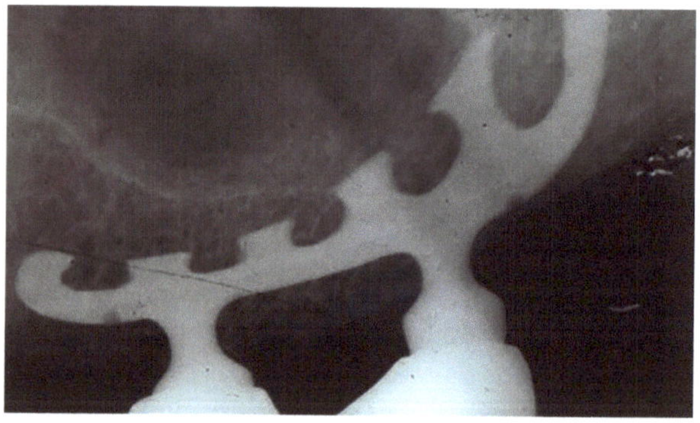

Figure 7.5. The principle of Combi implants in the posterior regions could not be based on an attempt at osseointegration (and because of the material from which it is made - tantalum), but more on the characteristics of subperiosteal implants with wings that rested on the periosteum of the alveolar ridge (work by the author of the book in 1975).

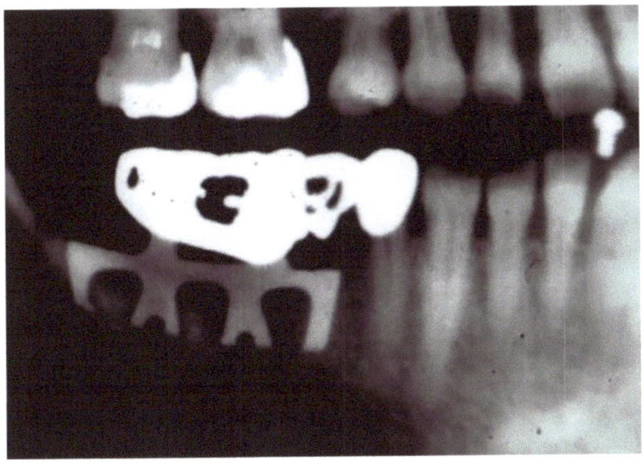

Figure 7.6. The first generation of open leaf Linkov implants. No consideration was given to possible osseointegration even though the material they are made of is titanium.

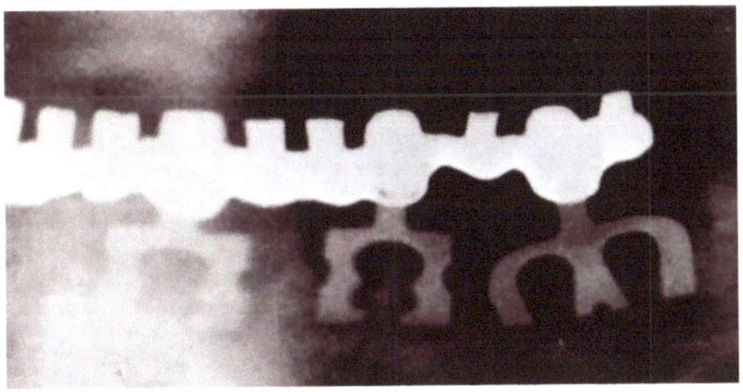

Figure 7.7. Different forms of open leaf implants had a destructive effect on the bone.

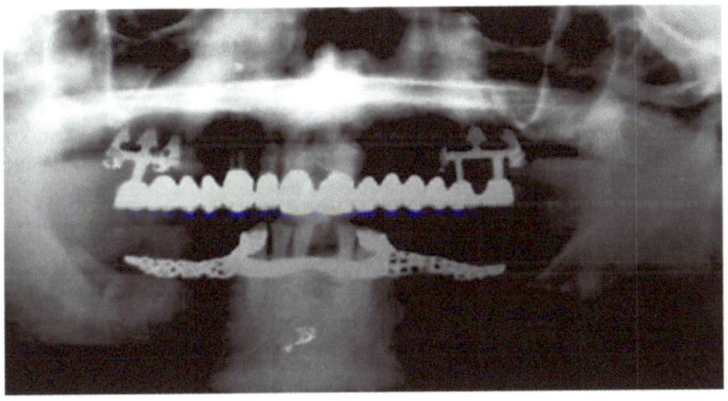

Figure 7.8. The first generation of Linkov's open implants indicated for the low floor of the maxillary sinus (author's work in 1973).

The American Leonard Linkow and the German Hans Grafelman also introduce the procedure of plasma treatment with titanium powder, i.e. applying titanium powder to the surface of the implant ("titanium-plasma") in order to help a more intimate and solid connection between the metal and the bone.

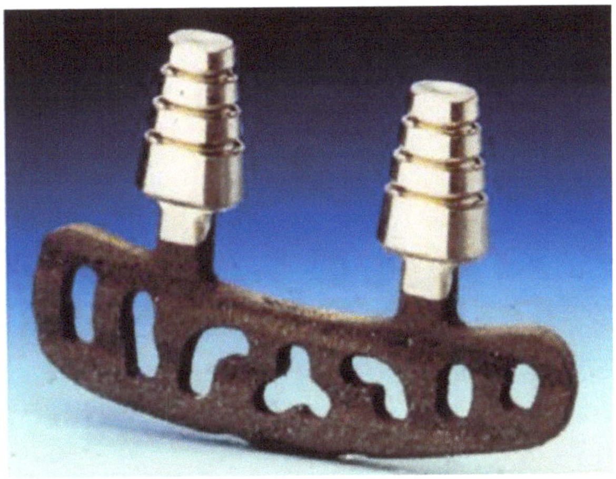

Figure 7.9. The fifth generation of closed Linkov one-piece sheet implants coated with "titanium-plasma". Even with the "V generation" Linkov leaf implants, the stability of the implant was not based on bone integration, but on the growth of new bone through the designed openings of the endosseous part of the implant.

The emergence of "plasmized" sheet endoseal Link implants marked the introduction of the fifth generation of sheet implants. Earlier generations of leaf implants underwent various changes in shape and design, which included both open and closed forms, as seen in Figures 7.6 to 7.8. The closed form was coated with plasma, as shown in Figure 7.9.

With the introduction of the term "titanium-plasma," the basic design of sheet implants remained unchanged; however, this term refers specifically to the treatment of the surface layer of the implant that interfaces with the bone. This part is coated with titanium powder, which consists of fine titanium particles. These particles are applied at high temperatures to the metal surface that contacts the bone. As a result, the titanium particles create pores on the implant's surface, facilitating faster growth of bone cells into these pores.

Many scientific meetings have long focused on determining the optimal pore size on implant surfaces for achieving the best connection between implants and bone. To address these questions, research groups dedicated to studying osseous integration have been established, uniting numerous dentists from around the world, including members of the French and German Associations for Implantology. The role of these professional scientific academies is to enhance understanding in the field, leading to the reevaluation of outdated concepts and the adoption of new insights in oral implantology.

Additionally, insights from the use of implants in orthopedics are drawn upon to extract valuable data regarding the relationship between bone and titanium. Dental implants are distinct from orthopedic and other types of implants due to their unique positioning in two environments: within the bone and the oral cavity. This duality allows for the potential penetration of saliva and bacteria, leading to the accumulation of soft deposits. These deposits can cause inflammation of the surrounding tissues, a condition known as peri-implantitis, which can ultimately result in implant failure.

Consequently, the method of processing the neck of the implant has been a longstanding topic of discussion and importance in the field. This issue remains relevant today. To promote successful integration, the design surrounding the implant neck and its clinical maintenance must facilitate effective biological closure where the implant meets the mucous membrane. This is essential to prevent the entry of saliva and bacteria, as well as the build-up of soft deposits and other contaminants in the connective tissue beneath the mucosa. If these contaminants are allowed to enter, they can lead to tissue inflammation around the implant.

French innovators were the first to propose various design solutions for the implant neck. One notable design is the implant featuring a zirconium neck. Because these types of implants have only recently been introduced, it is too early to determine whether zirconium offers any advantages over titanium at the neck interface. Further research will help us understand the biocompatibility of zirconium and whether it is superior to that of titanium.

Dental implants differ from orthopedic and other types of implants that are placed in the body because they exist in two environments: in the bone and in the oral cavity. This unique setting allows for the potential penetration of saliva and bacteria, leading to the accumulation of soft deposits that can cause inflammation of the surrounding tissues, known as peri-implantitis. This can ultimately result in the loss of the implant.

As a result, the processing method for the neck of the implant has been a topic of ongoing discussion and holds significant importance. This dilemma continues to be relevant today.

To ensure the longevity and health of the implant, the structural design around the implant neck, along with effective clinical maintenance, must facilitate adequate biological closure at the interface with the mucous membrane. This is essential to prevent the entry of saliva, bacteria, and other impurities into the submucosal connective tissue, which could lead to inflammation.

The French are pioneers in introducing various design solutions for the implant neck. One innovation includes implants featuring a zirconium neck. However, since these implants have only recently been introduced, it is still too early to draw definitive conclusions regarding the advantages of zirconium over titanium in terms of their interaction with the surrounding tissue. Future studies will determine the biocompatibility of zirconium and whether it surpasses that of titanium.

Primary fixation is the initial indicator of success and serves as the foundation for good bone integration. However, it is important to note that primary fixation of the implant is not always a reliable predictor of the procedure's long-term success and longevity. To achieve this, one crucial condition must be met: the prosthetic work must be well-planned and executed correctly. Poor prosthetic work can undermine even the highest quality implants.

Experience has shown that a successful oral surgeon or implantologist must also be a skilled prosthetist and periodontist. Simply placing an implant based on the availability of bone is not sufficient; it is essential to install the implant in the optimal location. Many beginners make the mistake of focusing solely on where bone can be found instead of where it is best to place the implant. Ultimately, the final prosthetic work should promote the processes of bone integration.

Applying the highest quality implants, often many dentists who have not entered into the secrets of oral implantology, ask the question: can the connection between the implant and the bone, after some time, loosen, that is, the implant be "rejected"? In other words, can an already integrated implant loosen after some time, i.e. that the osseous integration achieved is compromised?

First of all, every dentist should know that, especially in a conversation with a patient, the term "rejection" must not be used. Like any organ in the body, the implant can "get sick".

However, the term "diseased implant" refers to its environment (bone and tissues around the implant). If there is a disturbance of the previously good connection and function, or if there is a failure after a short or long time, and the implants showed excellent primary stability after installation, the reasons for the loss of the implants should be sought at two levels:

Conduct a detailed analysis of the patient, starting with an assessment of any systemic diseases. In relation to bone physiology, the metabolism of bone can be influenced by the duration that the implant has been in place. It is important to recognize that various diseases can affect bone metabolism, and these effects can manifest in the oral region as well. A disordered hormonal system that regulates bone metabolism does not necessarily indicate that a person is ill. The balance between bone creation (osteosynthesis) and decomposition (osteolysis) is in constant flux.

Examine any potential defects in the technological processing of the implant surface that is in close contact with the bone. Laboratories are available to analyze the quality of titanium to determine whether it is of second, third, or fourth grade quality.

The Swedish company Nobel-BIOcare provides detailed laboratory analyses for each lost implant. An experienced dentist with multidisciplinary knowledge often faces a dilemma when an implant fails: where should he look for the reasons behind the failure?

Are the causes localized microlevel issues, such as poor prosthetics, gnathological problems (especially with lateral movements of the lower jaw), or inadequate oral hygiene combined with heavy smoking? Or should attention be directed to other potential causes?

The human body functions as an indivisible unit, where each organ and organic system plays a crucial role in maintaining homeostatic harmony. Homeostasis refers to health and the balance of optimal conditions within the body's environment. Numerous organ systems, with the help of numerous regulatory mechanisms, maintain homeostasis, that is, health. Disturbance of homeostasis means that something is wrong in the function of the organism, which manifests itself as a disease.

The three main systems that participate in homeostatic regulation mechanisms are: the nervous, endocrine and immune. The knowledge that the immune system plays a very important role in maintaining homeostasis, i.e. human health, has been scientifically confirmed. In addition, there is almost no disease in which the immune factor is not more or less involved. It is no coincidence that during and near the end of the last century, as many as 15 scientists received the Nobel Prize for scientific contributions in immunology. The immune system is a collection of tissues, cells, and molecules whose primary function is to defend the internal environment of the organism and maintain homeostasis. There is no isolated operation of the immune system, but it is in correlation and interaction with all other physiological systems, such as the cardiovascular, neuroendocrine, gastrointestinal, respiratory, urogenital and musculoskeletal systems.

All these factors must be considered in surgical-implantology and periodontal procedures. Even the most experienced dentists have encountered cases where, despite correctly performed implants, the healing process does not proceed as expected.

It is a common tendency among patients with implants, who are satisfied with both function and aesthetics, to neglect regular check-ups. This is a significant mistake. Patients often make the same error after undergoing more serious periodontal procedures. Regular consultations with both the implantologist and periodontist are essential to assess the patient's condition and the level of plaque deposits through professional examinations. If insufficient oral hygiene is detected, patients should receive specific warnings highlighting the potential consequences.

Many patients only seek help when they experience pain. When pain occurs around an implant, it serves as a serious warning sign, indicating possible pathological changes around the implant itself. In many scenarios, the sensation of pain, which is transmitted through the spinothalamic pathway, can signal the need to prevent dangerous pathological conditions.

Due to the harmful effect of chewing forces, and most often due to incorrectly performed prosthetics (most often with the existence of occlusal gnathological problems), bone destruction can occur, which patients do not know, and only notice when the destruction process is in an advanced stage.

The purpose of dental implants is to restore the anatomical harmony in the mouth by integrating into the jawbone and replacing lost teeth with functional alternatives. This process aims to re-establish the physiological balance that was disrupted. However, the emergence of pain serves as an initial warning that the entire implant process may be at risk. It is important to note that the experience of pain associated with implants differs from that related to natural teeth.

A key question is whether the reflex transmission of pain around the implant, which occurs via the spinothalamic nerve pathways, is fully functional or diminished. This represents a significant drawback of implants when compared to natural teeth. In many cases, the sensation of pain from implants typically arrives with a delay.

These considerations have sparked further scientific inquiry, leading to the introduction of the term "bone integration." Free nerve endings, acting as receptors, detect every external influence and stimulus that might disrupt the body's homeostatic harmony, which refers to a normal physiological state, either in a specific area or within the entire organism.

Impulses are transmitted to the central nervous system, where all sensory sensations—such as hot, cold, sour, and sweet—are integrated and processed. The sensory perception of temperature, particularly the sensations of hot and cold, is especially significant with natural teeth. When it comes to dental implants, the lack of sensory transfer of heat is crucial. The ability to sense warmth, especially overheating, is vital for the longevity of the implant, as heat transferred through the metal can also be conducted to the surrounding bone. This issue has been a topic of discussion at numerous scientific meetings.

For this reason, using cement to fix the superstructure offers advantages as a thermal insulator compared to screwing. The adhesive layer helps to interrupt the unfavorable transfer of heat to the bone tissue. Dr. A. Kirsch was the first to address this thermal break by incorporating a movable Teflon ring between the implant body and the support in his IMZ implant design. His concept extended beyond just the thermal break, as the intramobile Teflon ring simulated the function of the periodontium. However, Kirsch's idea did not gain practical acceptance, and rightfully so, as it could become a preferred location for the accumulation of plaque and calculus, which is a vulnerable point in terms of resistance.

When examining nervous regulation during dental implant installation, the scenario is comparable to heart transplantation. Just like the heart, which operates independently of sympathetic and parasympathetic nerve influences, dental implants also lack intrinsic nervous regulation. In heart transplantation, attempts to connect the vagus and sympathetic nerve endings to the heart muscle have proven unsuccessful.

Natural teeth benefit from comprehensive physiological regulation and reflex responses to external stimuli. In contrast, dental implants, regardless of their biocompatibility with bone, do not possess the same intimate nervous regulation that allows natural teeth to respond to various external influences. This includes the ability to register sensations such as temperature (hot or cold), taste (sweet or sour), and responses to both static and dynamic forces experienced during chewing.

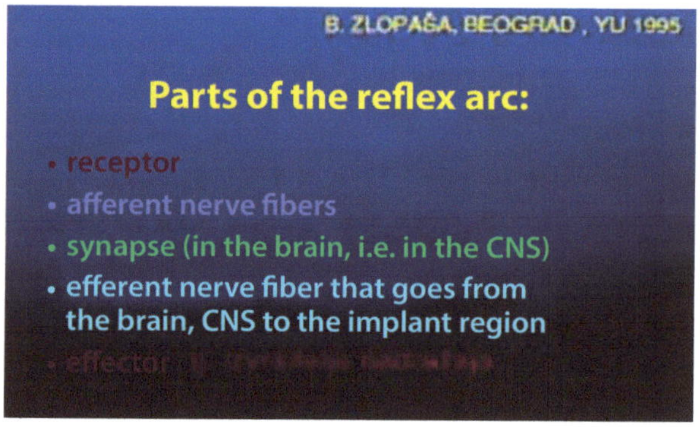

Figure 7.10. Parts of the reflex arc. (from the lectures of Dr. B. Zlopaša at international scientific symposia - Bremen, Liege, Dusseldorf, Bologna, Verona, the slide was translated into several languages).

For the realization of most reflexes, including the pain reflex, it is necessary to have the integrity of the reflex arc, which has the following parts:

1. receptors;
2. afferent nerve fibers;
3. synapse in the CNS;
4. efferent nerve fiber that goes from the central nervous system (CNS) to the region of the embedded implant;
5. effectors, i.e. executors of the order.

The question is: **is there a break in the reflex arc to the implant and the bone?**

A partial answer to this question and an explanation can be found in a comparison of an implant and a devitalized tooth. The situation is identical, except that the fate of a devitalized tooth is related to bone metabolism (homeostasis of calcium and phosphate, i.e. supplying the supporting apparatus of the tooth with blood, i.e. nutrients, so the devitalized tooth is subject to faster decay.

In both cases, **bone metabolism is of crucial importance, i.e. bone physiology, in the function of which three important hormones participate**:

- The first hormone to consider is **parathyroid hormone (PTH),** which is produced by the parathyroid gland and plays a crucial role in regulating calcium metabolism in adults. In contrast, the second hormone, calcitonin, has a minimal effect due to its osteolytic properties and its diminished significance in adults. Parathyroid hormone is essential for promoting osseous integration with implants.
- Another key hormone in bone metabolism is **calcitriol**, also known as vitamin D. It has a function similar to that of parathyroid hormone and is produced in the kidneys. The metabolism of vitamin D is vital for bone integration; insufficient vitamin D intake can lead to reduced bone metabolism, impairing the remodeling and restoration processes at the implant contact site. Since calcitriol influences calcium and phosphate homeostasis, kidney conditions pose a significant risk factor for implant placement. Additionally, the kidneys produce other important hormones, such as erythropoietin, which is crucial for maintaining proper erythropoiesis (the production of red blood cells), and renin, which is important for regulating blood pressure. A deficiency in calcitriol can lead to osteoporosis, while a lack of erythropoietin can result in anemia. Therefore, when investigating the causes of implant failure, it is important to consider not only the local jawbone region where the implants are placed but to adopt a holistic, multidisciplinary approach for a comprehensive understanding of the process.
- The third important hormone is **calcitonin**, which is produced by the thyroid gland. Calcitonin plays a crucial role in promoting bone formation, involving two types of cells: osteoblasts and osteoclasts.
  - Osteoblasts are the bone-building cells; they produce protein fibers, such as **collagen**, around which minerals are deposited. In contrast, osteoclasts create enzymes that break down bone tissue. The activity of these cells is synchronized by various hormones, including growth hormones, insulin, sex hormones, thyroid hormones, adrenal hormones, and cytokines, which act as "intercellular messengers."

The hormone calcitonin is more active in younger individuals and plays a crucial role in skeletal formation. During pregnancy, it helps protect the mother's bones from excessive calcium loss. In adults, however, calcitonin has a weaker effect, as it is countered by the parathyroid regulatory mechanism. This diminished effect of calcitonin increases the osteolytic activity of decomposing cells, leading to greater bone breakdown. Besides other influencing factors, calcitonin is significant in the development of age-related osteoporosis. Its primary function is to inhibit osteoclast activity and bone resorption. Together with parathyroid hormone (PTH) and calcitriol, calcitonin is essential for maintaining bone homeostasis.

These factors are important to consider in order to avoid risk factors and prevent unnecessary complications during implant placement, which could lead to failure.

Until recently, osteoporosis was regarded as a contraindication for implant placement. Although osteoporosis is a common condition today, some claims suggest it rarely affects or does not manifest in the upper and lower jaws. However, there is a lack of scientific evidence supporting these claims.

The rise in osteoporosis is influenced by increased inactivity, while the maxilla and mandible are in constant use**. However, clinical experience indicates that osteoporotic processes can also impact osseointegration, potentially weakening or jeopardizing the integration of dental implants with the surrounding bone. For instance, there is often a question regarding the loss of an implant that initially had good primary stability and successfully achieved bony integration, especially when a thorough analysis rules out all risk factors for implant failure. The assertion that osteoporosis does not affect bone metabolism around implants**

merits reconsideration, particularly as this disease continues to rise. Osteoporosis, recognized as a disease of modern civilization and exacerbated by lifestyle choices, is garnering increasing attention from the world's leading scientists.

The objective of scientific research is to find ways to stop or slow down the breakdown of bones, ultimately improving quality of life by preventing fractures and deformities. In relation to dental implants, early loss can occur if all other risk factors are eliminated; osteoporosis is a potential cause of implant failure and can deteriorate the integration between the implant surface and the bone.

Modern physiology needs to address this issue. The highest bone density is typically reached around the age of 35 and is maintained for about ten years before bone tissue loss begins around the age of 50. On average, women experience a loss of bone density six times more than men. The decline in estrogen and androgen hormone levels increases the likelihood of developing osteoporosis. Additionally, individuals with blonde hair, fair skin, and a slender build tend to show a higher susceptibility to osteoporotic changes. In contrast, Black individuals lose bone mass at a much slower rate than White individuals, even in old age.

Bone changes caused by osteoporosis happen when bone tissue breaks down by more than 25 percent. As a result, the bone becomes porous and hollow, making the installation of implants contraindicated. Engaging in increased movement and physical exercise is important for both prevention and therapy. If osteoporotic changes have occurred, the therapy will be tailored to the individual and will depend on the specific type of osteoporosis. It is essential for dentists to understand the challenges associated with this disease in order to effectively plan treatment and make informed decisions about implant placement.

Bone integration with immediately loaded implants

Efforts to improve the integration of dental implants with bone are ongoing in many scientific circles, which are continually seeking new solutions and conducting further research. It is well-established that the human body develops from a single cell that multiplies and differentiates. These processes lead to the formation of tissues, organs, blood circulation, and the nervous system. The body's functions work seamlessly together. For instance, as early as three weeks after fertilization, the heart begins to beat and pump blood, making it the first complete organ to perform its function, even when it is barely visible. It is astonishing how precisely each step in the development of tissues and organs is regulated, and how harmoniously these steps are coordinated to support the organism's overall development.

Tissue engineering aims to replicate the natural processes that lead to the development of tissues. The key player in this process is the stem cell, which acts as the primary architect of all tissues and organs. Scientists strive to create specific conditions for these cells that mimic those present during normal development, thereby encouraging them to form the desired new tissue.

When installing an implant, the question arises as to how and in what way to encourage and provide specific conditions for the formation of specific new tissues. Is one of those specific conditions, in addition to technological processing, the way and time of loading the substitute organ compensated by the bioinert material titanium from which the implant is made. If you are trying to make implants from zirconium and ceramics, practice has confirmed the advantages of titanium. In addition to replacing a lost tooth, restoring function to other "participants" in the restoration process (bone and soft tissues) is a permanent issue of scientific circles in oral implantology. In order to create tissue in the laboratory or stimulate regeneration in the organism, the only way is to "imitate" what happens in nature.

In order to achieve complete bone integration between metal (titanium) as an inert material and bone tissue, a very living and dynamic material, exposed to constant changes, science continues to investigate which implant surface treatment technology best achieves the biological integration of the implant surface and bone. That is why many authors claim that the term osseointegration does not mean "bonding".

In order to achieve this connection as best as possible, an answer to the question is sought: how long should we wait for the integration processes between the installed implants and the

bone to take place, and has the final position been formed?

The attitudes of implantologists and scientists have changed over time. At first, after the installation of Linkov leaf endosseous implants, it was thought that you should wait only three weeks from the day of implant installation. At that time, the author of this book supported and applied that attitude in his practice. Loaded implants with temporary acrylic bridges gave good results. All those types of implants were made of one part: the part that goes into the bone and the support (abutment), on which the crown is placed.

After the installation of the Linkov leaf implants, it became clear that leaving them unloaded would be a significant mistake. The support above the maxillary ridge, which replaces the missing tooth, was susceptible to lingual and lateral forces, along with the moments generated by these forces during the healing phase. If these forces exerted pressure too early, they could negatively affect the installed implant. Additionally, macroglossia could exacerbate the impact of unfavorable lingual forces and their moments.

In a short period, these adverse forces could compromise the primary stability achieved initially, leading to loosening and potentially the loss of the implant even before it was loaded. For this reason, one-piece leaf implants were loaded immediately upon installation, resulting in considerable success for that implant system at the time. The author draws insights from these experiences, which may not be covered in many textbooks, and is based on personal observations and failures.

The success of the insertion of leafy Link implants was checked during the surgical procedure by the achieved primary stability. Good primary stability with leaf implants, due to the large surface area of the implant, was pronounced. The implant was hammered into the created implant bed. This was considered to be the foundation for a successful outcome. Newly created bone grew through the perforations left on the endosseous part of the implant, which gave the implant additional stability. The integration of the surface of the endosseous part and the bone was not thought of, nor could it be achieved with earlier implant designs and the technologies of the time. Long-term survival in the bone was ensured by the newly formed bone growing through the designed perforations of the implant.

Since primary fixation must not be compromised, it can be affected by the action of lingual forces and their moments in the case of leaf implants. For this reason, the primary stability of leaf implants is supported by precise temporary prosthetic work that loads the bone immediately. This approach is believed to promote the healing period and, through favorable physiological action, stimulate the remodeling and growth of new bone through the designed openings on the surface that is in contact with the bone. The assessment and experience of the implantologist are crucial in this process. These one-piece implants are inserted into the bone during a one-stage surgical procedure.

Later, the installation of two-phase leaf implants began, and the waiting time from installation to definitive prosthetic rehabilitation varied from case to case and according to the doctor's attitude and assessment. The assessment of when to load a one-piece implant was variable, and this was also true for two-piece implants. The waiting period varied from three to six months, and sometimes it was longer. There was no established attitude, nor valid statistical data.

However, the practical experience gained with the use of leaf implants has shown, provided that good primary stability has been achieved, that even today the established forms of two-part implants with new technologies for processing the surface of the implant body and neck, especially in the lateral regions, should be primarily loaded.

The rationale for immediate loading is illustrated by the use of one-piece mini-implants in edentulous lower jaws. When implants equipped with retention clips are loaded immediately, they significantly stabilize total acrylic prostheses, even those that the patient has used for an extended period.

One-piece implants come with various surface treatments and allow for adjustments in support without generating heat that could affect the implant body. The portion of the implant that remains above the bone level, which is used for soft tissue attachment in certain systems, is processed using laser-lock technology.

In the front part of the lower jaw, reinforcing uncomfortable and unstable total acrylic prostheses with implants that include retention clips has proven to be a beneficial solution. Integration can also be achieved by connecting two or more implants using Dolder or Ackerman crossbars fitted with riders. Additionally, Teflon resilient rings are used to absorb adverse forces, thus aiding the integration process. (See Figures 7.11 and 7.12).

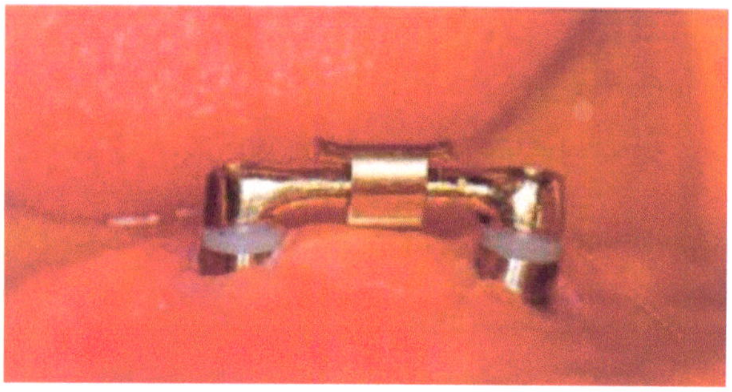

Figure 7.11. Dolder bar on two implants with retention-resilient riders and inserted Teflon rings.

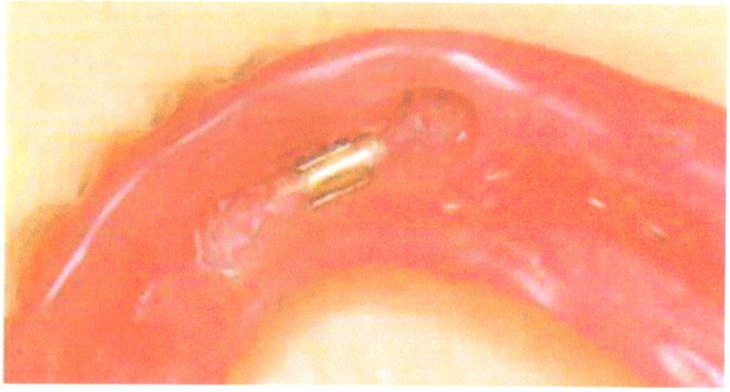

Figure 7.12. A rider embedded in the acrylic part of the prosthesis on two integrated implants connected by a Dolder bar.

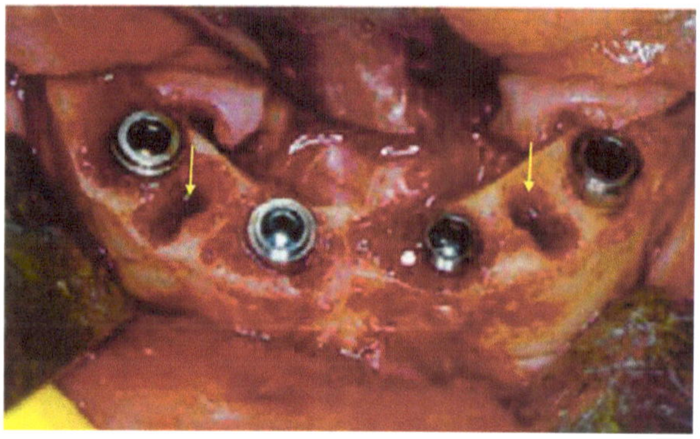

Figure 7.13. Replacement of diseased roots with implants embedded in a healthy part of the bone avoided the installation of implants in the alveoli of extracted teeth (yellow arrows).

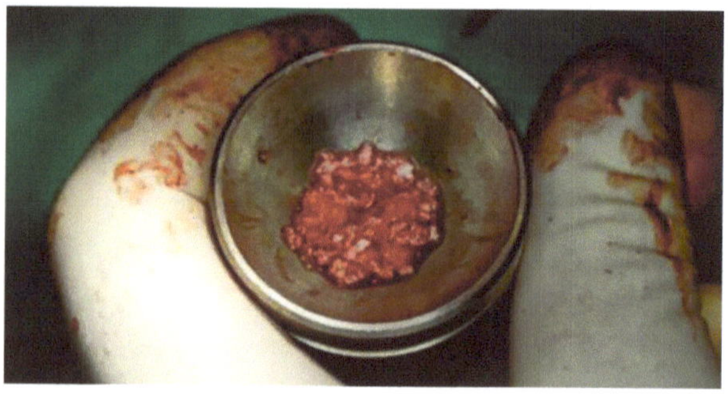

Figure 7.14. If immediate installation of the implant is planned after tooth extraction, it is necessary to preserve the alveolus. Assess whether there is bone resorption and to what extent and whether augmentation with a mixture of autologous bone and xenogeneic bone substitutes is required.

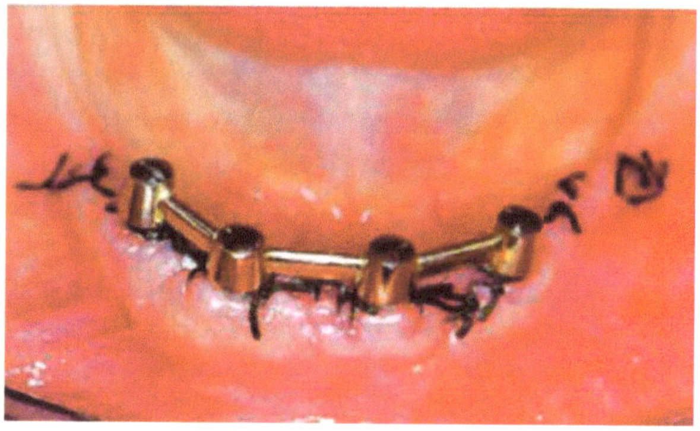

Figure 7.15. Dolder's crossbar worn on 4 implants (after soft tissue healing).

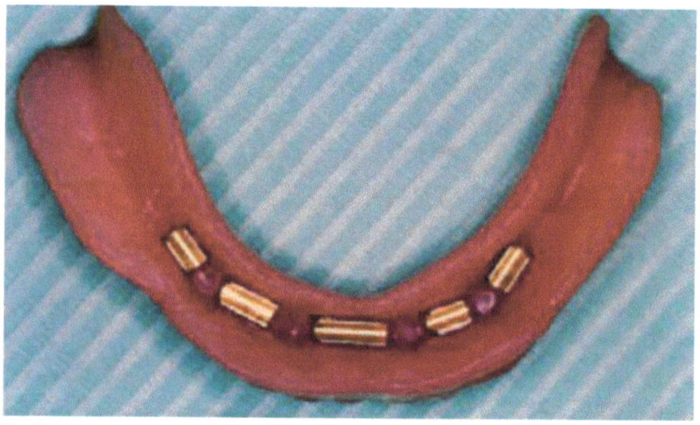

Figure 7.16. The most ideal solution is if there are conditions for the installation of four implants connected by a crossbar. Osseointegrated implants are a long-term solution for the stabilization of the lower total acrylic prosthesis.

Such a bar, on which special riders (clips) rest, fastens the movable and unstable total prosthesis, which until then "walked" in the patient's mouth. An anchored prosthesis, retained with buttons or crossbars, allows patients to bite off an apple.

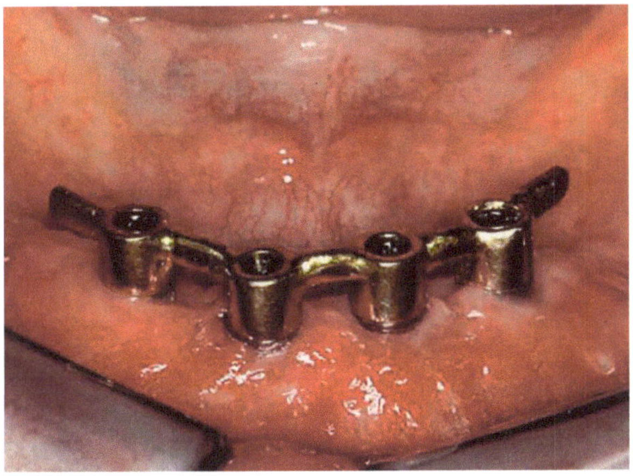

Figure 7.17. Case report after 5 years: successful bone integration, good oral hygiene - stable soft tissues.

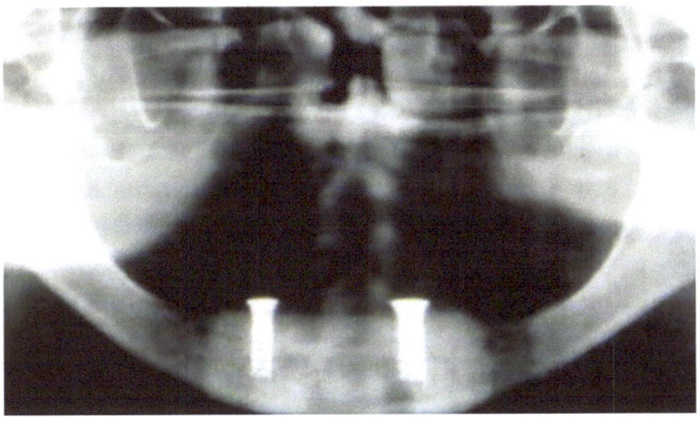

Figure 7.18. Two-part implants on which screw heads are visible, on which the retention matrix is placed, which is attached to the base of the acrylic prosthesis. The control image after 4 years shows a well-achieved bony integration in the frontal region of the lower jaw and the only possible implant-prosthetic solution, considering the extreme atrophy in the posterior regions.

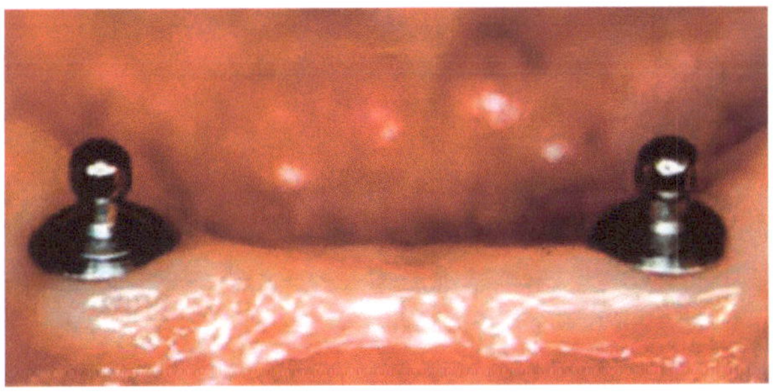

Figure 7.19. Endosseus (O-ball abutment) implants intended for stabilization of the lower total prosthesis. The design of the spherical heads enables the simultaneous retention-stabilization of the total acrylic prosthesis and resilient settling, promoting bone integration by the physiological stress of chewing forces and not jeopardizing the achieved one.

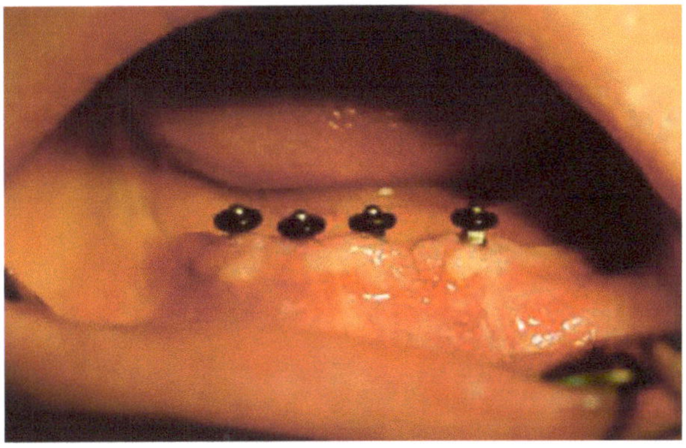

Figure 7.20. Rubber rings that enable resilient movements by amortizing the effect of forces on the implants, promoting bone integration by keeping the given forces within physiological limits.

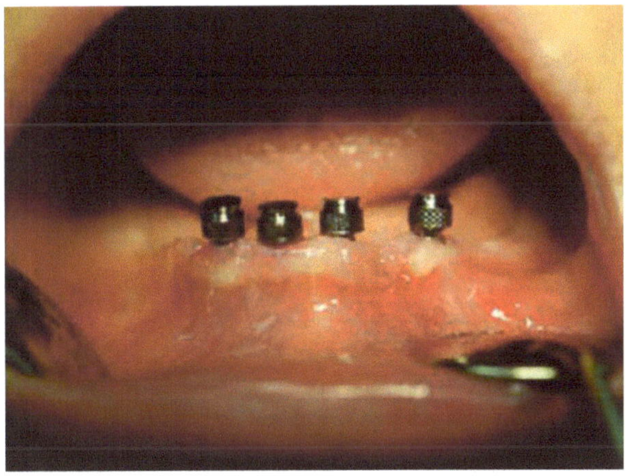

Figure 7.21. Appearance of retention clips on implants placed in the acrylic part of the prosthesis. Inserted elastic rings inside the retention clips (Figure 7.20) cushion the given chewing forces, thereby enhancing the osseointegration processes and protecting the achieved, which enables the biofunctionality of the implant.

Presentation of a case where good bony integration was achieved after immediate loading

The case that will be shown on the following pages is a very illustrative example of how the patient's wishes can be reconciled with a functionally maximally acceptable solution on immediately loaded implants. At the same time, the patient absolutely refused prosthetic rehabilitation with total acrylate prostheses upon arrival (Figure 7.22).

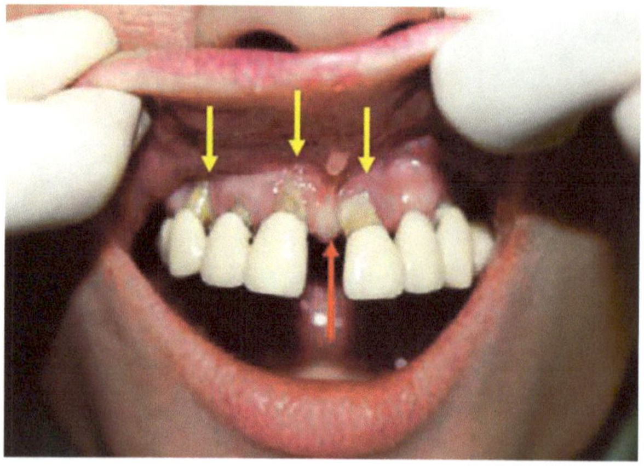

Figure 7.22. The first examination left a worrying impression (extreme recession and pathological root migration - yellow arrows). Maximally extruded teeth with frenulum to the middle of the ridge and a large diastema (red arrow).

Whenever a decision is made about the immediate installation of implants, the fulfillment of several prerequisites must be taken into account:

- The minimum length of the implant that is recommended for immediate installation and immediate loading, in accordance with prosthetic requirements, is 10 mm.
- The minimum diameter for immediate implantation by biomechanical and prosthetic requirements is 3.5 mm.
- The implant insertion torque must be at least 35 Ncm (35-55 Ncm).
- A lower torque (30 Ncm) can be tolerated provided that the implants are fixed with temporary prosthetic work.

The healing process begins from the moment the implant is inserted. The design characteristics and material quality of the dental implant have a decisive influence on the speed and quality of bone integration healing.

In this case, there were two possible treatment solutions:

The first solution involves augmenting the bone defects with a minimum healing period of at least six months for new bone formation. Following this, a two-phase delayed installation of the implant would be performed, with an additional wait of three to six months.

The treatment protocol would proceed as follows: First, the extraction of extruded teeth that are positioned outside the ridges would take place. Long-term periodontal disease has caused the destruction of the alveolar walls of the vestibular bone. After raising the flap, it is necessary to level the ridge, fill the bone defects with bone substitutes, and cover them with a collagen resorbable membrane. Once the flap is sutured and the implant is placed, the first phase of the surgical intervention would be complete. With the patient's consent, a temporary complete prosthesis may be created during this time. However, the drawback of wearing an immediate complete prosthesis during the healing period is the added pressure on the soft tissues and the augmented material.

After a waiting period of three to six weeks, the second stage of the surgical procedure will take place. During this stage, a circular incision is made to expose the implant caps, which will be replaced with components necessary for forming the gingival sulcus. This process once again requires some waiting time.

Once the gingival sulcus has formed, the healing abutments (also known as gingival formers) will be replaced with definitive abutments. An impression will then be taken and sent to the laboratory to prepare the planned prosthetic work. The definitive abutments will be adjusted in the lab to fit the mouth through a milling process, which involves fine-tuning their parallelism. After this adjustment, the modified abutments will be returned to the implants to establish the proper vertical dimension of the interjaw relationships.

Following this, the definitive abutments and caps will be reinserted to continue forming the gingival sulcus. It is important to note that the repeated removal and insertion of abutments can cause additional trauma to the peri-implant mucosal tissues, increasing the risk of irritation to the gingival sulcus and potential inflammation.

Throughout this process, a temporary upper total acrylic prosthesis is used, which can also affect the soft tissues. It is essential to emphasize that the procedures for removing and placing the abutments are repeated for all subsequent trials, further exposing the formed peri-implant tissues to iatrogenic swelling and the potential introduction of bacteria.

All this can jeopardize the aesthetic result, because the aesthetic result of the restoration depends on the condition and appearance of the soft tissues in the inter-implant spaces. Rehabilitation, in this way, significantly increases the cost of treatment.

Another treatment solution would consist in a complete change of the established protocol, due to shortening the time of the entire treatment procedure. The patient's wishes and impatience to have teeth as soon as possible were the main factors in thinking about how and by what method to achieve the set requirements. Due to the complexity of the case and the patient's requirements, the planning and treatment of the entire procedure is directed, contrary to the established protocol and theoretical recommendations, to the solution of two-phase implant placement.

Of course, all preliminary work: from the conversation and consultation with the patient, photographs as evidence of the condition from where it started, detailed anamnesis, initial analysis of the digital orthopantomographic image, analysis of the condition found on the plaster model, analysis of inter jaw relationships on the articulator and computerized 3D tomographic analysis, would remain unchanged in compared to the previously described protocol. The application of the stent would be absent, because due to the extreme pathological migration of the roots, it would have no purpose. All the bridges were removed from the plaster model, and the size and shape of the teeth were modeled using the wax-up method only as a guide so that the clinician, based on experience, would routinely assess where the implant should be installed, that is, how the axis of the implant should be directed and the parallelism of the support. The wax-up method also predicts future prosthetic work: the shape, size and position of the future artificial teeth, naturally coordinated with the color and harmony of the face.

However, in the presented patient, the protocol proceeded in the following order: after the removal of all bridges with pathologically extruded roots, the remains of granulation tissue were radically removed and the alveoli were preserved (Fig. 7. 23.)

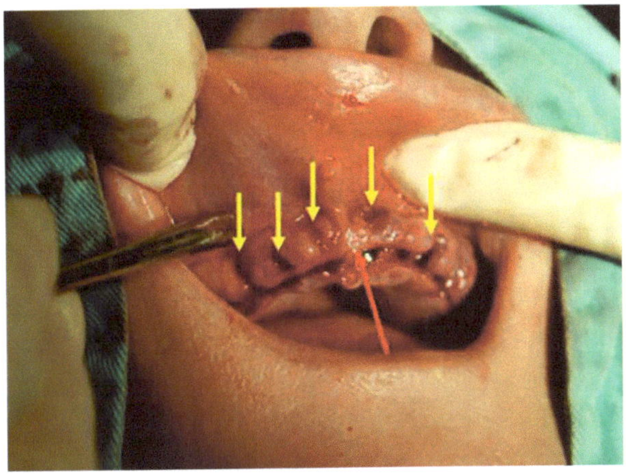

Figure 7.23. After placing the implant and shaping the alveolar arch with bone substitutes, the wounds of the extruded teeth were moved high into the fornix (indicated by yellow arrows), and a frenectomy was performed (red arrow).

Marking the position of the implant with a pilot drill and determining the direction of the bone preparation with a wider drill (2 mm) is the most important phase, not only of the surgical part of implant installation, but also of the entire implant-prosthetic treatment. It depends on the direction in which the row of seeds should be continued.

The alveoli, that is, the direction of the extracted roots could not serve as a landmark for the direction of bone preparation and the formation of the implant bed. Due to the long-term pathological migration of the natural roots, the bony lamellae of the alveoli are destroyed, whether it is the labial or buccal lamellae. In this case, there was a good amount of apical cortical bone above the tip of the migrated roots, as determined by computed tomography. The apical part of the skeleton mustn't be smaller than 2.5 mm.

So, marking with a pilot drill is the initial determination of the position of the implant as a replacement for the central incisors. The direction of the bone preparation is directed more towards the palatal and towards the mesial, due to the large diastema that existed, with a particularly strong frenulum. The spacing of the central incisors is increased by extreme pathological migration. Repair of the frenulum was necessary during the procedure. Previously, the position of the future artificial teeth was determined by the waxup method and this virtual indicator was used as a guideline for implant positioning. For this reason, the surgical procedure of installing the implant started from the central incisors, which is of crucial aesthetic importance due to the visual exposure of that part.

By marking the position of the bone with a pilot drill, bone preparation continued, while increasing the diameter of the drill (pilot drill, 2 mm, 2.3 mm, 3 mm and 3.2 mm), depending on the chosen diameter and length of the implant, determined on the basis of computed tomography indicators. The last drill must be narrower than the diameter of the implant, and how many millimeters the bone preparation should be continued depends on the evaluation of the bone quality. The use of a thread, experience shows, should be applied only at the beginning in the cortical part of the bone, up to 2 mm at most. Pay maximum attention to avoid overheating the bone. Continue the preparation with frequent interruptions with abundant cooling with physiological solution during preparation with drills of various sizes. Adjusting the rotation speed of the drill during bone preparation is extremely important in order not to overheat the bone. It is mandatory to place parallelism indicators in the prepared canals because achieving primary stability and establishing the parallelism of the supports are the foundations of both function and aesthetics, especially in the frontal region of the upper jaw.

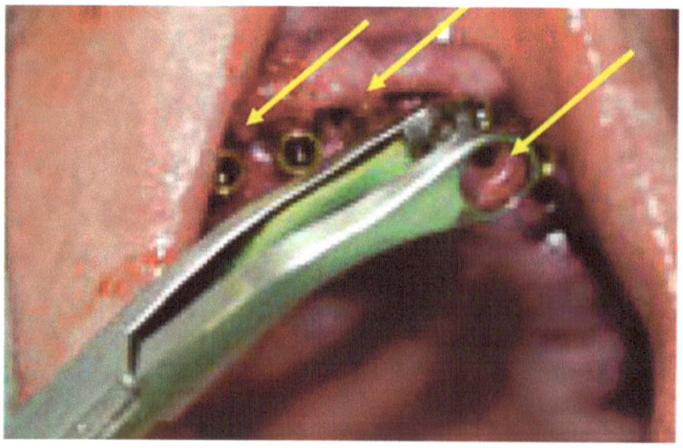

Figure 7.24. Special instrument with which the gingiva and interdental papilla are formed during the surgical procedure.

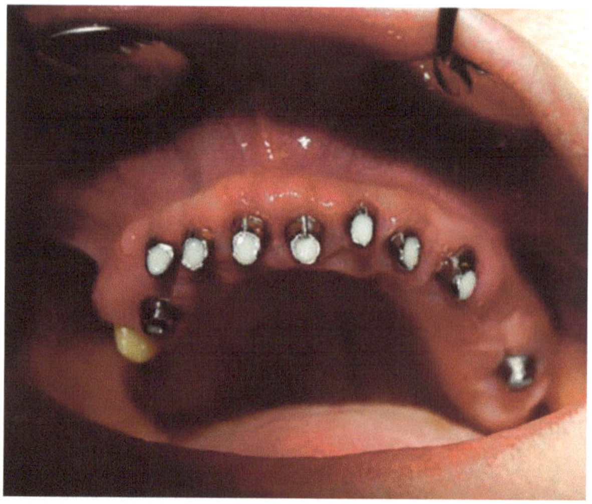

Figure 7.25. Condition after 3 months. At the same time: frenectomy, installation of implants, placement of definitive supports (instead of healing caps), formation of papillae and temporary prosthetic work.

Recently, several authors, including D. Tarnau and Salama et al., have suggested that the gingiva maintains a better shape around a definitive support (or abutment) that is tightened using a torque wrench. This method helps to avoid unscrewing and rescrewing the screw, which can create micro-cracks between the implant and the gingival former. Such micro-cracks can serve as sites for bacterial accumulation, increasing the risk of peri-implantitis.

After all the planned implants were installed, the abutments were tightened with a torque of up to 35 N, confirming the achieved primary stability. Using a special instrument (Fig. 7.24), the inter-implant mucosal tissues were shaped, and any destroyed papillae were restored. Subsequently, bone defects were augmented while simultaneously shaping the arch of the alveolar ridge.

Due to the mesial displacement of the implant bed for the central incisors, the distal parts of the alveoli—filled with coagulum—needed to be augmented with bone substitutes and covered with a resorbable collagen membrane. By gently compressing the sutured flap, the alveolar arch could be trimmed at the sites of the bone defects.

After that, an alginate print was taken for an immediate provisional fixed restoration. The situation after three months is shown in Figure 7.25.

When considering the complexity of the case and the patient's requirements, the question arises, which parameters determined the protocol for planning implant prosthetic treatment procedures?

One can never, based on one parameter, approach planning and any quality solution when it comes to the installation of implants. To solve the presented case, several parameters were needed in order to avoid an unwanted risk.

A significantly altered position of the teeth, with extreme migration in the upper jaw, with teeth outside the arch of the alveolar ridge of the upper jaw indicated extractions of loose teeth.

The patient wanted to have teeth as soon as possible due to professional obligations, refusing a mobile total prosthesis at all costs due to the urge to vomit.

Long-term torture with a mobile acrylate prosthesis in the lower jaw, which was retained with a wire hook for a loose tooth, caused the patient's refusal to have another unpleasant prosthesis in her mouth, despite the explanation that it was a temporary solution (pictures 7.55 and 7.56).

The case is complex for the following reasons:

- The labial bone lamella of the upper front is destroyed;
- High aesthetic demands of the patient;
- Due to the complete resorption of the labial and buccal bone lamellae, the arch of the alveolar ridge is destroyed;
- In the highly aesthetic region of the upper jaw, there was a risk that the bone support, crucial for the formation of soft tissues, was greatly weakened. The amount of bone and the distance from the papilla depended on the regeneration of the papilla, as well as the quality of the formation of the gingival sulcus around the support;
- Disturbed interjaw relationships are major risk factors for the success of the entire procedure.

The summary of the oral surgical-prosthetic intervention of the presented case, if it were performed according to the established protocol, would flow in the following order.

After the extraction of the extruded teeth, the wounds in the alveolar ridge were left exposed (see Figure 7.23). The augmentation procedure involved leveling the alveolar ridge by filling the bone defects with a combination of bone substitutes and autologous bone chips. To achieve an optimal aesthetic and functional outcome, the damaged arches of the alveolar ridges in both jaws needed to be reshaped. Throughout these procedures, the use of resorbable collagen membranes was essential. After covering the area with a flap and suturing it, we needed to wait 7 to 8 days for the stitches to be removed.

The next stage in the process involved fabricating immediate total dentures. However, the patient had struggled for years with a lower partial denture, which was retained by a single remaining tooth. This discomfort motivated him to seek the comfort of implant placement. Even though he agreed to wear total acrylic dentures, the transition from taking impressions to placing temporary total dentures on the unhealed soft tissues would pose additional trauma. Chewing with the prosthesis would compress it, altering the shape of the alveolar ridge.

It is clear that implementing this solution would necessitate a waiting period of more than 6 to 8 months to ensure that the bone was fully restored and stabilized before the installation of the implant.

From the point of view of the previous theoretical recommendations, the continuation of the protocol would be carried out in the following order: planning the implantation of the implant by computer tomography analysis, application of the wax-up procedure, determination of the position of the implant by the application of the stent, re-elevation of the flap, installation of the implant (in the marked places using the fabricated stent), placement of the caps for healing, suturing the flap. After removing the sutures, the waiting period for soft tissue healing and integration of the implant would continue for at least 3 months. During that time, the patient would continue to use total braces that would compress the bone and surrounding tissues. Then another surgical procedure would follow: uncovering the healing caps and replacing them with caps (healing abutment) to form a gingival sulcus around the neck of the implant and the support (abutment) of the prosthetic construction. If the prostheses would not fit well due to the changed conditions (leaving caps for the formation of gingiva), they should be supported. If it would not be possible to adapt the prosthetic plate to the placed gingival formers, direct underlayment in mouth would be a big mistake. Making a new temporary prosthesis would require repeating the entire prosthetic procedure (impressions, determination of interjaw relationships, tooth test, adjustment of occlusion, decubitus), which would be additional trauma to the bone and soft tissues, with additional cost. Taking an impression for definitive prosthetic work would require multiple repetitions of stages: removing the caps to form the gingiva and reinserting the definitive supports. After the impression was taken, the stages of prosthetic work would be repeated several times. So, during the production of prosthetic work, the soft tissues would be exposed to trauma several times; trial of metal structures and ceramic bridges, removal and insertion of caps for the formation of gingiva and supports. Plastic (teflon) supports are used to avoid trauma to soft tissues by removing and placing the supports, which is an additional cost for the patient.

The conclusion is that the choice of implantology therapy protocol was influenced by the patient's desire to have teeth as soon as possible, along with their explicit refusal to wear a total prosthesis. As such, the implant-prosthetic treatment plan should have been tailored to achieve bone integration through alternative methods. Given the complexity of the case, the outcome relied heavily on thorough planning and careful consideration of all risk factors. Ultimately, the success of each solution depends on the foundation upon which it is built.

Relying only on the orthopantomographic image can give a false spatial impression, and prevent good initial planning and the start of the implant-prosthetic procedure. Also, the check of augmentation after a certain time must be performed based on a computerized tomography, because there is no insight into the volume of the bone on the orthopantomographic image. Computed tomography gives a realistic image of where and how the ridge was really augmented. (see also chapter 12 - "The future of diagnostics"). Taking into account the above, the authors (B. Zlopaša and T. Zlopaša) realized the metho dom of immediate installation of implants with immediate loading according to the set plan of the entire treatment. At the same time, bone defects were filled, by shaping the ridge and alveolar arch with bone substitutes mixed with autologous bone, which was covered with a collagen resorptive membrane.

The course of treatment in the upper jaw is explained in pictures 7.32 to 7-53.

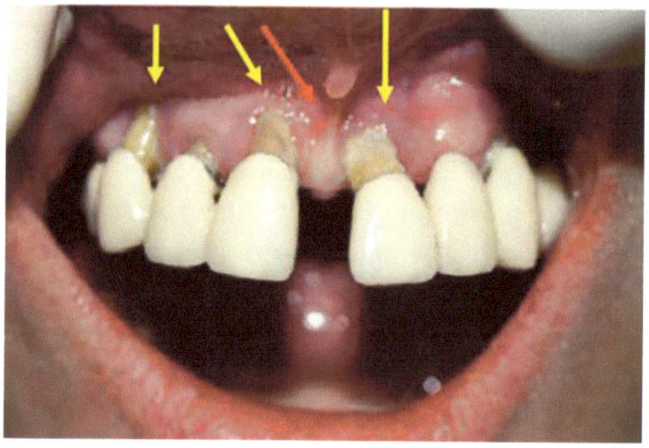

Figure 7.26. Low inserted frenulum, root positions and destroyed buccal lamella are the factors that direct the plan of the entire implant-prosthetic treatment.

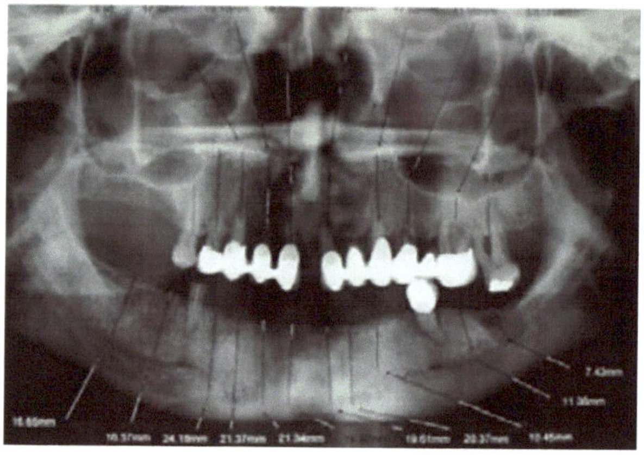

Figure 7.27. Computed tomographic representation of the resolved case of both jaws.

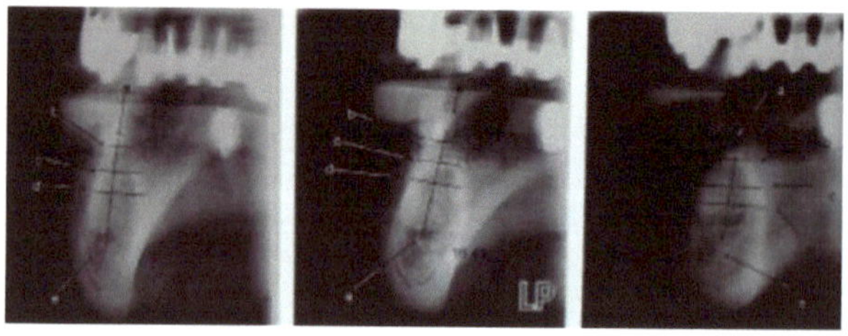

Figure 7.28. Computed tomographic image of the dimensions of the available bone, on the basis of which the implant-prosthetic treatment plan is set.

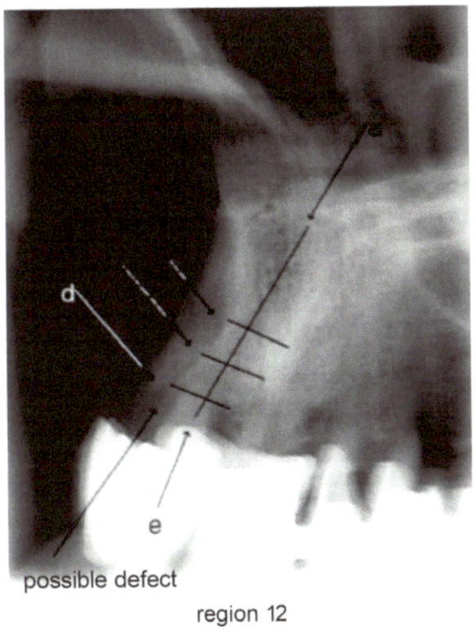

Figure 7.29. Tomographic analysis, cross section of vertical and horizontal alveolar bone, dimensions of the 12-alveolar ridge region for selection and positioning of implants.

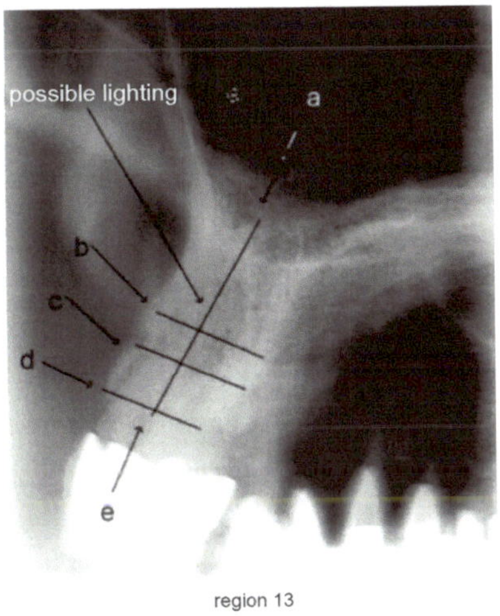

Figure 7.30. Radiological 3D analysis of region #13 does not confirm the details, but marks them as "possible".

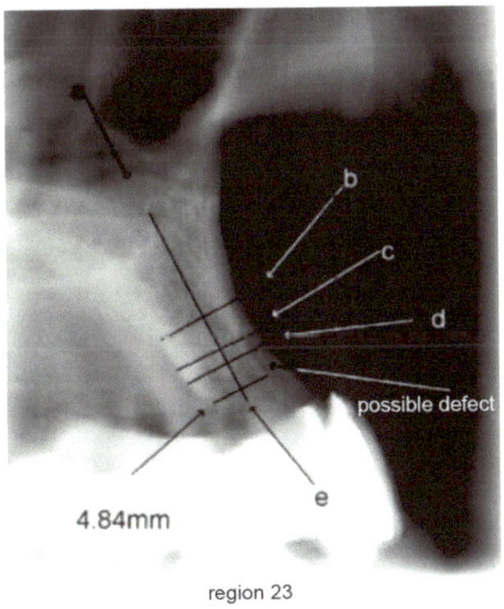

Figure 7.31. 3D analysis of region 23 indicates a "possible" defect - the actual condition is determined by a surgical procedure.

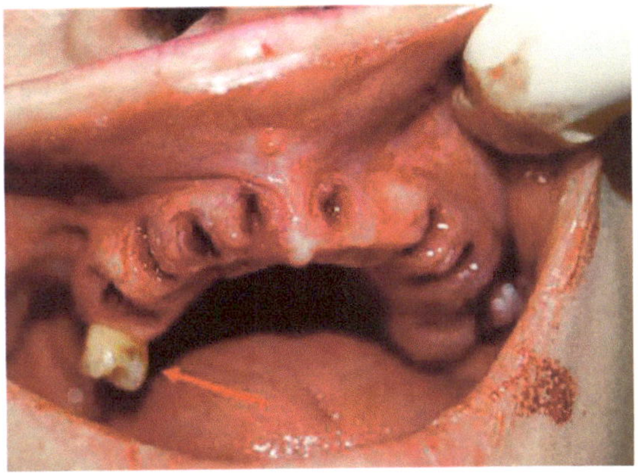

Figure 7.32. All loosened teeth were removed, a solid premolar was left in order to avoid, in this case, an unnecessary and lengthy procedure of raising the sinus floor, which is also the patient's request.

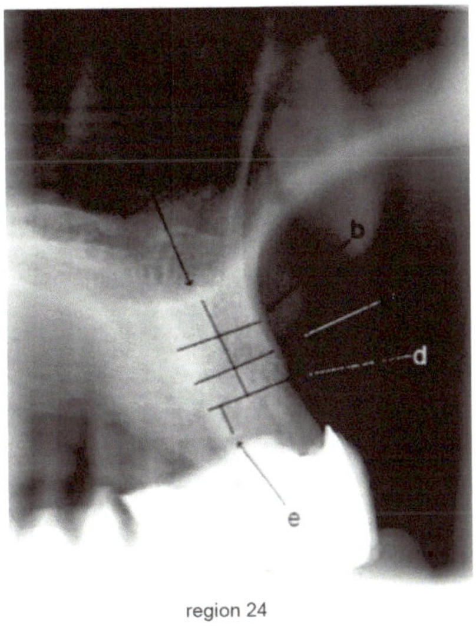

Figure 7.33. 3D analysis determines the choice of implant dimensions (diameter and length).

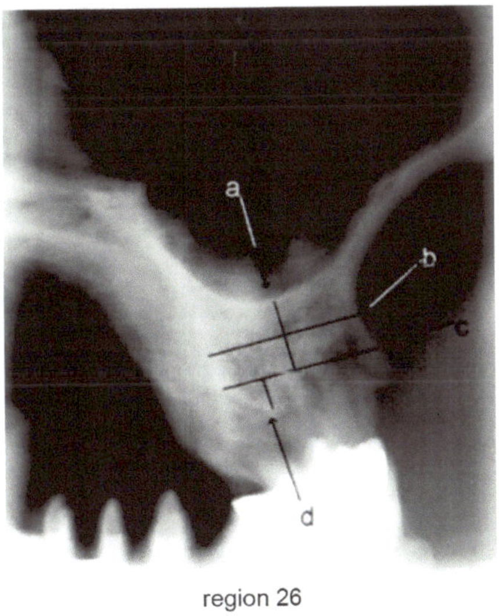

Figure 7.34. 3D analysis of region 26 suggests the choice of the widest diameter implant.

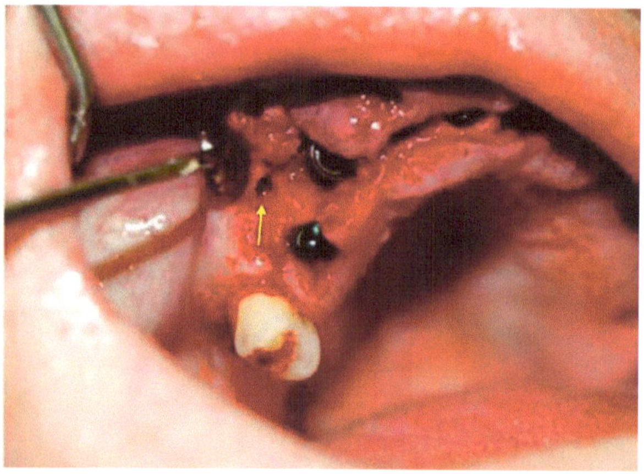

Figure 7.35. Aesthetic risk, the position of removed pathologically migrated teeth in the fornix can be seen. A strong frenulum extends from the middle of the ridge - frenectomy performed. The course of treatment depends on the degree of primary stability achieved. The installation of the implant was started by marking the position of the implant at the place of the central incisors (11,12). The implant at the position of the first premolar (14) is placed in the compact part of the bone towards the palatine. Completely destroyed buccal wall of the first premolar (you can see the position of the buccal root - yellow arrow). In order to achieve good primary stability, it was necessary to shape the arch of the alveolar ridge by augmentation with bone substitutes mixed with autologous bone, and to position the implant more palatally.

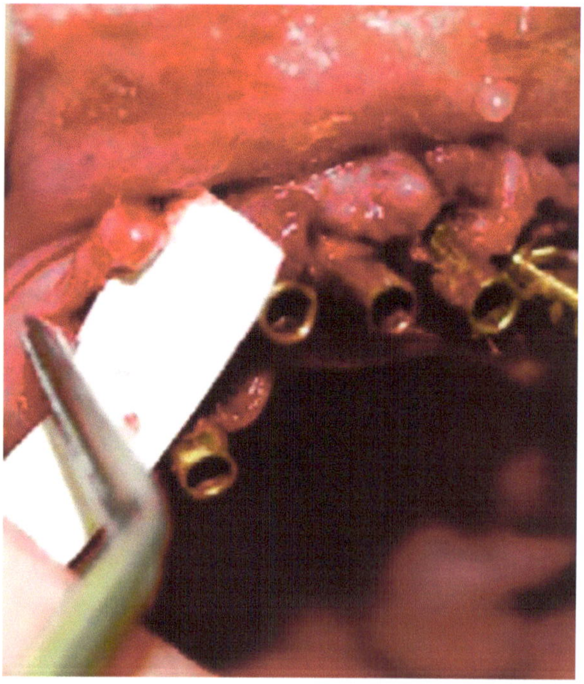

Figure 7.36. Shaping of the alveolar crest with bone substitutes with simultaneously placed definitive supports (abutments), instead of healing caps, enables faster, better and more correct formation of the peri-implant mucosa.

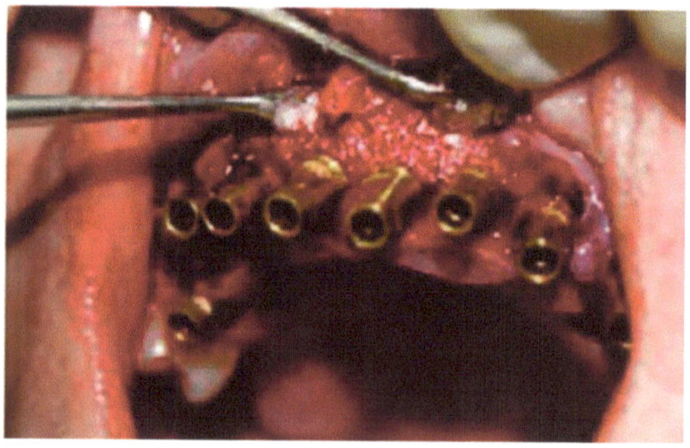

Figure 7.37. Placement of collagen resorbable membrane over augmented material - bone substitute.

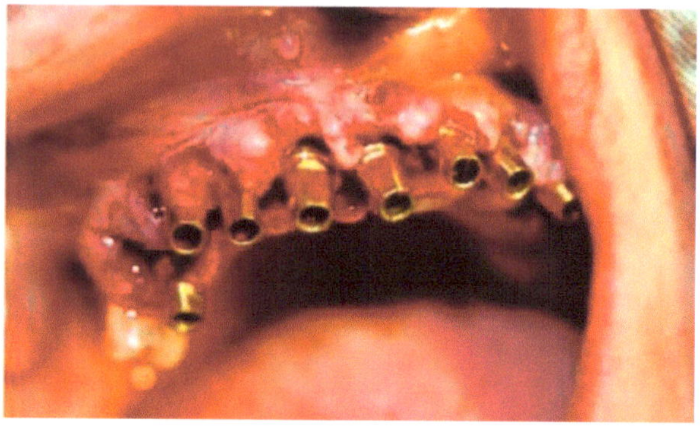

Figure 7.38 illustrates that healing and the formation of peri-implant soft tissues and papillae around definitive supports (abutments) is preferable to using caps for healing and covering the implants. The use of caps requires reopening the surgical incision, which means revealing and positioning the components necessary for the formation of the gingival sulcus. This not only prolongs the treatment process—since the screw must be removed and replaced on the abutment—but also increases the risk of subsequent infections in the microcrack between the implant and the support. This viewpoint is based on the author's experience.

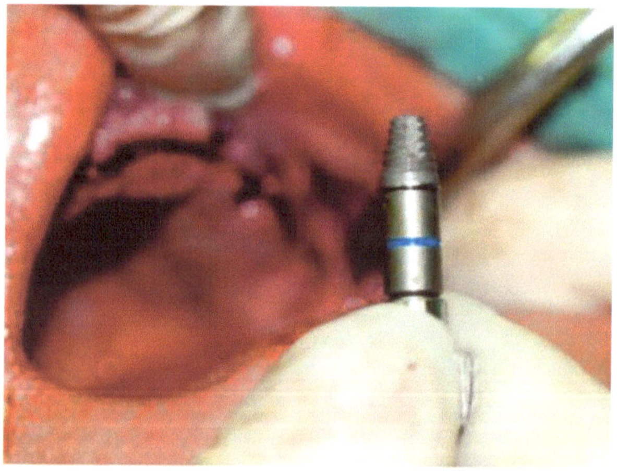

Figure 7.39. Implant with a wide diameter of 6.25 mm, length 10 mm.

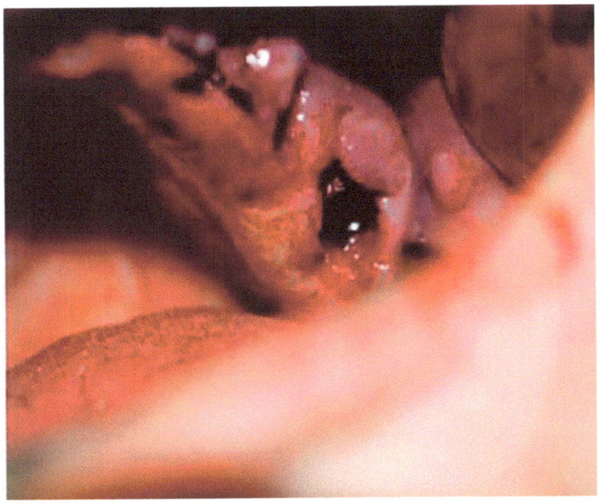

Figure 7.40. The implanted "spare" implant of the widest diameter (6.25 mm.) The quality of the cancellous bone walls (D4) required supplementation with a bone substitute and the application of a resorbable membrane. Delayed healing and weight bearing required after 6 months.

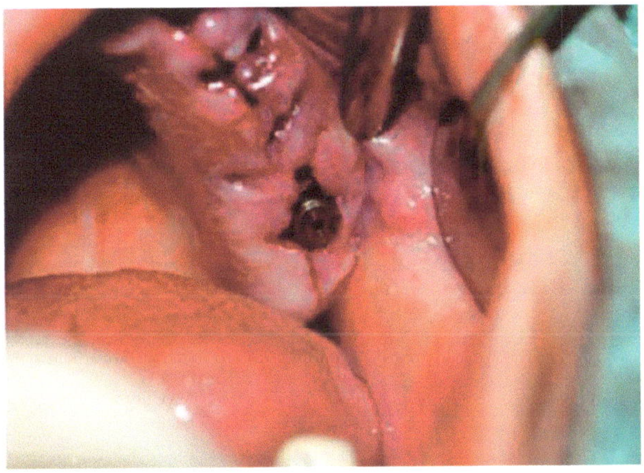

Figure 7.41. A wide-diameter implant installed in the lateral region with a gingiva-former in place. The assessment is that it is not immediately burdensome.

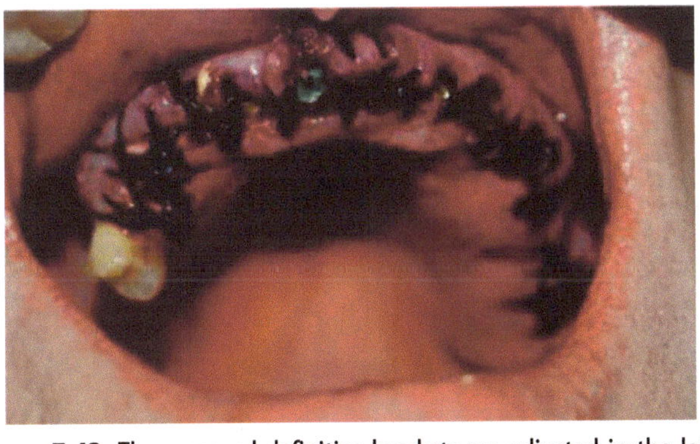

Figure 7.42. The removed definitive brackets are adjusted in the laboratory and a provisional prosthetic work is made on them (acrylate on a metal base). The arch of the alveolar ridge was formed by augmentation.

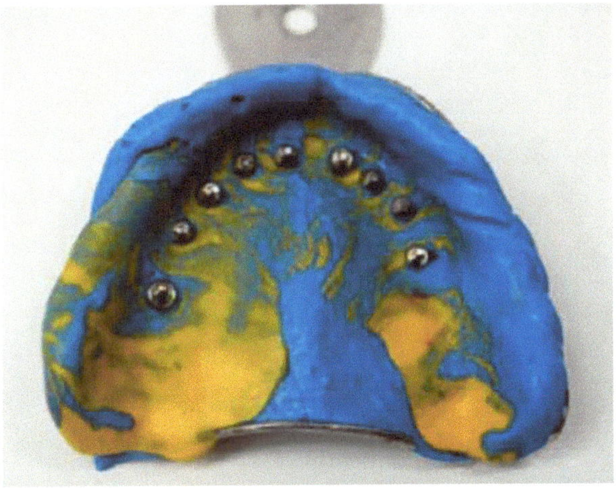

Figure 7.43. Transfers for transferring the position of the implant enable the precise transfer of the position of the abutment (support) to the plaster model (Figure 7.45).

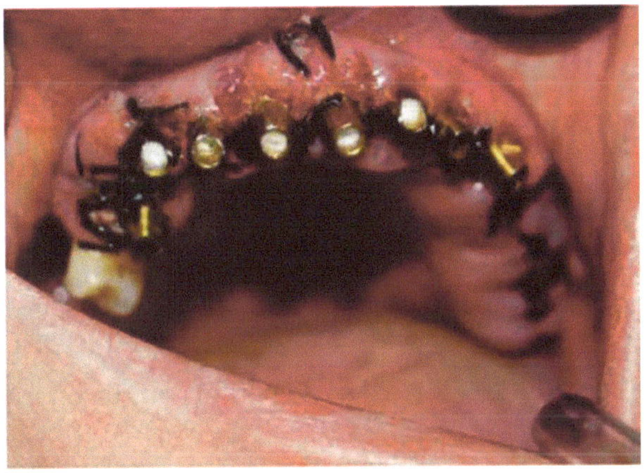

Figure 7.44 shows the brackets after laboratory processing, which involves adjusting their parallelism, shortening, and shaping the frontal part. Once the adjustments are made in the laboratory, the brackets are returned as prosthetic supports for both the provlslonal and future definitive superstructures.

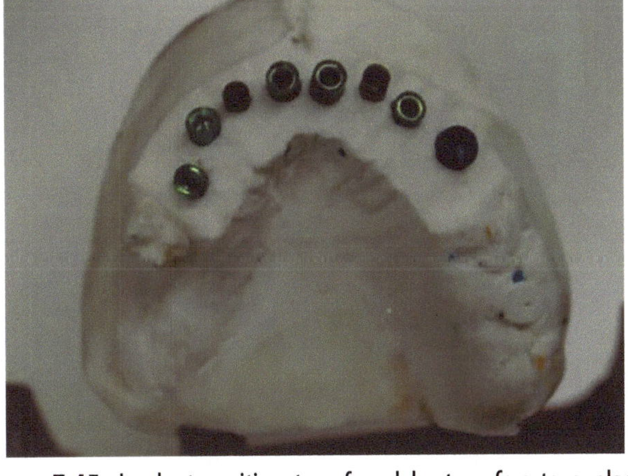

Figure 7.45. Implant position transferred by transfers to a plaster model for making a provisional bridge.

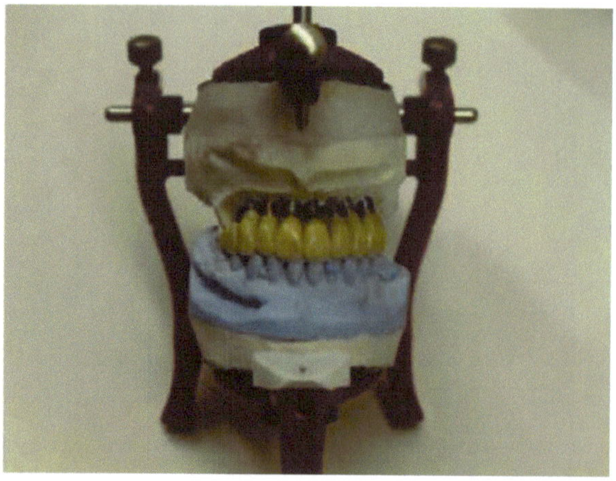

Figure 7.46. The provisional restoration must be performed precisely, especially in the neck area, in order not to compromise the healing of the soft tissues. Pay special attention to the establishment of occlusion and remove any existing premature contacts on certain parts of the temporary prosthetic work.

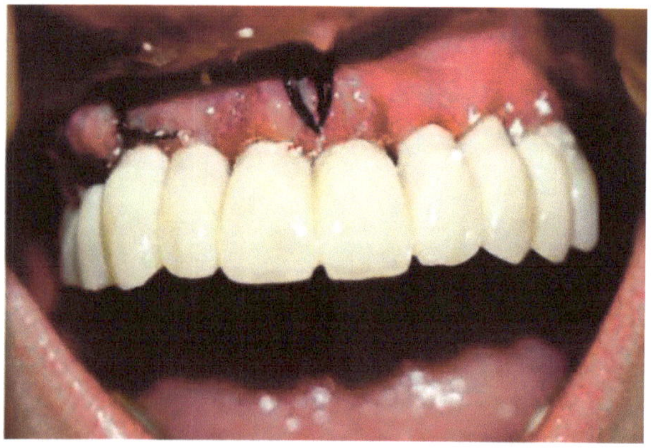

Figure 7.47. A fixed temporary bridge in acrylate placed immediately after implantation. The appearance of the original fixed prosthetic work 7 days after the installation of the implant (seams are still visible). The patient is an avid smoker, which can be seen in the temporary prosthetic work (Figure 7.48).

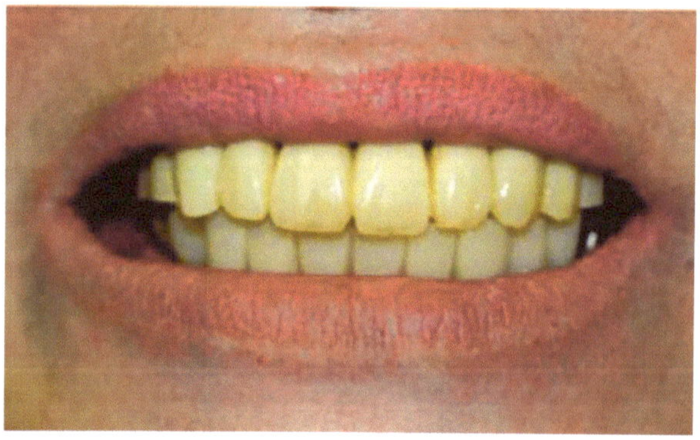

Figure 7.48. The patient's requests to enable the optimal performance of professional duties (lawyer) were met, and the fixed temporary bridges in both jaws enabled the acquisition of self-confidence and security of communication. Compare the appearance of the provisional bridge with the conditions in pictures 7.32 to 7.38.

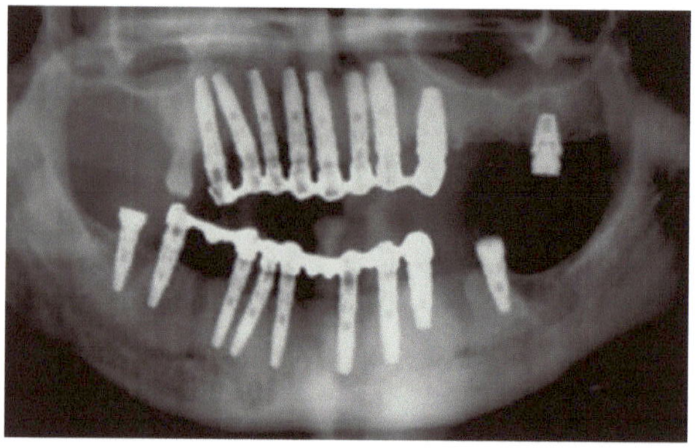

Figure 7.49. Control shot immediately after immediate loading with temporary acrylic bridges on a metal base. Due to the evaluation of the bone quality during implant installation (below 25 N - insufficient primary stability), the implant in the lateral region is not immediately loaded. A longer period is needed to achieve good integration.

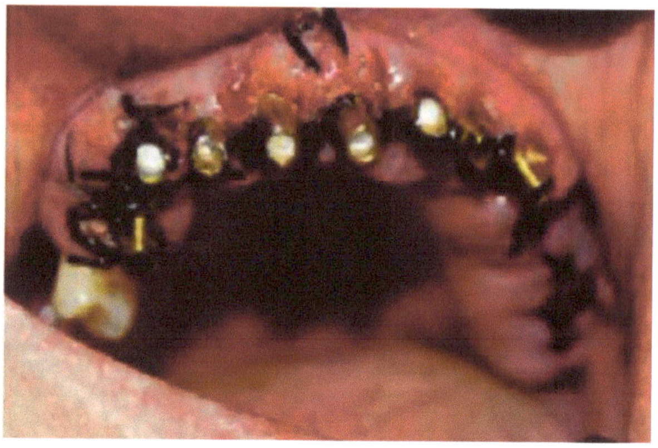

Figure 7.50. Preparation for primary loading by making a precise provisional bridge. At the position of the first premolar on the right, augmentation was performed with autologous bone mixed with xenogeneic granulate and covered with a collagen resorptive membrane.

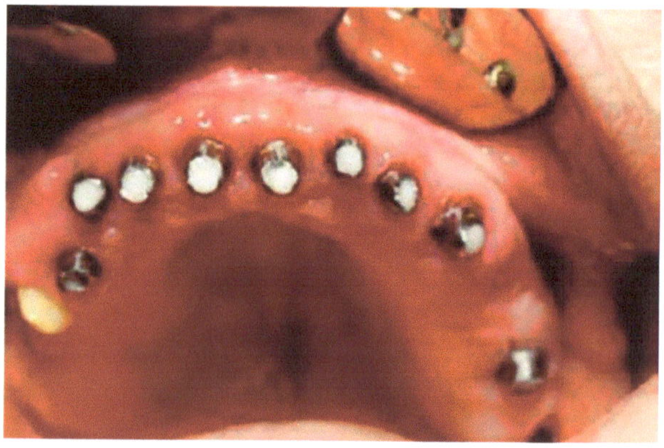

Figure 7.51. Appearance of the alveolar arch shaped by augmentation after 6 months, with primarily loaded and well integrated implants. At the position of region 14, due to the destroyed vestibular alveolar bone, the implant is positioned more palatally, which was corrected by prosthetic work.

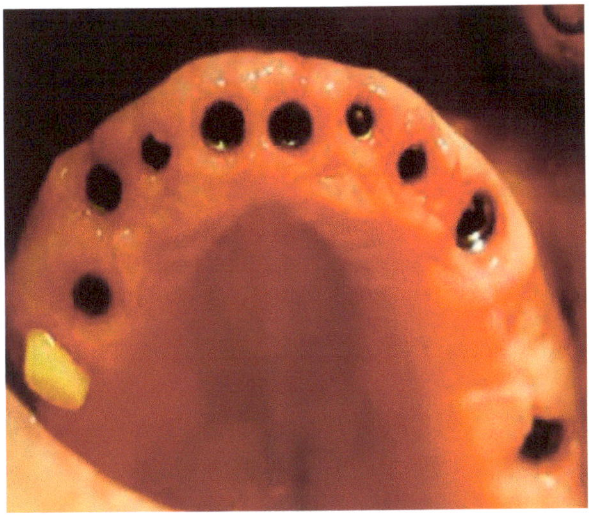

Figure 7.52. The appearance of an arch formed by augmentation, with formed gingival sulci around definitive supports. Appearance of the peri-implant mucosa (absence of inflammation) with an inter-implant formed papilla.

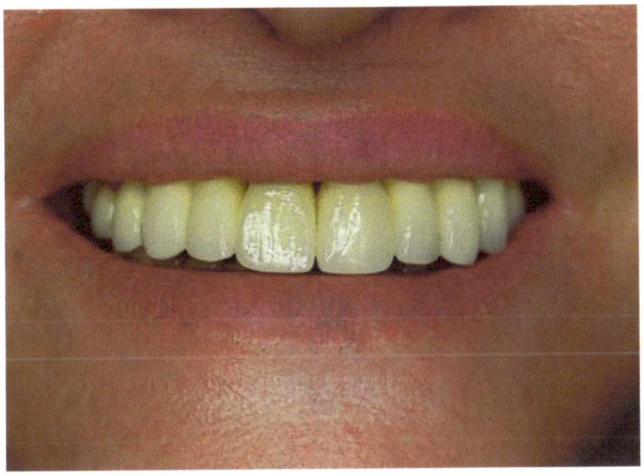

Figure 7.53. A successful functional and aesthetic result of an extremely complex case. (Compare with Figures 7.26 to 7.48).

Immediate installation of implants in the lower jaw in the same patient

In the same patient, the procedure protocol required a different approach in the lower jaw than the one used in the upper jaw.

Tomography showed favorable basic parameters for implant installation, i.e. sufficient horizontal dimension and height of the alveolar bone (pictures 7.54 and 7.57). The advantage of the available bone, the shape and arch of the alveolar ridge dictated the implant installation procedure. Unlike the procedure in the upper jaw, where it was necessary to fill bone defects with augmentation, shape the alveolar arch of the ridge, and raise the flap, in this case, it could be avoided. The sufficiency of the available bone in all three dimensions made it possible to use implants of standard diameters and maximum lengths. In addition, by avoiding raising the flap, trauma to the soft tissues was reduced, thus creating the conditions for faster integration.

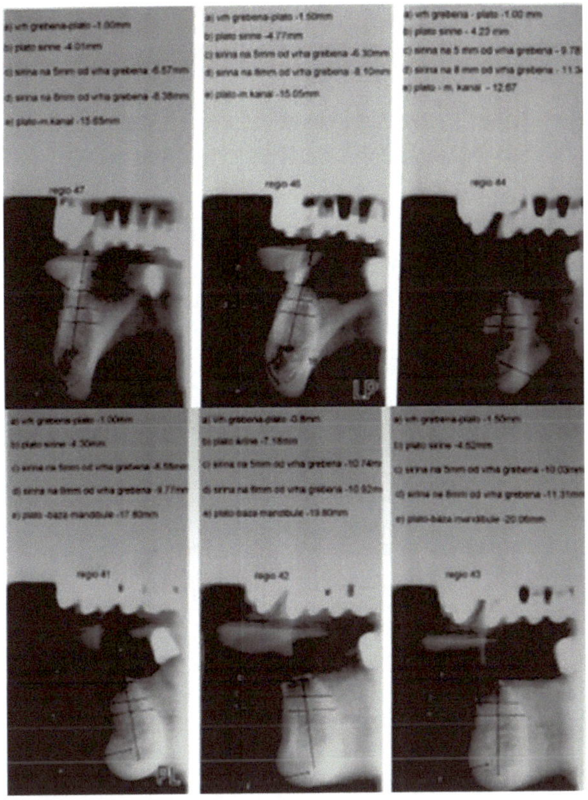

Figure 7.54. The measured sections of the alveolar ridge in the upper and lower jaw determine the length and diameter of the implant.

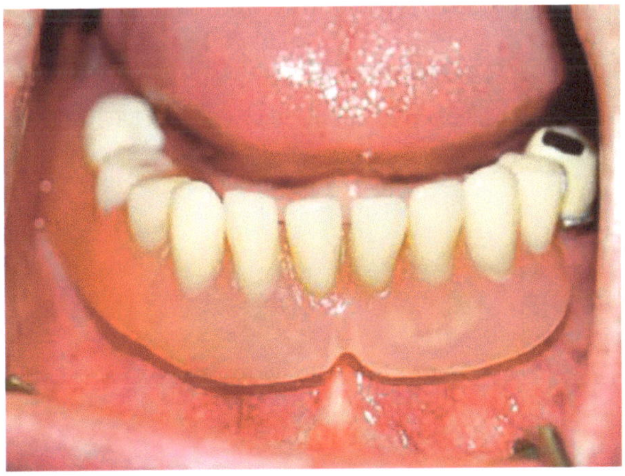

Figure 7.55. After the loss of teeth, through periodic and partial removal of bridges and extraction of teeth in the lower jaw, the practicing dentist, at one time, decided on an uncomfortable solution with a partial prosthesis, which the patient had been using for several previous years.

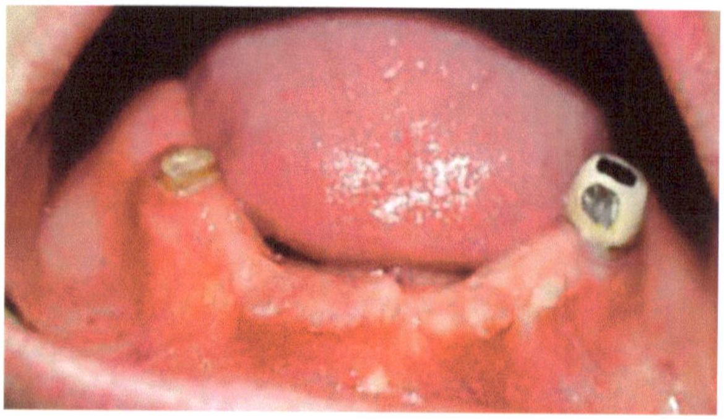

Figure 7.56. The remaining premolars were cut from the bridge, for which an acrylic prosthesis was retained with wire hooks.

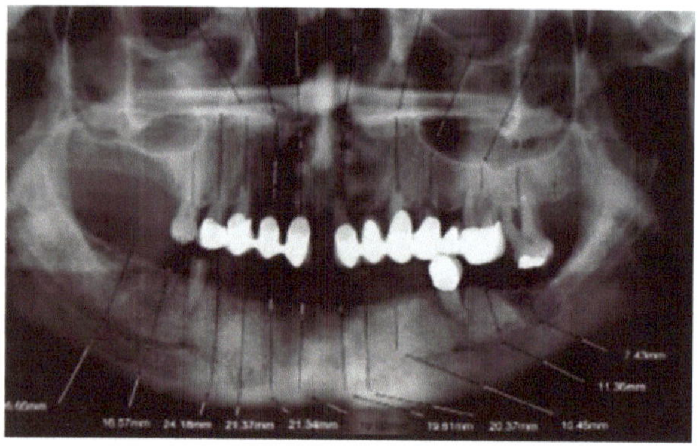

Figure 7.57. Results obtained by tomographic analysis in relation to anatomical structures.

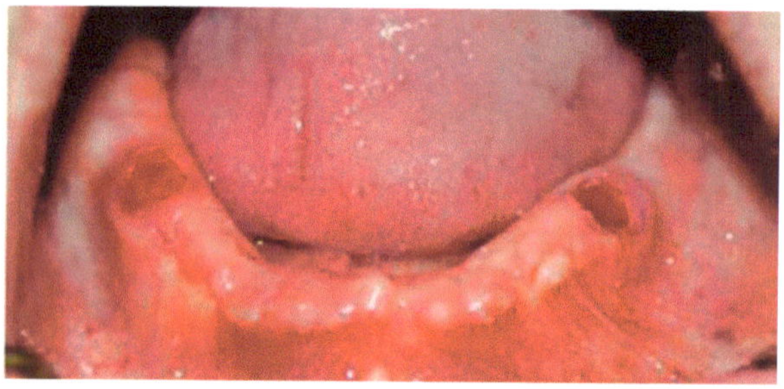

Figure 7.58. Presentation of the condition after extraction of loosened teeth. Express request of the patient - not accepting a total acrylate prosthesis even as a temporary solution.

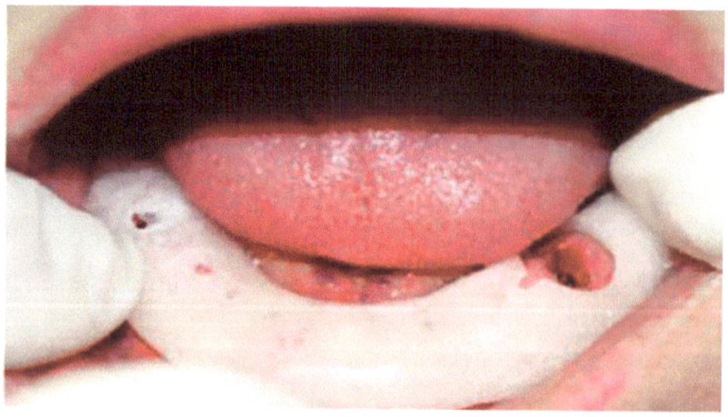

Figure 7.59. Previously, the appearance of the future prosthetic work was modeled in wax on the plaster model of the lower jaw, and based on the position of the teeth, the position of the implant was determined, marked on the stent.

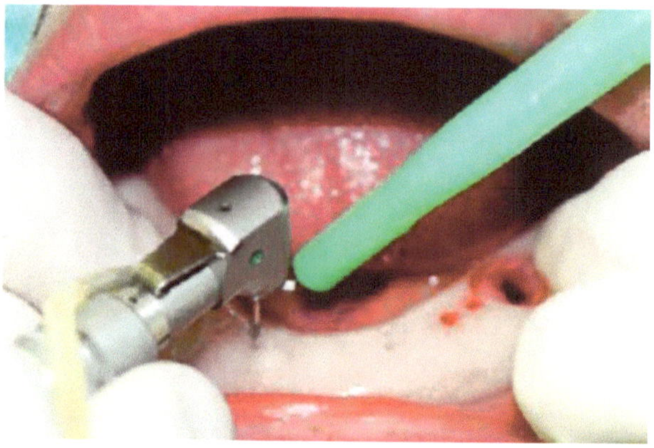

Figure 7.60. Marking the position for installing the implant with a pilot drill.

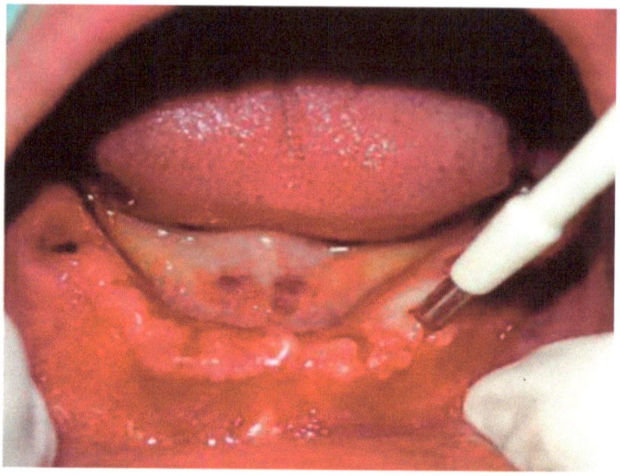

Figure 7.61. Plugs of mucosal tissue removed by suturing with a special instrument can be used simultaneously as a graft in places where there is a lack of soft tissue.

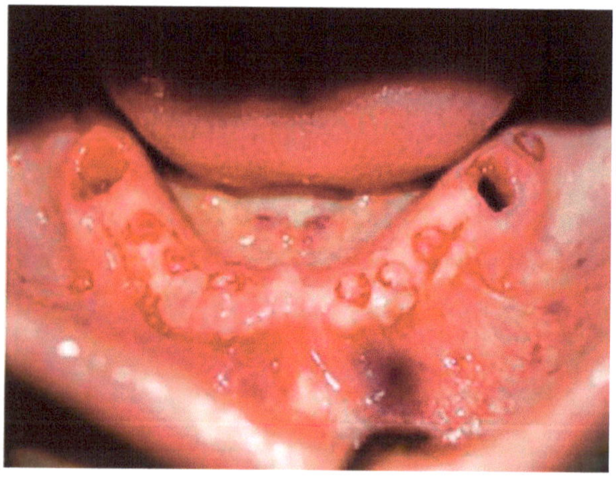

Figure 7.62. After a detailed tomographic analysis and wax-up performance, the position of the implant was determined.

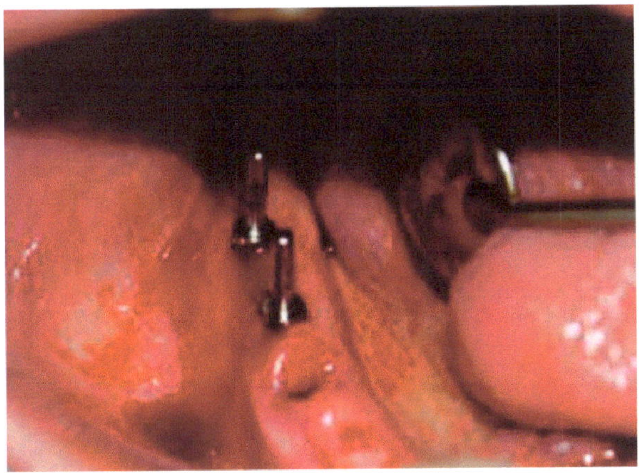

Figure 7.63. Control of the paralysis of the implant tray.

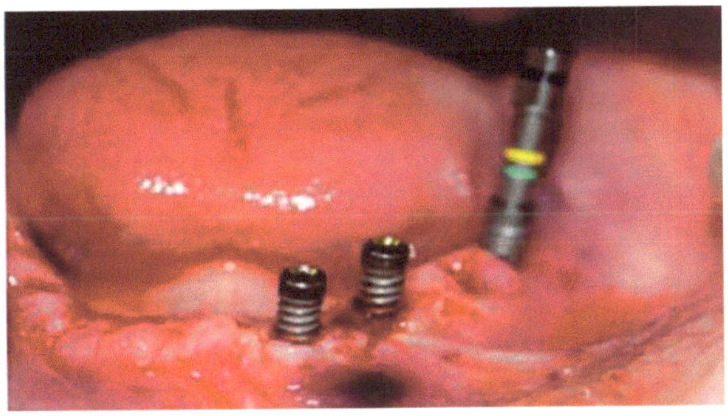

Figure 7.64. In the lower jaw, after a detailed tomographic analysis, it was estimated that the installation of the implant can be performed without raising the flap. Implant placement started in the frontal region by predicting the aesthetic outcome.

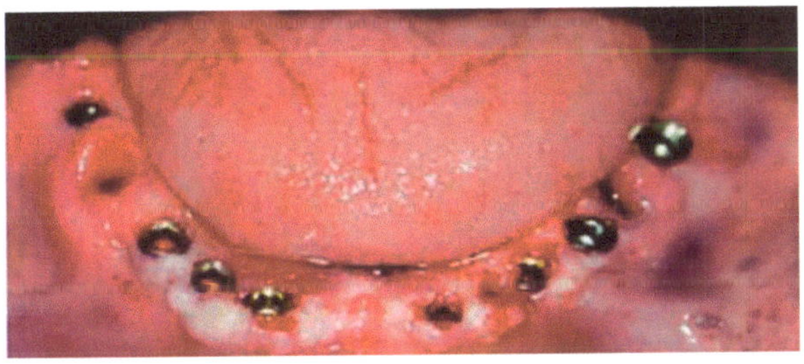

Figure 7.65. Implants are not inserted into the alveoli of extracted teeth.

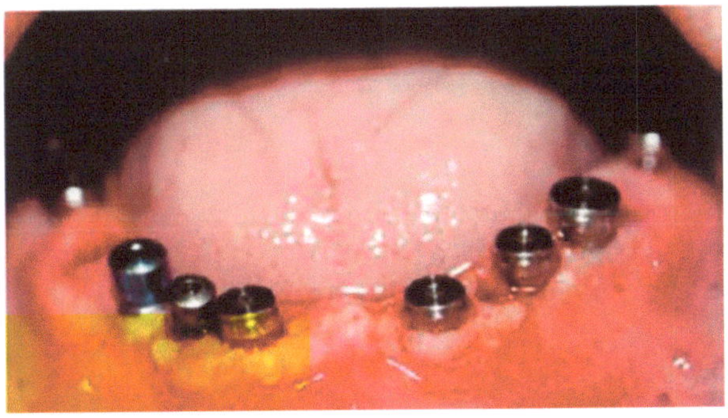

Figure 7.66. Temporarily placed gingiva-formers (healing caps) while precise provisional prosthetic work is made in the laboratory on supports (abutments) processed in the laboratory.

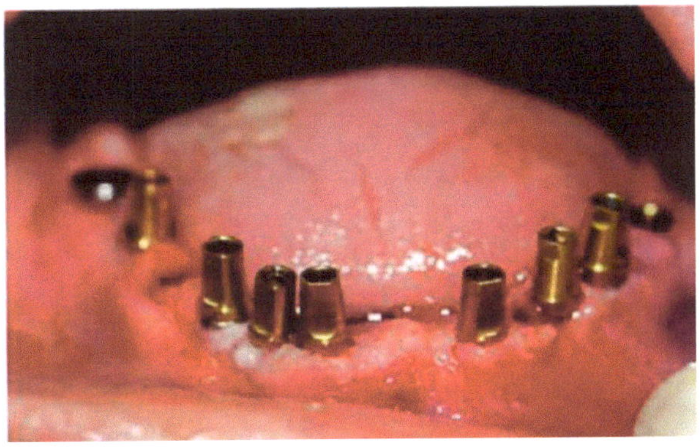

Figure 7.67. Placing and leaving definitive supports is best for healing and formation of peri-implant tissues. Never shorten and adjust the brackets directly in the mouth due to heat transfer to the implant and bone (it would jeopardize the osseointegration processes).

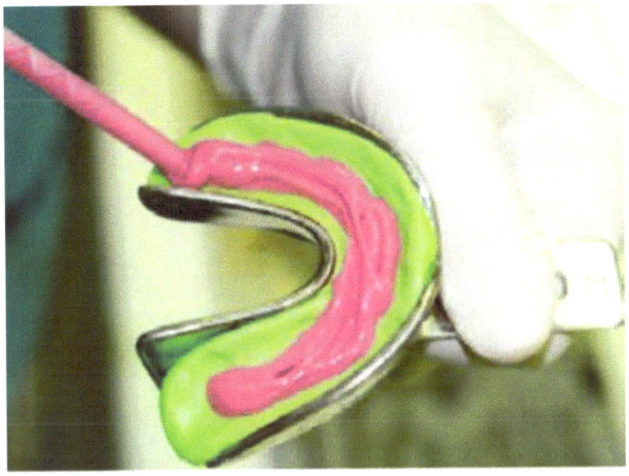

Figure 7.68. Taking the first and second impressions simultaneously or with monophasic silicone materials intended exclusively for taking impressions in oral implantology.

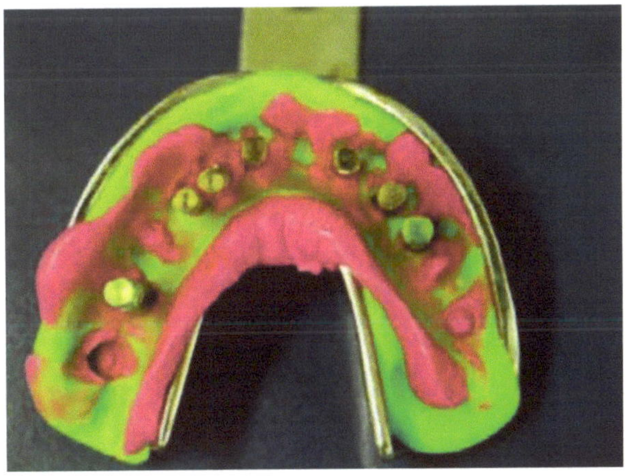

Figure 7.69. Placed analogues - one-stage impression taking for provisional restoration.

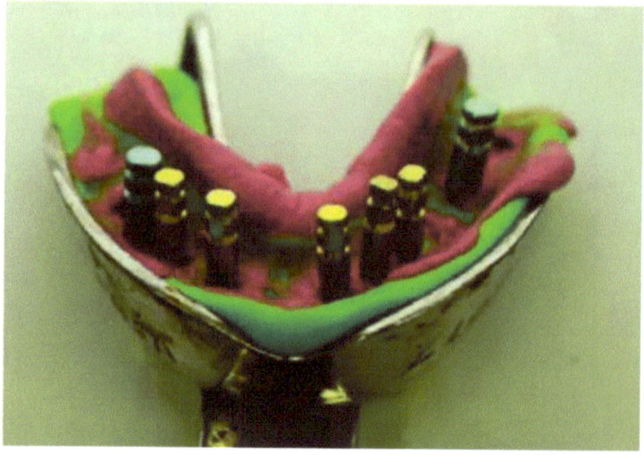

Figure 7.70. The position of the analog in the impression shows both the parity and the position of the implant.

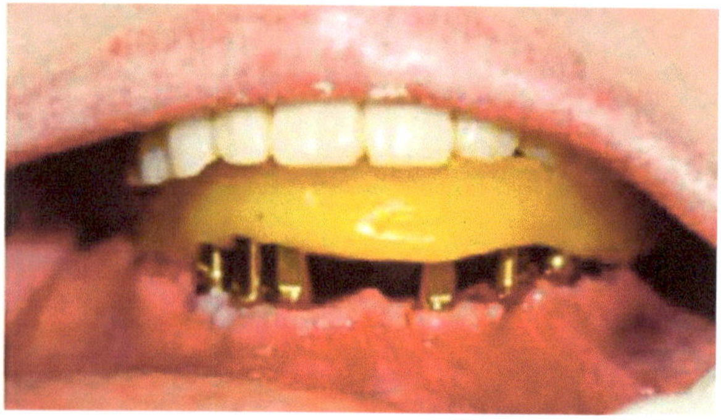

Figure 7.71. Determination of vertical dimension for temporary compensation.

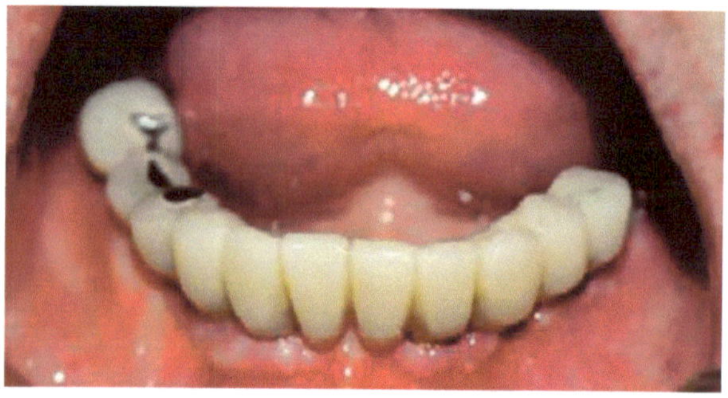

Figure 7.72. Temporary provisional acrylic bridge placed on immediately loaded implants.

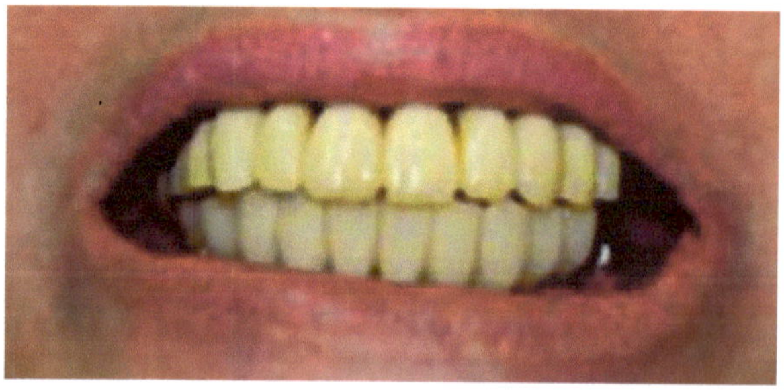

Figure 7.73. It is important to stimulate osseointegration with preliminary precise work. Temporary rehabilitation in this way creates comfort for the patient opposite to that which would be provided by a mobile acrylate prosthesis, and healing would have a different course.

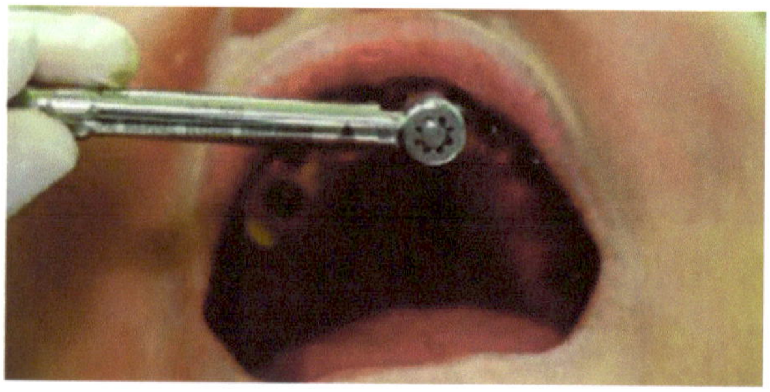

Figure 7.74. The stability of all implants was checked with a special dynamometric wrench (Dynatorq torque wrench), as well as the connection of the support (abutment) and the implant.

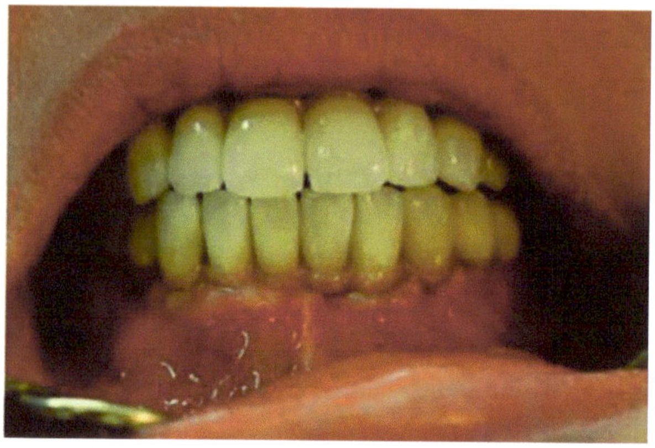

Figure 7.75. Appearance after 6 months imitating the gingiva with the orange color of the surrounding tissues.

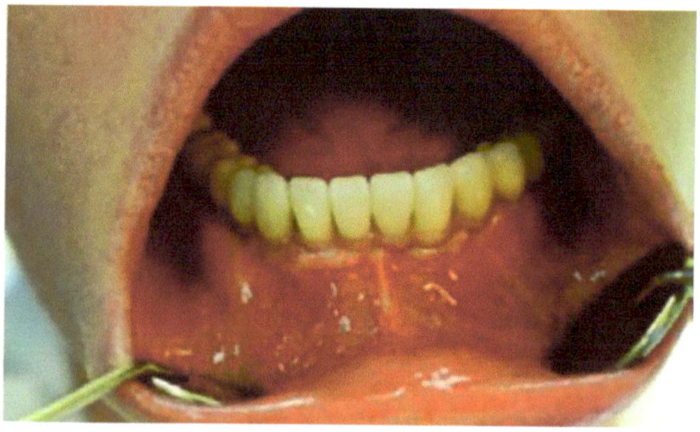

Figure 7.76. After 12 months, the patient's request to replace the part of the porcelain imitating the gingiva with tooth color was fulfilled, in order to improve aesthetics (Figure 7.83).

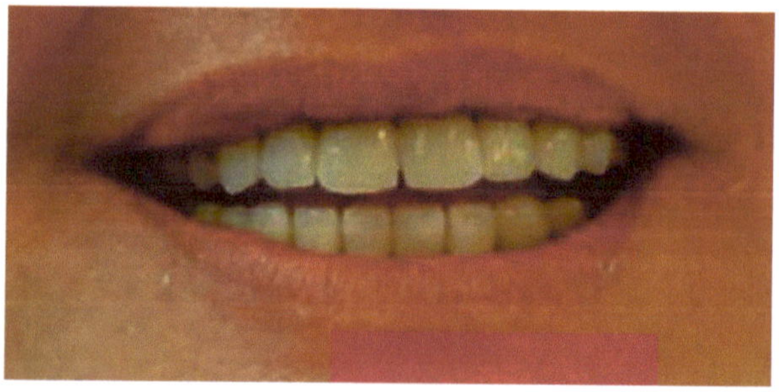

Figure 7.77. Aesthetic requirements are fully met.

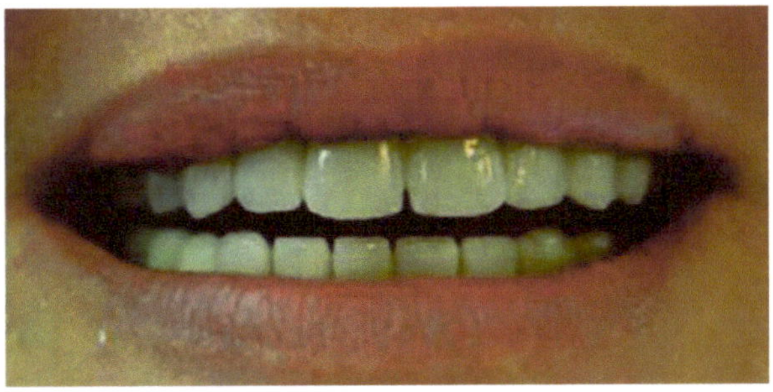

Figure 7.78. Achieving good function is also a fundamental condition for successful implant placement.

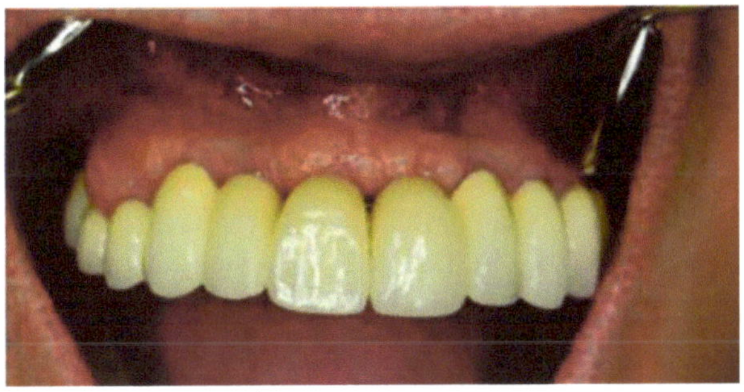

Figure 7.79. Check after 24 months. Compare with the initial state (Figures 7.26 and 7.87).

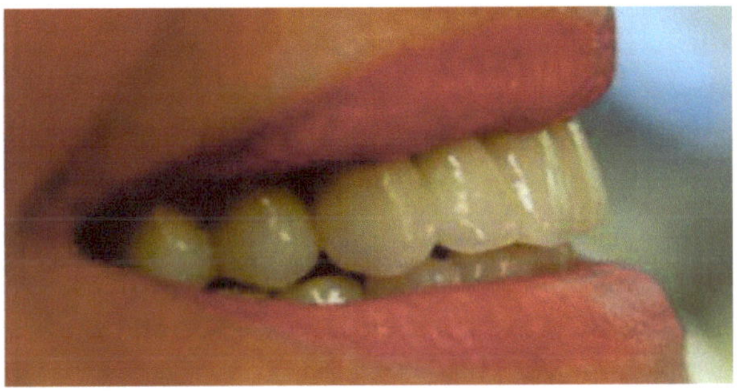

Figure 7.80. Canine-guided occlusion. Special attention is paid to the lateral movements of the lower jaw.

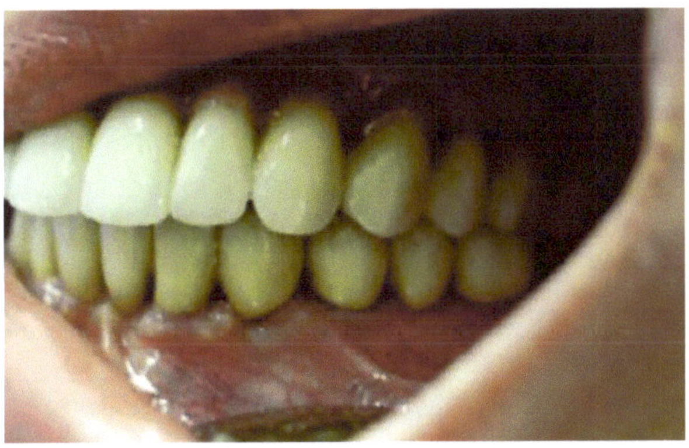

Figure 7.81. Control after 24 months, radiographic images and the objective state of the mouth, check the degree of bony integration and healing of soft tissues. Occlusion control checks and controls the direction of occlusal forces. Checking the occlusion during lateral movements of the lower jaw, periodic controls, is essential to promote and preserve the achieved integration.

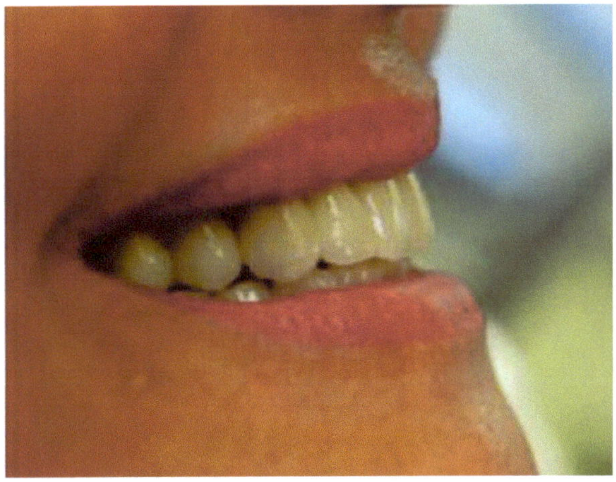

Figure 7.82. Profile view of the patient. A favorable smile line and lip shape make the aesthetic result exceptional.

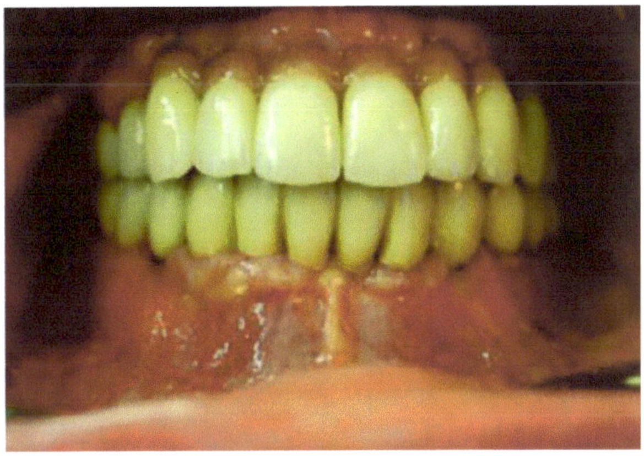

Figure 7.83. Finally, occlusion is the most important factor for maintaining the overall harmony of the masticatory system. Repeated prosthetic work in the upper jaw after 24 months, stabilized bone support and soft tissues - improved aesthetics. (Shown in Figures 7.79 and 7.85).

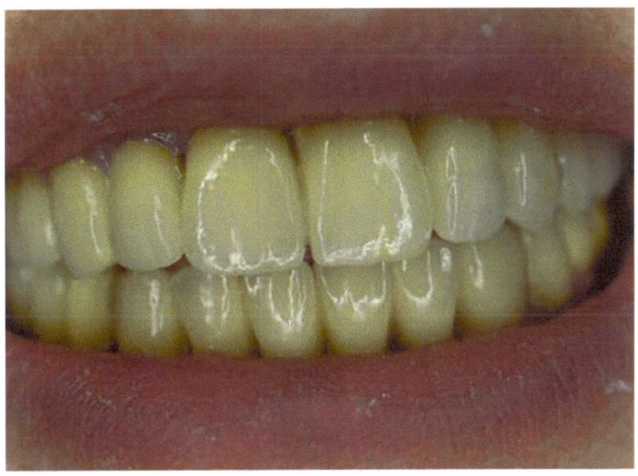

Figure 7.84. After complete stabilization of the soft tissues and achieved osseointegration, after 24 months the prosthetic work was repeated in order to achieve a better aesthetic result.

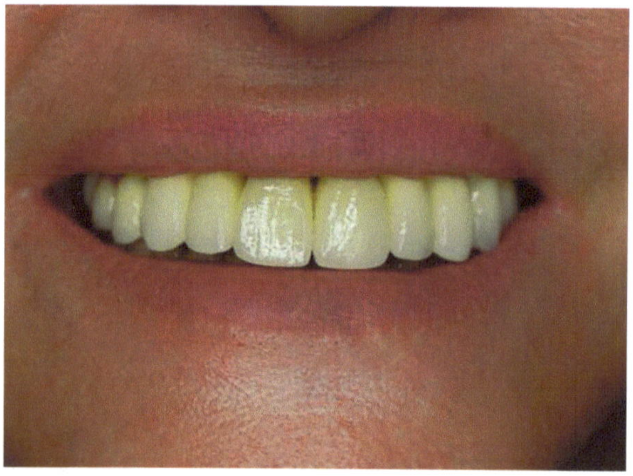

Figure 7.85. Successful aesthetic outcome of an extremely complex case.

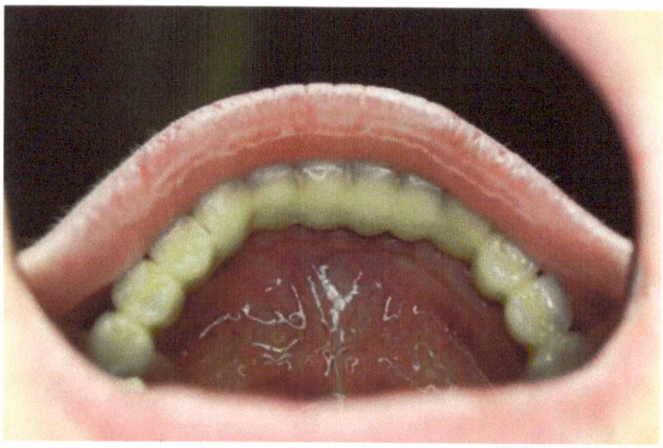

Figure 7.86. Appearance of definitive prosthetic work lingually. Laboratory error in making definitive prosthetic work in the lower jaw, lack of a metal collar in the neck part of the implant, which enables better maintenance of oral hygiene. Work repeated Figure 7.87.

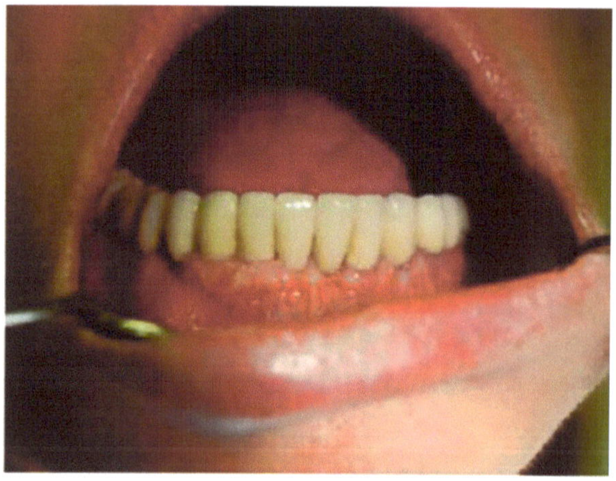

Figure 7.87. After 18 months, the patient's aesthetic request was met again by creating a bridge without gingival imitation, which was made possible by well-integrated bone support and stabilization of soft tissues. Compare the functional and aesthetic result with the initial state of the patient.

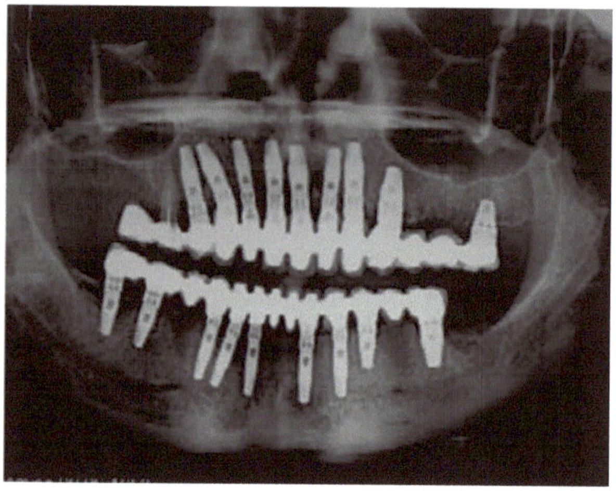

Figure 7.88. Control shot after 6 years. The result of immediate loading - good bone integration.

Solving the mentioned complex case shows the scope of modern implantology. The demands of the patients are increasing, and the patience is decreasing. Most of the patients want to get their teeth as soon as possible, to recover their damaged nature, to chew food well, and to look good. If the immediate installation of implants and their loading was successful in such a complex case, a similar procedure is all the more justified in cases with a smaller number of implants, especially in the case of single-tooth implantation.

To approach the solution of such a complex implant-prosthetic rehabilitation, it is not enough to have routine knowledge of performing the implantation. Sufficient presence of available bone does not have to be a reliable parameter for a successful procedure outcome. For the predictability of a successful outcome, fundamental knowledge of anatomical structures and their possible variations, bone physiology, prediction of the process of bone integration, and prosthetic, gnathological, and biomechanical laws are necessary. Experience is only one of the important factors that reduce the risk of the entire operation. However, the risk does not have to manifest itself in the first or second year after the completed implant-prosthetic rehabilitation, but also later, which is why the periodic check must be focused on occlusal events and maintenance of oral hygiene. If the occlusal developments are not aligned with the gnathological principles, even though good bone integration has been achieved after a certain time, unfavorable complications in the peri-implant space and subsequent peri-implantitis are possible.

The course of rehabilitation in the lower jaw is shown in pictures 7.54 to 7.73, and the complete result of implant-prosthetic rehabilitation is shown in pictures 7.76, 7.77, 7.78, and 7.86.

The presented cases lead to a conclusion that derives from the results of experience, seeking an answer to the question: what decision, plan, and method should be applied to achieve the intended goal?

Fulfillment of all requirements of implant-prosthetic rehabilitation depends on several factors. The method that was applied in the presented case was used for the following reasons.

The patient's primary request was aesthetics, with a note that she does not want a movable total acrylate prosthesis even as a temporary solution. Considering her current condition, her professional obligations, and her desire to have her teeth immediately, it was necessary to think carefully about which path to take to reach the goal set by the patient. Considering all the risk factors, good planning was the foundation of the entire operation. Of course, experience was an added advantage. In the current situation, the most important thing is to estimate the required volume of bone to achieve good primary stabilization of the implant, supported by augmentation that would shape the arch of the ridge to achieve aesthetics. You should always keep in mind what will happen in the coming years. Soft tissue recessions are also possible, which are usually difficult to resolve and threaten the achieved aesthetics. It is very important to create a good bone base with soft tissues. The presented solution meets the patient's expectations in terms of aesthetics and good function. However, the long-term success is based on good bone integration of the implant. The author of the book justifies the correctness of immediate implant installation and immediate loading with the following facts: if it takes a certain amount of time to induce new bone tissue through augmentation and bone shaping, why shouldn't the integration processes of the implant surface and bone take place simultaneously with immediate loading. By putting the implant into operation as soon as possible, i.e. by restoring the lost function of the bone, physiological processes are also supported - physiological stress on the surrounding bone. This is also clearly stated by Wolff's Law, which was stated a long time ago. Its principles are increasingly recognized today, both in orthopedics and oral implantology, when it comes to bone healing and integration with bioinert materials such as titanium. The author's position also justifies the replacement of joints in orthopedics (knee and hip), because a patient with an artificial knee or hip must walk the day after surgery.

The author discussed this topic at several foreign scientific symposia and congresses.

Limiting factors for achieving osseous integration

By inserting the implant into the prepared bone bed, the implant firmly anchored in the bone after implantation is exposed to chewing forces. This mechanical interaction - the primary stability of the inserted implant in the prepared bed is the first step towards the formation of new bone around the implant, and the final goal can be predicted after the first step is the creation of secondary stability of the implant, that is, the achievement of bone integration.

Scientific research and practice have proven that there are several limiting factors that influence the achievement of primary implant stability.

The three main influencing factors for achieving primary stability are:

- **The first factor is the implant design:**
  The details of the design allow greater stability in different clinical situations, which depends on the overall design of the implant, starting from the morphology, inclination, and spacing of the threads. The biofunctionality of the implant depends on the design; reception of maximum forces with the full support of the available bone.

- **Surgical procedures:**
  The simpler the surgical procedure, the faster and better the bony integration will be. Preservation of biological characteristics of the recipient (bone) and preservation of vascularization will promote faster and better bone integration.

- **Bone density is a decisive factor for the success of bone integration:**
  Although there is a balance between bone density and bone integration, with less vascularized bone, the favorable conditions for the success of bone integration are less favorable than in bone with better vascularization. Very dense bone is more favorable for achieving good primary stability, but there is a greater risk of vertical bone recession.

Knowledge of bone types is extremely important for successful implantation and achieving good bone integration.

There are several classifications of the quality of the available amount of residual bone in total edentulous and edentulous regions. These classifications facilitate a faster and easier assessment of the characteristics of the recipient (bone) and the planning of the entire implant-prosthetic rehabilitation. At the time when the author of the book was installing implants, the only classification of bone types that was respected was the classification by Karl Misch, which lasted for a long time.

Knowing the characteristics of bone types, enables an easier choice of bed preparation and implant placement procedures with a prediction of the quality of primary stability. The type of bone and achieved primary stability are key factors for the selection of procedure protocols and the planning of implant loading.

Lekholm and Zarb (1985) proposed a classification of bone quality of "zero" to "fifth" type about cortical and trabecular bone, and this classification is the most widely used today. According to this classification, it is possible to measure bone density, using the measurement unit Hounsflied Units (HU). The measurement unit HU for bone types ranges from 1000-1500 HU. According to this classification, bone density measurements are possible with a CT scanner and CBCT software. See chapter 12.

Bone architecture and the relative ratio of cortical and trabecular parts are the parameters that determine the classification of bone type. The Lekholm and Zarb bone type classification contains new bone types, such as "type V" and "type 0", which complement the traditional classification (K.Misch), improving its clinical utility. Classifications of bone types aim to clarify the amount of available bone. Available bone width is the distance between the outer surfaces of the buccal and lingual cortical lamellae. The width is variable from the top to the bottom of the ridge. The length of available bone is variable in anatomical structures.

Identification of the bone in which the implant is to be inserted is extremely important for the success of planning the entire implantological treatment, starting with drilling the bone to prepare the implant bed, as well as determining the diameter and length of the implant. By evaluating these parameters, we can determine the guidelines for the application of different surgical techniques and the implant loading protocol by the type of bone.

All these parameters are shown in Figures 7.89 and 7.90) Bone type classification according to Lekholm and Zarb:

Type 0

This type of bone is characterized by the highest density of corical bone (density 1200 to 1500 HU) and poor vascularization, which limits the possibility of bone regeneration. Due to poor vascularization, this type of bone is subject to greater bone resorption, which is why crestal bone preparations must be avoided. When preparing the implant bed for "type 0", the diameter of the prepared bed must be 0.2 mm smaller than the diameter of the selected implant. Immediate implant placement can be applied, but should be avoided in the aesthetic region due to possible bone recession.

Type 1

Despite the strong cortical bone (1000-1200 HU), "type 1" is characterized by better vascularization than "type 0", and due to the greater presence of cancellous bone, operations on the crestal part of the bone are possible, and the possibility of bone tissue regeneration is much better. The diameter of the bone drilling for implant insertion should be 0.2 mm smaller than the diameter of the implant to be inserted. This type of bone is favorable for immediate implantation.

Type 2 and Type 3

These two types of bone are characterized by: high-quality cortical bone that ensures primary stability of the embedded implant, and the cancellous bone structure enables good blood supply to the bone tissue around the implant (bone density 500-1000HU) promoting bone regeneration, which in this type of bone has a favorable prognosis. This type of bone is suitable for immediate implant placement. Bone drilling, given the high density of cortical bone, can vary, and the diameter of the drilled bone should be 0.2 to 0.4 mm smaller than the diameter of the implant being inserted. In relation to the body and apex of the implant, this difference should be 0.4 to 0.6 mm.

Type 4

This type of bone has a low bone density (400 to 500 HU), and is characterized by thin cortical bone. This type of bone requires the installation of implants with the largest possible diameter in order to achieve primary stability, and at the same time, it is necessary to use implants with a larger surface of the endosseous body of the implant, in order to create the conditions for successful bone integration. With this type of bone, the achievement of primary stability is usually not successful, and it does not guarantee that there will be no micro-displacement of the implant during the healing and bone integration process. For this reason, the diameter of the implant must not be less than 5 to 5.5 mm. The diameter of the prepared bed must be 1 to 1.5 mm smaller than the diameter of the implant.

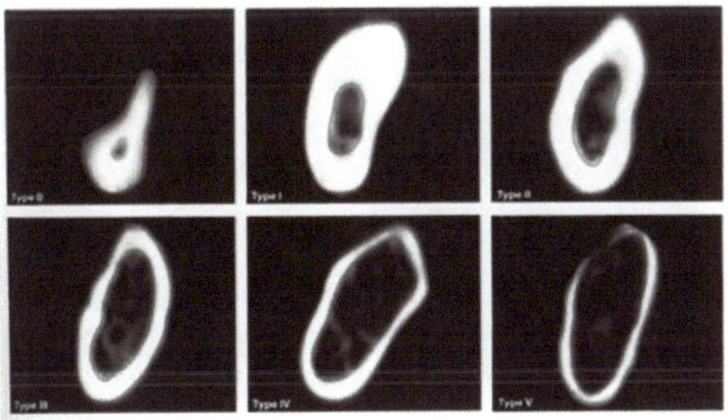

Figure 7.89. Classification of bone types in the lower jaw.

Type 5

This type of bone is characterized by low bone density (less than 400 HU), which is why immediate installation and immediate loading should not be applied. Two-phase surgical implant placement is indicated. Bone drilling with a drill should be reduced to a minimum to very thin cortical bone, use quality implant systems that ensure self-injury. Postpone and monitor the loading protocol in the lower jaw for at least 4 months, and in the upper jaw for at least 6 months.

For this type of bone, implants with the widest diameter (5.5-6 and 6.25 mm) are indicated. The last bone drilling, and only at the beginning, as already emphasized, should be 1.5 to 2 mm less than the diameter of the implant. Classification of bone types (modified by Lekholm and Zarb) shown by CT scan. The part corresponding to the cortical bone is marked to represent its relationship with the bone marrow (in the upper and lower jaw).

Type 0: This type of bone can be said to be the most coronary bone characterized by a tendency towards bone resorption; the loss of 1-1.5 mm of crestal bone is shown in the video. However, as this type of bone is extremely poorly vascularized and highly dense, bone drilling must be performed with particular care to avoid compression and overheating of the bone. Augmentation with autologous bone blocks (solit crest) should not be applied in this type of bone, because the outcomes can be catastrophic. Type 1: This type of bone is similar to type 0, but with better vascularization, which provides the possibility of increasing bone volume by augmentation.

Bone types 2 and 3 are ideal for increasing the horizontal and vertical dimensions of the alveolar bone by augmentation. In bone types 4 and 5, implants with a wide diameter are used with the aim of improving the primary and secondary stability of the implant. The length of the implant in these bone types is less important (and can vary between 5.5 to 6.5 mm), while the diameter of the implant is crucial and is 5.5-6 or 6.25 mm.

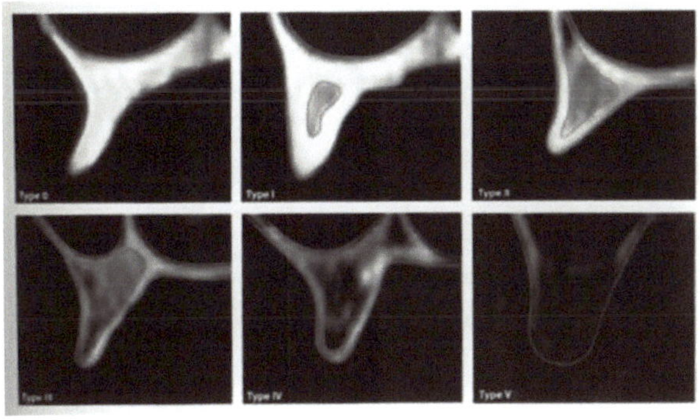

Figure 7.90. Classification of bone types in the upper jaw.

Secondary stability: from mechanical retention to osseous integration

After the implantation of the implant in the living bone tissue, biological processes occur at the molecular and cellular level. All the molecular and cellular events that are caused by the installation of the implant will result in the transition from primary stability to secondary stability when it can be said that the implant is integrated with the bone tissue.

To understand this dynamic, biological process of bone integration, it can be summarized in the following steps:

1. By forming a blood clot (hematoma), interrupting the blood supply in the first few hours, it causes a decrease in pH due to a decrease in oxygen and partial pressure (pO2), the partial pressure of carbon dioxide (pCO2) increases. Figure 7.91.

   Absorption of proteins and media to the surface of the implant will occur. Biomolecules with the highest specificity on the surface of the implant form the first single anatomical layer on which other molecular layers will be built.
2. By releasing and activating biomaterials from the tissues surrounding the implant, and blood circulation activates this process with cytokines. These cytokines are of different types and each of them has a specific function. A cascade of these mediators will stimulate cells to respond by: migration, differentiation and proliferation. The results of this activity will form a hematoma, inflammatory and multipotent mesichymal cells in the space between the implant and the bone tissue. This process takes 2-4 days. Figure 7.92.
3. Cell migration, differentiation and proliferation will result in neoangiogenesis and formation of granulation tissue with the presence of fibroblasts, revascularization and formation of loose connective tissue (from one to 4 - 6 weeks) Figure 7.93
4. At the end of the process, the differentiated cells will turn into osteoblasts, which starts osteogenesis. The bone woven by synthesis will form new bone and result in osseous integration. Figure 7.94.

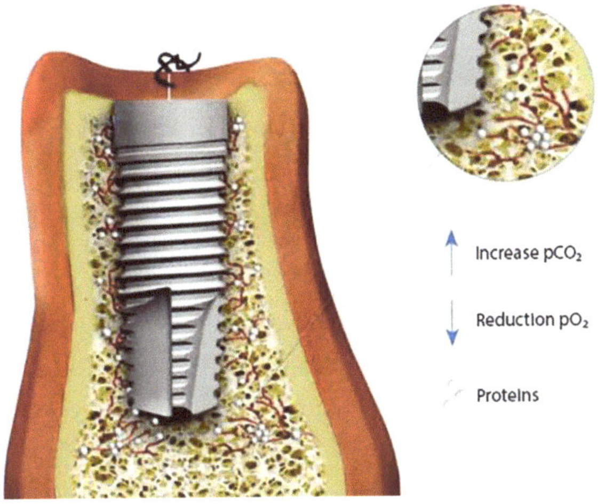

Figure 7.91. Presentation of the process after implant placement; The pH value decreases due to a decrease in the value of oxygen (p02) and an increase in carbon dioxide (pC02). During the first hours, proteins are released from the blood cells that are absorbed onto the surface of the implant.

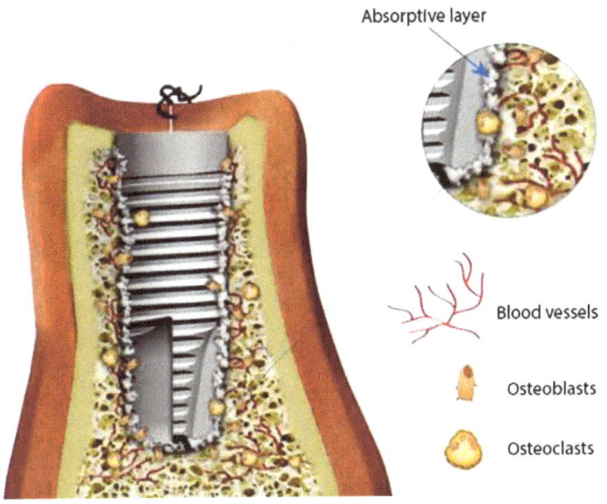

Figure 7.92. Display of the beginning of the cell reaction, i.e. creation of new ones (angiogenesis) and migration of cells.

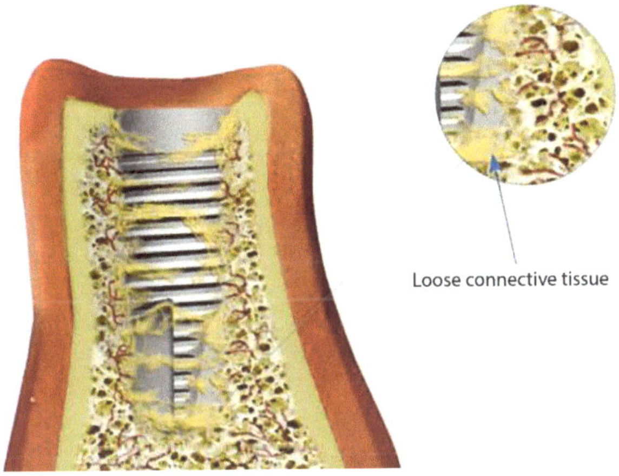

Figure 7.93. Showing the beginning of the formation of loose connective tissue that will later replace bone tissue.

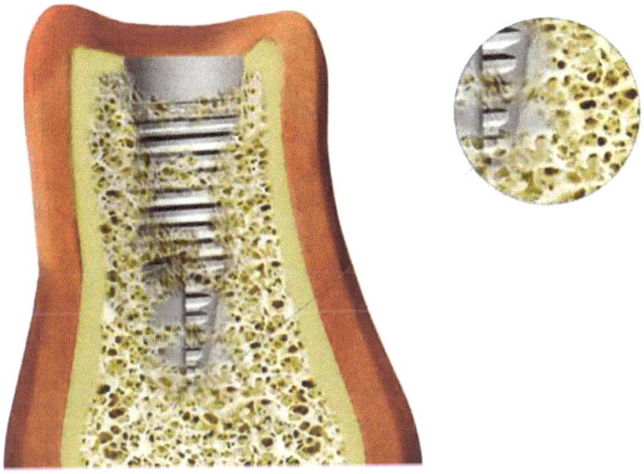

Figure 7.94. Presentation of the final formation of new bone around the implant and achieved bone integration.

Conclusion

To integrate into the surrounding tissue, the implant must have basic properties: BIOCOMPATIBILITY and BIOFUNCTIONALITY.

Biocompatibility means that the material from which it is made is chemically and biologically inert to be accepted by the surrounding tissues.

Biofunctionality determines the implant design and the design details that limit the absorption of forces within physiological limits. The result of biofunctionality can be verified by clinical and histologic evidence.

For the success of bone integration, it is important to determine the bone availability in the regions intended for implant placement. Extreme caution is required when assessing the bone supply in the maxilla due to the existence of several anatomical structures of different sizes. The cortical lamella in the maxilla is thinner, less thickened and more porous than in the mandible. The bone supply in the retromolar regions is always sufficient and can be used for augmentation procedures.

Scientific research finds that the bioelectric phenomenon also plays a role in bone integration; the load induces the creation of a piezoelectric effect in the bone. As a consequence, the tension of the implant on the bone has the effect of creating a potential difference that indicates microcurrent. These normal physiological events lead to the differentiation of mesenchyme cells into fibroblasts, osteoblasts and vitreous. In the part of the negative pole, osteoblasts accumulate, creating new bone. At the opposite pole, vitreous crystals accumulate and the bone is resorbed. By compressing the implant on the trabecular bone, a negative pole is created, which leads to the formation of new bone. In the process of bone integration, osteoblasts accumulate around the negative pole, because the pH is in the process of bone integration, osteoblasts accumulate around the negative pole, because the pH in this area is more basic than the pH in the body fluid. The osteoblast enzyme (alkaline phosphatase) works best in a weak basic environment. Alkaline phosphatase from osteoblasts is thought to cleave phosphate compounds from the interstitial fluid, creating numerous intermediates and free phosphates. Free phosphate combines with calcium to form calcium phosphate, which is the basis of new bone building and bone integration. (Figure 7.94).

Simultaneously with the regeneration of the supporting (bone) tissue, epithelial cells migrate to the surface of the wound to cover and line it. Due to the "contact inhibition", the epithelial cells do not migrate over the entire length of the implant. Epithelial cells proliferate and migrate until they come into contact with other normal epithelial cells or collagenous connective tissue, which acts as an effective contact inhibitor for the epithelium. Thus, as the epithelial cells move in an apical direction, they come into contact with healthy connective tissue collagen fibers that stop the migration. If the connective tissue of the collagen fibers is infected or inflamed, epithelial cells can grow around the implant due to necrosis of the connective tissue, which can manifest itself in the achieved bony integration with peri-implantitis and loss of the implant.

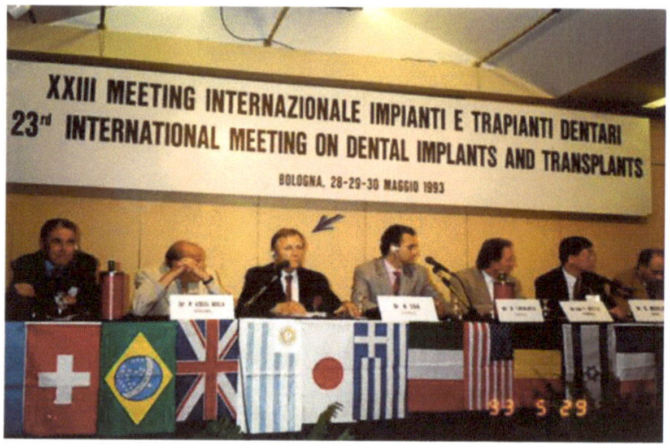

Figure 7.95. Dr. Zlopaša chairs the international scientific symposium (Bologna, 1993).

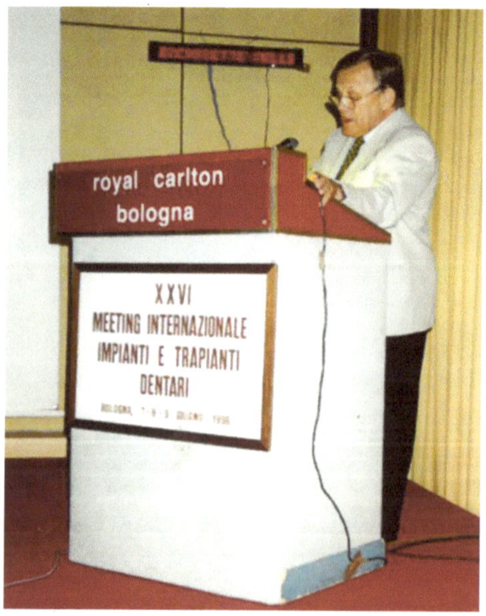

Figure 7.96. Presentation of the author of the book on bone integration at a time when opinions were divided (Bologna, 1989).

8

Temporomandibular Joint And Occlusion

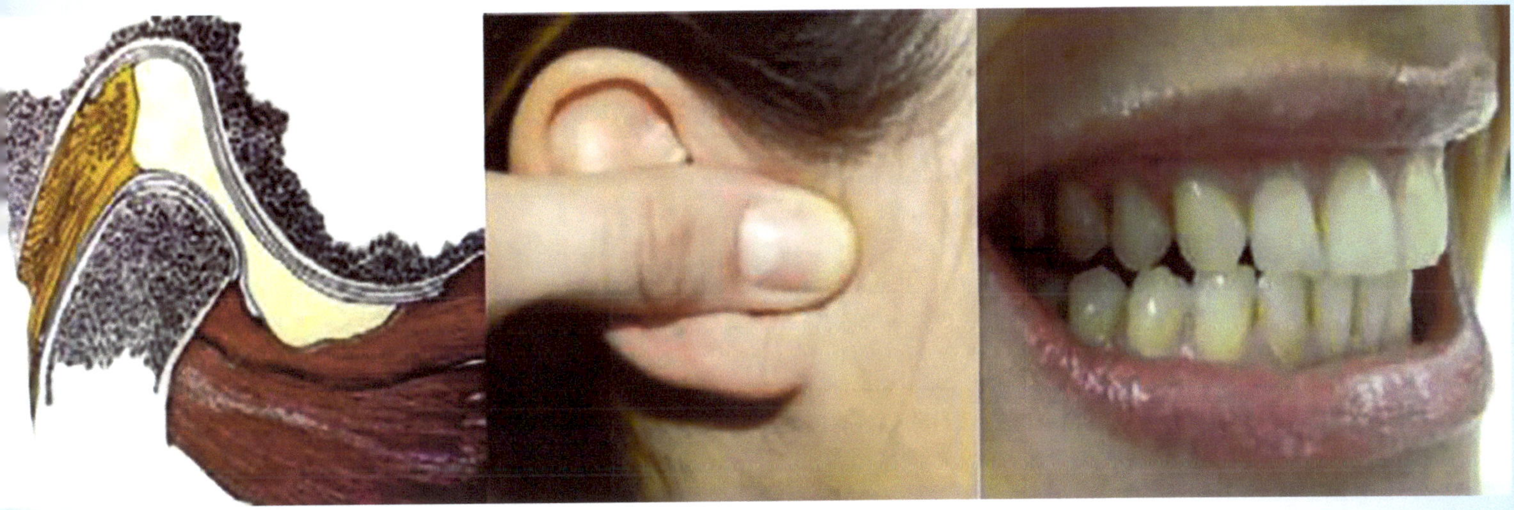

The function of the temporomandibular joint (TMJ), its physiology and pathophysiology, as well as the dynamics of the masticatory system, represent one of the most fascinating basic chapters in all of dentistry. Optimal oral health requires anatomical and functional harmony, occlusal stability and natural aesthetics. Knowing the details of the function of the entire masticatory system is necessary to understand orofacial harmony or its imbalance. This is important in order to know how pathological changes in one segment can affect the entire masticatory system. In the treatment of the resulting changes, diagnosis is the key to success, and for this reason it is very important to analyze in detail the reasons for the imbalance of orofacial harmony, which are often the result of changes in the TMJ.

Loss of teeth, whether it is partial or total toothlessness, disrupts the interjaw relationships, which disrupts orofacial harmony. Bringing it back into function, by restoring certain parts of the masticatory system (prosthetic works, whether the restoration is performed in the classical way, or by installing implants), requires detailed knowledge of this issue.

Implant placement, as an oral surgical procedure, is much simplified thanks to new techniques and, for an experienced practitioner, it is only the first step towards successful rehabilitation. But, all the actions that follow after that (establishing interjaw relations in an ideal position, which also achieves an ideal occlusion) are important factors that will affect the longevity of the installed implants and maintaining the health of the TMJ, i.e. maintaining the orofacial harmony of the masticatory system. A crucial condition for this is a good knowledge of gnathological principles.

When it comes to implant restoration, knowledge of gnathology and establishment of good occlusion and articulation is a priority knowledge for a successful outcome in creating physiological harmony of the entire masticatory system. Occlusion is not only the physical contact of biting surfaces in the resting phase, but also implies coordinated functional interaction between various parts of the masticatory system. Occlusion (contact of occlusal surfaces in maximum intercuspation) and articulation (intercuspular relationship during movements of the lower jaw) are not only static and dynamic relationships between teeth, but also all other tissues of the masticatory system.

For this reason, every dentist, whether he is an oral surgeon or a prosthetist (according to the author of the book, these two are inseparable in practice), must have a good knowledge of the principles of occlusion (gnathology) in order to harmonize the dental arrangement of prosthetic works with the aesthetic and functional requirements of the entire masticatory system.

For successful predictability, the fabrication of prosthetic work must ensure the smooth and harmonious function of all movements of the lower jaw. Predictable clinical success, when it comes to embedded implants, depends on the decision of the therapist what kind of occlusion will be achieved by making the prosthetic structure and whether he should maintain or change the existing state of occlusion.

When it comes to establishing or reconstructing an occlusion, there are general principles that apply regardless of the type of prosthetic work and the clinical situation:

1. achieve a maximally symmetrical distribution of contacts in the position of maximal intercuspation;
2. achieve axial or maximum possible axial loading of natural teeth or implant supports;
3. achieve an acceptable occlusal balance;
4. enable lower jaw movements without traumatic interference and premature occlusal contacts;
5. determine the individually acceptable vertical dimension of occlusion and free occlusal space.

All components are important in any prosthetic rehabilitation, but occlusion is one of the most important factors of successful implant-prosthetic treatment due to the unique relationship between living bone tissue and integrated alloplastic material. By not fulfilling these principles, the harmony of the masticatory system can be disturbed, with more serious consequences, which are first manifested by pathological changes in the TMJ.

An imbalance of harmony can be caused by one or more pathological changes in the TMJ. When creating an individual plan, the dentist must recognize the masticatory disorder and what causes it.

In order for a dentist to be competent in solving the resulting changes in the changes in the TMJ, he must be a "doctor of the masticatory system", points out one of the greatest gnathologists today, Peter E. Dawson, wanting to emphasize that a perfect knowledge of the TMJ is also necessary. Gnathologist Peter

Thomas, with whom the author of the book studied this issue, emphasized the same position much earlier.

Both of these gnathologists point out that there is a very small percentage of dentists who know the TMJ well, and for that reason they are not competent in solving the pathological changes in it. This is especially important when disturbed interjaw relationships are restored by placing implants.

Dawson believes that in order for a dentist to understand the function and pathophysiology of the TMJ, he should be able to draw it (Figure 8.1), just as he can draw the root of a tooth lying in an alveolus in detail. This principle of TMJ knowledge testing shows how well we are able to understand its function.

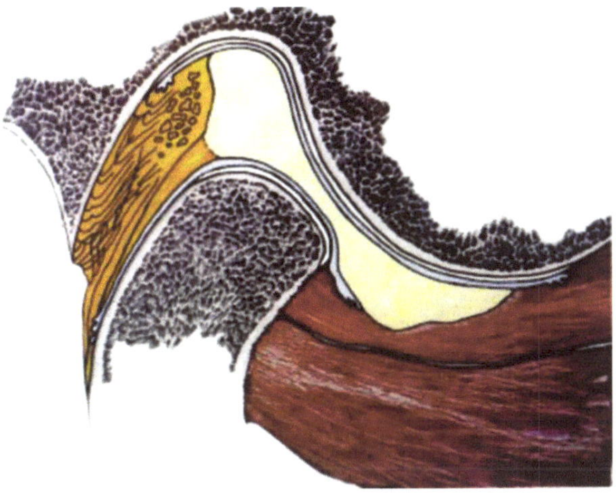

Figure 8.1. A schematic representation of the TMJ with which Dawson recommends checking basic knowledge of the joint.

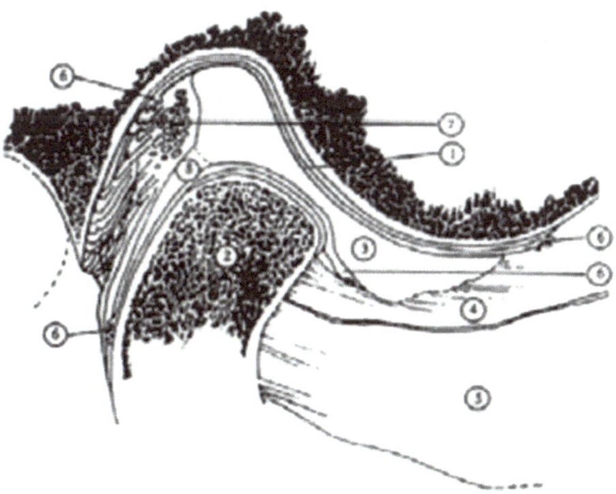

Figure 8.2. Lateral section view of the TMJ: 1. eminentia articularis. 2. condyle 3. disc (pay attention to the biconcave shape of the disc so that the convex part of the condyle and the convex part of the eminence fit intimately. 4. m. pterygoideus medialis 5. m. pterygoideus lateralis 6. synovial tissue. 7. retrodiscal tissue that connects the disc to temporal bone 8. lateral ligament that connects the disc to the condyle.

Dawson believes that every dentist should remember this picture. A clear visualization of the TMJ anatomy makes it possible to analyze the problem of the joint itself. The correct interpretation of X-rays and other images depends on the ability of memorized images (Figures 8.1-8.3). No specialty in dentistry can be practiced at the highest level without understanding the relationship of teeth to other parts of the masticatory system, including the TMJ. The masticatory system must function in harmony (Figure 8.3). Neuromuscular harmony depends on structural harmony of occlusion and TMJ. The smooth functioning of the masticatory musculature is mostly dependent on this relationship, so this relationship is always of key importance for diagnosing conditions in the TMJ and planning therapy.

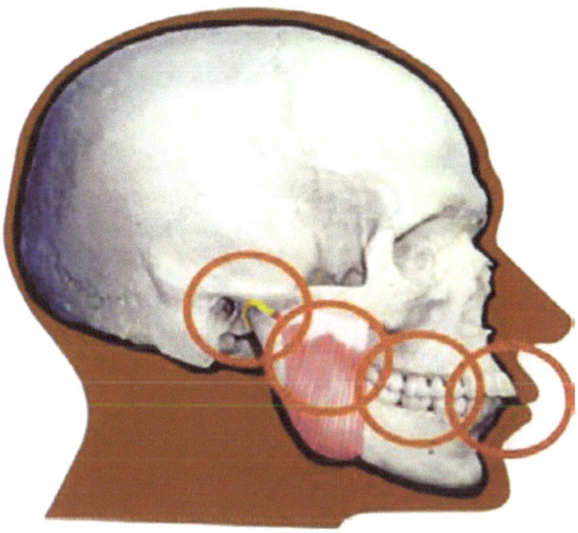

Figure 8.3. Implantology treatment will be considered successful if the harmony of the entire masticatory system is achieved (P. Dawson).

Teeth are only one part of the masticatory system. If they are not in harmony with other parts of the overall masticatory system, disharmony will occur, which can manifest itself in various ways.

Knowing and understanding the function of the masticatory system is the key to success when the lost natural teeth need to be replaced with prosthetic work, especially if it is done on embedded implants.

Occlusal relationships are unlikely to be assessed until it is established that the TMJ joint is in harmony.

It is not possible to establish a perfect occlusion, that is, that the intercuspular relations are in maximum intercuspation, if there are changes in the TMJ.

Disturbance of harmony most often begins with disturbed occlusion, from the simplest to the most complex. Occlusal disharmony is manifested by dysfunction of the TMJ, namely.

Certain forms of malocclusion (open bite, overlap of frontal teeth of the upper jaw greater than 4 mm);

- unstable occlusal contacts of the teeth during lateral movements of the lower jaw;
- the presence of occlusal disturbances (mediotrusion side of the molar),
- Early loss of molars;
- Poor occlusal modeling of the biting surfaces of artificial crowns.

Dentists who ignore the relationship of occlusion with the position and condition of the TMJ can only guess when diagnosing changes in the masticatory system, which are often accompanied by pain of lesser or greater intensity when chewing.

Dysfunction of the temporomandibular joint (TMJ) is based on a change in the relationship between the articular disc and the condyle, and is manifested by the following phenomena:

- shape deviation (defects on the articulating surfaces and disc thinning and perforations);
- disc dislocations (dislocation with reduction and dislocation without reduction);
- Dislocations of the condyle-disc complex (hypermobility and dislocation of the condyle);
- Inflammation of soft structures in the TMJ itself (capsulitis and retrodiscitis);
- Degenerative diseases of the TMJ (osteoarthrosis);
- TMJ ankylosis.

Okeson (1989) explained that the imbalance of joint structures is caused by biomechanical factors:

- the condyle does not occupy a physiologically optimal position in the articular pits;
- The condyle cannot be placed in central occlusion in the position of maximum dystoposition;
- the relation of joint structures is disturbed;
- the condyle moves relative to the disc in order to take a more stable position;
- Translational movements between the disc and the condyle cause microtrauma. Such an unstable relationship between the condyle and the disc by permanent microtrauma eventually leads to the perforation of the disc and its dislocation, which is a more severe form of TMJ disease (Okeson 1989, Ash 1996 and Carisson, Magnusson 2000.

Therapy of temporomandibular dysfunctions (TMD) is very complex and often requires a multidisciplinary approach to treatment. In addition to dental procedures and occlusion correction, cooperation with neurologists, psychiatrists, physiotherapists, or otorhinolaryngologists is sometimes required. Occlusal therapy is primarily used in the treatment of TMJ disease.

- Reversible occlusal therapy with splints in combination with physical therapy. The goal of therapy is to eliminate the symptoms of the disease. Indications are extracapsular and intracapsular dysfunctions.
- Surgical therapy: trauma, tumors, ankylosis, adhesions, disc ruptures. Surgical therapy is in the domain of maxillofacial surgery.

In certain cases, drug therapy can also be carried out, by administering corticosteroids, analgesics, non-steroidal anti-inflammatory drugs, anxiolytics (diazepam 10 mg) or antidepressants (amyzol 25 mg).

Physical therapy consists of certain exercises prescribed by the therapy protocol. This type of therapy includes thermotherapy by placing compresses in the joint region and cryotherapy.

Another modality of physical therapy is the use of ultrasound:

- By increasing tissue temperature, blood flow is enhanced;
- Micromassage increases the elasticity of collagen fibers;
- Ultrasound increases the permeability of the cell membrane, which removes the inflammatory exudate.

As already emphasized, TMD therapy is very complex and sometimes requires the involvement of several specialties. In order to determine adequate therapy, an accurate diagnosis of TMJ disease must be made and causal treatment must be carried out.

Making a diagnosis begins with an examination of both joints: the ability to open the mouth as much as possible (no less than three crossed fingers) and whether opening the mouth is accompanied by pain.

The causes of pain and limited opening of the mouth can be:

- Inflammation and spasm of the masticatory muscles;
- Disturbance of the relationship between the disc and the condyle;

The examination should determine whether there is deviation or deflection of the lower jaw when opening the mouth. Deviation of the middle of the lower jaw occurs due to spasms of the upper bundle of the lateral pterygoid muscle and anteromedial dislocation of the disc. Deflection of the middle of the lower jaw occurs due to an intercapsular disorder in one of the TMJ.

It should also be determined how much movement there is in lateral occlusion (maximum 8 mm). The appearance of pain and limited lateral movements of the lower jaw may be the result of inflammation and hyperfunction of the upper bundle of the lateral pterygoid muscle and anterior dislocation of the disc.

The possibility of protrusion should also be checked - the maximum protrusion is from 8 to 10 mm, the sensitivity and pain of the TMJ should also be checked when palpating the side wall of the TMJ and the back wall of the TMJ capsule.

- Auscultation of sounds in the TMJ - intercapsular dysfunctions
- Sound effects in the TMJ (clicking, skipping) due to anteromedial disc dislocation, and crepitations indicate degenerative changes in the TMJ.

Based on the parameters presented during the examination, a diagnosis of TMD and disharmony in the functioning of the TMJ is made.

Dentists who ignore the importance of the TMJ cannot be successful in creating prosthetic works, whether they are anchored to natural teeth or implants.

If the clinician does not have thorough knowledge of occlusion and gnathology, he is not competent to diagnose the resulting changes in the TMJ. Likewise, dentists who ignore the relationship of occlusion with condyle position and condition in the TMJ can only guess at what the problem is. And the problems can be different: pathological changes in the joint itself, loss of natural teeth or implants, masticatory muscle pain, various types of orofacial pain, etc.

Knowledge of occlusion is an absolute requirement to understand what is needed to keep the overall masticatory system in harmony. If he understands this, the clinician will then succeed in achieving a peaceful neuromuscular harmony of the masticatory musculature.

The analysis of the neuromuscular system is an integral part of the dental examination, and in some cases also of the neurological examination. The peaceful functioning of the masticatory musculature depends on the harmonious relationship between occlusion, articulation and TMJ, so this relationship is always of key importance for diagnosing changes and planning rehabilitation.

Disorders of the masticatory musculature in which the opening muscles (external pterygoid muscle, mylohyoid muscle and geniohyoid muscle) are affected limit the opening of the mouth to about 40 mm, and the cause of the limitation is pain.

Restricted mouth opening of less than three fingers is one of the contraindications for implant placement (see chapter "Risks in Oral Implantology.

Back in 1934, otolaryngologist Dr. James Costen observed the connection of a series of symptoms that appeared in the area around the ear, caused by changes in occlusion. At first these observations were not accepted. But the works of the American otorhinolaryngologist attracted the attention of dental circles, and then the use of splints for raising the bite began.

In the 1950s, significant research on this problem began, and in the 1960s and 1970s, research attention was focused on occlusion as the primary factor in the development of progressive disorders in the TMJ. In the 1980s, attention was paid to the intercapsular causes of disorders in the stomatognathic system, and only recently has the complexity and multifactorial nature of the causes of temporomandibular dysfunctions (TMD) been increasingly pointed out.

Over time, the terminology of TMJ disorders has changed. They were first called Costen's syndrome, after the author who first described TMJ disorders, then TMJ dysfunction and TMJ functional disorders. Other authors proposed different terms: myoarthropathies, myofascial dysfunction syndrome, temporomandibular pain dysfunction syndrome and others. In the end, the majority of authors considered all these terms too exclusive and finally a general term was proposed - craniomandibular dysfunction (CMD). The term temporomandibular imbalance (TMD) can also be found in the literature. Occlusion is conditioned by various decisions of the therapist, and in order to achieve perfect occlusion and satisfy aesthetic requirements (setting of teeth, precise position and shape), one must know the formula of perfect occlusion.

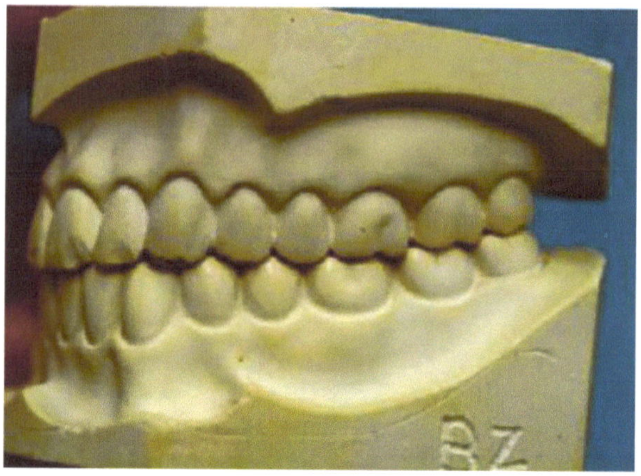

Figure 8.5. Ideal intercuspal relationship.

What is the formula for perfect occlusion?

Assuming that the explanations are clear and the knowledge is complete about the relationship between occlusion and masticatory musculature, a vision of how to achieve perfect occlusion in rehabilitation should be created.

The following picture (Figure 8.4) should be remembered as the perfect occlusion formula.

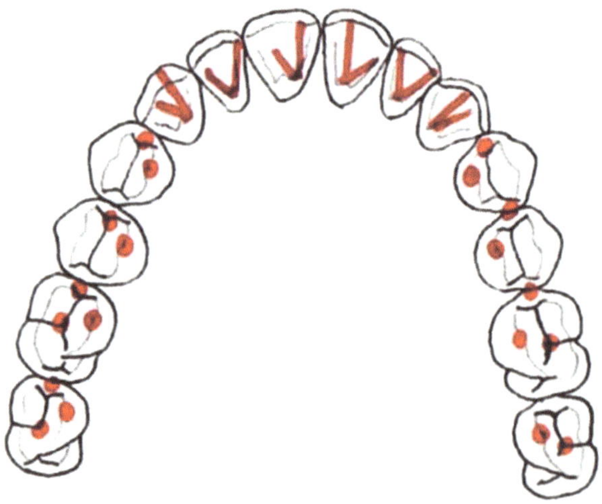

Figure 8.4. Dawson's perfect occllusion formula.

The first step is to achieve the same intensity of contact on all teeth at the same time when the condyles are in the maximum physiological disposition, that is, when the condyles and discs are completely in their sockets. The contact on the lateral teeth is at the tips of the cusps (in the picture shown as red dots).

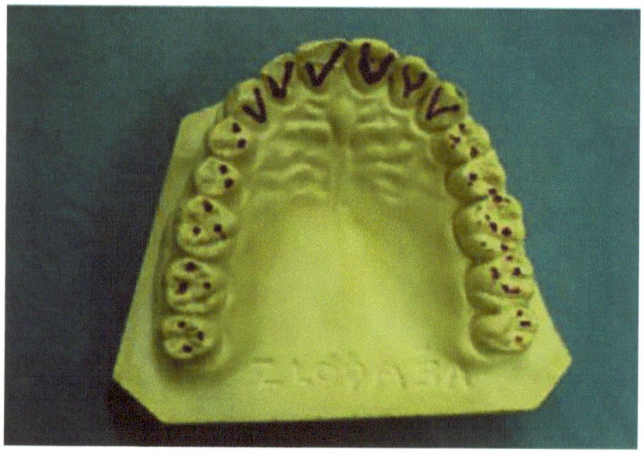

Figure 8.6. Overview of the gnathological formula of occlusion.

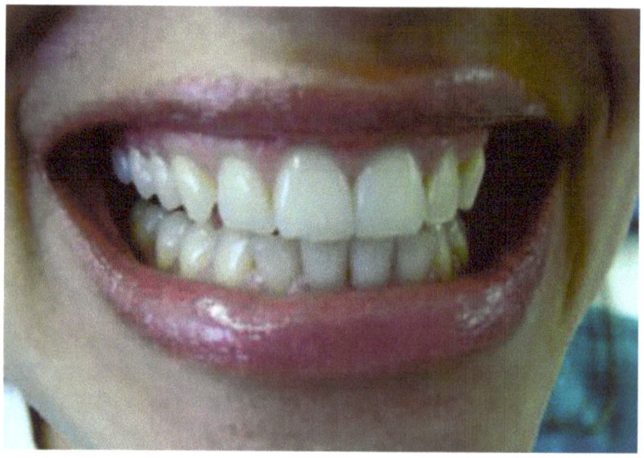

Figure 8.7. The ideal ratio of canine-guided occlusion in natural teeth.

The lines on the front teeth show the condylar contact from the central relation to the incisal edges if the lower jaw moves forward and laterally.

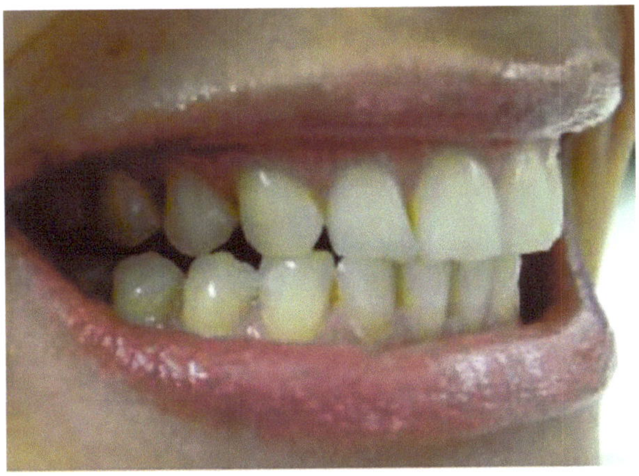

Figure 8.8. Canine guidance position of contacts on the balance side.

The perfect occlusion formula (Figures 8.4- 8.7) is checked using indigo-articulation papers placed between perfectly occluded arches. Firm closed contacts by movements of the lower jaw and tooth scraping, contact marking should be dotted on the occlusal surfaces of the molars and premolars, and linear on the palatal surfaces of the frontal teeth. It is very important to register premature contacts with occlusal markers (foil 8- 19 microns).

The formula represents the contacts in the central relationship and the disocclusion of all lateral teeth at the moment when the lower jaw moves out of central occlusion (Figures 8.7-8.9).

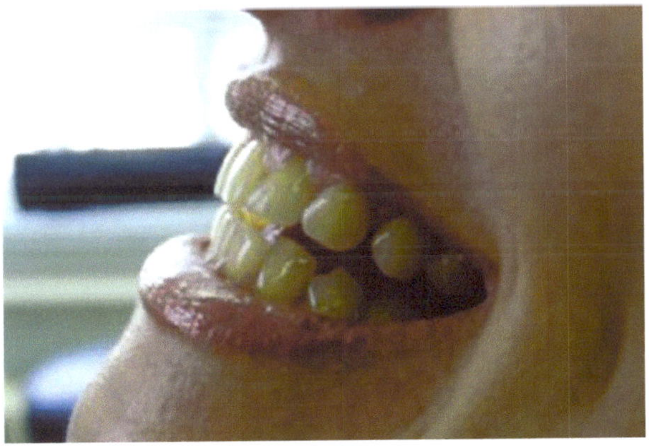

Figure 8.9. The initial stage of development on the balance side and separation of the lateral teeth during all excursions.

The anterior teeth (anterior guides), together with the condylar path, are responsible for the separation of the lateral teeth during all excursions (Figure 8.9). The reason for the separation of the lateral teeth is because at the moment of lateral separation, almost all the levator muscles are switched off, so that the forces acting on both the TMJ and the front teeth are significantly reduced. If the crowns of the front teeth are anchored on the implants, this detail should be given special attention, especially in patients prone to parafunctional movements.

For the effect of creating a calm neuromuscular balance, it should be additionally emphasized that it is impossible to overload the lateral teeth during movements, even if the patient has pronounced bruxism. This condition is maintained exactly as long as the anterior guides remain stable and the TMJ is healthy. That is the goal of perfect occlusion!

With perfect occlusion and articulation, everything is balanced in the TMJ. The condyle-disc assembly is intact and undamaged and has a self-centering effect on the disc (Figures 8.13a and 8.13b).

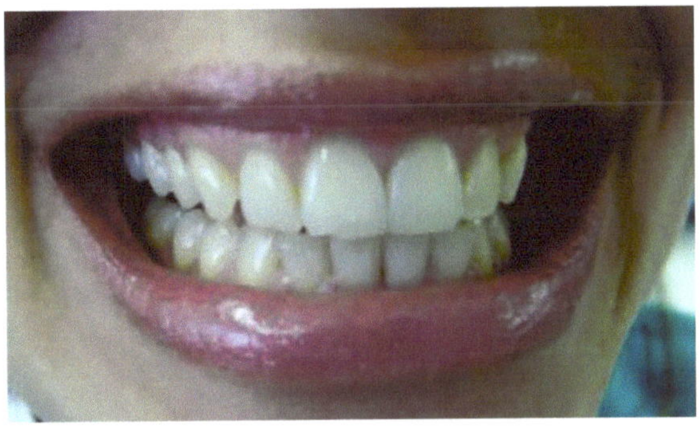

Figure 8.10. Position of central incisors during canine guidance.

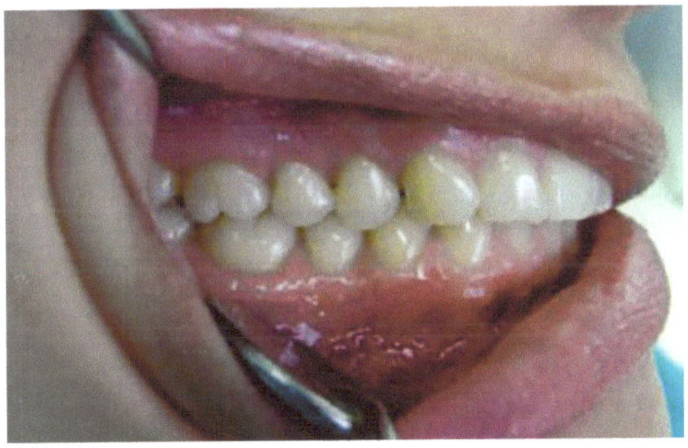

Figure 8.11. Ideal antagonist relationship in central occlusion.

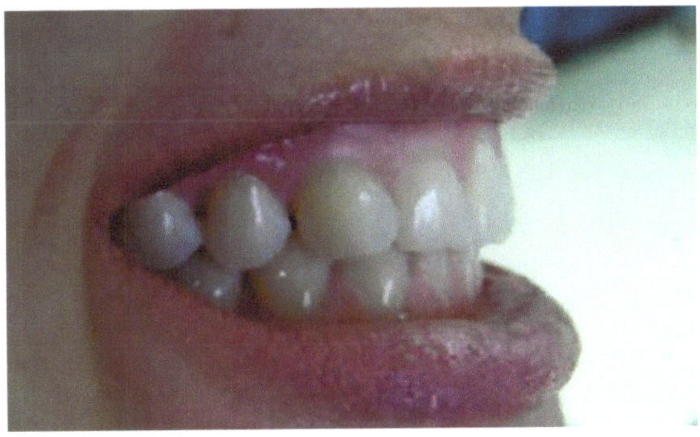

Figure 8.12. Ideal contact relationship of central incisors in central occlusion.

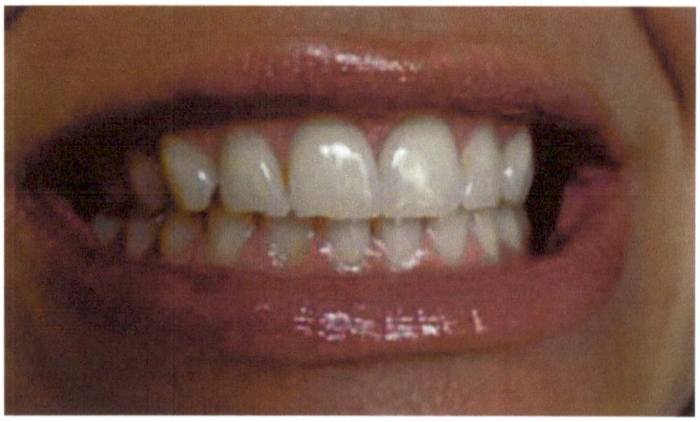

Figure 8.13. Ideal relationship in central occlusion.

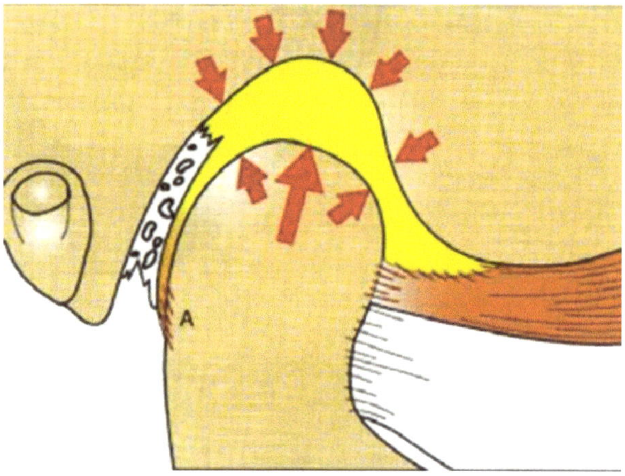

Figure 8.13a. An intact, undamaged condyle-disc complex enables self-centering of the discs. Contrary to belief, that the condyles will slip from the rear edge of the disc, if the TMJ is not supported by teeth, dislocation of the disc is not possible and the disc will not be displaced if its ligaments are preserved, as well as the biconcave shape of the disc is not deformed - unchanged. In addition to the self-centering shape of the disc, the posterior ligament extends from the disc and attaches at the back of the condyle. It serves as an inelastic connection that prevents the disc from dislocating forward, i.e. from displacing the disc anteriorly.

In a deformed TMJ, in order to obtain the balanced relationship shown in the previous images, the type and degree of adaptation should be determined before addressing the relationship between occlusion and TMJ.

The temporomandibular joint is the most adaptable joint of all the joints of the human body. It is the most burdened in its function, and yet it is the least likely to get sick (Scherzer, Otorhinolaryngology).

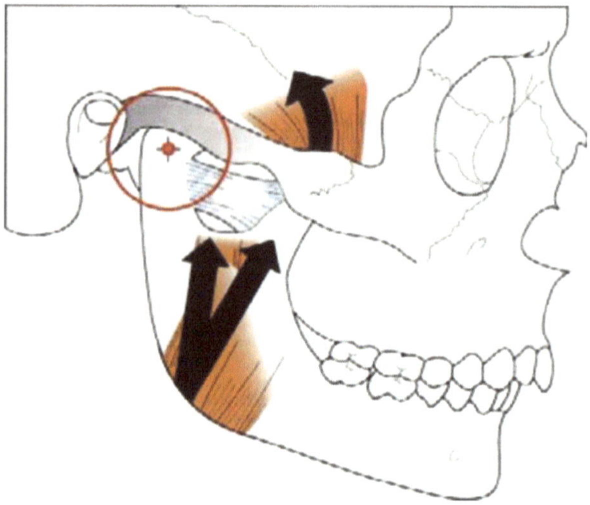

Figure 8.13b. Registration of the terminal hinge axis is evidence that the condyles rotate around a fixed axis. The goal of achieving an adapted central position is the same as with the central relation and represents complete relaxation of the lower external pterygoid muscle. If the joints in that position can receive loads without effort, good results of occlusal therapy can be expected. - Dawson.

Occlusion analysis requires standard instruments and procedures performed in practice. We perform complete control of occlusion and articulation with articulating indigo papers on which a layer of color is applied on one or both sides. Articulation foils are 10 to 40 microns thick. In addition to the colored ones, there are also uncolored articulation papers (thickness about 8 microns), resistant to tearing, which makes them ideal for fine checking of contacts with antagonists (Figures 8.14-8.19).

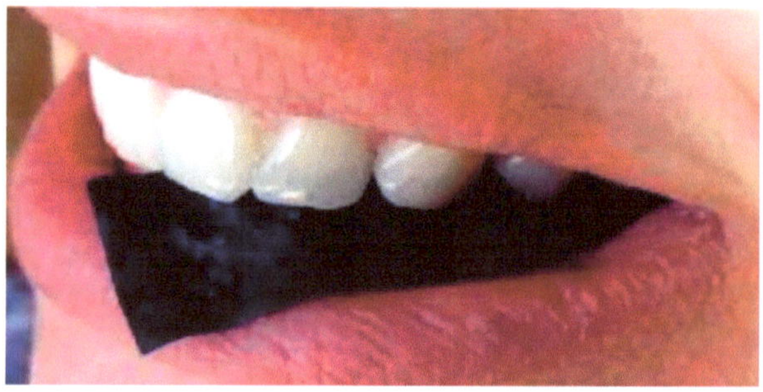

Figure 8.14. Registration of occlusion on the balance side.

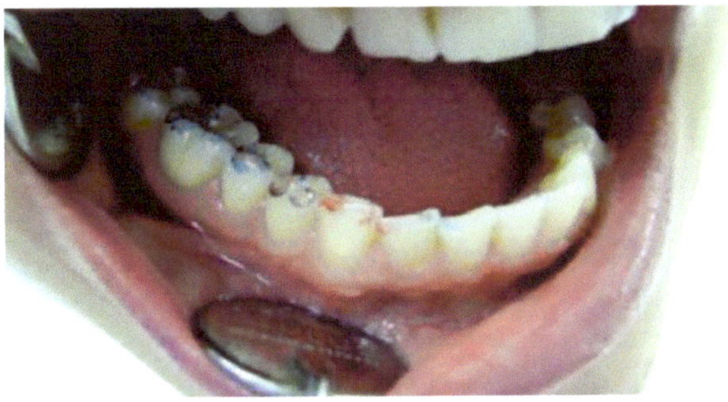

Figure 8.15. Antagonist contacts by canine guidance (red color).

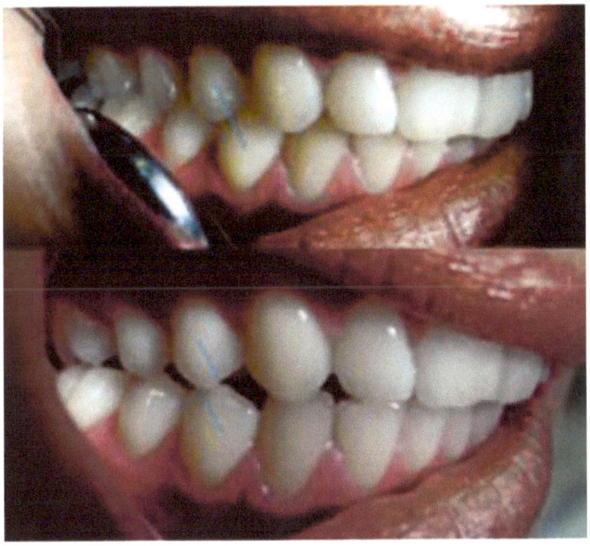

Figure 8.16. Representation of canine-guided occlusion and position of lateral tooth contacts.

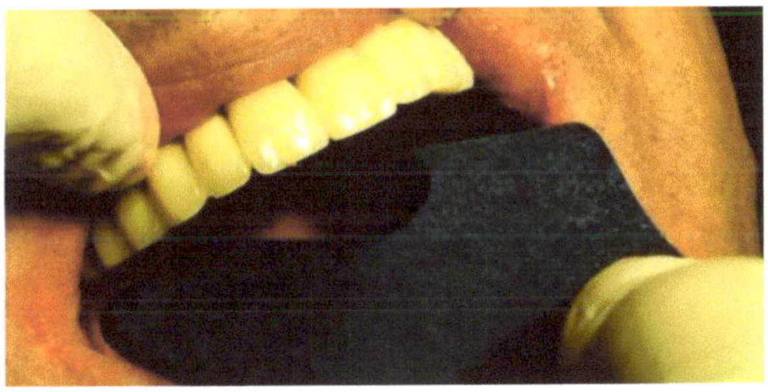

Figure 8.17. Registration of occlusion on the working side - bilateral toothlessness restored by fixed prosthetic work placed on implants.

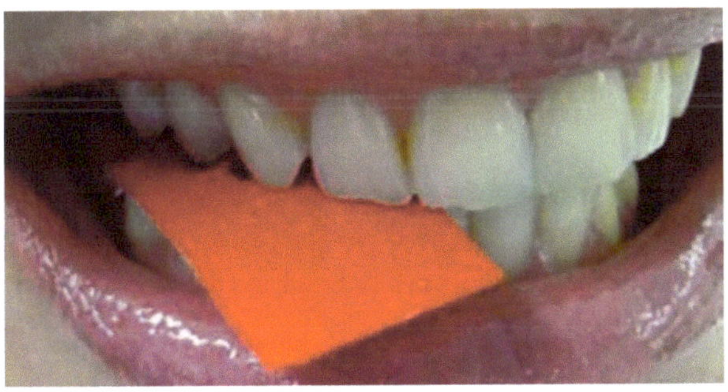

Figure 8.18. Registration of canine-guided occlusion.

Movements of the lower jaw can be expressed as deviations and deflections. Deviation of the lower jaw is a deviation from the straight path when opening the mouth and returning to the medial line when the mouth is maximally open.

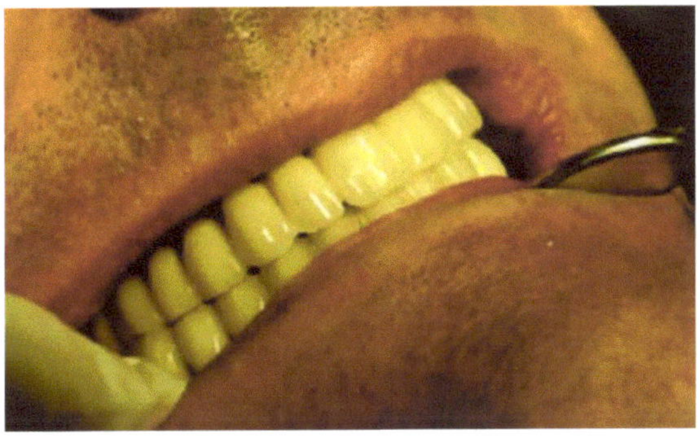

Figure 8.19. Established balanced occlusion with suprastructures on implants in case of total edentulism.

In the gnathological procedure of establishing an ideal occlusion, we use a combination of two papers of different colors (for example, blue and red) in order to distinguish the contacts formed in the position of maximum intercuspation from the contacts formed during eccentric movements of the lower jaw (Figures 8.20-8.24).

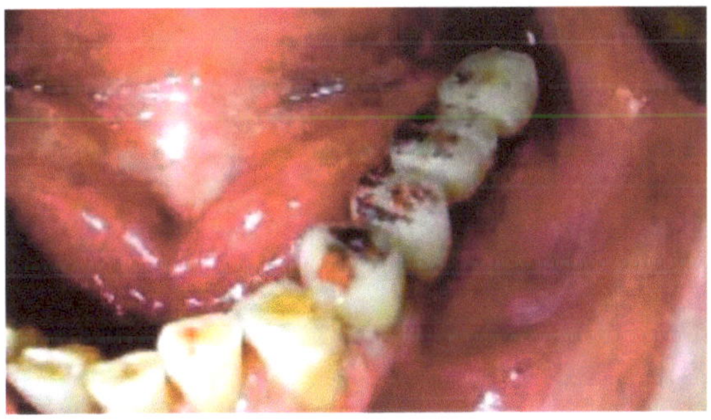

Figure 8.20. Registration and correction of stronger contacts (blue-red color) of the occlusion of the bridge supported by implants (regions 35, 36, 37).

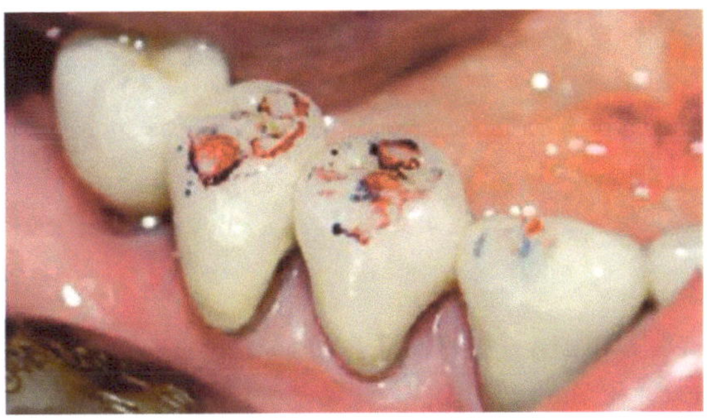

Figure 8.21. Marking of contacts during lateral movements - emphasized coloring - premature and too strong contacts.

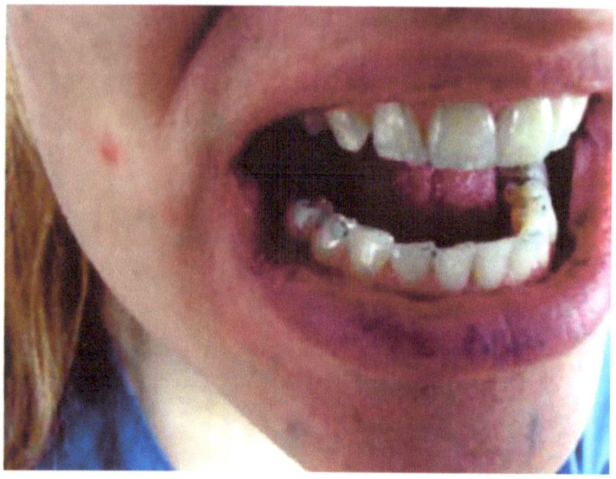

Figure 8.22. Registration of contacts on the balance sheet.

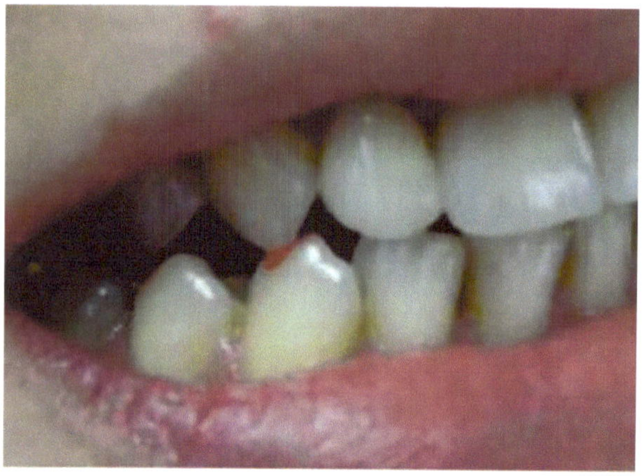

Figure 8.23. Guiding the occlusion with the canine - marked contact position in red.

Deflection is turning the lower jaw to the side without returning to the medial line when the mouth is maximally open.

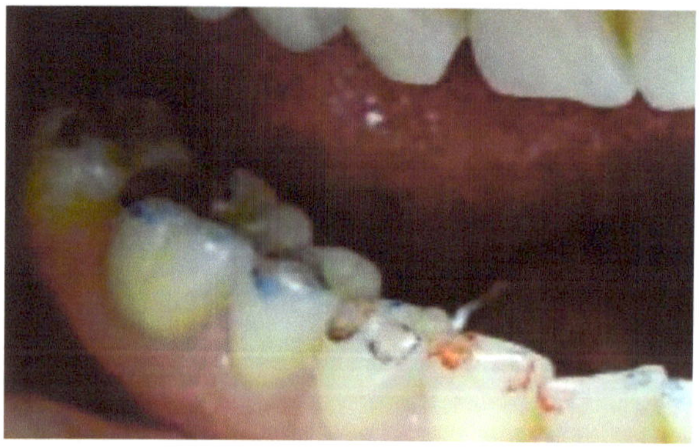

Figure 8.24. Marked contacts on the working side in the initial stage of canine guidance.

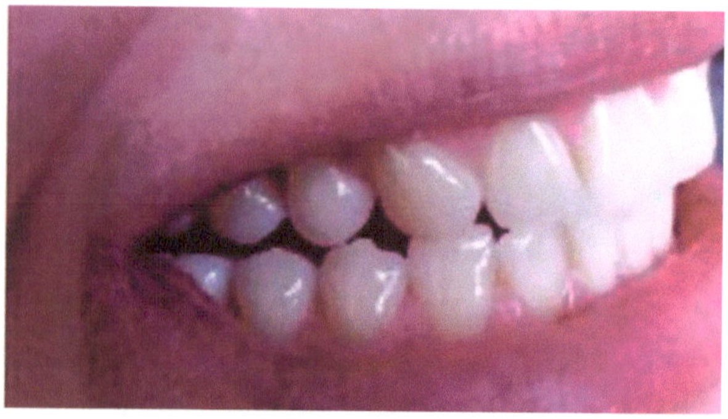

Figure 8.25. Position and contact of canines in natural teeth.

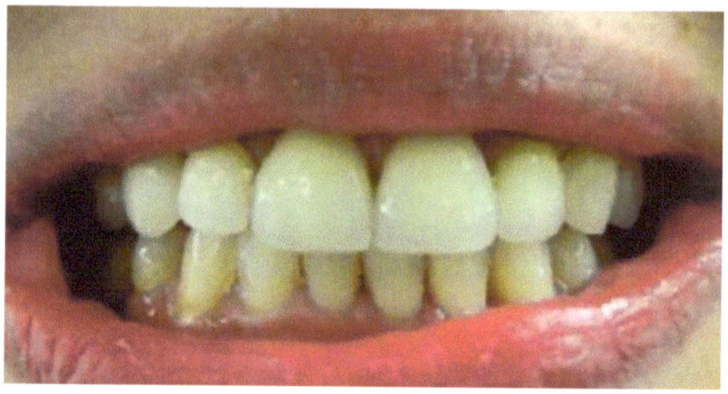

Figure 8.26. The relationship of occlusal contacts and the large overlap of the frontal teeth can be manifested by changes in the TMJ.

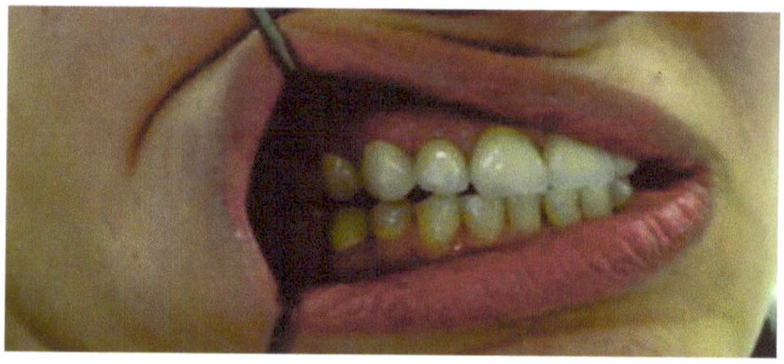

Figure 8.27. Displaced position of the canines towards the distal required the positioning of the implants in order to achieve good aesthetics.

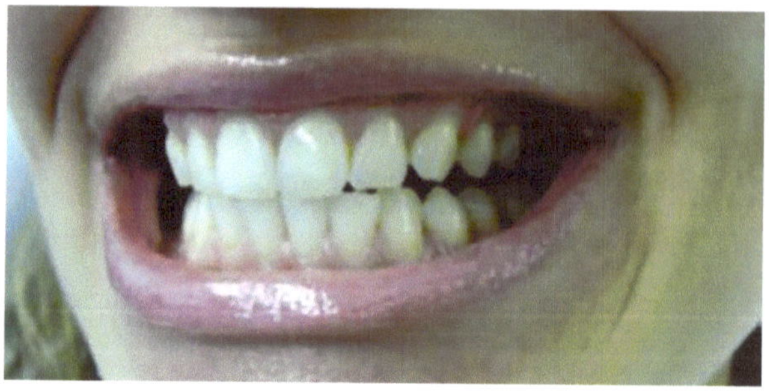

Figure 8.28. Movements of the lower jaw in protrusion, contact is lost on the working and ballast side.

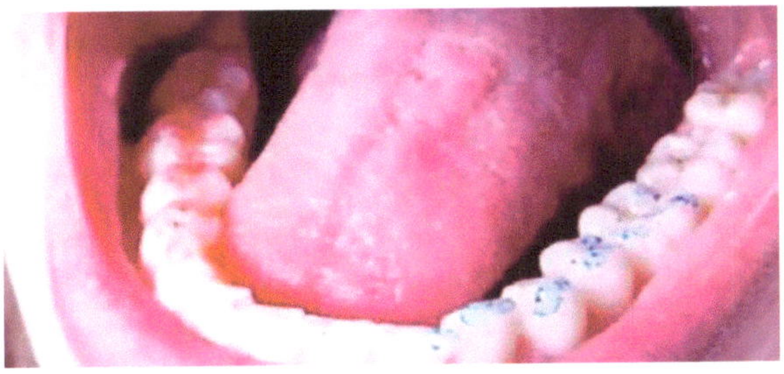

Figure 8.29. Maximum opening and closing of the mouth, marking of occlusal contacts and gnathological alignment shows ideal harmony in the TMJ.

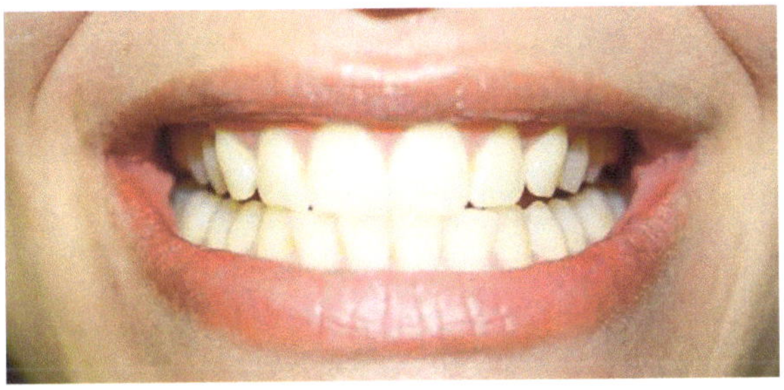

Figure 8.30. When the condyles move from the central relationship, forward movements of the mandible guide the palatal surfaces of the upper incisors and the incisor surfaces of the lower jaw. The condyles translate forward, and the lateral teeth lose contact.

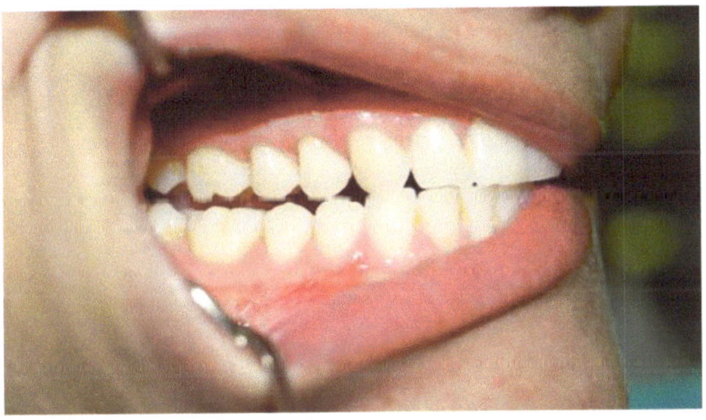

Figure 8.31. During the protrusive movement, the lower jaw moves forward, leading to the palatal surfaces of the upper incisors and front incisors of the lower jaw, which in the ideal occlusion of this movement determines the TMJ and front teeth, and the lateral teeth lose contact (view on the working side).

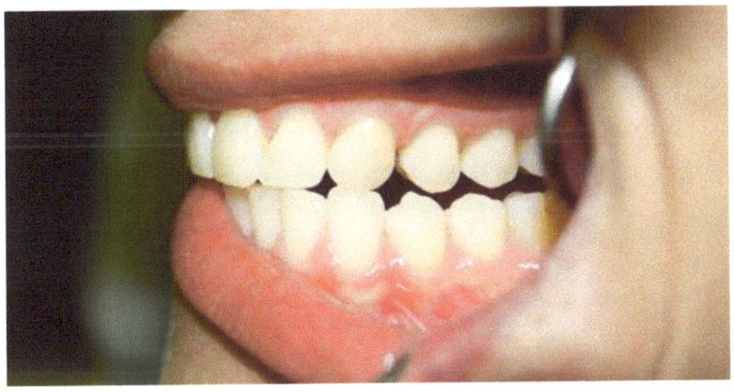

Figure 8.32. Changes in the anatomy of the TMJ and anterior teeth can influence changes in the shape of mandibular movements. Display of the position of the side teeth on the balance side.

While deviations in a milder form are a normal occurrence of imperfections in muscle coordination and congruence of joint bodies, deflections are almost always a sign of a unilateral pathological process in the muscles or TMJ.

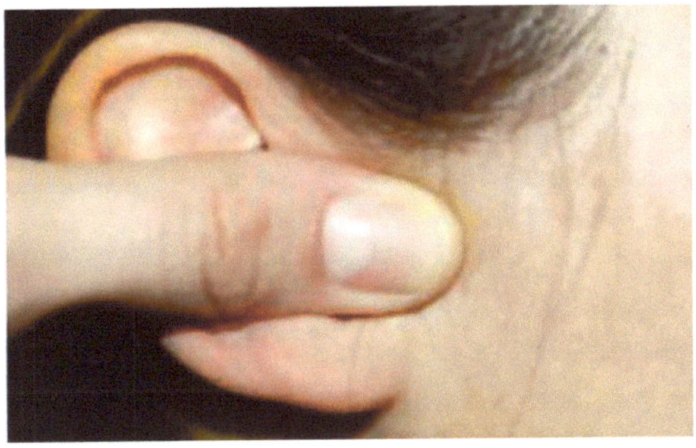

Figure 8.33. Palpatory checking of the condition of the joint.

The most common signs and symptoms of dysfunction in the TMJ are:

- pain that spreads through the temporomandibular region, accompanied by a headache;
- The pain spreads to other parts of the face;
- pain is especially felt during movements of the lower jaw;
- limited opening of the mouth;
- Deflection of the middle of the lower jaw when opening the mouth and
- Sensation of sound in the TMJ during movements of the lower jaw (crepitations, clicking, skipping of the condyle).

Pain in the TMJ is tested by palpation by using the tips of the fingers to find the poles of the condyle (about 13 mm in front of the tragus), and we will precisely locate them if the patient opens and closes the mouth slightly. We examine the pain of the disc-condyle complex with light pressure. By rotating and positioning the finger backwards with the mouth maximally open, we can provoke pain that occurs as a result of changes in the capsule itself and on the back side of the disc (Figure 8.33).

Painful compression of the retrodiscal tissue (Fig. 33a), i.e. the posterior part of the disc, is not treated in the same way as acute bone disease (A), although both disorders (B) (Fig. 33b) are classified as intracapsular disorders.

The image of the arthrogram of a normal joint shows an extension of the color and in the front part of the condyle limited to 2-3 mm. The anterior border of the color represents the attachment of the upper lateral pterygoid muscle to the discus (1). Everything in the lower part of the joint borders the contour of the lower part of the discs. A normal disc has a concave lower part (2). Joint sounds are a good diagnostic indicator of intracapsular disorders of the disc-condyle complex. They are examined clinically by palpation and stethoscope.

In recent times, electronic stethoscopes, which have the ability to more accurately record, reproduce and analyze the sound signal, provide significant help. The two most common sounds are clicks that occur when the condyle passes over the posterior band of the disc. It is important, along with the sound, to pay attention to the moment of its appearance during the opening of the mouth because it indicates the extent of the anteromedial luxation of the disc.

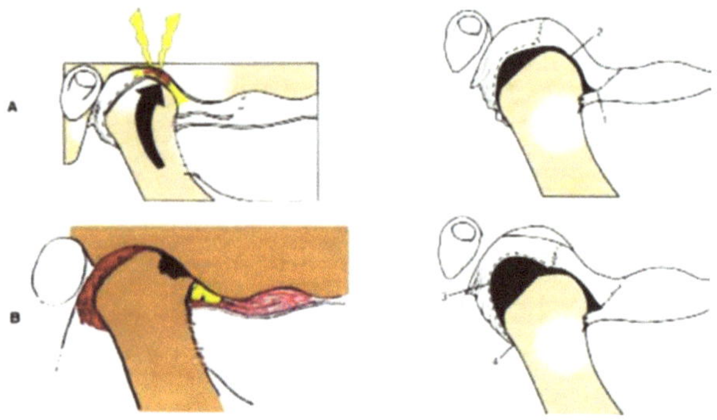

Figure 8.33a and 8.33b. Painful compression of retrodiscal tissue (A) is not treated in the same way as acute bone disease (B). Both disorders, both bone and tissue, are classified as intracapsular disorders (P.E.Dawson). The filling of the lower joint space borders the contour of the lower side of the discs. B - as the condyle moves forward the disc rotates towards the top of the condyle allowing the paint (black) to spread over the loosened ligament that attaches to the back of the condyle.

All this must be accompanied by a detailed analysis of the occlusion.

Just as we can perform an occlusion analysis in the patient's mouth, we can also perform an occlusion analysis in the articulator. In both cases, errors are possible: in the patient due to his reduced cooperation due to discomfort and pain in the TMJ and moist environment in the oral cavity, and in the articulator due to incorrect transmission, or the use of an inadequate articulator. Therefore, the recommendation: before the procedure, when occlusion correction is needed, both analyzes should be performed in the mouth and in the articulator, and the results must be consistent. In order to meet these requirements, the level of knowledge of dental technicians needs to match the level of knowledge of therapists. The author's experience shows that implant treatment failures are more often the result of poorly executed prosthetics than mistakes made in the operative technique of implant placement.

However, when it comes to natural teeth and implants, the transfer of the positions of ground teeth and embedded implants to impression materials is quite different. In order to achieve this, when transferring the exact position of the implanted implants to the laboratory, i.e. to the articulator, the exact position of the implant during impression taking must be ensured by transfers that are different for each system.

It should be emphasized that, in our conditions, mistakes made in the laboratory are very common, and most often they are difficult to correct for the following reasons: poor knowledge of dental technicians and the use of weak articulators.

Some laboratories even use occluders for the same purpose, which is an absolutely unacceptable variant. The first fact that we observe when examining the occlusion in the mouth is the presence or absence of harmonic antagonist contacts.

The absence of harmonic contacts in the position of habitual occlusion, whether it is partial or total toothlessness, is called malocclusion. Acute malocclusion occurs due to an acute disorder (most often muscular) in the jaws in which the occlusion was normal or disturbed by poor prosthetic work. Chronic malocclusion is most often the result of gradual tooth loss or orthodontic anomalies that take time to develop.

Important factors that influence the evolution of temporomandibular dysfunction (TMD) are the height of the occlusion and a series of orthodontic anomalies that can be observed when checking the occlusion with articulation papers. In the case of pronounced orthodontic anomalies, the installation of implants should be planned with caution in a patient with partial edentulism.

This clearly explains why it is so important to understand how the TMJ and anterior guides work together and what keeps these two determinants in a healthy state. With this preliminary knowledge we are enabled to gain a deeper understanding of TMJ.

Craniomandibular joint

In order to understand many events in the oral cavity, primarily the function of the TMJ, knowledge of the craniomandibular relationship, its anatomical content and functional complexity is necessary. This is of particular importance for understanding many events in the oral cavity, especially when, through the installation of implants and prosthetic works, the disturbed natural state is to be re-established in functional harmony.

The craniomandibular joint consists of two symmetrically positioned temporomandibular joints that function as a whole.

With intact interjaw relationships with natural teeth, all complex movements of the lower jaw, when opening the mouth, are first manifested by physiological events in the joint itself. Events continue by making contact between the teeth of the antagonist in the state of central position, that is, in the phase of statics - rest, and making contacts in the phase of dynamics - articulatory movement, or free jaw movement.

All this happens in physiological balance. A good knowledge of the anatomical structures of the jaw joint and its function, in case of prosthetic restorations, whether the supports are natural teeth or implants, is a basic prerequisite that all movement events in the TMJ can and must be transmitted and simulated in the articulator.

In order to understand the "joint" (housing) of the articulator, one must know the temporomandibular joint, both from an anatomical and a physiological point of view (Figure 8.26). Movements in the housing (joint) of the articulator must approximate the movements of the condyle in the TMJ.

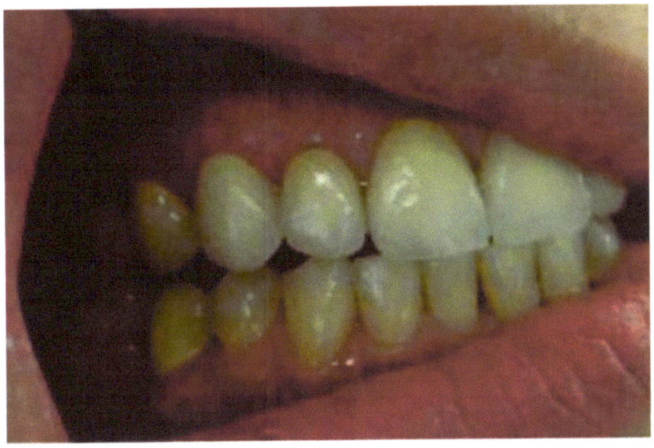

Figure 8.34. Prosthetic work on implants. Positioning of implants in the upper jaw (position depends on the available bone) displaced canines in relation to antagonists in the lower jaw.

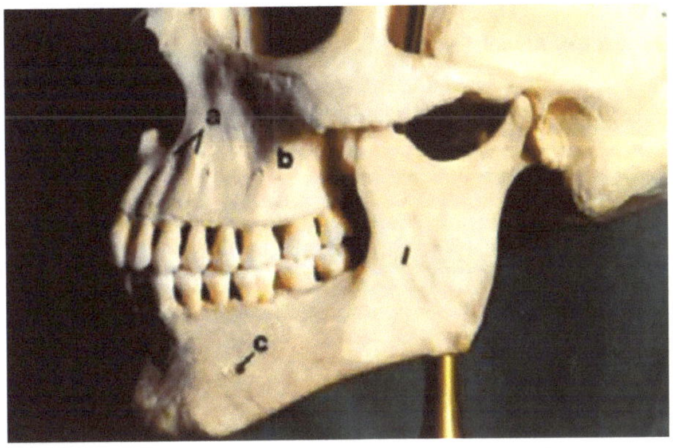

Figure 8.35. The position of the condyle in central occlusion.

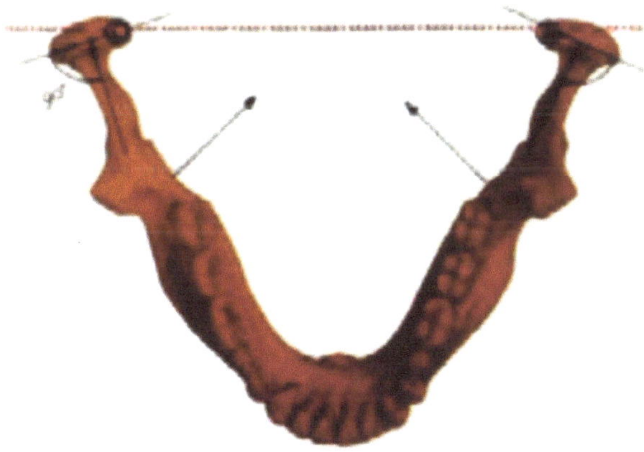

Figure 8.36. The medial poles of the condyles are the only points that would provide a fixed axis of rotation because the condyles are not parallel to the horizontal axis. This means that the lateral poles of the condyles must move translationally, even when the medial poles rotate around a fixed axis (as is the case in central relation, that is, in central occlusion).

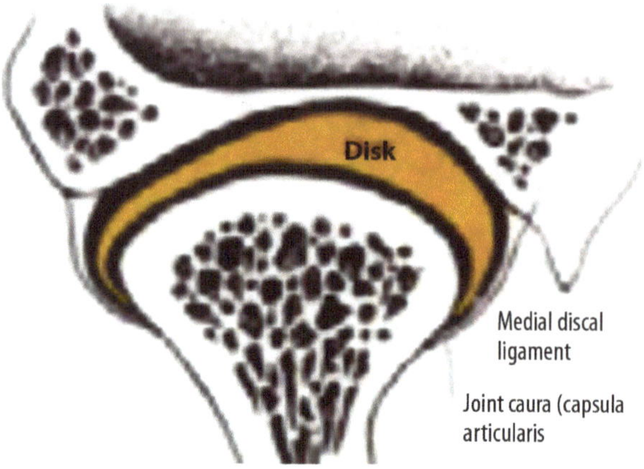

Figure 8.37. The condyle and disc assembly is placed in the most central and highest position by compression of the medial third of the condyle and disc assembly to the medial tip both triangle pits. In order to provide resistance to the action of m. pterygoides towards the inside and upwards, the pits are strengthened by a strong bony support which is directed in the direction of the load. The front surface of each condyle at the same time it presses the last slope of the eminence (protrusion).

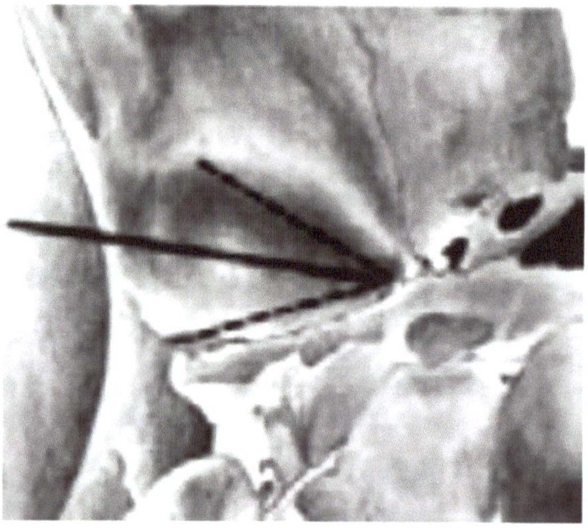

Figure 8.38. Additional proof that the horizontal axis passes through the medial ones poles of the condyle, is in a triangular fossa, the top of which is directed towards the medial fossa semi. If the horizontal axis would go through any part of the condyle, but not through the medial pole, there would be translational displacement of the medial half around the fixed axis of rotation, which is incompatible with the "V" shape of the pit.

Anatomical structures of the TMJ consist of:

- articular fossa (fossa mandibularis ossis temporalis);
- condylar process that has a head and a neck (condylus mandible);
- articular disc - discus articularis;
- articular capsule (capsula articularis);
- joint ligaments (ligamenta articularia).

The articular surface consists of the anterior and superior sides, which are covered with highly elastic fibrous tissue. The articular disc is in the form of a single biconcave plate, sandwiched between the articular surfaces and circularly attached to the condyle of the mandible by the anterior and posterior bands and collateral ligaments. The articular disc divides the temporomandibular joint into upper and lower synovial cavities, which act as separate units during joint function.

The basic movement of the lower jaw is manifested in the temporomandibular joint by rotation of the condyle, which takes place in the lower joint space between the condyle and the articular disc, and the transmission of condylo-discal movements takes place in the upper joint space along the entire articular surface of the temporal bone.

The **fossa mandibularis ossis temporalis** is located at the basal part of the squama of the temporal bone. The posterior, extra-articular part of this fossa is formed by the tympanic part of the temporal bone, and the anterior, articular part is formed by the horizontal part of the squama of the temporal bone. Only the squamous part of the fossa mandibularis is part of the temporomandibular joint.

Fossa articularis consists of a posterior concave part and an anterior convex part that forms the entire articulation surface. The articulation surface of the temporal bone, viewed as a whole, is saddle-shaped, unlike the articulation surface of the condyle, which is ovoid in shape.

Articulating surfaces of the TMJ are not always equal, neither in shape nor in surface, which is one of its specificities.

The articular tubercle is located on the outer part of the floor of the zygomatic arch and represents the attachment point of the temporomandibular ligament. It does not enter into the composition of the articulation surface of the temporal bone.

The articulatory surface of the mandible is formed by the upper and anterior surfaces of the condylar process of the mandible. The condyles of the mandible are ovoid in shape, although morphological variability is very common. The longer axis of the condyles is at right angles to the ramus of the mandible (Figure 8.36), and the condyle of the mandible is convex in all directions, more in the anterior-posterior direction and less in the medio-lateral direction.

The smooth articulating surface of the condyle is directed forward and upward so that, viewed from the side, the condyle looks as if it is slightly bent forward.

The sides of the condyle are bulging and are called the poles of the condyle. The articular disc and the inner part of the temporomandibular ligament are attached to the outer pole of the condyle, and the medial fibers of the articular capsule are attached to the inner pole of the articular disc. The lateral pterygoid muscle attaches to the front of the neck of the condyle.

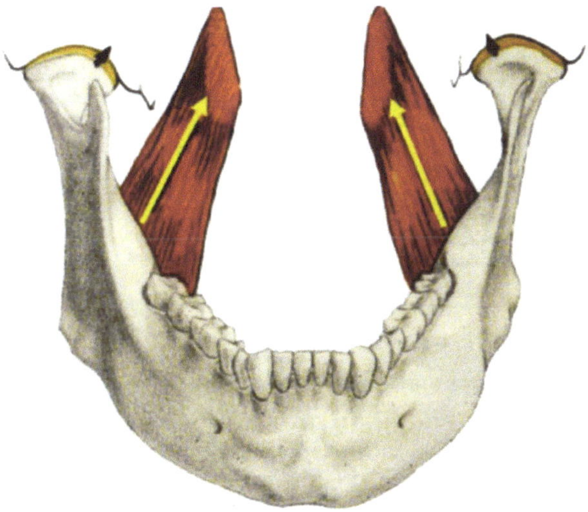

Figure 8.39. Medijalni pol kondila u sadejstvu sa kontrakcijom unutrašnjeg pterigoidnog mišića zauzima središni položaj u centralnoj relaciji. Kondili u centralnoj relaciji pričvršćeni su medijalno, a da bi bile moguće lateralne kretnje donje vilice moraju se spuštati prema dole. Ovakav centralni položaj se dešava istovremeno sa najvišim položajem kondila. Zaustavljanjem medijalnog pola kondila sprečava se da se donji bočni zubi u horizontalnoj ravni pomere ka medijalnoj liniji, koja je glavni anatomski oblik koji omogućava normalnu zakrivljenost okluzalne ravni. Ovo objašnjava zašto nije moguće odmah započeti lateralne kretnje iz centralne relacije.

The **discus articularis** is a biconcave cartilaginous articular plate, inserted between the articulating surfaces of the temporomandibular joint. The articular disc is composed of dense and hard fibrous tissue with islands of cartilage cells, which makes it flexible, allowing easy adaptation of its shape to the articulating surfaces of the joint in various phases of mandibular movements. The articular disc, on the periphery, is thickened and fused with the articular capsule (capsula articularis) at its deepest side, and is thin in the middle. The disc relieves the pressure of the condyle on the mandibular fossa of the temporal bone (articular fossa) during chewing and serves as a movable articular tubercle.

The **articular capsule** forms the envelope of the entire joint, or capsular ligament. The fibrous joint capsule, with its upper end, is attached to the edges of the articular fossa, and with its lower part to the neck of the condyle. The posterior attachment of the capsule has thickened, covering its edge and the entire anterior surface of the postglenoid process. On the anterior side, the capsule and disc have fused. There are two capsular ligaments formed by thickening of the fibrous membrane of the capsule articularis and three fascial ligaments formed by thickening of the fascia.

The external connection has a triangular appearance, with its base turned towards the lower edge of the apple-shaped process of the temporal bone, and its tip towards the outer side of the neck of the condyle.

The fascial connections are the sphaenomandibular ligament, which starts from the spine of the sphenoid bone and ends at the tongue of the lower jaw. This connection was created by the thickening of the interatrial fascia. Ligamentum stylomandibulare was formed by the thickening of the masseteric fascia, and starts from the tip of the styloid process to the angle of the mandible. The pterygo-mandibular suture extends the hamulus pterygoideus to the mylohyoid line, and was created by the thickening of the bucco-pharyngeal fascia. Fascial connections, even though they are distant from the joint, prevent excesslve openlng of the mouth and reduce the possibility of dislocation of the jaw joint.

The temporomandibular joint is strengthened and wrapped by articular ligaments.

From the aspect of joint function and stability, the most important roles are played by: collateral discal ligaments, capsular and temporomandibular ligaments, and there are also two accessory joint ligaments: sphaeno-mandibular and stylo-mandibular.

Ligaments play a major role in joint protection, they are made of dense collagen connective tissue and are not elastic. Ligaments do not actively participate in joint functions, but act as passive stops, i.e. stoppers that limit the movements of the condyle and disc. Excessive stretching of joint ligaments causes pain.

Collateral ligaments attach the disc to the medial and lateral poles of the condyle. They are responsible for rotational movements in the joint that take place between the condyle and the articulating disc, but do not allow translational movement of the disc on the condyle.

The anatomical and functional specificities of the craniomandibular joints and neuromuscular regulation allow the lower jaw a wide range of movements, from basic to very complex.

The basic movement in the jaw joints is the rotation of the condyle. It takes place in the lower joint space between the condyle and disc, with the transfer of the condylo-disc complex, which takes place in the upper joint space, along the entire joint surface of the temporal bone.

Movements of the lower jaw, as already written, can be basic and complex movements.

The basic movements of the lower jaw include opening and closing the mouth, then forward movements (propulsion or protrusion), backward movements (retropulsion or retrusion), laterally directed movements (left and right laterotrusion) and the movement of returning from the lateral position to the central position.

These very complex movements, which are created by a combination of basic movements of the mandible, perform all physiological functions of the lower jaw: chewing, swallowing, speech, facial movements, and of course parafunctional movements.

Apart from opening the mouth, all other movements of the lower jaw can take place in the creation of contacts between antagonist teeth, calling them contact - **articulation or sliding movements**.

Movements of the lower jaw without contact of antagonist teeth are called **free jaw movements.**

Central occlusion can be defined in several ways. The position of the central occlusion is the position of the relationship between the lower and upper jaw, where the upper and lower teeth are in contact. The position of the contacts is determined by maximum intercuspation, which is achieved by the morphology of the teeth that are in contact. Central occlusion can also be defined by the position of the condyles, when they are in the position of maximum dystoposition, i.e. in the most cranial physiological position of the condyles at a certain value of bite height. Extreme excursions that the lower jaw can make in a certain direction occur without the participation of joint structures. Anatomical determinants limit the movements of the lower jaw to articular or posterior and occlusal or anterior. In articular guidance there is an influence of the temporomandibular joint, and in occlusal guidance we have the influence of the lingual surfaces of the upper front teeth and the internal inclinations of the leading cusps of the lateral teeth on the movement of the lower jaw.

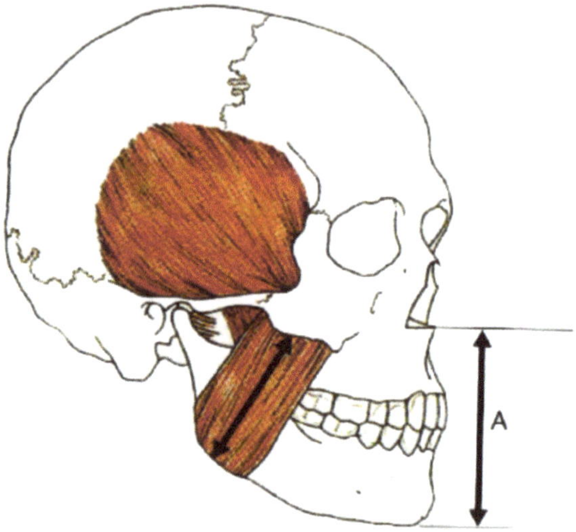

Figure 8.40. The repetitive contracted length of the levator muscles determines the vertical dimension of the bite (A)

The symmetrical trajectory of both condyles during protrusion and mouth opening is designated as the **sagittal condylar trajectory**.

The inclination of the sagittal condylar path, in relation to an assumed plane of the skull (Kamper's plane), determines the characteristics of the protruding movement of the mandible, and it depends on several factors: the angle, shape and convexity of the sagittal condylar path.

Depending on the type of occlusion and the relationship of the front teeth, the mandible during protrusion can be **incisally guided (see the perfect occlusion formula)**, or the lingual surfaces of the lateral incisors and canines are also included in this function, when it comes to guiding by a group of front teeth.

The position of central occlusion, i.e. when maximum intercuspation is achieved, is the initial and final position of all mandibular movements. It is the reference position of the lower jaw from which all other movements of the mandible are analyzed.

The limits of movement of the lower jaw are characteristically different in size and shape for each person and are easy to analyze.

The execution of normal movements of the lower jaw is regulated by numerous factors that initiate, program, control and limit these movements. All these factors have the common name determinants of jaw movements and are divided into: anatomical and physiological determinants. Anatomical structures of the craniofacial skeleton and jaw complex that guide and direct, or limit the movements of the lower jaw are called anatomical determinants of jaw movements.

With prosthetic restorations, it is important to establish an **articulatory balance**, which is a balance between the correct dental row and the ability of the surrounding tissues to resist pressure forces. With a proper, natural, intact row of teeth, articulation movements are performed without interference and effort, because the mutual relationship is coordinated, so that during horizontal lateral movements of the lower jaw, the opposing teeth do not interfere with each other during contact.

With such articulation balance when the lower jaw moves in any position, the tooth contacts are distributed in several points. This achieves an even distribution of the pressure of chewing forces on the jawbone in the TMJ through the teeth, and then the teeth are said to have **Ideal articulation**, or **articulation balance. This articulation balance must also be achieved when it comes to solutions with implants.**

Free movements are those that do not reach the boundary of the polygon where the teeth are not in contact, and which exist in all unconscious and reflex movements.

One should always strive to achieve a perfect occlusion formula (see pictures 8.4, 8.5, 8.6 and 8.10, 8.11).

Articulatory movements can be symmetrical and asymmetrical.

Symmetrical articulation movements are movements of protrusive and retrusive gliding. Protrusive sliding occurs when the mandible moves forward to direct incisor contact, and repressive sliding is the opposite, and occurs when the mandible moves backward from the position of central occlusion.

Asymmetrical articulation movements are lateral and latero-protrusive sliding. During lateral sliding, the mandible moves to the right or left side. The side towards which the mandible moves is the working side, and the opposite side is the **non-working or balance side.**

Lateral protrusive sliding of the mandible is a combination of protrusive and lateral sliding movements. Articulating movements of the mandible are dental contact movements, during which the antagonists maintain contact.

In addition to these, there are also so-called border and free movements. **Limit movements** are obtained when the mandible performs all possible extreme movements (maximum opening and closing).

One should always strive for occlusal events in prosthetic works to be close to the perfect occlusion formula!

9

Occlusion Analysis In Lateral Teeth

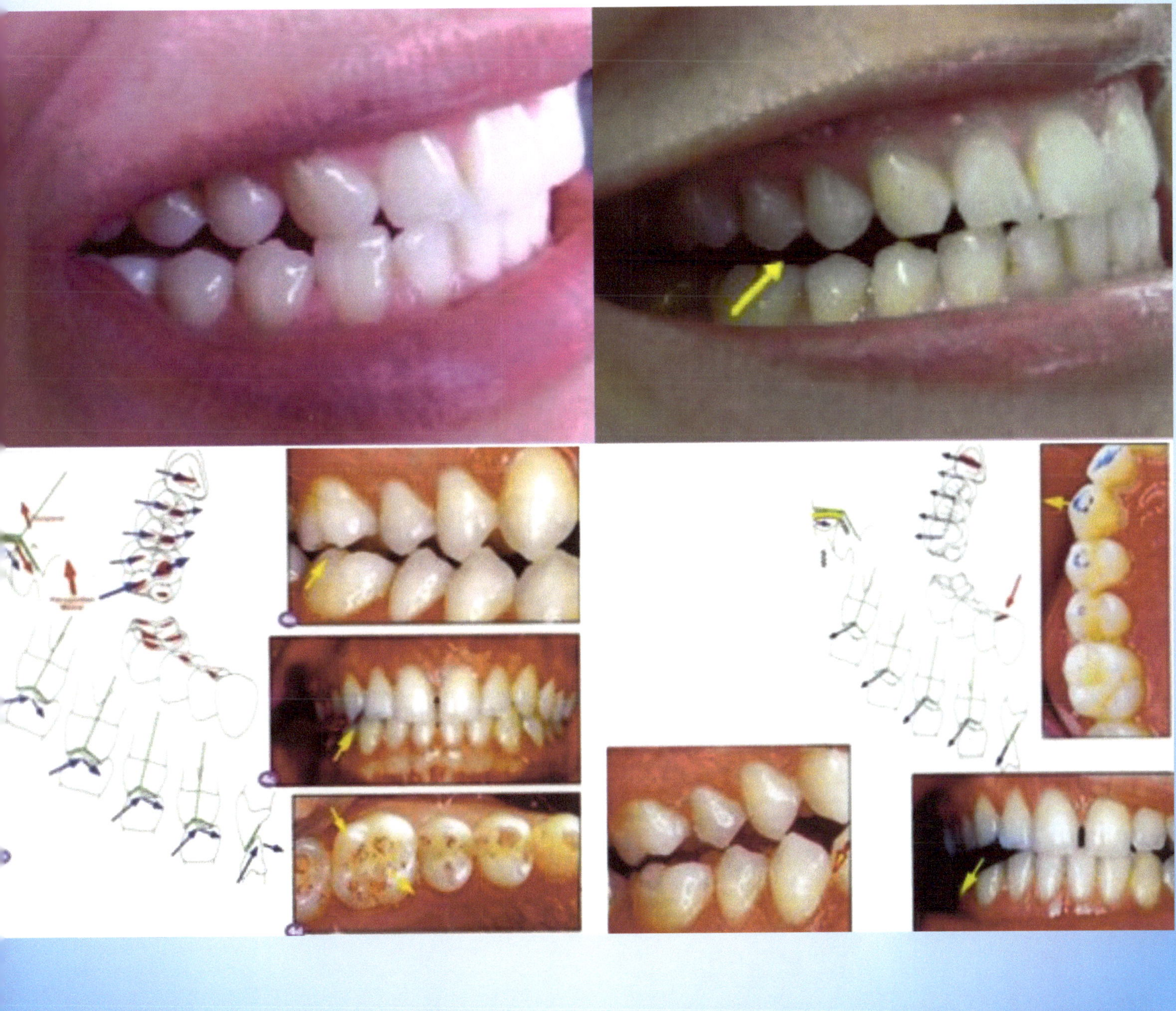

Comparison of clinical conditions and articulator conditions

The relationship between clinics and laboratories is extremely important for the successful outcome of prosthetic, and especially the entire implant and prosthetic procedure. Since prosthetics is one of the important factors in the success of implant placement, and is closely related to all problems and possible risks, implant-prosthetic rehabilitation should be given special attention from the aspect of prosthetics.

Curricula for students of dentistry and specialist education at our educational institutions, implant placement and prosthetic restoration are studied as two strictly separate disciplines. However, in practice, for a dentist involved in practical implantology, prosthetic rehabilitation is more often a complex procedure than the implant placement itself. For this reason, it seems to me that this chapter belongs to prosthetics as much as it belongs to oral implantology.

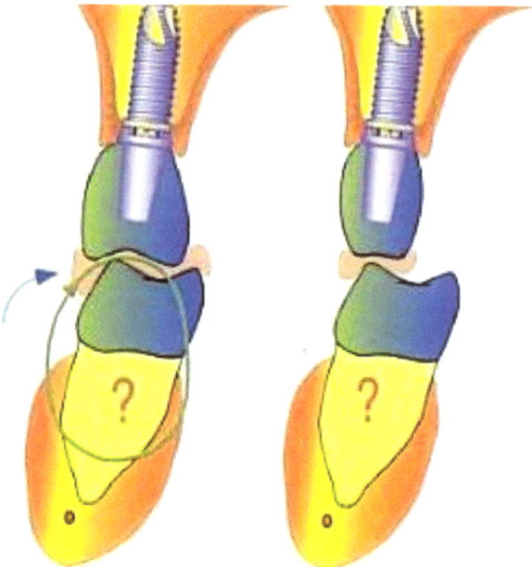

Figure 9.1 The question that requires an answer: by laboratory shaping of the occlusal surfaces of the artificial crowns, did we direct the forces of chewing at lateral movements axially?

When it comes to the issue of occlusion and natural teeth, especially when it comes to restorations on implants, the practitioner is faced with the following questions after the implant placement:

How to establish an occlusion in the mouth and perform an analysis of the occlusion at the lateral mandibular calluses when it comes to mutual nodule contacts in the chewing cycle phase (Figure 9.1), especially if the implants are immediately put into operation, i.e. if they are under immediate load. This is especially important due to the fact that the axially received forces are evenly decomposed into the bone around the implant (Figure 9.2);

- What are the possibilities and limitations of articulators in reproducing this functional kinematics?
- With which and what kind of articulators in the laboratory does our associate, a dental technician, realize our imaginary project?
- Also, the question arises, is the evolution of common conceptions of occlusion necessary when it comes to dental restorations carried by implants?

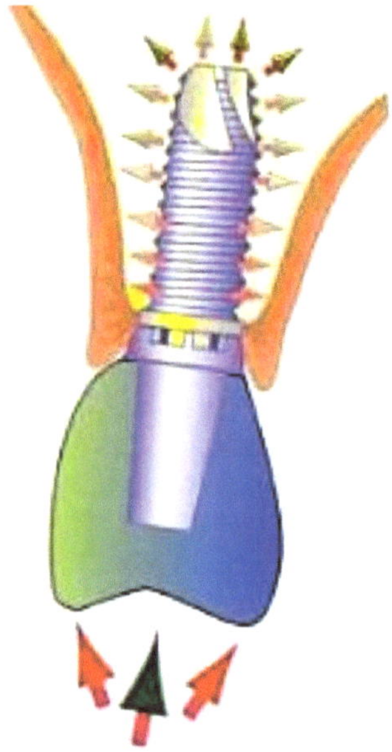

Figure 9.2 The axial force reception results in their uniform decomposition, reducing them to physiological limits of action.

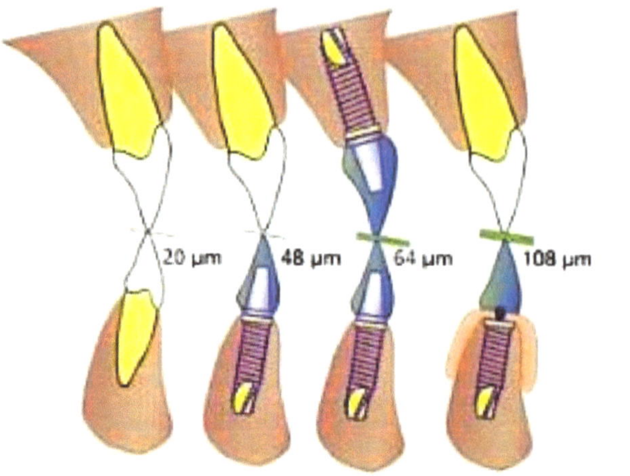

Figure 9.3 Schematic representation of the mobility of the root of the natural tooth and the depreciation of the set forces in relation to the implant.

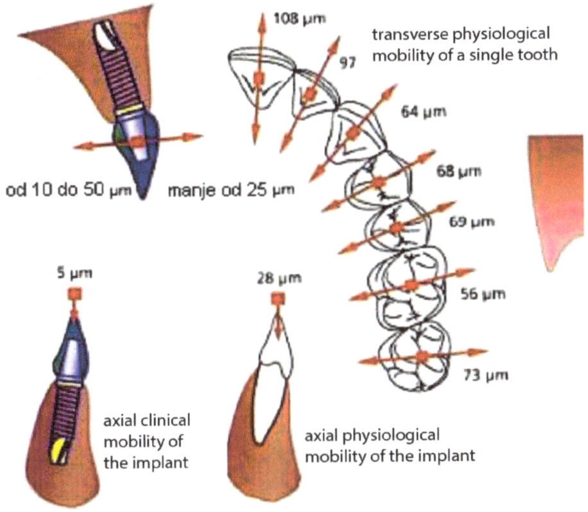

Figure 9.4a The clinical median mobility of the implant is definitely lower than the median physiological mobility of the natural tooth.

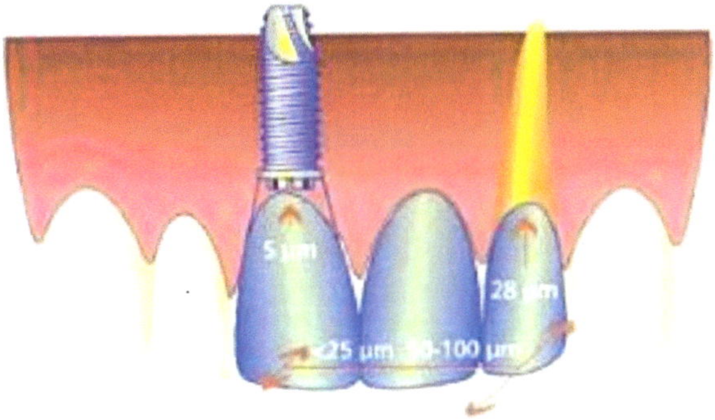

Figure 9.4b A comparison of the axial clinical mobility of a natural tooth in the axial and horizontal directions.

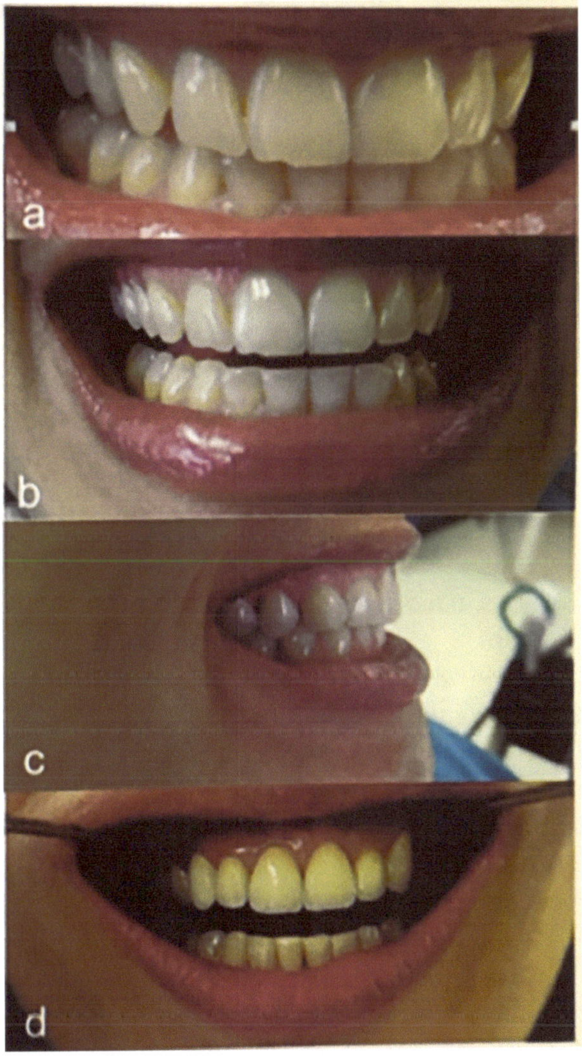

Figure 9.5. Occlusions of maximum intercuspation in natural teeth (a,b and c) and mass intercuspation in patients achieved by prosthetic fixed restorations on upper jaw implants (d). This example indicates in two concurrent patients how important prevention is from the earliest age, i.e. Monitoring the development of dentition in the oral cavity.

These are questions that are asked not only by the prosthetist but also by the oral surgeon. The importance of these questions is also shown by the fact that they were first asked by a group of oral surgeons (Lore, M. Le Gal and Lando), which confirms the opinion that these two dental disciplines are actually one, when it comes to prosthetic rehabilitation on implants.

However, the same questions can be asked by a periodontologist, due to the recognition of the effect of favorable and unfavorable forces on the entire supporting apparatus of the natural tooth. For each pre-set question, an analytical answer should be sought. There are numerous and different papers and publications regarding the approach and analysis of occlusion in lateral mandibular movements. From the abundance of literature, 2 streams of thought emerge, mainly based on 2 theoretical concepts, the theory of balanced occlusion and the theory of occlusion exclusively guided by the canine, and some authors indicate this as a function of the canine.

The theory of more balanced occlusion substantially developed at the beginning of the last century under the Influence of researchers such as Christensen, Gizzy and Monson. Already during the twenties, the works focused on the research of the mandibular cranial position, that is, on the central relationship, which led to the emergence of the gnathology school. One of the central definitions of collision is that it is an occlusion when the condyle is in maximum disposition from which lateral movements are possible.

At first, and until the mid-50s of the last century, the pioneers of the gnathology school advocated the theory of balanced bilateral occlusion in natural teeth.

A few years later, after the first observations described by Amiko (Amico) regarding the occlusion of the lead canine during the eccentric movements of the mandible, the gnathology school gradually began to recommend the conception of a mutually protected occlusion.

In this conception, the entire clinical procedure was aimed at establishing canine (cuspid) function. Until then, the relationship of teeth with lumps is observed exclusively from the aspect of statics. However, it should be said that the initiators of this conception (that the patient also performs lateral movements guided by cuspids), did not predict the role of occlusal lumps in establishing occlusal balance guided by the cuspids. The ideal status of the preserved balanced ideal ratio in the mouth is schematically shown in Figures 9.6 and 9.8.

However, on such a conceptual development, it can be noted that some essential facts are neglected: neuropsychological and kinetic components of the actual chewing function. Namely, the movements and contacts of the teeth with lumps, during the last phase of chewing, before swallowing a bite of food, are the consequence of a kinetics that is completely opposite to the kinetics of lateral movements that is usually required from the patient in the analysis of occlusion.

On the other hand, there are also muscle actions, and thus mandibular conditions that arise from them, which is not the same. The literature dealing with the chewing function is extensive, so it is quite logical to ask the question: why have the authors of many publications not put into practice the consequences of such approaches?

The author spent some time with Peter Thomas (USA), studying the concepts of gnathology set by this most famous gnathologist today. General directions and conceptions of gnathology were accepted in practice due to the ease of clinical application. However, if the kinetic problems posed by the cuspid sectors were studied through the leading function of the canines, would not this conceptually proposed functioning be oversimplified?

It is on this question that a group of oral surgeons (Lore, Le Gali, Lando) tries to present their views on some developmental perspective, answering a question, such as a clinical analysis of the lateral movements of the mandible.

It should be emphasized how important it is to know this issue for an implantologist, because this is also noticed by a group of oral surgeons (if it is in the domain of prosthetics), suggesting what kind of articulators should be used.

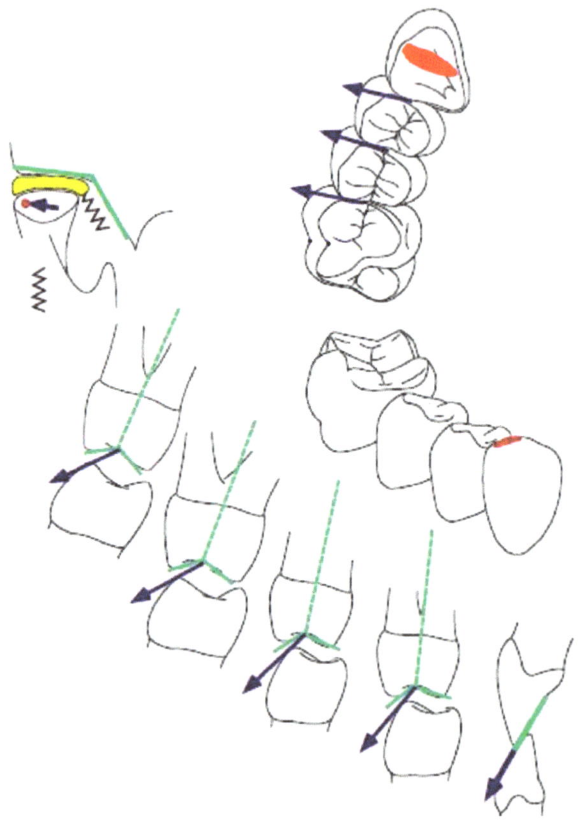

Figure 9.6. The direction of the forces of occlusal contacts in the centrifugal movement passes from the occlusion of maximum intercuspation. Side teeth lose all sliding contact (Figures 9.8 and 9.9), indicated by blue arrows. The yellow arrows indicate the initial position of the lumps of the occlusal relations in the centripetal movement and the position of the condyle (see Figures 9.8,9.9, 9.10, 9.13, 9.20, 9.32 and 9.51).

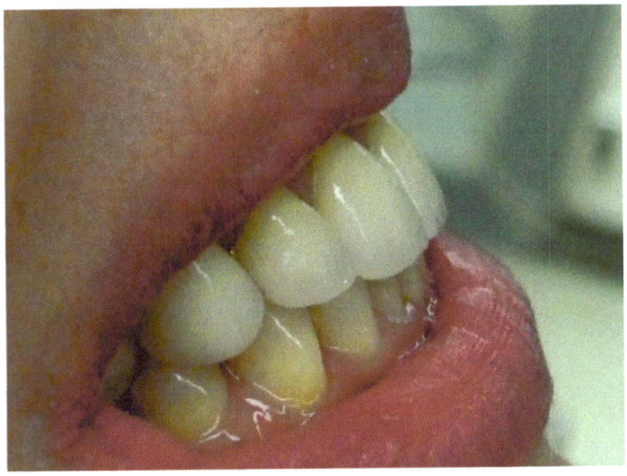

Figure 9.7. Canine teeth are teeth with the longest roots, which therefore tolerate the loads caused by lateral movements well, taking on this role by protecting the incisor and the back teeth. This ratio should also be applied when installing implants at the canine site by selecting a longer implant.

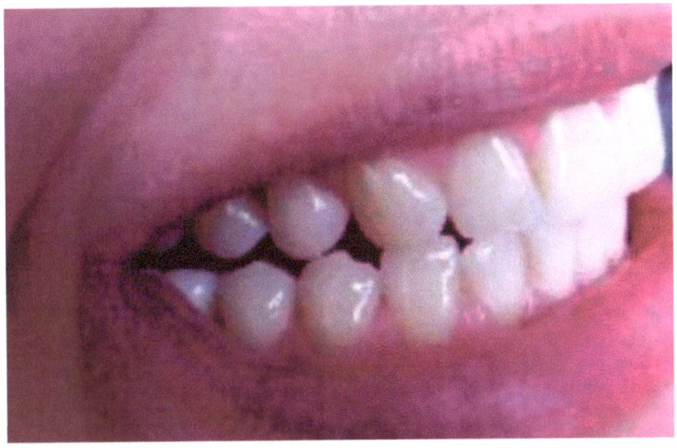

Figure 9.8. When guiding with a canine tooth, premolars and molars take a sliding position and lose contact on the working side. This is achieved by an ideal occlusion and mutually protected type of occlusion. Mutual protection is manifested in the protection of the frontal teeth at maximum intercuspation of the protection of the lateral teeth at the lateral movements of the lower jaw.

Through a study of a clinical case that otherwise corresponds to the criteria of normality of the occlusal scheme (Figure 9.9.), lateral occlusal trajectories, observed in the mouth, and comparison with trajectories generated by articulators were compared (Figure 9.14). Due to this comparison, models of the same patient were placed in two different types of articulators: one articulator was classic, from the family of so-called semi-adaptive articulators of the second generation (Figures 9.26 and 9.28), and the other, the articulator was with significantly better characteristics as for example the articulator Reverse (Figure 9.24).

On the classic articulator (Figure 9.26), it is not possible to obtain a lateral centrifugal movement contacts to the initial stage of the process. The analysis of occlusion on models in a classic articulator is different from the analysis of the condition in the mouth. The clinical analysis of the oral occlusion should precede the analysis of the articulator occlusion. Here, too, it should be emphasized that the models of functioning are very accurately depicted by the patient, and not by the mechanical system, the articulator, which is activated in the laboratory! Namely, it seems that lateral movements, which are usually required in the patient when voluntarily performing movements of the mandible, transferred to the kinematics of handling articulators, actually become centrifugal movements from the position of maximum intercuspation, and not the transmission of nodule contacts in lateral movements.

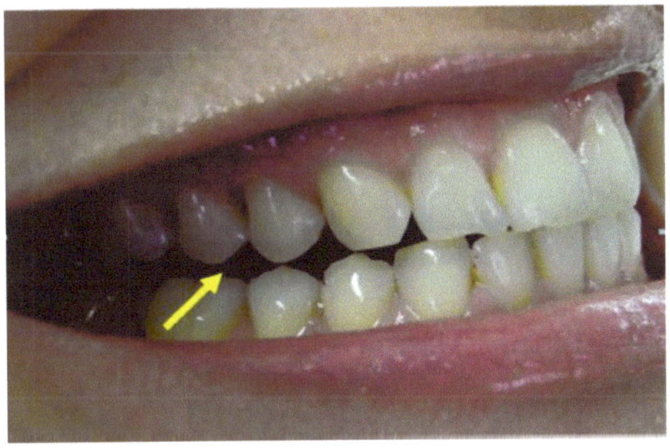

Figure 9.9. During lateral movements within canine control, premolars and molars on the working side lose contact. The paradontia of the posterior teeth is adapted to the reception and withstanding of strong vertical loads, but is not resistant to lateral forces. In contrast, the paradontium of the front teeth tolerates vertical loads in lesser amounts, but compensates for the horizontal forces generated by the protrusion.

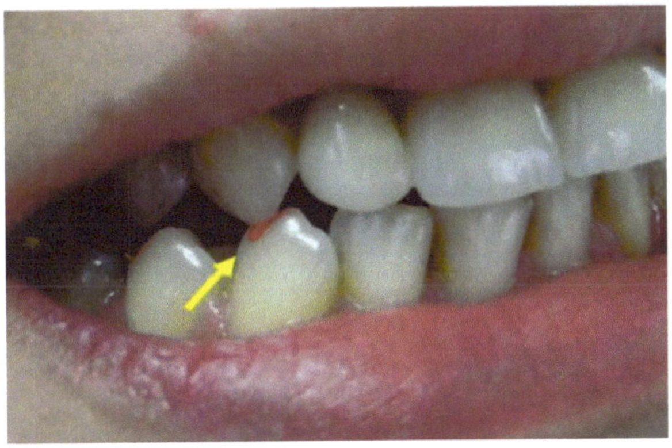

Figure 9.10. Group management of occlusion is considered to be a subtype of canine management, that is, a form that occurs when the canine lump loses contact slightly (Figure 9.10 and 9.13)

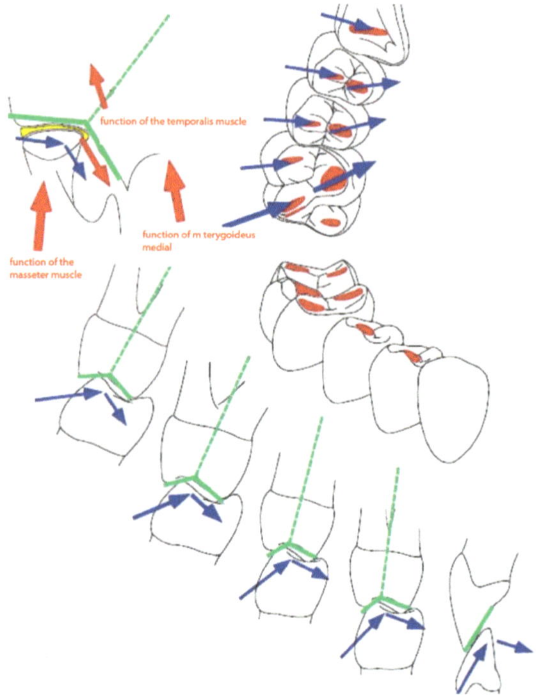

Figure 9.11. Schematic representation of occlusal guidance in opening and closing movements of the chewing cycle on the right side before and after the passage of maximum intercuspation (as seen in figure 9.13)

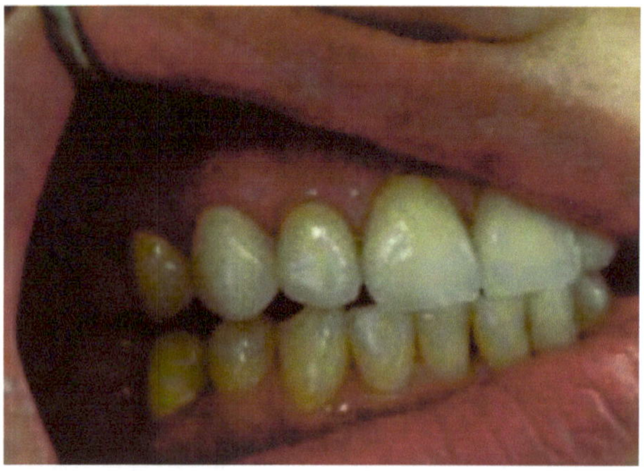

Figure 9.12. The initial phase, registration of canine guidance on the right side is often difficult to achieve with prosthetic work on implants.

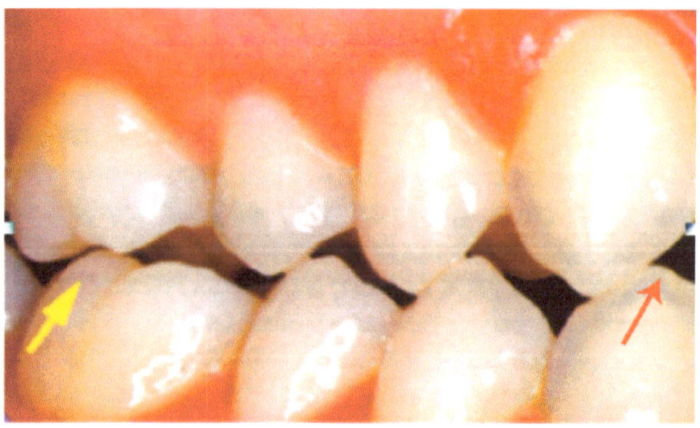

Figure 9.13. The yellow arrow indicates the initial position of the lumps of occlusal relations in the centripetal movement, and the cycle of movements towards the occlusion of maximum intercupation continues, and the canine gently loses contact.

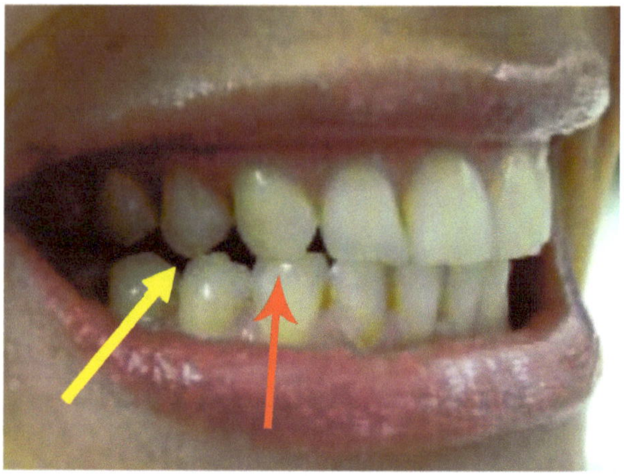

Figure 9.14. Group guiding of the occlusion is considered a subspecies of canine guiding, that is, a form that occurs when the canine lump loses contact slightly (red arrow), 1 and 2 premolars assume the role of guiding (yellow arrow)

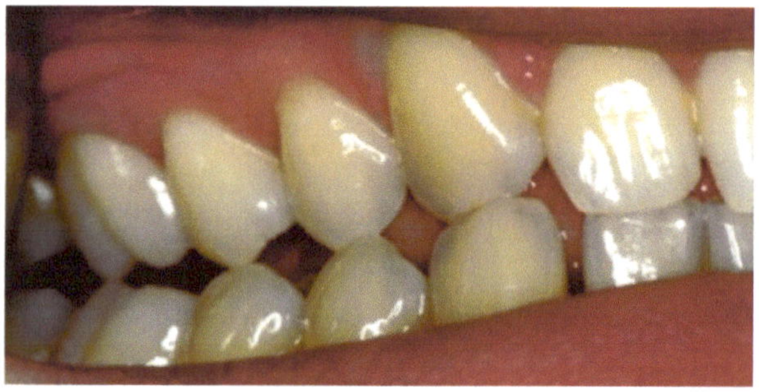

Figure 9.15 Display (schematic see Figure 9.11) of occlusal guidance in right-hand chewing cycle opening and closing movements (before and after passing maximum intercuspation). The occlusal guidance is maximal on all occlusal surfaces, and the articular relationships are changed by the function of the muscles (red arrows of Figures 9.11 and 9.21 a) to adapt to the situation of as close as possible to the lumps of the lateral teeth (Fig. 9.13). Condillar kinematics during the chewing process initiation phase corresponds to a direction that is higher and curved upwards and backwards, and the muscle functions in that kinematics are indicated by red arrows.

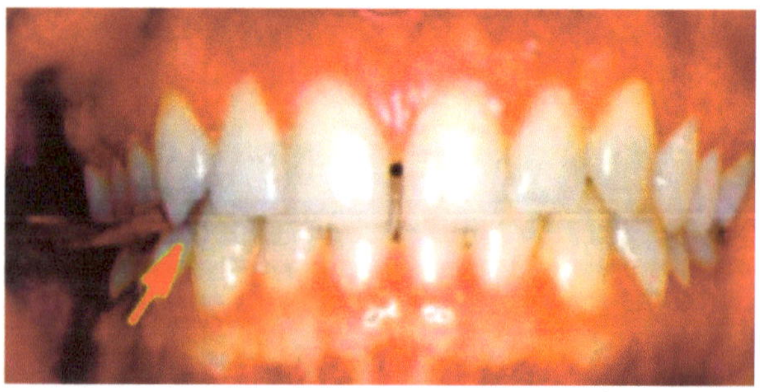

Figure 9.16. Position of the canines in the initial phase of the lower jaw movement cycle

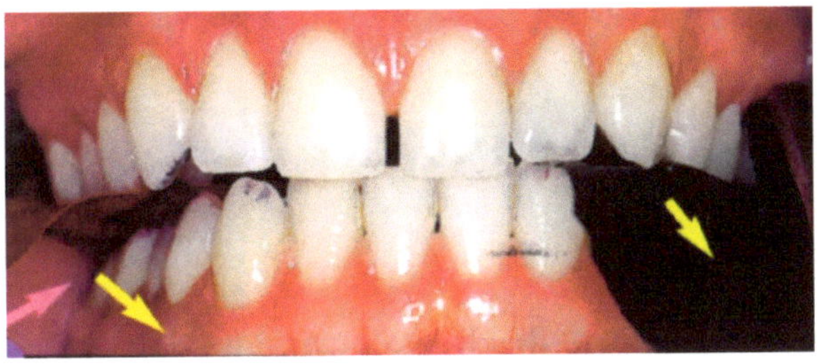

Figure 9.17. Registering the entire occlusal contacts in the chewing phase: red indigo paper on the working side, and blue indigo paper registers the opposite lateral balance side.

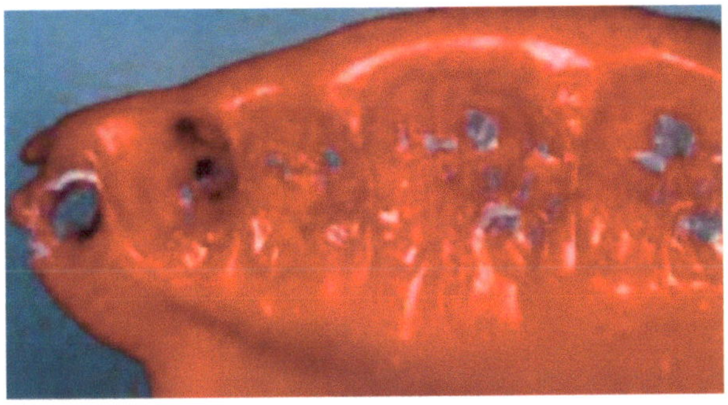

Figure 9.18. Chewing the polymer on the right side provides visibility of the occlusal contacts.

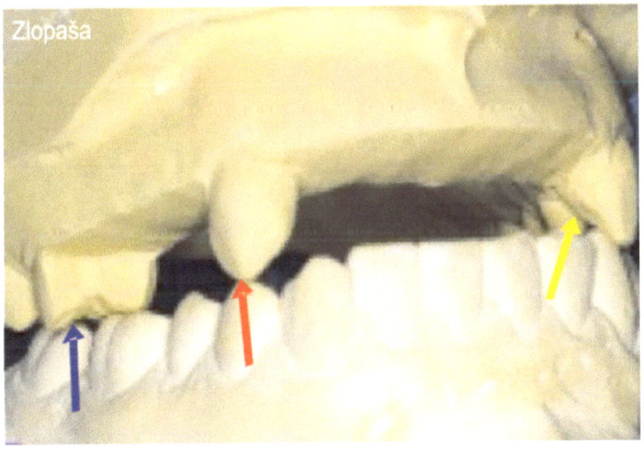

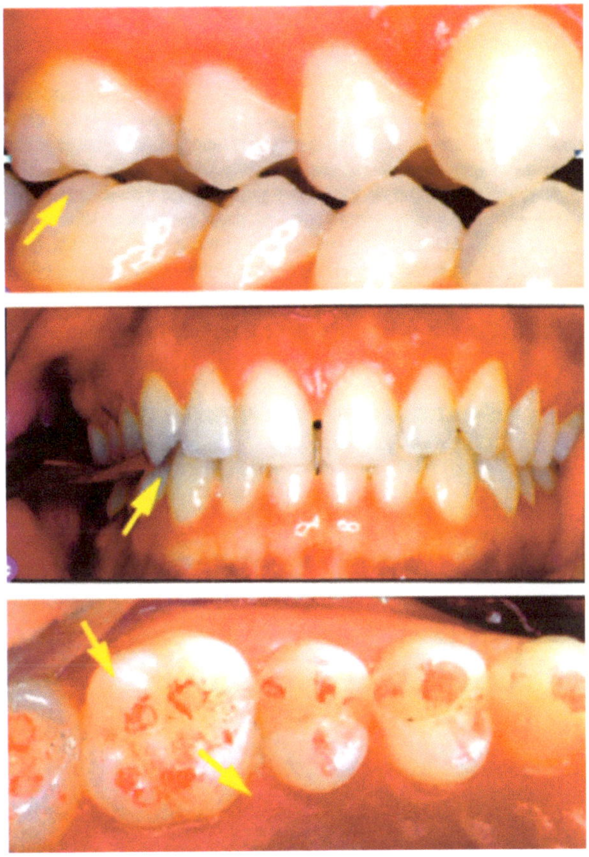

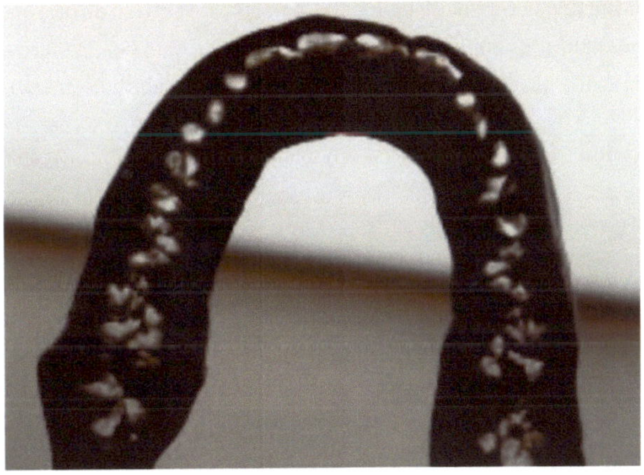

Figure 9.19. Registration of occlusal contact cycles by chewing polymers (alu-wax). The visibility of the perforations shows the dynamics of the occlusal contacts.

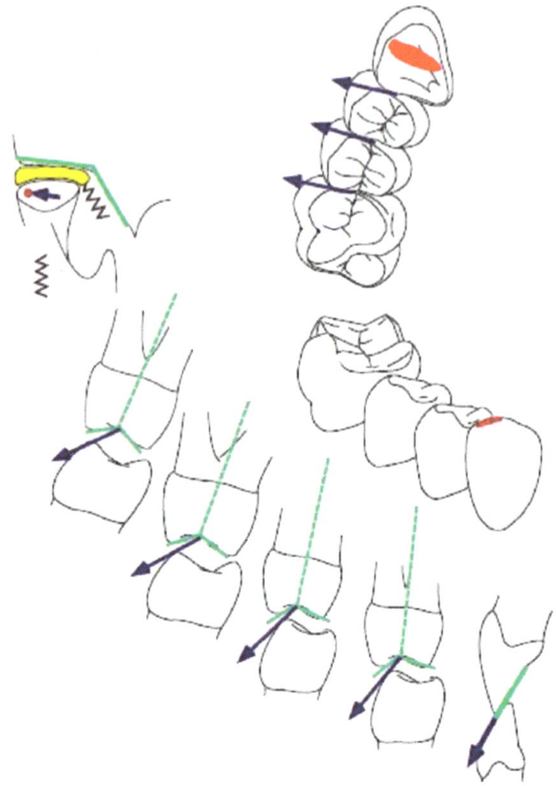

Figure 9.20. The modified model (by removing the central incisors and premolar) shows the initial phase of the opening of the chewing cycle and the role of canine guidance on the working side (red arrow) and the position of the canine support on the balancing side (yellow arrow), as well as the position of the bucomasial cusp of 1 molar (blue arrow).

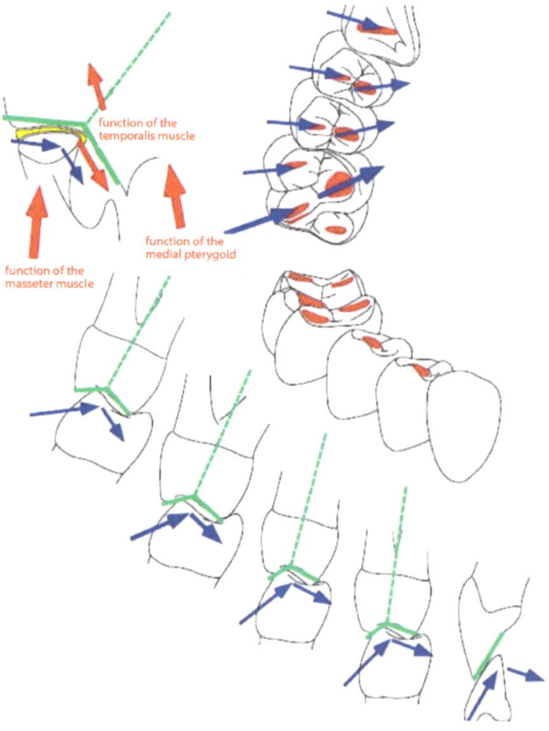

a

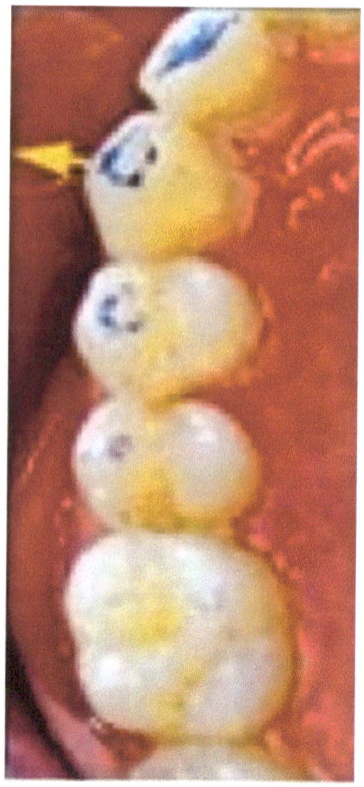

b

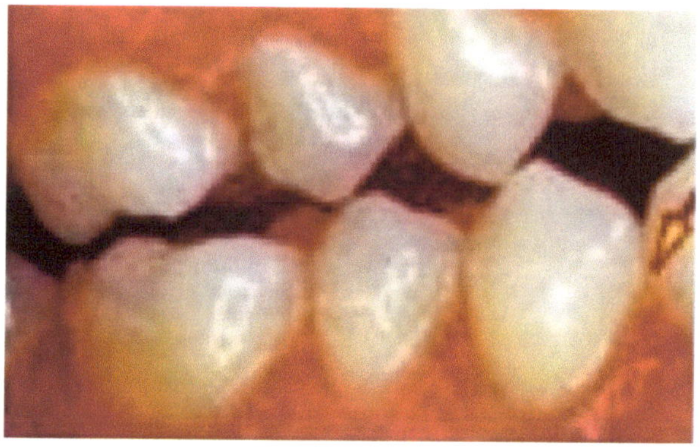

c

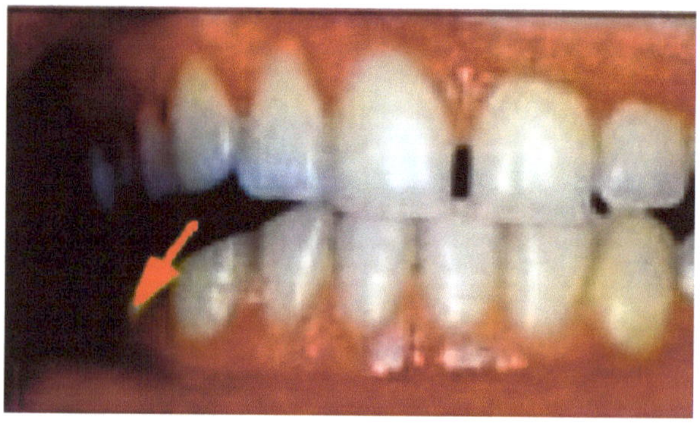

d

Figure 9.21. In lateral movements on the working side, all teeth are in contact, while on the non-working side, all teeth are in dissocclusion.

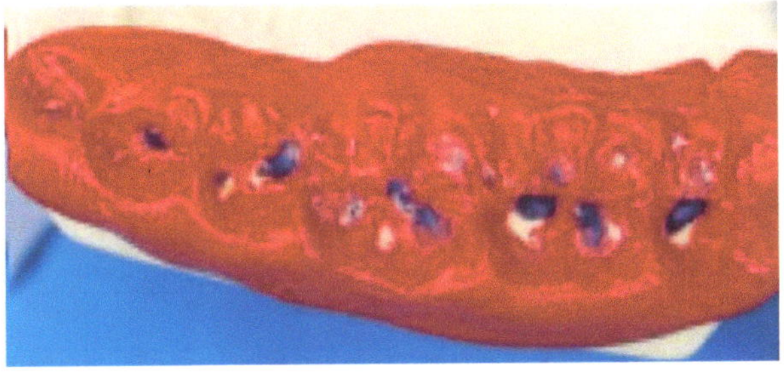

Figure 9.22 The perforations (blue) show the position of the contacts in group guidance - the canine loses contact. By simulating the problems of lateral movements of the mandible, using articulators, clinical conditions observed during chewing, answers to some of the pre-set questions are given with certain suggestions as to what new articulators should be applied.

Dento-dental kinematics in transverse lateral movements (centrifugal)

Dento-dental kinematics (nodule contacts) in transverse motion (centrifugal) will be best explained by the scheme shown in Figure 9.30. As can be seen in the picture, the front teeth, primarily the canine, provide lateral guidance that does not use real muscle strength and lifting activity. The temporo-mandibular articular complex, therefore, is not exposed to the action of musculoskeletal attachments. In this type of motion, condylar kinematics is essentially transversal.

In the case of functional occlusion, it has been shown that the movements observed during the occlusive phase of the chewing process, on the chewing side, have a centripetal direction, that is, the direction opposite to the direction performed in the laboratory on the articulator. Such a difference in direction between functional and kinematics, which is centripetal, and movements when testing lateral movements, which are centrifugal, originates from different occlusal conditions at the level of nodular sectors. These differences can be explained by comparing the muscular activities that characterize these two types of movements, as well as the adaptation of the temporomandibular articular region to the need to approach the occlusal surfaces during lateral movements. The difference that affects these occlusal relationships of the nodular sectors, in both situations, can be shown using articulation indigo paper (Figures 9.35-9.46).

Dento-dental kinematics in the occluded phase of the chewing process

In order to better register muscle activity, the patient may be asked to chew a polymer (Alu-wax, Utile Plaster) that is previously softened in warm water. The perforations that occur during chewing are good evidence of the effect of occlusal contacts during chewing (Figures 9.18, 9.19 and 9.22). This is extremely important for checking the occlusal balance, especially when it comes to implants. In this way, with this type of material, the boundary movements of the chewing can be registered and thus it is possible to easily determine the parameters of the condylar housings of the articulator.

It should be noted, regarding the guidance of canines or the anterolateral sector on the balanced, non-working side, the opposite of the working side: these contralateral dental elements represent an effective support

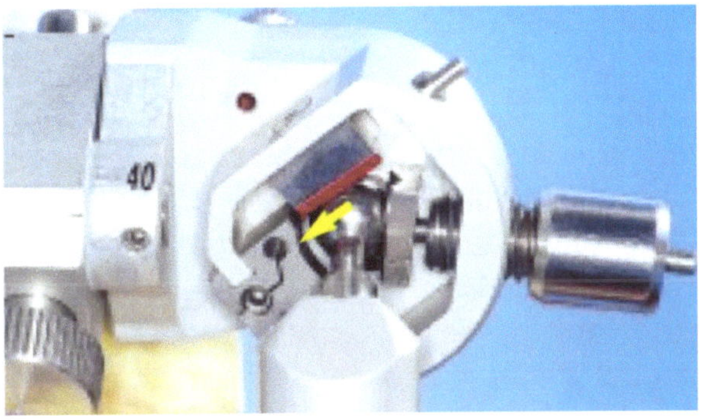

Figure 9.23. The condillar casing of the adjustable articulator is set to allow the establishment of occlusal contacts of the opening of the chewing cycle. This position of the ball and simulates the position of condyle movement from top to back as occupied by condyles when this happens on the working side.

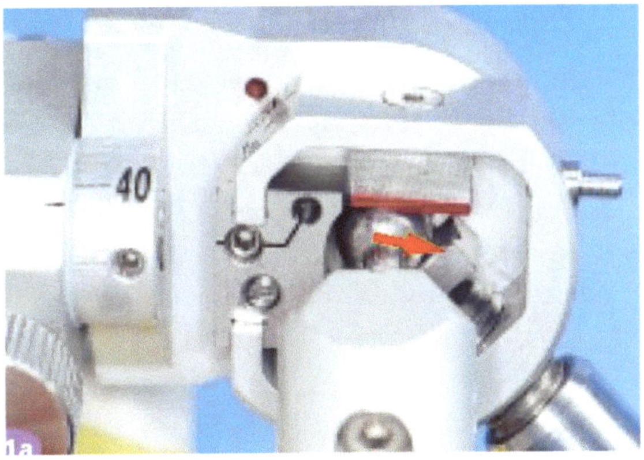

Figure 9.24. The condylar housing of the articulator reverse red line shows the rear wall that does not allow the condylar ball to descend

from up and back (red arrow), and such a position is taken by the control when opening the chewing cycle on the balance side.

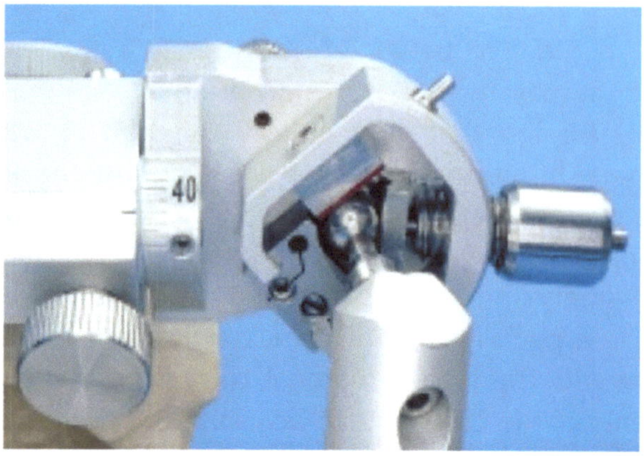

Figure 9.25. Such adjustable articulators, by adjusting the details in the housing itself, can quite accurately mimic the occlusal kinematics of closing the chewing cycle specific to each patient.

Supports muscle activity when chewing and crushing food. Here too, we have a subtle activity of the muscular system that, by positioning the mandible on the non-working side in a significantly anterior position, facilitates the leading contact of the opposite side in the closing phase of the chewing cycle. Here, in this very functional context, the term "canine guidance" finds justification!

In addition, it is important to emphasize that it will be easier for the patient to achieve a simulation of centripetal movements of closing the cycle on indigo paper if 2 pieces of paper are inserted in the canine area on the opposite side (Figures 9.16. – 9.17).

It has been shown that the analysis of lateral movements and contacts in cases of occlusal disorders is very delicate, especially if prosthetic work is performed on implants. Particularly important is the registration of premature extraordinary strong contacts, which is shown in Figures 9.33, 9.35, 9.38, 9.48, 9.49.

In lateral centrifugal movements, it is not possible to obtain contacts of the initial phase of the chewing process on the classic articulator. Occlusion analysis on models in the articulator gives different observations from those in the mouth.

It should be known that, in addition to chewing stimulation, articulation paperis used to imprint traces of functional guidance on the occlusal surfaces of the lateral teeth. It is distinguished by "excessive guidance", which shows excessive functional contacts (which prevents harmonious guidance) and "insufficient guidance", which is similar to the absence of functional guidance, or reduced functional guidance on a lump, tooth or group of teeth.

When analyzing the occlusion of lateral movements, it should be known whether it is performed on a semi-adjustable or fully adjustable articulator. With a fully adjustable articulator, the functional contacts of the lumps can be simulated accurately (Figure 9.52). If there is "excessive guidance" or premature contact, it is corrected by subtraction, while "insufficient guidance" requires additions to establish contacts that are verified by the appearance of functional guidance at their level.

The possibilities of simulating lateral movements in the laboratory also have certain limitations. Lateral movements of the mandible have two periods of dento-dental phases of the chewing cycle, before and after passing through the occlusion of maximum interspersion, and they should be observed separately (Figure 9.53 – 9.57).

Simulation of the closure phase in the chewing cycle has been given far greater attention, which has also affected the development of equipment in parallel with knowledge, while it seems, chewing cycle opening phase, inverted from the working movement described by Bennett, was less considered. The reason for this dual attitude, according to the author of the book, probably lies in the direction of movement analysis, both at the occlusal level and at the condylar level, which is opposite to the direction of actual movement on the working side!

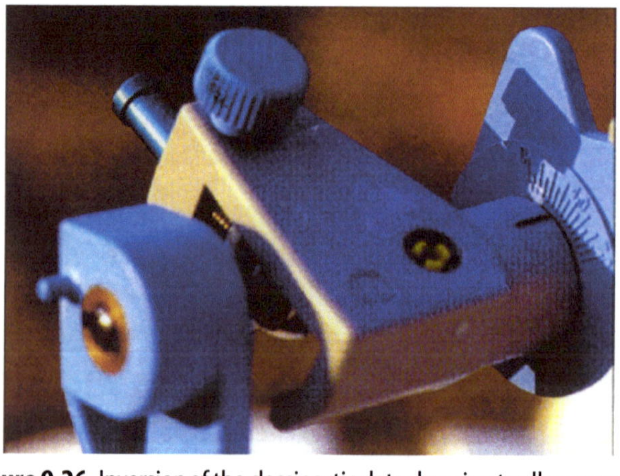

Figure 9.26. Inversion of the classic articulator housing to allow upward and backward movement of the condylar ball.

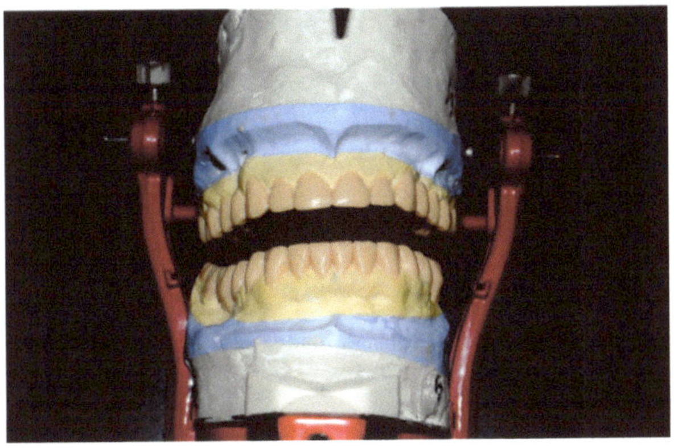

Figure 9.27. Articulators on which it is not possible to simulate lateral movements.

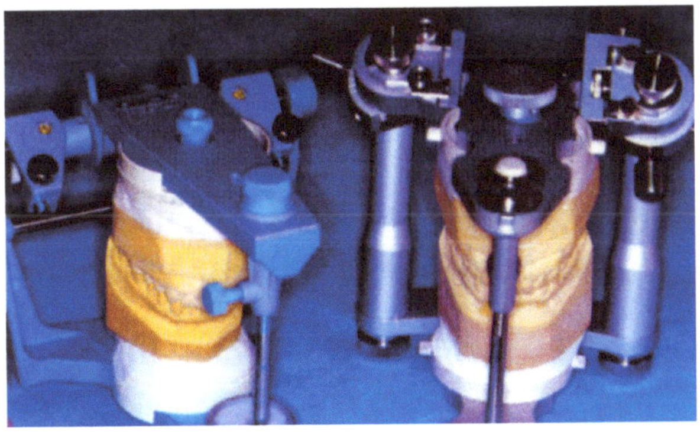

Figure 9.28. Semi-adjustable articulators in which it is not possible to simulate the events in the joint and dental contacts that exist in the mouth.

Kinematic data are quite different, as shown by the works of Landin (Lundeen) and Gibz (Gibbs). The direction of movement of the working condyle during the opening phase of the chewing cycle is much more oriented backwards and upwards, than during its analysis of laterality testing movements. For this reason, special attention is paid to the possibilities of simulating occlusal contacts in the opening phase of the chewing cycle: observing the lateral sectors placed on the testing articulator reveals the possibility of matching the functional contacts. However, the results obtained are not exactly appropriate to the events that exist. This lack of reproducibility is associated with the conception of a part of the housing (joint) thanks to the articulator, which transversally directs the movement of the condylar ball on the articulator, without the possibility of raising it and pulling it backwards. He tried to refine the articulator housing with various "small modifications", but this was really not applicable in everyday practice. There are very few articulators that can reproduce this phase of the chewing cycle simulation approximately to reality. While the simulation of the closing phase of the chewing cycle corresponds to the capabilities of most articulators, preferably the usual condylar parameters are regulated with the necessary precision, in the meantime the simulation of the chewing cycle creation phase is subject to many approximations. There are articulators (such as "Reverse") where the programming of the articulator housing can be performed based on clinical registrations, which makes it possible to simulate very accurately all the more functional dental contacts that can be observed in the mouth.

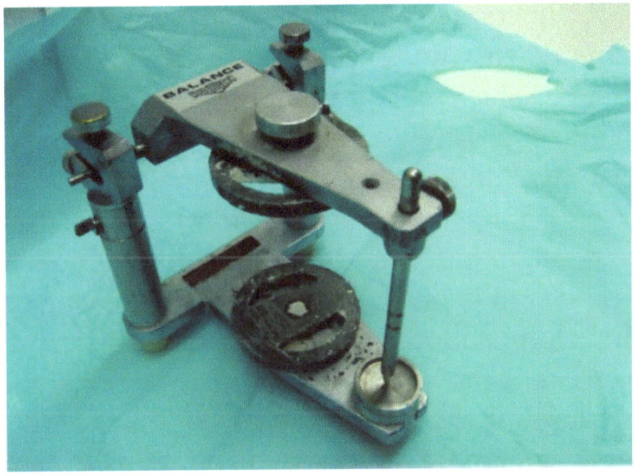

Figure 9.29. Articulators as mechanical devices reproduce the exact individual movements of the lower jaw and between the jaw relationships. The difference between occluders and articulators is that articulators can also reproduce lateral movements. Fully adjustable articulators can be fully adjusted by adjusting the movements of the lower jaw: articulated inclination, condyle angle, lateral condyle paths, vertical folding of the front teeth and angle.

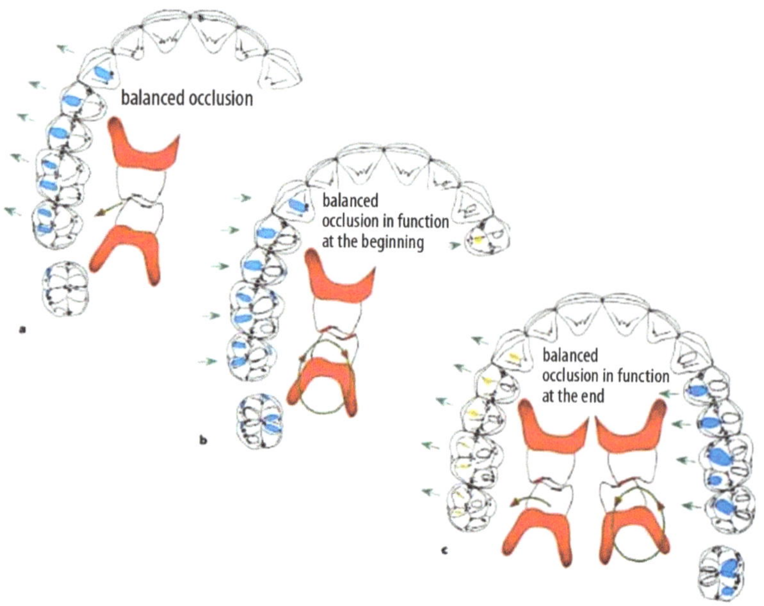

Figure 9.30. Schematic representation of balanced occlusion a) position of intercuspal contacts in function at the beginning of the chewing cycle, i.e. lateral movements of the mandible (b), and position of contacts in function at the end of the balanced occlusion cycle (c).

What should be remembered when analyzing the occlusion in lateral movements?

A functional approach to mandibular movements, where a fine analysis of occlusal trajectories is required, which is of great importance when it comes to implant prosthetic rehabilitation, requires the necessary evolution in our behavior, both in clinical practice and in the laboratory, according to the author of the book. In order to achieve the desired goal, it is necessary to know the realities of the chewing function beforehand, also predicting the occlusion protocol in lateral movements in clinical conditions, taking into account the differences of the observed kinematics depending on the direction of execution of these movements. In order for the articulator occlusion analysis to be consistent with the clinical findings, it is necessary to consider the simulation results very carefully. Thanks to the articulators used by most of our dental technician associates, the desired effect cannot be achieved. It should be sought that the rational use of state-of-the-art articulators, with knowledge of the mechanical system on which they are based, tries to obtain the best possible reproduction of the characteristics of kinematics inherent in each patient. According to some very important theories, the implant should be loaded in a different way than a natural tooth. Dentists with many years of experience who have been involved in implant placement, when asked the question of how to load the implant, and how to load a natural tooth, the practice found an answer. A different load mode for the adaptation period of the tissue should be sought in the formation of occlusal surfaces of prosthetic temporary work of a much softer material than ceramics, and zirconium should be avoided. The formation of occlusal surfaces is extremely important for the integration process, especially in the first 6 months the control of the established balanced occlusion must be done precisely. This is easily feasible in practice if very thin articulation paper is applied. Using very thin articulation paper with a slight closing force in the central occlusion, only a slightly pronounced imprint of the contact is outlined on the implant crowns, while on the adjacent natural tooth, these marked imprinted signs of contact would be significantly stronger. In the simulation phase in the laboratory, the implant crown, or its occlusal surface, should be formed in such a way that only axial contacts are present, and thus the reception of the most favorable forces of the chewing cycle.

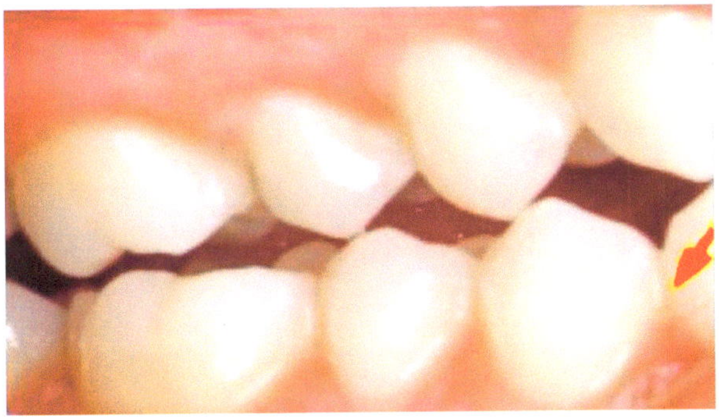

Figure 9.31. Canine guidance and sliding position of side teeth on the working side.

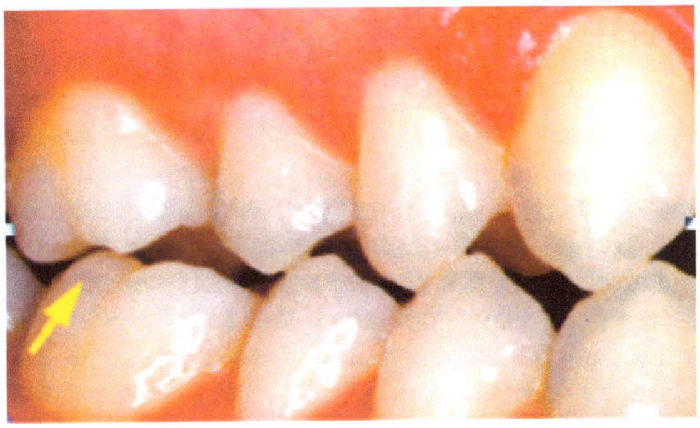

Figure 9.32. Occlusal relations in the centripetal cycle opening movement according to the conception of maximum occlusal contacts. The lateral teeth are in the sliding contact.

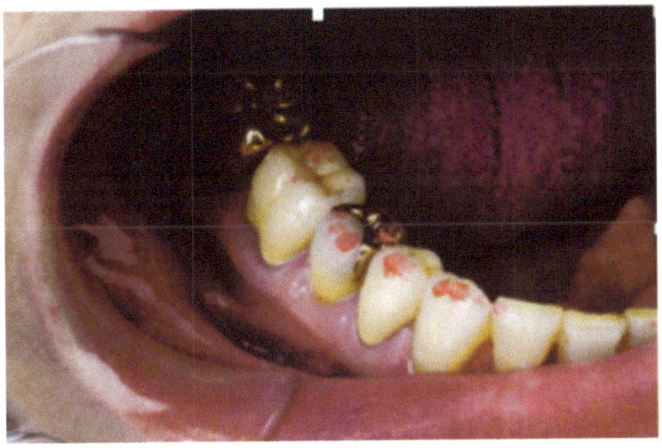

Figure 9.33. Registering premature contacts.

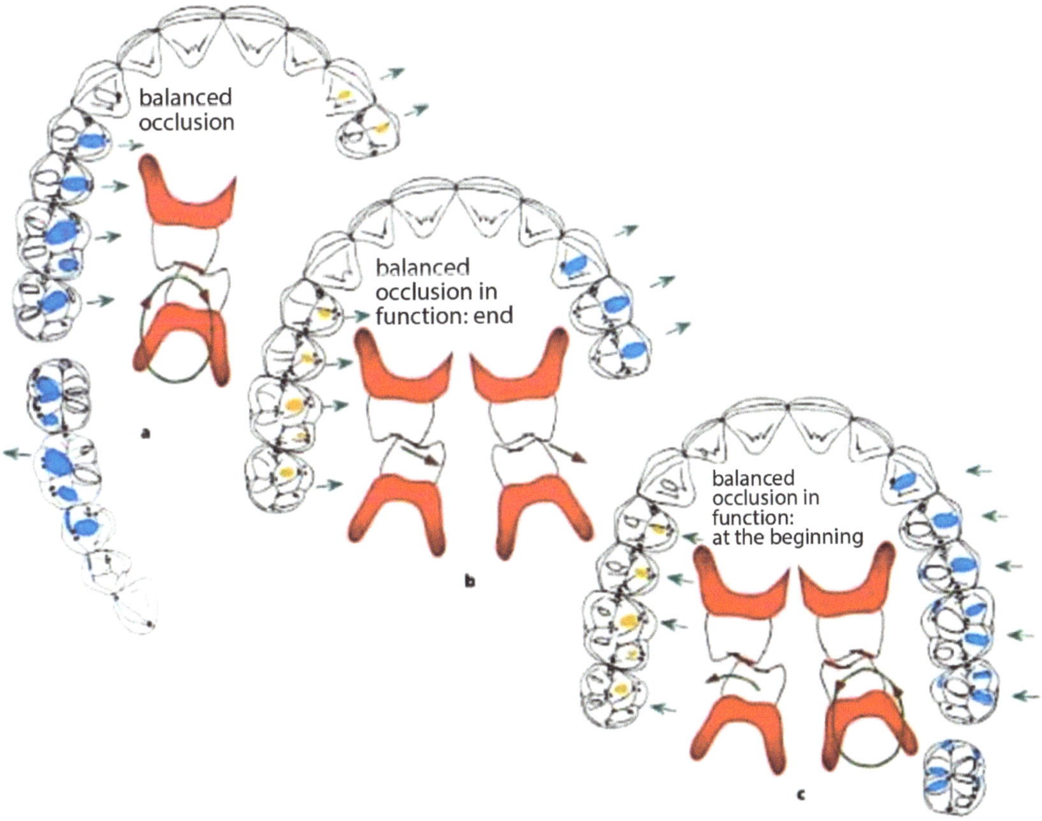

Figure 9.34. During mastication, the external sides of the palatine nodules are in dynamic contact.

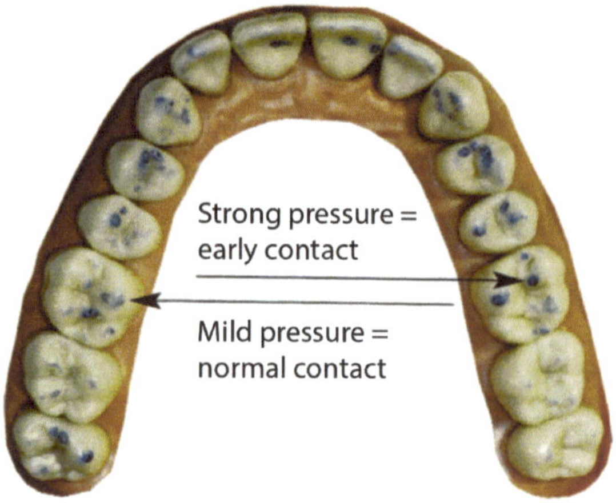

Figure 9.35. Marked point with the upper arrow; the intensive trace of the indigo paper shows premature contact, and a milder coloration of the trace, normal contact.

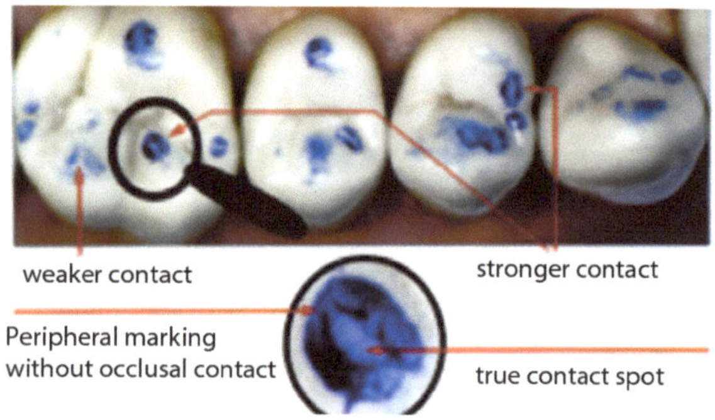

Figure 9.36. The display of occlusal traces by guiding will be best registered using Bausch articulated indigo paper of a certain thickness.

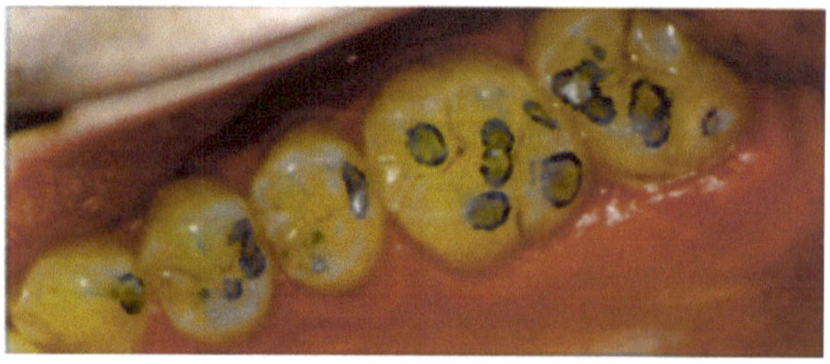

Figure 9.37. Registering balanced occlusal contacts.

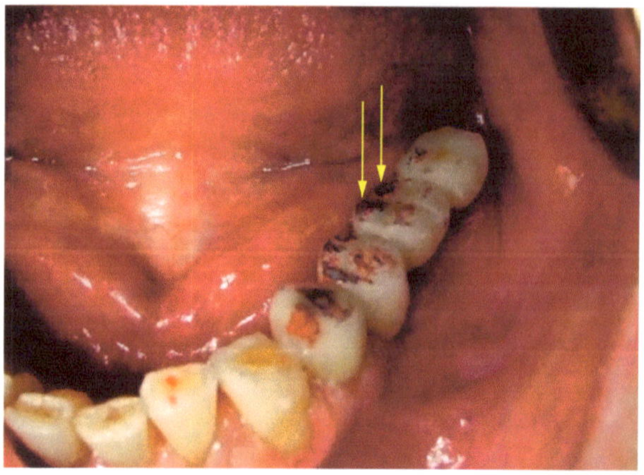

Figure 9.38. Removal of premature contact - prosthetic work on implants.

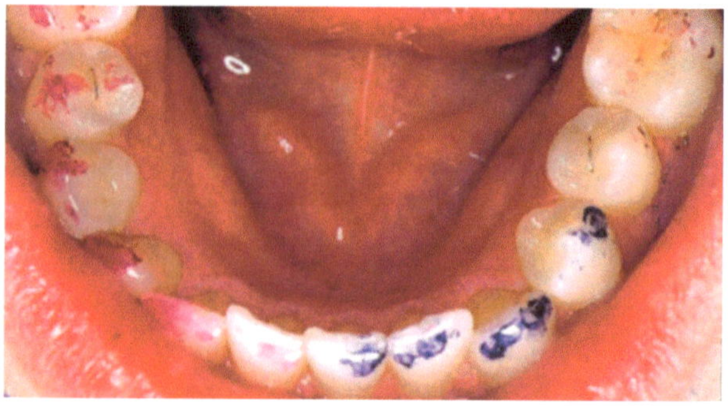

Figure 9.39. Traces of the sliding position of the side teeth on the working side (red) and the position of the canine contact on the opposite balance side (blue)

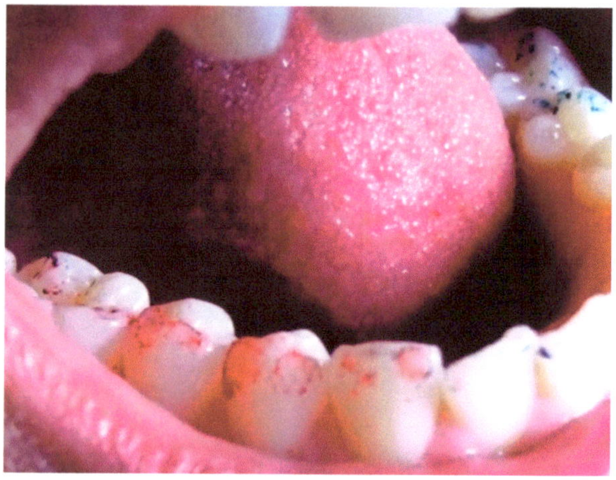

Figure 9.40. Contacts in balanced ideal occlusion of natural teeth on the right working side.

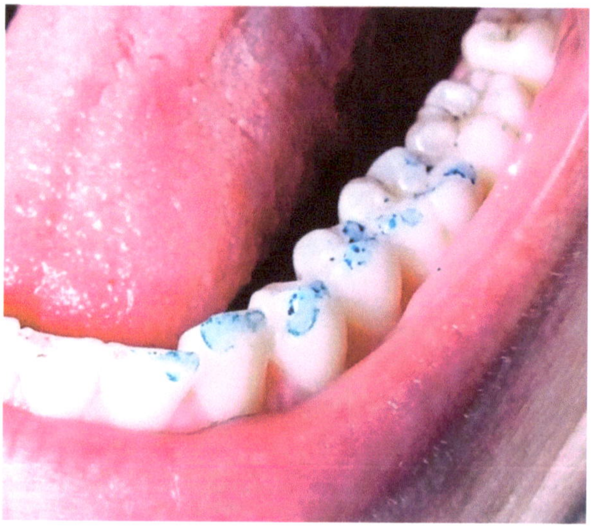

Figure 9.41. Evenly colored marks on the left side show a balanced ideal occlusion

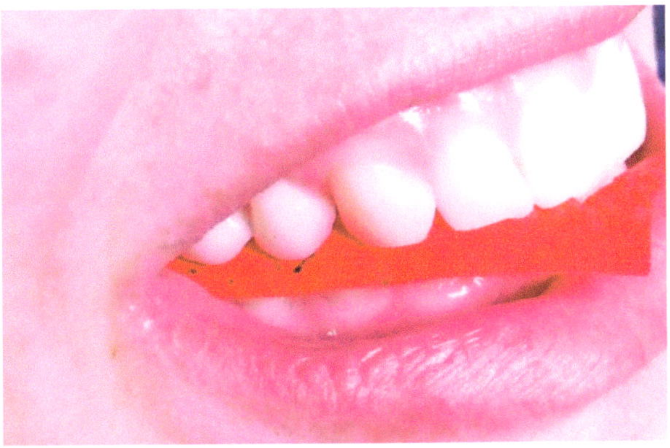

Figure 9.42. Registering contacts on the working side on the right.

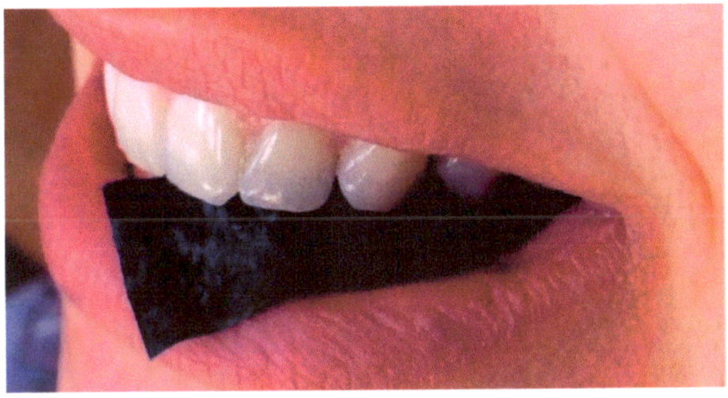

Figure 9.43. Registering on the left balance side.

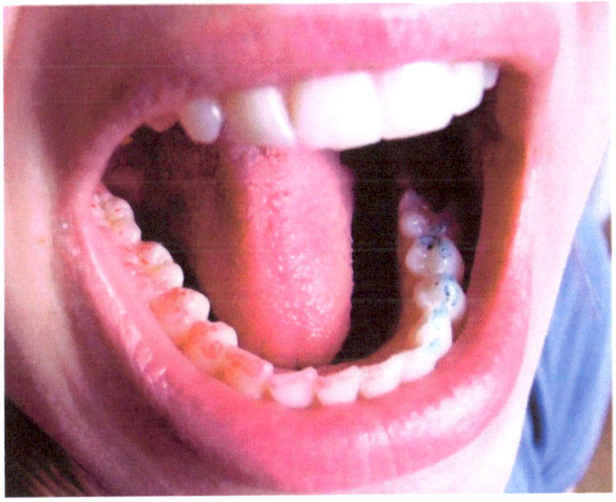

Figure 9.44. Traces of indigo paper in balanced occlusion (red on the working side and blue on the balancing side).

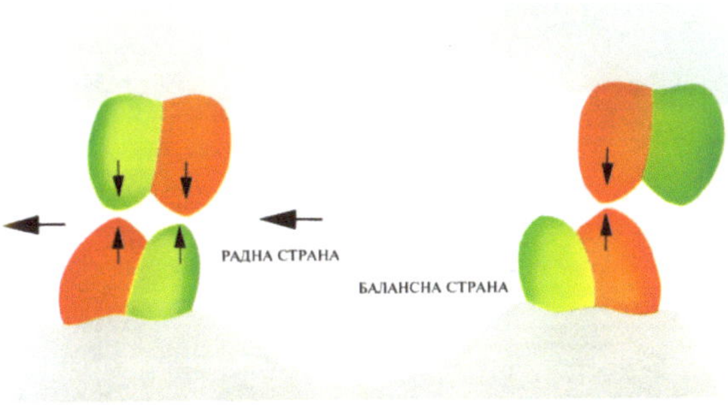

Figure 9.45. Schematic representation of the working and balancing side.

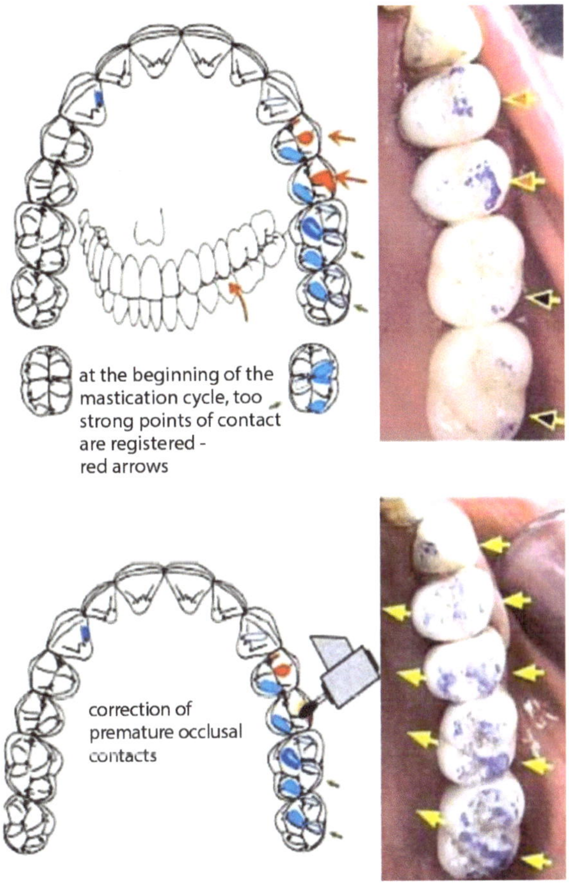

Figure 9.46. Correction of premature and too strong occlusal contacts after registration with indigo paper.

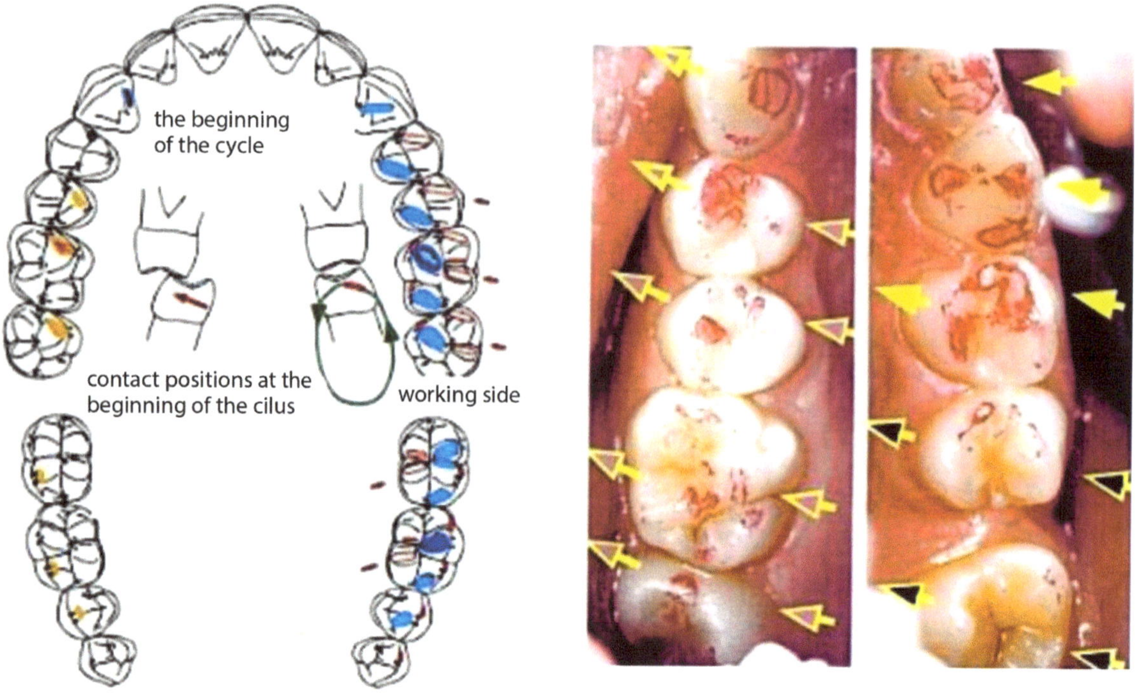

Figure 9.47. The contact registration scheme at the beginning of the masticatory cycle on the work side (marked in blue), and in the images with yellow arrows indicates the position of the contacts at the beginning of the cycle. Yellow-black arrows indicate the loss of lateral contacts.

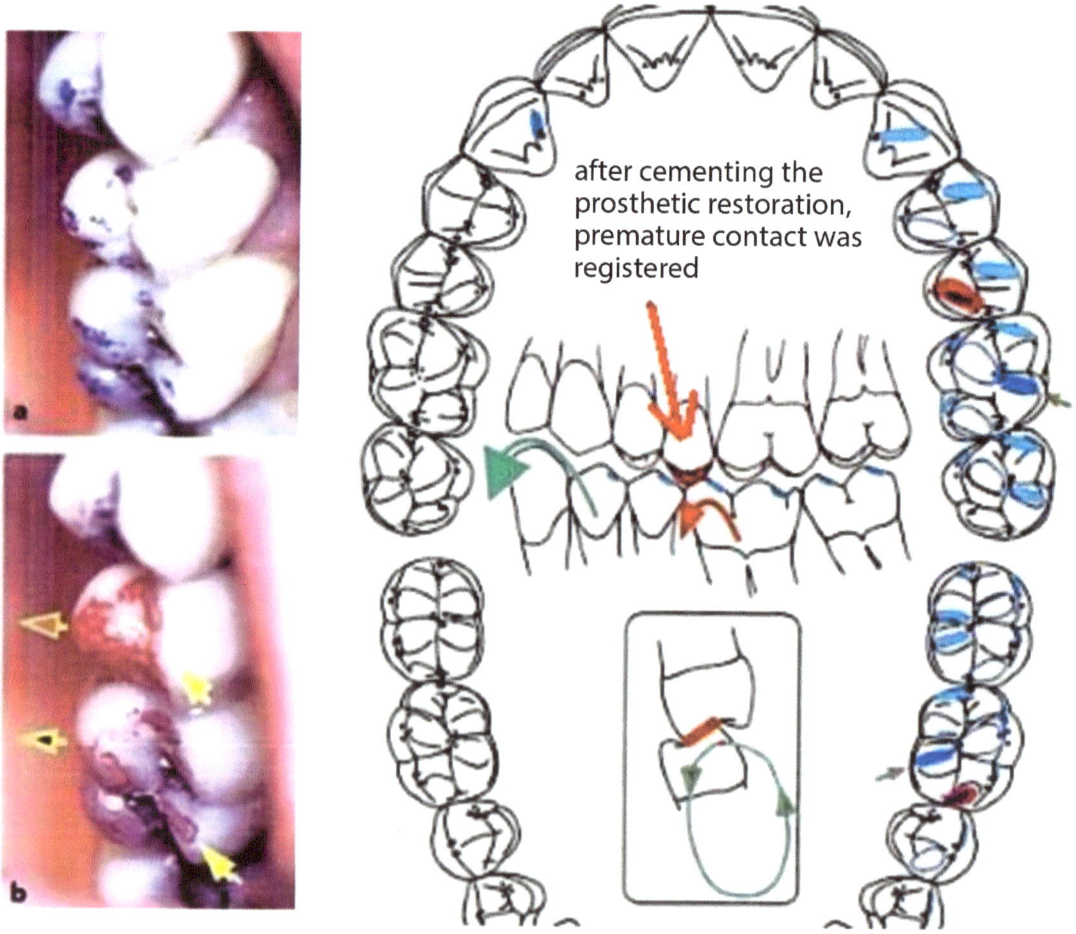

Figure 9.48. Registering premature extraordinary strong contacts (red arrows) after cementing the prosthetic work.

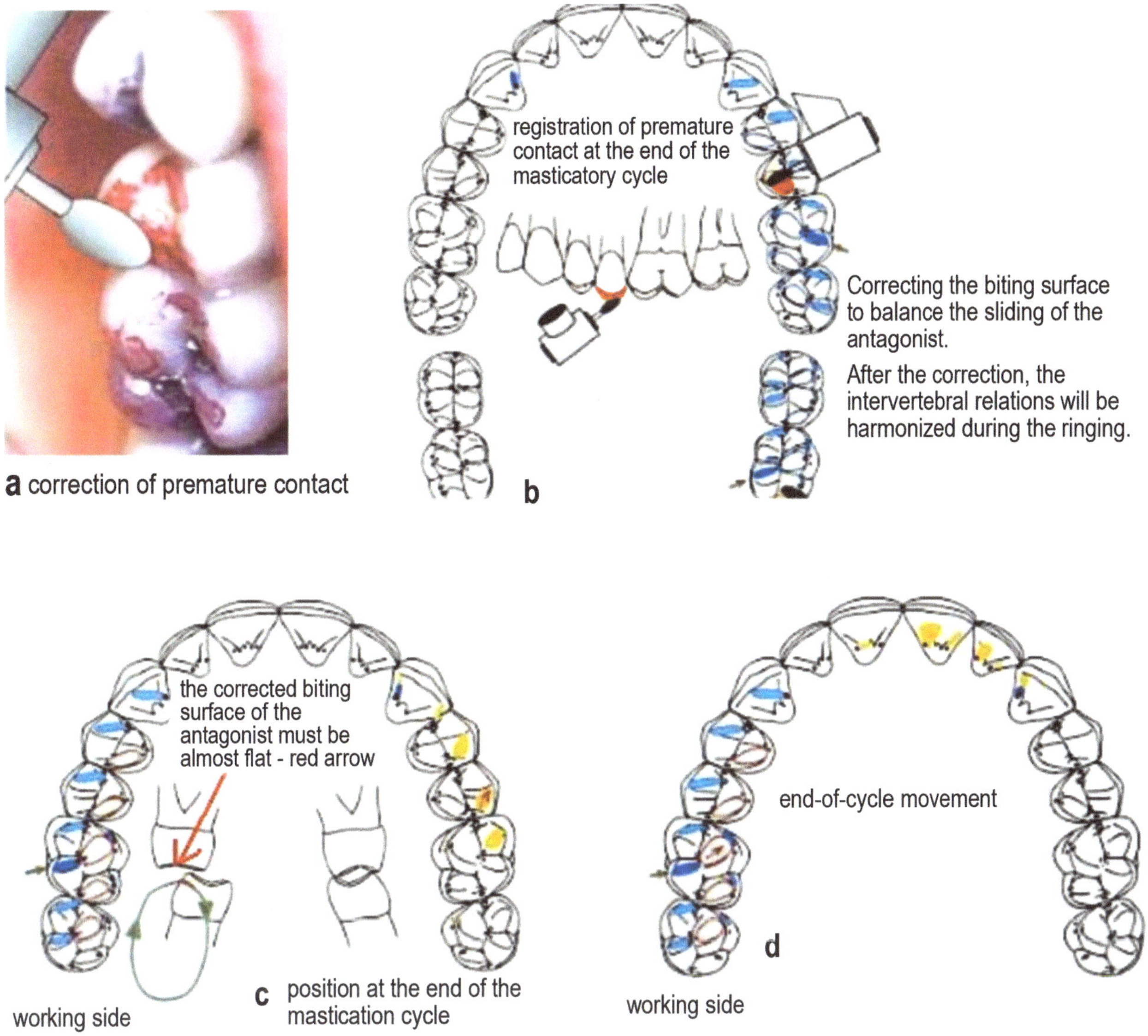

Figure 9.49. Correction of occlusal surfaces, overstressed lumps should be adjusted in accordance with gnathological principles, so that in lateral movements of the lower jaw, the given forces act evenly within physiological limits.

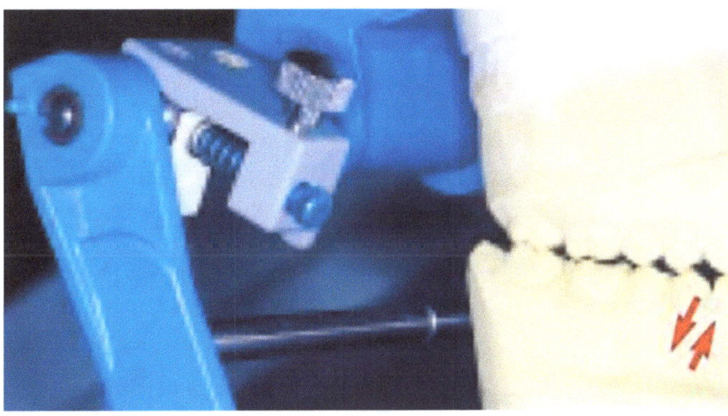

Figure 9.50. Lateral centrifugal movements to the right, shown on the classic articulator. It is not possible to get the contacts of the initial phase of the chewing cycle (red arrows). The analysis of occlusion on such an articulator gives different observations than those in the mouth.

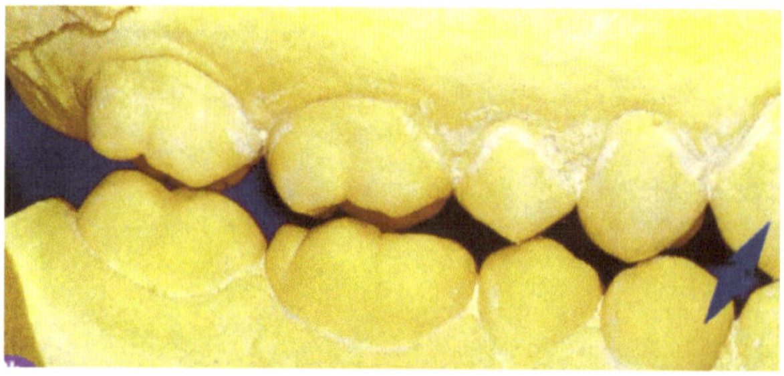

Figure 9.51. Differences on the plastered model in the classic articulator from the state in the mouth (Figure 9.9).

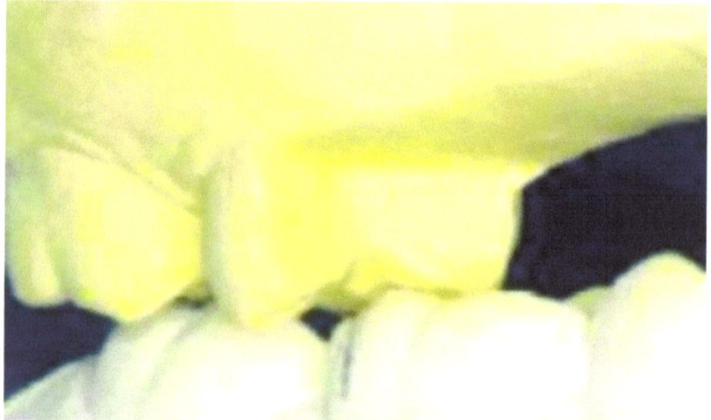

Figure 9.52. With a good articulator (such as Reverse), it is possible to achieve a simulation of the ratio of occlusal surfaces such as in the mouth at the level of the first molars in the laboratory. This relationship enables the articulator housing (condylar tilt, curve selection and Bennett wing angulation).

Conclusion

- Lateral movements of the mandible can be accompanied by functional dental sliding contacts, especially during chewing.
- Occlusal but prosthetic conceptions offer various ways of treating dental contacts in lateral movements.
- Analysis of occlusal contacts in the mouth during lateral movements leads to different observations depending on whether the movement is centrifugal or centripetal.
- Occlusion analysis of lateral movements performed in mouth cannot be reproduced on outdated traditional articulators without modification of the condylar housing (joint) of the articulator.
- The condylar housings (articulator joint) must be designed so that they can perform an analysis of the occlusion of lateral movements in the laboratory by simulating the chewing cycle in the mouth.
- Knowledge in these areas is necessary for both the implantologist and the dental technician. The architect designer - implantologist and the contractor - dental technician must be in maximum coordination.

Glossary of used terms:

Functional occlusal contacts: dental contacts (antagonist contacts) and guidance that occurs during the food chipping, chewing and swallowing phases.

Work side: chewing side (alternating one-sided function). Indicates both the occlusal contacts and the musculoskeletal parts of the chewing machine.

Non-working side: the opposite side to that on which the chewing is performed.

Opening the cycle (of chewing): the initial dental phase of the chewing cycle that contributes to the acceptance and tearing of food by the lateral teeth.

Centrifugal movement: indicates the direction of movement of the mandibular point that moves away from the medial sagittal planes during the lateral movements of the mandible.

Centripetal movement: indicates the direction of movement of the mandibular point approaching the medial sagittal plane during lateral sagittal movements of the mandible.

Closing the cycle (chewing) the final dental phase of the chewing cycle that contributes to the crushing of food with the lateral teeth.

The following images are pictorial conclusions and representations of important occlusal events in lateral movements of the mandible

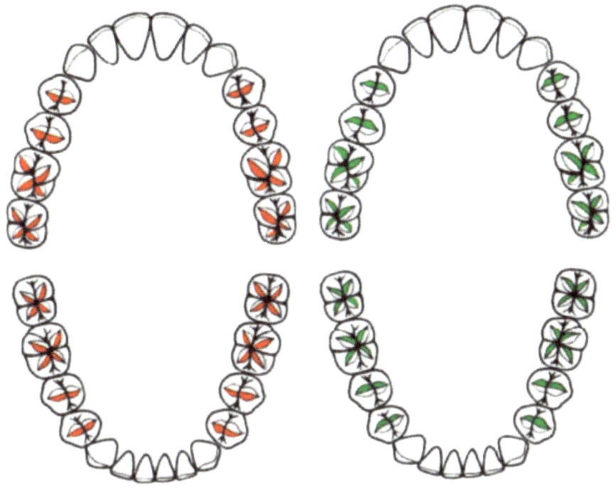

Display of registration of intercuspid contacts on the working (red) and balance side (green). Look at the picture 9.30

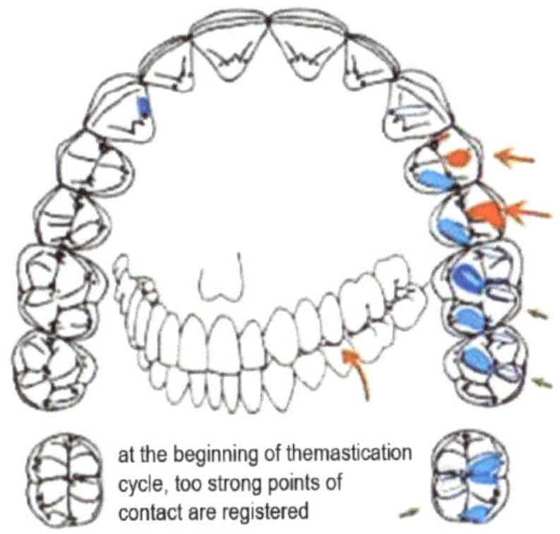

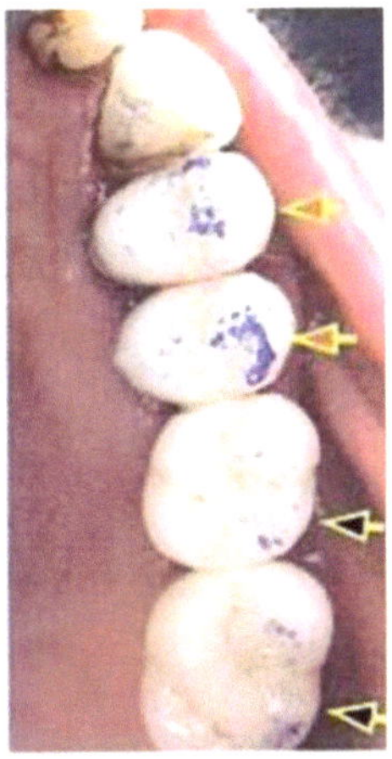

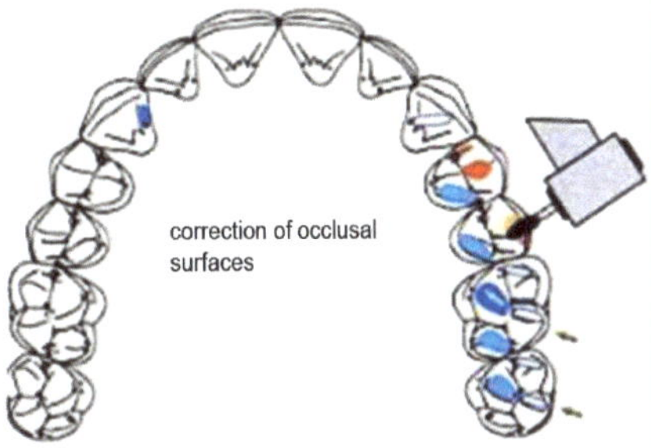

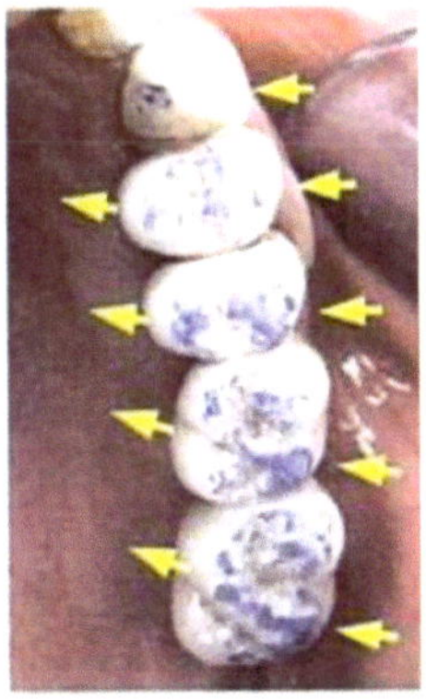

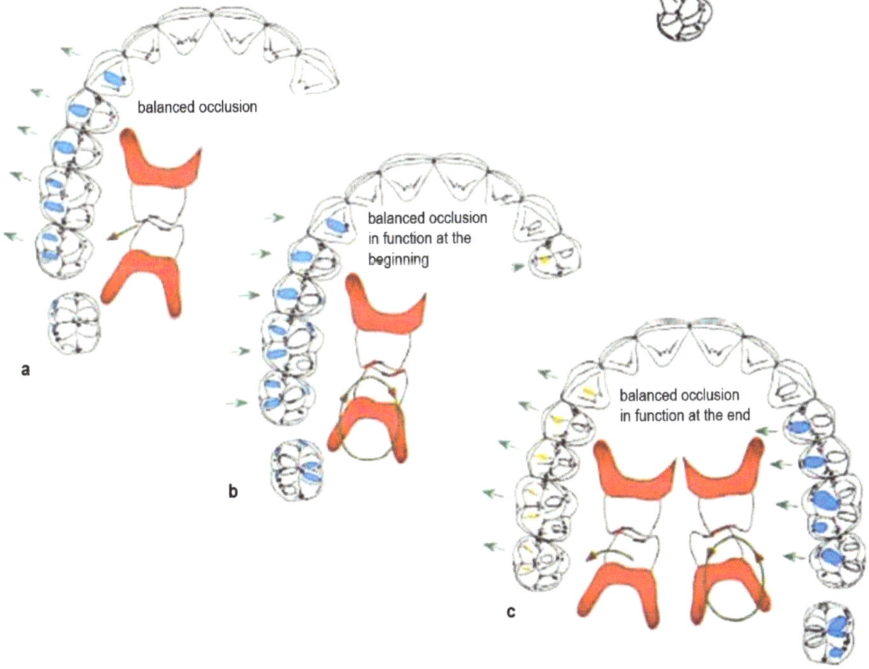

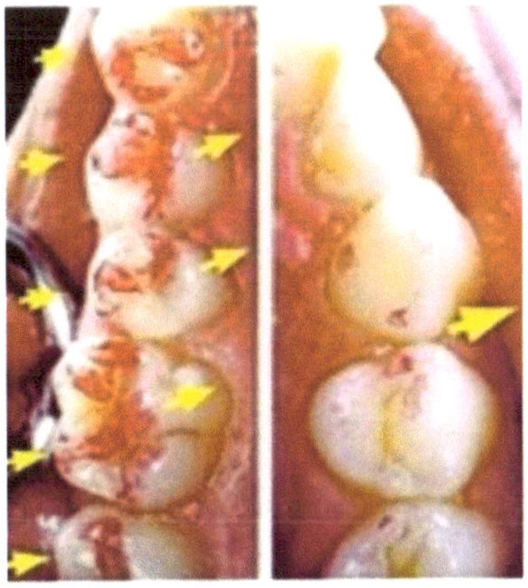

Figures 9.53. – 9.57. Blue colored lumps on the bite surfaces indicate occlusal contacts in lateral movements of the lower jaw on the working and balancing side.

10

Bone Tissue Augmentation With Bone Substitutes

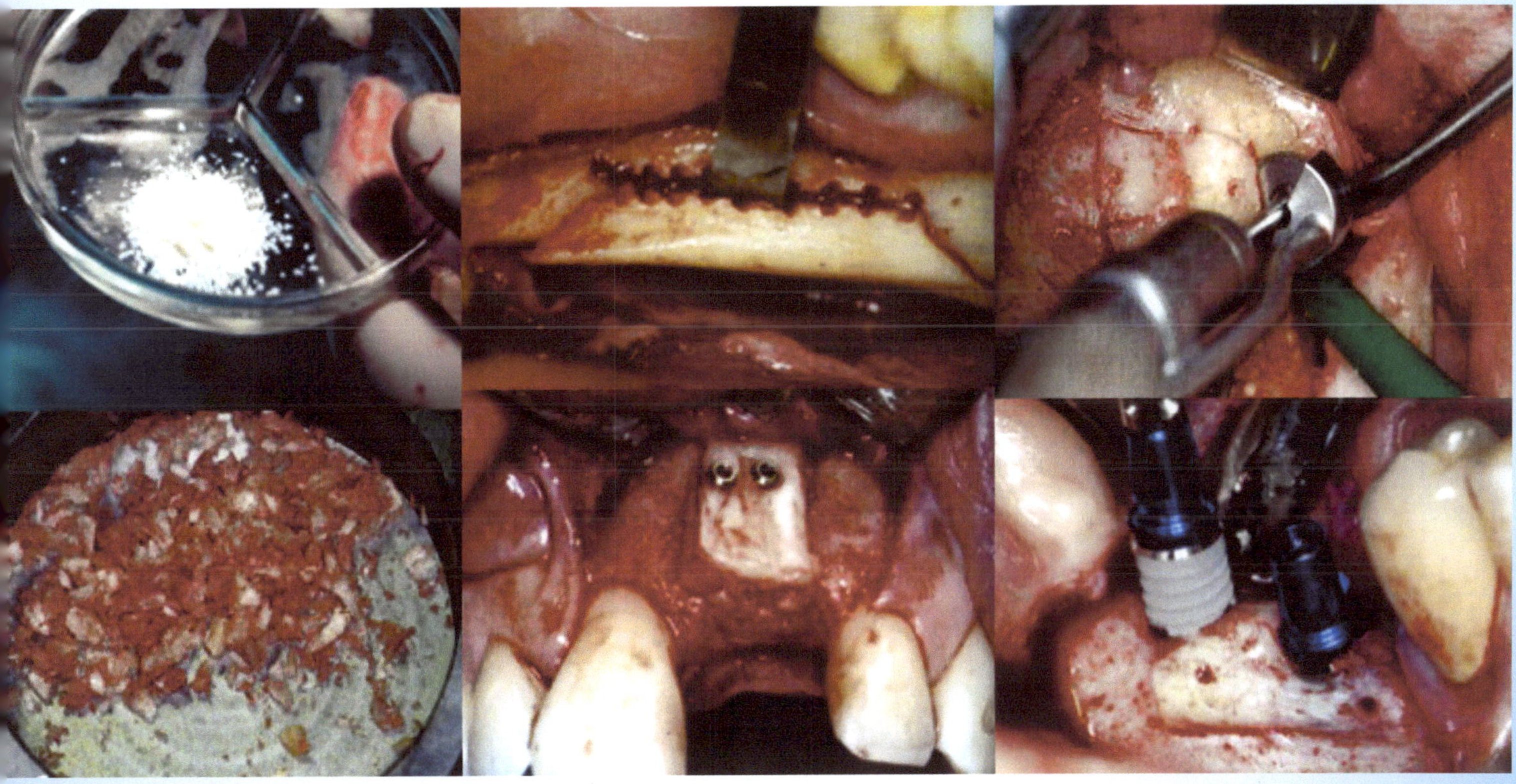

In order for the oral surgical procedure of implant placement to be optimal, there must be a fundamental condition - that there is sufficient bone in the place where the implant is to be placed. If this condition is not met, then implant placement loses all meaning. The existence of satisfactory horizontal and vertical bone dimensions is a basic prerequisite for a successful implant placement result. The first step in fulfilling this prerequisite - creating a favorable implant bed - begins with tooth extraction and alveolus care.

Tooth extraction inevitably results in the loss of a portion of the alveolar bone that is connected to the periodontium. The greatest loss is observed on the bone walls of the alveoli. Since tooth extraction most often destroys the buccal wall of the alveoli, this leads to a reduction in the horizontal and vertical dimensions of the alveolar bone. Accelerated processes of resorption of the alveolar bone walls occur in the first three months after extraction. The resorption processes are most evident on the labial walls of the alveoli of the front teeth of the upper jaw.

The extent of the loss of bone walls of the alveolar socket mostly depends on the extraction technique. The most important thing is to perform the extraction with minimal trauma. Many years of experience confirm that in places where the root has been resected, the vestibular lamella is most often missing.

If an implant procedure is planned at this site, it is necessary to fill the fresh alveolus with bone substitutes, most often Bio-Oss collagen. The collagen granules can be ideally shaped by molding. Covering with a BioGide membrane will create ideal conditions for creating an implant bed. This alveolus preservation procedure is not only manifested by preserving the alveolar bone, i.e. the alveolar ridge, but also prevents collapse and preserves the volume of soft tissue.

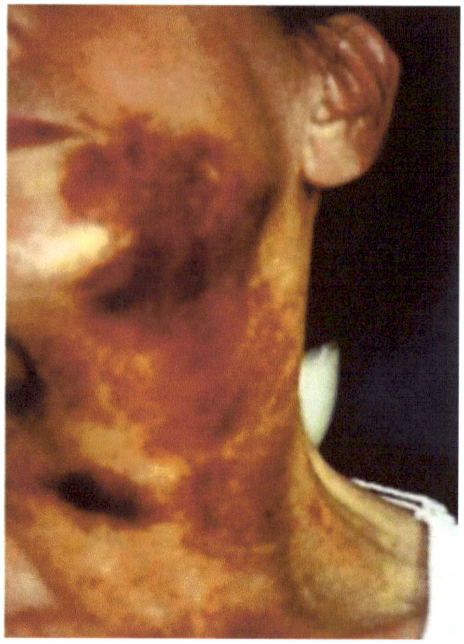

Figure 10.1. Extensive hematoma after augmentation with xenogeneic bone substitutes. (Fouad Khoury, Augmentattive Verfahren in derlmplantologie, 2008.)

The above confirms that replacing lost bone is becoming increasingly successful. However, despite the enormous progress in the development of bone substitute materials, there are still questions that the practice needs to answer.

Despite the improvements in new techniques and good results, replacing lost bone can often be a complex procedure, and it should not be forgotten that with any augmentation procedure there is always a risk of infection and failure. As an unwanted consequence of more extensive augmentation, a hematoma may occur, which can affect the entire face, oral cavity, and even the neck (Figure 10.1).

For this reason, oral implantology should provide an answer to something that began in the 17th century - the first attempt to restore damaged and lost bone dates back to that time. To better understand augmentation, it is worth recalling when and how it began.

The first documented bone transplant was in 1668. J. Janszon van Meekeren described the successful transfer of a dog's calotte to a human skull to compensate for a bone defect. It took 225 years, or rather, until 1893, when J. Barth described the first histological investigation. The transplanted bone failed, but he proved that it left a backbone, which was infiltrated by new, vital cells. Barth described this process as a "latent replacement" of the bone defect.

After that, it took a long time for the replacement of lost bone by augmentation to reach its present level.

True modern augmentation began only in 1980, when Brenemark installed the first endoosseous implant in grafted bone. Intraoral grafts appeared in the early 1990s. Dahlin introduced GBR in 1988. Over the next 10 years, attempts began with successful results, but the techniques were very demanding. Collagen resorbable membranes only appeared in the late 1990s. Bone substitute engineering is experiencing a great rise, and the market is increasingly offering more and more. However, replacing lost bone by augmenting alveolar ridges is a field that science still needs to shed light on. Oral implantology also has to provide many answers that have not yet been fully obtained in the field of bone regeneration.

Oral surgery and periodontology are improving operative techniques every day, enriched by the offer of a considerable number of different bone substitute materials for clinical use. Despite this, there is no definitive opinion on which material is the most optimal for the replacement and reconstruction of lost bone.

Recently, a combination of platelet-derived growth factor with beta-tricalcium phosphate has been attempted. This synthetic, inorganic, bioactive material has osteoinductive potential and promotes the filling of bone defects. There is no verification through practice and a definitive position yet, because the growth factors need to be harmonized or approximated as they occur in natural law.

"Bone substitute" materials have become the basis of three major sections of the industry, primarily bone substitute manufacturers who are able to generate huge revenues and use a marketing approach to find as many indications as possible, which in many cases is absolutely unnecessary and often unsuccessful. The application of bone substitute materials also requires the application of membranes. Many improvements are to be expected in this direction, with even greater certainty of success. Everything that nature has created has its reason, and everything that she has created is in perfect harmony. Man has not yet managed to achieve this harmony, but he has often managed to repair what has been damaged. When it comes to reconstructing bone in places where nature has not designated a place for it and where it never existed, the task of science is to clarify many dilemmas. Overcoming, until recently, insurmountable obstacles, such as unfavorable anatomical structures (sinus cavities), is today a solvable problem. Sinus lifting represents a significant advance in oral implantology (Figures 10.2-10.4). New systems are increasingly appearing on the market that simplify the sinus lift technique. But if bone is replaced in a place where nature did not intend it, and this procedure "corrects" nature, a logical question arises: to what extent can we reconstruct bone and fill the maxillary sinuses with different materials and of different origins?

Understanding the physiological role of the paranasal cavities and their connection with the surrounding anatomical structures (nose, eyes, brain, bronchi, lungs), the question arises of establishing the doctrine in oral implantology - to what extent and in what quantity should the sinus cavities be filled with building materials for bone replacement, whether of autologous, allogenic, xenogeneic, or alloplastic origin.

Materials that are not of human origin, but rather from donors of a different species, are called xenogeneic or heterologous materials, which also have the following advantages: they are easily sterilized, easily stored, and available in unlimited quantities.

Likewise, for allogeneic or homologous materials, which are of human origin, advantages are also highlighted: high biological value, biocompatibility, as well as osteogenetic and osteoinductive properties.

Osteogenesis is attributed to the ability to create new bone with the help of surviving bone graft cells. Osteoinduction is the creation of new bone in which an inorganic skeleton of material implanted in the sinus cavities enhances new bone formation three-dimensionally. The process is completed by mineralization with the ingrowth of blood vessels and osteoprogenitor cells.

To date, there is no clear position in oral surgery as to which material is osteoinductive and to what extent, and whether it is osteoinductive at all.

It is also not known exactly at what rate the building material is resorbed, and at what rate new bone is created, and to what extent.

Since there are no clear answers to these questions and since there is a lack of a doctrinal position, it has happened that the filled sinus cavity completely ossifies after implant placement.

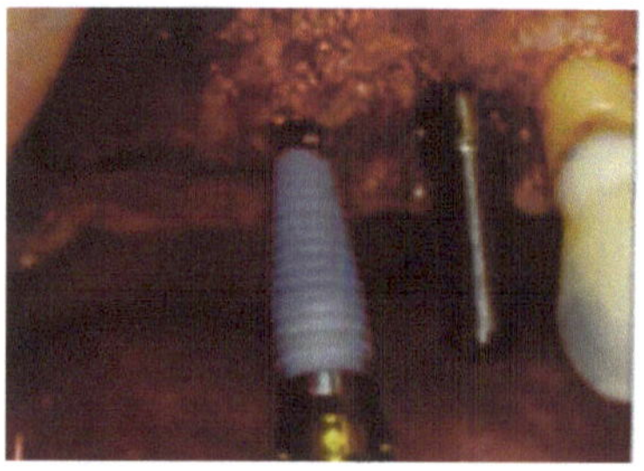
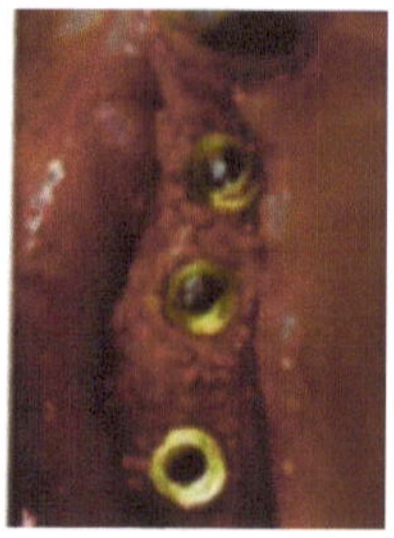

Figure 10.2. Sinus floor elevation. Alveoli filled with bone replacement and placement of implants.

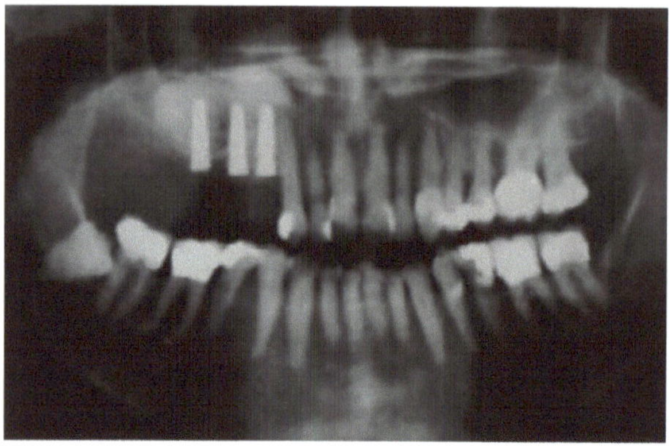

Figure 10.3. Display of ossification of sinus cavities after sinus lifting and positioning of three implants.

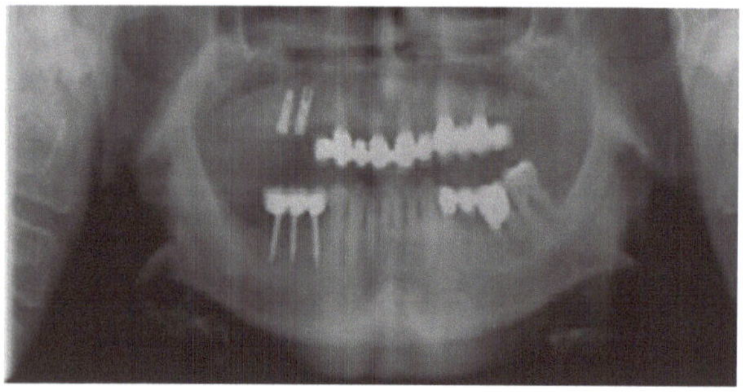

Figure 10.4. Implants installed after sinus lifting, procedures and implants with a narrow diameter (3mm) installed in the sharp ridge in the lower jaw. Condition after 8 years.

These questions deserve the attention of science and must be answered in the future. Despite the above-mentioned thinking, the development of oral implantology on a scientific basis has fully fulfilled its original functional requirement: that a person can eat and chew food well, but the second, aesthetic one has also been achieved. The third, no less demanding and important one has also been achieved - the return of self-confidence and a smile, which is the basic expression of psychological satisfaction.

Very often in practice, the clinician encounters cases where, due to anatomical changes in the alveolar ridge, caused by atrophy, the planned treatment with implants cannot be achieved.

An experienced clinician must initially accurately recognize and determine the location of bone volume deficiencies in order to decide on the need for alveolar ridge reshaping (Figure 10.5). When assessing bone volume and quality, the future planned reshaping of the alveolar ridge with bone substitutes and implant placement in that location must be taken into account - the newly formed bone should meet all biomechanical requirements and withstand all functional and parafunctional loads.

The strength and load forces that will act on the changed shape of the alveolar ridge, i.e. the newly formed bone, will crucially depend on the way the implant is placed and on the optimal choice of implant (diameter, shape, titanium quality and surface treatment of the implant and the region in which the forces act). For example, in the molar region the load forces acting on the bone are almost ten times stronger than the forces in the frontal region. This fact must be taken into account as a risk factor when performing augmentation.

Based on many studies, it has been shown that the load is affected by the shape of the jaw and the strength of the masticatory muscles. This must be carefully assessed when making a decision to use these procedures, primarily for the repair of anatomical structures with bone substitutes.

The activity of the load forces during mastication also depends on the type of food - these forces are usually greater, because they last longer, than the forces in parafunctional loads. Parafunctional movements, or loads, are influenced by several factors, depending on the person, stress, life trauma, etc. This must also be taken into account. Parafunctional forces are usually of lower intensity and shorter duration. This information should not be omitted from the medical history.

Despite all the professional doubts, bone augmentation with bone substitutes is increasingly being used in oral implantology. Augmentation in the anterior regions is most often conditioned by aesthetic requirements, and in the posterior regions by biomechanical reasons.

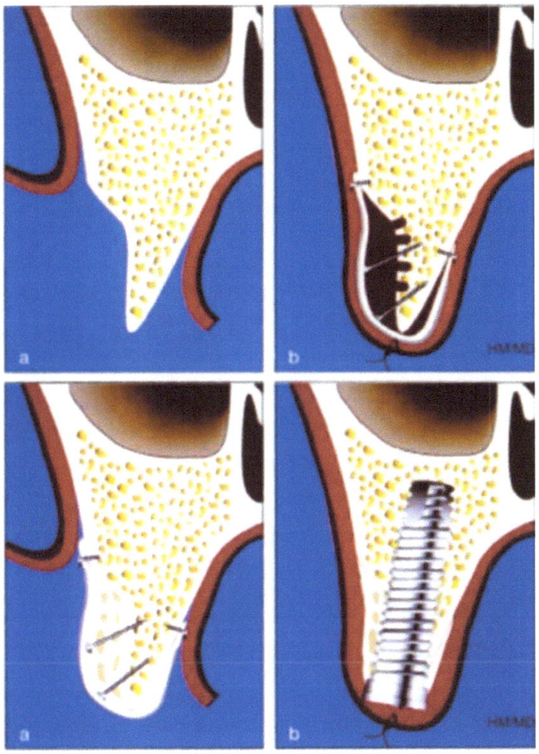

Figure 10.5. Schematic representation of guided tissue regeneration in jako pointed narrow alveolar ridge (a). Augment placement (b), newly formed bone (c) and installation of an ideally oriented implant eight, when there is enough bone base.

The main criteria for assessing the necessary augmentation are:

1. the relationship of the ridge to the future position of the tooth (of implants);
2. quantity and quality of bone;
3. functlonal and parafunctlonal load.

BASIC PROBLEMS

Anterior region in the upper jaw:

a) aesthetics;
b) loss of alveolar bone width and height;
c) thin lamellar bone.

Lateral region of the upper jaw:

a) sinus position;
b) biomechanical problems;
c) aesthetic problems (sometimes).

The most common problems in the upper jaw are loss width and height of the alveolar ridge and sinus enlargement. Problems in the front region of the lower jaw are loss width and height of the alveolar bone, and in the lateral region; mandibular canal, mental foramen and biomechanical problems.

The front regions in the upper and lower jaw are subject to aesthetic and biomechanical rules, while the lateral regions are primarily biomechanical.

Substitutes for bone (an established term in practice "artificial bone"), are applied in periodontology as much as in oral implantology, which requires more detailed knowledge properties of ideal substitutes for bone.

Almost insurmountable obstacles to the installation of implants are overcome with bone substitutes, narrow alveolar ridge and shallow maxillary sinus floor. The biggest trap for the most experienced clinicians is still today the shallow floor of the maxillary sinus, and the treatment of raising the sinus floor by implanting a bone substitute is a permanent risk with a sometimes uncertain outcome, although recent progress in this area has been increasing in favor of predicting success with augmentation. By what method and in what way will the sinus floor be raised, whether by augmentation with grafts (a graft is a material used for the reconstruction of body parts with bone block or granules), a closed or open approach, or an osteotomy technique with or without rafting (Figure 10.6). The procedure depends on the assessment of the case and the dentist's experience, which will be discussed in more detail in this chapter.

Characteristics of an Ideal Bone Substitute

1. **Osteointegration** - the ability to chemically bind to the bone surface without an intermediate layer of connective tissue.
2. **Osteoconductivity** – the ability to support and enable bone growth.
3. **Osteoinductivity** - the ability to cause differentiation of pluripotent mesenchymal cells into osteoblasts and osteocytes, respectively.
4. **Osteogenetic potential** – ability to form new bone by osteoblastic cells present in the bone substitute itself.

OSTEOGENESIS is the process of formation of new bone tissue by osteoprogenitic cells located in the bone graft, surviving transplantation, proliferating and differentiating into osteblasts.

Bone marrow elements ensure fusion of osteoinductive proteins of potential osteogenic cells and local blood vessels.

OSTEOINDUCTION is the grouping of adjacent undifferentiated mesenchymal stem cells at the site of graft application and differentiation into chondrocytes and osteoblasts or osteocytes.

Factors that affect osteoinduction are:

- bone morphogenetic protein (**BMP**);
- platelet growth factors;
- fibroblast growth factors;
- interleukins;
- growth factors that stimulate blood vessel growth.

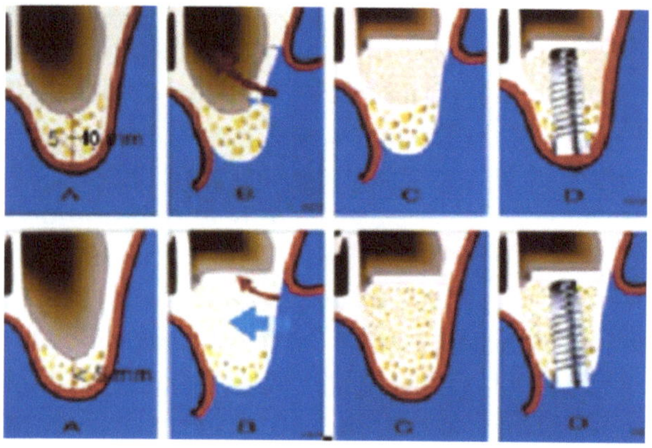

Figure 10.6 Top row: Raising the sinus floor with bone replacements, so that the required bone height (A) is doubled, opening and raising the buccal bone wall (B), forming a new sinus floor by placing the bone replacer (C), the immediate positioning of the implant (D).
Bottom row: Sinus floor lifting with delayed implant placement from 6 to 8 months: bone height of the alveolar ridge is less than <5 mm (A), formation of a new sinus floor with a bone substitute (B), new bone formed after 6-8 months (C), implant installed

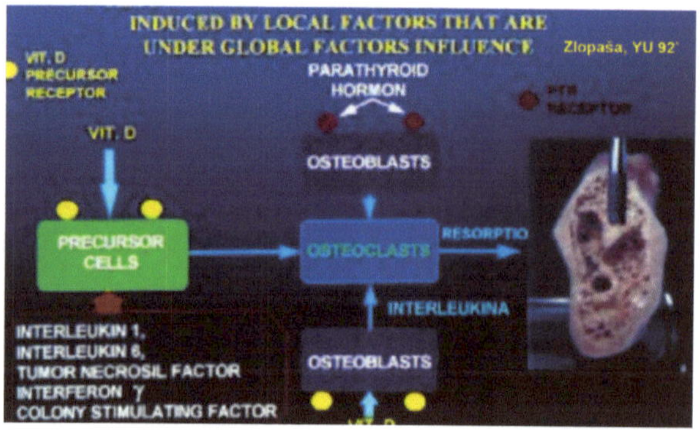

Figure 10.7. Schematic explanation of bone metabolism and factors involved in this physiological process with reference to the processes of augmentation and osteointegration. (From the lecture of the author of the book at the world symposium of implantologists in Bologna. 1992.)

OSTEOCONDUCTION is the growth of vascular tissue and mesenchymal stem cells into the graft structure.

OSTEOINTEGRATION is a process of close i.e. direct bonding of implant, i.e., the graft, and the bone tissue of the host, without the mediation of connective tissue.

Bone replacers can be:

- autografts;
- allografts;
- xenografts;
- synthetic materials;
- composite grafts or mixtures.

Autografts have all the characteristics of an ideal transplant. The disadvantages are the limited number of grafts and the morbidity of the site of administration.

Allograft is a transplant taken from a biologically same host species, but genetically different, determined by the HLA (human leukocyte antigen) system.

Allografts can be:

- Fresh
- frozen,
- frozen dried,
- mineralized,
- demineralized.

Allografts have:

- Osteointegration;
- osteoconductivity,
- osteoinductivity.

Allograft preparation is carried out:

- By physical and ultrasonic processing,
- By ethylene oxide treatment
- By antibiotic treatment
- by eliminating the spore with the help of gamma rays,
- by eliminating the allograft antigen component
- By enhancing the body's immune response,
- preserving the biological and mechanical properties of graft.

The biggest problem and danger of allografts is the possibility of HIV virus transmission.

Xenografts represent bone grafts obtained from other biological species.

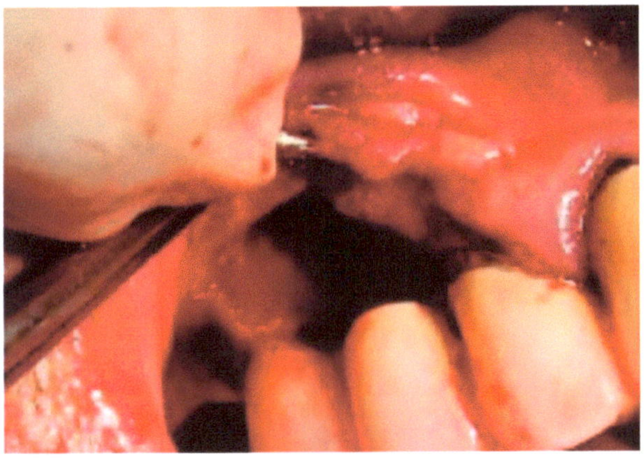

Figure 10.8. Cystic bone destruction in the premolar area.

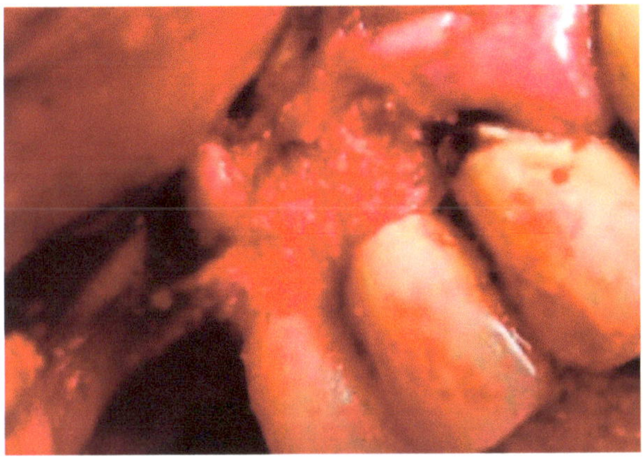

Figure 10.9. Filled bone cyst with Bio-Oss collagen covered with resorbable BioGide membrane.

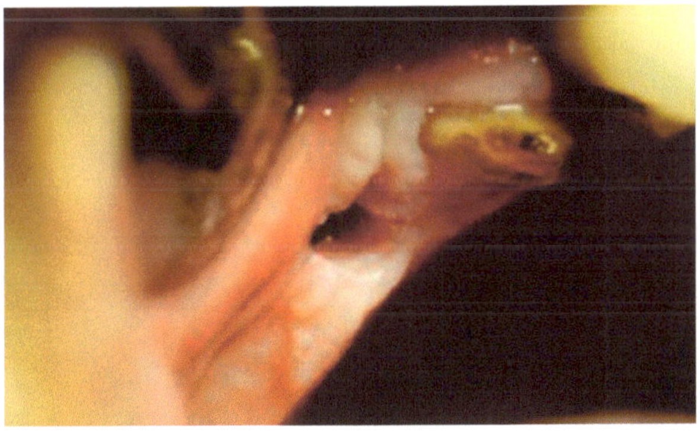

Figure 10.10. Embedded implant in augmented bone (Figures 10.8 and 10.9) after 8 months well formed kertatinized part of the gingivae.

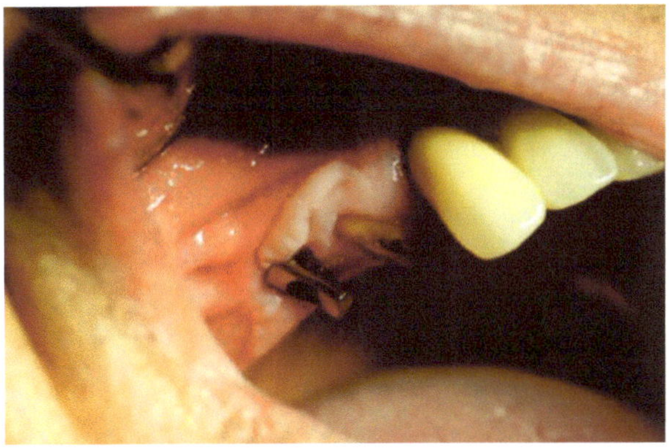

Figure 10.11. Mounted bracket on the implant embedded in the argumented part of the bone after 8 months.

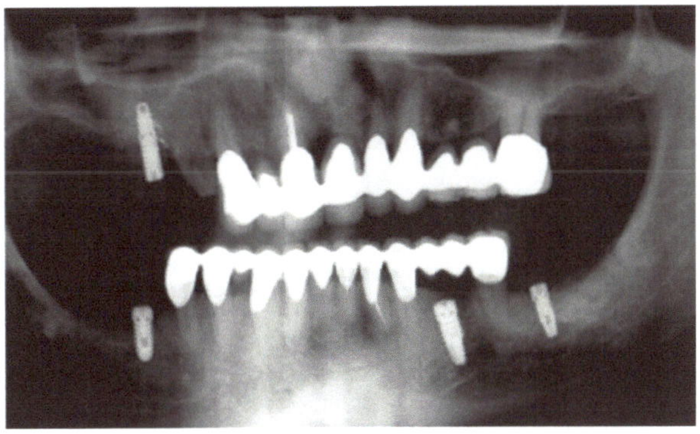

Figure 10.12. Follow-up scan after 8 months. See Figure 10.8.

Bio-Oss is one of the most commonly used bone replacers that is very often used before implant placement (Figures 10.8. to 10.12. It is a deproteinized bovine bone mineral obtained by removing all organic matter. The particle size of the material is from 0.25 to 1 millimeter, which favors osteogenesis. By implantation of autologous bone, the percentage of newly formed bone tissue after 6 months is 40%, and after implantation Bio-Oss is approximately the same (39%).

In autologous bone augmentation, the remaining amount of transplantation is 18%, while in Bio-Oss it is 31%. Such data on success percentages are most often marketing and unreliable.

The exact time of complete resorption of BioOss has not been determined. The data from the literature are different. Some authors believe that complete resorption takes about 14 weeks, and Tarnau and Salama prove that complete resorption of Bio-Oss occurs after 44 months.

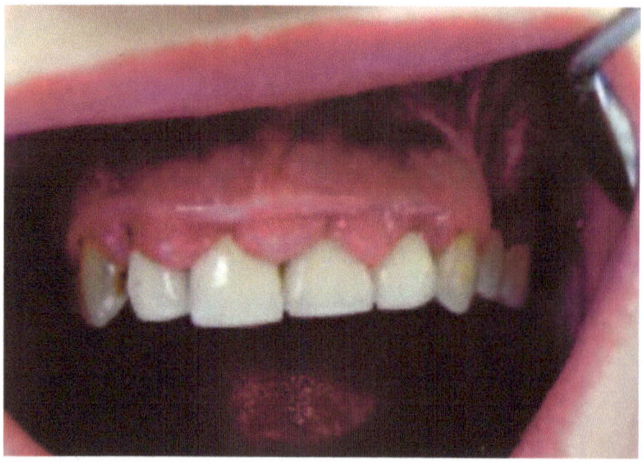

Figure 10.13. Poor prosthetics make it impossible to maintain good oral hygiene with the consequences of periodontal disease and bone destruction.

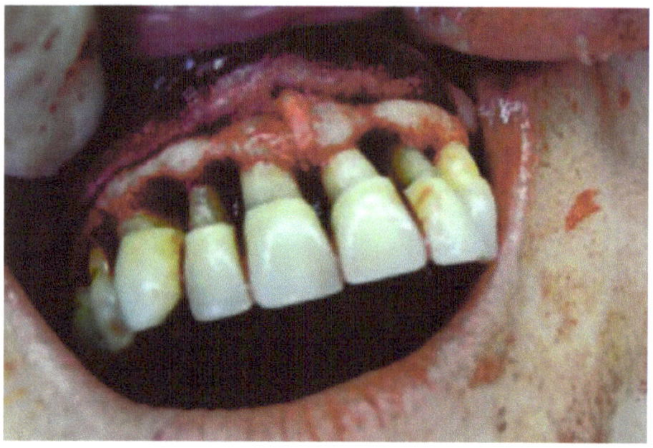

Figure 10.14 Major bone defects caused by wide crowns in the tooth neck.

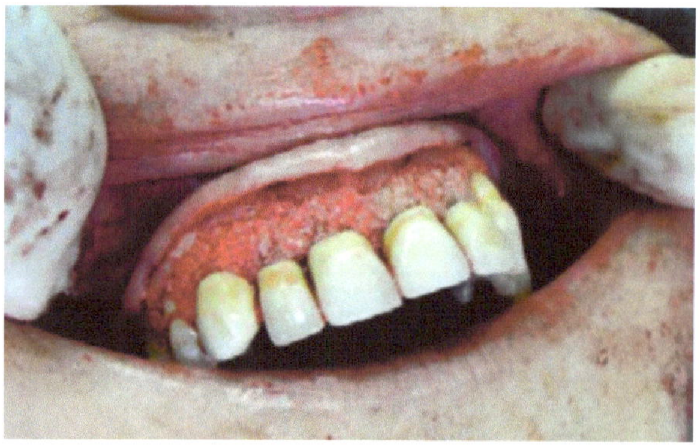

Figure 10.15. Replacement with Bio-Oss collagen covered with BioGide collagen membrane.

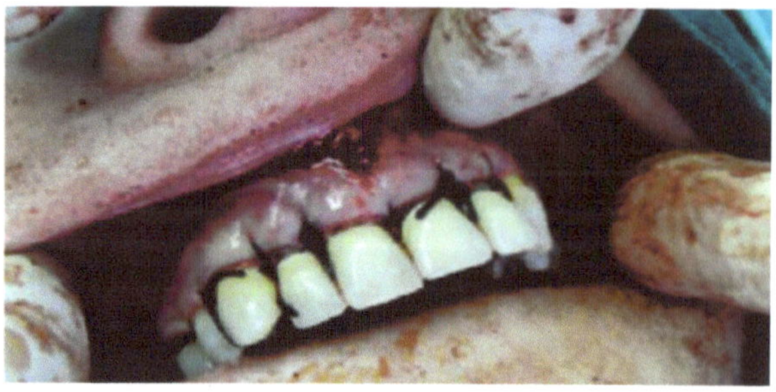

Figure 10.16. It is necessary to replace imprecise metal ceramic crowns with temporary ones in the composite.

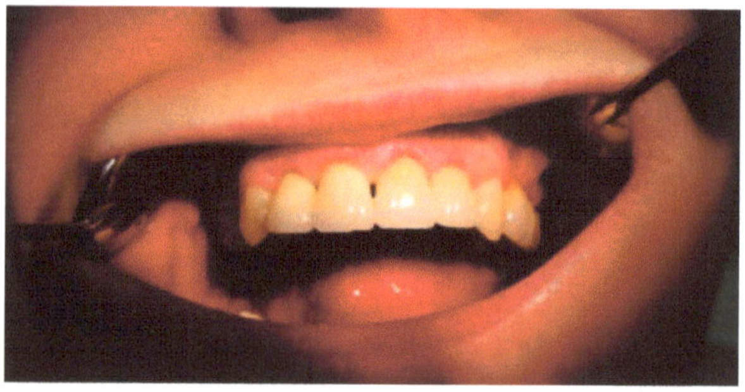

Figure 10.17. Replaced the most precise metal-ceramic crowns with temporary ones in the composite. Required waiting time (at least 8-12 weeks) for fully healed soft tissues and the production of definitive prosthetic works.

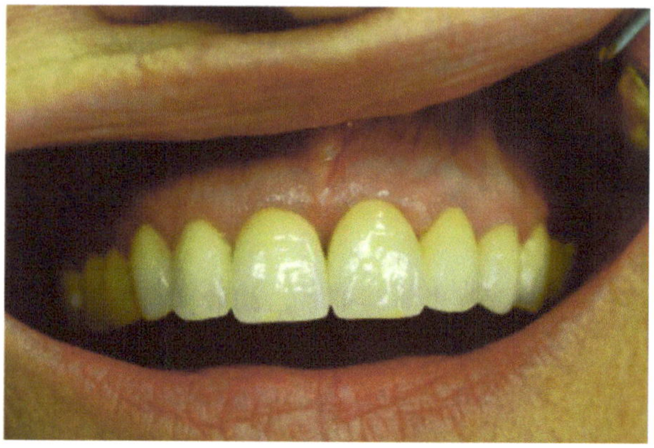

Figure 10.18. After the surgery and the placement of the bone substitute, the reconstruction and preservation of the papilla is extremely important. Successful outcome.

Bio-Oss Collagen is applied in periodontology and for guided regeneration of bone tissue and for filling larger bone losses (Figures 10.13.-10-14).

There are other bone substitutes:

Hydroxyapatite (e.g. Pro-Osteon) is obtained from sea corals by complete removal of organic components. The pore size, from 45 to 100 microns, is favorable for good osseointegration. Characteristics of hydroxyapatite:

- dimensionally unstable,
- non-absorbable,
- mixture with 25% autologous bone achieves better dimensional stability.

CHITOSAN is obtained from the crab skeleton. **GUSUIBU** is derived from Drynaria Fortunei. **RED ALGAE** that are chemically processed into hydroxyapatite.

Synthetic materials as bone substitutes

These materials possess the following characteristics:

- osteoconductivity
- osteointegration
- biocompatibility
- specific hardness and modulus of elasticity, as well as pressure resistance comparable to that of the host's spongious and cortical bones.

A large number of course alternates can be found on the market whose marketing announcement is often unrealistic, resulting in failures (Figures 10-20-10-21 and 10-22).

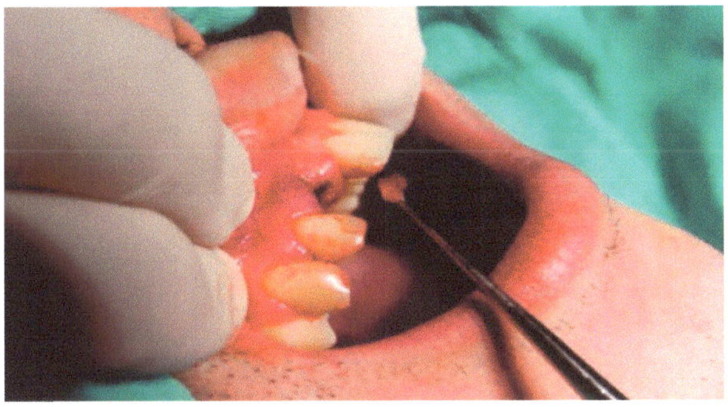

Figure 10.19. Preservation of the alveoli after tooth extraction for immediate implant placement.

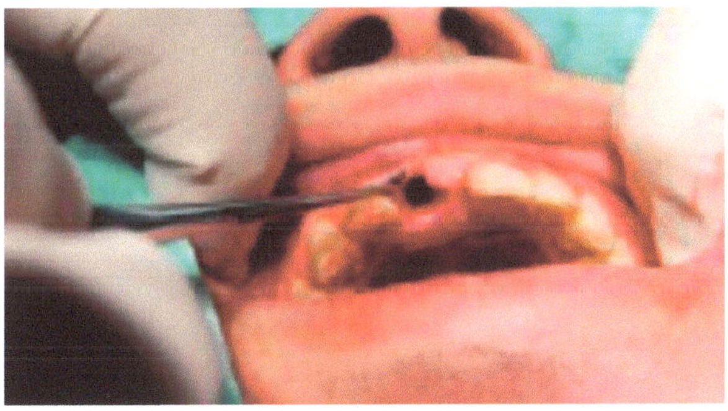

Figure 10.20. Prepared alveoli for graft placement.

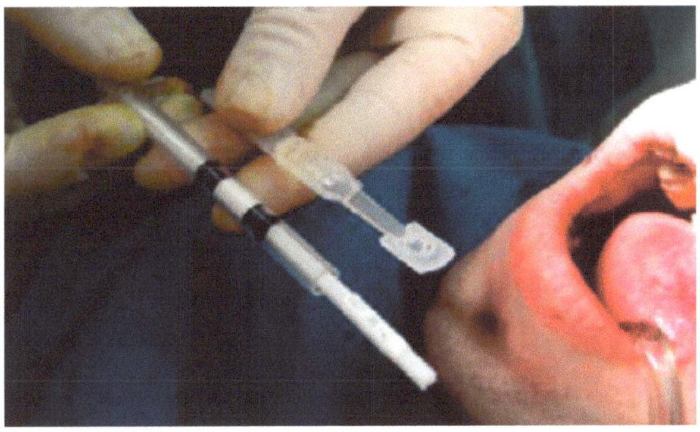

Figure 10.21. Easy-graft augmentation resulted in failure. The results were the opposite of marketing compliments.

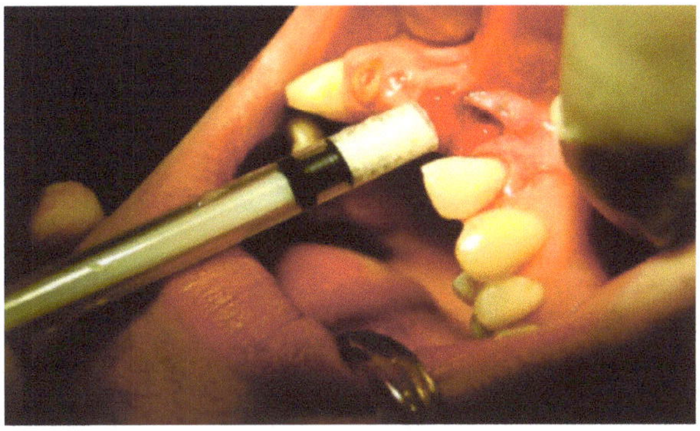

Figure 10.22. The manufacturer's marketing recommendation is that the application of a collagen resorptive membrane is not required.

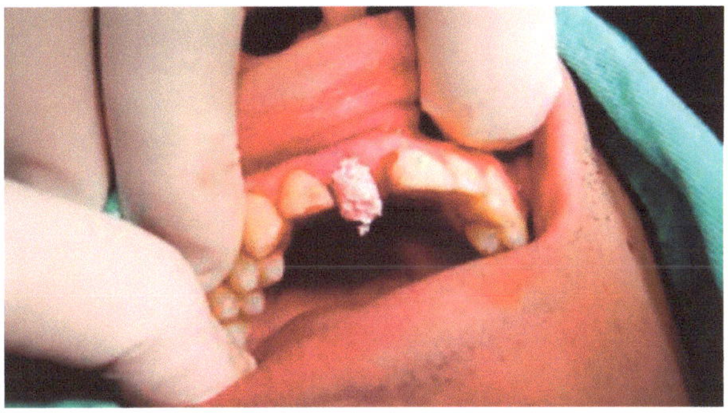

Figure 10.23. Placement of beta-tricalcium phosphate graft after tooth extraction. Outcome failed.

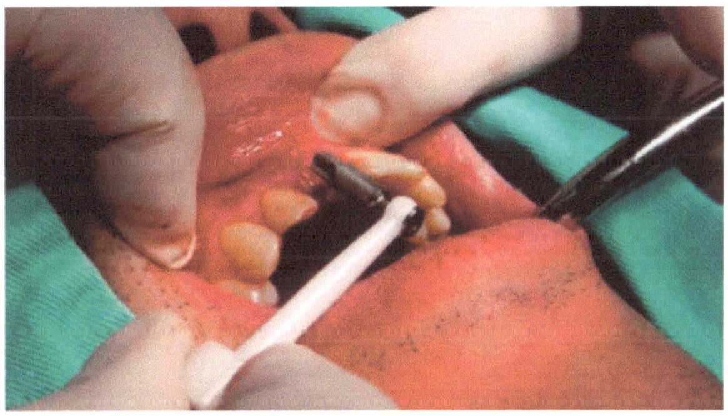

Figure 10.24. Implant placement after augmentation with beta tricalcium phosphate. Experience confirms that the use of this material as a graft is a failure, and at the same time warns to be wary of the manufacturer's marketing praise.

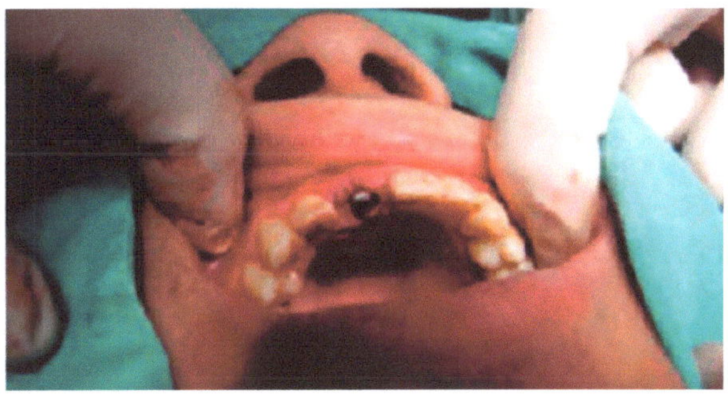

Figure 10.25. Implant placement completed. Delayed waiting for healing (two-phase method).

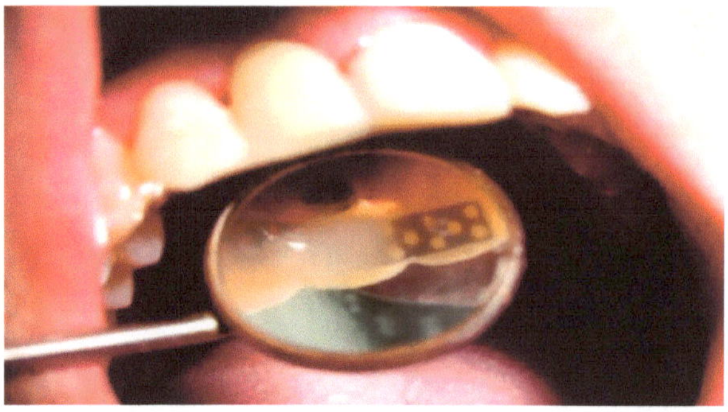

Figure 10.26. Temporary tooth restoration attached with adhesive composites to adjacent teeth. Failed augmentation with betatricalcium phosphate. The application of the marketing "hit" – "Easy-graph" ended in failure. The launch of this bone deputy is a failure (after all, the author is an engineer, not a biologist).

Types of synthetic materials:

1. bioactive glass,
2. glass ionomer,
3. aluminium oxide,
4. calcium salts (sulfate phospate, alpha and beta),
5. synthetic hydroxyapatite.

1. **Bioactive glass** also contains silicon dioxide, calcium oxide, phosphorus pentoxide, and sodium oxide. This type of material is characterized by:
   - Exceptional firmness,
   - formation of a strong bond with host tissue via hydroxyapatite crystals.

2. **Glass ionomer** is characterized by the following characteristics:
   - porous and highly osteoconductive.
   - appropriate modulus of elasticity and pressure resistance,
   - is not absorbed.

3. **Aluminum oxide** – Aluminum ions are neurotoxic.

4. **Calcium sulfate** is characterized by:
   - Biocompatibility;
   - Osteoconductivity;
   - Unique ability to stimulate osteogenesis;
   - very fast resorption.

   Calcium phosphate is characterized by:
   - Biocompatibility;
   - Osteointegration;
   - Osteoconductivity through the formation of hydroxypatite on its surface.

   Alpha-tricalcium phosphate contaminated with saliva leads to a gigantocellular inflammatory reaction. Beta-tricalcium phosphate is often used, is extremely osteoconductive and absorbs very quickly.

5. **Synthetic hydroxyapatite** has a porous, non-porous, ceramic and non-ceramic form. They are characterized by good osteointegration (coating around the implant).
   In the future, we should expect:
   - new technologies
   - better understanding of platelet growth factor and other bone healing processes.

Seek to preserve the good and remove the undesirable properties of each new material.

Conclusion:

The result of augmentation is based on the following parameters:

1. the reconstruction location;
2. the size of the defect;
3. the objectives of the project;
4. the patient's condition and wishes;
5. knowledge of bone grafts.

Bone substitutes have found a very wide application in periodontology in guided bone regeneration. For the success of the implants installed in the augmented region, there is also valid evidence published in the journal Quintens-senze internationale:

- Chiapso et al. (2009) prove that success of installed implants in the augmented region is the same as in pyriform bone.
- Pjettursson et al. (2008) record the success of the installation of implants in the augmented region of 96.3% up to 99.8% after 3 years.
- Giovani et al. (2010) evaluate the success after 15 months of 92.5%.
- Cricchi et al. (2010) prove the success of augmented region with 98.7% after 6 years.

Augmentation can be:

- horizontal augmentation of the alveolar ridge due to insufficient width,

- Vertical augmentation of the alveolar ridge due to insufficient height.

Techniques for horizontal augmentation of the alveolar ridge are:

- GBR (granulated or block grafts)
- Bone distraction
- Bone splitting.

To perform horizontal alveolar augmentation ridge there are two approaches: simultaneous and two-phase. The two-phase approach is much more demanding and more complex, because it requires time, patient understanding and patience.

The two-phase approach of horizontal augmentation applies in the following cases:

- advanced ridge resorption;
- ridge width less than 4 mm;
- the existence of bone defects with only one wall.

Favorite places:

- frontal region of the upper jaw, aesthetically sensitive zone
- lateral segments of the lower jaw with a sharp (razor-like) ridge.

Vertical augmentation of the alveolar ridges is used for insufficient height of the alveolar ridge and poor quality of the cancellous bone (D3 and D4) in the lateral regions of the upper jaw. **Vertical augmentation ensures satisfactory anatomical conditions for safer implant installation. (Fig 10.28)**

Vertical increase of bone mass can be done by using a transplant or by using a substitute for bone with collagen resorptive membranes.

The widest and most successful application of materials for augmentation of the alveolar ridges was shown by:

- autologous bone;
- beef deproteinized bone (BDB);
- bovine deproteinized bone mixed with autologous bones;
- human deproteinized bone;
- human deproteinized bone mixed with autologous bone.

Application Of Bone Grafts

Bone grafts can be in the form of bone blocks or bone granules.

Vertical and horizontal augmentation are possible performed with bone block grafts that have the following advantages:

- mechanical resistance to pressure of soft tissues,
- the degree of vascularization depends on the shape and composition
- collagen membrane slows down vascularization,
- perforation of the cortex accelerates revascularization,
- revascularization is slower in compact bone, but also resorption (60% in 6 months),
- after a few years, they are replaced by a new bone.

The characteristics of granulation bone grafts are:

- greater osteoinductive and osteoconductive potential,
- less formation of osteogenic cells,
- weaker mechanical stability,
- faster resorption.

There are 3 types of granules: ground bone, bone shavings, and bone chips.

Summarizing the characteristics of both, the question arises: which is better, block graft or granulation graft?

A larger bone volume is achieved with a block graft. With the application of granulated grafts, fibrous encapsulation can often occur which is manifested by micropigmentation due to impaired revascularization.

For a successful outcome of both, firm fixation is crucial.

In the case of cortical bone augmentation, it is extremely important to perforate the cortex in several places, because this allows bone marrow cells to grow into the graft faster. Perforation of the cortical bone also facilitates angiogenesis.

Summarizing the advantages of all substitute materials for bone, autogenous bone grafting is unparalleled for the following reasons:

- genetically identical tissue;
- the donor and recipient regions are in the same place;

- embryologically identical tissue;
- the best, safest and cheapest material.

However, taking grafts, especially blocks, either from the chin, retromolar trigone or thigh (crista iliaca), is not a simple surgical procedure.

The application of bone substitutes and collagen membranes is a proven successful procedure.

The best combination is 50% bone substitute mixed 50% with autologous bone. Good results are also achieved with a combination of 80% substitutes for bone mixed with 20% autologous bone.

Vertical enlargement of the alveolar ridge with a low floor of the sinus cavity (sinus-lifting) can be performed with several procedures - open or closed procedure, with the use of block-graft or granulation graft.

The most acceptable method for practice is the osteotomy technique, for which the following prerequisites must be met: that the subantral dimension is at least 4-5 mm, that the sinus floor is flat, and most importantly, the dentist's experience.

Sinus lift with closed osteotomy is performed when the height of the available alveolar ridge bone is at least 4 to 6 mm.

Another way of applying the osteotomy technique is osteotomy condensation, which consists of the following procedures:

- careful elevation of the floor of the sinuses with osteotomy simultaneous bone condensation;
- preparation of the bed with osteotomes;
- after the graft is inserted, the procedure can continue with implant placement;
- also, to raise the sinus floor up to 3 mm often no grafting required - waiting time required is 6 to 8 months. It is very important that the implant has a wider diameter (4.1 mm x 10 mm). The success rate after 1 year is 100%.
- Osteotomy technique without grafting, confirmed by experience and bibliographic data after 3 years, the success rate is 100%.

When it comes to applying the osteotomy technique with or without grafting, there are still dilemmas.

Schimidlin et al. (2008) and Nedir et al. (2010) thinking that grafting is not necessary because of the osteogenic potential of the membrane with a barrier role.

However, Petrusson et al (2008 and 2009) show that grafts should be used because a larger amount of bone is obtained, and the result is predictable.

During augmentation, whether it is larger or minor bone defects, quality of surface treatment implant has a great influence on the entire process. The influence of the quality of the machined surface of the implant from is of crucial importance, especially with augmentations of larger bone defects with transplants taken from different parts of the body (pictures 10.28-10.29 and 10.30).

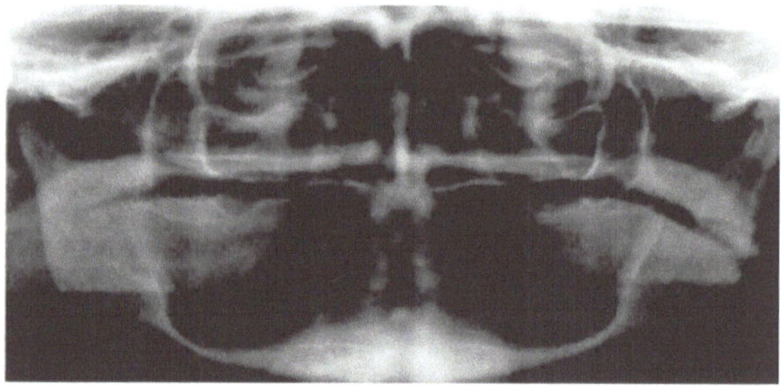

Figure 10.27 Extreme bony atrophy of the ridge of the lower jaw pre augmentation. Always a risky procedure with an uncertain outcome patient morbidity.

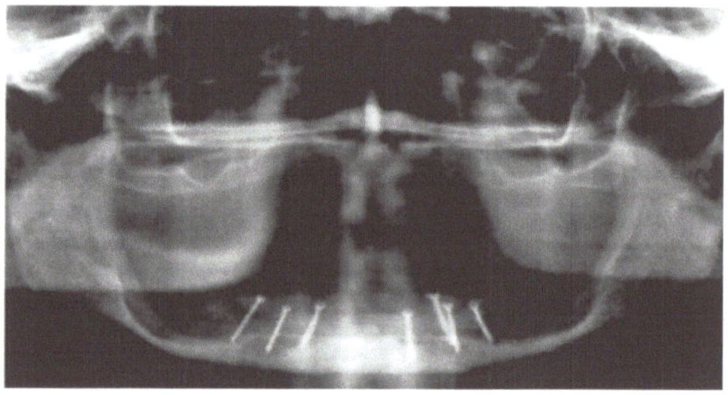

Figure 10.28. Radiological control after bone augmentation blocks fixed with titanium screws.

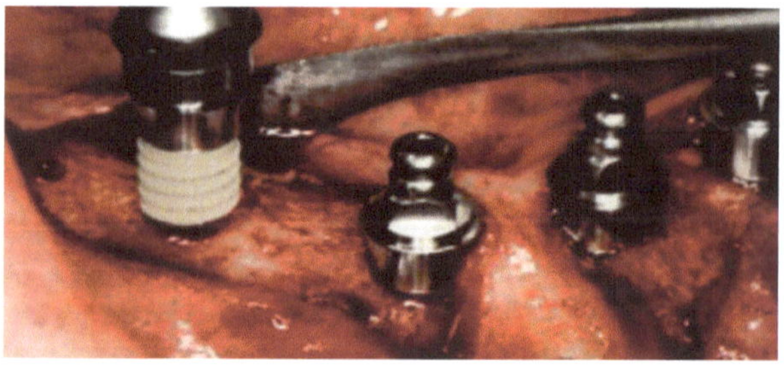

Figure 10.29. After removing the titanium screws, they were installed implants in the augmented area 4 months after augmentation.

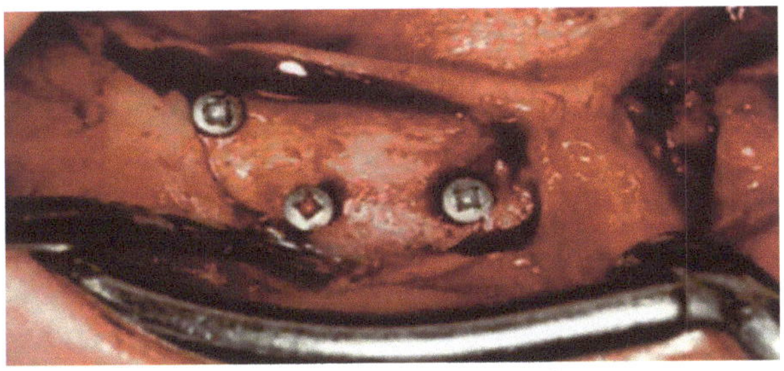

Figure 10.30. Initial contact of the implant surface with blood during installing the implant in the augmented part of the bone is the first step accelerates the integration with the bone of immediately loaded implants.

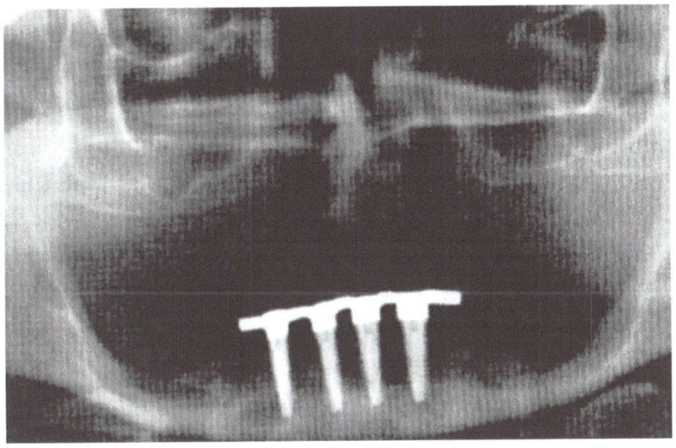

Figure 10.31. Radiological control 2 years after implant placement. Stably formed bone relationship between the cervical part and the microstructural endosteal part of the implant, which is accompanied by good formation of soft tissues as a barrier against the onset of peri-implantitis.

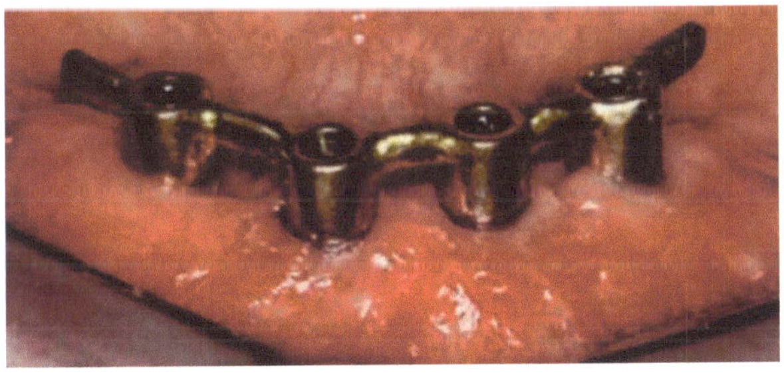

Figure 10.32. Appearance after 6 months of immediately loaded implants. Healthy and keratinized gingivae around the implant.

When bone destruction is greater on a smaller area, usually after the loss of one of the central incisors in the frontal region of the upper jaw, rehabilitation that begins with augmentation of the bone defect is extremely complex. The outcome of the treatment depends on the extent of the defect; whether it is possible by the procedure of placement of a xenogenic bone replacement or whether the use of an auto-transplant taken from the retromolar region where a sufficient amount of available bone allows it, covered with a bone substitute with the application of collagen of the resorptive membrane is required. The formation of stable soft tissues and an aesthetically successful outcome depend on the quality of bone support achieved (Figures 10.33. – 10,37).

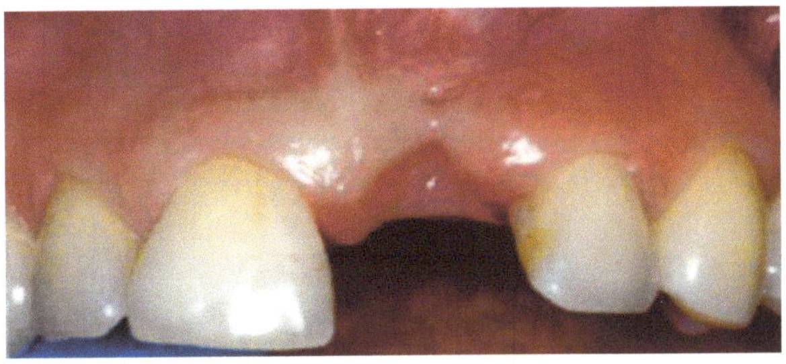

Figure 10.33. Central incisor deficiency (#21) with greater bone and soft tissue loss. In cases where the lamellar bone wall has been destroyed, in addition to compensating the lamellar bone for bone substitutes, soft tissues must also be shaped by the guiding procedure.

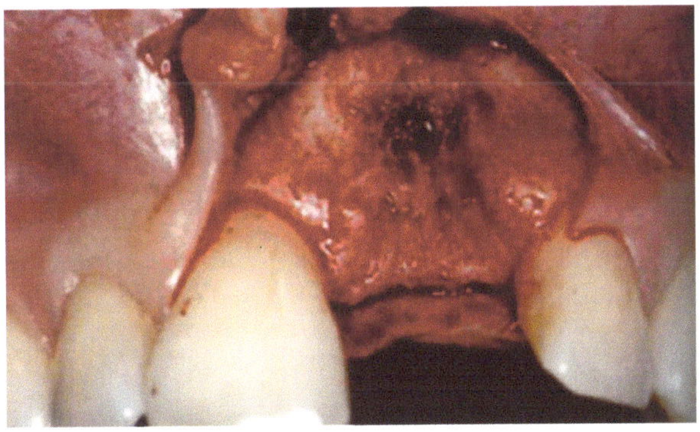

Figure 10.34. By detecting the lobe, a clear overview of the extent of the bone defect and destruction in the area of the root apex is obtained.

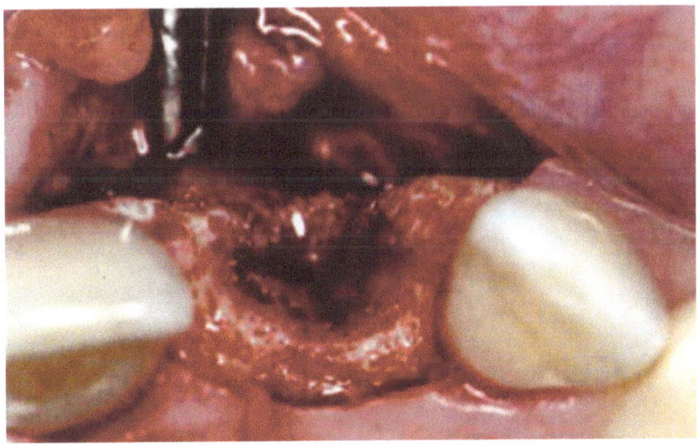

Figure 10.35. Display of occlusal defect and lamellar bone.

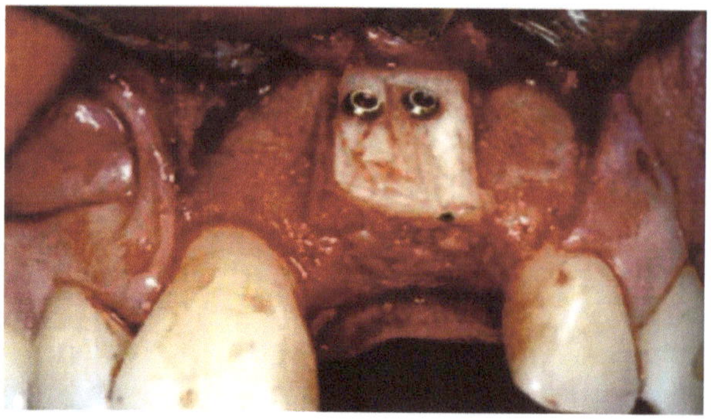

Figure 10.36. Reconstruction of the bone defect with an autotransplant block taken from the retromolar region of the mandible, fixed with titanium screws.

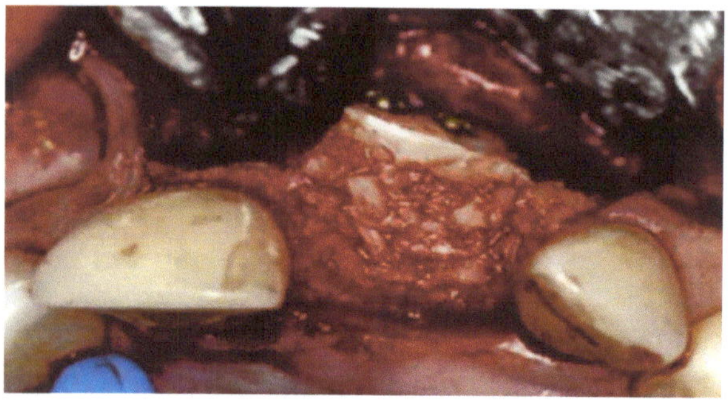

Figure 10.37. Occlusal appearance of additional bone substitutes and on the bone autologous block covered with collagen receptive membrane. Healing waiting time of at least 6 months.

Examples of treatment of complicated cases in the frontal region of the upper jaw

Extremely large gingival recession (Class IV) with complete destruction of the vestibular lamellar bone (Figure 10.42) represents the most complex, but also the most attractive procedure from the aspect of augmentation, mucogingival surgery and implant-prosthetic restoration.

The etiology of this mucogingival destruction and the complete destruction of the vestibular lamellar bone can be multicausal. It is extremely important to determine the causes of this anomaly, in order to plan the entire therapy procedure and predict the success of future implant prosthetic restoration. The causes of such large recessions can be different: coronally inserted frenulum, congenital anomaly of the alveolar bone such as dehiscences, orthodontic anomalies manifested by a malposition of the tooth and malocclusion, phenotypic properties of the gingivae (thin and gracile gingivae), overemphasized alveolar jugs and the use of hard nylon brushes. According to many authors, the most up-to-date view of the causes of recession with greater gingival destruction, thanks also to the resorption of the vestibular bone lamella, is based on hereditary genetic causes. This is especially true for malformations of the vestibular bone lamella. In the presented case, the recession that reaches to the apical part of the exposed root, with complete resorption of the vestibular bone lamella, is based on hereditary genetic causes. This is especially true for malformations of the vestibular bone lamella. In the presented case, a recession reaches the apical part of the exposed root, with complete resorption of the vestibular bone lamella. It is caused by malposition of the frontal teeth in the lower jaw with the consequences of disturbed occlusion. In this type of gingival recession, an attempt to bridge with a free mucous graft would result in failure, as the survival of the free mucous graft would be impossible due to the avascular surface of exposed root. Treatment in this way should not even be attempted. The recession in the presented case is too wide to establish adequate and collateral circulation of from adjacent medial and distal vascularized regions between which the transplant would be placed. Given the distance of the vascularized borders of the mucous tissue, due to the large width of the gingival recession, the central parts of the mucous autotransplant most often necrotise.

In this particular case, the establishment of collateral circulation with the apical mucosa would be unsuccessful, because it is too far away to establish adequate nutrition of the coronary and central parts of the muco-gingival transplant, which would result in transplant necrosis. Collateral circulation can come from three sources: mesial, distal, and apical. In the presented case (Figure 10.38), all three sources of blood circulation of the mucous transplant are endangered. In situations of wide recessions in which complete resorption of the vestibular lamellar bone has not occurred, collateral circulation from the lateral regions is insufficient, but the blood supply coming from the apical zone most often allows the transplant to be adequately nourished. In the presented case, in the apical part, there is inflammation with visible granulations, a large area of recession and a pronounced convexity of the exposed root. Attempting to reconstruct the gingivae with mucogingival surgery over the bare root would result in absolute failure. Therefore, removing the diseased tooth and preparing the region for implant placement is the only correct solution with a long-term successful result (Figures 10.39-10.45)

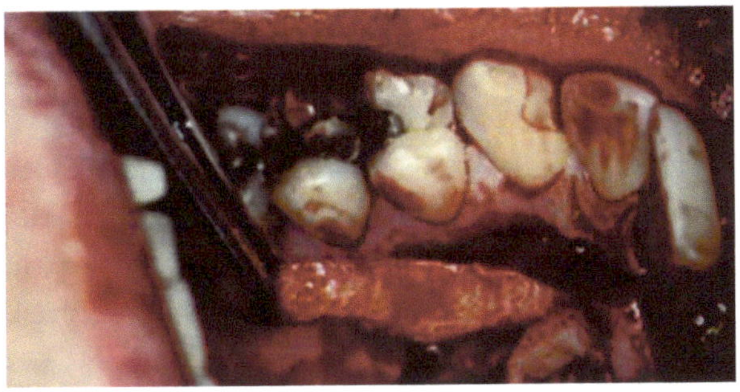

Figure 10.38. Prepared the lobe on the palate in 2 layers so that by reaching the edges of the incision, the wound was later well closed.

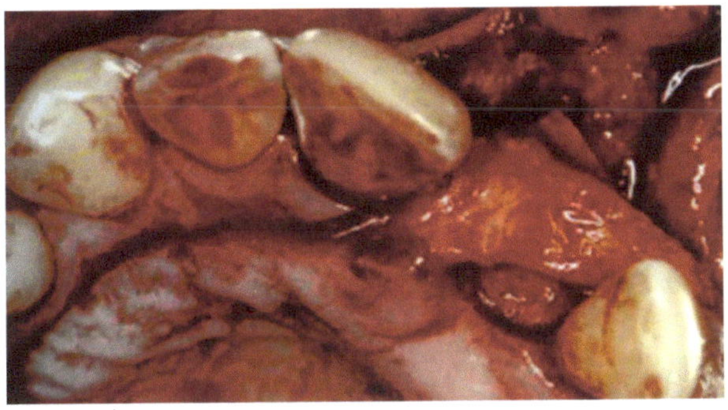

Figure 10.39. Covering the augmented ridge vestibularly with 2 layers - detected lobe and transplant of submucosis and periosteum taken from the palate. Closure of the wound from the vestibular side.

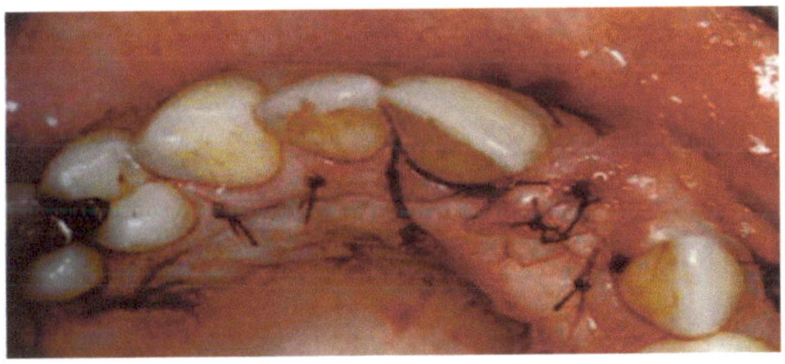

Figure 10.40. Wound closure using a free and raised lobe and a transplant taken from the palate.

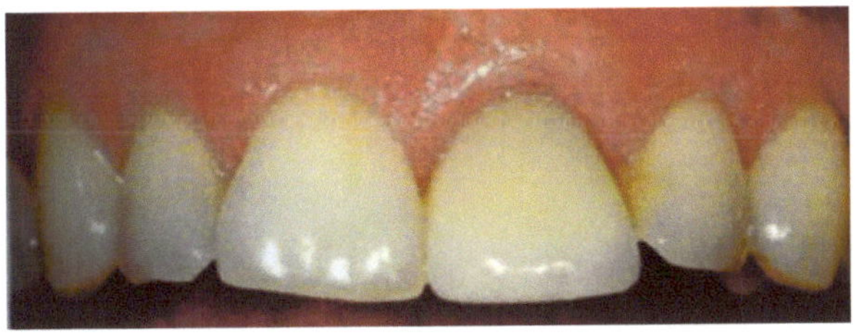

Figure 10.41. Clinical appearance after 4 years, after prosthetic restoration. Good appearance of soft tissues without visible scars.

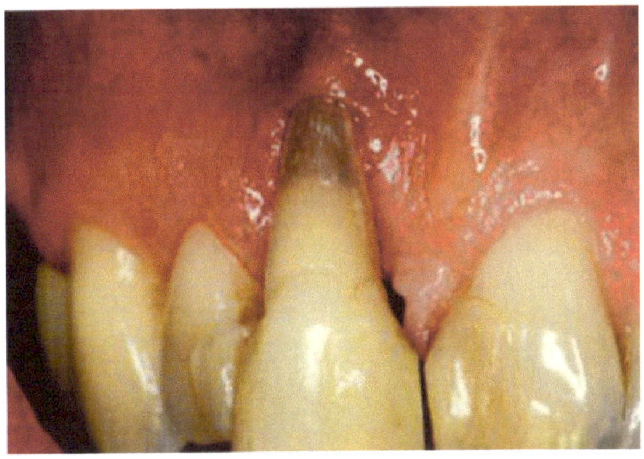

Figure 10.42. Extreme recession of the gingivae with an exposed root of the central incisor, followed by resorption of the lamellar bone. Gingival recession is defined as the migration of the gingivae apically in relation to the enamel-cement border and represents the degeneration of soft and bone tissues of the mucogingival complex, which occurs under the influence of etiological factors: periodontopathy, unfavorable biotype of the gingivae, weakened vestibular bone lamella, tooth malposition, traumatic occlusion, iatrogenic factors, use of hard brushes.

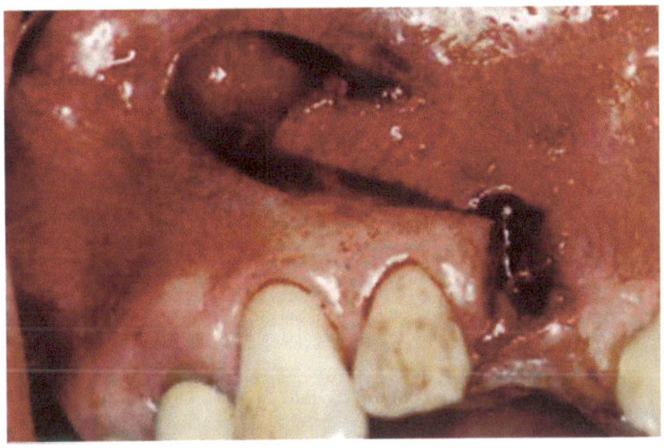

Figure 10.43. Removed central incisor (#11). The semi-circular cut on the vestibular side simplifies the easier movement of the full-thickness lobe.

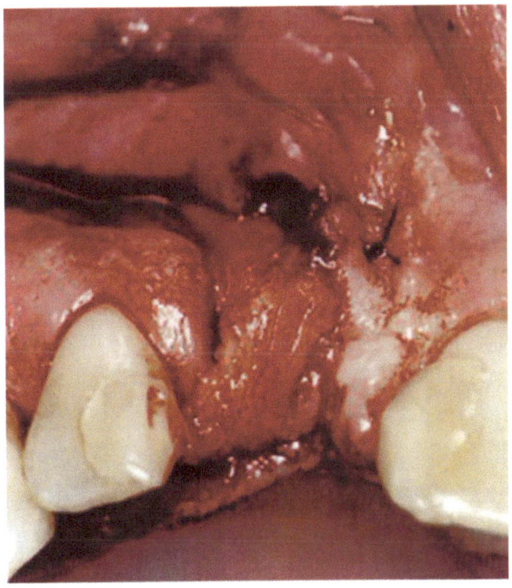

Figure 10.44. Positioning of the lobe with the stem by rotating towards the prepared palatal lobe, thus covering the region of the argued defect.

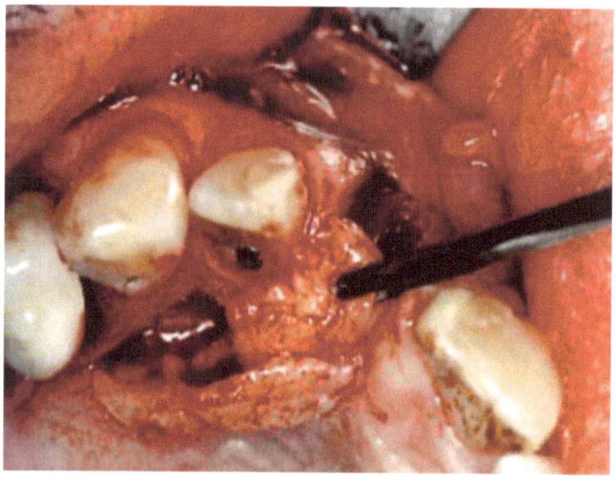

Figure 10.45. Preparation of the palatal lobe with the connective tissue stem allows its displacement to cover the region of the defect to be augmented.

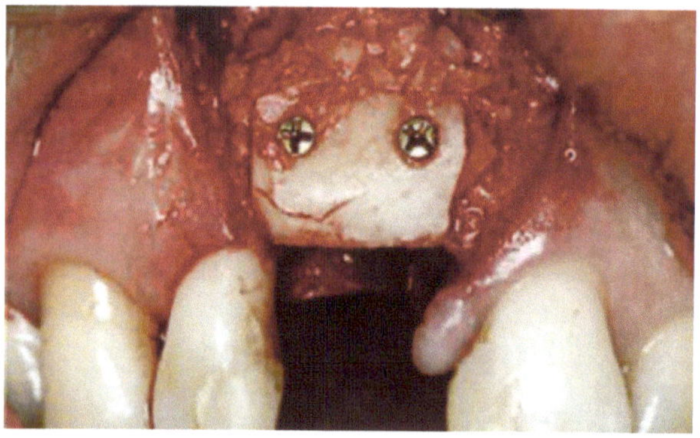

Figure 10.46. Filling in the bone defect with a block, taken from the chin fixed with titanium screws, supplemented with Bio-Oss autologous bone filings. Covering the augmented region is done with connective tissue, rotating the vestibular lobe of full thickness. The waiting time for removal of titanium screws and implant placement requires at least 3 months of waiting. A period of at least 6 months is required for complete healing of hard and soft tissues.

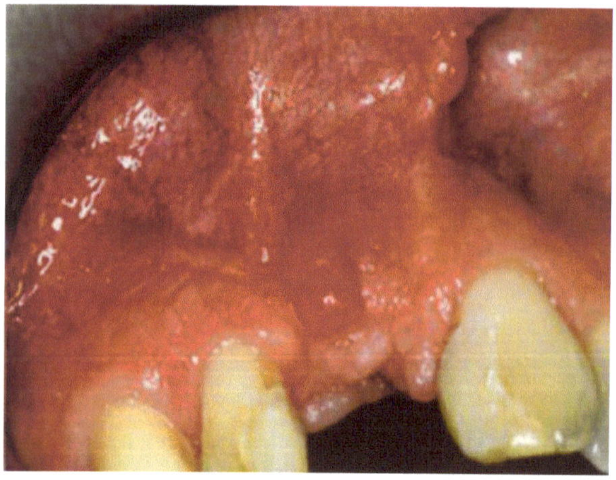

Figure 10.47. Clinical appearance of the augmented region of fully graded soft tissues with no visible scars after 8 weeks.

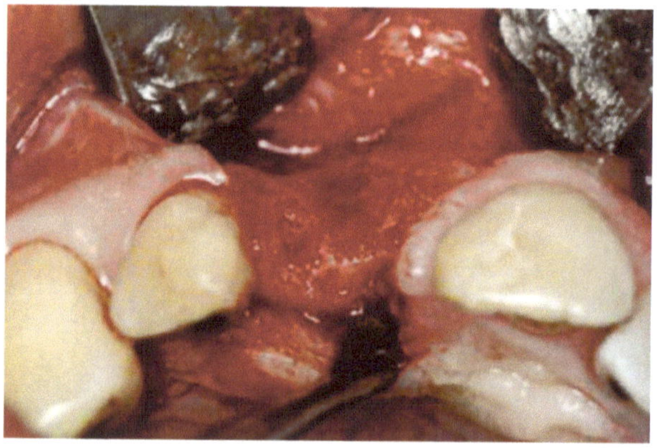

Figure 10.48. Lobe lift after complete healing of connective tissues. Appearance of healed alveolar bone with bone block and bone substitutes.

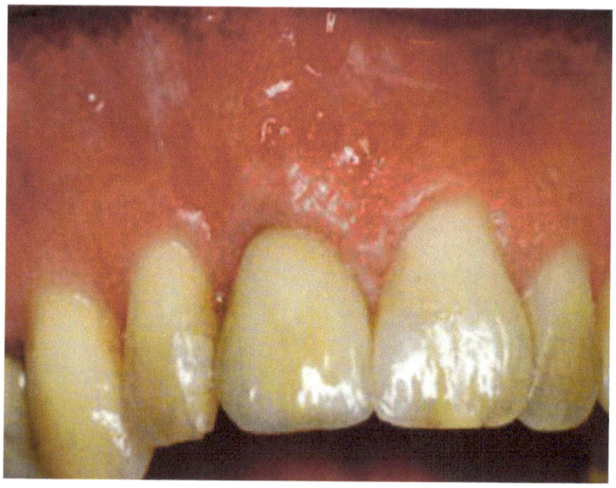

Figure 10.49. Clinical appearance 8 years after the restoration of the bone defect by augmentation and implant placement. Lateral incisor (12) and central incisor (21) repaired with composite seals. Definitive prosthetic crown on the implant. Soft tissues healed without visible scar.

Treatment in case of vertical root fracture

When managing alveolar bone defects in the frontal part of the upper jaw, aesthetics is of particular importance. An interesting solution to provide an augmented part of the alveolar ridge is to use the periosteum from the palate as a membrane that is placed vestibularly on the augmented part of the alveolar extension. For vertical root fractures (Figure 10.50.) There is a recession of the gingivae and the formation of abundant granulation tissue along the entire length of the fracture line, which endangers the nutrition of the vestibular alveolar bone lamella due to the interruption of vascularization and is a progressive pathological process. The complexity of the etiology of this mucogingival pathological progressive process can be caused multicausally. In the etiology of gingivae recession most common and greatest pathological effect has extensive occlusal forces, i.e. traumatic occlusion. Gingival recession causes complete destruction of periodontal tissues. In vertical root fractures, too, the destruction of periodontal and bone tissues is accelerated. Vertical root rupture most often occurs after endodontic treatments: over-expansion of the root canal, "foss rut" canal, failed resection, etc. The growth of granulation tissue along the length of the fracture line leads to avascularization of the region around the roots and accelerated destruction of the tissues surrounding the roots.

A root with a vertical crack should not be attempted to heal. By delaying tooth extraction, the destruction of soft and hard tissues is increasingly progressive, which makes the treatment extremely complex and prolongs the treatment time. Figures 10.51-10.54 show a possible therapeutic plan that includes tooth extraction, bone defect augmentation and subsequent implantation.

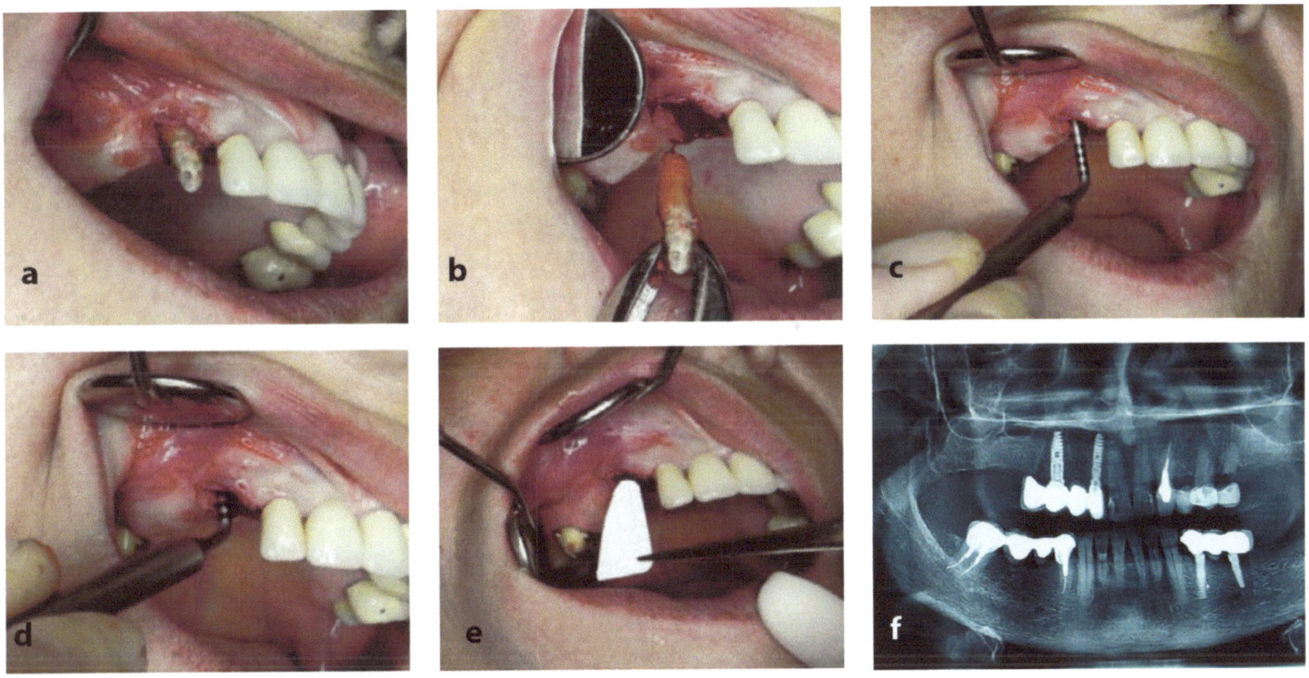

Figure 10.50. Due to the vertical fracture of the canine root, the lamellar bone (a) has been completely destroyed. After tooth extraction and radical preservation of the alveolar wound (b) and measuring the depth of the bone defect of the lamellar bone (c and d), it is necessary to perform augmentation with a bone substitute and using the collagen resorptive membrane (e). The waiting period for healing is from 6 to 12 months. After 12 months, 2 implants were implanted with a successful outcome. The patient was proposed to install 3 implants, which he did not accept.

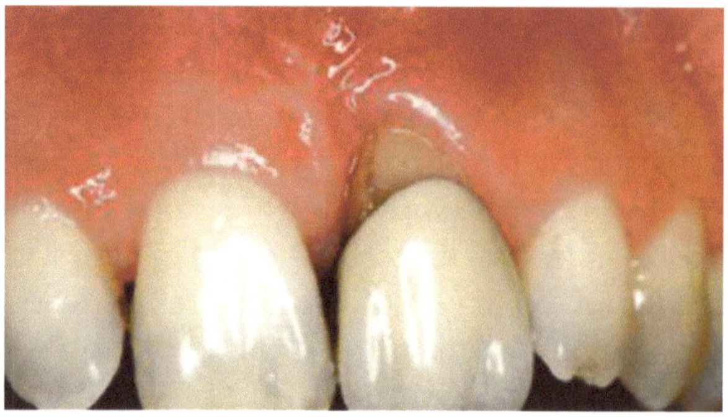

Figure 10.51. Display of vertical fracture and roots with consequences of recession and gingival inflammation.

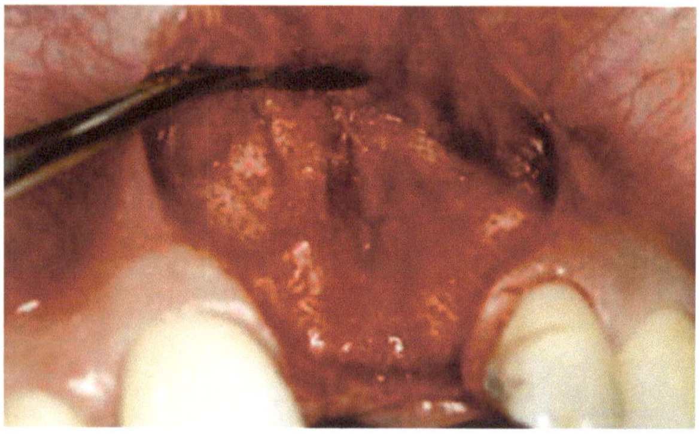

Figure 10.52. After tooth extraction and lobe lifting, a completely destroyed vestibular lamellar bone can be seen.

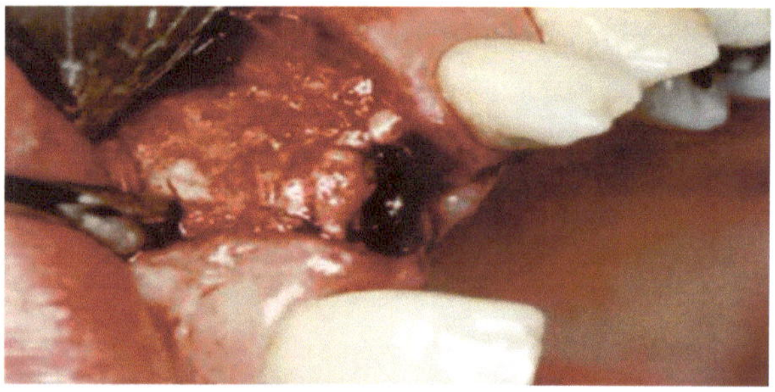

Figure 10.53. A standard diameter implant was implanted, supplementing the lamellar part with bone substitute granules, covered with a collagen resorptive membrane.

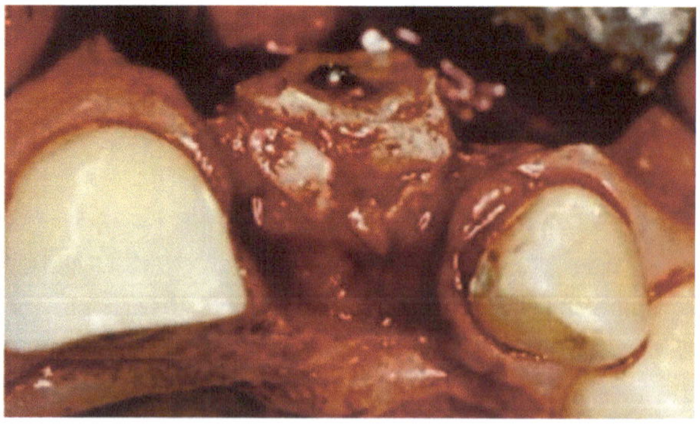

Figure 10.54. Bone defect reconstruction performed by augmentation with autologous bone taken from the retromolar region of the mandible, supplemented with collagen bone substitutes.

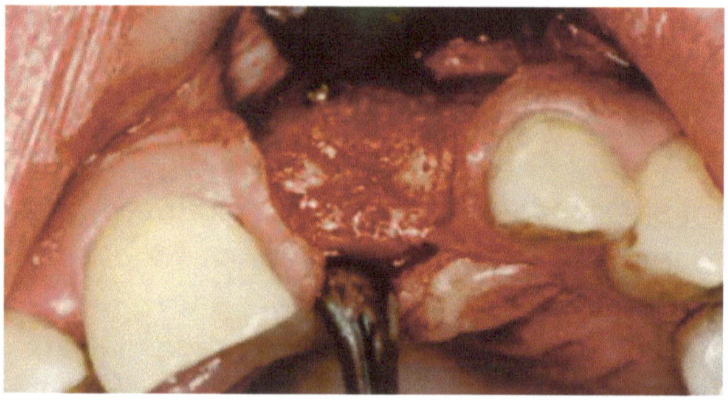

Figure 10.55. By raising the lobe, the condition is displayed after 6 months.

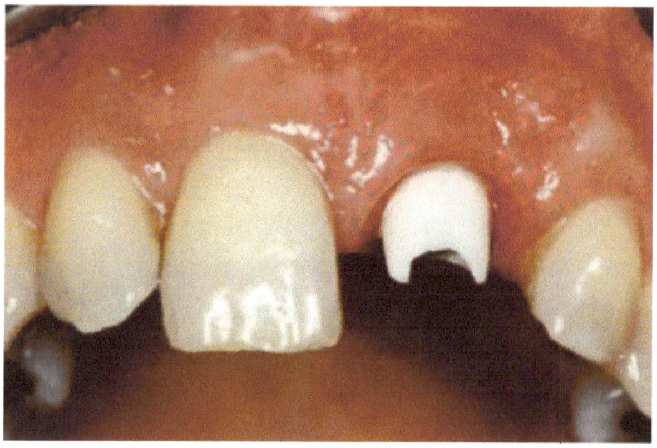

Figure 10.56. Compensation of the central incisor removed due to vertical root cracks. A titanium abutment was first placed on the implant, on which a provisional crown was placed. After 4 months, install the zirconium abutment. The final result of successful guided regeneration of soft tissues and alveolar bone, periodontal tissues were also regenerated. The clinical outcome of the presented case of reconstruction of periodontal infracostal defects proves that the method of tissue regeneration has a predictable and well-achievable function and aesthetic result with reconstructed and regenerated interdental papillae.

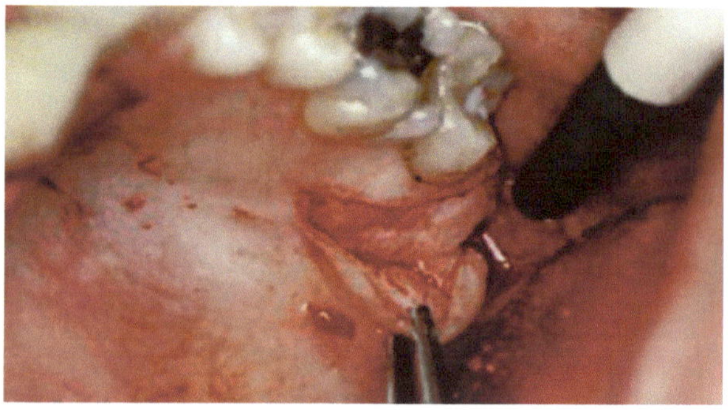

Figure 10.57. Taking a connective tissue transplant from the upper tuber forks.

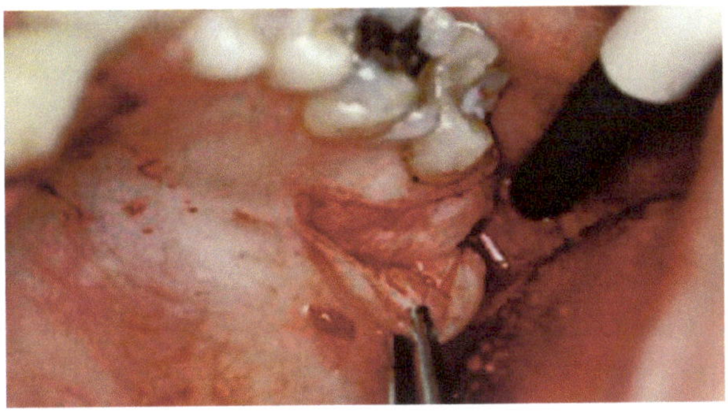

Figure 10.58. The positioned graft from the maxillary tuberosity and the formed vestibular flap should be sutured without tension.

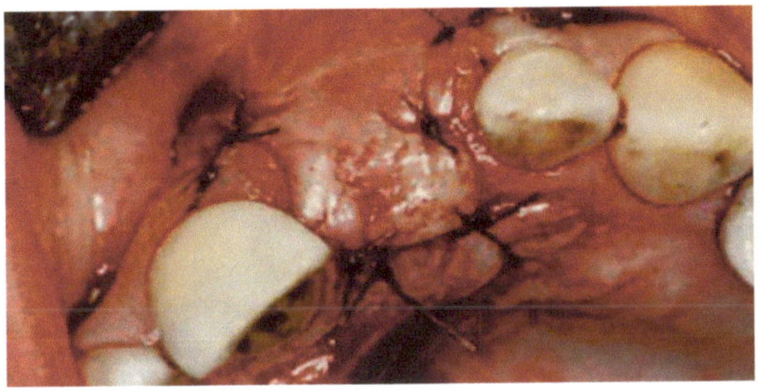

Figure 10.59. Mucoperiosteal graft positioned palatally, and by rotating the vestibular lobe, the augmented region is covered without tension.

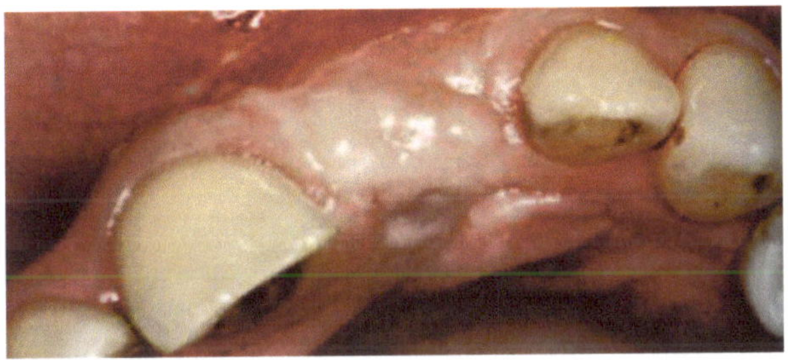

Figure 10.60. Clinical appearance of well-formed soft and hard tissues by aqueous tissue regeneration with the reconstruction of the alveolar bone. All prerequisites for a successful installation of the implant have been created—sufficient horizontal and vertical dimensions of the alveolar ridge enable predictable aesthetic and functional success of the entire procedure.

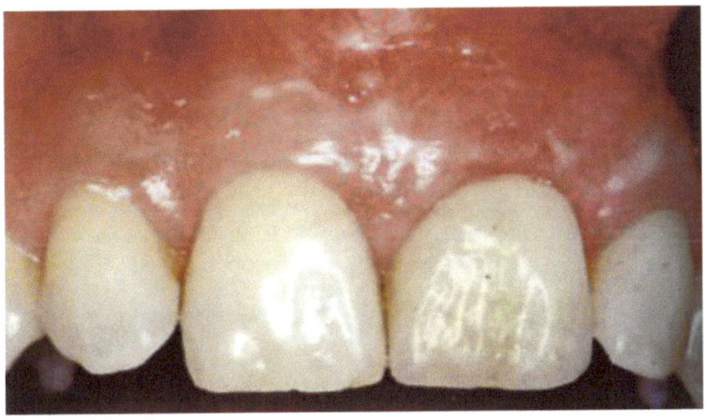

Figure 10.61. The situation after 10 years of treatment. Realized perfect harmony of the reconstructed tissues, without visible scars and a healthy appearance of the interdental papillae was obtained.

Single tooth restoration

When it comes to replacing an individual tooth, especially in the frontal region, patients are becoming increasingly demanding and put the doctor in a dilemma of how to meet their requirements to compensate for a lost tooth without waiting. The complexity of the solution is greater if the bone defect on the vestibular side also needs to be compensated. The process of lamination of soft and hard tissues requires waiting time for healing. However, if it is required that implant placement and augmentation should be performed at the same time, and the implant should be implanted with immediate load, this depends on the assessment of the physician and his experience. Modern oral implantology and newer understandings allow such requirements to be successfully resolved. In many cases, the author succeeded! The starting point for justifying this attitude is Wolf's rule told in orthopedics 100 years ago, today, due to enormous technological progress, it is becoming more and more relevant "the bone should be loaded as soon as possible and its impaired physiological function restored".

As many of Tesla's ideas have not yet been fully realized, and in the future Wolf's rule is likely to grow into Wolf's law, it is completely being realized with technological advances in the surface treatment of implants and bone substitute materials. In orthopedics, when installing an artificial knee and titanium hip, Wolf's rule is the basis of therapy. Patients must move the day after the implant placement of the replaced parts of the organ, in order to put the bone under immediate load. The author's position is that Wolf's rule has full confirmation in oral implantology.

When talking about augmentation in oral implantology, an example of a bone substitute is preferred. For example, Bio-Oss is a natural bone material that is successfully applied both in oral implant placement and in periodontal surgery. In this natural bone substitute of bovine origin, all organic matrix is chemically completely removed, so the material is immunologically inert Bio-Oss and similar bone substitutes are produced in the form of a substrate or a compact block.

By technological processing (sterilized by dry processing), their chemical structure is fully compatible with bones of human origin, and their macroscopic and microscopic structure is similar. In order to achieve the best possible therapeutic results in the reconstruction of bone defects by augmentation, the implanted bone replacement material should be placed so that it is always in contact with the surface of the bone that has good vascularization. The placed material is gradually modelled by tissue osteoblasts and osteoclasts. Bio-Oss (there is also an offer of similar materials on the market) as an implant material in the treatment of infracostal defects where it is necessary to install an implant and in the treatment of infracostal defects in paradontiuml, it is used in combination with the method of passive regeneration of periodontal tissues and the application of guided Tissue Regeneration (GTR) principles. The principle of directed tissue regeneration assumes that periodontal ligament cells possess the regenerative potential to form a new attachment. Guided Tissue Regeneration (GTR) is based on various types of mechanical barriers covering bone and periodontium, which is achieved by applying bioactive collagen resorptive membranes or periosteum tissue grafts (Figures 10.43-10.45). Passively "guided" soft tissue regeneration encourages the formation of a new attachment on the newly regenerated alveolar bone.

The quality of the newly created connection on the cervical part of the implant depends on the technological treatment and the cervical surface of the implant. Today, more and more attention is paid to this problem to achieve the best possible aesthetic result. In many implant systems, the way the cervical part and the implant are processed is different. Implant neck processing is not only important for achieving the best possible attachment of epithelial and connective tissue, but also from the biomechanical aspect of receiving intense forces on the implant.

The above confirms the position of the author of the justification of the immediate load. Treatment of soft and bone tissues at the same time is based on the accelerated development of material technology that compensates for bone defects, thus significantly expanding the indications: treatment of infracostal defects in the periodontium, reservation of the alveolar ridge after tooth extraction, contouring of the alveolar ridge by augmentation, as well as the procedure of the once insurmountable impediment for implant placement - lifting the low sinus floor. Thanks to these materials, this obstacle was removed by the application of "sinus-lifting", and at the time when the author began to practice oral implantology, this was not even considered.

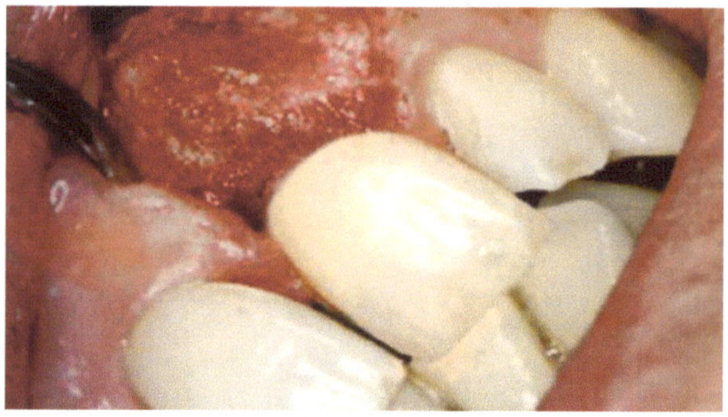

Figure 10.62. After tooth extraction, an implant was implanted into the preserved alveoli. After 3 years, there was a milder gingival recession caused by the resorption of one part of the lamellar bone. Due to the high line of a person's smile, the aesthetic defect was noticeable. It was necessary to lift the lobe to see the resorption size of the lamellar bone.

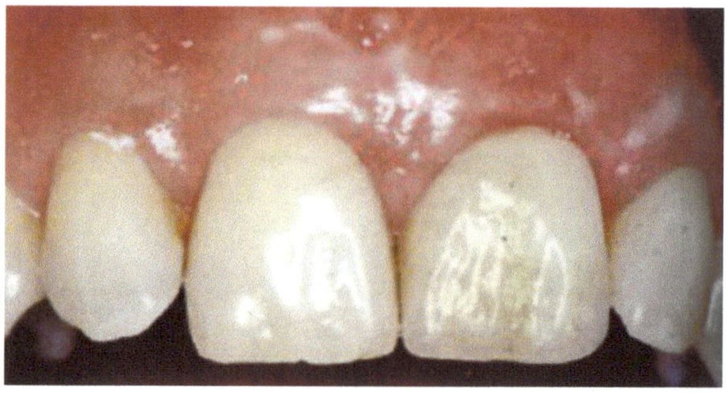

Figure 10.63. The treatment procedure was performed by lifting the mucoperiostal lobe at full thickness. The lifting procedure was performed by semilunar incision. The incision of the interdental papillae, which were left as a whole, was avoided. After augmentation with bone substitutes using a resorptive membrane, the lobe is drawn over the cervical part of the crown. Avoiding capturing by incision of the interdental papilla, sewing allowed better formation of the gingival edge and preservation of the papillae in their entirety.

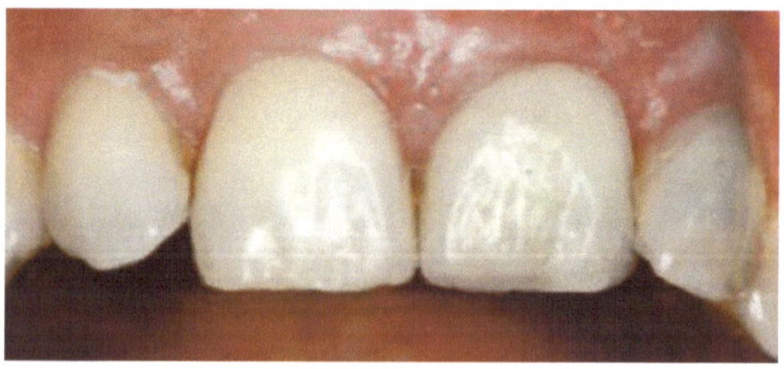

Figure 10.64. Definitive appearance after 12 months. Regenerated interdental papilla.

With large resorption of the vestibular lamellar bone, especially in the apical part it happens that during the preparation of the bone for the implant beds, perforation of the lamellar bone wall occurs, and a smaller part of the bone lamella remains attached, indicated by the yellow arrow (Figures 10.65-10.66). In order to create favorable conditions for implant placement, it is necessary to perform augmentation of the alveolar bone.

The non-resorbed part of the lamellar bone is significant in the augmentation process. Which type of augmentation will be applied depends on the size and bone defect. Good results in certain cases can be achieved by using bone substitutes mixed with autologous bone filings, and in larger defects or a very narrow ridge, augmentation must be performed with bone blocks taken from the chin or from the retromolar region.

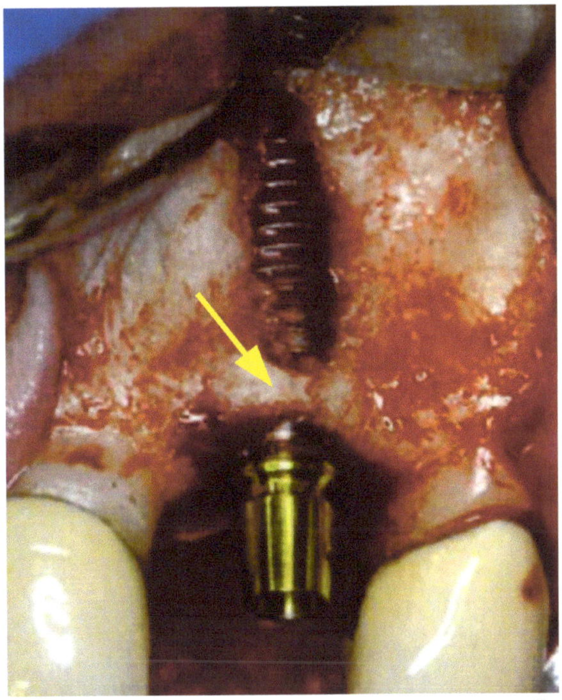

Figure 10.66. Lamellar bone fenestration, standard diameter implant. Primary stability achieved palatinally. With a sharp titanium boron, with abundant cooling, the implant threads on the vestibular side are removed, thus increasing the space for graft covering. The spared part of the bone (yellow arrow) is extremely important for the success of the augmentation procedure.

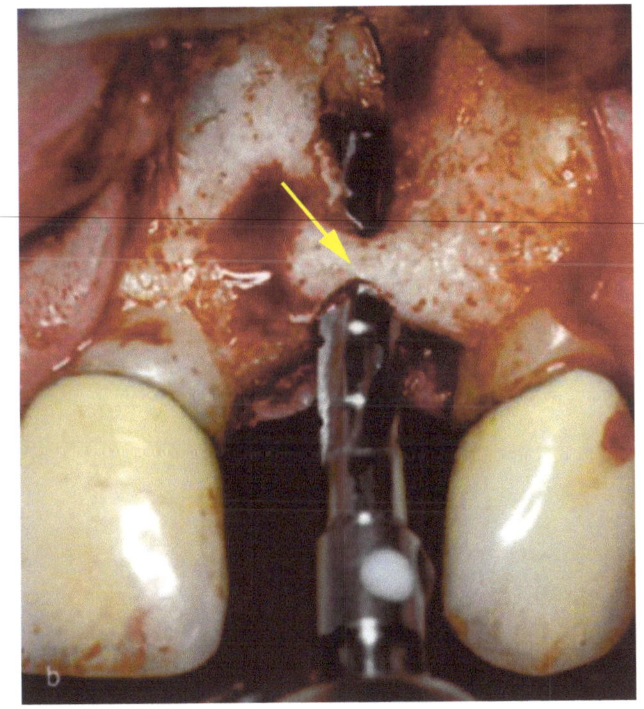

Figure 10.65. Fenestration in the central incisor region (#21). Anamnestic data indicate that tooth loss after root resection.

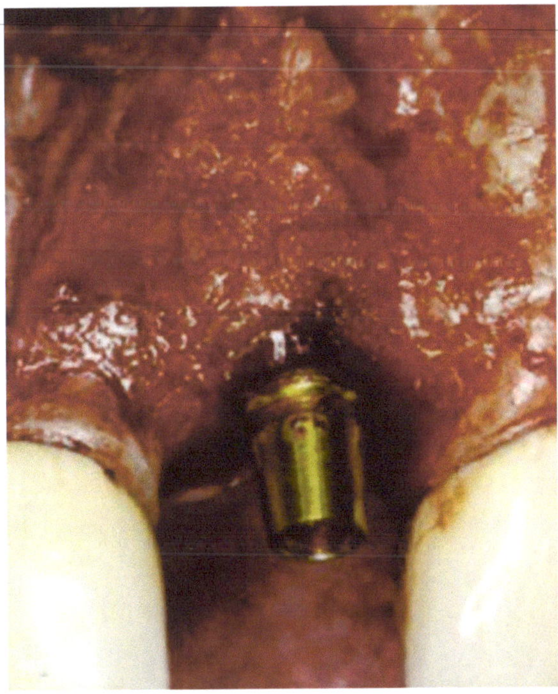

Figure 10.67. Covering bone defect and implants with bone substitutes mixed with autologous bone filings, covered with a block of graft taken from the chin and tuber maxilla. (Figure 10.68.)

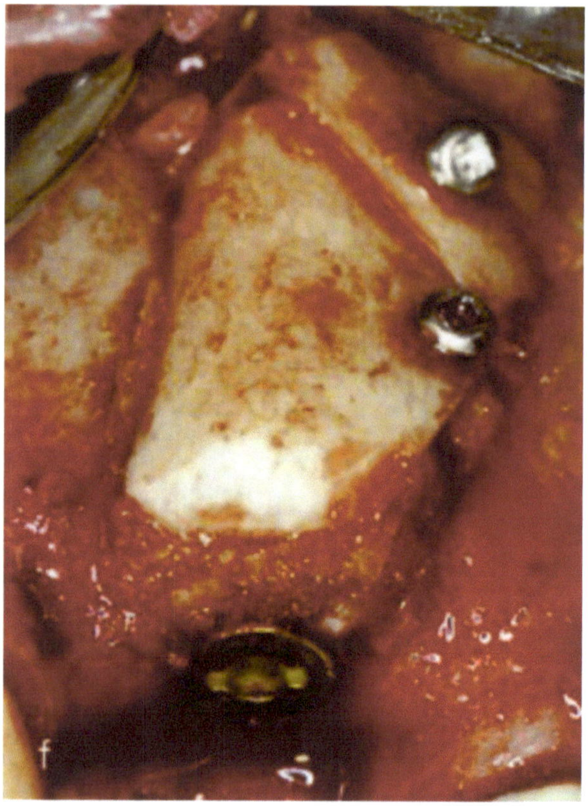

Figure 10.68. Part of the implant is covered with a mixture of Bio-Oss and autologous bone. Due to the size of the defect, the bone block transplant was taken from 2 parts, from the chin and tuber of the upper jaw, and fixed with titanium screws. By covering the augmented region with a flap, the implant is immediately loaded with a tentative acrylic crown.

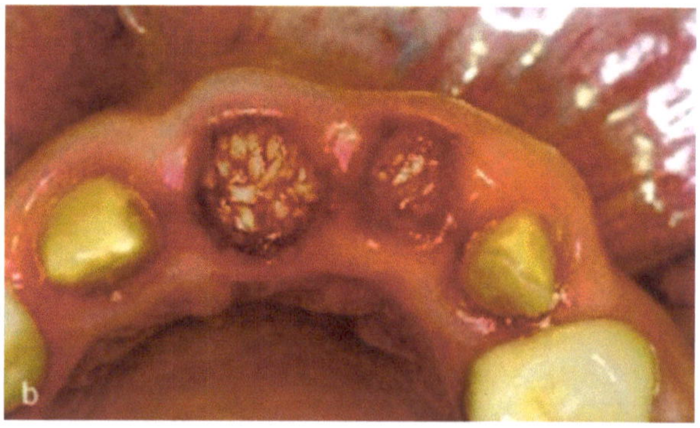

Figure 10.69. After the atraumatic extraction of the once resected roots of teeth #21 and #22, augmentation with bone substitutes is necessary. Appearance of alveoli filled with bone substitutes.

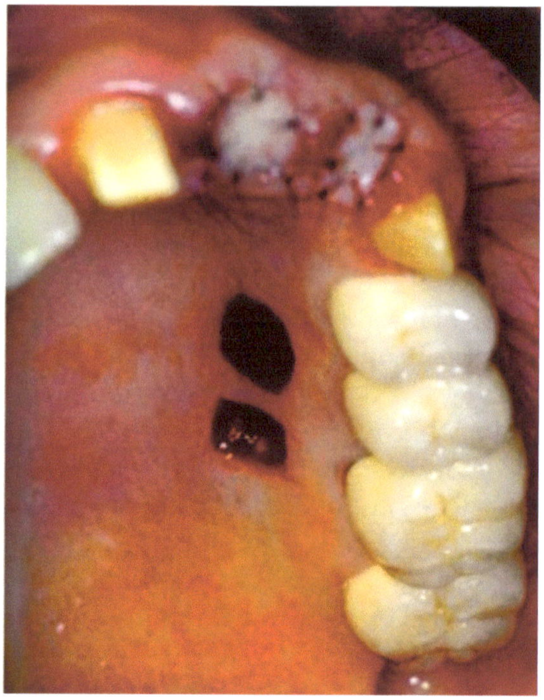

Figure 10.70. Wounds after taking transplants from the palate.

Regions of once resected roots, after tooth loss, are a poor substrate for implant placement, because the bone in the resected region never fully regenerates. If the resection removes most of the root, there is also resorption of the lamellar bone in the part of the resected root. Also, it completely destroys periodontal tissues in the resection area, which is manifested by impaired vascularization, so that the resorption of the vestibular lamellar bone progresses. With this in mind, after atraumatic extraction of the central and lateral incisors (Figures 10.69.), the anterior lamellar bone wall is completely resorbed. In order to compensate for the absorbed vestibular lamellar bone and retain the existing shape of the alveolar ridge, the alveoli of the removed tooth need to be filled with collagen bone substitutes.

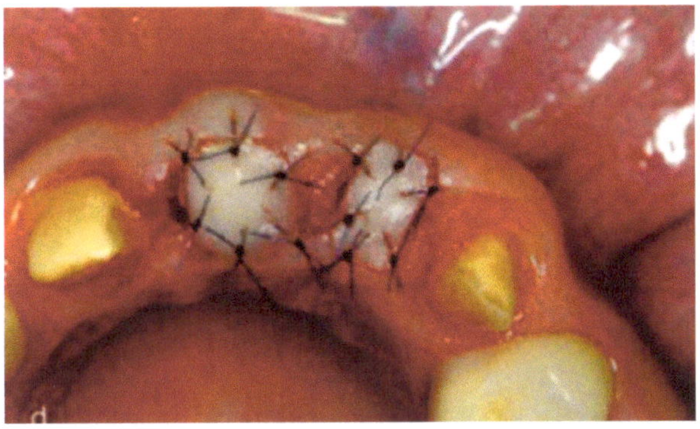

Figure 10.71. Sewn transplants.

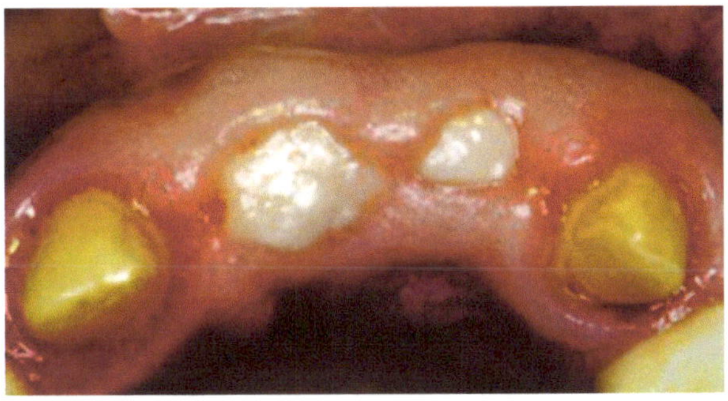

Figure 10.72. Postoperative status after 3 months.

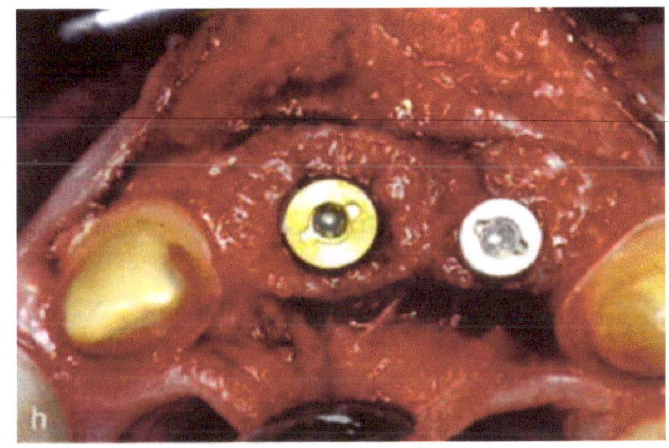

Figure 10.73. Occlusal appearance of regenerated alveolar bone with preserved contours around the implant.

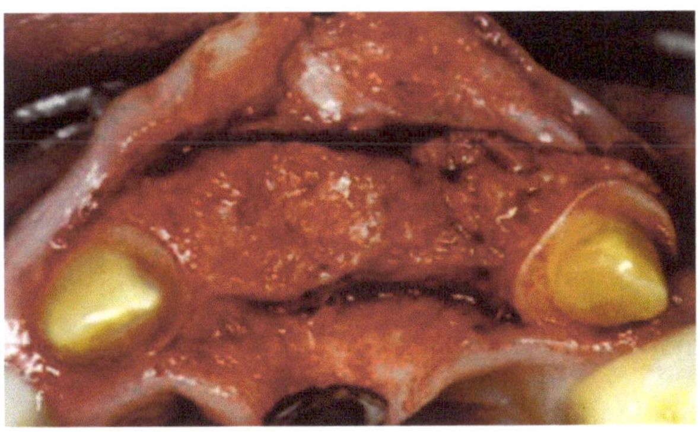

Figure 10.74. Regenerated alveolar bone 6 months after augmentation.

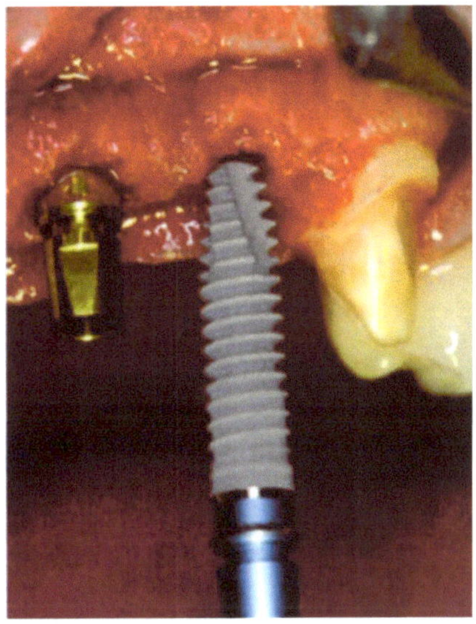

Figure 10.75. Installation of the implant in the regenerated bone of the alveolus after augmentation.

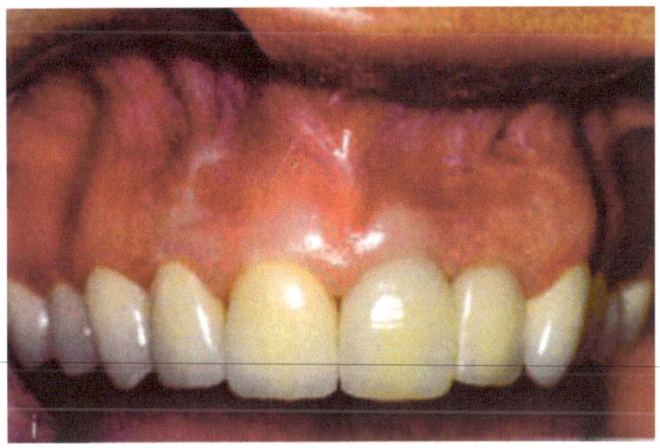

Figure 10.76. Definitive prosthetic work.

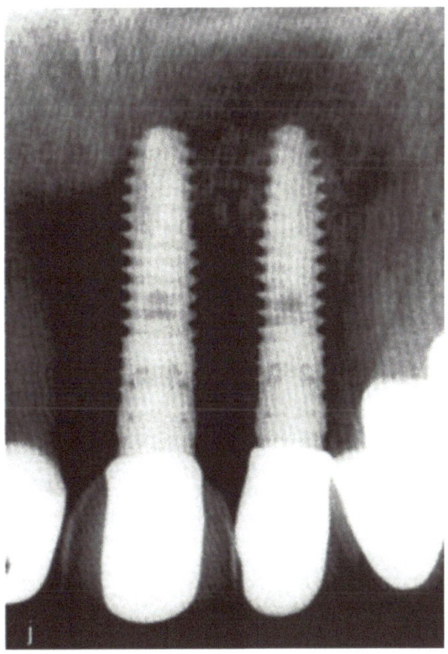

Figure 10.77. Control X-ray after 3 years.

Sinus-Lifting

3 decades ago, many bone areas were an insurmountable obstacle to implant placement. One of the insurmountable obstacles to implant placement was the low sinus floor. The first attempt to overcome the anatomical obstacle posed by the sinus cavity was made by Leonard Linkov, one of the creators of leaf implants. He designed the so-called "fifth generation" of leaf implants in 64 forms, and only 12 for bypassing the sinuses. Surgical entry into the maxillary sinus and lifting of Schneider's membrane was neither considered nor attempted. Linkov addressed the sinus obstruction by approximating the design of the implant according to the sinus boundaries (Figure 10.78.)

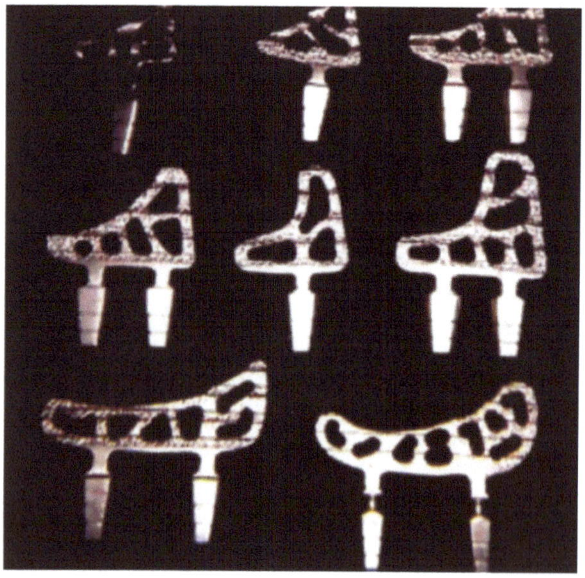

Figure 10.78. Linkov's leaf implants adapted to the boundaries of the sinus cavity.

It must be emphasized that at that time, the placement of leaf implants was adapted to the sinus cavity, i.e. the floor of the sinus. The implant placement was arbitrary, routine and depended solely on the physician's experience. The implant was designed so that its stronghold starts from the tuber of the maxilla, where most often the amount of available bone was the largest (Figures 10.79-10.81). From the tuber maxilla, the implant extended along the length of the sinus floor provided that the thickness of the residual alveolar bone allowed it (minimum 6 millimeters).

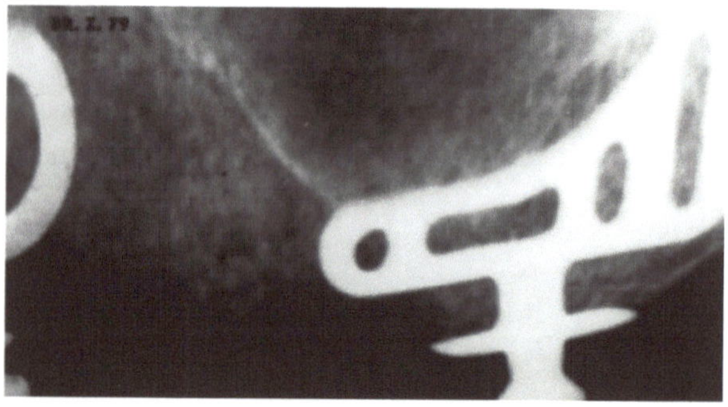

Figure 10.79. Linkov's tuber implant with subperiostal backrest (work of the author 1977.)

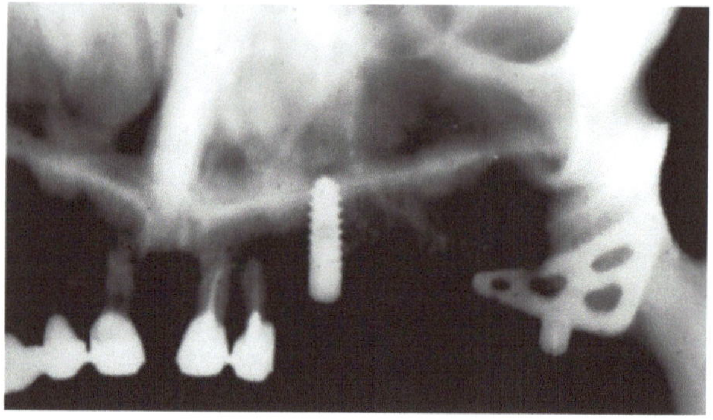

Figure 10.80. A combination of Pit-Easy and a leaf implant adapted to the anatomical structure of the maxillary sinus. (work of the author 1979.)

At that time, the greatest precaution was devoted to the preservation of the Schneider membrane, which was at the same time the biggest obstacle and a great risk of implant placement.

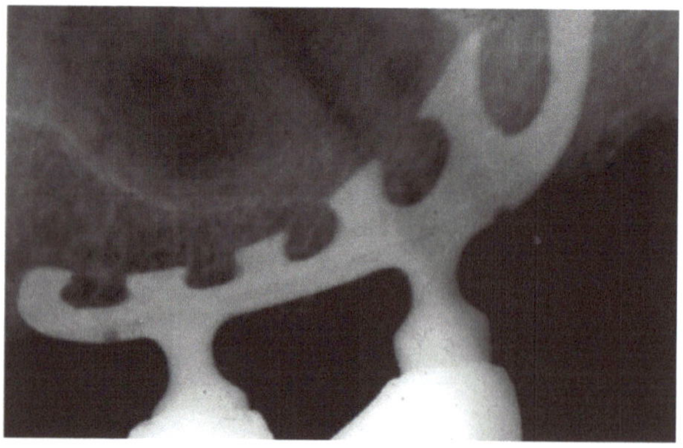

Figure 10.81. A leaf implant was implanted along the length of the sinus drop. (work of the author 1979.)

The next step of implant placement in the sinus cavity was done by fenestration of the bone wall from the vestibular side. Opening of the so-called surgical window, which involves raising the bone block, is a very aggressive method accompanied by postoperative pain and larger swelling. Due to the inaccessibility and poor visibility of the operative field, the patient is forced to keep his mouth as open as possible with great strain. The masseter muscle is a strong closure, and keeping the mouth open at maximum for a long time required straining of the entire masticatory musculature and temporomandibular joint, which manifested as greater fatigue of the patient, and the operation was accompanied by pain and dizziness. The amount of graft was not dimensioned, so ossification of the entire sinus cavity often occurred.

In any case, due to the above reasons, this method probably goes into the oral surgical implantological past.

The disadvantages of conventionally applied sinus-lifting methods are:

1. difficulty accessing the sinus,
2. non-transparent operational field,
3. frequent perforations of the sinus floor membrane when lifting,
4. difficulties in the preparation and separation of parts of the autogenous bone,
5. frequent inability to achieve good primary implant fixation, especially in poor bone quality.

In order to avoid all the negative sides and previous surgical techniques, especially opening the window from the vestibular side and closing it with a larger bone block, a method of vertical approach has been developed – the so-called osteotomy sinus lifting technique.

But the osteotomy technique also has major drawbacks. The application of the osteotomy technique was performed blindly, and the result was based solely on the routine and experience of the dentist. Incidents of Schneider's membrane perforation are very common because there is no insight into its lifting during the procedure by inserting the osteotome, especially if the force of insertion is undosed. In fact, the osteotomy technique, despite having a vertical approach, is among the inaccurate and aggressive methods, because the force of the osteotome inserting is routinely arbitrary. Also, the inserting of osteotomas caused, in addition to pain, dizziness due to shaking of the labyrinthine fluid of the inner ears.

By applying any of the aforementioned methods, the success of the sinus lift procedure is related to the thickness of the cortical bone of the sinus floor. In the case where the sinus lift is performed by a vertical procedure, which is the case with the osteotomy method, we find two cortical bones (bicortical path).

The alveolar part of the cortical bone has less compactness than the cortical part of the sinus floor bone. The success of sinus lifting treatment is based on the technique of the procedure to enter the cortical part of the sinus floor bone, which has a relatively higher compactness without injuring the Schneider membrane.

In the early 1980s, the first works dedicated to raising the Schneider membrane appeared (Drettner B. 1980.) and determined its depth, which on average ranges from 0.13 to 0.5 mm.

Group of authors (Moss-Salentia L. & assoc. 1985.) notes that the mucous membrane of the maxillary sinus can be easily separated from the bone, as there are almost no elastic fibers.

Group of authors (Rosenberg and Closslet 1982.) concluded that after tooth extraction and graft introduction, after 24 to 35 days, there is a complete attachment of epithelial tissue to the grafted material.

The authors Del Fabbro and Testory (2004) concluded in their research with vestibular fenestration methods, that by simultaneously lifting the sinus membrane and implanting implants, the results are the same as with delayed sinus lifting and waiting periods for implant placement. Conclusions were made after 6 months from the procedure. These authors suggest the advantage of simultaneous sinus lifting and implant insertion. In their research, they conclude that the survival rate of implants is 90% to 97% successful.

Group of authors (Friber, Sennerby, Grondahl & assoc. 2002.) has repored the results of the osteotomy technique after 3 years and the percentage of Schneider membrane perforations.

Authors Buchner A. Kleeinbeinz J. & assoc. 2005.) described the biological and biomechanical condition after the lifting of the sinus membrane and implant placement using the osteoma application technique.

Palma VC, Lundgern & assoc. 2006.), by experimenting on monkeys, had shown the results of bone regeneration and implant integration when lifting the sinus membrane. This group of authors noted that bone contact with the Schneider membrane resulted in the formation of new tissue, especially in the space where the hematoma was formed. Their conclusion is that the maxillary mucosa has osteoinductive potential.

The same group of authors (2008) reported on the results of simultaneous lifting of the sinus floor membrane and implant placement with a new surgical technique - sinus floor augmentation.

The results of their research comparing cases in several patients 6 months after the implantation of autogenous grafts came to the conclusion that Schneider's membrane in contact with autogenous graft has osteoinductive potential.

Wood RM. and Moore DL. 1988.) published the results of the lifting of the sinus membrane by grafts of autogenous bone and the result is that the entire maxillary sinus is coated with mucous membranes about 1 mm thick. These authors conclude that sinus membrane perforation causes complications.

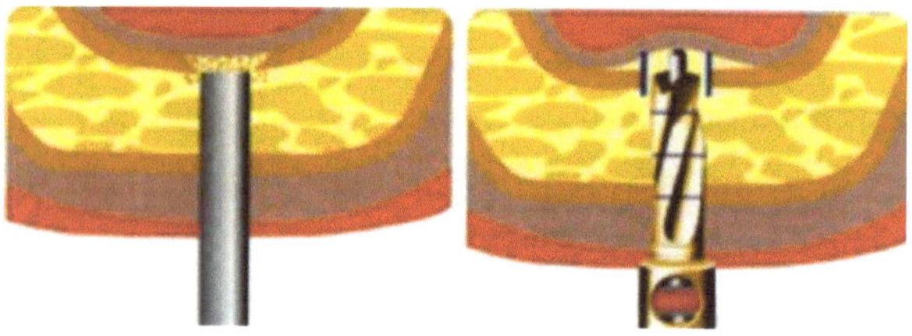

Figure 10.82. Osteotomy SLD technique

Advantages Of Sinus-Lift Drill (Sld) Technique

In cases where the thickness of the residual alveolar bone is less than 3 millimeters, the spongiogenic part of the bone practically does not exist because there has been a fusion of the alveolar cortical bone and the cortical part of the bone of the sinus floor.

Using the sinus-lift drill (SLD) technique, even in cases where the height of the alveolar bone is less than 3 mm, the sinus membrane can be safely lifted and the graft and implant installed at the same time (Figure 10.78.). The lifting of the sinus floor with the SLD technique exceeds all previous ones. Due to the ease of application, speed and simplicity, with the high safety of preserving the Schneider membrane, there is a major shift in the development of oral implantology.

The essence of this method is based on a hydraulic effect based on the laws of physics on the incompressibility of liquid media since the fluid is pressurized indoors. The pressure exerted by injecting the liquid indoors is consistent in all directions.

By injecting saline through the prepared borehole of the sinus floor bone, uniform compression is performed equally in all directions and the Schneider membrane is raised upwards (Figure 10.83). The lifting of the membrane, i.e. the gradual separation from the cortical bone of the sinus floor, must be soft and gradual, using special drills and devices (Figures 10.82. and 10.83).

The new concept of sinus lifting with a hydraulic effect, based on the fluid pressure that separates the membrane from the cortical bone of the sinus floor, compared to conventional methods, is incomparably easier for the patient. Conventional techniques required the use of more instruments than the SLD method where everything was simplified. The uniform pressure of the liquid in the confined space is provided by a specially designed syringe and tube that prevents the return of the material to be injected (Figure 10.83 and 10.88.) After separating the membranes with saline, the graft is placed in the newly opened space, and the injected graft can all be suppressed by the osteotome.

After graft material insertion, the implant diameter selection should be accurately evaluated to achieve good primary bicortical fixation in the bicortical alveolar bone. This is very important for the initial fixation of the implant.

The recommendation for the application of the SLD method consists in the simplicity, speed and safety of the entire procedure, which is an absolute advantage over all other techniques.

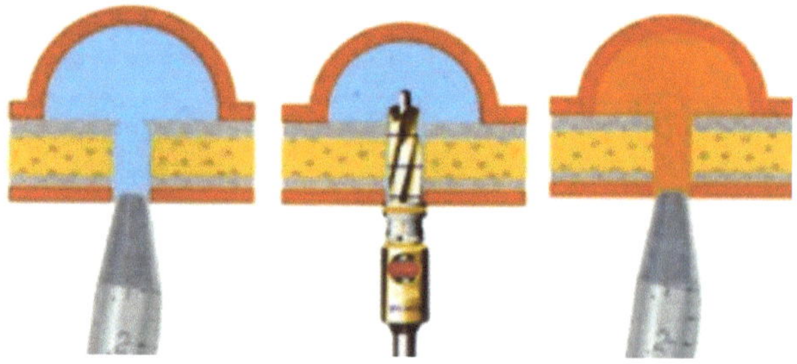

Figure 10.83. Schematic of the concept of hydraulic lifting of the sinusoidal floor membrane.

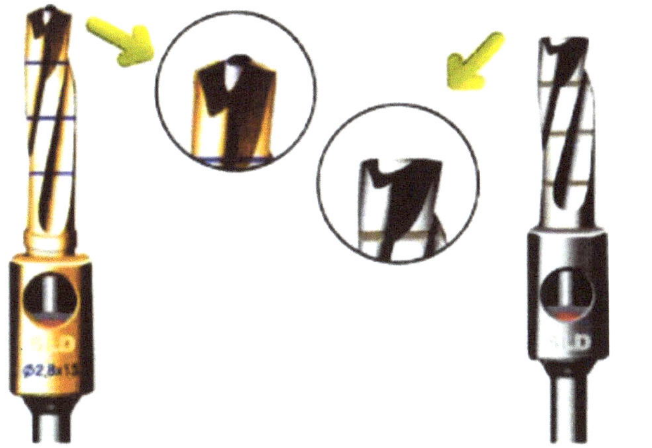

Figure 10.84. Drill, bone reamer, which enters the bone of the sinus floor. In the drill, a device is designed that reduces the blowing force of the bone in contact with the membrane.

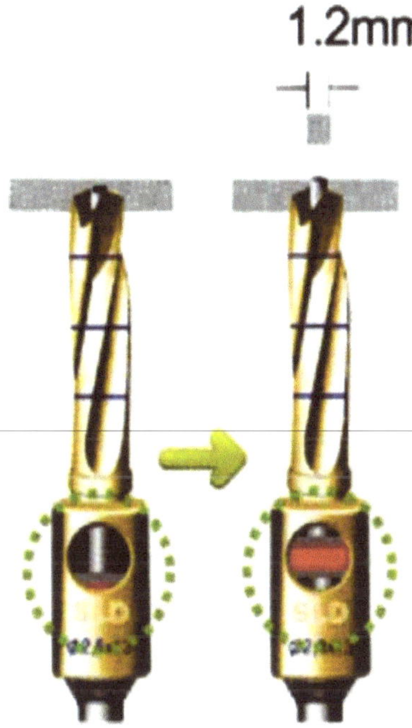

Figure 10.85. The identification device is a safety device that prevents incidental breaches of the sinus membrane,

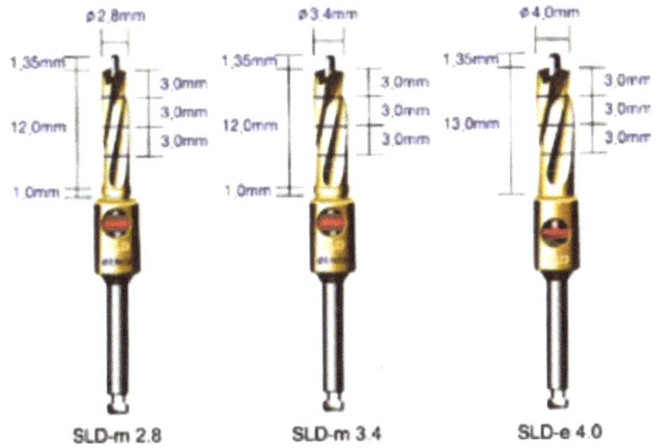

Figure 10.86. Dimensioned drills SLD methods.

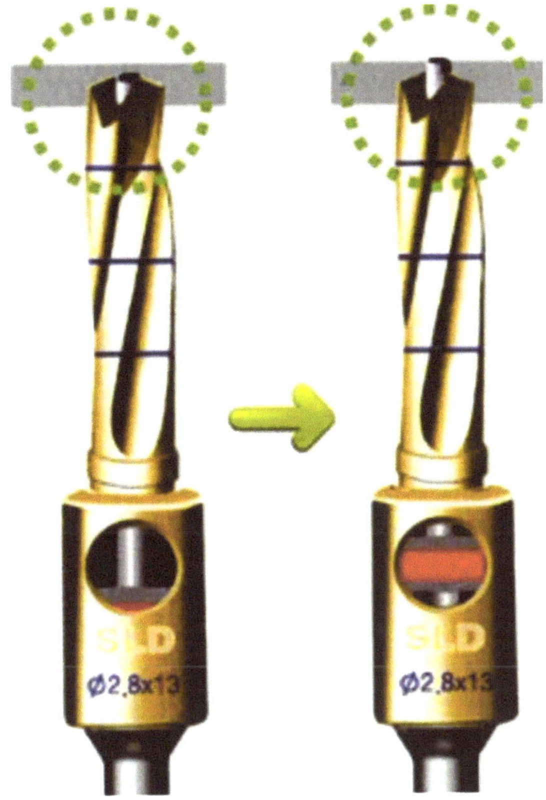

Figure 10.87. A special device inside the drill activates the safety wand to ensure the inviolability of the membrane.

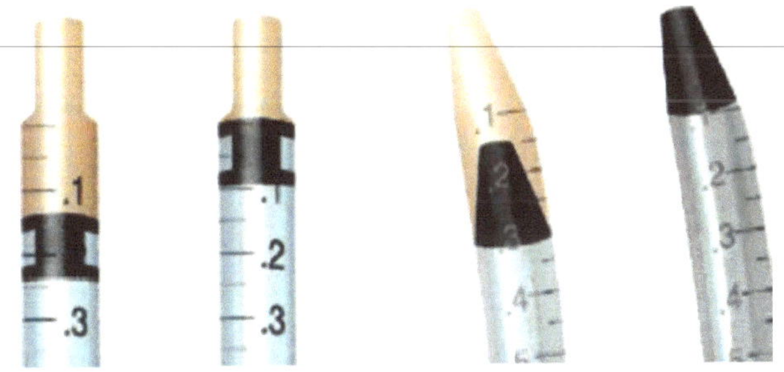

Figure 10.88. Standard syringes and syringes designed for SLD, the SLD syringe has the same diameter of 2.8 mm as the SLD drill, and differs from the classic syringe in that the grafted material is easily marketed without lagging. The maximum capacity of the SLD syringe is 1 ccm.

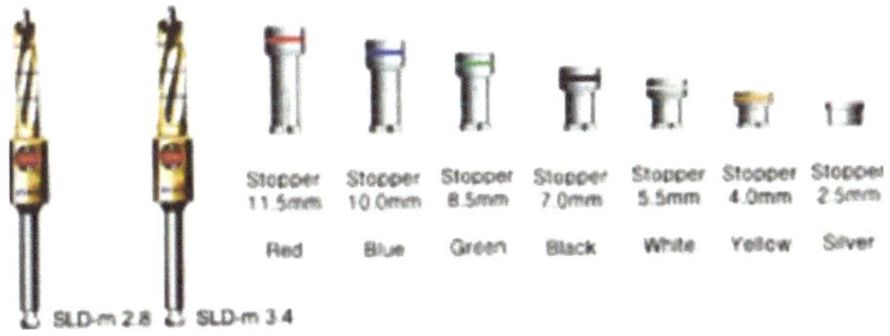

Figure 10.89. 7 types of stoppers of different diameters and lengths.

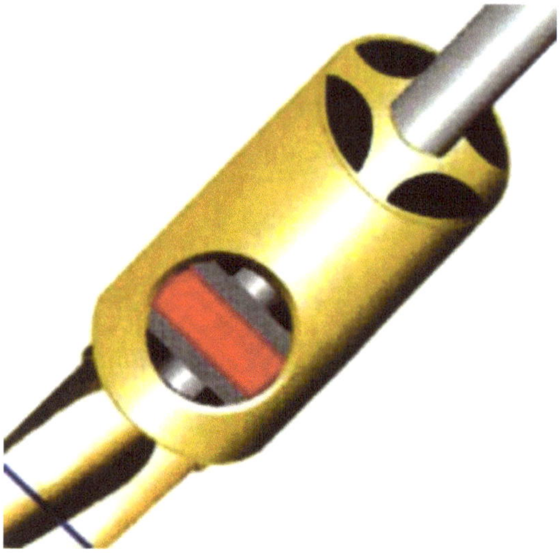

Figure 10.90. At the bottom of the SLD drill there are four openings for cleaning, and in the upper part three that enable easy cleaning and sterilization disinfection.

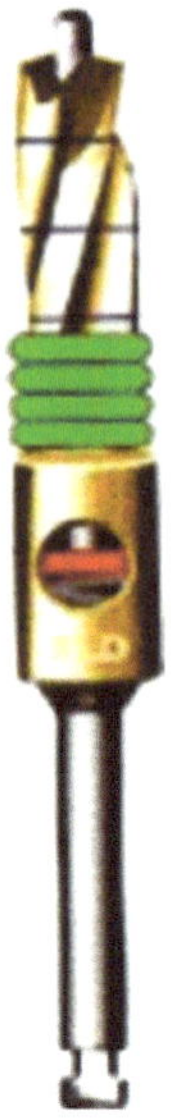

Figure 10.93 Elastic stopper.

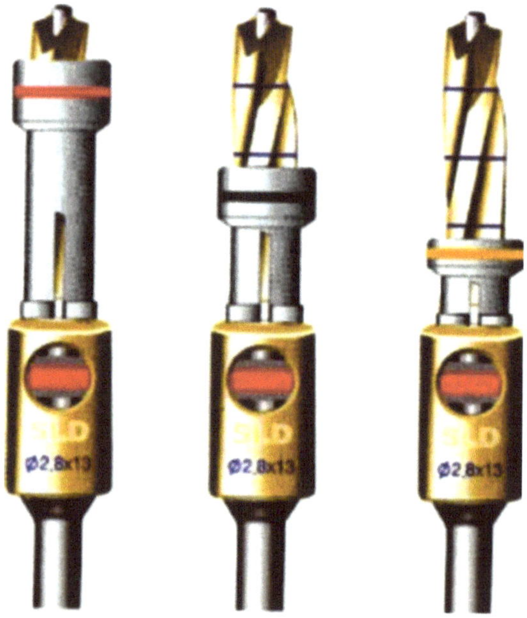

Figure 10.91. Stoppers are placed on the drills, in order to prevented unwanted perforation of the sinus floor membrane.

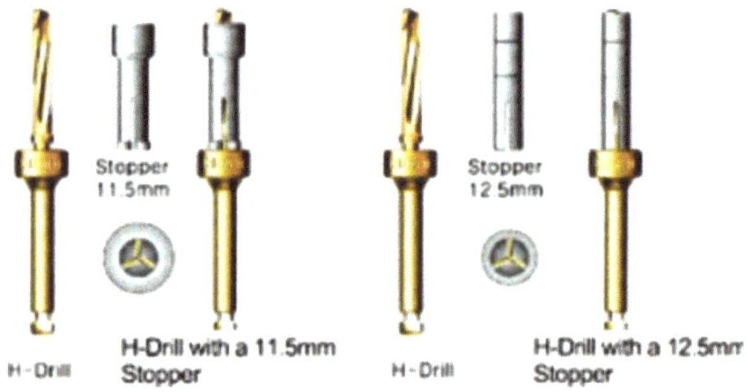

Figure 10.94 H-drill for entry and H-drill for dissection of cortical alveolar bone of the sinus floor less than 3 mm thick. 11.5 mm stop.

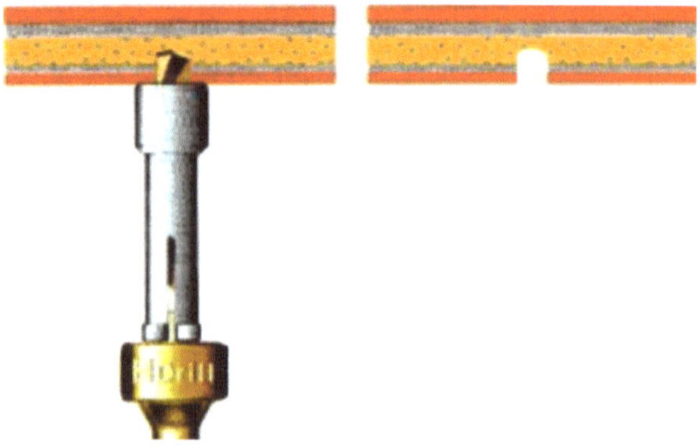

Figure 10.92. H-drill with stop.

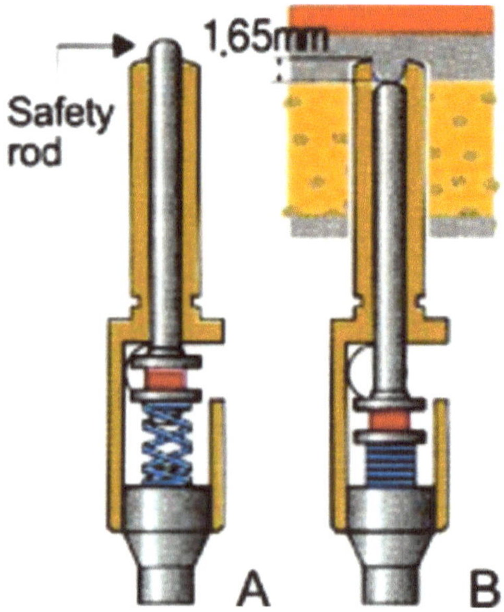

Figure 10.95. Cross-section of the internal structure of the SLD drill (A). Enlarged section of the SLD drill (B) with a diameter of 1.65 mm during drilling of the floor of the maxillary sinus with a rod protrusion.

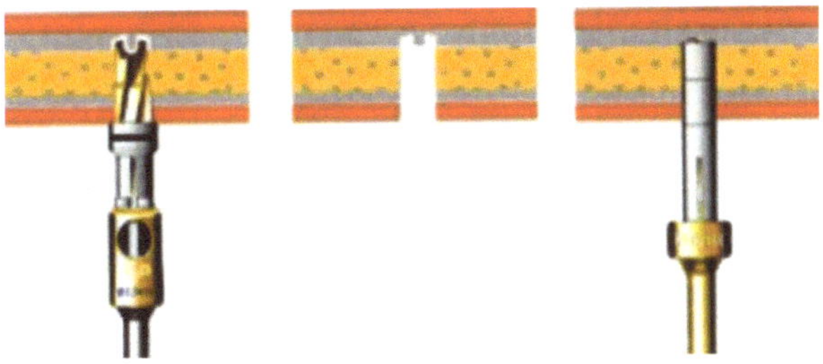

Figure 10.96. Cortical bone reamer. Movable part of H-drill (H-drill)

Sinus Drill Lifting Clinical Application Protocol

The application of the SLD technique for sinus-lifting is very simple and does not require lifting of the solution, and the lifting of the sinus membrane is enabled by the use of SLD drills and the application of a hydraulic effect. Placing the building material without the use of autogenous bone facilitates the procedure.

Various methods have been used in raising the sinus floor, and it must be recognized with great risk and unpredictable outcome. The SLD technique exceeds the entry into the bone of the sinus drop, lower speeds should be used to prevent the drill from slipping. With raising the sinus floor, various methods have been applied, and it must be recognized with great risk and unpredictable outcome. The SLD technique surpasses the previous methods already by significantly reducing tissue trauma.

Preliminary phase (10.97) It starts with the use of H-drill (Figures 10.92. and 10.96), when the speed is greater than 50 revolutions.

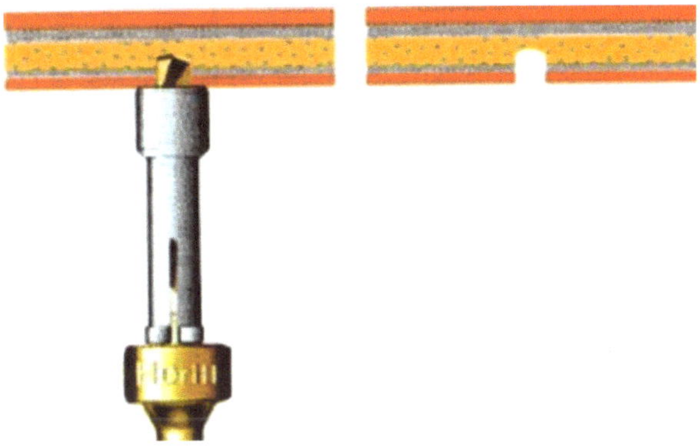

Figure 10.97. Preliminary phase. Marking the position of bone drilling using the SLD technique, using an H-drill bit (Figure 10.95) with stopper (stop-gap).

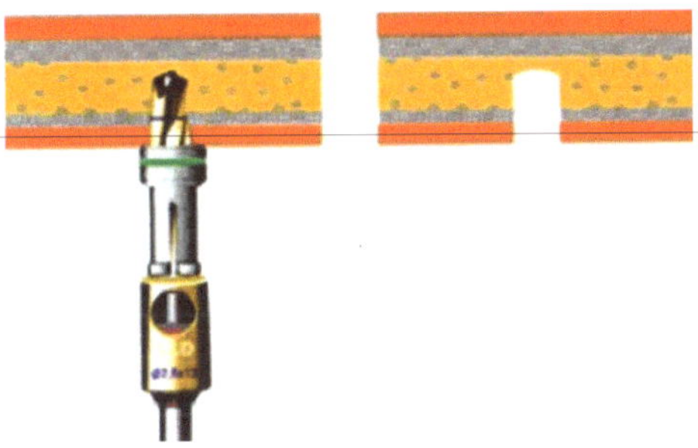

Figure 10.98. Display of phase 1.

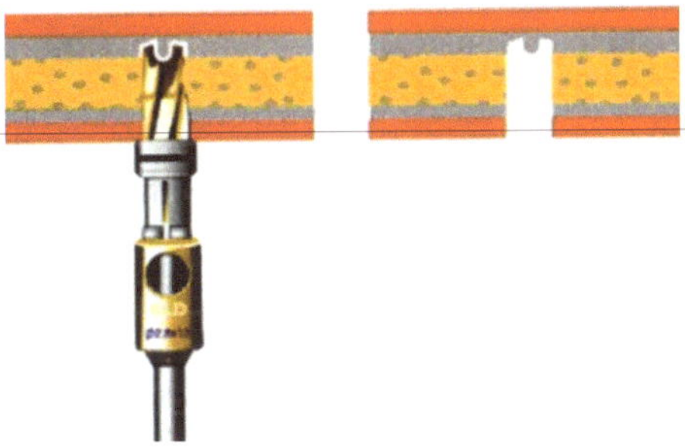

Cortical bone reamer appearance of the punctured bone to the sinus floor membrane.

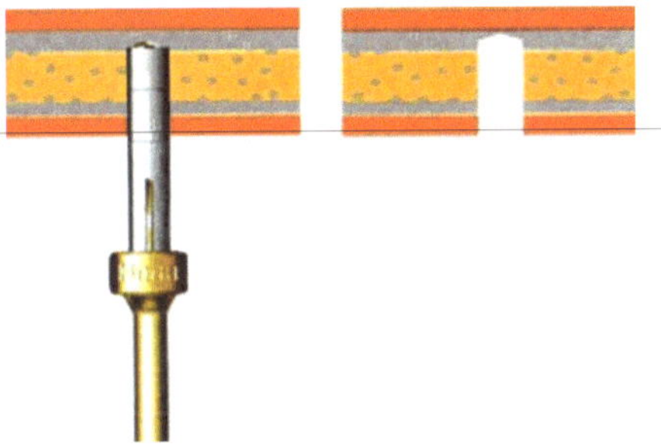

Display of H-drill and perforated bone to the sinus floor membrane.

If a 2.8 mm drill was used in the initial stage of the SLD procedure, the drill would slip. Therefore, in the initial, preliminary phase, a stopper (limiter-stopper) of 11.5 mm is used (Figures 10.89, 10.931, 10.92, 10.95, 10.98). This is especially true in cases where the height of the alveolar bone is less than 3 mm. In such cases, an 11.5 mm stopper should be installed on the H-drill to prevent it from slipping. With the stopper in place, it is easily drilled into the bone and enters the sinus.

Phase 1

Initial SLD speed is greater than 50 rpm/1000RPM). At this stage, a 2.8 mm stopper is placed on the SLD drill to reach the sinus floor safely (Figures 10.89-10.92). In this phase of entering the bone of the sinus floor, lower speeds should be used to prevent the drill from slipping.

Phase 2

At this stage, drilling of the sinus floor bone continues with slow revolutions and careful monitoring of the identification device (Figure 10.85.) Drilling should continue with stopper changes of 1.5 mm, then from 2.5 mm to 11.5 mm. Stoppers ensure entry into the sinus cavity without perforating the membrane.

Phase 3

At this stage, in order to avoid protrusion, an H-drill with a stop of 12.5 mm is used. It is necessary to apply the procedure with the mode of two-speed revolutions, faster and slower mode. By using a 12.5 mm stopper inserted on the H-drill, protrusion into the maxillary sinus is prevented. In cases where the height of the cortical bone of the sinus floor is less than 1.65 mm or in cases where the cortical bone is somewhat softer, the drilling procedure is continued with a low-revving H-drill.

Phase 4

At this stage, the H-drill with the attached stop enters the maxillary sinus activating the 1.2 mm safety rod. Entering the sinus, it separates and elevates the membrane from the cortical bone of the sinus floor (Figure 10.99).

The drill continues to rotate, but remains in the bone, and only the safety rod penetrates the sinus. The device is designed to raise the membrane without perforation. The safety rod lightly touches the membrane, and the drill bit remains in the bone. In cases where the sinus floor membrane is strongly attached to the cortical bone, it must be manipulated more carefully, and the movement of the red line on the identification device should be monitored. During the drilling of the bone and the penetration of the drill into the sinus, the red line on the device should not be visible (Figure 10.100). If the red line on the identification device is raised, the drilling process should be stopped and saline solution should be injected into the well with a specially designed syringe.

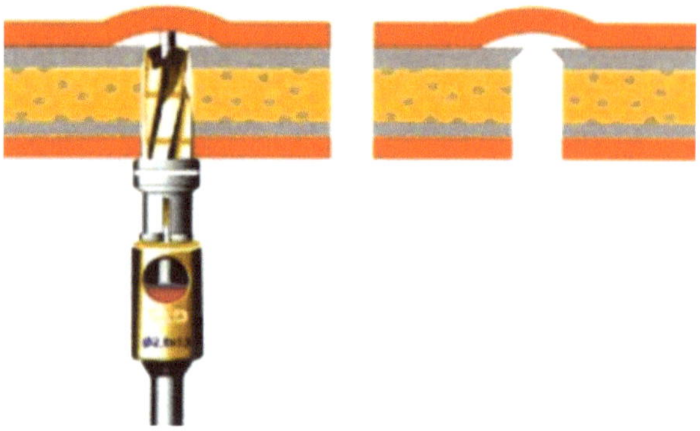

Figure 10.99. Elevation of the sinus membrane from the cortical bone

Phase 5

A syringe adapted to SLD technology is placed in the drilled opening of the sinus floor. By injecting 1 to 2 cc of saline, the pressure on the sinus membrane increases slightly (Figure 10.94). The pressure of the fluid causes the sinus membrane to separate from the cortical bone of the sinus floor and swell slightly. The course of the bone drilling must be closely monitored on an identification device (Figure 10.95), and the lifting and separation of the membrane from the sinus floor is achieved by the pressure of the saline. At this stage, the sinus membrane must not be perforated, which is easily determined by injecting the saline, because the syringe plunger suddenly slides more easily.

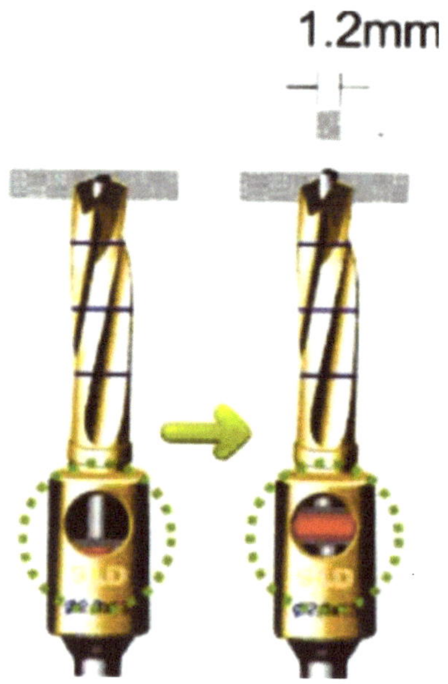

Figure 10.100. Identification drill.

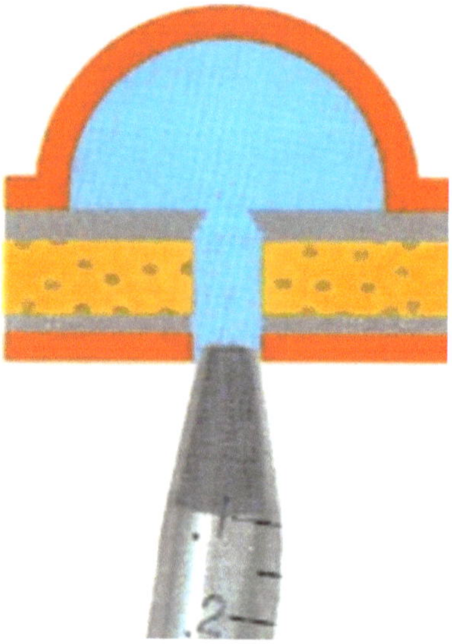

Figure 10.101. Elevation of the sinus floor membrane by injection of saline.

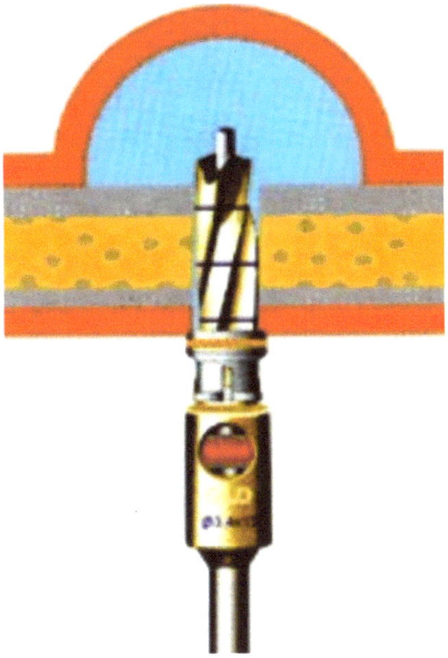

Figure 10.102. Sinus membranes by saline injection

Phase 6

This phase consists in processing the sinus floor opening with a smaller claim of 50 rpm (Figure 10.96.). Since the sinusoidal floor membrane is optimally elevated (by the hydraulic effect of saline), additional drilling and refinement of the sinusoidal floor opening can be safely continued. Additional drilling should be carried out with a small and short-term force of 1 to 2 seconds, which will be enough to continue the procedure.

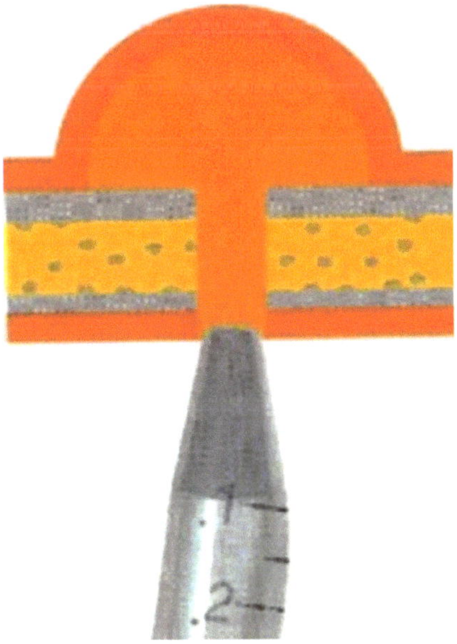

Figure 10.103. Injection of collagen replacement bone graft material

Phase 7

Only the graft injection technique procedure is performed gradually from multiple times, injecting under pressure with a syringe designed for the SLD technique (Figure 10.96.). Due to the hydraulic effect, the membrane is already separated from the cortical bone of the sinus floor, and the injection of graft material will raise the membrane in the form of a dome, targeting the places where the implant should be placed. The amount of graft material to be injected depends on the arrangement and number of implants. In any case, the primary stability of the implant in the part of the cortical bone should be achieved.

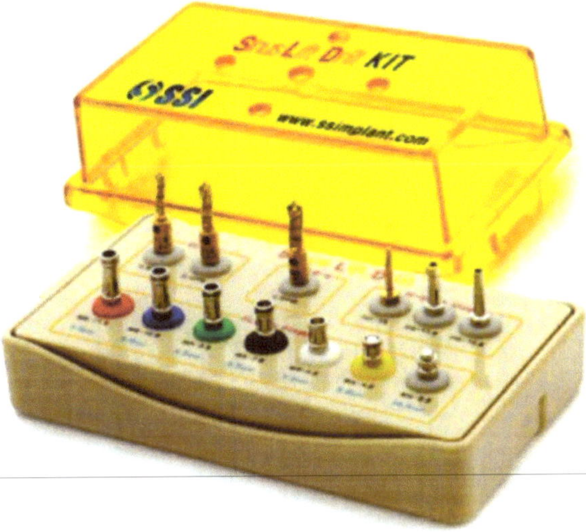

Figure 10.104. Set of SLD techniques.

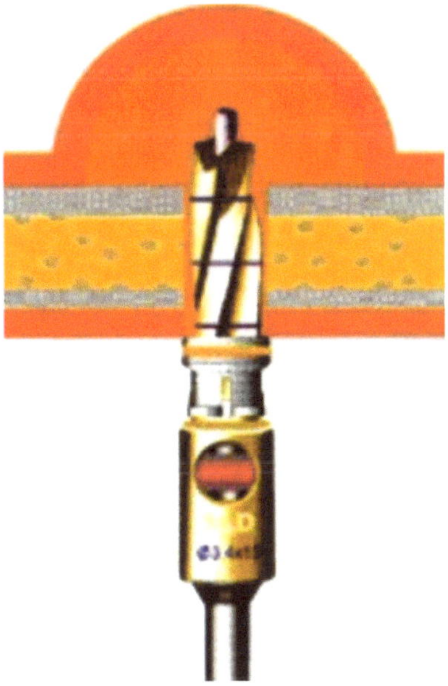

Figure 10.105. Final drilling and rinsing of the cortical bone opening with a torque of 50 rpm.

Phase 8

Depending on the size of the implant (diameter and length), the final phase of cortical bone drilling is performed with the appropriate diameter of the SLD technique bur. This phase is usually neglected, but it is very important. In this phase, the bone opening is expanded and all remaining drilling material is rinsed with saline. If all remaining drilling material is not removed, it may remain between the implant surface and the bone wall of the drilled hole, which hinders osseointegration. For this reason, rinsing with saline is extremely important.

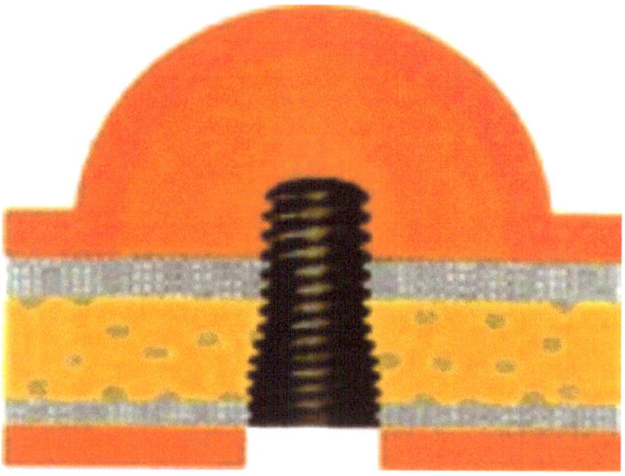

Figure 10.106. Installation of the implant in the space of the raised sinus membranes.

Phase 9

This phase (Figure 10.106) of the SLD technique is the placement of implants using bone compactness, and the selection of implant diameter is of utmost importance in order to achieve bicortical primary fixation with the SLD technique.

Summary

The basic principle of the SLD technique is to precisely and safely drill the cortical bone of the sinus floor and lift the sinus membrane without damage, i.e. without perforation, using a small number of instruments.

A special advantage of the SLD technique is that it does not require raising the mucoperiosteal flap from the vestibular side and opening the window by cutting a block of the sinus wall. The procedure is performed vertically, and there is no need to raise the alveolar ridge flap.

One of the key factors in the SLD technique is that the opening in the floor of the maxillary sinus, made with the SLD drill, should be the same size as the drill blade and the diameter of the syringe for injecting the saline solution and the building material (bone substitute).

The sinus membrane is raised by the pressure of physiological solution through the created opening. It follows in the same way graft injection process. Insertion of the graft is performed slowly, without resistance, and continues with the injection graft until resistance occurs. If resistance occurs, with a drill, with a lower number of revolutions, you should continue 1-2 seconds for the opening to expand and continue insertion graft to make the sinus membrane safe raised.

In short, the SLD technique involves two steps: the first is the injection of saline solution, and the second is the insertion of bone substitute. Both procedures are safe for preserving the sinus membrane.

Figures 10.107 and 10.108 show various cases where implant placement was performed after sinus lifting using the SLD technique.

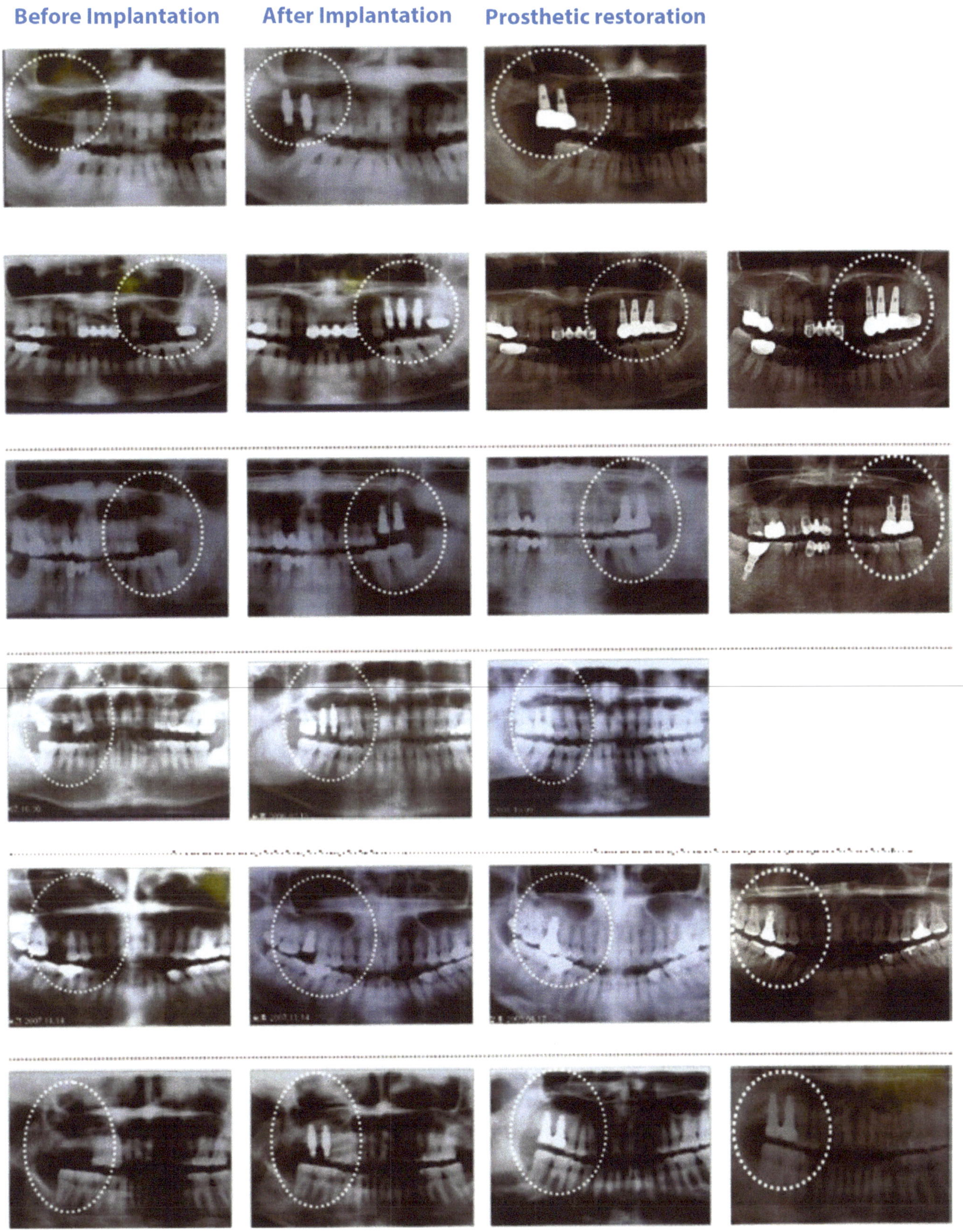

Figure 10.107. A presentation of several cases in which the SLD (Siinus Lift Drilli) technique of sinus floor membrane elevation (sinuslifti) without mucoperiosteal flap elevation was successfully applied.

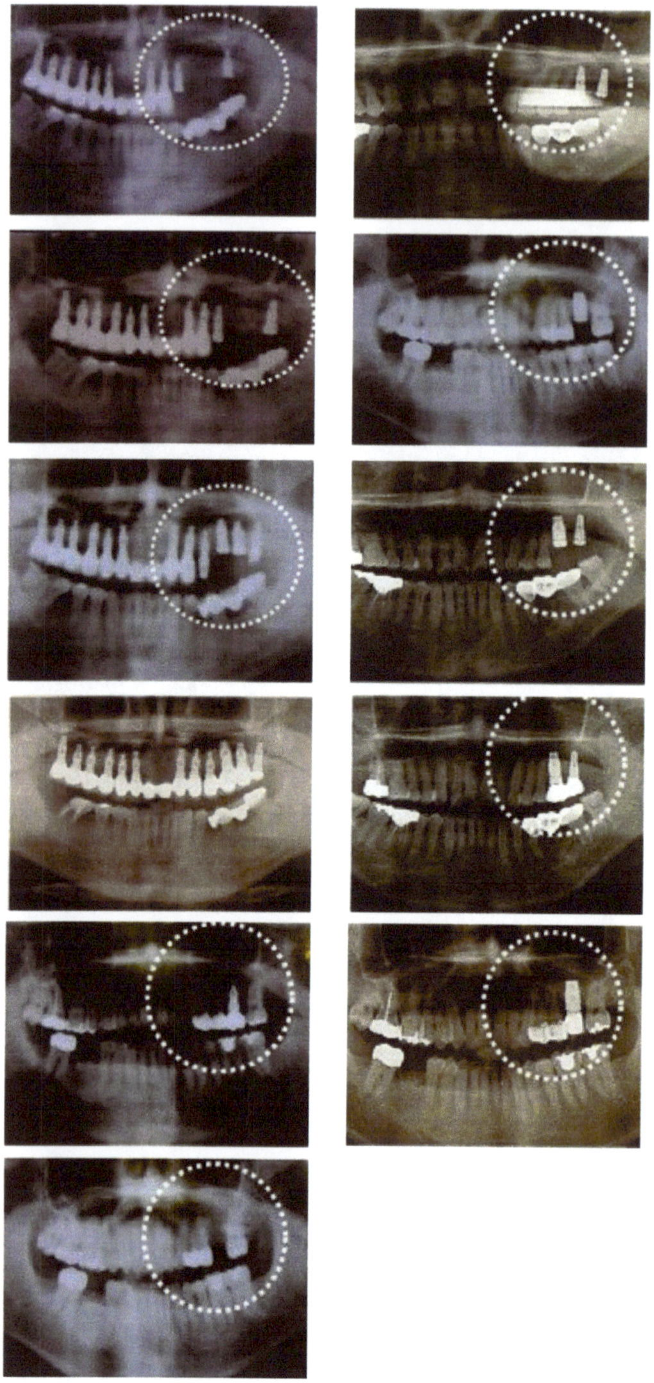

Figure 10.108. Results of successful implantation after application of the SLD technique by lifting the sinus membrane and placing the graft.

Sinus-lifting by applying a hydraulic effect through the implant canal

When there is a need for implant placement in the molar region of the maxilla, sinus augmentation in more than 50%, and even more than that, is indicated. Pneumatization of the maxillary sinus is accompanied by pronounced atrophy of the alveolar bone of the sinus floor, and the vertical dimension, height, decreases below 4 millimeters. A common surgical sinus lift procedure was to open the bone wall of the sinus from the vestibular side. However, as emphasized repeatedly, this way of lifting the sinus floor also involves complications: considerable trauma to the patient and usually a long recovery with pain, swelling, and local bleeding. However, the most common complication of sinus lifting was perforation of Schneider's membrane.

How to simplify the sinus lifting procedure and how to install an implant in the area of lost molars, where the cortical bone of the sinus floor is less than 4 millimeters, is still a great challenge. Today, there is a large selection of routine surgical methods of augmentation and reconstruction expressed by bone destruction in certain regions of the alveolar ridge, and if the methods are good, there are some certain limitations.

When it comes to the augmentation of the maxillary sinus floor, new implantable sinus lifting technologies are also being published, which enable the safe lifting of Schneider's membrane, placement of graft with immediate implant placement, but there is still a lack of valid statistical data on the percentage of success.

The relatively newer method for safely lifting the Schneider membrane is based on the same principle as the previously described SDL technique of lifting the sinus floor membrane by hydraulic pressure. The procedure begins with careful entry of the appropriate auger into the bone of the sinus floor without injury to the mucosa. In the literature, this process is also commonly defined as hydraulic sinus condensation.

With this method, the authors state, the separation of the membranes from the sinus floor is safe. The hydraulic effect of separating the membrane from the cortical bone is achieved by injecting 3cm3 of saline with air through the implant channel (shaped as the letter L - Figure 10.109.). The injected fluid creates a hydraulic pressure that is uniform to all parts of the membrane. With even hydraulic pressure from below, the membrane lifts everything up, forming between the graft placement area (bone deputies, Figures 10.117 and 10.121).

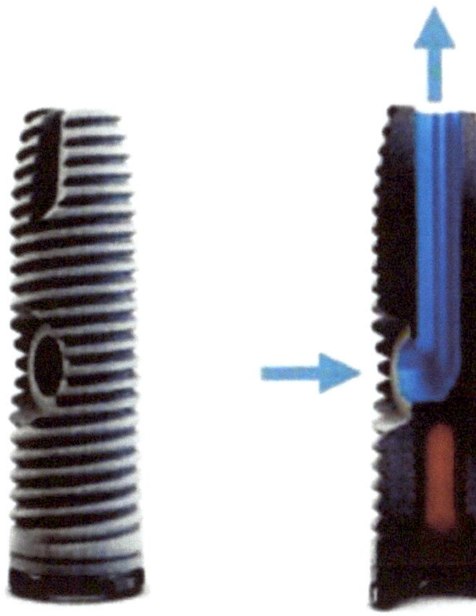

Figure 10.109. An implant with an internal curved duct through which saline is injected.

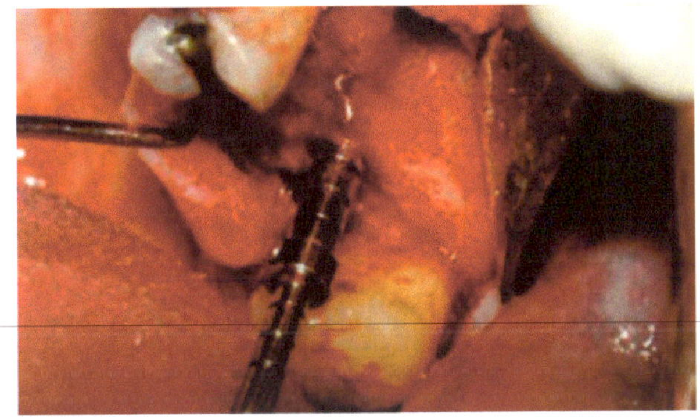

Figure 10.110. Assessment of implant positioning with careful entry of osteotomas into the bone.

Hydraulic lifting of the membrane is a safe and secure method because the pressure is equally distributed over the entire membrane, so that its perforation does not occur despite the splitting of capillary blood vessels which, after graft injection and implant placement, will restore its physiological function. This procedure is determined as the hydraulic condensation of the sinuses. The duct within the implant is designed to block the possibility of bacterial contents from the oral cavity communicating with the sinus interior during healing and after prosthetic work has been completed. A new iRaise-Maxillent implant is used for this method. This implant corresponds to the principle of hydraulic action on the sinus floor membrane using an internal channel to achieve a hydraulic effect.

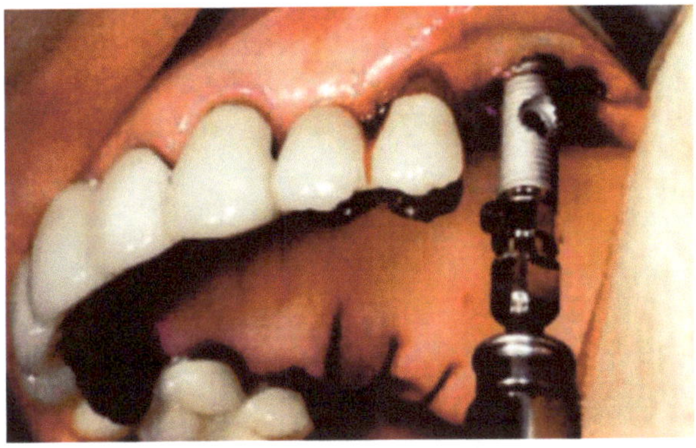

Figure 10.111. Implant positioning with accessible saline injection port.

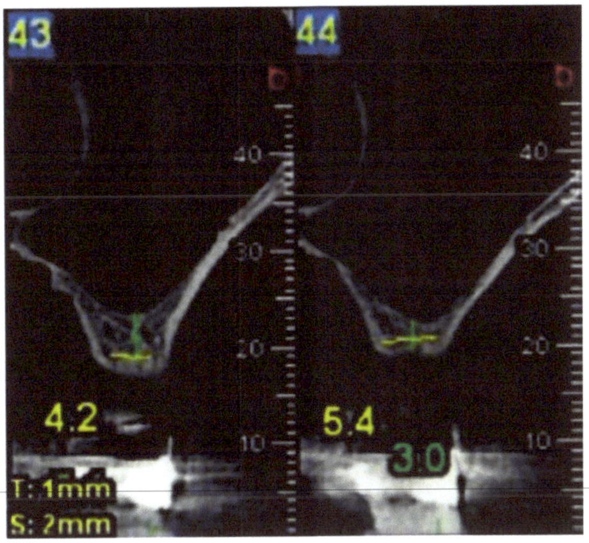

Figure 10.112. Radiographic view of regions 26 and 27 before sinus floor membrane lift.

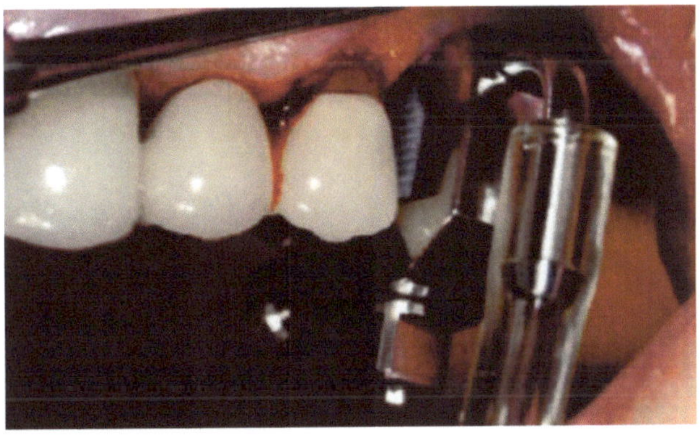

Figure 10.113. Adjusting the device for injecting saline and separating the membrane from the cortical bone - through the implant opening.

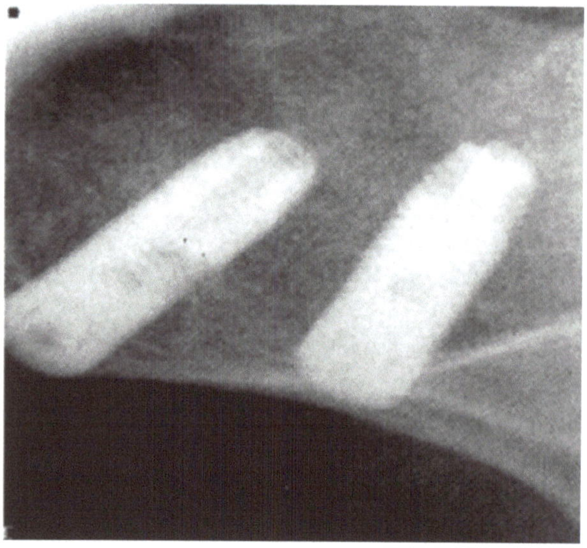

Figure 10.114. Placed "iRaise-Maxillent" implants simultaneously with the insertion of a graft (bone substitute) in position 26 and 27.

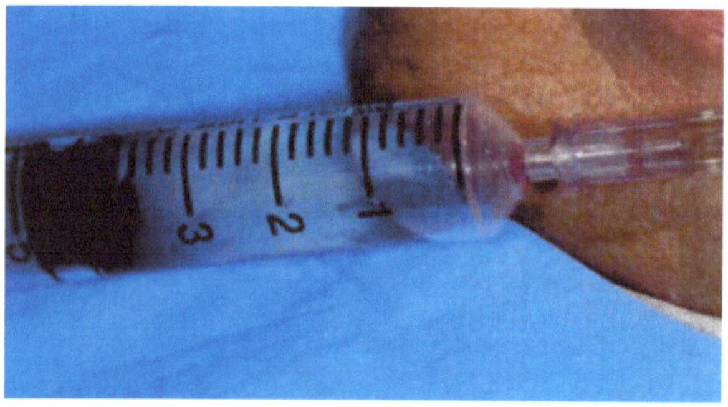

Figure 10.115. Extraction of injected saline with slight traces of blood after separation of Schneiderian membrane from the sinus floor.

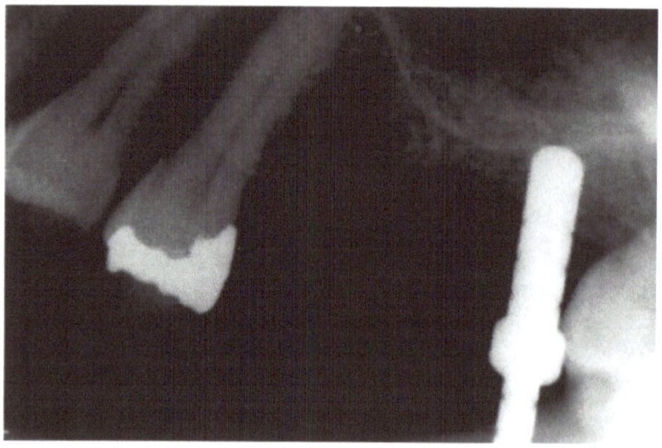

Figure 10.116. Osteotome checking of the height of the sinus floor bone and the proximity of the membrane. Radiographic analysis (by RVG method) before the procedure is extremely important.

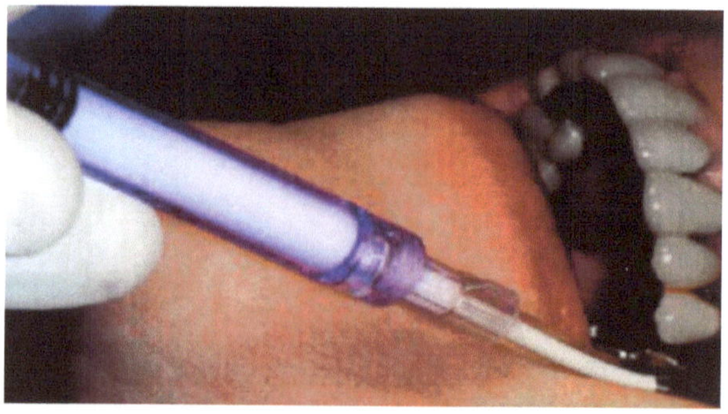

Figure 10.117. Injecting the graft into the formed space between the separate membrane and the cortical bone of the sinus floor.

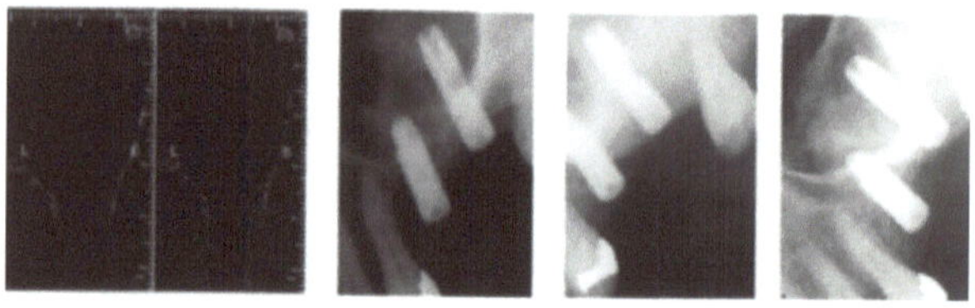

Figure 10.118. Radiographic CT scan before the procedure, after immediate implantation, after 4 months and after 8 months,

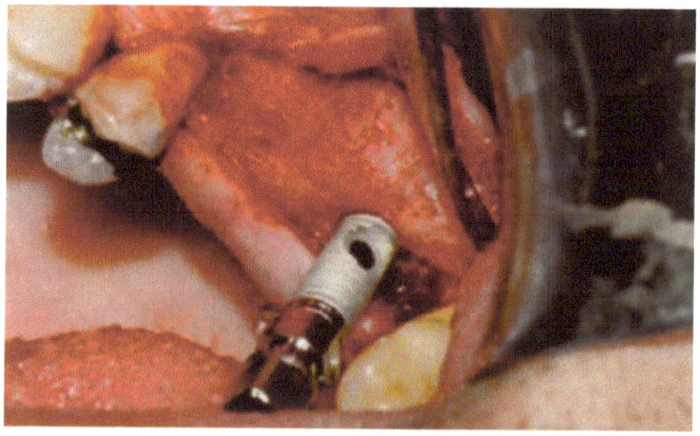

Figure 10.119. Lifting the flap from the buccal side and inserting the implant into the prepared opening. Bleeding from the opening confirms that the implant is touching the sinus floor membrane.

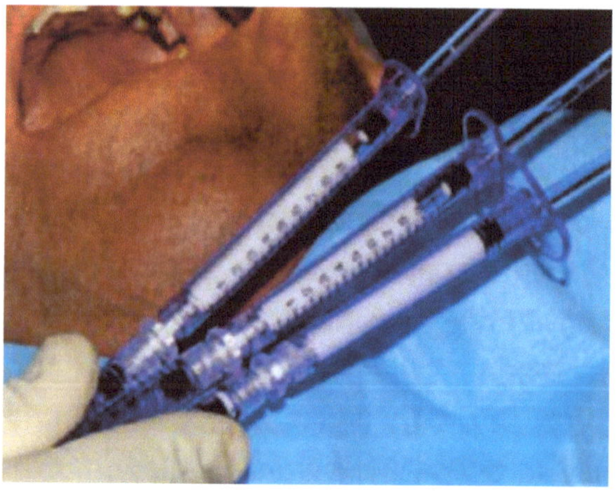

Figure 10.120. Prepared bone replacements in the amount of 3ccm in the spikes through which the graft formed space between the raised membrane and the cortical bone of the sinus floor is placed through the opening and the implant duct.

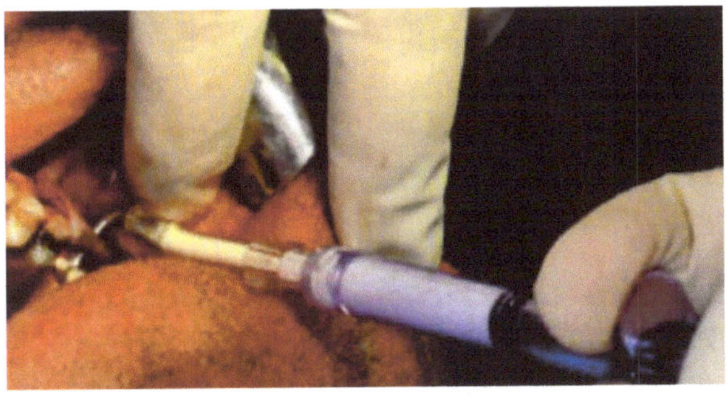

Figure 10.121. Prepared Graft Injection

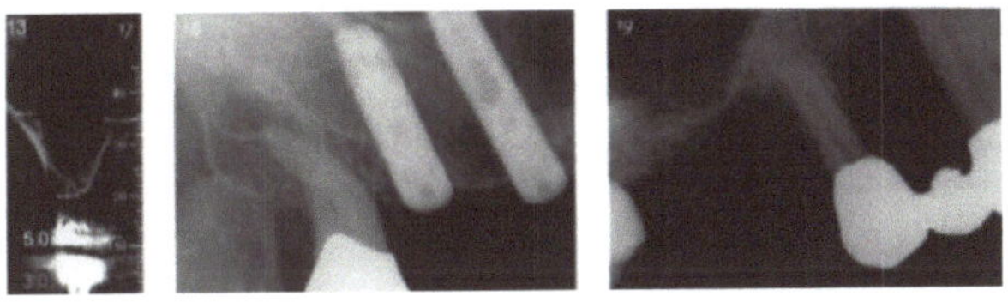

Figure 10.122. Radiographic representation of the bone thickness of the sinus floor 3mm, the situation after the placement of graphite and implant placement.

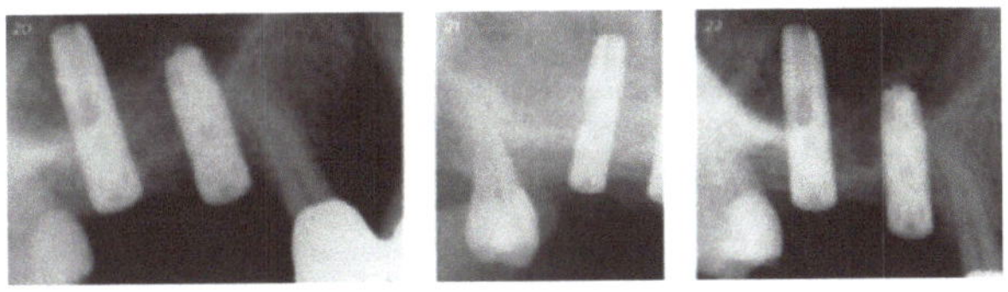

Figure 10.123. Radiographic representation of bilateral sinus lifting and implant placement. Situation after 4 months and after 8 months.

Conclusion

The described methods of sinus lifting with immediate implant placement are aimed at: simpler surgical approach, less trauma, faster healing, and faster recovery of the patient. Removal of the injected saline solution from the sinuses, mixed with traces of blood (Figure 10.115), is a clinical indication that the solution has come into contact with the membrane, intersecting the tiny blood vessels that vascularize the membrane and the cortex of the sinus floor. The ease of the procedure is enabled by the design of the connector, and it is also simple to manipulate when inserting a dosed graft in the amount of 3 ccm, with the same implant placement.

Antibiotic prophylaxis (amoxicillin 500 mg) is mandatory before the intervention. with clavulanic acid and maintaining oral hygiene by rinsing the mouth with solutions with chlorhexidine gluconate or Curasept solution at a concentration of 0.12%.

The described methods of sinus lifting with immediate implant placement will confirm that they become a routine procedure in everyday practice, although we still do not have sufficient performance statistics.

Augmentation of the alveolar ridge of the mandible with extreme atrophy

A few decades ago, the biggest challenge in oral implantology was how to restore the patient's chewing function. And the patients' demands were consistent with the range of oral implantology at the time.

However, today the requirements of patients have also been significantly expanded, even in those cases where the possibilities of implant placement were not even considered. Hence, at one time, an attempt to resolve such cases was with subperiostal implants which after a short time ended in failure. However, patients' request to establish function was primary. Today, even with extreme atrophy of the alveolar bone (Figures 10,124 and 10,129) and unfavorable anatomical relationships, endosseus implants can be installed, and uncomfortable mobile prostheses can be replaced with fixed prosthetic work. Today, patients' requirements are so expanded that, despite the requirement to establish a good chewing function, the requirements to achieve aesthetics also dominate in parallel. Patient requirements have also been extended in cases where the alveolar bone resorption process has progressed significantly with significantly altered dimensions of the alveolar bone in the vertical and horizontal direction of less than 4 mm, which also have a repercussion on the aesthetic appearance of the patient.

Reimbursement of local bone defects in certain regions is most often a routine procedure. But the overall restoration of the alveolar ridge by augmentation in the horizontal and vertical direction is still an extensive and complicated procedure. For example, in the patient shown, for the restoration of the alveolar ridge, it would be necessary to take bone block transplants from the thigh, with the addition of bone substitutes with a collagen resorptive membrane. The whole procedure would represent an extremely complex team surgical procedure, but from the point of view of routine practice and is closer to theoretical considerations, than feasible procedures in practice. However, there are cases in the literature where similar methods of alveolar ridge restoration have been applied. Experience shows that even with the most successful major alveolar ridge reconstructions, it is not possible to meet the aesthetic requirements of the patient with fixed prosthetic works, as the restoration of the profile would not meet the patient's expectations regarding aesthetics.

Today, it is possible to augment at least part of the ridge in a much simpler way, and after immediate implant placement, successfully prosthetically care for the patient with a significant improvement in aesthetic appearance (Figures 10.124. and 10,132)

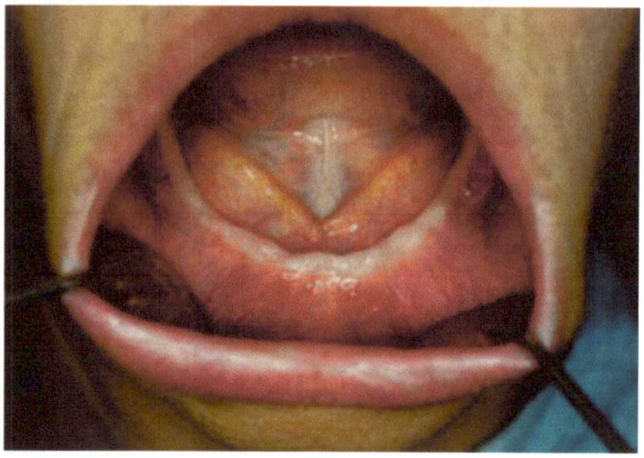

Figure 10.124. Extreme resorption of the alveolar ridge: in the horizontal direction (crestal part 1 mm), and in the vertical direction 10.2 mm. In similar cases of oral implantology, today it can meet the aesthetic and functional requirements of the patient with fixed mobile reimbursements supported by implants.

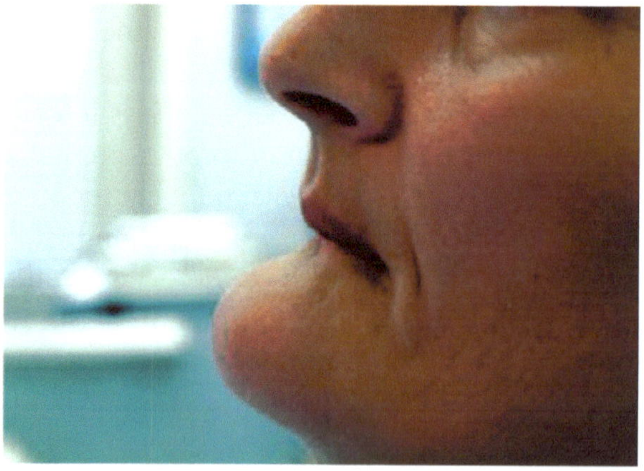

Figure 10.125. The influence of more extreme atrophy of the alveolar bone and ridges in the horizontal direction of 1 mm, and in the vertical direction of 10.2 mm affect the positions of the lips and the aesthetic appearance.

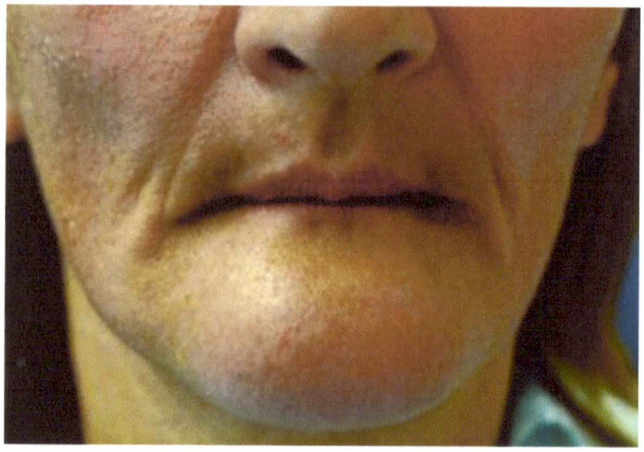

Figure 10.126. In similar cases where the parameters of the available bone (extremely reduced horizontal dimension of the alveolar bone) the patient's demands for fulfilling the aesthetic requirements with fixed prosthetic works are unrealistic. The eventual use of augmentation by the PRF method (blood plasma enriched with platelet and leukocyte growth factors) is currently a long-term procedure, still in the research phase.

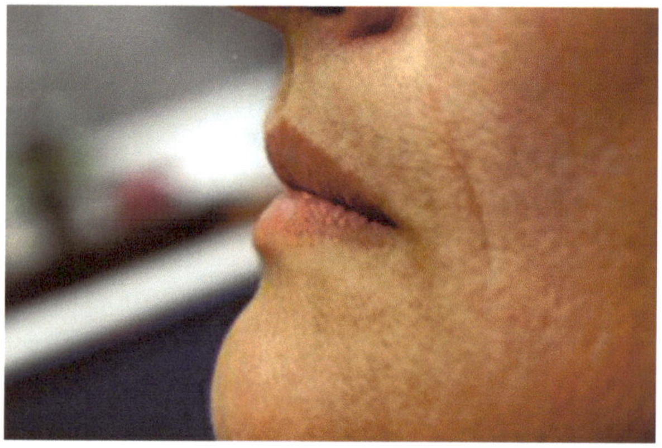

Figure 10.127. Profile of the same patient (compare with Figure 10.125).

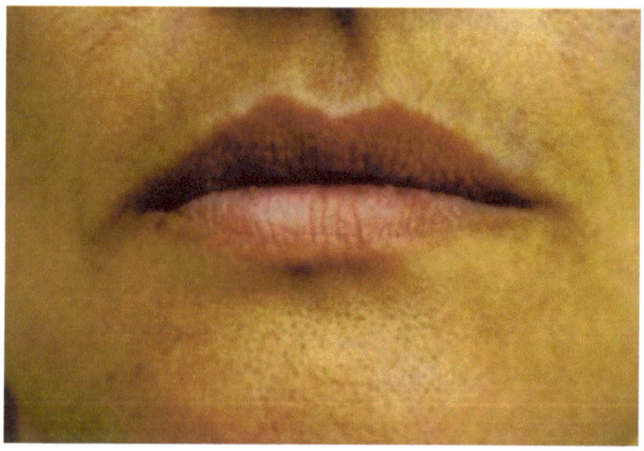

Figure 10.128. Front view of the same patient. Compare with Figure 10.126.

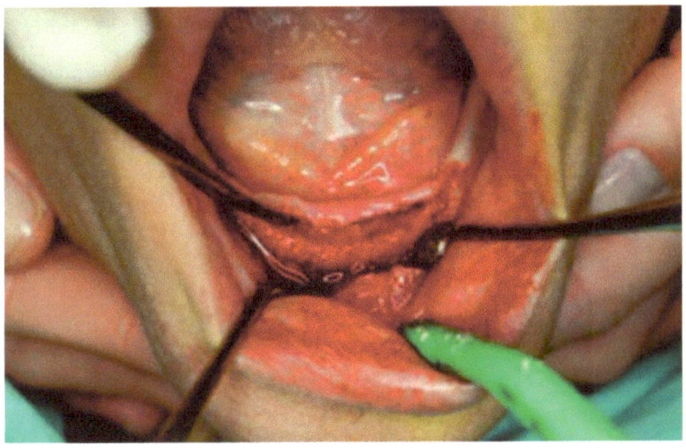

Figure 10.129. By lifting the flap, an insight into the actual condition is obtained: dimensions and quality of the bone. The disadvantage is also increased by a thick layer of mobile tissue along the entire length of the crestal bone. It happens thatthe local finding deviates significantly from radiographic measurements.

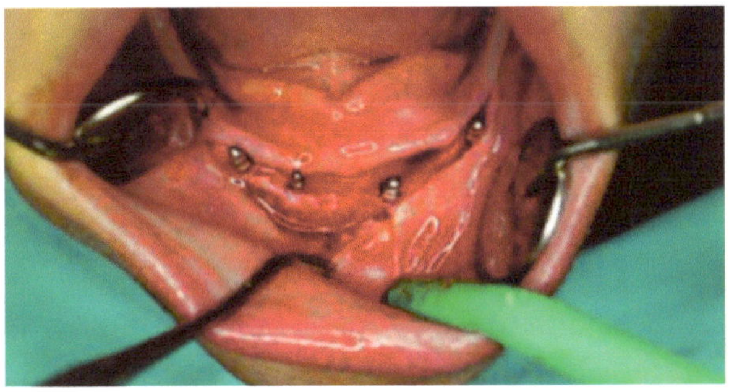

Figure 10.130. Implant placement with retention clips, and the width of the ridge is increased by augmentation with bone substitutes.

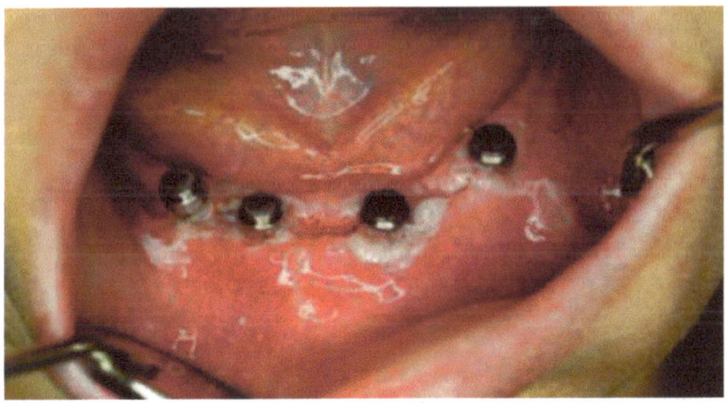

Figure 10.131. Laser treatment of soft tissues 10 days after implantation.

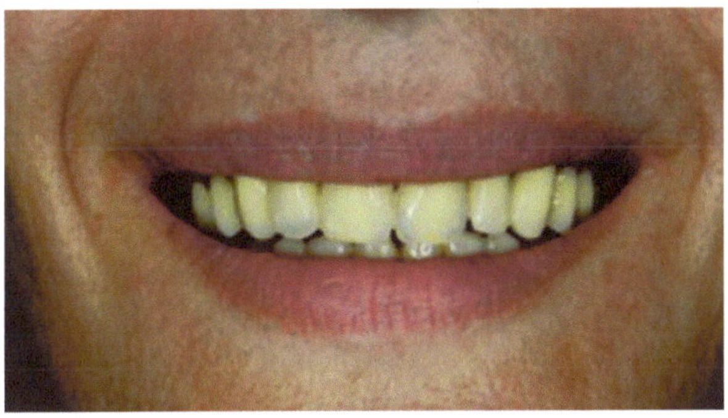

Figure 10.132. Prosthetic work anchored on immediately loaded implants. The patient's aesthetic requirements are met.

PRF (PLATELET REACH FIBRIN)

Since the time when the author began to deal with implant placement and to write this book, the progress of oral implantology from that period until today has been immeasurable. This is the value of what is written, because it shows the continuity of the development of this branch of medicine, without which it is unthinkable today to treat a disability in the oral cavity, in the first place by implant-prosthetic procedures. If the PRF method had been discovered at the time of treatment of many of the cases presented in the book, it is likely that many of the cases would have been treated differently.

What is the essence of this method?

The essence of this method is the enrichment of blood plasma with platelet and leukocyte growth factors, as well as numerous cytokines. Today, the PRF method is used in everyday medical practice to accelerate wound healing. Indications for obtaining both connective tissue and horizontal and vertical bone volume. The PRF membrane is beginning to find increasing application in oral implantology and periodontology and to change the soft tissue biotype. By last technological preparation of graft (sandwich technique) and using I-PRF (injection membrane), fixing the prepared graft mach (mesh) membrane, bone volumization can be achieved for safe implant placement. The same application of this method can be used in cases of alveolar bone fenestration, predominantly in destroyed lamellar bone wall and alveolar ridge concavity. The position of the author of the book is that it should still be accepted with some reservations because many cases have not yet been fully followed up and documented. In any case, by exchanging experiences with practitioners, in all treated cases, a much better effect resulted in obtaining a higher quality tortuous complex (formation of the exit profile of the gingiva and resolution of mucogingival resesions).

What is the concept of this method?

The concept of PRF is based on centrifugation of the patient's blood in anticoagulant-free tubes. At the end of centrifugation, a fibrin clot with a multitude of platelets is separated from the other shaped blood elements.

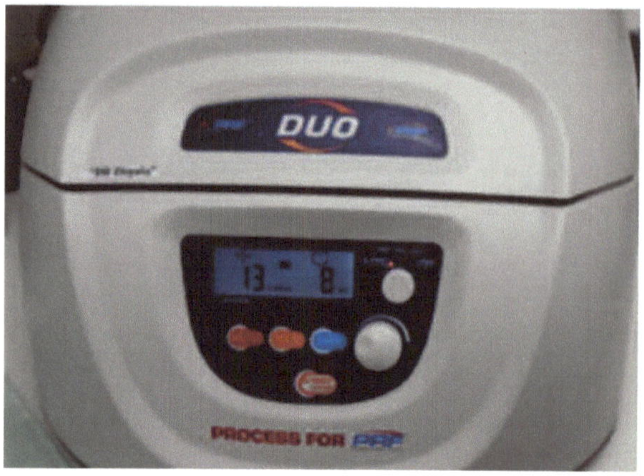

Figure 10.133 Patient blood centrifuge device in tubes.

This fibrin clot is called Riche Fibrin Platelet or PRF, it gradually and over a long period of time releases growth factors and cytokines into surrounding bone or soft tissue. The main goal of growth factors that are released is to accelerate the healing of soft tissues as well as the healing of bone.

Many studies and publications available prove the success of PRF application in a wide field of indications: general surgery, maxillofacial surgery, oral surgery with oral implantology (implants, bone augmentation, periodontal surgery, extraction and extraction wounds, sinus lifting...), orthopedics of the jaws, cosmetic and dermatological surgery, facial aesthetics... Such wide application when it comes to oral implantology, however, decades of experience suggest that it should be accepted with reserve, waiting for scientific confirmation.

The basic difference between PRF membranes, which arose in 2001. according to the blood centrifugation protocol for 14 minutes at 1300 rpm, and A-PRF according to the centrifugation protocol for 8 minutes at 1300 rpm, is in the presence of leukocyte growth factors. A-PRF was obtained by examining the contents of the tubes under a microscope, leukocytes were deposited at the bottom of the tube due to their large mass. Based on this observation, a conclusion was reached; by reducing the centrifugation time, there will be a significant increase in the number of leukocytes that will remain on the surface of the tube.

Leukocyte growth factor, which has been proven in recent scientific studies, directly affects the production of BMP2 protein, which is considered to be one of the most significant invoices for bone morphogenesis. A wide range of indications for the application of PRF in everyday practice today a large number of scientific studies published in more serious and highly cited world scientific journals.

What is the role of growth factor?

Growth factors belong to proteins or steroid hormones that play a dominant role in wound healing. These factors communicate with cells through special prescriptions located on the cell surface and are responsible for cell differentiation, growth, and proliferation.

There are over 150 different growth invoices that have been investigated so far.

Effect of growth factors on wound healing

In modern practice, there are several products that lead to wound healing and that are obtained from human tissue by purifying or recombining different growth factors. However, PRF belongs to autologous platelet preparations, autologous proteins, and is a platelet concentrate formed by centrifugation that separates blood components. Numerous growth factors play different roles in wound healing, but vascular endothelial growth factor VGEF stands out as particularly important because it is responsible for neoangiogenesis. **Neoangiogenesis is the formation of new blood vessels,** and newer scientific methods have proven that signs of neoangiogenesis occur as early as 24 hours after PRF membrane administration. Studies performed with concentrated platelets since 1998. PRP (Platelet Reach Plasma) and PRGF (Plasma Rich in Growth Factors) were not on the market until 2001. when the first research on PRF was published. The main difference between PRF and all other so far made preparations of concentrated platelets is in the presence of anticoagulants.

Namely, the natural pathway of hemostasis, necessary for the healing of any wound, takes place in 3 basic stages: narrowing of the blood vessel, the formation of a platelet plug and blood coagulation.

The narrowing of the blood vessel occurs due to the sympathetic response, whereby there is a local and contraction of the blood vessel muscles in response to injury and secretion of vasoconstrictive substances. After that, platelets accumulate and coagulate, forming a fibrin clot. Platelets can produce their growth factors only after coagulation. The released growth factors also lead to new angiogenesis and cell stimulation, and the ultimate outcome of this physiological process is manifested by wound healing. Knowledge of the natural process of hemostasis, preparations of concentrated platelets used as a wound healing aid should not have anticoagulants in their composition. The above text explains the biological significance of the PRF membrane and its physical properties such as: solid consistency, elasticity, stickiness, shaping and light application, contribute to increasing application in a wide field of indications.

By extracting the patient's blood using a specially designed system for drawing blood into the tubes and centrifuging the blood, physiological coagulation occurs within the tube, in which PRF remains at the end of centrifugation, i.e. a fibrin clot and exudate consisting of plasma and adhesive proteins (Fig. 10,134)

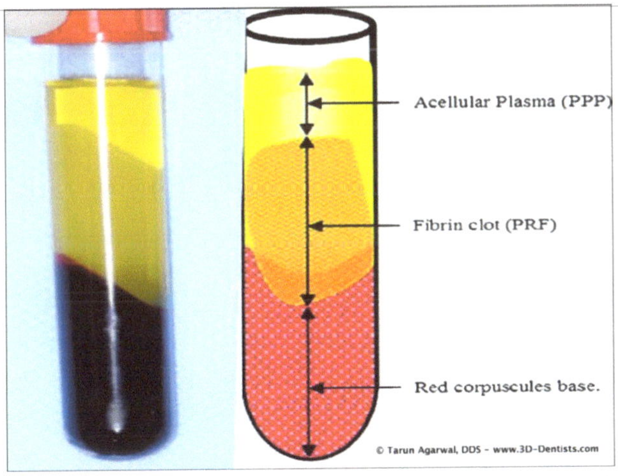

Figure 10.134. Appearance of the tube after centrifugation and schematic representation of the contents of the tube

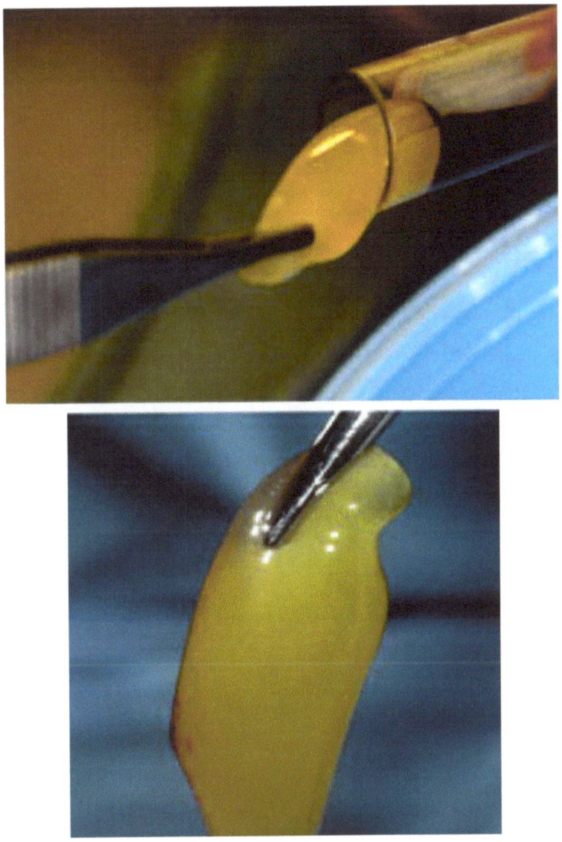

Figure 10.135. Appearance of PRF COLT after centrifugation

PRF by composition represents 100% platelet concentrate and 50% fibrin

Fibrin in PRF is a tentative extracellular matrix that is responsible for the slow release of platelet growth factors.

The fibrin clot obtained by centrifugation is called a "membrane" and can be stored for use in various forms depending on the indication: pressed, plug-shaped, quilted membrane, chopped for ease of administration shredded mixed with bone replacers.

Difference between PRF and PRP

Both preparations contain a similar concentration of platelet growth factors, but there is a significant difference in the amount of leukocyte growth factors.

Growth factors in A-PRF are released slowly, for a longer period of time, because they are attached to the fibrin mesh, while in PRP growth factors act very briefly, because anticoagulants are used to obtain them and thus fibrin is broken down. Therefore, there is a difference in the consistency of the preparation, due to the presence of a fibrin clot, the membrane can be pressed, chopped, shredded or shaped as needed while the PRP is only in a liquid state.

I-PRF preparation

I-PRF (injectable PRF) is a preparation obtained without additives, without anticoagulants, automatically contains a high concentration of leukocytes, and a clot is formed immediately after injection. Because of these properties, it is used for direct injection into tissue and for mixing with various bone substitutes. It binds granular bone substitutes into a compact mixture and gives them dimensional stability while avoiding material scattering, which is very important in horizontal and vertical augmentation procedures, in case of raising the sinus floor if perforation of the sinus floor membrane occurs...

Difference between I-PRF and PRP

The main difference between I-PRF and I co-PRP is in anticoagulants that are not used to obtain I-PRF and in the concentration of leukocyte growth factors, monocytes, neutrophils and lymphocytes (Fig.10.144)

	i-PRF	P.R.P.	
Leukocytes	14.420/mL	680/mL	1/20
Monocytes	121/mL	2/mL	1/60
Neutrophiles	4.270/mL	100/mL	1/40
Lymphocytes	8.590/mL	540/mL	1/20
PLATELETS	690.000/mL	632.000/mL	

Figure 10.136. The table shows the ratio of growth factors between I-PRF and PRP. All parameters are richer in PRF than in PRP. I-PRF is an improved membrane rich in fibrin, in contrast to I-PRP it has a slight fibrin content.

Indications for use

PRF membranes first found application in general surgery where they are most commonly used to cover pressure ulcers and open vulnerable surfaces in diabetics, and only later they began to be used in oral surgery, periodontology and other branches of dentistry.

Indications for the use of PRF membranes in oral surgery:

- alveolar preservation after tooth extraction
- alveolitis therapy
- rehabilitation of gingival recessions
- conservative therapy in the closure of some oroantral communications
- sinus floor lift
- accelerating bone healing
- perforation overlap
- window covering
- as a biomaterial
- bone augmentation
- wound healing
- periodontology
- immediate implant placement
- single-phase implant placement protocol whether a sulcus former, temporary crown or prosthesis is used, the membrane is placed as a collar.
- Treatment of peri-implantitis

It should be emphasized that the application of a PRF membrane can replace some of the grafting materials that it can completely replace the collagen membrane where there is an indication for its application.

With the use of a PRF membrane in addition to everything that has been used so far for grafts, it can be freely used in excess bone substitute and to work is already hyper-corrected even in the case that there are no conditions for passive suturing of the lobe after augmentation, the membrane can be left exposed and the wound can secondarily epithelialize.

When installing the implant, commented in the area where growth factor (PRF membrane) was added as an addition to a bone replacement, during the preparation of the implant bed, better bone vitality is clearly observed clinically.

When preparing the opening in an augmented area where growth factors have not been used, most often there is either too hard bone, so it is necessary to use all diameters of borers and bone notches to the end of the prepared opening to avoid graft breakage, or if there is too soft bone where it is necessary to use a short borer or to use it only halfway through the opening. When preparing the opening in the augmented area where bone growth factors were used, it shows solid compactness.

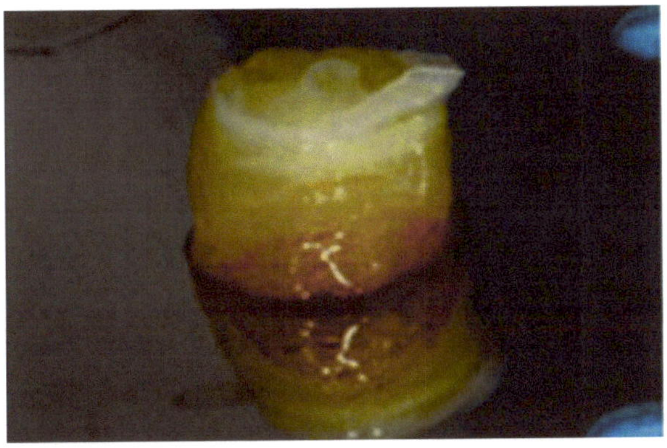

Figure 10.137. PRF membrane as "PUNCH". The appearance of the membrane is pressed in the form of a cylinder used for application in post-extraction wounds and in alveolith therapy.

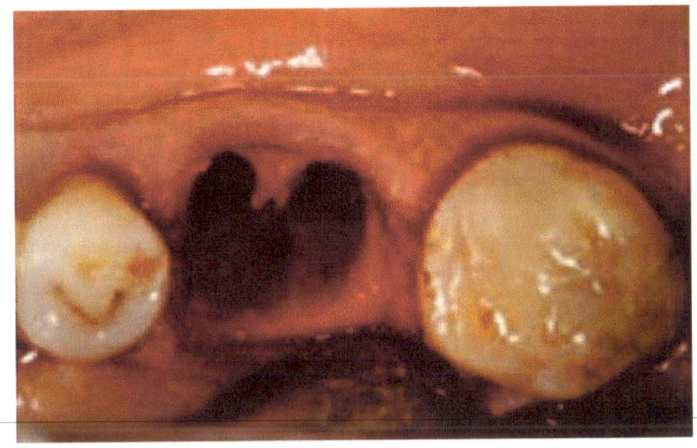

Figure 10.138. Appearance of extraction wound with bone tissue destruction

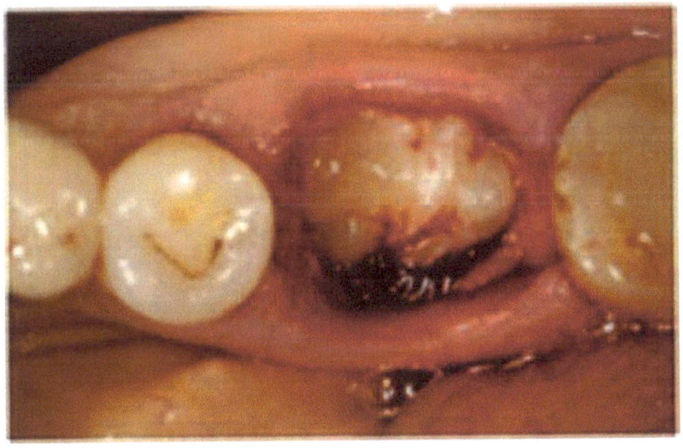

Figure 10.139. Placed pressed fibrin clot in the form of a cylinder (PUNCH).

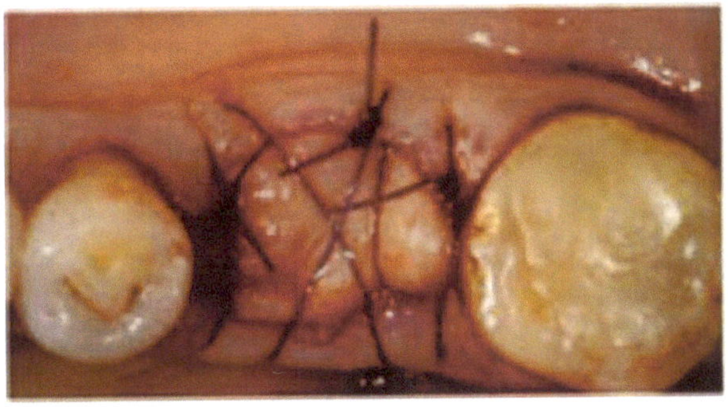

Figure 10.140. Sewn PRF membrane.

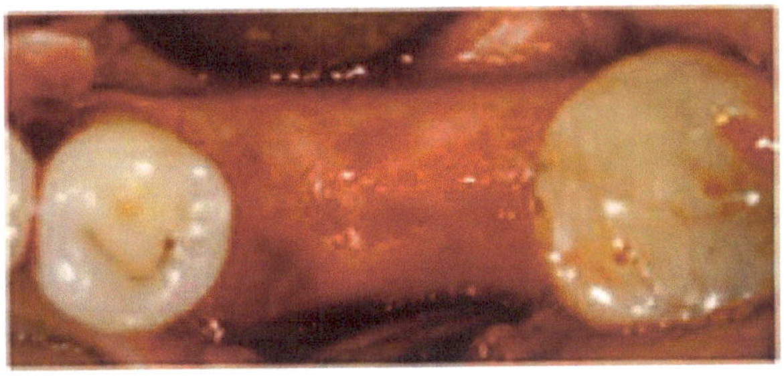

Figure 10.141. Appearance of the shaped alveolar ridge after 6 months. Increased bone volume in horizontal and vertical directions.

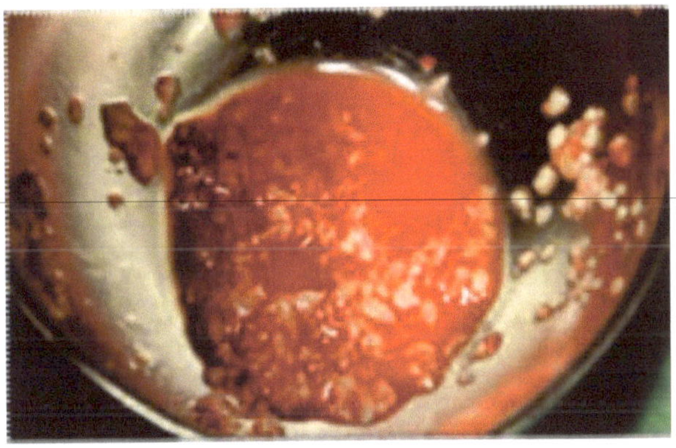

Figure 10.142. PRF membrane, comminuted, mixed with bone substitute prepared for augmentation.

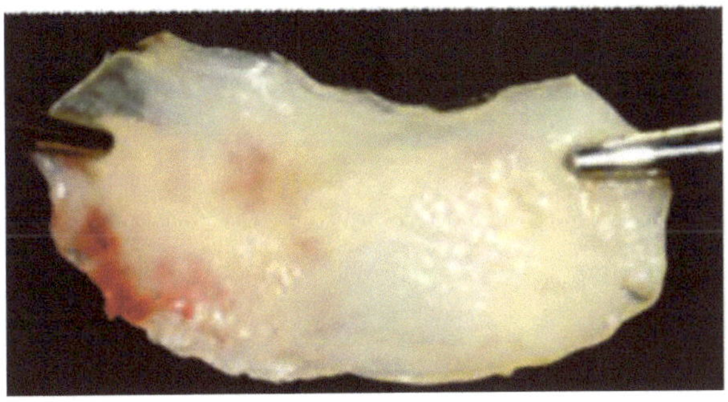

Figure 10.143. Appearance of PRF membrane after pressing.

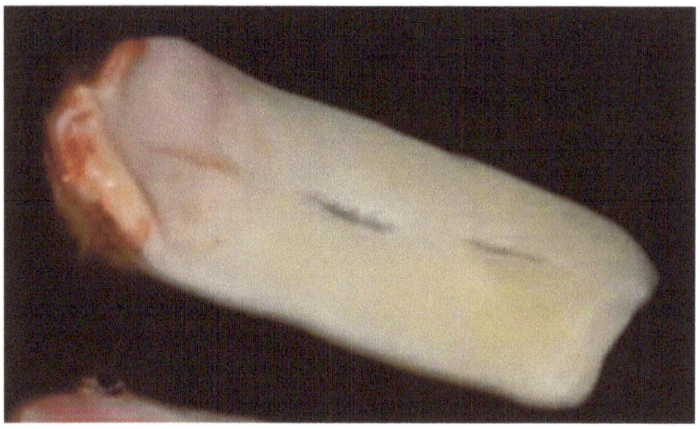

Figure 10.144. -PRF membrane averaged to be able to multi-layered application.

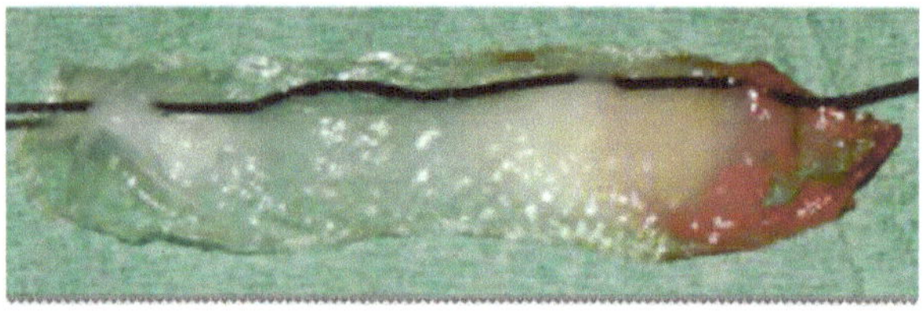

Figure 10.145. Stitched PRF membrane to help provide stability of the application to the surrounding soft tissues.

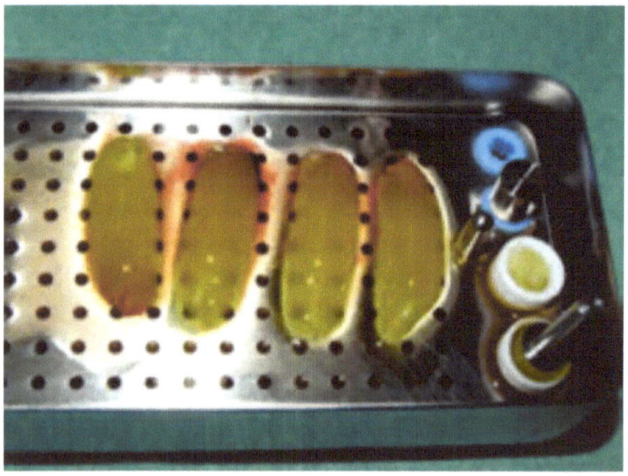

Figure 10.146. Appearance of separated COLTS obtained after centrifugation prepared for pressing, after which the membrane is obtained.

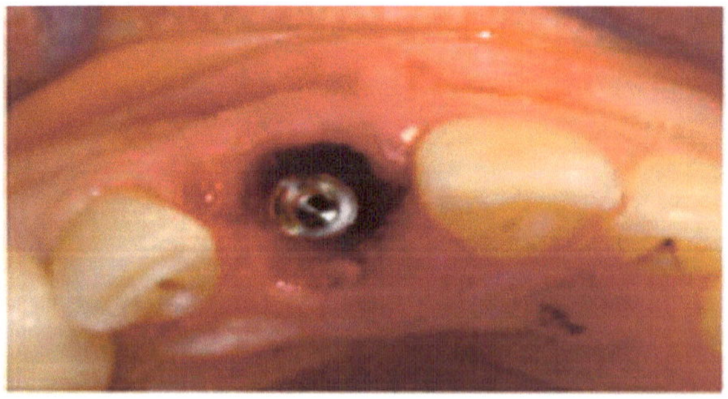

Figure 10.147. PRF membrane placed around the definitive abutment.

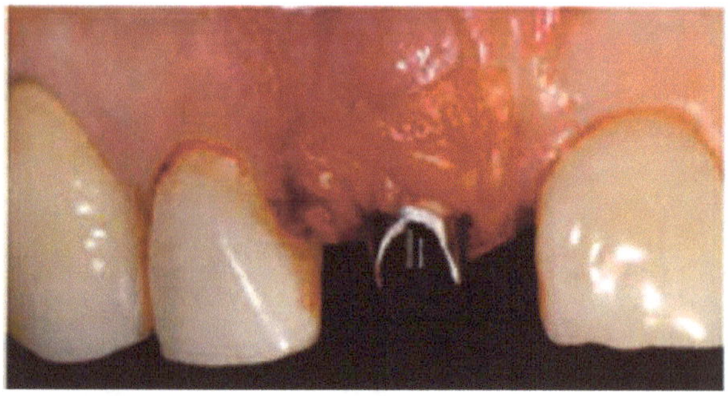

Figure 10.148. Placed PRF membrane.

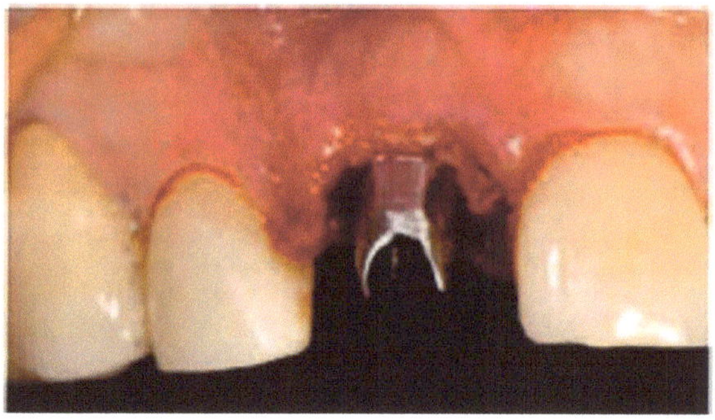

Figure 10.149. Appearance of the placed PRF membrane from the vestibular side.

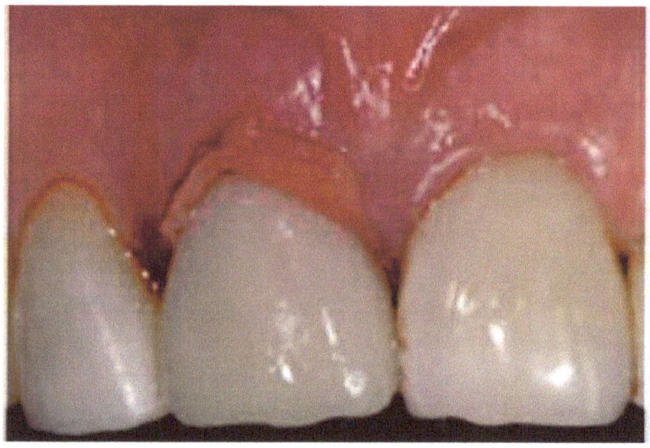

Figure 10.150. Treatment of gingival recession with PRF membrane.

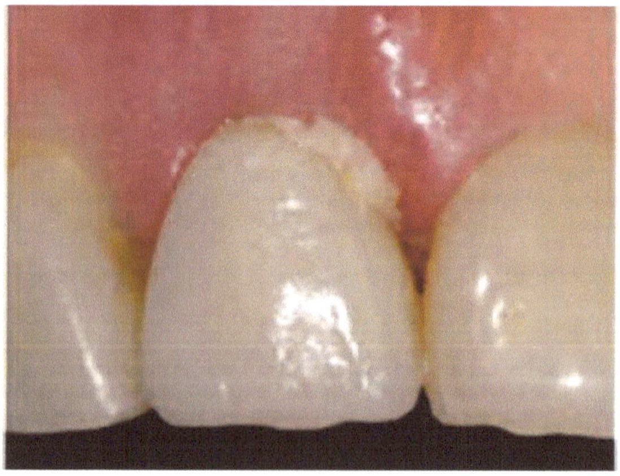

Figure 10.151. Appearance of the healing phase after two weeks.

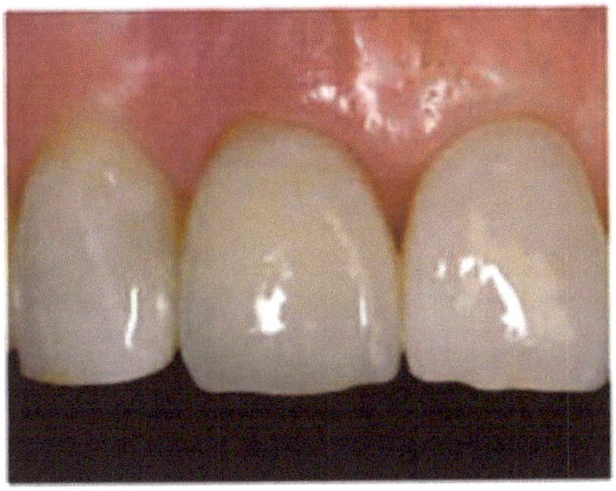

Figure 10.152. Healed gingiva using PRF. Appearance of healed gingiva after 3 months.

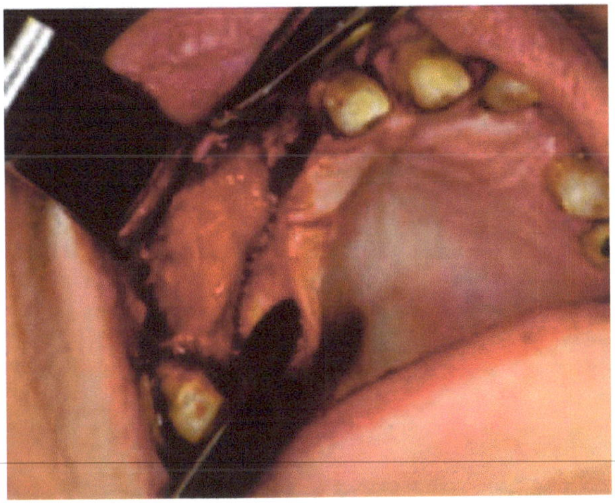

Figure 10.153. Appearance of bone destruction in the canine region(13).

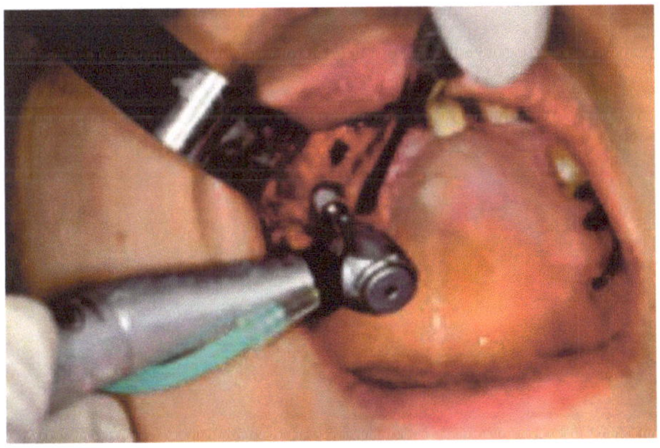

Figure 10.154. Implant site preparation in a region of sufficient bone after augmentation and application of PRF membrane mixed with bone substitutes.

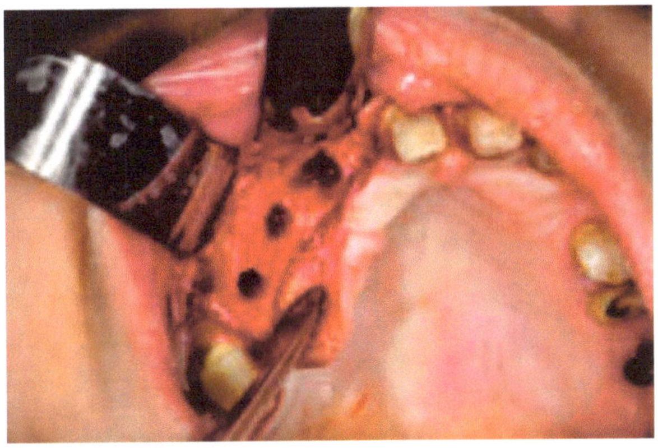

Figure 10.155. Prepared sites for endosseous implants.

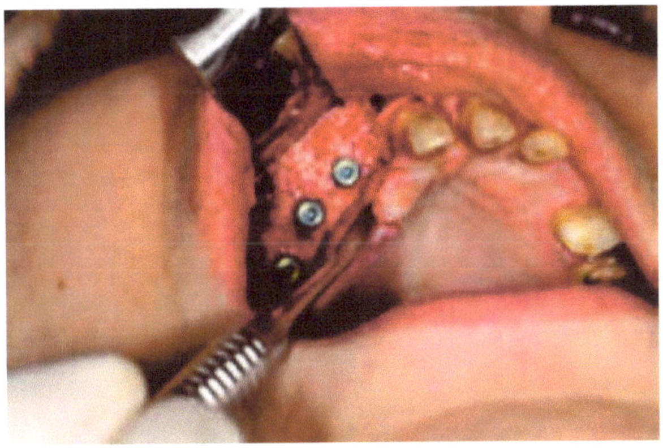

Figure 10.156. Placed contents of the extruded PRF membrane mixed with bone substitutes (Figure 10.142)

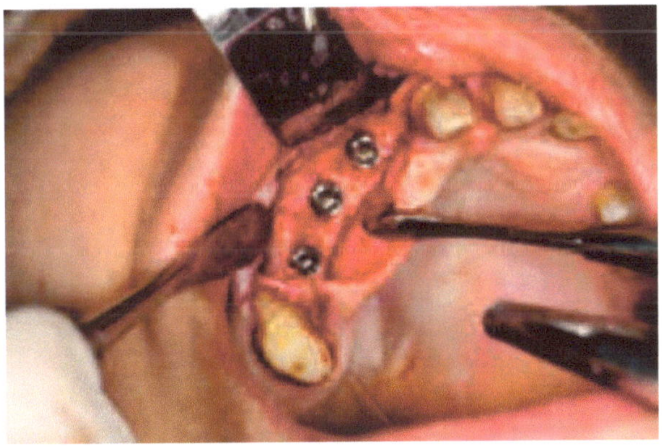

Figure 10.157. Appearance of the formed alveolar ridge after 8 weeks..

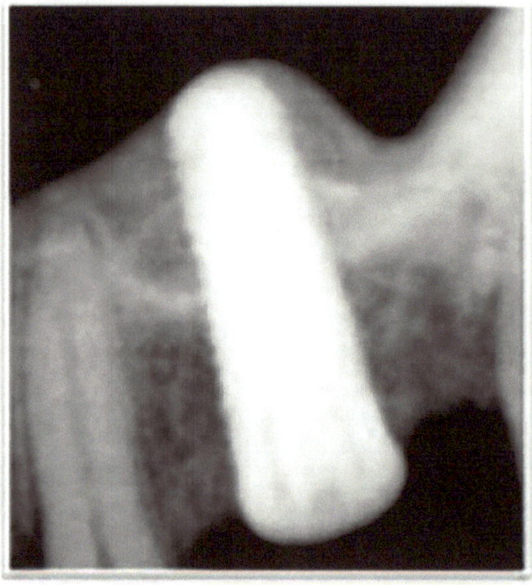

Figure 10.158. Immediate implant placement with PRF pressed membrane.

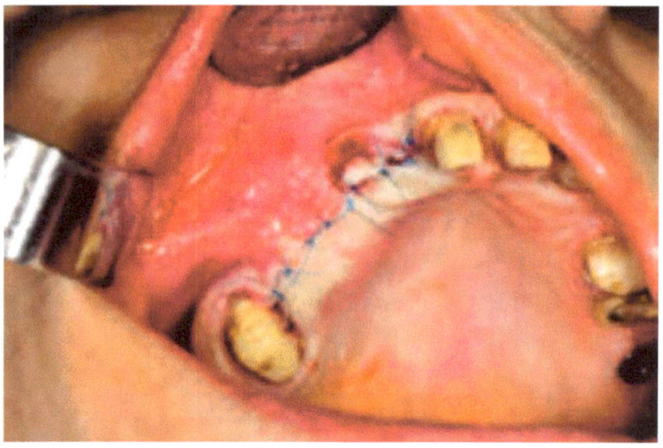

Figure 10.159. Alveolar ridge augmentation with extruded PRF membrane mixed with bone substitutes.

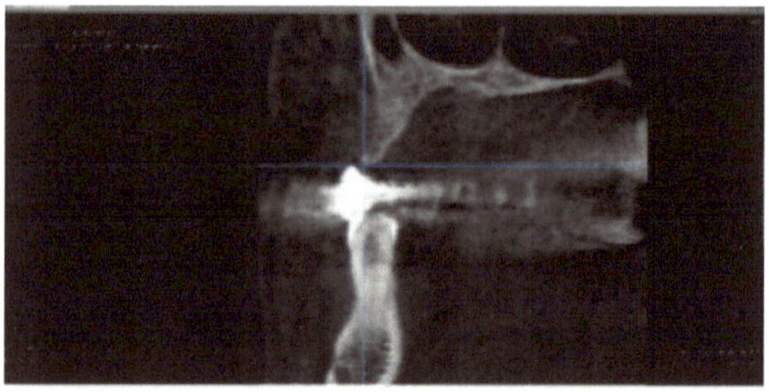

Figure 10.160. Appearance of the resorbed part of the alveolar ridge bone Before applying PRF, a mixture is made by grinding the PRF membrane with bone substitute, ready for placement.

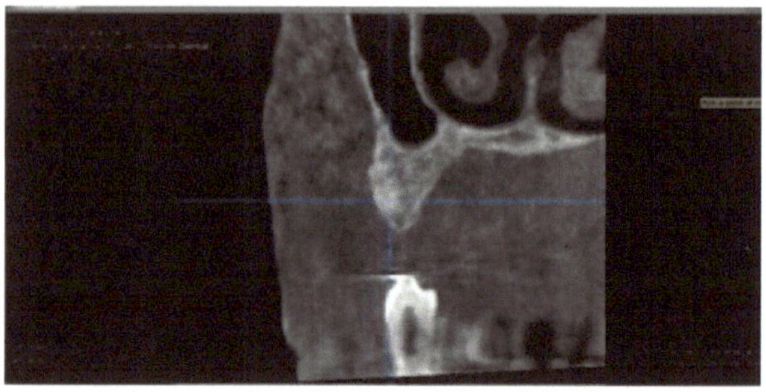

Figure 10.161. After placement of PRF, the crushed membrane mixed with bone substitutes.

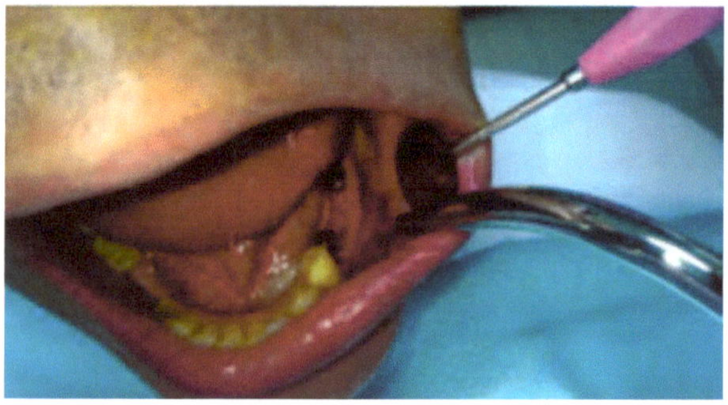

Figure 10.162. Appearance of a narrow alveolar ridge.

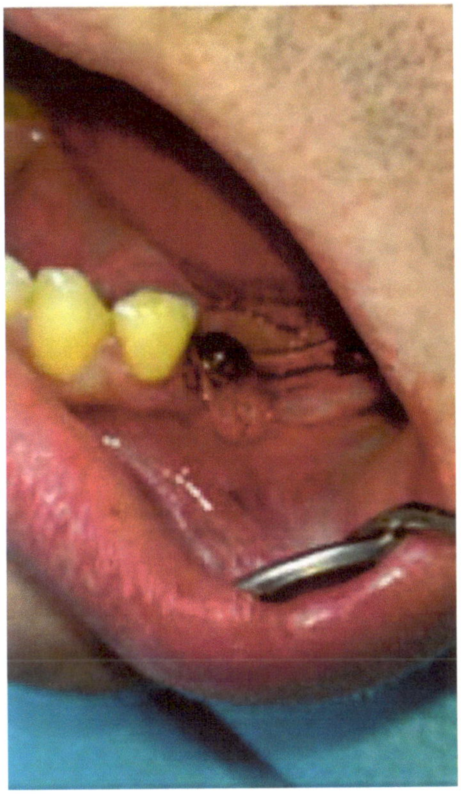

Figure 10.163. PRF membrane ready for placement around immediately placed implants with alveolar ridge augmentation.

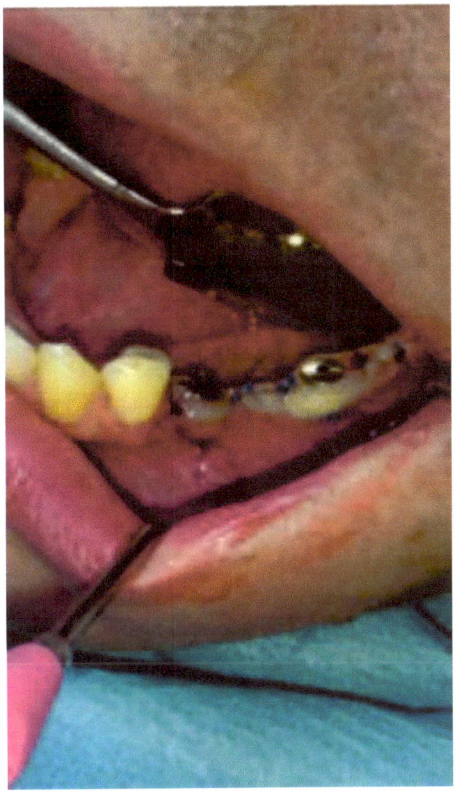

Figure 10.164. Increasing the dimensions of the bone ridge vertically and horizontally.

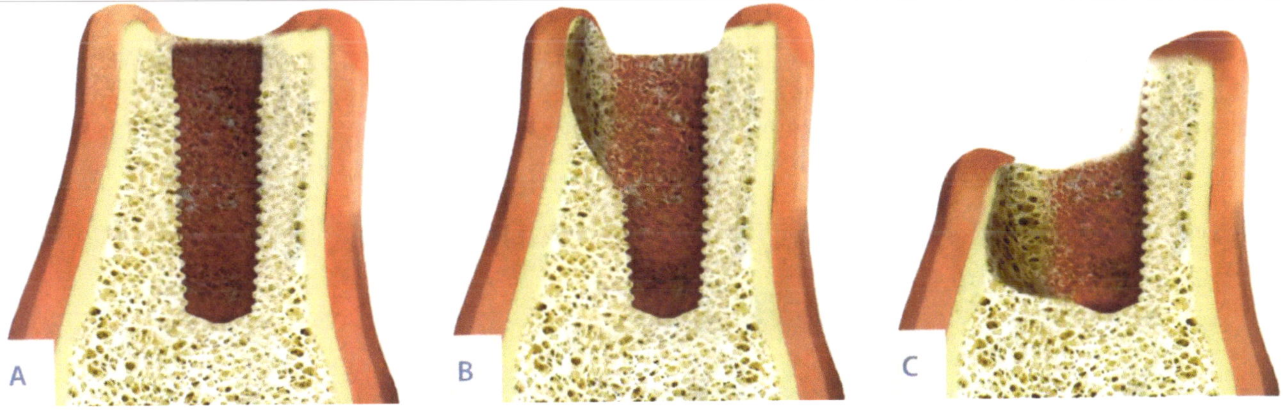

Figure 10.165. Schematic representation of defect shapes and defect augmentation procedures using the PRGF method. a) Vertical bone loss. Treatment procedure is insertion of a new implant of a wider diameter. b) Crater-shaped bone defect. Treatment procedure, retain the implant, perform defect augmentation with a bone substitute covered with a collagen resorbable membrane. c) Larger horizontal bone defect. Treatment procedure, perform bone defect augmentation with a bone substitute covered with a collagen resorbable membrane, wait at least 6 months before implantation.

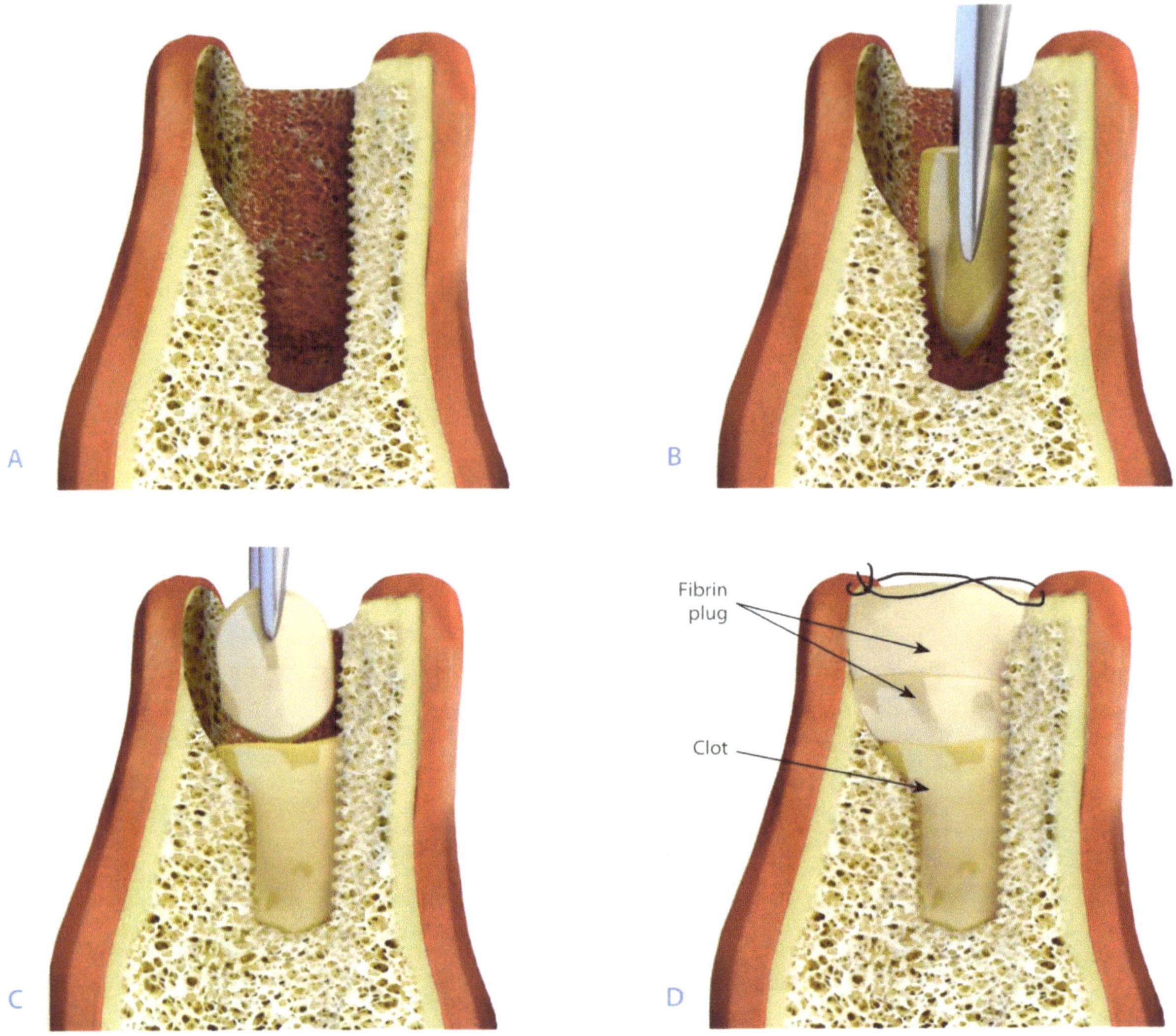

Figure 10.166. a) site after implant explantation. b) placement of a collet at the bottom of the site. c) placement of a fibrin collet obtained by fractionation. d) The placed fibrin and PRGF collet will result in regeneration of the bone defect for safe implant placement (Figure 10.172). (Source: E.Anitua)

CLINICAL CASE

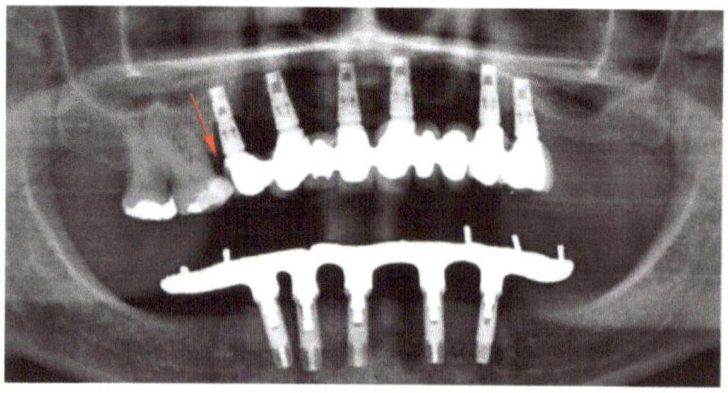

Figure 10.167. Peri-implantitis region #15

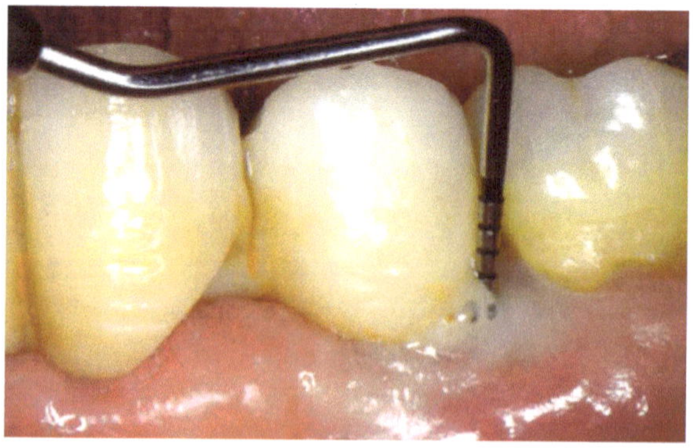

Figure 10.168. Probing diagnosed a peri-implant pocket with suppuration 10 mm deep - Implant explantation performed.

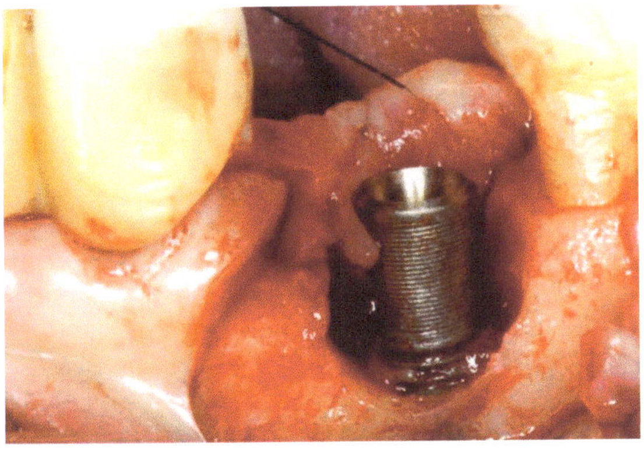

Figure 10.169. Appearance of the condition after flap elevation. Removal of granulation content and treatment of the implant surface with titanium brushes.

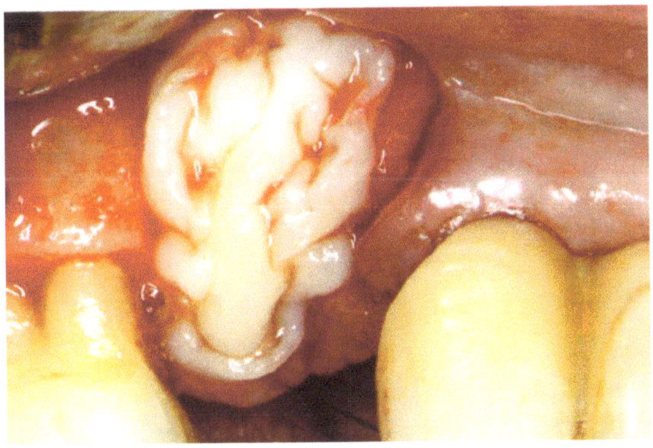

Figure 10.170. Illustration of a placed PRGF graft for bone defect regeneration.

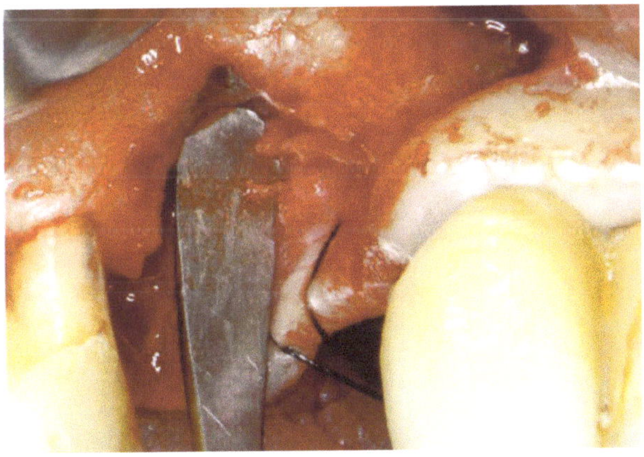

Figure 10.171. View of the regenerated defect after 6 months.

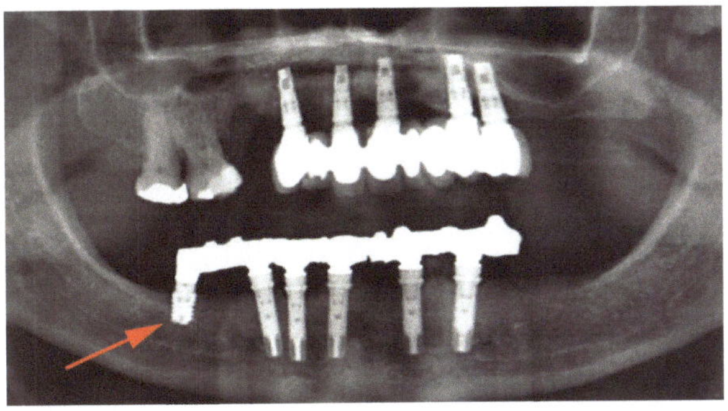

Figure 10.172. View of regenerated bone in region #15. In the lower lateral region (red arrow). implanted implant with a wide diameter of 6mm and a length of 8mm. Reconstruction of the prosthetic work was performed by shortening the hanging member, eliminating the biomechanical risk factor.

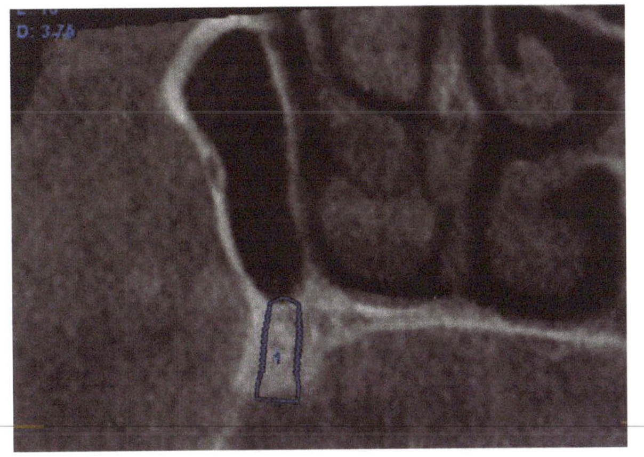

Figure 10.173. CT scan of a fully regenerated bone defect. Conditions created for safe placement of a larger diameter implant.

Conclusion: Finis Opus Coronat

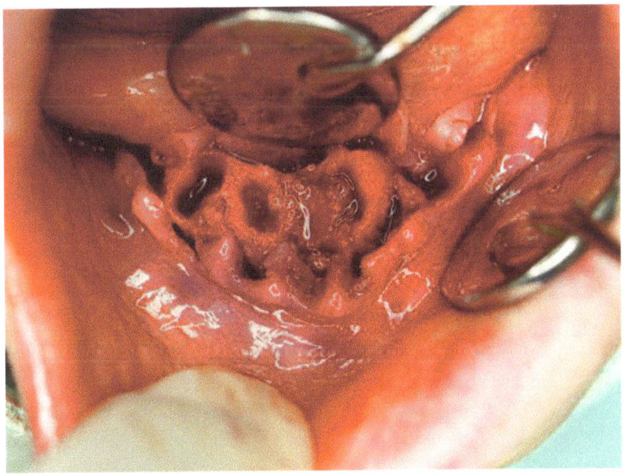

Figure 10.174. Major bone defects make implant-prosthetic rehabilitation extremely complex. Replacement of the lost bone is the first step of the set treatment plan, and for the predictability of the outcome, the experience is dominant.

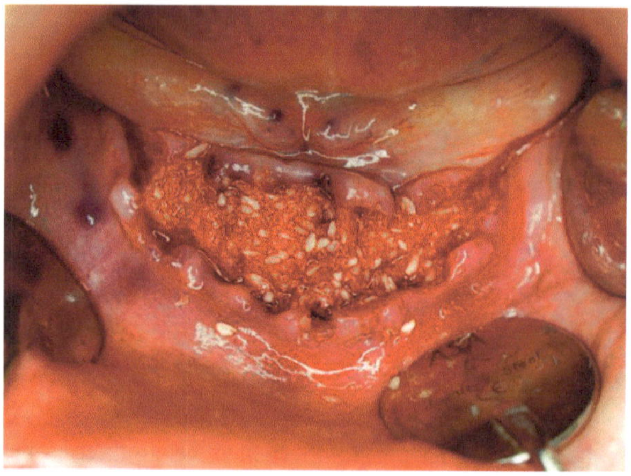

Figure 10.175. Bone substitute augmentation mixed with autologous bone filings. Replacement of lost bone is the basis of the predicted outcome of implant-prosthetic rehabilitation.

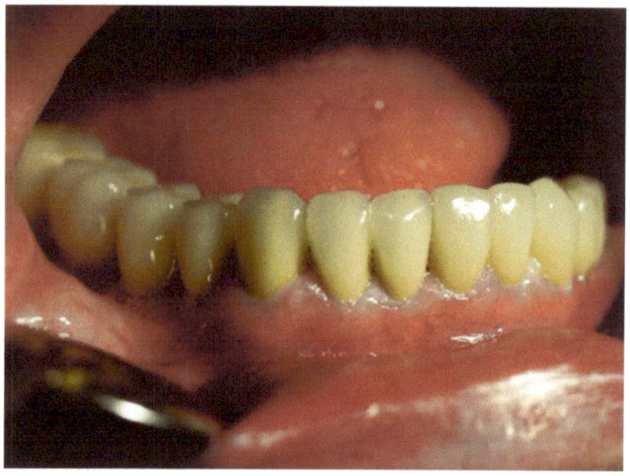

Figure 10.176. Overview of the situation after 24 months. Extensive augmentation restored the arch of the alveolar bone with extremely high quality bone support, which resulted in stable healing of soft tissues around the implanted implants and good bone integration.

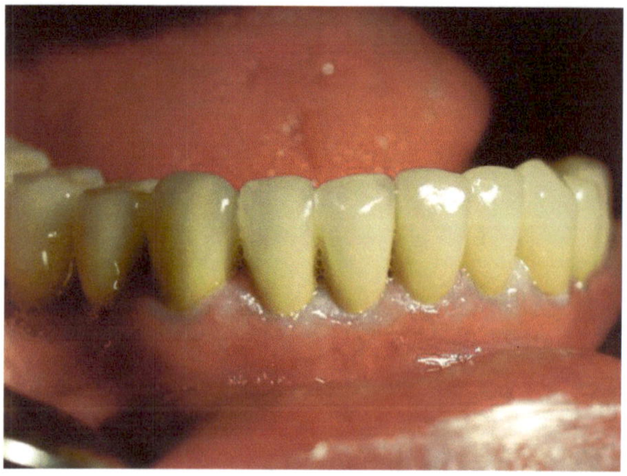

Figure 10.177. The patient also contributed significantly to the successful outcome, by trusting patience and maintaining oral hygiene. Overview of the situation after one year (work of T. Zlopaša and B. Zlopaša).

Postoperative complications of augmentation

Postoperative complications of augmentation can be hematoma and candidiasis.

Hematoma can manifest in the oral cavity, face, and neck (Figure 10.1).

The manifestation of hematomas on the face and neck is an aesthetic problem. In the oral cavity, they are manifested by blueness of the mucous membrane and pain. The pain can be intense with difficulty swallowing.

The postoperative complication of augmentation is manifested in the oral cavity by a fungal disease, candidiasis (Candida albicans), characterized by pain and soft deposits on the tongue, mucous membrane of the oral cavity, on the gums. It can manifest itself on the pharynx with white deposits. Deposits are most pronounced on the tongue. Removing white deposits on the tongue by scraping is a painful procedure with consequences of tongue bleeding. Candidiasis is accompanied by a decrease in immunity. Candida albicans is present in the mouth in minimal amounts. If cnadidiasis is not treated immediately, it can turn into a chronic condition with tendencies to spread to the digestive tract and is very resistant to treatment.

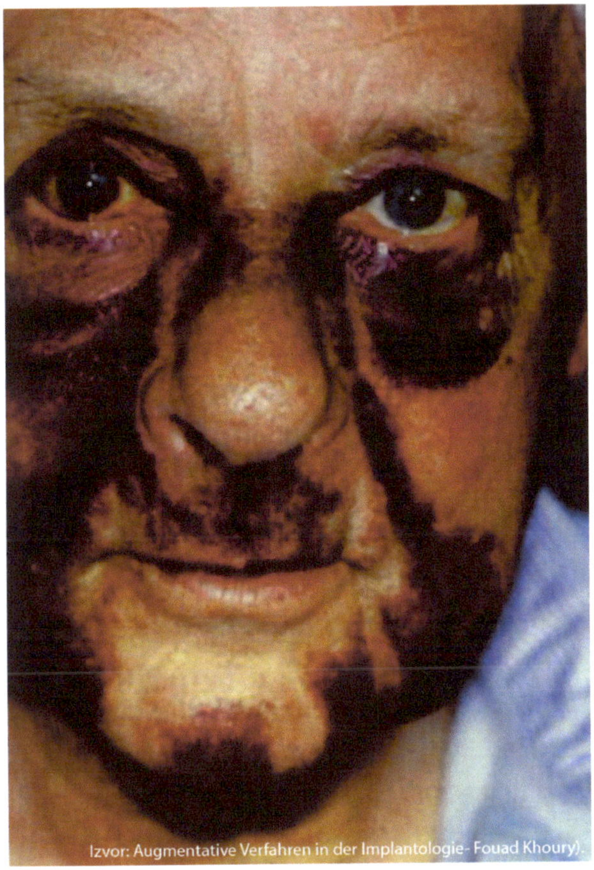

Figure 10.178. Postoperative complication of augmentation, hematomas manifested on the face. Aesthetic problem.

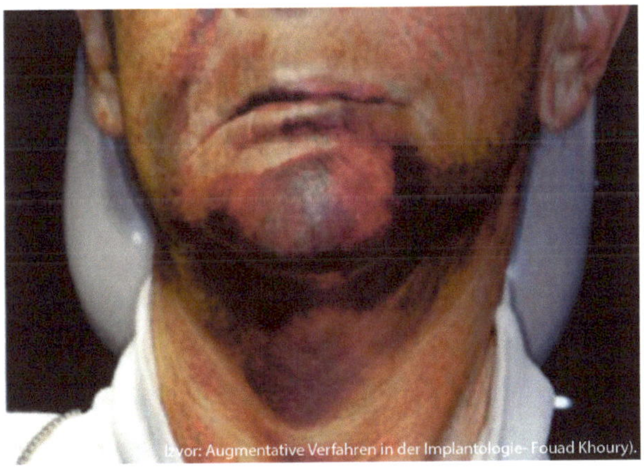

Figure 10.179. Postoperative complications of augmentation: formation of a hematoma with manifestations on the face, chin, extended and on the neck.

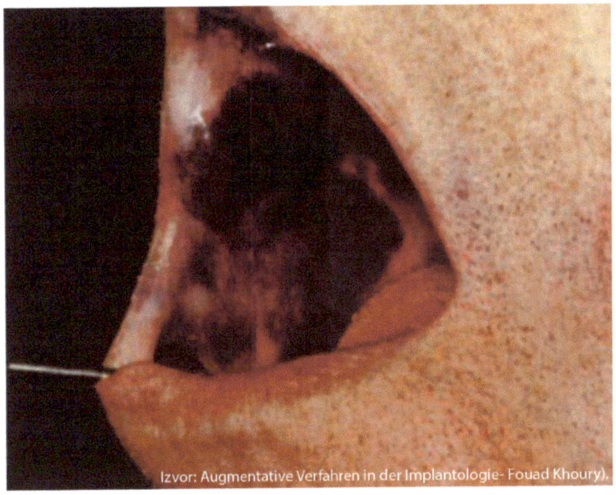

Figure 10.180. Postoperative complications of augmentation with the manifestation of hematoma in the oral cavity, affecting the mucous membrane of the oral cavity, tongue, pharynx, and can also affect the respiratory organs. Difficulty swallowing. Urgent therapy is indicated.

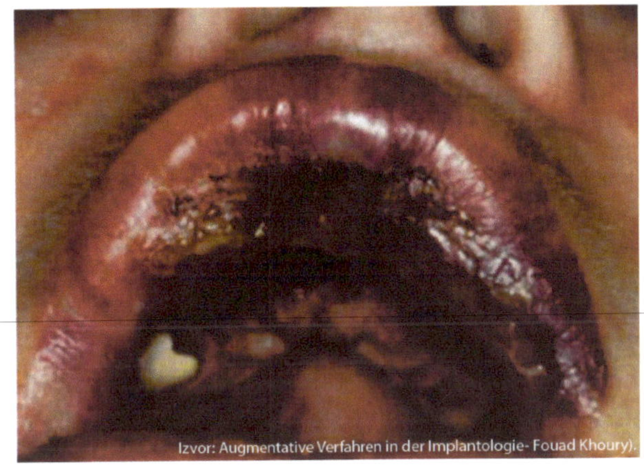

Figure 10.181. Hematoma manifested after augmentation.

11

Importance Of Biomechanical Laws In Oral Implantology

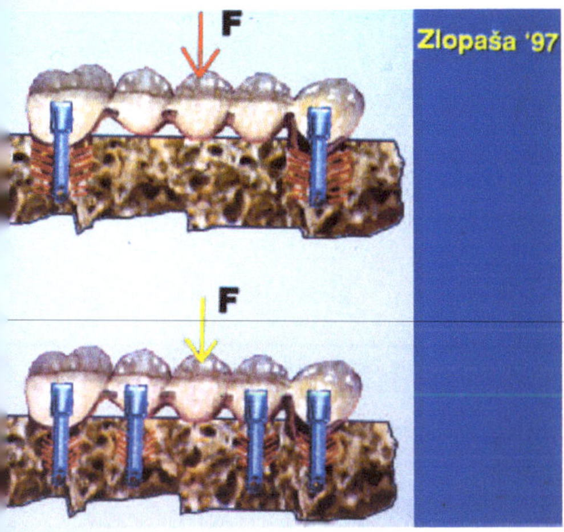

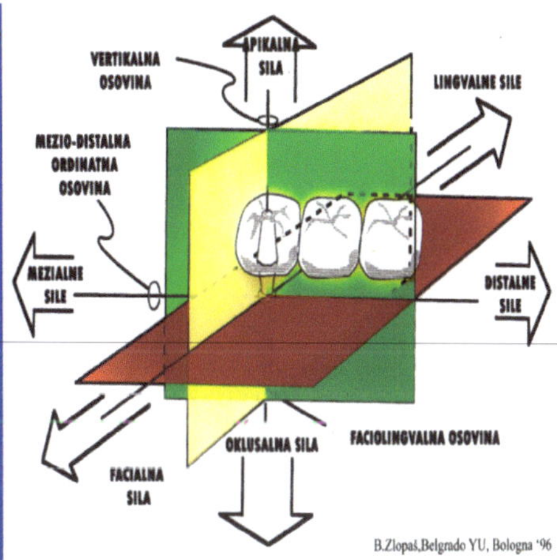

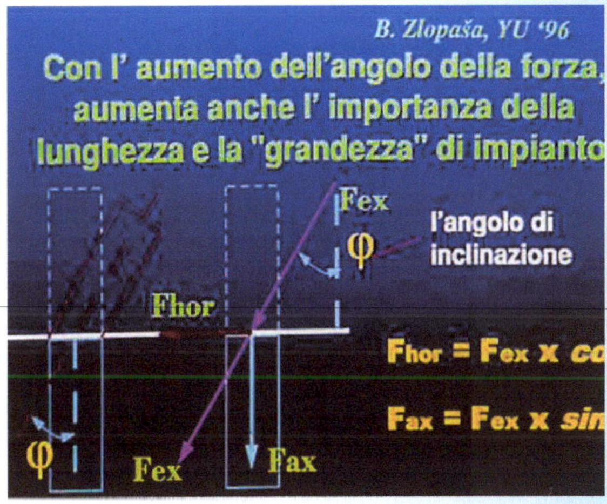

Biomechanical considerations in oral implantology largely follow simple mechanical rules, which are based on the principle of leverage and the initial, primary, anchoring of the implant in dense bone or bone of poor quality, i.e. well or badly chosen bone. Knowledge of these simple mechanical rules enables the implantologist practitioner to make a correct assessment. It facilitates the achievement of several important factors, for example: primary stability, strategic positioning of the implant, a better understanding of the functional behavior in the oral cavity, limiting habits, (bruxism) and the like. The primary value of the implant is the quality of the material from which it is made (grade of titanium quality) and the technology used to process its surface. The speed and quality of the integration process largely depend on the technology used to process the surface of the implant made of biocompatible material. Good bony integration of the implant and the bone makes the implant completely replace the role of the natural tooth. Assuming the role of natural teeth, implants are exposed to the action of different forces to which natural teeth are exposed, and this factor should be taken into account so that eventual failure is not explained by lay explanations, such as "bad integration" or "rejection" of the implant.

Many reasons lead to implant failure and even loss of integrated implants after a certain time. It happens that even with implants that initially showed good fixation and a high degree of bone integration, subsequent overloading of the implant compromises the entire project. Around the implants where there was good bone and a solid connection with it, the first symptoms of peri-implantitis appeared, which would be followed by loosening and loss of the implant with a significant loss of bone around the implant. From the above, it can be concluded that many complications and failures of implant installation are the result of poor planning and excessive loading of the implant by poor prosthetic work.

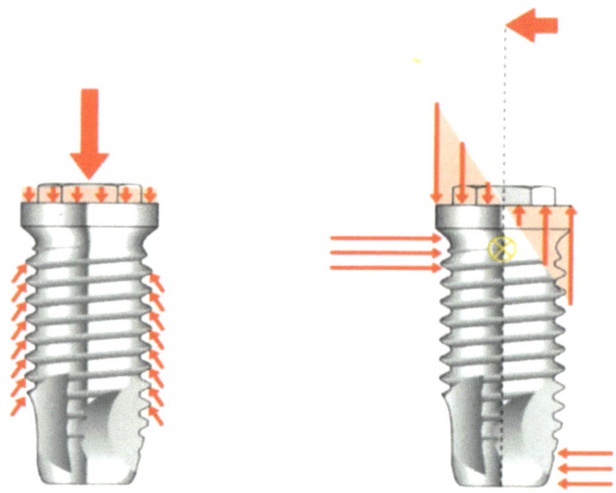

Figure 11.1. Action of forces on the implant. a. Axial force; b. horizontal force.

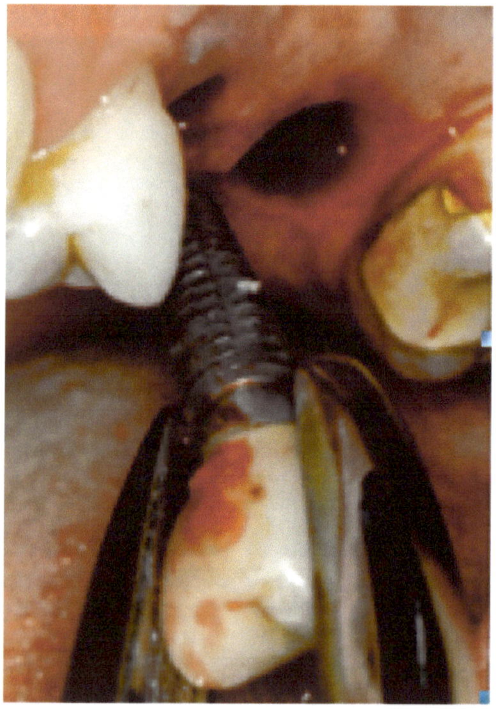

Figure 11.2. The reasons for implant loss should be sought in overheating of the bone during preparation, as well as biomechanical imbalance due to the influence of unfavorable forces and their moments on the bone. The surface of the extracted implant in the picture shows that no bony integration has been achieved.

Most often, the implant is lost without any pain or other clinical symptoms, characteristic of inflammatory pathology. (Figure 11.2).

If the axial force acts along the axis of the implant (Figure 11.1a), the stress of the forces around the implant will be evenly distributed, and thus will be distributed on the threads around the neck of the implant. If, on the other hand, the forces act in a horizontal direction, then there is an attack moment on the bone (Figure 11.1b). The moment of force is the product of the force and the arm on which it acts (M = F x L) - the greater the force (F), the greater the moment; likewise, the longer the arm (L) on which the force acts, the greater the torque. The greater the length of the installed implant, the less stress from the bending moment, i.e. transverse, unfavorable forces on the bone.

The majority of experienced doctors noticed that the reason for the occurrence of peri-implantitis in a large percentage was not the result of accumulated plaque, but the effect of unfavorable chewing forces directly on the implant.

Non-observance of biomechanical requirements, i.e. the principle of breaking down the received chewing forces, causes excessive stress on the bone and surrounding tissues, manifesting later in the loss of the implant.

In a natural tooth, the biomechanical laws are harmonized in the way that nature itself did it. Due to this alignment, as well as the elasticity of the connection between the teeth and the bone, the pressure of the load is transmitted evenly. In such a balance of load reception, each tooth, individually, receives and carries its part of the load, and through the contact points, the pressure is distributed evenly. When a tooth is lost, whether one or more teeth, the biomechanical and biostatic balance is disturbed. In the classic method of replacing lost teeth, their role is taken over by adjacent teeth-replacement carriers. When one tooth is lost, especially in the lateral region, one supporting tooth cannot take over the role of the adjacent one, i.e. of a lost tooth, as in the case of a "suspension bridge", the second tooth must be included in the prosthetic construction as the anchor point of the future bridge, due to biomechanical laws - to exclude the effect of the lever. For this reason, replacing a lost tooth with an implant is fully justified.

Is bacterial plaque the primary cause of peri-implantitis and implant loss?

Bacterial plaque is one of the primary causes of periodontal decay and natural tooth loss. On the other hand, it should be pointed out that the experience of the author of the book and a careful study of the literature show that the primary clinical connection between the accumulation of bacterial plaque around the implant supports, i.e. the neck of the implant, and the loss of the implant has not been proven. Only a small number of clinical trials show a relationship between minor peri-implant bone loss and bacterial plaque build-up.

Many implantologists have investigated the causes of implant loss, analyzing their cases; it was observed that a third of the placed implants (34%) are lost in places where the bone structure is less favorable - type 4 bones.

Overload: the primary risk factor

Many authors, based on personal experience, have come to the conclusion that overloading is the primary reason for bone loss around implants. Most of the conclusions prove that overloading is the most serious risk factor that compromises the integration of bone and implant.

Variable biomechanical effects

Variable biomechanical effects that cause occlusal overloads are conditioned by various factors:

- bone base (quality and quantity);
- implant post - abutment (length, surface diameter, slope, geometry, number and position);
- prosthetic typology (fixed, movable, partial, materials);
- occlusal function (muscular activity, macroglossia, dysfunction);
- parafunctions, antagonists and inter-jaw relations.

Scientific data on the mutual interaction of these factors and their interaction with the bone base are still very limited.

For the above reasons, the question arises whether when making fixed prosthetic work, the implant supports should be loaded with the extension that forms the arm of the lever.

The intensity of unfavorable masticatory forces on the implant itself depends on the length of the extension (lever arm) and contact with the antagonists. By increasing the angle at which the force acts, the force acting on the implant also increases, which is compensated by the length and diameter of the implant, which is shown schematically in Figure 11.3 (from the lecture at the World Congress of Implantologists in Bologna).

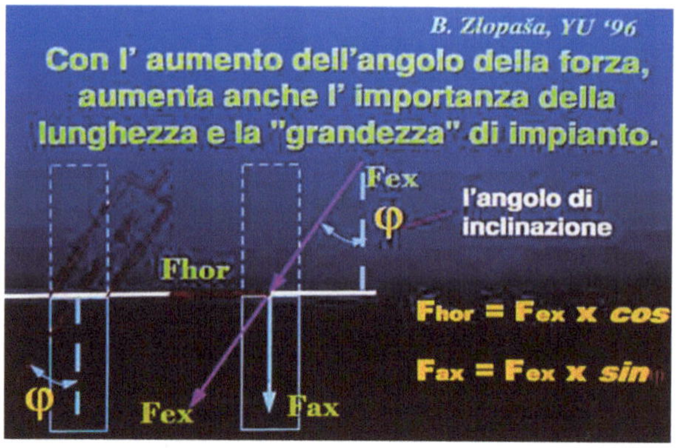

Figure 11.3. By increasing the angle of action of the force, the importance of the length and width of the implant increases. The greater the force angle, the greater the shear force at the same force intensity. A force acting at an angle increases its intensity. Horizontal forces that load the implant at an angle cause adverse stretching forces.

Respecting biomechanical principles, with strict control of the occlusal scheme and contacts, fulfilling the prerequisites to position the implants parallel, without tilting the supports, can significantly reduce possible adverse loads. The schematic diagram (Figure 11.3) shows one of the important biomechanical requirements: the length and diameter of the implant depend on the angle at which chewing forces act.

Complications caused by biomechanical reasons

Complications caused by biomechanical reasons are most often manifested at an early stage. Therefore, it is most important to consider load control during the initial period, to prevent further weakening of the bone's properties as a support for the implant bed. It is necessary to indicate and remove unfavorable occlusal factors, thus meeting the biomechanical requirements and establishing the implant-bone balance. This allows faster bone recovery. To achieve this, all previous information must be used to adequately design the implant reconstruction. First, the diameter and length of the implant are taken into account from a biomechanical point of view. First of all, we need to visualize the design of the future final prosthetic reconstruction - its dimensions and occlusal contacts in function. It is necessary to take into account anatomical limitations, which will affect the number and position of implants, which must be harmonized with biomechanical requirements. The balance between wishes and the ability to fulfill all biomechanical requirements must be observed in the earliest phase of implantological treatment planning.

During the design process, an experienced implantologist can predict, identify, and evaluate different risk factors and see the effect of their action on each of them.

It is necessary to think and predict, to plan such a prosthetic construction that can enable a possible change of the treatment plan, for example, by adding one more implant or adjusting the prosthetic work and occlusal scheme in a given case.

If complications appear after the implant treatment, the biomechanical risk factors should be considered again, in great detail, and the entire treatment should be adapted to the given situation to eliminate the causes of the problem.

If overload occurs, warning signs should be noticed before complications lead to failure. Warning signs should not be ignored, but, on the contrary, with great care, analyze and discover the causes of the warning and know how to solve the resulting problem. For example, in practice, it happens that the therapist is not at home: has the thread weakened, or has the screw loosened, or has the thread fractured, the prosthetic structure loosened, or has the implant loosened: an intraoral recording will help determine one of the above causes.

It is not enough to strengthen or replace weakened components, it is much more important to determine the cause of the resulting complication and eliminate the reasons for their existence in time. The opposite view can lead to even greater failure. By observing the risk factors from a biomechanical point of view, the specific situation can be modified: by removing the hanging members, adding new implants, modifying the occlusion and reducing the non-physiological stress on the implants.

Biomechanical risk factors can be classified into four types:

1. **geometric risk factor** - the number of implants, their position and the geometry of the prosthetic work;
2. **occlusal risk factor** - lateral contacts with enormous movements of the mandible and dysfunctional habits;
3. **risk factor of bone** - implant relationship - reliance on newly formed bone and absence of good primary stability, incorrect choice of implant diameter, which is significantly smaller than it should be. Or, if a wide-diameter implant is surrounded by an insufficient amount of bone, which jeopardizes all the physiological processes of that part of the bone;
4. **technological risk factor** - lack of compliance with the prosthetic solution (appropriate size of the crown, height, size of the occlusal surface) and the method of fixing the prosthetic superstructure.

Signs of overload: Recognizing the symptoms of overload during clinical function is extremely important to prevent complications that would cause implant loss.

The presence of a large number of these factors manifests itself as a risky situation for the implant itself, prosthetic work or both.

Geometric risk factors and biomechanical requirements

Risk factors:

- number of implants;
- using implants with a wide diameter;
- connecting the implant with the natural tooth;
- placement of implants in a tripod configuration;
- presence of added hanging members - negative effect of leverage;
- implants placed for the retention of the prosthesis;
- presence of retention clips (buttons);
- implants used for the retention of dentures with telescopic crowns;
- excessive height of the prosthetic reconstruction - crown and body of the bridge.

Number and arrangement of implants

In order to meet the biomechanical requirements, the number of implants is very important. The ideal number of implants in a given clinical situation depends on the set plan (Figure 11.4):

a) whether implants are installed in case of total or partial toothlessness;
b) whether the prosthetic restoration will be anchored only on implants;
c) whether the prosthetic restoration will be anchored on implants and connected to natural teeth;
d) when connecting implants to natural teeth, the number of implants depends not only on the number of remaining teeth, but also on the type and quality of the teeth, that is, on the state of the periodontium.

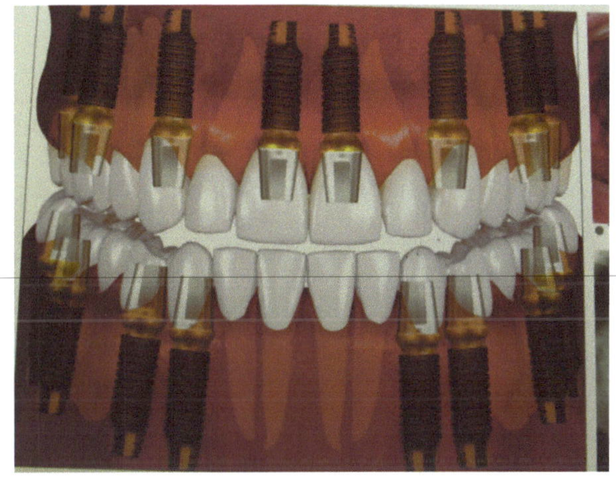

Figure 11.4. The future of the entire implant procedure depends on the number of implants, arrangement and occlusal compliance.

Application of implants with a wide surface area

By using implants with a wider surface, the mechanical properties are increased, because a greater resistance is created to the chewing forces that are transmitted to the bone. However, if wide-diameter implants are applied in the lateral region of the lower jaw, if the implant is not surrounded by a sufficient amount of bone, due to poor vascularization, accelerated marginal bone resorption and overloading of the implant, and even its loss, may occur, especially if during installation performed and minimal thermal trauma to the bone.

One of the most important conditions for good bone integration is primary stability. If the implant is primarily stable, with the added value that the implant's surface in contact with the bone is treated with the best technology, there will be a faster apposition of the newly formed bone tissue around the implant. Primary stability can be achieved with a detailed surgical protocol and bicortical implant positioning. In partially edentulous regions, it is often difficult to achieve primary stability due to poor bone quantity and quality. To avoid this problem, in practice, the conception method of using a wide-diameter implant is often proposed, whose larger volume can better activate the cortical bone, and such a choice is also favorable from a biomechanical point of view. Even today, however, there are different opinions, without fundamental scientific clinical data, regarding the real benefits of using wide-diameter implants.

It is not uncommon to think that implants with a diameter greater than 4.6 mm should not be inserted where the bone has sufficient length (Figure 11.5).

Why?

In a natural tooth, good blood supply is supported by the periosteum, the periodontal artery and the artery of the apex of the tooth, because that part has the best blood supply. That blood supply is somewhere around nine tenths in the spongy bone component, and a very small part, one tenth, in the cortical part of the bone. Apart from mechanical immobility at the beginning of the stability assessment, and in order to support it with possible augmentation of any type, the presence of sufficient blood supply is very important.

In oral implant surgery, in places where the periodontal artery is missing, the blood supply is supported only by the periosteum and blood vessels of the alveolar ridge. That is why it is important to have a favorable relationship between the bone density and the diameter of the implant diameter: only essential periosteal blood supply and adequate cancellous bone density can guarantee the establishment of biological exchange, the establishment of homeostasis necessary for tissue healing. With a natural tooth, we have good homeostasis, but by our actions we must establish a homeostatic balance of the milieu where the implant lies.

Implants of the widest diameter can be used in cases where we have sufficient width and a small height of the alveolar ridge (Figure 11.6).

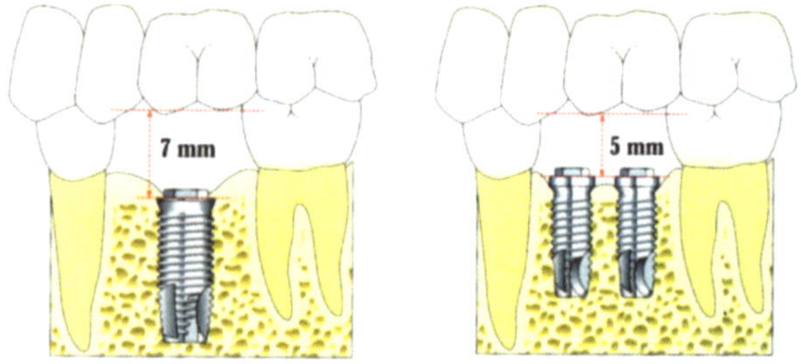

Figure 11.5. The ideal minimum height with antagonists must not be less than 7mm. In places where the relationship with the antagonists is less than 5 mm, increase the number of implants of standard diameters.

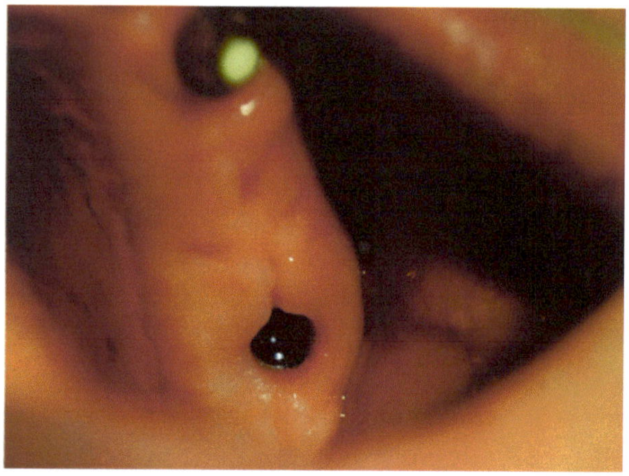

Figure 11.6. The use of the tuber due to the reception of masticatory forces requires implants with wider diameters.

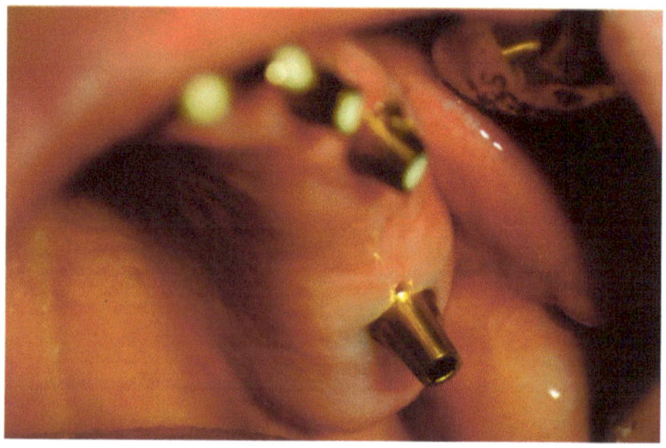

Figure 11.7. Od planiranja protetskog rada, njegove izvedbe, okluzalnih površina i bočnih kretnji donje vilice, zavisiće prijem i razlaganje sila žvakanja. Široki dijametar protivteža transverzalnim nepovoljnim silama i momentima tih sila.

Biomechanical consideration of implant diameter

In deciding which diameter to choose, a certain amount of spongiosa in the vestibular and oral parts must always be taken into account. This parameter of the amount of bone also determines the diameter of the implant. In patients with a thin bone ridge or a mesiodistal space of less than 7 mm, it is preferable to use an implant with a slightly smaller diameter.

This attitude is justified, not only to obtain good primary stability necessary for a faster and favorable reparative process at the point of contact between the bone and the surface of the implant, but also that, from a biomechanical point of view, there is a counterbalance to the possible occurrence of transverse adverse forces (Figure 11.7).. It happens that potential problems with the bone are overlooked in the pre-surgical planning, which is noted during the installation of the implant itself, after which it is necessary to perform an augmentation of only a few millimeters, with the placement of a membrane, using abundant periosteal blood supply.

In cases where there is a dilemma as to which diameter to choose, for example in the area of molars, it must be taken into account that the occlusal forces are the strongest in that place. Likewise, replacing a canine with a narrow-diameter implant is a wrong decision.

Choosing a wide-diameter implant in places where the anatomical bone quantity conditions are not favorable, and there is insufficient interdental space, or insufficient height in relation to the antagonists, can be a wrong decision from a biomechanical point of view. A single implant, with the possibility of the widest diameter, does not rehabilitate the existing crown-root relationship (Figures 11.8-11.10). Since the task of the implant is to replace the missing natural root, in cases where the mesiodistal space is wide due to the movement of adjacent teeth, from the aspect of biomechanics, the most logical solution is to replace the molar roots with two implants of a narrower or standard diameter (3.25 mm) and , if possible, perform immediate loading with a provisional crown made of soft material (acrylate). The assessment of which load will be applied depends on the experience of the doctor.

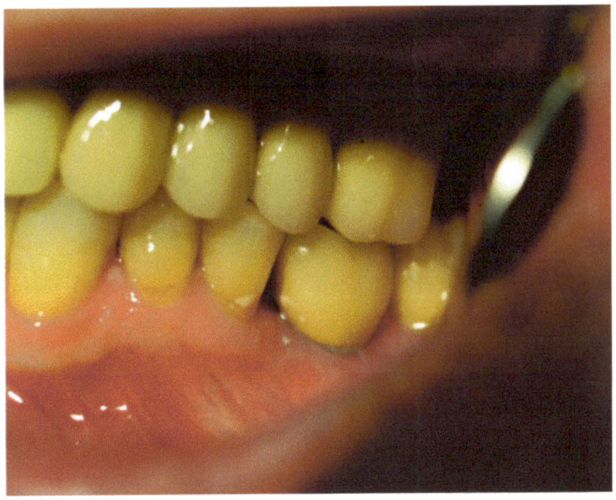

Figure 11.8. A narrow alveolar ridge and mesiodistal space determine the implant type, length and diameter.

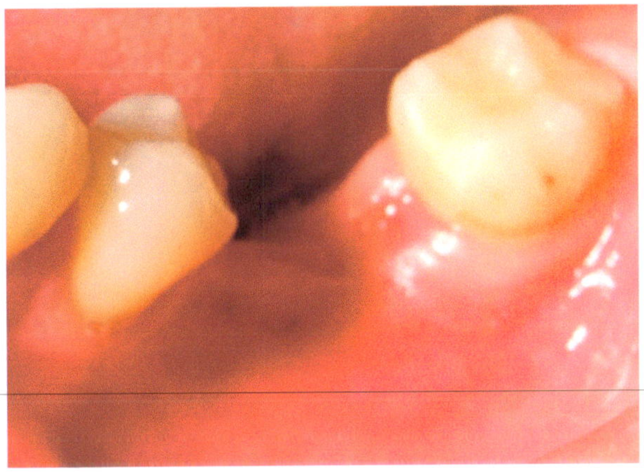

Figure 11.9. From a biomechanical point of view, in the case shown in the previous picture, the installation of two implants with a diameter of 3 mm may be a more favorable solution.

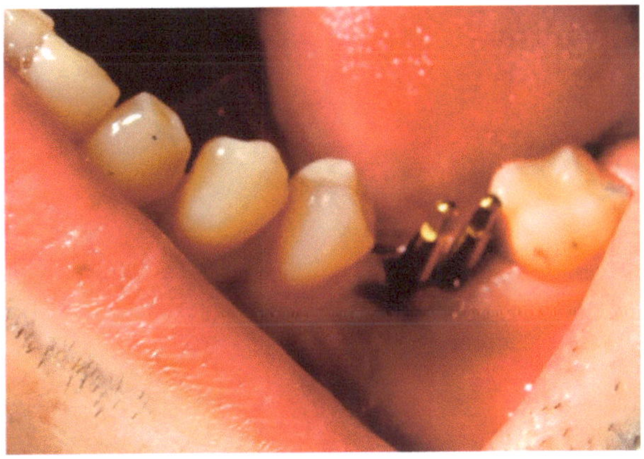

Figure 11.10. Alignment of occlusal events also stimulates the integration of the implant with the bone.

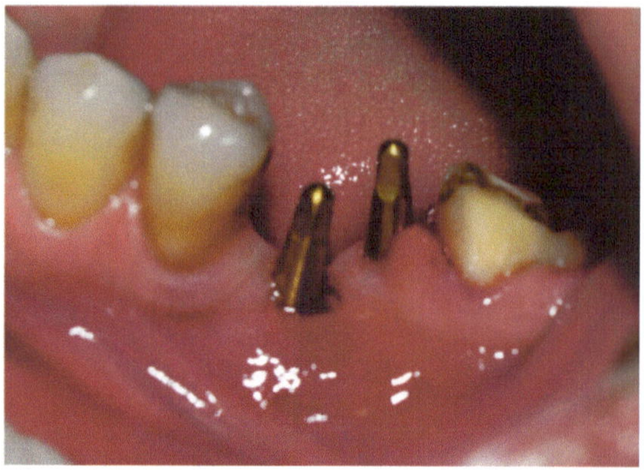

Figure 11.11. Installation of two implants without raising the flap. Tomographic indicators of the width and height of available bone were missing.

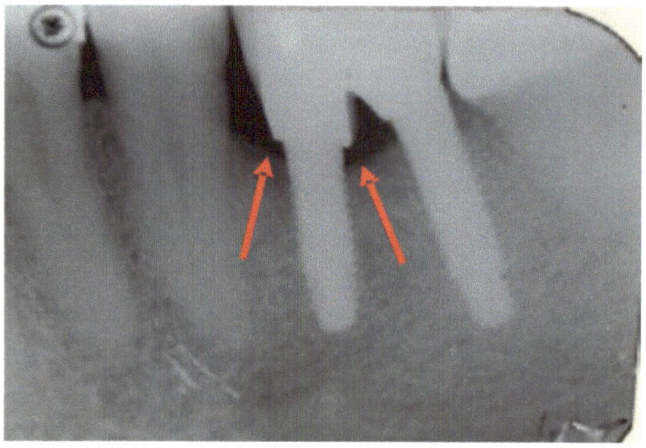

Figure 11.12. Implants of narrow and standard diameters in the lower jaw - control image after 6 years.

Bone resorption around the implant in region 36 in Figure 11.12 is caused by crown edge protrusion and plaque deposition. There is no bone resorption in region 36.

The situation in the mouth depends mostly on the prosthetic solution, which includes the installation of implants, but with respect for biomechanical laws (Figure 11.14).

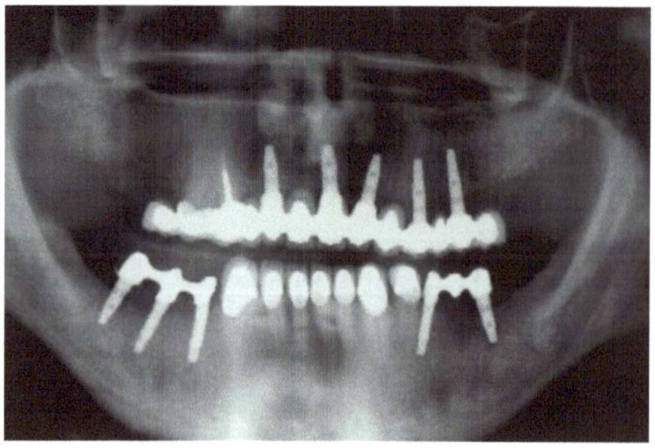

Figure 11.14. The state of the existing teeth determines the prosthetic rehabilitation plan and bonding with implants without the addition of hanging members. In the upper jaw, on the left side, a hanging member was added for aesthetic reasons, and due to the lack of an antagonist, it has no effect on the reception of chewing forces. On the right side, adding one member and bonding with the remaining teeth can be the wrong combination. Embedded implants in region 16 and 17 after sinus lifting.

The length of the crown is determined by the vertical distance between the occlusal plane and the tip of the residual alveolar ridge. The greater the vertical bone resorption, the longer the length of the crown will be, and the length of the implant will be shorter, which is unfavorable from a biomechanical point of view, but can be compensated for by choosing a wider implant diameter, or vice versa.

The most favorable relationship is where the maximum height of the alveolar ridge is maintained, when the most favorable relationship between the length of the crown and the body of the implant can be restored; that the body of the implant lying in the bone should be twice as long as the length of the crown. In this case, the adverse effect of horizontal rotating forces and their moments on the implant body is reduced. A 1:1 ratio is tolerable, and if the ratio of the clinical crown to the implant body is greater in favor of the clinical crown than the 1:1 ratio, the action of the moment of force through the lever arm will cause an increase in inclination, twisting and rotation of the implant body around its axis, resulting in accelerated loss of the implant.

For example, in cases where the alveolar ridge is between three and four millimeters wide and of sufficient height, above 12 mm, 15 or above 18 mm, it is not possible to install an implant with a standard diameter of 3.5 mm or 3.75 mm, because it would fenestration of the implant thread occurred either from the vestibular or oral side. When fenestration occurs, the primary stability is insufficient, so an additional surgical procedure is necessary with the installation of a bone substitute with bioactive membranes, which prolongs the healing time and thus the bone integration process. This procedure also increases the cost of the intervention. In such cases, the subsequent biomechanical events after the healing period during mastication, the reception and dissipation of forces, must be strictly taken into account.

The use of implants with a reduced diameter (3 mm) is advantageous for narrow and high alveolar ridges, because they contain less cancellous bone, which enables better primary stability of the implant. Misch and Judi (1990) stated that narrow alveolar ridges are compact (most often bone type D2) and favorable for the installation of reduced-diameter implants and for immediate loading (Figures 11.15-11.20).

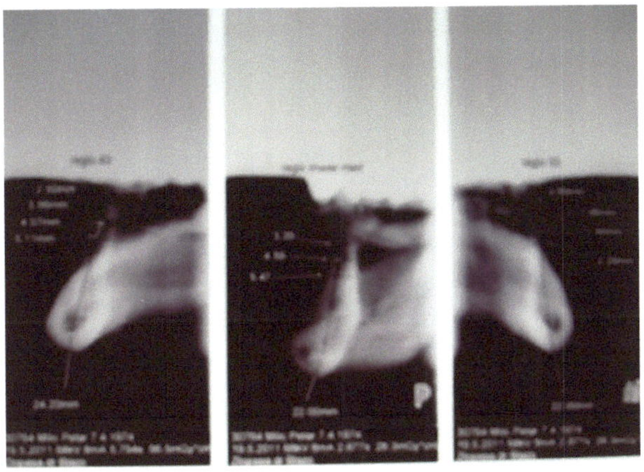

Figure 11.15. Details of the tomographic analysis of the patient shown in the following images.

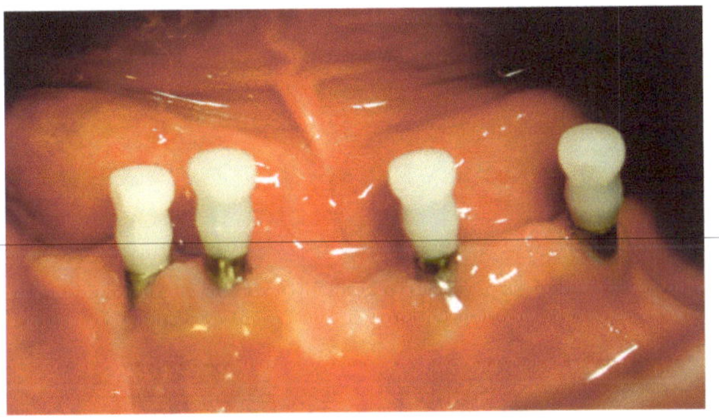

Figure 11.16. Unfavorable conditions due to premature tooth loss (34-year-old patient) narrow the indications for the restoration method.

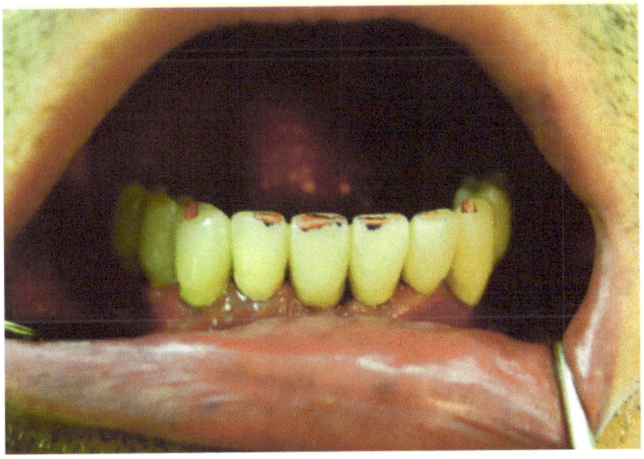

Figure 11.17. There are two possibilities: a total acrylate prosthesis on the atrophied ridge or fixed work (which was the express request of the patient).

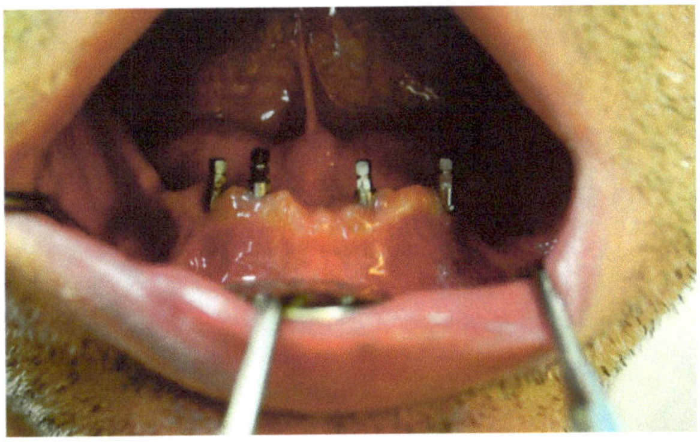

Figure 11.18. The only possible solution - application of implants with narrow diameters and maximum lengths (18 mm).

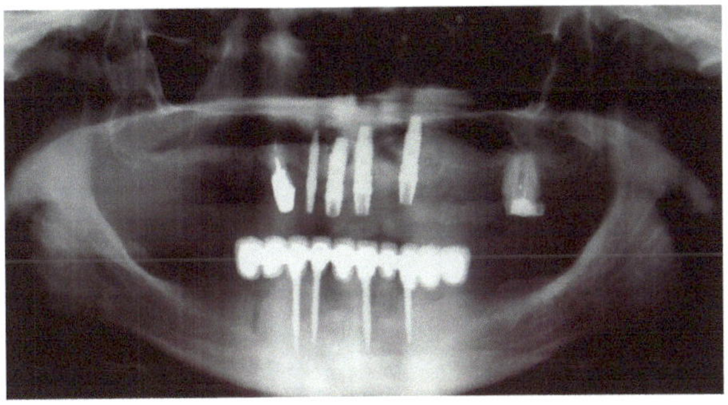

Figure 11.19. Risk - remaining teeth and eventual fracture of the implant. Fulfilled patient requirements. Suggested replacement of remaining teeth with implants.

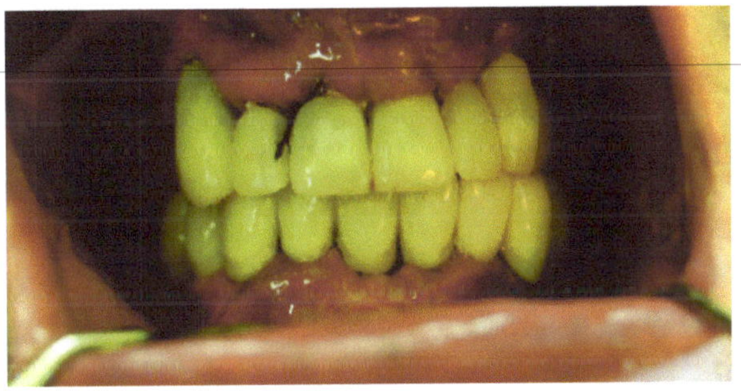

Figure 11.20. The therapy plan is determined by the patient's financial situation.

The suitability for achieving good primary stability of the implant is the proximity of the vestibular and oral cortex. The decrease in the height of the alveolar bone, which occurs due to the resorption of the alveolar ridge, causes an apparent increase in the width of the alveolar ridge. The author's experience confirms that more cancellous bone is present in the wider part of the alveolar ridge, which reduces the possibility of achieving good primary stability of the implant. In that case, if the biomechanical requirements for the even reception and distribution of chewing forces are not met, the integration processes will be endangered. For this reason, the mentioned parameters, in certain cases, clinically justify the use of narrow-diameter implants.

One should always keep in mind a series of "precautionary" measures that, in fact, protect biological and mechanical structures from the action of unfavorable forces. In cases of wide-diameter implants (Figure 11.21), the dimension of the artificial crown may be larger than the diameter of the implant, in which case the occlusal load vectors will allow bending moments in all directions.

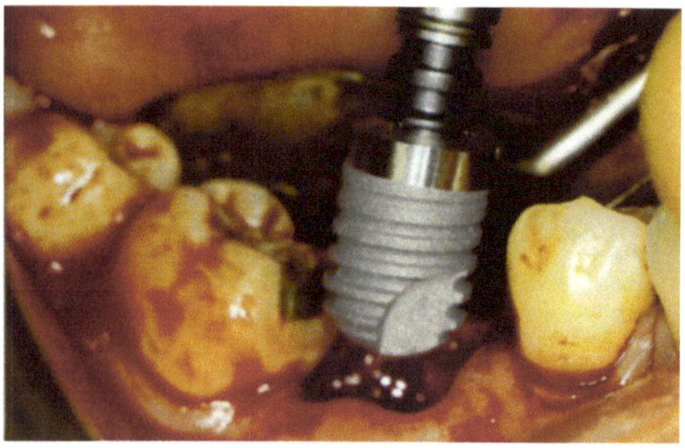

Figure 11.21. Installation of a wide-diameter implant in the place where the occlusal forces are the strongest in the molar region.

For this reason, often, the occlusal surface must be significantly reduced and the occlusal contacts must be placed on the inside diameter of the implant. An occlusal relief that is wider than the diameter of the implant determines the eccentric contacts that occur more often during mastication or parafunctional movements. In addition, the concentration of forces (of normal or reduced intensity) that arise during daily chewing activities are closely related to the width of the occlusal relief (Figures 11.22- 11.24). Mitigation of the action of forces and produced unfavorable moments forces a significant reduction of the crown, and to reduce the action of transverse forces, the morphology of the cusps must not be overemphasized but, on the contrary, significantly reduced.

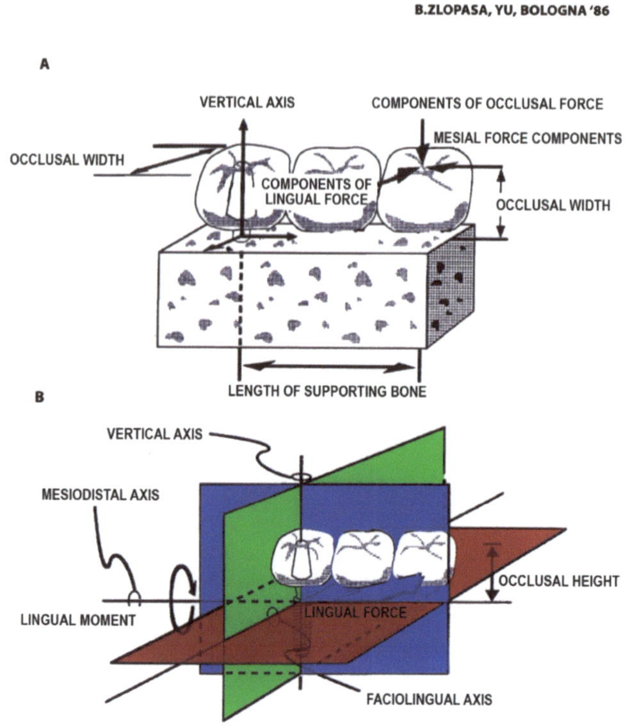

Figure 11.22. Schematic representation of the action of vertical forces on the implant depending on the occlusal width of the crown and the length of the support (implant), which determines the occlusal width and height of the added members that are exposed to the components of occlusal forces, vertical and horizontal, as well as the action of lingual and facial forces and their moments. The occlusal height can affect the vertical of the load moment. The occlusal height serves as a moment arm to the force directed along the facial axis. The force component can be directed along the mesiodistal axis. Lingual force can also indicate a twisting moment in the implant neck if applied along the cantilever. (According to Karl Misch).

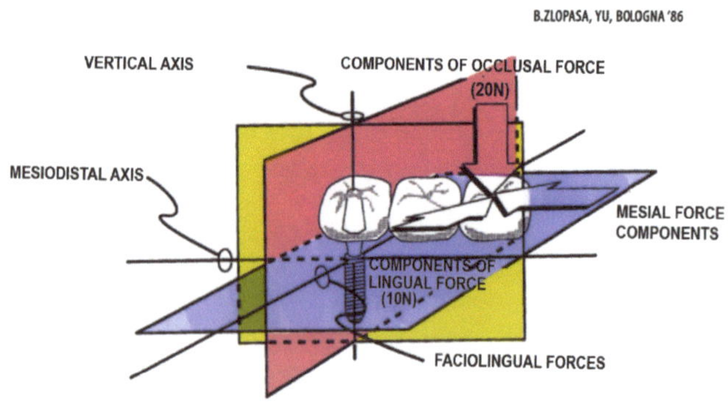

Figure 11.23. Given forces with enough available bone produce less load moments on the crestal part of the bone, in contrast to the situation when there is far less available bone. The occlusal height of the crown and the height of the cusps can affect the resultant of the load

moment. The height of the crown must be formed in proportion to the effect of these forces.

Considering all these points of view, it can be concluded that the effect of unity between teeth and implants is still not sufficiently clarified. But, despite the theoretical dilemmas, practical experience confirms a long-term successful relationship.

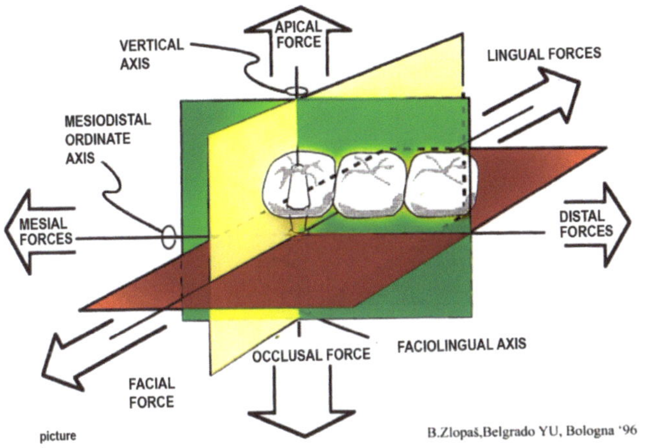

Figure 11.24. The load moment tends to induce rotation in three planes (clockwise and counterclockwise rotation). Six moments result on these three planes: lingual transverse, facial transverse, occlusal, apical, facial and lingual.

Bonding of implants with natural teeth

This issue is still being debated today with very different points of view. Most conclusions are made based on theoretical knowledge, and far less based on experiences verified through practice.

Many views consider bonding natural teeth and implants as risk factors. That point of view could be justified by the fact that natural teeth in the alveolar bone are approximately ten times more mobile than implants and that by combining these two systems, with different mobility and elasticity, when acting and receiving chewing forces, there is a risk due to an unbalanced load between the two supports. However, it is important to say that this risk factor is often combined with other geometric factors (lack of support, added hanging extensions that act as levers). The length of the extension depends on the force with which the unfavorable moments of force will act. In addition, if two or more implants are connected to a natural tooth, the ankylosing stiffness of the implant causes the implant itself to take the majority of the load.

Another point of view is that, due to the difference in mobility, tying the natural tooth to the post of the immobile implant, ankylosingly attached to the bone, can endanger the periodontal tissues around the natural tooth, and thus the survival of the implant itself. This is explained that the immobility of the implant and the mobility of the natural tooth can cause a leverage effect and the action of shearing forces (pulling), overloading the implant.

On the other hand, there are also claims that partial immobilization of natural teeth, tying them to an immovable implant, can cause atrophy of the periodontal structures of natural teeth.

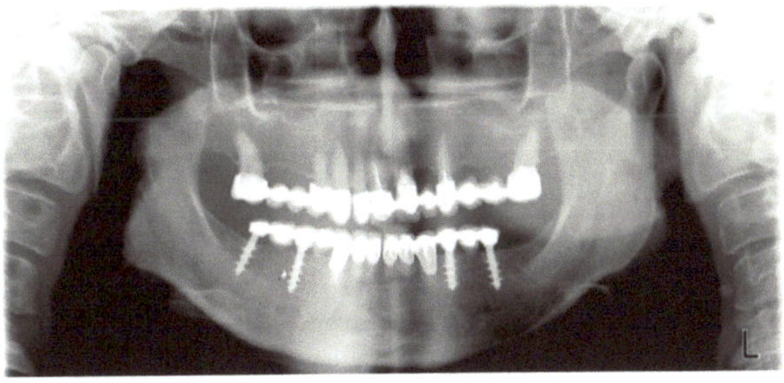

Figure 11.25. Balanced occlusion, separation of prosthetic work in the midline of the mandible make Tramonti implants stable with slight marginal bone loss (Work completed in 1992. Control shot March 2012).
Figure 11.25. Balanced occlusion, separation of prosthetic work in the midline of the mandible make Tramonti implants stable with slight marginal bone loss (Work completed in 1992. Control shot March 2012).

The possible benefit of bonding implants and natural teeth can be justified by several facts, and this possible benefit lies in the following:

a) distribution of occlusal load on natural teeth
b) the possibility of reducing the number of necessary implants.

Despite the fact that many studies have been devoted to this issue in the rehabilitation of partial edentulism with implants, it is difficult to obtain valid results on the percentage of success due to the lack of clearly defined success assessment criteria. Some authors described these criteria, but in many studies the only criterion for assessing success was the survival of the implant.

All clinical trials on natural tooth-implant bonding described no difference in survival among rehabilitated cases with separate implants or among cases with implants bonded to natural teeth. Experience confirms that if the condition of the anchor teeth is good and if the occlusion is balanced (Figure 11.25), then such a connection is justified and long-lasting.

However, there is only one prospective study published first by Gunny and then by Olson where two types of bridges were performed on the same patient: on the one hand, using two implants with three elements, and on the other hand, one implant and one natural tooth that were connected by a bridge, also with three elements. The three-year and five-year results showed that there was no significant difference between the two differently connected sides for implant survival.

Experience, however, suggests that implant bonding and telescopic crowns should not be used to compensate for the different mobility between periodontal bonding and implant stiffness.

Many authors have observed the phenomenon of constant subsidence of natural teeth that are connected by a prosthetic structure to implants. A prospective study of thirty-one implantologists showed that only 3% of such settlements were due to different mobility of teeth and implants.

The subsidence occurs in the first year under the prosthetic load and can reach up to 2 mm, but cases of significantly greater subsidence, several millimeters each, have been recorded.

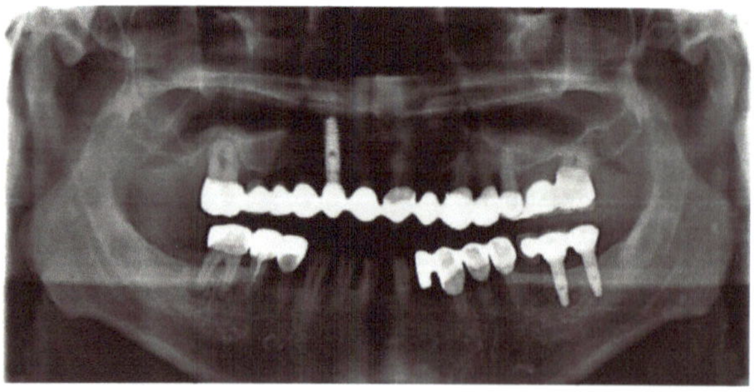

Figure 11.26. View of the attachment of the implant and the natural tooth in the upper jaw (Pit-Izi). Condition after twenty years in the upper jaw and after 11 years in the lower jaw, in which the load is only on the implants (Nobel Biocare Replace implant). The duration of implants in the bone is influenced by the fulfillment of biomechanical laws.

The cause is not clear, but it is assumed that it was caused by various mechanisms, which may arise from the following reasons:

- atrophy of the periodontal connection;
- presence of detritus in the interior of the coupling;
- reduction of return elastic capacity, prevention of mobility of periodontal tissue around the teeth due to friction (shearing force) caused by bonding with the implant;
- bruxism, bending of the metal structure and movement of the lower jaw.

Some studies try to explain this subsidence by the fact that the supports of the prosthetic work differently survive the energy waves caused by the impact force of the occlusal forces, creating a leverage effect and overloading the implant posts.

In prosthetic restorations, whether it is solutions where the supports are only implants or a combination of bonding with a natural tooth, the most important thing is to create conditions for chewing forces to be directed along the axis of the implant (Figure 11.26-11.30). Therefore, it is necessary, already in the pre-surgical planning, to determine the exact position of the implant, that is, its place and the direction of the axis of the implant; that is, align the positioning of the implant with the position of the natural tooth, which nature has already done.

In order to create a predictable success in bonding the implant and the natural tooth, it would be advisable to carry out the prosthetic restoration in two stages: as a provisional, but precise, and definitive.

Temporary prosthetic work performed lege artis would be useful for several reasons: placement of a definitive abutment instead of a cap to form a gingival margin around the implant, thus avoiding subsequent opening and re-trauma of the soft tissues (Figures 11.31-11.37).

In order to avoid initial overload, the contacts of the occlusal surfaces must be formed in such a way that the cusps are not emphasized, avoiding even the smallest oblique planes on them (see Figures 11.27 and 11.28).

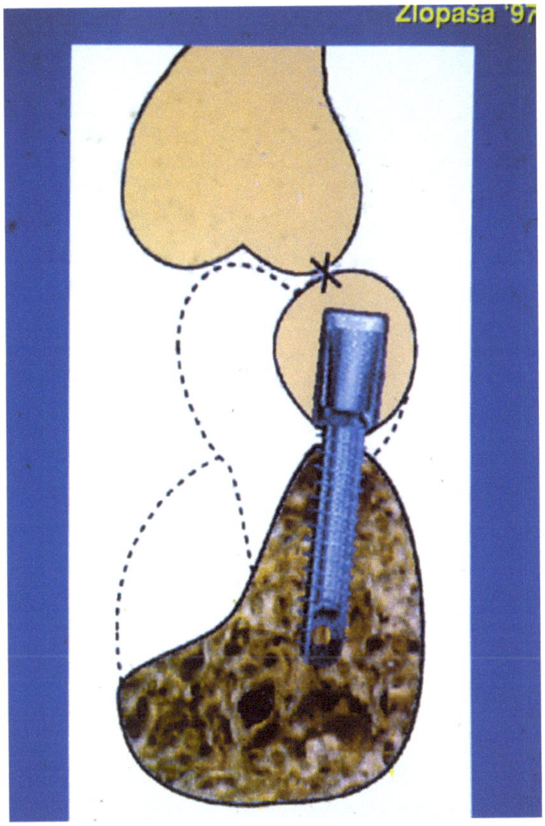

Figure 11.27. Adapt the shape of the crown to the movements and trajectories of the antagonist in order to direct the forces of action axially. If the contacts were on the palatal cusp, then the load would be off the axial axis.

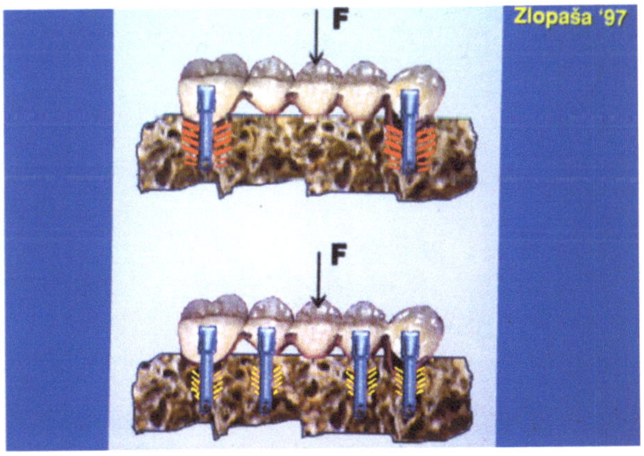

Figure 11.28. The number and arrangement of supports, the occlusal width and the height and inclination of the cusps determine the magnitude of the force on the bone schematically. Increasing the number of supports reduces the intensity of forces on the bone.

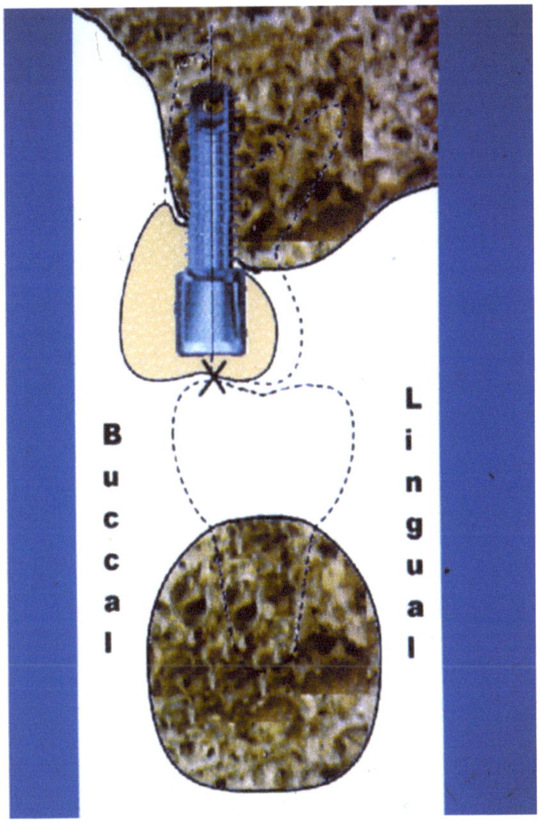

Figure 11.29. Prosthetic design creates conditions for receiving favorable axial forces and eliminating horizontal forces and their moments. Care must be taken to ensure that the buccal cusp of the lower teeth lies in the central fissure of the antagonist. When the buccal cusp is in the central fissure, load forces act favorably, axially - along the axis of the implant.

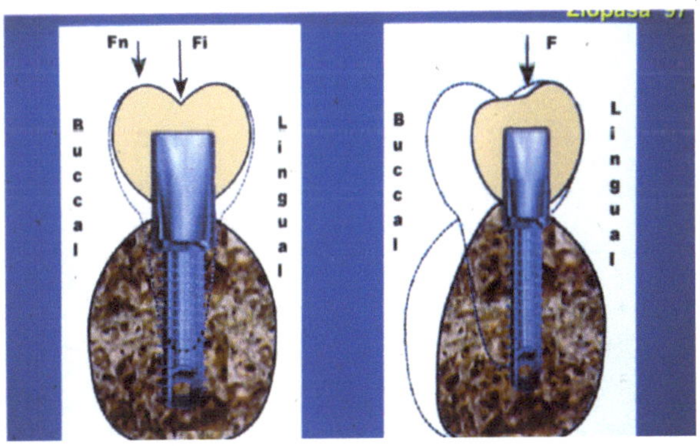

Figure 11.30. The intensity of the forces that will be received and distributed depends on the shape of the crown, the slope of the shape of the cusps. By shaping the crown on the implant, the necessary conditions (width of the crown, height and inclination of the cusps) must be created to direct the extra-axial forces towards the axial direction.

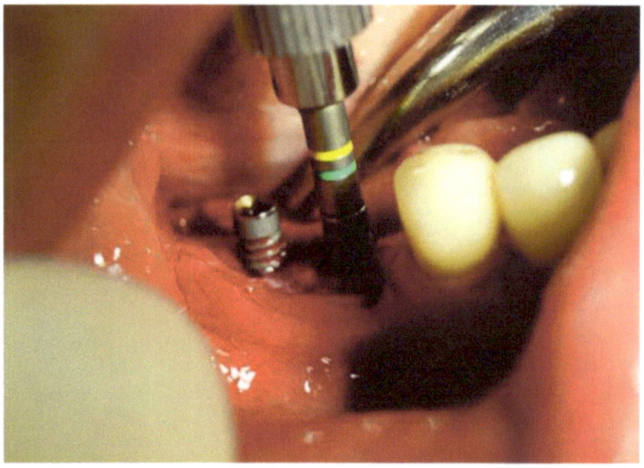

Figure 11.31. Choice of implants (height and diameter). Success is determined by: implant placement with as little aggression as possible, choice of position, type of load and quality of performed prosthetic work.

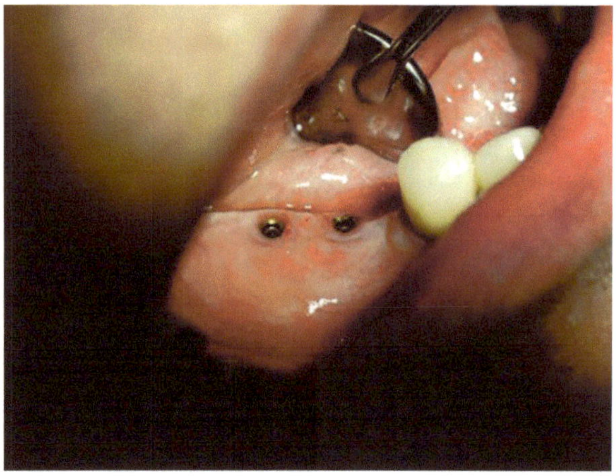

Figure 11.32. Healing after immediate stress. Definitive abutments were placed instead of caps for healing and gingival formation.

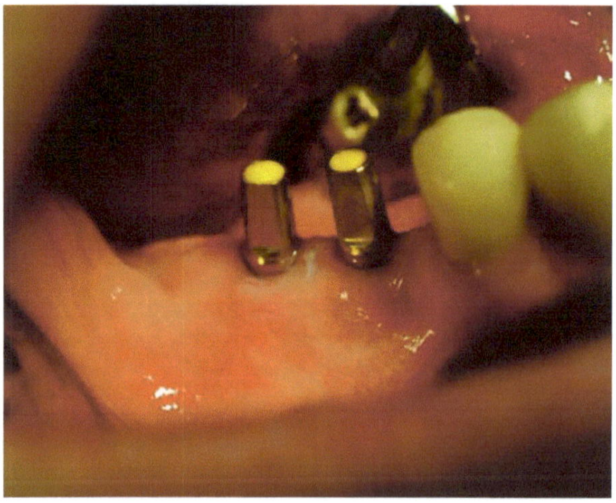

Figure 11.33. The appearance of a formed gingival margin with definitive abutments, which avoids the use of healing caps and other surgical procedures. Appearance after 6 months. B. Zlopasa, YU, '92.

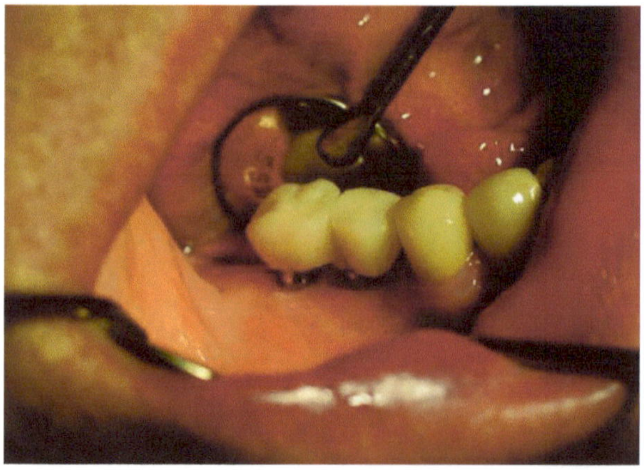

Figure 11.34. Display of installed implants on which definitive abutments are placed and immediately loaded with provisional crowns. Temporary prosthetic work should be placed in a slight subocclusion.

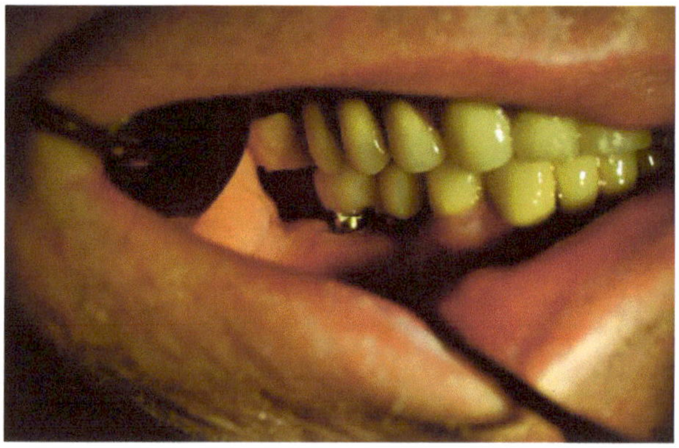

Figure 11.35. Implants immediately loaded with provisional prosthetic work placed in mild subocclusion.

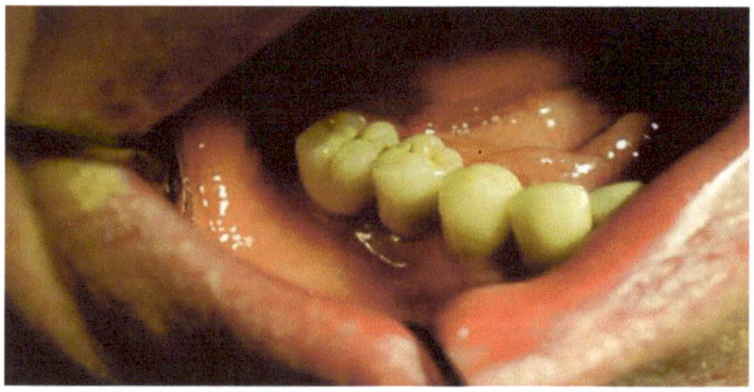

Figure 11.36. Definitive work after 6 months. Cusps modeled according to gnathological princes by the absence of oblique planes.

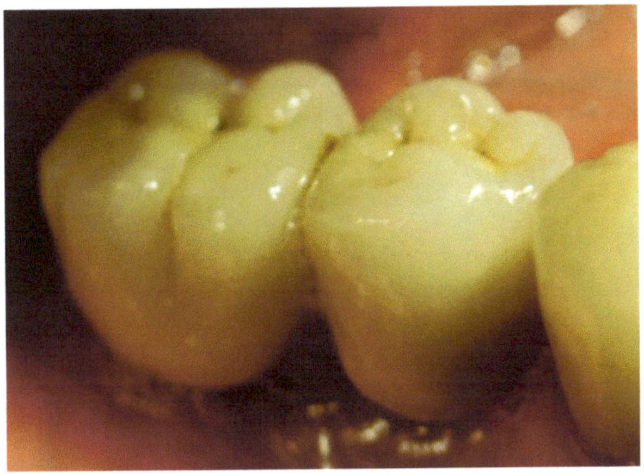

Figure 11.37. The morphological appearance of the crowns and the shaping of the cusps, which are adapted to the lateral movements of the lower jaw. By avoiding the oblique planes of the cusps, the forces are directed axially, and the horizontal ones are neutralized. High cusps create large moments of forces that cause adverse horizontal forces; lower cusps during lateral movements of the lower jaw create smaller force moments, and if the surface is flat, only pressure forces on the peri-implant bone tissue are created in the central axis.

In this way, we achieve dento-dental contacts only during chewing, and in fact those functional rhythmic stimuli would additionally affect the capacity of bone remodeling.

Provisional compensation creates conditions for progressive bone loading, which would exhaust the regenerative capabilities of reparation found in a metabolic state of slowed turnover due to lack of loading. The vascularization of this living tissue is best stimulated by the natural physiological load of the bone around the implant. Physiological processes cannot be stimulated in the amorphous material from which the implant is made, but the tissues around the implant can be stimulated. The biocompatible substance from which the implant is made (in this case, titanium quality) can stimulate the osseointegration of bone cells. Likewise, when we consider the load as a stimulating factor for the regenerated part of the bone, care must be taken in the dosage of that load, i.e. implant system on the bone.

How to implement it in practice?

Experiences, confirmed through many years of practice, say that the dosing of physiological load in the healing phase should be done with provisional prosthetic works made of a much softer material, i.e. less hard and more elastic than porcelain. Physiological load dosing on implants will not be optimal with materials such as zirconium due to its high hardness and inelasticity.

What it means in practice?

In order to understand these processes in oral implantology, we should remember the laws that apply in general orthopedics and Wolff's law, which is over 100 years old - that the physiological load of any bone in the body stimulates the osseointegration processes. Therefore, depending on the dentist's assessment, it is desirable to load the implant immediately, and experiences prove good results.

Why is it important to restore bone function so quickly? The function is established by the macroscopic and microscopic elements of the bone (Wolff's law). Without good blood circulation, there is neither fast nor good regeneration. Nutrition of the bone depends partly on the arteries, but also on the muscles, periosteum and all the surrounding tissues, which make up the trophic unit, that is, the functional unit. Wolf's law, that bones should be restored to function as soon as possible, despite the fact that it was stated 100 years ago, with the development of the quality of the material (titanium) and surface treatment with laser technology that comes into contact with the bones (artificial hip and knee), it was applied as a principle of treatment. Classic orthopedics meant lying down for a long time, at least six weeks, and even up to three or more months, in order for the bone healing process to take place. It is precisely the early loading of the segments that shortened the healing time of the bone with better quality callus.

And why is callus of better quality?

Many experimental studies have shown that the shorter time of callus formation is due to early physiological stress and that the callus heals faster and with better quality.

The load improves the local vascularization of the regenerated bone, confirming the postulate: that without good vascularization there is no good regeneration and healing.

If orthopedists dose the early physiological load by moving patients through the hospital corridor and exercises, this justifies the position that dental implants should be loaded as soon as possible by chewing, speaking and moving the masticatory muscles. If the load is dosed with a provisional restoration made of acrylic or composite, the occlusal morphology of the provisional can be gradually corrected, until the characteristics corresponding to the planned occlusal scheme are obtained.

According to some authors, the load on the implant should, at least in the first stage, be different from the load on the natural tooth. It is very easy to do in practice, by correcting the occlusion with a very thin articulating paper, a slight closing movement in the central occlusion. On the implant crowns, a barely noticeable contact would remain, while on the adjacent natural tooth, the impressions of the contacts would be much more pronounced. Care should be taken to ensure that the imprints of the contacts on the implant crown are directed exclusively towards the axial direction of reception of masticatory forces. By modeling high blood vessels, a steep oblique plane is created, on which vanaxial forces act, reducing the resistance of bone tissue. High bumps increase the angle at which the forces act (Figures 11.27 to 11.30) destructively. Bone has the least resistance to horizontal forces, which are increased by high cusps.

It is important to try to achieve occlusal contacts at multiple points, using articulating papers in multiple colors. In practice, this approach to occlusal adaptation is the most realistic and achievable. The bite can be very usefully checked using aluminum wax (pictures 11.39 - 11.42). Based on such a check, the state of occlusion can be faithfully mapped and unwanted contacts can be observed (pictures 11.44 - 11.46, 11.47, 11.48).

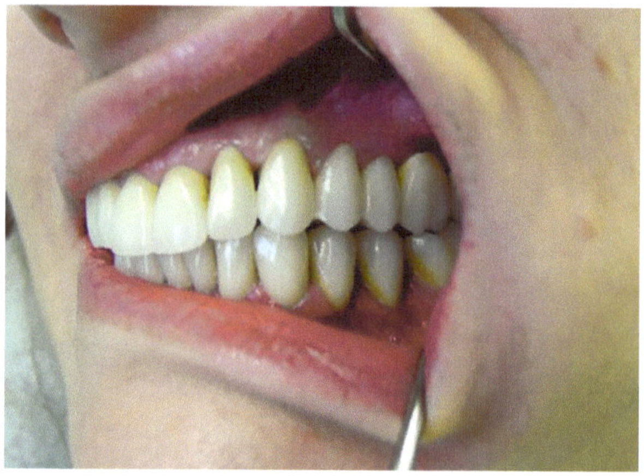

Figure 11.38. Excessive fulfillment of the patient's aesthetic requirements - emphasis on sharp high bumps in the lateral regions during lateral movements of the lower jaw increases the adverse effect of horizontal forces and their moments. Bone is the least resistant to the intensity of these forces.

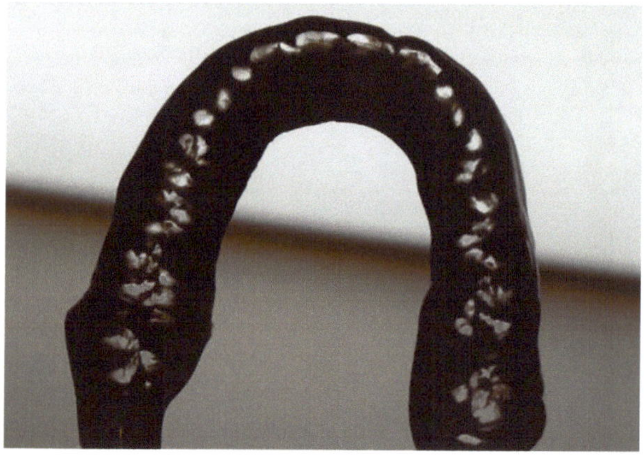

Figure 11.39. The best way to check the occlusion formula is by biting into aluminum wax. Premature and too strong occlusal contact would be manifested by aluminum wax perforation.

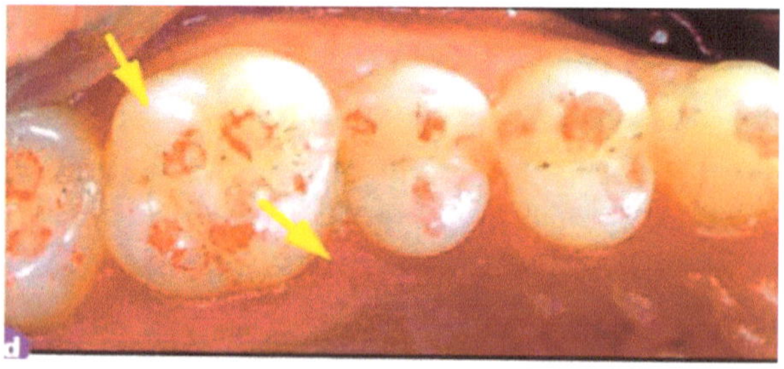

Figure 11.40. Even staining in all movements reflects good occlusion.

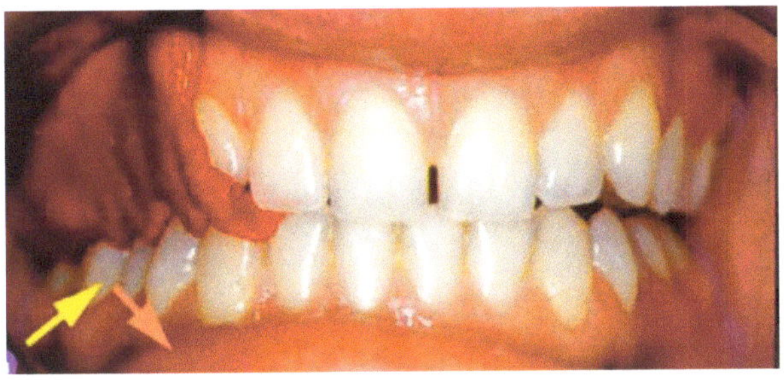

Figure 11.41. The relationships on the working and balance sides are checked with elastic aluminum wax.

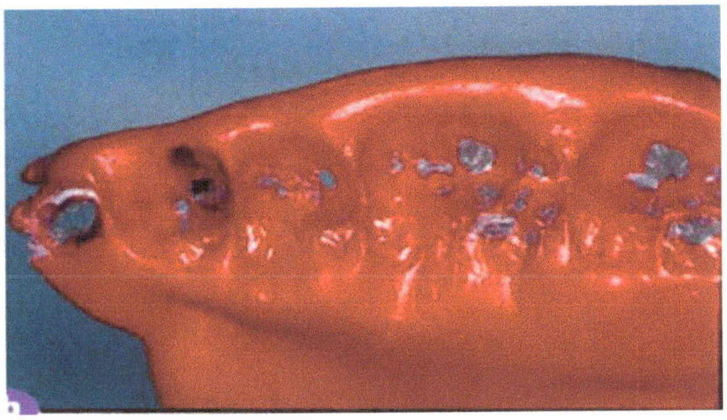

Figure 11.42. Mapping of the occlusal state.

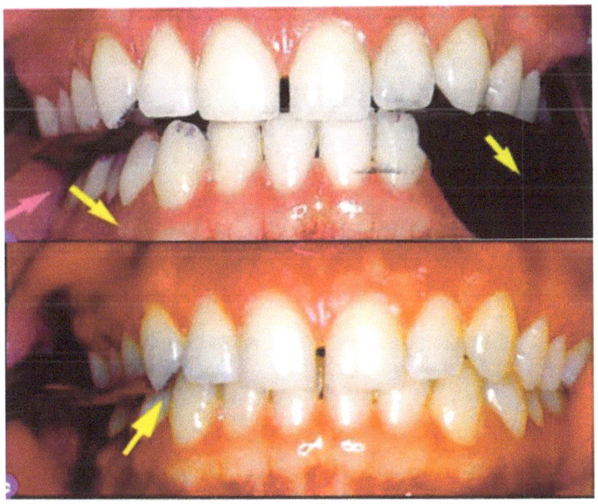

Figure 11.43. Checking occlusal contacts with articulation papers of different colors, canine-guided occlusion and articulation (yellow arrow) and molar relationship (pink arrow) on the working side and canine position on the balance side.

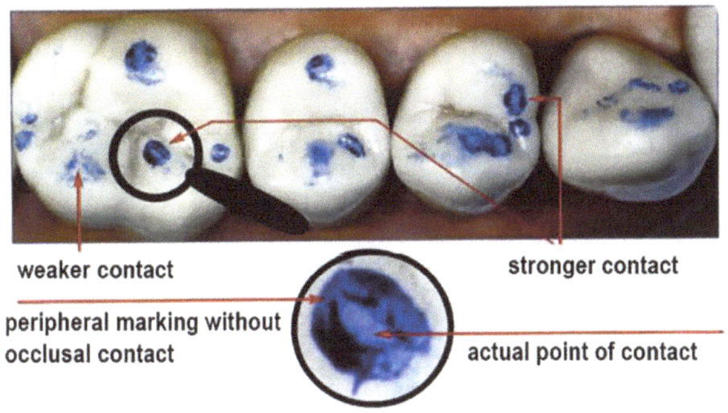

Figure 11.44. Description of the appearance of occlusal contacts to which maximum attention should be paid when checking and registering occlusion. Mapping of occlusal contacts.

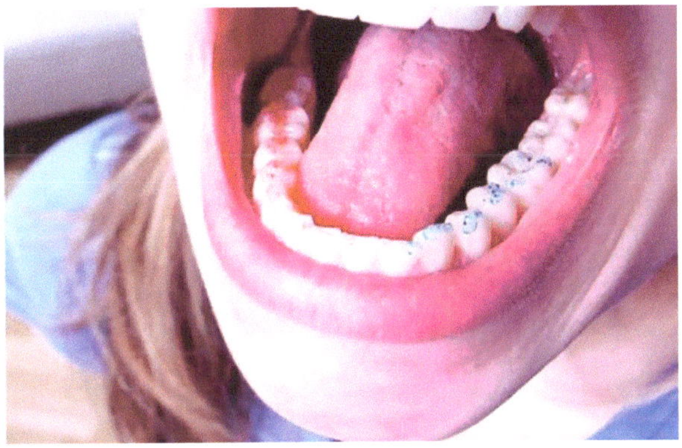

Figure 11.45. Ideal contacts both on the working side and on the balance sheet.

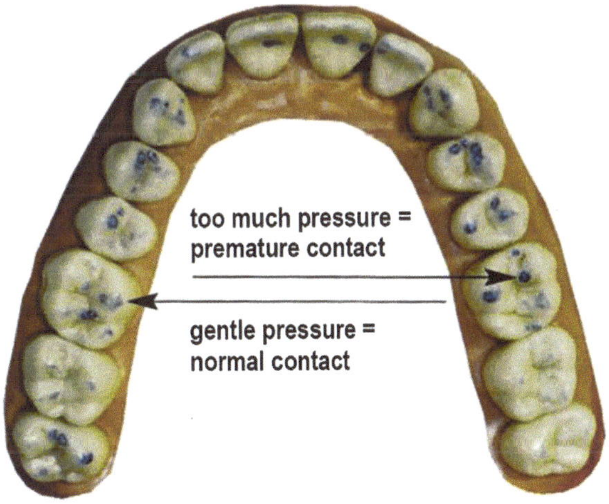

Figure 11.46. An extremely important check in practice.

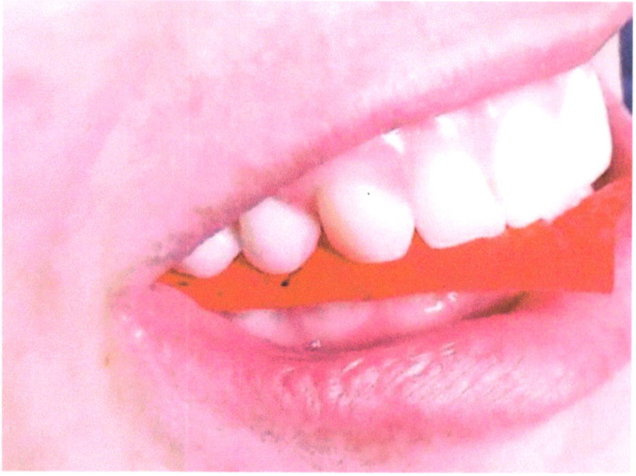

Figure 11.47. The examination requires time, patience and establishing good cooperation with the patient during the examination. Relaxation of the patient is essential.

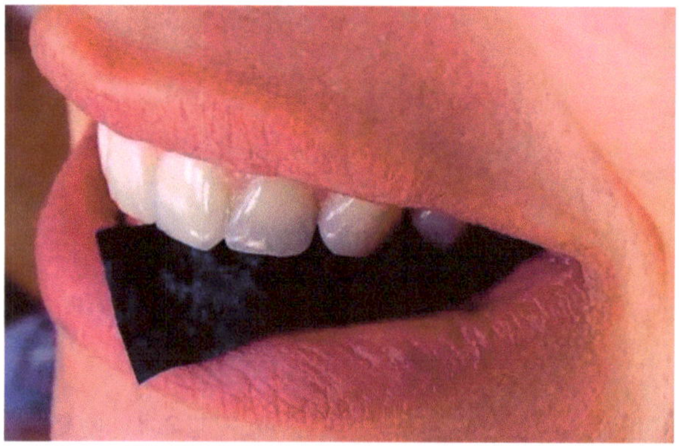

Figure 11.48. Check with different thicknesses of articulation papers.

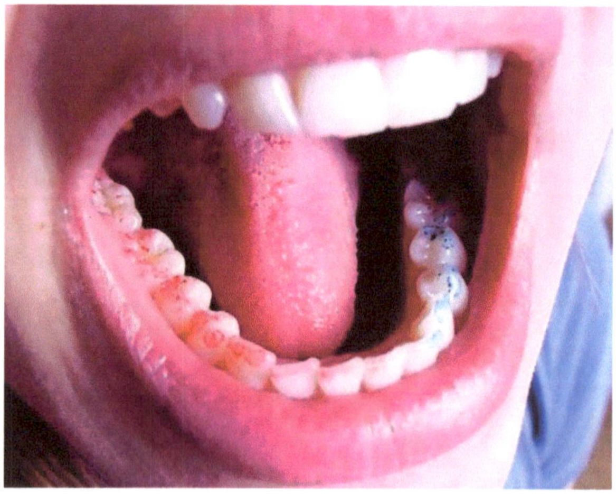

Figure 11.49. Ideal interjaw and intercuspular relationship on the working and balance side.

Theoretical conclusions say that the mobility of a natural tooth is different from an implant, but it is still uncertain whether such data (Figure 11.50) can be transferred to clinical practice in the presence of physiological load.

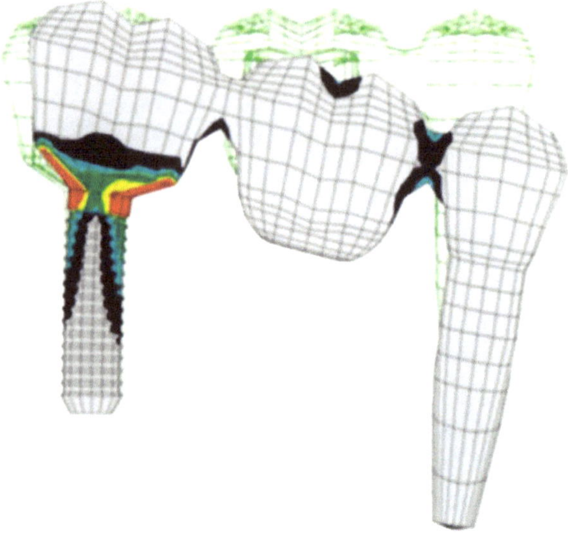

Figure 11.50. Theoretical presentation of the rigid, ankylosing immobility of the implant and the relationship with the natural tooth (analysis by Dr. Laurent Pierissnard, Paris V University).

Some in vivo studies say that during normal chewing activity, with the correct distribution of forces, no unwanted events were observed on any of the prosthetic work supports.

The physiological forces of chewing in short intervals - discontinuously, are insufficient to allow tissue fluids (lymph and blood) to flow out of the implant environment, that is, to change the already established homeostasis. Therefore, it is possible to compare the real intrusion unit of a natural tooth with the elastic deformation of titanium, jaw bone and biotechnical structures that construct the prosthetic superstructure.

Starting from the assumption that the unity between the implant and the bone, the absence of elastic supporting tissue, often obliges the practitioner to approach a specific way of establishing occlusal relations and to bear in mind that lateral movements (on which a separate chapter is dedicated due to its importance) in the mouth are never identical to those which are regulated in the articulator, although the pre-surgical planning phase was performed very cautiously. One must always go through a very delicate "clinical phase" of repair. At this stage, we do not have at our disposal a precise instrument of "zero density" or density equal to the values of periodontal baroreceptors.

Therefore, it is necessary to call the patient again for an examination. With lateral movements of the mandible, using very thin articulating papers, care should be taken to ensure that the contacts are not only on the crowns that carry the implants. If the contacts on the implants are more emphasized, then the corrections become very difficult. The patient, especially in the first correction, very often does not immediately give precise answers about discomfort or a positive state. It means that it is often impossible to get any specific warning sign from the patient that would give us information about the obtained occlusal scheme.

During the creation of definitive prosthetic work, risks of overloading should be immediately avoided and conditions should be created to immediately promote bone adaptation to the implant, leaving about 0.1 mm outside the occlusion.

When it comes to bonding natural teeth and implants, it can be concluded that the basic parameters for such bonding are:

- Teeth with a good prognosis and minimal mobility and implants with excellent bone integration.

Planned work must leave the possibility of independent removal of certain parts of it in case of unforeseen and unwanted events. This is made much easier by the latest elastic fixing materials - firm connection and easy removal (picture 11.51).

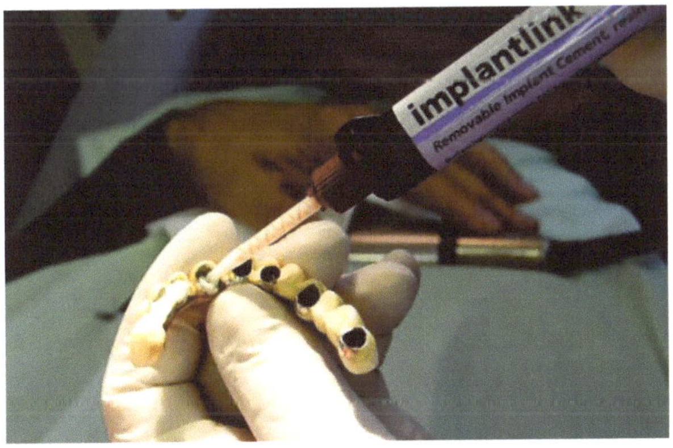

Figure 11.51. The latest adhesive materials enable good fixation, but also easy removal of the prosthetic work, enabling the test of time for the entire procedure and easier elimination of possible omissions and complications.

Anticipation of possible future events should be a determinant of the planning of prosthetic work, which should be planned and carried out so that it is possible to make the necessary changes very easily in case of failure of the role of any of the support elements.

However, it should always be kept in mind that one of the reasons justifying the use of such a connection (natural tooth-implant), i.e. reducing the number of implants, is the financial factor of limitations on the part of the patient.

According to some authors (Misch), the application of bonding implants below 10 mm in length to a natural tooth, even in the mandible, where the success rate is as high as 98%, is not justified. However, many authors have positive experiences with such binding, especially if a wide-diameter implant is used (7.5 mm long and 4.6, 5.6 or 6 mm wide).

In any case, there are many dilemmas, especially if the height of the alveolar ridge is very low, which has recently caused the relaunch of the so-called "basal" ("disk") implants, about which the reader will find a special overview and thinking of the author of the book.

However, experience has confirmed in many cases that the application of implants below the previously indicated length due to the proximity of some anatomical structures (mandibular canal, mental foramen, narrow crestal bone, etc.) often does not have a good prognosis.

Tripod implant positioning (with three-point, triangle configuration)

Of particular importance, from the aspect of biomechanical principles, is the method of positioning the implant in the lateral region. Insertion of the implant along a straight line in that region enables the adverse effect of lateral forces in the sense of destruction, bending of the implant. Conversely, if the implants are placed in a tripod (triangular) configuration, those unfavorable lateral forces will be mostly neutralized by receiving favorable axial forces (Figures 11.52-11.54). However, the possibility of tripod positioning of the implant depends on the width of the alveolar bone and is sometimes difficult to achieve in practice.

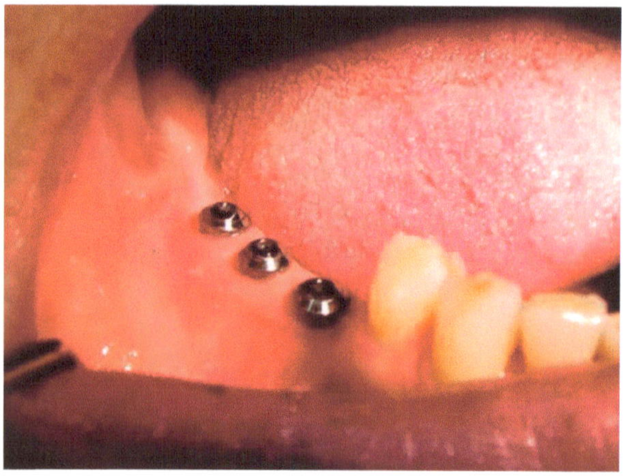

Figure 11.52. The tripoid positioning of the implant for static biomechanical reasons depends on the shape of the alveolar ridge and the quality of the bone. The configuration of three implants in a geometric plane (one line) increases the stress of the load on the bone.

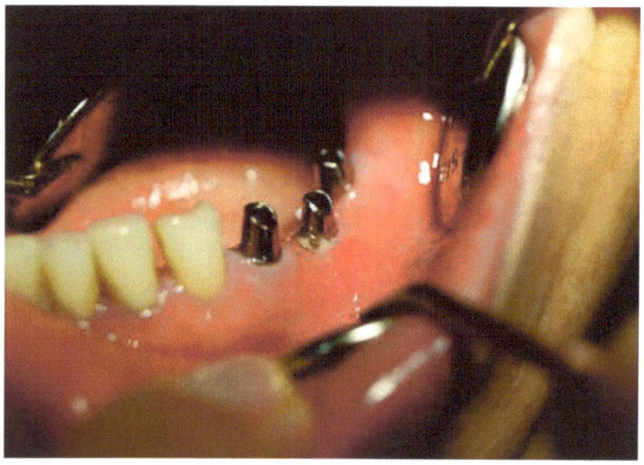

Figure 11.53. The tripoid position of the implant is important so that the action of axial forces remains within the triangle to prevent twisting and bending from adverse forces (Figure 67).

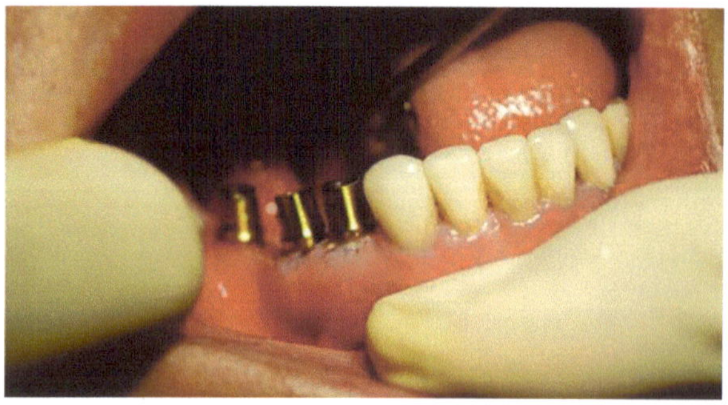

Figure 11.54. Nobel Biocare Replace implants immediately installed and immediately loaded, positioned in a tripoid geometric line.

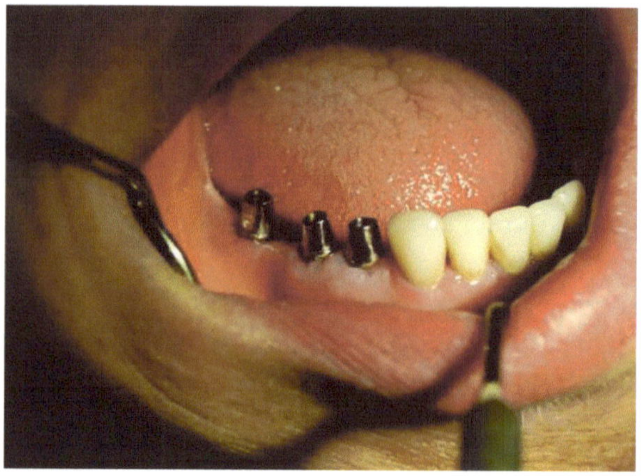

Figure 11.55. Presentation of the appearance of the formed gingiva around the abutment three months after immediate installation and loading. By typoid positioning of implants and creation of temporary precise prosthetic work in acrylate, with unemphasized cusps, chewing forces are directed axially, which enhanced osseointegration processes and healing of soft tissues.

Schemes of treatment methods in these cases and the possibility of tripod arrangement of implants are shown in the following pictures.

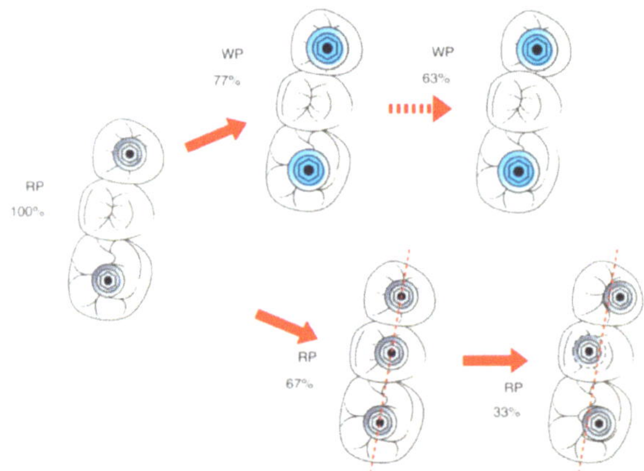

Figure 11.56. Display of the prosthetic solution on implants of standard diameters (SP) with three elements in different implant positions. Two SP implants loaded with crowns and one member in between cause 100% bone stress. Two SP implants loaded with crowns and one hanging member cause stress on the bone of 200%. Three SP implants placed in the geometric plane cause a load stress of 67%. Three SP implants placed in a tripod (triangular) position cause a stress load on the bone of 33%.

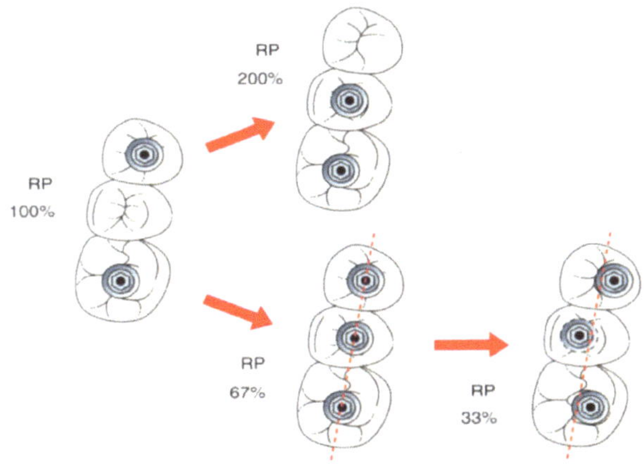

Figure 11.57. Two SP implants cause 100% bone load stress. The two wide-diameter (WB) implants cause stress loads on the bone between 77% and 63%. Three SP implants placed in a geometric plane cause a stress on the bone of 67%. Three SP implants positioned tripoidally reduce the stress on the bone to 33%.

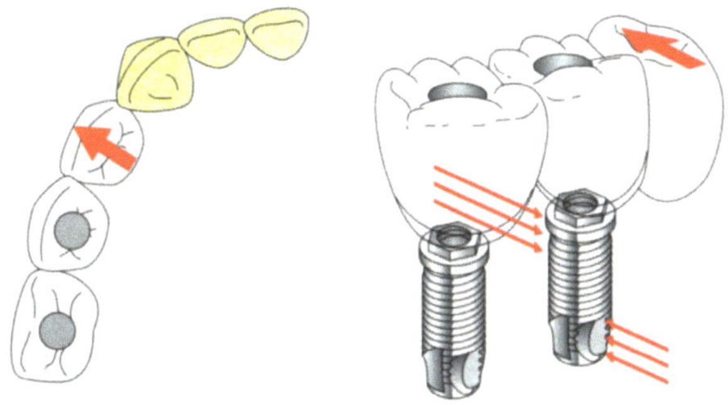

Figure 11.58. The direction of action of the forces on the extensions (hanging elements) increases the unfavorable stress forces on the implant, and thus on the bone.

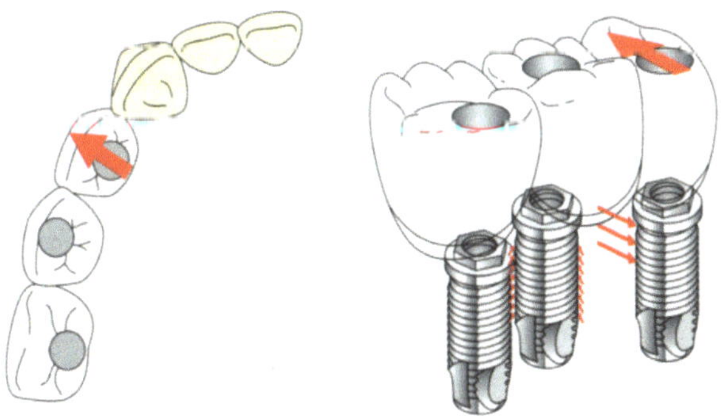

Figure 11.59. The forces that act in the surface of the triangle on the three points of support, and are not in a geometric line, do not have an adverse effect in terms of twisting the implant.

Prosthetic extension (hanging limb - "appendix")

The presence of prosthetic extensions in any clinical situation is always a risk factor.

Each added extension increases the overall risk. For example, load two implants in the lateral region with the addition of an extension, according to many authors, is not permissible due to unfavorable stress forces on the implant (Figure 11.58), especially if there are additional biomechanical risk factors.

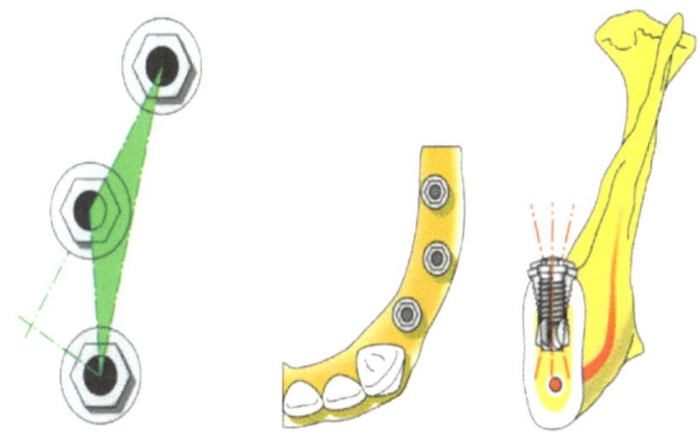

Figure 11.60. Preferred positioning of the middle implant 2 to 3 mm in the buccolingual direction to keep the forces of action within the triangle.

Implants placed as a counterweight to the prosthetic restoration center on them

Excessive height of the prosthetic structure

When planning prosthetic work on an implant with a crown, strict attention must be paid to the relationship between the length of the implant and the height of the crown - the height of the constructed crown must be less than the length of the implant or at least equal. For this reason, it is considered inadvisable implanting implants shorter than 10 mm, especially in the molar region. This attitude has recently been somewhat modified. There are implant systems of adapted diameter on the market, for cases where the height of the alveolar ridge is below 7 mm - the shorter the implant design, the wider the diameter of the implant, which requires sufficient width of the alveolar bone. But this system was not widely used in practice.

If anatomical restrictions require the installation of short implants and if the intraocclusal space is favorable, the biting surfaces of the anchor crowns on short implants should be slightly excluded from the articulation, transferring the load, if possible, to the function of the canines.

The functional load that the implant can transfer to the bone tissue largely depends on the clinical relationship between the implant and the crown.

Occlusal forces in the molar region can be three to four times stronger than in other regions, and very often the available bone in that part is unfavorable both in terms of quantity and quality. This must be taken into account when planning prosthetic rehabilitation with implants.

In order to understand the biomechanical laws in oral implantology, one must know the laws of physics, when it comes to the directions and points at which chewing forces act, as well as the intensity and duration of the action of those forces. The point of attack is where the force acts. The place where the force acts depends on: force intensity, stress and torque.

The direction and point of attack on which the force acts belong to the group of the most important characteristics of forces. The most favorable load force is the vertical force that acts physiologically along the longitudinal axis of the implant. The vertical force, due to its action along the length of the implant, is accepted by the large area of the peri-implant bone tissue, and because of such force action, the bone offers the greatest resistance.

What and how much the effect of vertical forces will be on the implant also depends on the shape of the occlusal surface of the prosthetic crown, that is, on the relationship of the cusps and their contact with the antagonists. The cusps on the occlusal surface of the crown supported by the implant affect the distribution of the forces received by the implant into vertical and horizontal components. The most unfavorable forces are shear forces that act in a plane along the entire length of that plane.

The disadvantage of shearing forces is that they can act on a certain pressure by stretching and tearing the object on which this action is directed. Shear stresses are strongest in an inclined plane at about 45 degrees to the direction of the force. This is important for the correct formation of the cusp and its oblique planes on the occlusal surface of the artificial crown by gnathological principles. For example, if on an artificial crown, the inclination of the oblique plane of the cusp is greater, the horizontal component of the force is that much greater. The effect of horizontal forces is directed towards smaller surfaces, and therefore they have a less favorable impact compared to vertical forces. Horizontal forces of lower intensity, the bone tissue around the implant can compensate, but when these forces exceed the limit of tolerance, there are unwanted consequences in the peri-implant area of contact between the bone and the implant, which is manifested by the breakdown of the bone. In the biomechanics of the oral cavity, there are the same biomechanical relationships in natural teeth, and these events are especially important when it comes to bone implants.

The oral cavity is an extremely dynamic milieu, both from a physiological and biochemical, as well as from a biomechanical aspect. In this extraordinary dynamic, histological renewal of tissues is constantly taking place. In the dynamics of the oral cavity, in addition to constant renewal, we also have the constant establishment and maintenance of oral homeostasis.

We can observe that dynamic in two phases:

a) resting phase, and
b) the active phase, due to the dynamic mobility of the lower jaw.

The lower jaw can be in two positions: in the static position when it is at rest during sleep, and in the dynamic phase, that is, in the chewing phase. Both jaws in both phases are exposed to the constant action of forces transmitted to the bone via the roots of the teeth or implants. To understand the dynamics of the oral cavity, it is necessary to clarify some terms. Statics is the science that looks at forces in equilibrium, when there is no movement.

Dynamics considers the balance of forces in the phase of movement. In both phases of receiving forces (statics and dynamics), the balance of these forces must always be achieved, because active forces act from several directions, and receiving forces, balance inertial, i.e. retroactive forces. Force is proportional to mass and acceleration. Active forces deform the object on which they act, until retroactive forces appear, which bring the active forces into equilibrium. From the theoretical consideration of the action of forces, the action of active forces is endless, and something must stop them.

Force is defined by four parameters:

1. force intensity;
2. the place on which the force acts, which in mechanics is called the "point of attack";
3. the direction of the force, i.e. its direction;
4. the angle at which the force acts.

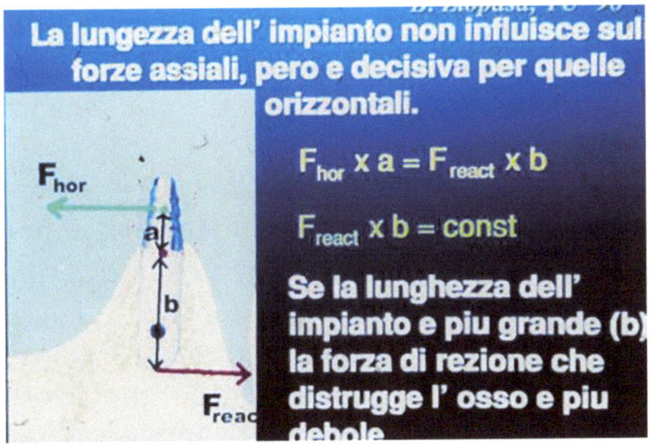

Figure 11.61. The reception of axial forces does not depend on the length of the implant, but the intensity of the effect of horizontal forces will depend on the length of the implant, how much these forces will be weakened. Translated: The length of the implant is not decisive for receiving axial forces. If the length of the implant is greater (b) the forces and directions of the destructive forces on the bone are weaker.

The intensity of the force can be variable, and when it comes to implant loading, the direction of the force, i.e. its direction, is extremely important. In order to achieve long-term survival of the implant in the bone, it is necessary to precisely define how much intensity and to which place and in which direction the force acts. When we have a defined direction, then the direction of action of the force can be on several sides, and it is also important whether that force has the effect of tearing-shearing or pressing, that is, whether these forces push or pull the object on which they act.

In dental literature, the authors call these forces differently: torsional forces, twisting forces, turning forces, or bending forces...

The effect of the force at the point of attack (which happens constantly in occlusion) is manifested by the deformation of the body on which the force acts. At the same time, the deflection of the body depends on the intensity of the force and the hardness of that body. The deformation, that is, the deformation of the object on which the force acts, always tends to be responded to by the retroactive force, which is proportional to the force of the attack. It stops within the limits of the part on which it acted.

The point of attack of force plays an important role when it comes to natural teeth, but it is even more important for restorations on implants. The point of attack of occlusal forces on premolars and molars lies in the occlusal surfaces, and the intensity of various force moments depends on the width of the occlusal surface. The moment of the force is the product between the force and the arm, that is, the moment is the product of the intensity of the force and the distance from the point of attack to the point for which the moment is sought.

Due to the law of balance, a given moment must be balanced by another moment of force of the same magnitude, but in the opposite direction.

A load moment (Figure 11.62) tends to induce rotation in three planes: clockwise and counterclockwise rotation. The load moment on these three planes results in six moments: lingual-transverse, faciotransverse, occlusal, apical, facial and lingual.

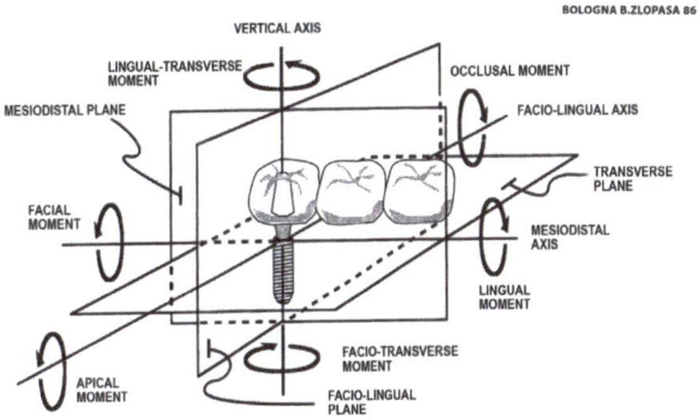

Figure 11.62. Forces acting on the implant can be from several directions. The intensity of the action of the force moment depends on the length of the arm and the slope of the extension (hanging elements). The intensity of the produced moment depends on the inclination and the length of the arm. A longer arm produces more torque. The load moment induces rotation in three planes. Clockwise rotation in these three planes results in six moments: transverse-lingual, transverse-facial, occlusal, apical, facial and lingual.

As already mentioned, the essence of statics is the consideration of forces at rest, while dynamics is the consideration of the action of forces in motion. The basic law of statics is that the sum of all forces, from all directions, should be in balance, i.e. at zero. It means that the action of the active force must be balanced by the same amount of reactive force from the opposite direction. By changing the position of the attack point, i.e. by influencing the point of attack, we can influence the distribution of load forces. The goal is to focus the greatest load on the part that can best receive and bear the force acting on it.

Events in the oral cavity are in constant dynamics between the movement of the mandible, the force of the oral musculature and the tongue. In order to meet favorable biomechanical requirements, restorations on implants must be designed in such a way that they bring the effect of every force from all directions into balance, as is the case with a natural row of teeth.

The attack points of the forces on the front teeth in the upper jaw are located on the palatal surface (see the occlusion scheme in the TMJ chapter), and on the lower ones on the vestibular surface of the teeth. The point of attack is achieved at the point of contact with the antagonists. Observing the point of attack, when it comes to compensation on the implant, is of great importance for the ultimate success, because knowing the position of the point of attack of the force, with a certain vertical load, can mitigate the size of the unfavorable horizontal component of the force, by shaping the appropriate slope of the cusps.

A force whose point of attack is formed at an angle in relation to the body of the implant has an unfavorable moment of force (the moment for a given point is the product of the force and the arm, ie the distance from the line of action of the force to the given point). Unfavorable force moments can be in different directions (Figure 11.62). The greater the angle of the arm (lever), the greater the intensity of the force on the lever. The arm on which the force acts (see Figure 11.58), in this case it is the added hanging tooth in the drawing that has no support on another point, and the lever is the implant located in the bone.

There are numerous factors that depend on the strength and duration of the intensity of force action. The strongest constant forces act when the condyles are in the maximum physiological distal position, i.e. in central occlusion. In central occlusion, the teeth contact in the terminal stage of chewing and during swallowing, and these contacts are relatively short, but the attack points are pronounced. How bone tissue will adapt to these forces and receive them within the limits of physiological stress depends on many factors. Under physiological conditions, the natural series of teeth is exposed to forces of varying duration and intensity. On the one hand, the forces of the cheek musculature act, and on the other, the forces of the tongue. Forces of different duration appear as intermittent and continuous forces, so their mechanisms of origin and action are different.

Intermittent forces act for a short time, are of lower intensity and are absorbed by the surrounding tissues. These forces include chewing and swallowing forces and last about 18 minutes during the day, and this time does not interfere with the maintenance of healthy bone and peri-implant tissue.

Continuous forces act for a long time, are of the same intensity and occur as a consequence of poorly performed prosthetic work. They are mostly destructive, and they also occur in parafunctions, clenching and grinding of teeth, being continuously transmitted to the peri-implant tissues, and depending on the intensity and duration, manifest themselves as pathological changes in the peri-implant environment.

Immediate load

Most dentists assess the loads of implants immediately after their installation with great caution and indecision. However, many authors, for a reason, call immediate loading progressive loading.

What is the optimal period when the implant should be exposed to the action of favorable forces, is a question that is answered from different points of view.

All research has shown that axially directed forces of occlusion are best transferred via the implant to the bone, and it can be said that this progressive loading is advisable, because in the early phase of healing, i.e. bone tissue remodeling after operative trauma, prevents the appearance of microcracks between the implant and the bone. In order to reduce the early loss of bone around the implant and the early loss of the implant, according to Mish's thinking, immediate loading - progressive loading promotes the formation of new bone, ie. its complete organization into a compact built bone. Such progressive loading will make the implant permanently stable and all subsequent actions: prosthetic work, occlusal design, type of material, will not be able to affect the loss of bone around the implant, as well as the loss of the implant itself.

Another study confirms the thoughts of K. Misch. The behavior of the implants during immediate loading and the behavior of the bone around the implants that were not immediately loaded after the implant placement were investigated. Digital X-rays showed an increase in bone density in the crestal area by 40% in implants that were immediately loaded. This study was based on a detailed analysis and control of occlusal forces under immediate loading. In all examined cases, it was proven that early loading increases biological and physiological stress, stimulating the formation of bone density during the healing period and significantly reducing early bone loss around the implant.

There are many conflicting opinions regarding early loading, when it comes to assessing whether to load the implant immediately or leave it covered for several months. Which method will be used depends on the experience, good judgment and courage of the implantologist. The justification of immediate loading (long ago stated by Wolff's rule in orthopedics) is proven in cases where there were exclusively risk factors. The patient's aesthetic request was not made, nor was it important, which can be seen in the following pictures (pictures 11.63 - 11.70).

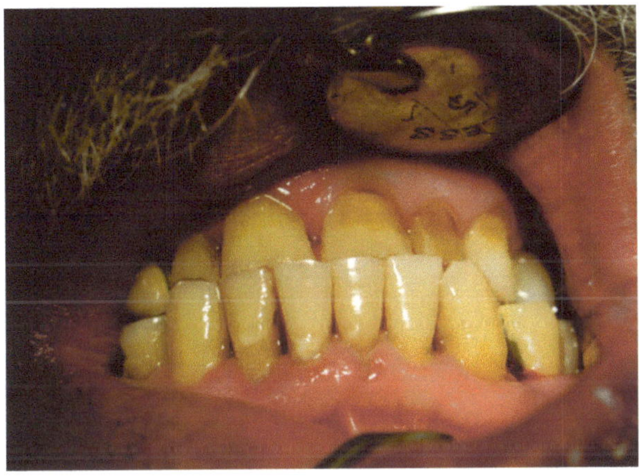

Figure 11.63. Fulfillment of biomechanical requirements is primary.

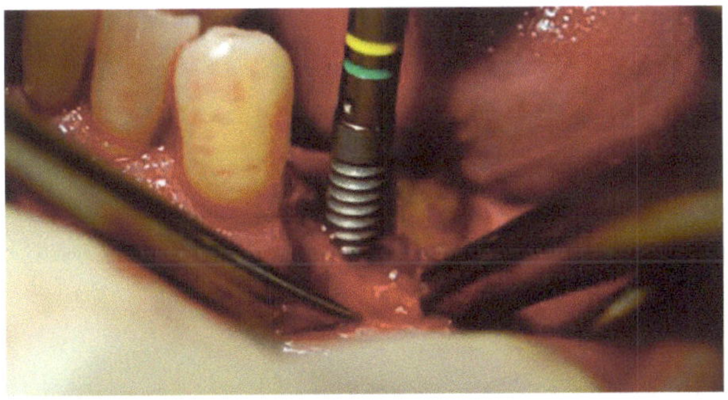

Figure 11.64. During implantation, the implant must not be wetted with saline solution or touched with gloves.

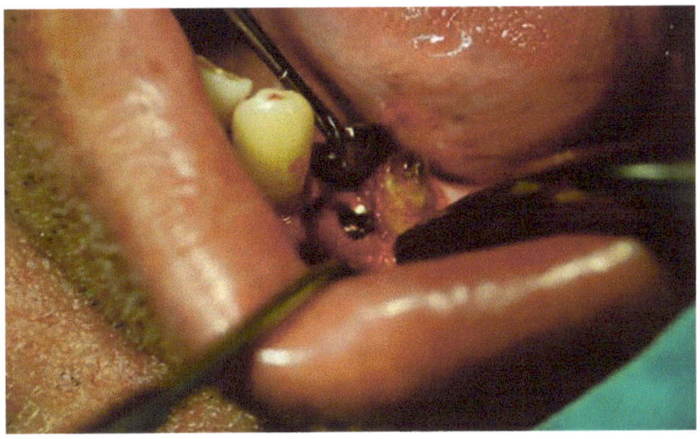

Figure 11.65. Placed implant on the left side in the lower jaw with good primary fixation - preparation for immediate loading.

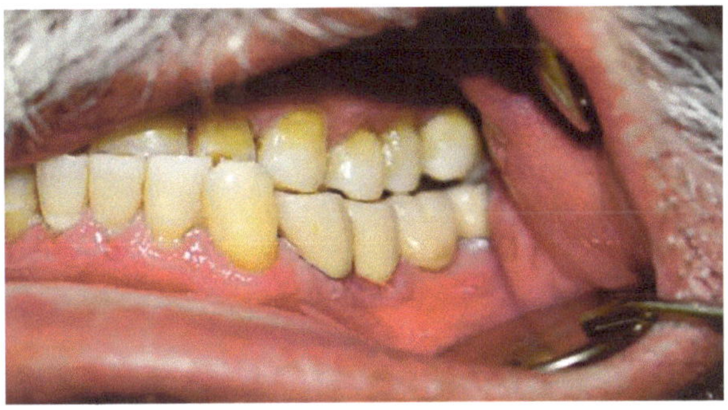

Figure 11.66. Establishing a good occlusion in this patient is the most important success factor.

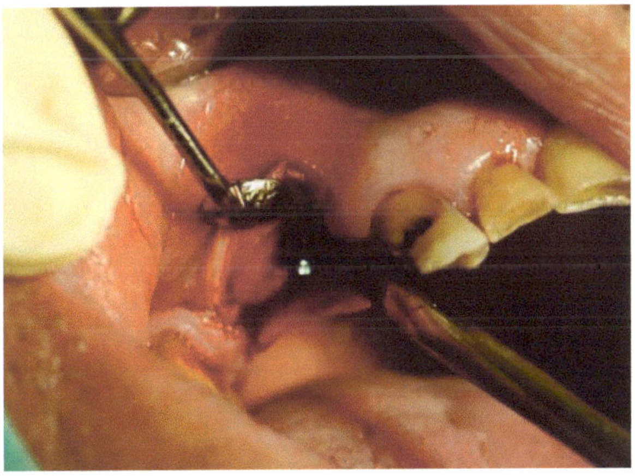

Figure 11.67. Insertion of an implant in the same patient on the right side in the upper jaw.

In this case, the only requirement was functional - good chewing of food. The implants are immediately loaded with temporary restorations in mild subocclusion, with bite surfaces in metal and with accentuated inter-implant spaces for good maintenance of oral hygiene.

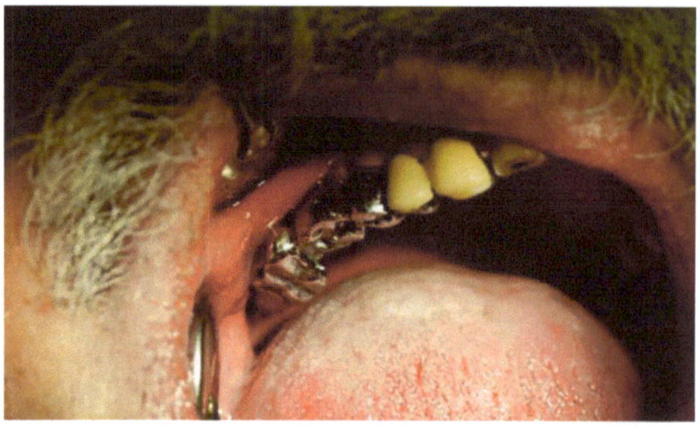

Figure 11.68. A temporary restoration adapted to the situation in the mouth. Aesthetics are neglected at this point.

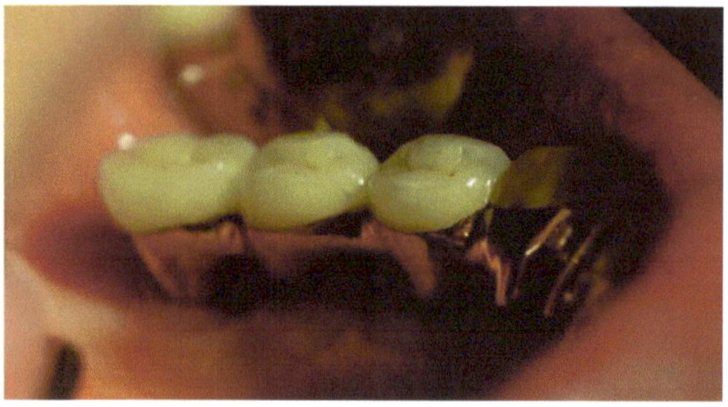

Figure 11.69. Definitive work is adapted to good occlusion and easier maintenance of oral hygiene around the implant.

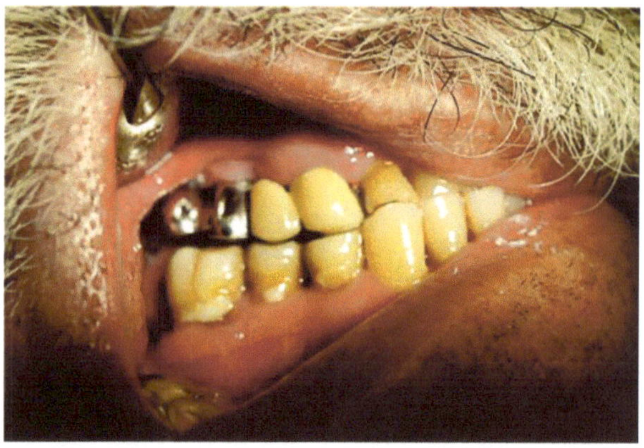

Figure 11.70. Due to unfavorable occlusion, a provisional bridge with bite surfaces in metal was left in mild subocclusion.

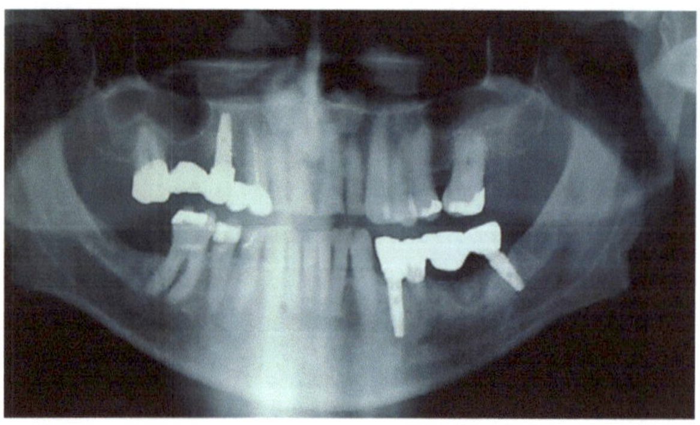

Figure 11.71. Control image after 8 years of immediately installed and immediately loaded implants.

Occlusal overload, whether immediate or delayed, may initially result in marginal bone loss, and if the point of attack of occlusal forces is off-axis of the implant, complete loss of osseous integration will occur. If the traumatic occlusion is combined with inflammation of the surrounding tissues, bone deterioration is accelerated. In order to neutralize unfavorable forces, we can look for a solution on two levels: in reducing the biting surface and the circumference of the crown so that the point of attack is along the axis of the implant, or in increasing the number of implants so that the reception of forces is evenly distributed (see Figure 11.53).

Marginal bone loss in the first year

Claims why the greatest marginal bone loss occurs in the first year after implant placement have not yet been fully clarified. The most likely cause is occlusal events, depending on the occlusal load present.

The reader of this book will notice that the author inseparably considers prosthetic and oral surgical developments. In all textbooks, these two branches of dentistry are completely separated. And the way of specialization is different.

An oral surgeon at the faculty (at our place) studies exclusively oral surgery, including oral implantology, and a prosthetist studies prosthetics. However, the daily practice of these two branches of dentistry, administratively completely separate specialties, unites them into one.

For example, occlusion is much more than the physical contact of maxillary and mandibular tooth surfaces and prosthetic work, whether on natural teeth or implants. Occlusion, in fact, represents the coordinated functional interaction of different tissues of the masticatory system that differentiate, model, remodel, decay or renew. **Therefore, occlusion is not only a static and dynamic relationship between the contact of the biting surfaces of the teeth, occlusion is also a relationship between the tissues of the masticatory system.**

For this reason, the dentist who deals with the installation of implants must know that prosthetic work should restore harmony between the aesthetic and functional requirements of the masticatory system. Successful implantation should be followed by well-planned and successfully performed prosthetic work, which will establish harmony with the surrounding structures and ensure the smooth and harmonious function of the lower jaw. Experiences confirm that for predictable clinical success, diagnosing occlusion and establishing it is a more complex procedure than the procedure of implant installation itself. The doctor's decision whether to maintain or change the existing state of occlusion has a crucial influence on the integration process of the implant surface and the bone.

Research by K. Misch and colleagues showed that the effect of occlusal forces decreases later, increasing the bone's resistance to those forces, which means that after the first year there is a functional adaptation of the oral musculature to prosthetic work, which also reduces the effect of occlusal forces. After a certain time, the bone reacts to all these events by increasing the density around the implant. Over time, by increasing the functional unity of all relevant structures in the oral cavity, the success rate of the implant procedure increases.

Effect of masticatory forces in relation to implant neck design

Where to look for reasons for failure? What should be considered in advance to avoid failures?

These are questions to which we must have an answer before the procedure begins.

Designing the neck of an implant is increasingly given importance due to biomechanical requirements and soft tissue relationships. The reception of various forces and their distribution and transmission to the bone depends on the design of the door. It was believed that a polished, smooth and flat neck conducts shearing forces, while the rough surface of the neck and the angled neck receives and transmits compressive forces that the bone can withstand best. The smooth neck of the implant can affect crestal bone loss. Cortical bone is stronger against compressive forces, but is 30% weaker against tensile forces, and 65% weaker against shear forces compared to compressive forces.

At one time, it was believed that the smooth and polished surface of the implant neck results in shear stresses in the region of that implant. In contrast, the implant neck at a greater angle to the surface increases contact with the bone, causes favorable compression and tension components on the bone, and thus reduces the risk of bone loss. Significant crestal bone loss, up to 3 mm, was observed in implants with a long, smooth, machined neck region.

More and more doors are being processed by creating nano threads with special technologies. Bone loss has been clinically proven to be most common above or below the first thread in some implant designs. Bone growth above the thread during healing is noticeable in the second phase; however, after prosthetic loading, bone loss occurs up to the first thread, after the first year of prosthetic loading.

In many biphasic implant systems, the gap between the implant platform and the first neck thread varies from 1-3 mm. Bone loss is not related to the length of the implant, but may be related to the design of the implant neck, as it changes shear forces into compressive force components, which the bone is most resistant to.

This explains the example of implanted implants, one with a smooth, and the other with a rough design in the neck area. The smooth-necked implant was placed at the level of the crestal bone, while the other implant was placed 1.5 mm below the level of the crestal bone. After 6 months, the bone level remained unchanged with the first implant, while bone loss occurred with the second implant. It was shown that the bone loss in the second implant was due to the reception of forces that caused biological deformation, which was related to the design of the neck of the implant.

It was found that, regardless of the type of implant, there is an early loss of crestal bone in the healing phase, i.e. in the first year, unlike the following years, where the loss of crestal bone is slowed down, and in some cases almost non-existent.

Possible causative factors for early crestal bone loss can be found in: surgical trauma, occlusal loading and peri implantitis, microcracks between the implant and the abutment, and the design of the implant neck.

The following conclusion can be drawn from all this: in implantology, there are two basic principles of implant installation - below the bone level or at the level of the bone level (in two phases).

In a large number of implant systems that are installed in two stages, after a certain time of the implant's stay in the bone and after the implant is connected to the abutment, there is a microcrack between the two parts. This microcrack can be above and below the level of the edge of the alveolar bone. This phenomenon exists only in two-phase implant installation; with one-piece implants, which are installed above the level of the bone edge of the alveolar ridge, there is no microcrack in which bacterial content can be retained.

The Branemark school suggests placing the implant below the bone level. Branemark's team recommends installing the implant, i.e. the first stage, below the level of the bone, in order to avoid the influence of unfavorable forces chewing during bone healing and remodeling, considering that during that time the implant should only be in contact with the bone, without the influence of oral musculature, tongue movements, etc.

Some research has shown that in the microcrack between the implant and its extension, the abutment, which has already been emphasized, can be a place for the penetration of granulation tissue and the accumulation of bacteria, one of the causes of peri-implantitis. Research has also shown that with embedded two-phase implants, bone formation in the marginal part largely depended on that microcrack. With Branemark's two-phase implants, installed below the bone level, in the first year, the marginal bone loss was about 2 mm, in contrast to the one-piece implants immediately loaded, where the bone level remained unchanged in the same period.

There are implant systems where the microcrack between the implant and the abutment is avoided, so in the second phase the abutment is not screwed but cemented, and thus the microcrack is filled with cement (Bonne system). The author's experience suggests that the placed abutment should not be unscrewed. The more times it is unscrewed and re-inserted, the formation of peri-implant tissue is prevented, and by repeated unscrewing and screwing, in addition to traumatizing the soft tissues, the possibility of infection of the peri-implant tissues increases.

Experience shows that installation at bone level is more optimal, and instead of placing healing caps (gingiva formers, Figure 11.52), by placing definitive abutments, the soft tissues will be better formed, of course with immediate loading. (pictures 11.53 to 11.55).

The issue of screwing or cementing the superstructure on implants

The issue that was discussed the most, when it comes to the definitive fixation of the compensation (suprastructure) on two-phase implants, is the choice of the method to be applied: screwing or cementing.

Until recently, there were no data or opinions in the literature that would show that one of these two techniques is superior to the other, as far as retention is concerned.

Those who are in favor of cementation emphasize the following advantages: the aesthetic effect is far better, also the occlusion, greater ease and lower manufacturing cost.

When screwing is used, the imperfection of the superstructure can be reduced by unscrewing the screw with which it is attached to the implant (Figure 11.72). It happens that the inaccuracy of the suprastructure can cause continuous tension on the screw, transferring it to the peri-implant part of the bone. After a certain time, the superstructures that were screwed to the implant could loosen by unscrewing the screws, which could happen again.

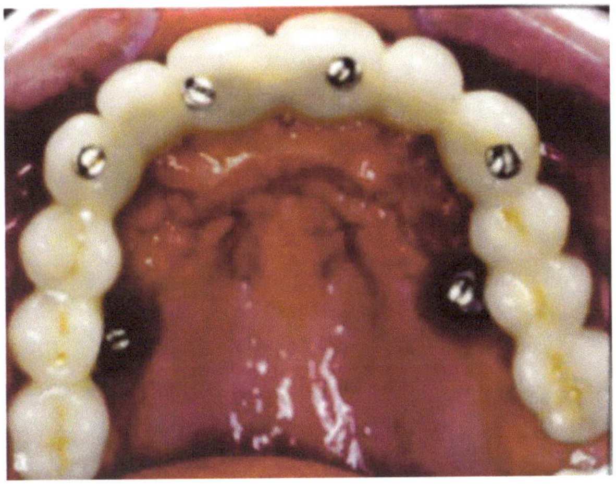

Figure 11.72. There are dilemmas: should you screw the work or cement it? Both solutions have advantages, depending on the case.

The advantages of cementation are that the inaccuracy can be partially compensated by creating a different thickness of the adhesive material in the different parts where the inaccuracy was observed when making the restoration. For this reason, cementing the prosthetic work is far more justified, especially with "Removable Implant Cement Forte", which enables easy removal of the prosthetic work.

In this conclusion, it is very important to check the possible tension caused by different biomechanical conditions because it can compromise the long-term success of already osseointegrated implants. In any case, it is far more justified to apply the cementing method, which has many advantages over screwing the implant superstructure. When the superstructure is screwed, during the establishment and adjustment of the occlusion, there is a risk of destruction of the screw head, which can lead to major problems.

Today, there are means for definitive cementing of prosthetic work, with the same characteristics as materials for temporary work in the mouth: good fixation and easy removal, and one such material is implantlink semi (Removable Implant Cement). This type of fixation of prosthetic work should be considered definitive, with the favorable characteristics of means for temporary fixation, such as Tempbond, Provicol, etc.

This method of fixation is particularly advantageous for immediate loading, and it also has the advantage that the stability of the implant can be checked occasionally by easy removal, which was an advantage of screwing, but very often also a big disadvantage, because it can lead the clinician to a dilemma: is it loosened implant or screw.

One-piece implants (diameter 3 mm and 3.2 mm) are fixed exclusively by cementation. For example, with one type of one-piece implant, the support of the prosthetic work is made of soft metal, and a special drill is attached to each implant, with which possible correction - shortening, adjusting the slope - can be easily performed without the risk of overheating, i.e. transferring heat through the implant to bone. Such a one-piece implant has a neck designed to favorably receive masticatory forces and, due to the one-piece abatement and implant, there is no microcrack as a possible site for bacterial plaque deposition. The great advantage of such implants is that, due to the surface treatment with Laser-Lok technology, we speed up the healing of the surrounding tissues, and the faster the healing, the more firmly the implant is integrated with the bone.

The standard dimension of 3 mm (existing lengths of 10, 12, 15, 16 and 18 mm) is extremely advantageous in cases where there are anatomical limitations due to insufficient width of the alveolar bone. Due to the emphasized processing of the surface that is in contact with the bone in the form of a gutter, by achieving exceptional primary stability and progressive (immediate) loading, we provide the patient with great convenience by quickly setting up prosthetic work, both functionally and aesthetically.

Summary

When it comes to the installation of implants, experience and bibliographic knowledge from the professional literature say that in oral implantology more and more importance is attached to biomechanical events in the oral cavity. Essentially, implantological treatment is based on two basic components: the biological component - the relationship between the tissue and the implant that surrounds it, and mechanical components.

With the loss of natural teeth, the broken harmony that requires restoration with implant treatment has a path: office-laboratory, laboratory-office.

Provided that the first stage of that journey - the surgery, met all the requirements of the implant installation protocol, the stage of creating the laboratory part is extremely important because it can completely cancel the first stage - the surgery.

Every structure that is realized in the laboratory is planned to be subject to the load of masticatory forces. The goal of performing the laboratory part is that the compensation is constructed in such a way that it reduces these forces to the physiological limits of action on the bone.

Any structure subject to load can, for certain reasons, be overloaded, which results in complications. If we divide these forces and determine one as functional, which stimulates bone integration, and the other as dysfunctional, whose effect is the opposite, we must take into account the biomechanical requirements so that dysfunctional forces do not prevail with the prosthetic design.

If the implant had good primary stability in the first phase, by overloading, the bone loses its support properties, and thus the entire procedure is endangered. For this reason, it is most important to discover the causes of this happening at the beginning, so that the implant-bone connection has time to establish the balance of the bone integration process, which will be maintained during function by the action of favorable chewing forces. The clinical approach to the analysis of biomechanical factors begins with planning the treatment, defining the load during the initial period, in accordance with the geometric and occlusal load factors, as well as defining the support capacity in accordance with the load capacity of the bone. Ultimately, the foundation for all these developments is laid by the clinician. The foundation is all the more stable if it knows biomechanical laws better.

The fulfillment of biomechanical laws begins with the selection of the implant, diameter and length, which will neutralize the forces in horizontal directions, increasing the attacking moment of the force on the implant, that is, on the bone. For example, the longer the length of the implant insertion into the bone, the lower the bending stress, i.e. the action of adverse transverse forces on the bone. With the square of the length, the intensity of the attack moment is weaker.

For example, if the length of an implant lying in the bone is 8 mm compared to a 16 mm implant, the 8 mm implant is subjected to four times greater stresses than the 16 mm long implant. Another example, comparing the reception of stress forces on a 10 mm long implant with a 14 mm implant, then the "ten", is twice as unfavorable as far as stress forces are concerned.

Among the various biomechanical factors that influence occlusal overload, the factors that are crucial for the survival of the implant in the bone should be singled out: bone substrate, quality and quantity of bone, length, diameter, design and technological processing of the implant neck.

Several pictorial representations of the basic postulates of biomechanics

The following figures will illustrate some of the basic rules of biomechanics (Figures 11.74-11.76, 11.88 and 11.89).

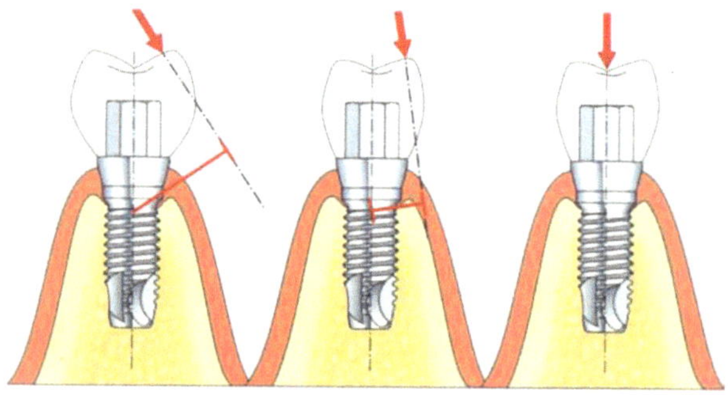

Figure 11.74. The greater the lateral contacts and inclination of the cusps, the greater the twisting moment. Whether the acting force will be a function of biological stimulation, or will lead to pathological changes depends on the slope of the cusps (oblique plane). It should be kept in mind that when it comes to the resultant of several forces in the mouth, they always act simultaneously. The morphological shaping of the occlusal surfaces depends on the direction in which the forces that act will be directed during the function and with what intensity on the oblique plane of the cusp. If the bump is higher, the inclined plane is steeper, the horizontal component of the force will be higher. The location of the attack point of the force also depends on the shaping of the occlusal surface, i.e. the occlusal contact. When it comes to receiving and dispersing forces during extreme lateral movements of the lower jaw, axial load is one of the basic attributes of physiologically optimal occlusion. The strength of horizontal forces is greater if the teeth on which the force acts are closer to the TMJ. A feature of physiological optimal occlusion is the role of the front teeth, i.e. canines, in guiding the lower jaw during eccentric lateral movements of the lower jaw, which protects the lateral teeth from overloading.

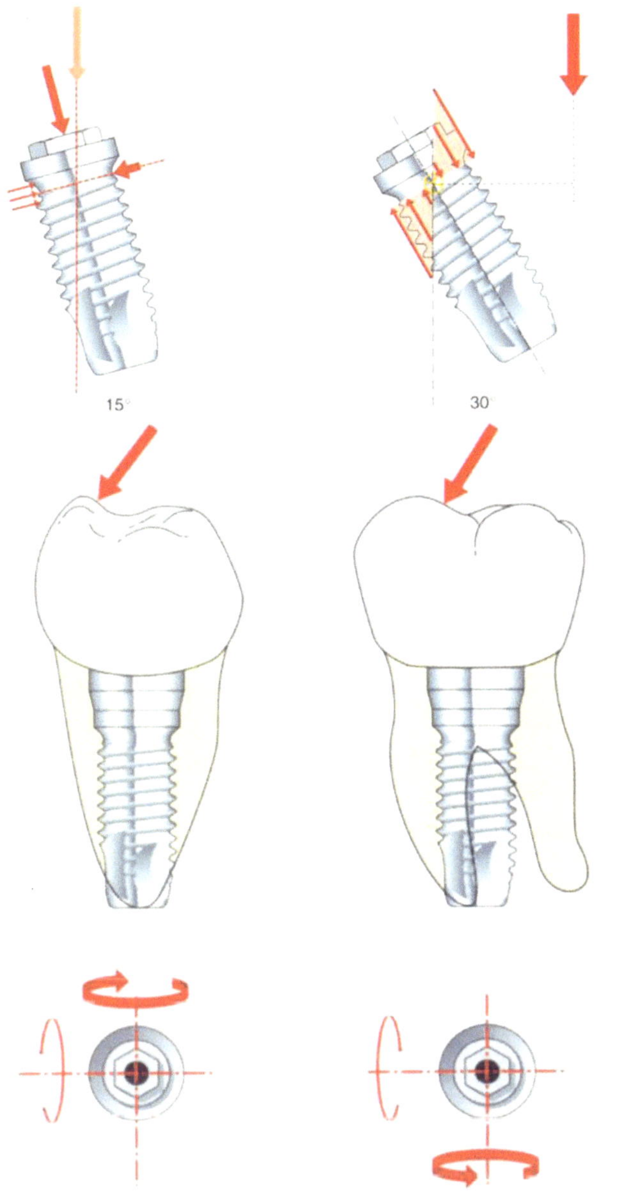

Figure 11.75. The direction and position of the implant in the bone is important from the aspect of biomechanical events. A tilt in the buccolingual direction should be avoided, when the superstructure on the abutment does not follow the axis of the implant, because it leads to bending and an unfavorable effect on the bone. The farther the force acting on the inclined implant is from the axis of the implant, the greater the stress and the attack points of the twisting moment. If the slope does not exceed 15°, the stress and twisting is less. An inclination of 25° and 30° produces greater stresses, and an inclination in the bucco-lingual direction will create insurmountable problems. When it comes to replacing one tooth, a molar, the crown is significantly wider than the diameter of the implant, which can lead to a twisting moment in all directions.

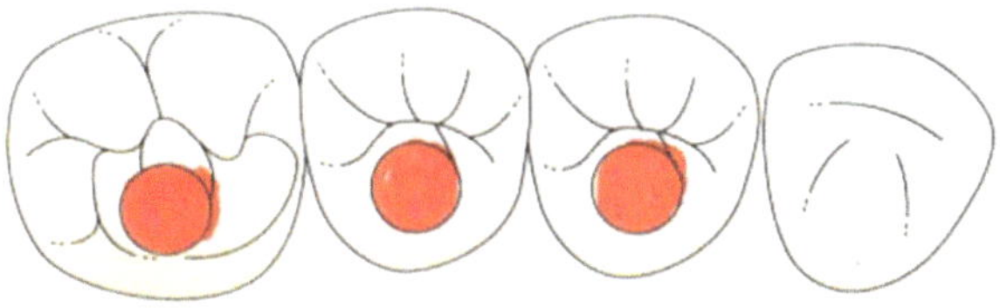

Figure 11.76. Placing the implant in the geometric plane produces a higher stress load on the bone. Cutting the implant thread into the cortical part of the bone creates the most favorable conditions for the stability of the implant - reception and transmission of forces.

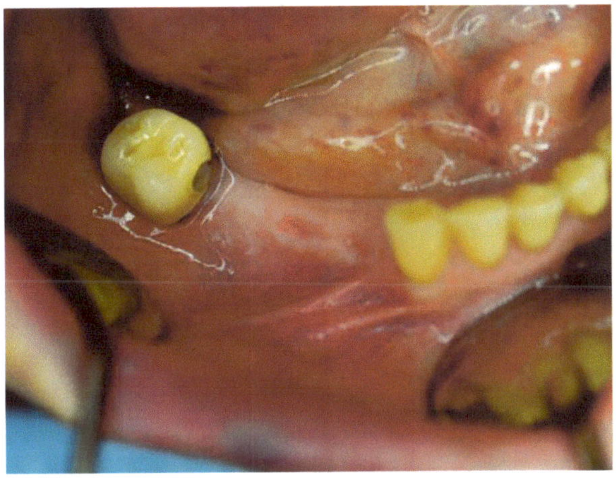

Figure 11.77. Initial state of unilateral toothlessness. Before deciding whether the implant placement will be performed with or without raising the flap, it is necessary to determine the position of the implant placement.

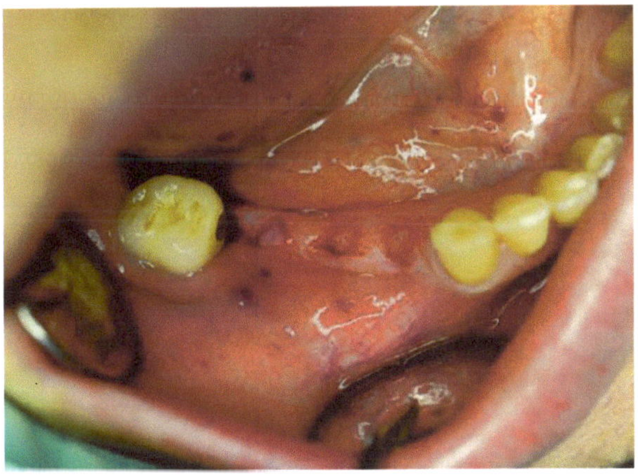

Figure 11.78. Marking the implant position is extremely important so that the implants are installed in the tripoid position (Figures 11.78 to 11.85).

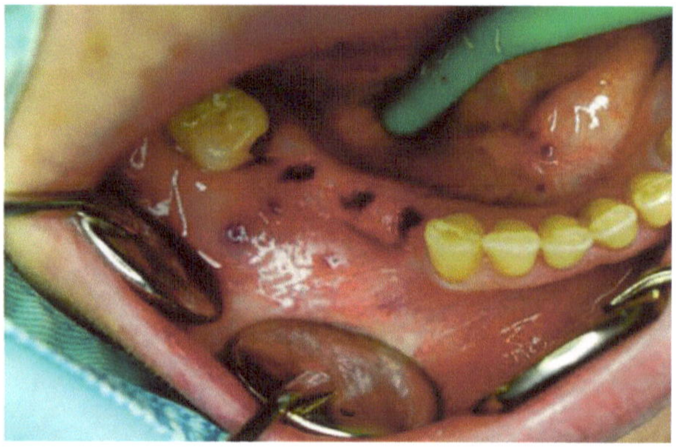

Figure 11.79. With a special instrument, the position is prepared for the immediate installation of the implant without raising the flap.

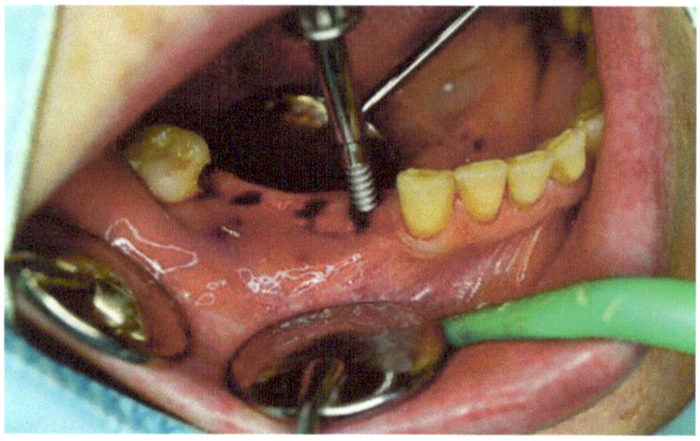

Figure 11.80. Installing the implant without raising the flap is a relief for the patient, and the healing of the surrounding tissues is faster with less trauma.

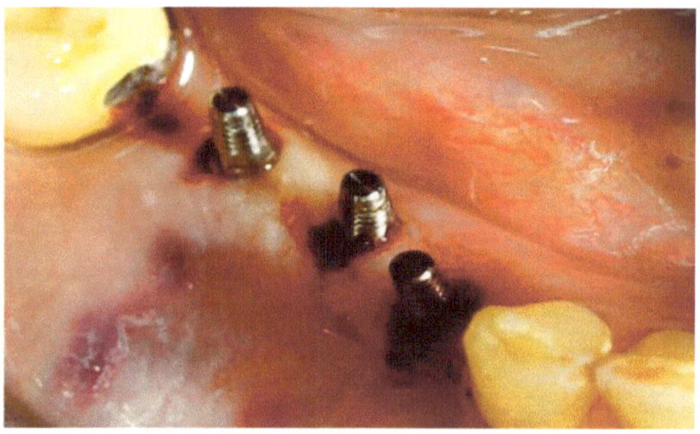

Figure 11.81. Immediately installed implants without raising the flap placed in the tripoid position immediately loaded, leaving the possibility of soft tissue healing (Fig. 11.86) until the creation of a precise provisional bridge in acrylate.

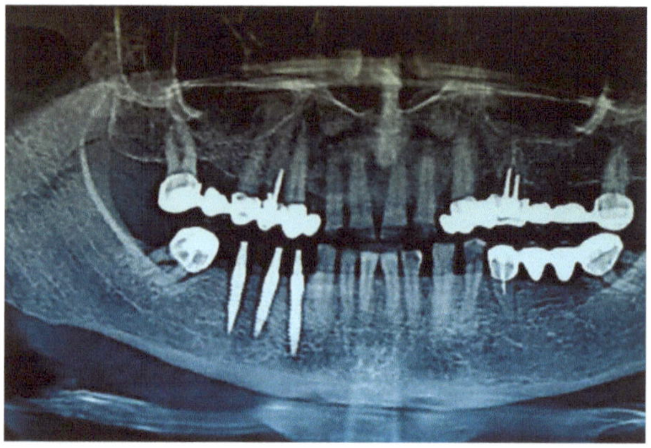

Figure 11.82. Control shot after the immediate installation of a reduced-diameter implant.

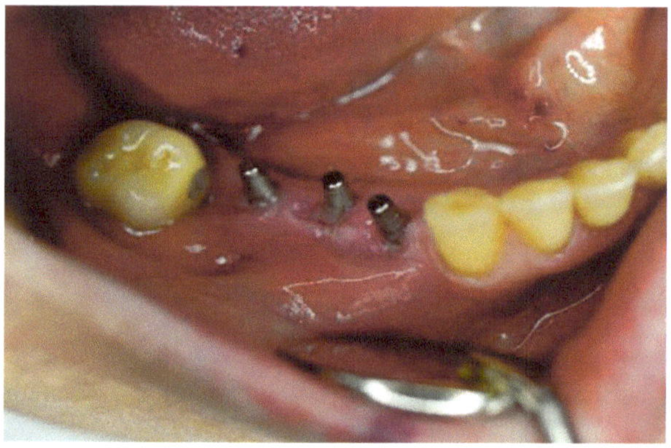

Figure 11.83. Appearance of healed tissues after ten days.

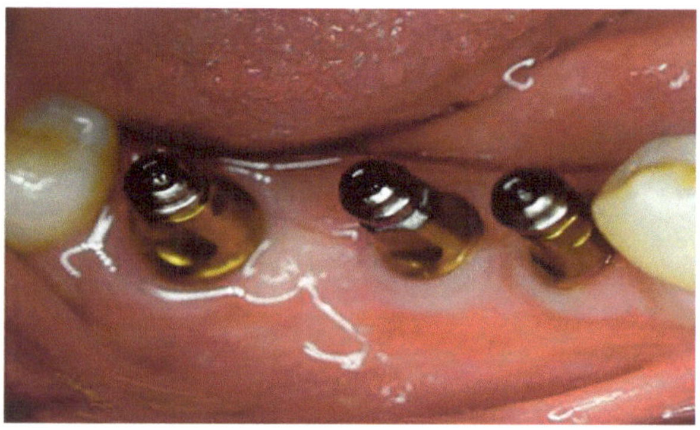

Figure 11.84. Appearance of healed soft tissues in implants immediately placed without raising the flap in the tripoid position, appearance of healed tissues after three weeks.

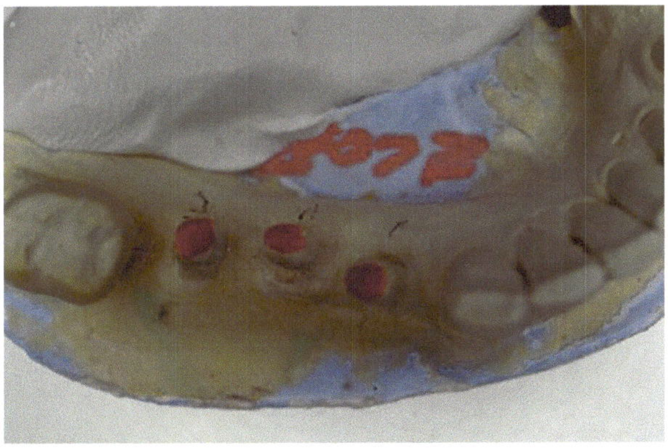

Figure 11.85. Display of the position on the plaster model for making a temporary acrylic bridge.

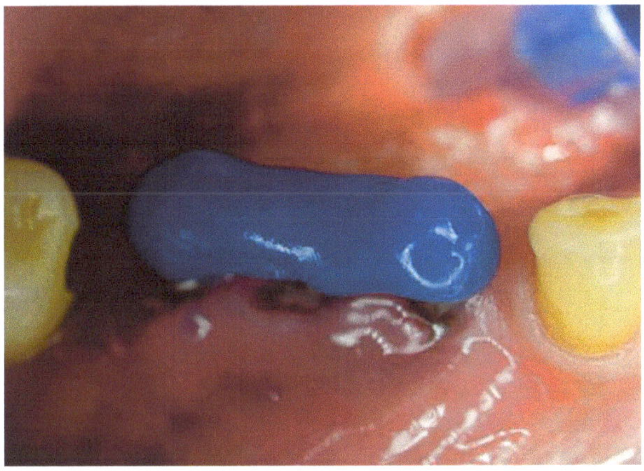

Figure 11.86. Temporary protection with self-polymerizing composite, left the possibility of smooth healing of soft tissues for ten days until the fabrication of a provisional acrylic bridge.

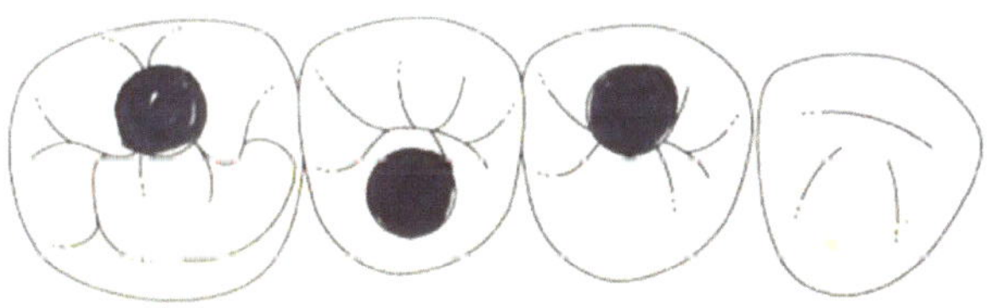

Figure 11.87. The tripod configuration of the implant allows a large part of the load forces to be received along the axial axis of the implant, minimizing the effects of stress and torsion.

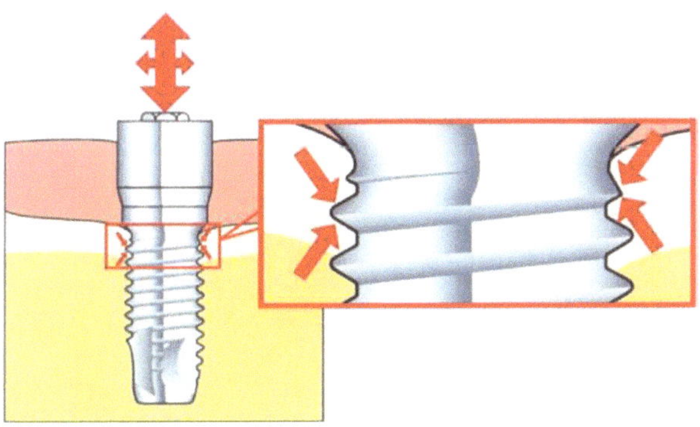

Figure 11.88. Axial load induces compression as the most favorable type of load and uniform reception of forces on all threads.

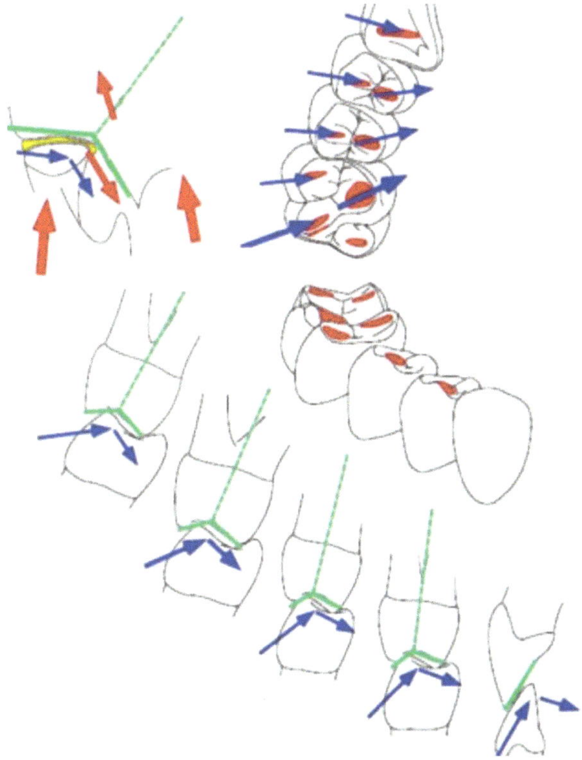

Figure 11.89. Schematic representation of occlusal contacts during lateral movements of the lower jaw - the reception and transmission of chewing forces depends on the inclination of the cusps and the manifestation of these movements in the TMJ.

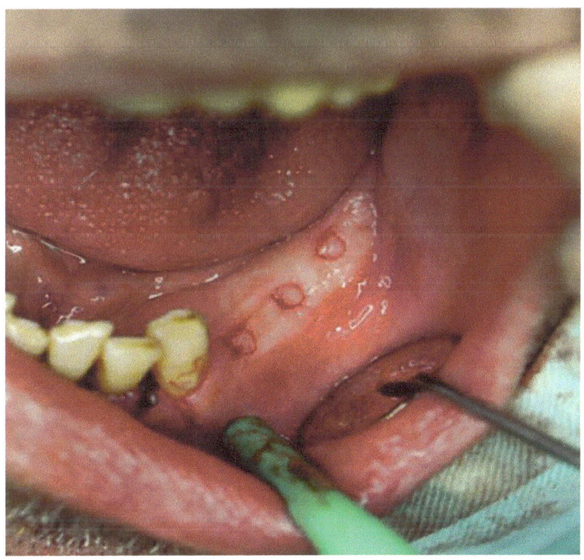

Figure 11.90. Immediate installation of implants without raising the flap in certain positions - patient morbidity is reduced and the time of the entire implant-prosthetic treatment is shortened.

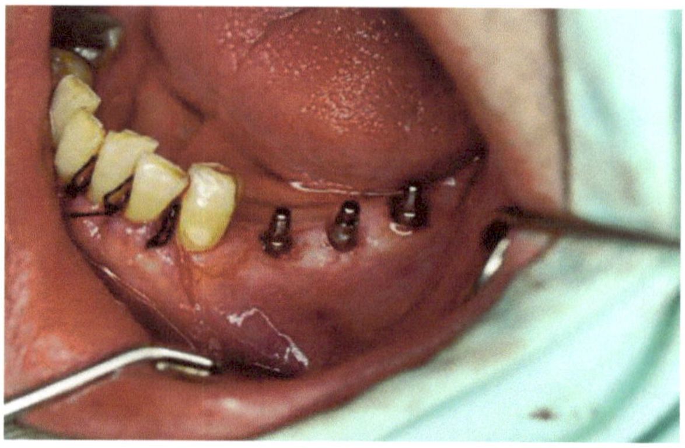

Figure 11.91. Implants immediately installed without raising the flap. Periodontal treatment performed at the same time. Tripoid positioning of the implant with achieved good primary fixation, it is necessary to immediately load temporary prosthetic work, which promotes osseointegration processes followed by patient comfort during the healing period.

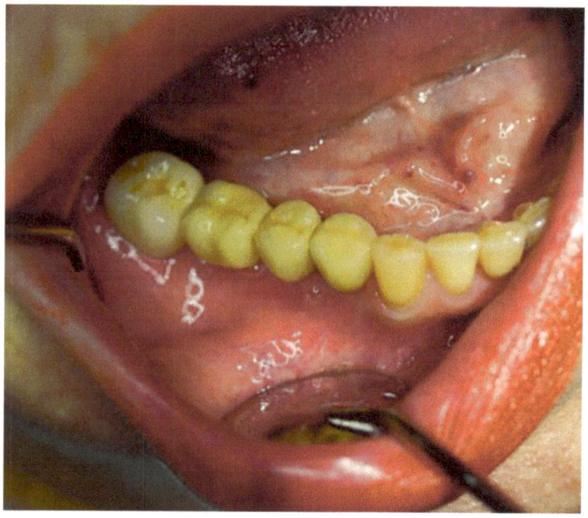

Figure 11.92. Definitive prosthetic work must be performed by fulfilling gnathological requirements. Appearance of well-healed soft tissues.

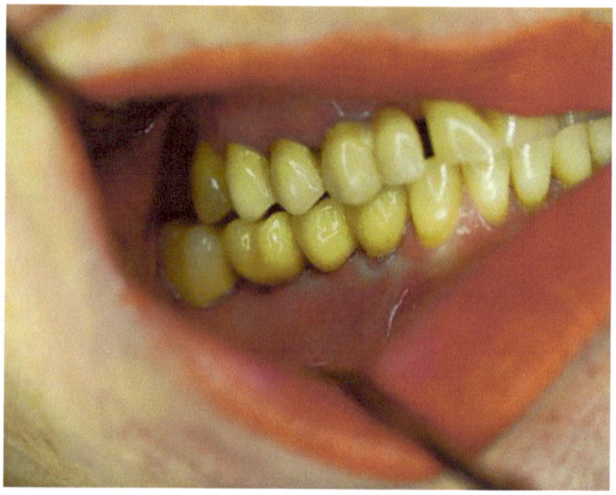

Figure 11.93. Appearance of healed soft tissues after six months. The inclination of the cusps adapted to the lateral movements of the lower jaw It was necessary to shape the cusps of the antagonist of the prosthetic work performed in another office to harmonize them with the lateral movements of the lower jaw.

12

The Future of Diagnostics in Oral Implantology

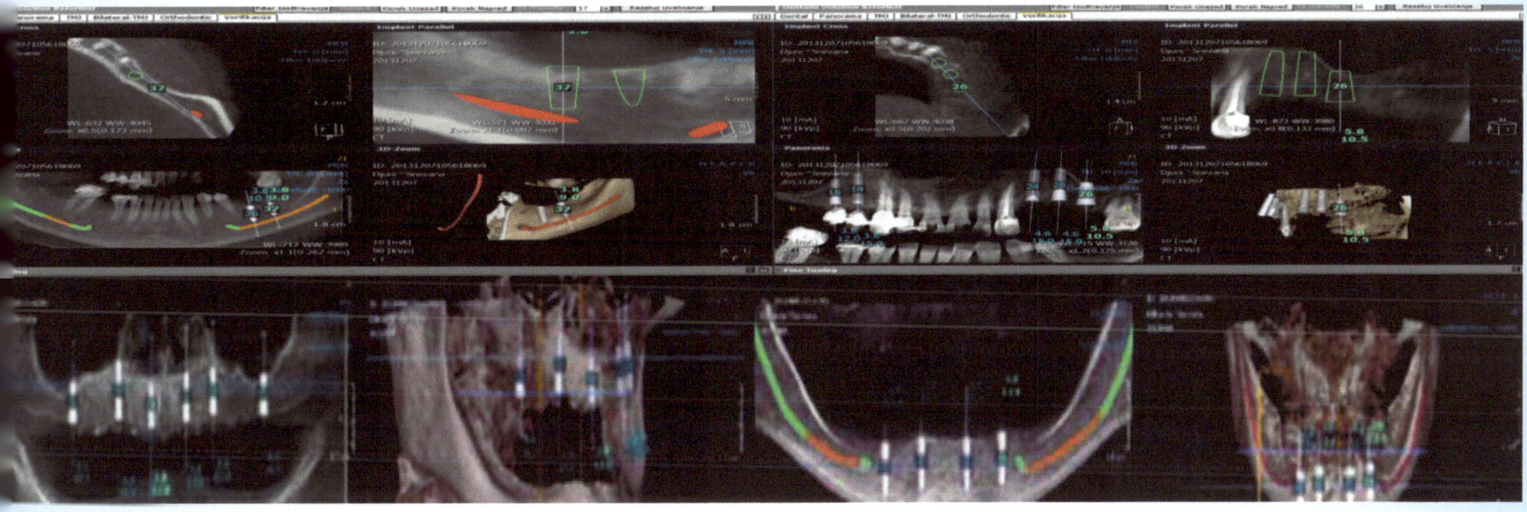

In the period of only two decades ago, the diagnosis of X-ray images has advanced a lot. At one time, dentists had at their disposal mostly conventional methods, insufficient for good diagnostics and planning. However, the first step towards successful implant therapy is good planning. Sometimes the plan was made on the basis of intraoral and classic, orthopantomographic imaging, often with unclear details (Figures 12.1-12.10.)

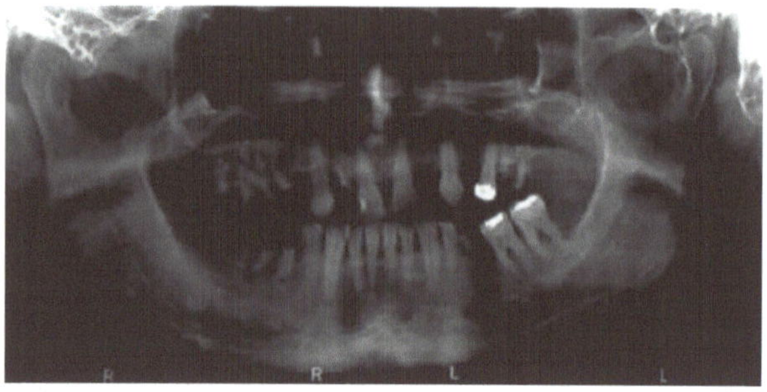

Figure 12.1. Indistinct orthopantomography.

Even today, such a way of visual presentation cannot be ruled out, but for modern implantology planning, especially when the dimensions of the bone bed cannot be determined by conventional X-ray techniques, additional techniques are increasingly being developed that provide great relief to implantologists. Three decades ago, radiographic images were worked exclusively on the basis of conventional methods, orthopantomographic images, which was always a considerable risk, because the poor quality of the images was an aggravating circumstance for planning.

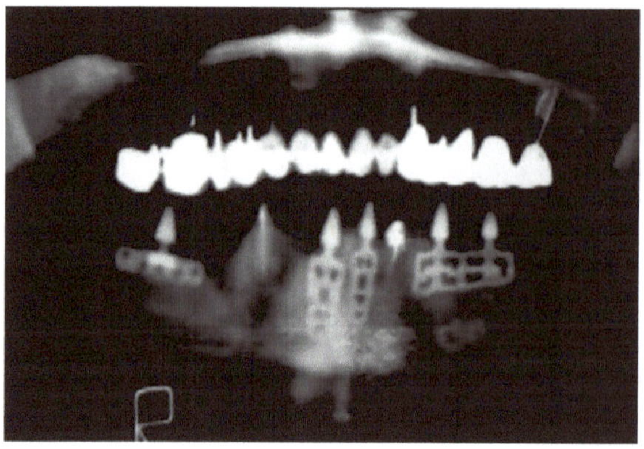

Figure 12.2. Embedded one-piece leaf implants.

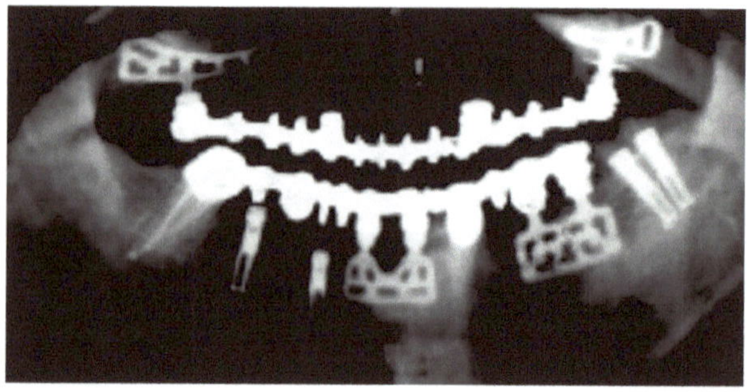

Figure 12.3. In the upper jaw, one-piece Linkov implants of the V generation (tuber implant on the left). In the lower jaw, a combination of cylindrical and Linkov-closed implants of the V generation.

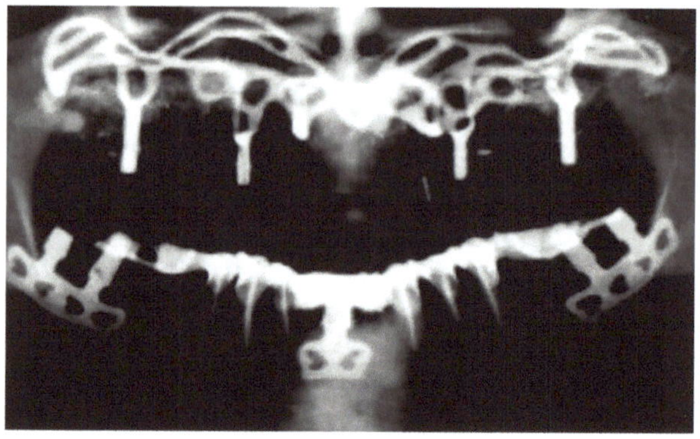

Figure 12.4. Subperiosteal implant in the upper jaw and leaf implants in the lower jaw. Unclear anatomical structures as in the previous picture.

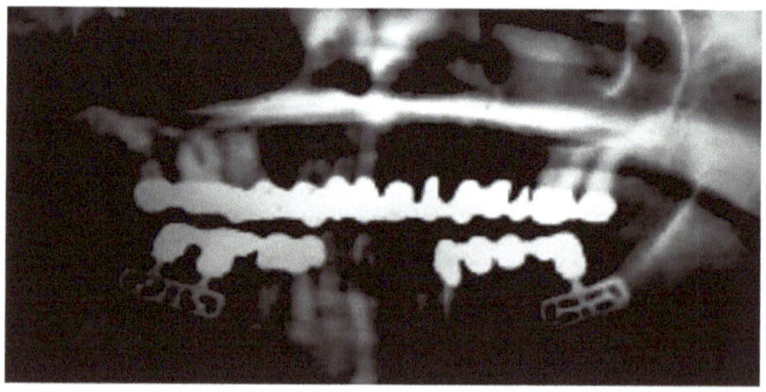

Figure 12.5. Linkov implants in the lower jaw. In the video, the anatomical structures are unclear. Implant placement was performed almost randomly.

For the pioneers of implantology, a few decades ago, it was much more difficult to precisely position the implants based on the unclear radiographic images of the time. Figures 122.1-12.10 illustrate the risks with which implant placement was performed due to poor X-rays. By comparing with the following pictures, the reader of these lines will get a clearer idea of future diagnostics. The safety of implant placement, the predictability of success and the possibilities of precise planning today are unmatched compared to the past.

From the attached radiographs from two decades ago, it can be concluded that the boundaries of the maxillary sinuses, mandibular canal and mental foramen were never clear. Implantological procedures were performed routinely. Therefore, it is clear that the implant placement procedures were accompanied by risk. A special risk was the installation of implants in the vicinity of the mentioned anatomical structures. The experience of the dentist, then, was dominant for the successful outcome of the implantation procedure. Digital technique has significantly advanced radiographic analyzes in clarifying anatomical details compared to earlier orthopan tomographic images.

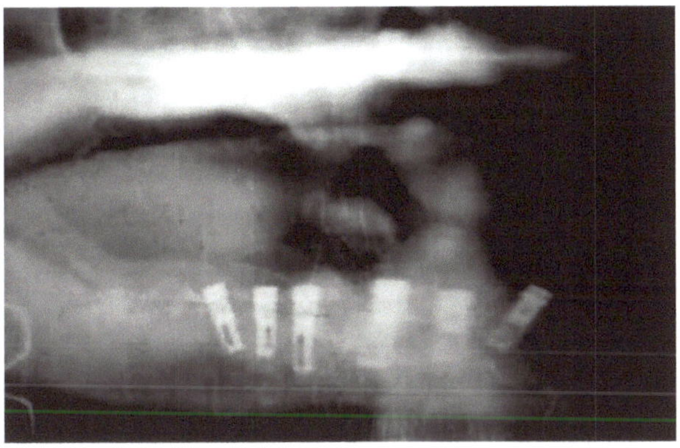

Figure 12.6. The poor quality of the anatomical presentation made implant placement risky.

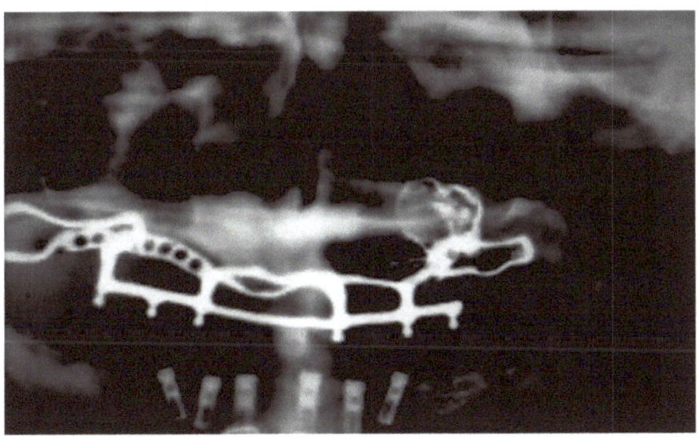

Figure 12.7. Such and similar orthopantomographic recordings dominated in the eighties of the last century.

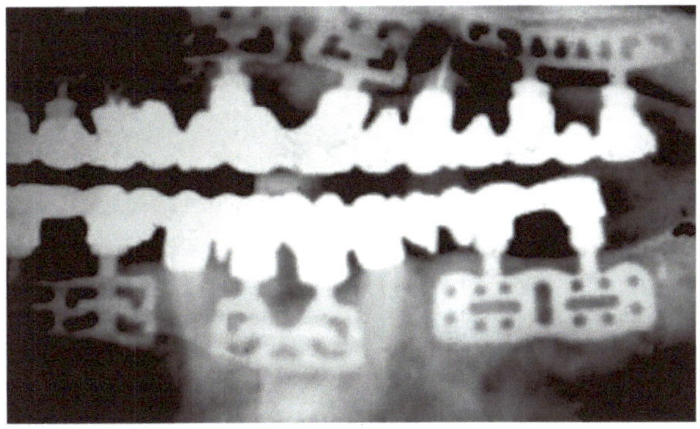

Figure 12.8. Resolving bilateral edentulism in the upper and lower jaw with V generation Linkov leaf implants.

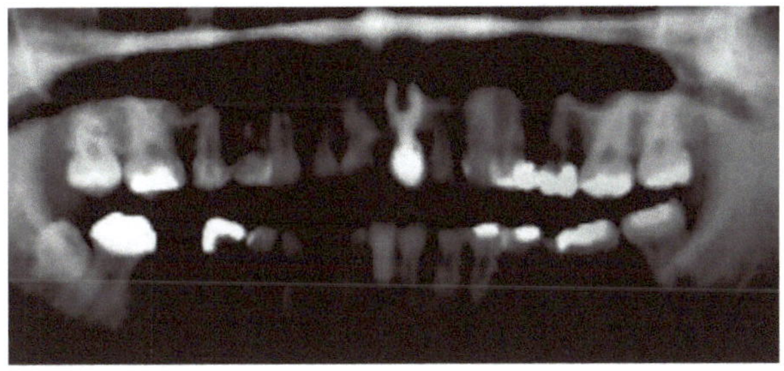

Figure 12.9. Replacement of the central incisor in the upper jaw with a one-piece leaf implant (author's work in 1976).

In the mid-1980s, significant improvements were made, but still insufficiently precise, when it comes to anatomical structures, which are extremely important for the safe installation of implants.

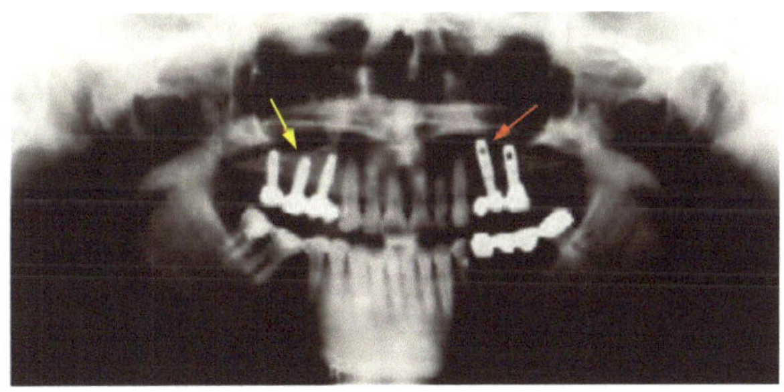

Figure 12.10. Cylindrical implants in the upper jaw. On the right, cylindrical implants coated with hydroxyapatite (yellow arrow), and on the left, Pit-Easy (red arrow) implants (author's work in 1983).

Today, the very rapid development of digital technology offers the possibility of storing data and transferring it to programmable devices. The devices are equipped with sensors and optical devices, and today all of this is offered within dental diagnostics, therapy and planning in everyday practice.

Over the past years, technical, and especially computer-supported, procedures within dental diagnostics and therapy have advanced significantly. Constant innovations in the field of digital technologies promise that this technology will also be significantly improved in the future. The advantage of these technologies becomes even more important with certain programs in everyday practice, not only because it saves the precious time of the therapist, but also because all achievements are multifold useful for the patient himself.

The precision that can be achieved with new procedures in diagnostics and planning has advanced significantly. The greatest contributions from the field of computerized diagnostics were made at the beginning of the 21st century, although even then it was established that experienced oral surgeons did not exceed deviations of 2-3 mm during routine implant placement, and the maximum error during navigation was still in the range of 0.6 up to 0.8 mm.

However, today all dentists have at their disposal portable X-ray devices with digital intraoral sensors, which allow them to achieve a very good diagnostic quality of intraoral X-ray images (Figures 12.11-12.16) and to display them immediately on the display X-ray device or a portable color LCD screen high resolution. In addition to the X-ray display, these devices enable additional actions, such as zooming in on the image, adjusting the lighting contrast, depositing several hundred images on an SD (Secure Digital) memory card, and opening folders for each patient. The transfer of the intraoral recording to the computer is possible wirelessly using the "Bluetooth" technique.

After the X-ray images are transferred to the computer, they can be analyzed on a large screen, zooming in on individual details, adjusting contrast and lighting, and all actions can be permanently saved in the patient folder using any application for manipulating X-ray images.

A big advantage of portable X-ray devices is that the radiation dose is almost negligible for the doctor and the patient.

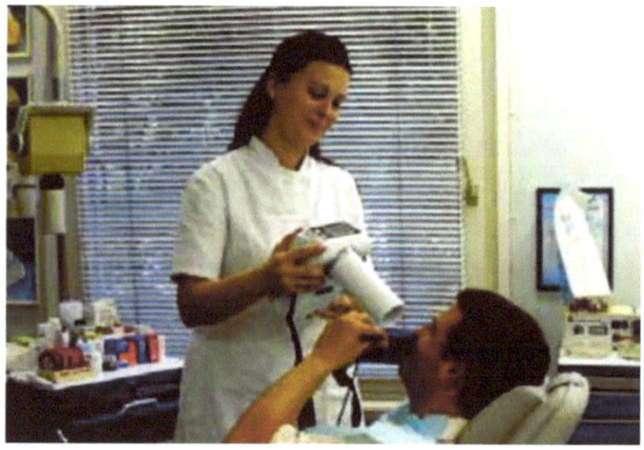

Figure 12.11. Modern portable x-ray with negligible radiation. Despite this, protective aprons should be used for both the patient and the doctor (from the "Dr. Zlopaša" office).

With a short exposure of 0.02 or 0.03 sec. high-quality images are obtained, which is extremely important during implant installation, when several control images need to be taken.

With classic x-rays for intraoral imaging, the exposure time, compared to portable x-ray devices, is fifty to one hundred times longer. The longer the exposure time, the higher the effective radiation dose and vice versa. Manufacturers of portable x-ray devices announce that the new generations will have an even shorter exposure time, with the condition that digital intraoral sensors are used, because classic x-ray films will be less and less used.

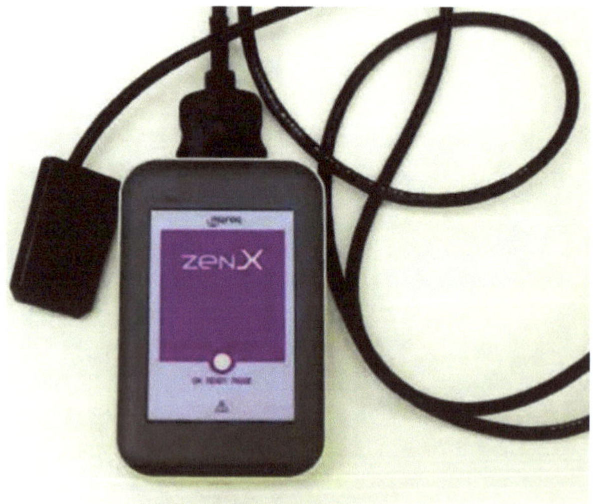

Figure 12.12. Digital intraoral sensor (RVG)

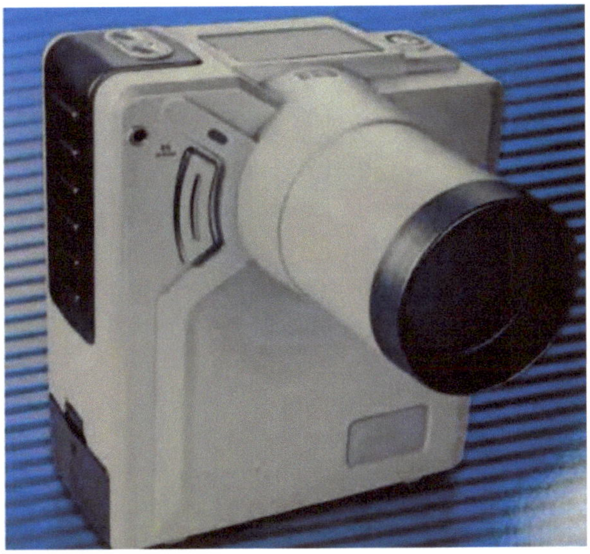

Figure 12.13. RVG tube display - there are two tube lengths.

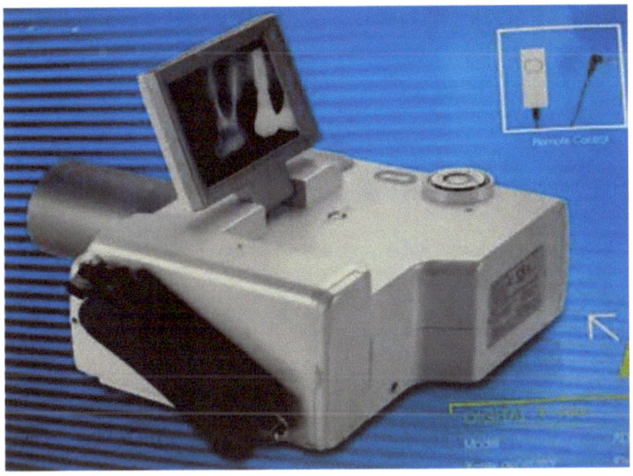

Figure 12.14. The last generation of portable x-ray devices where the recorded area is immediately displayed on the screen.

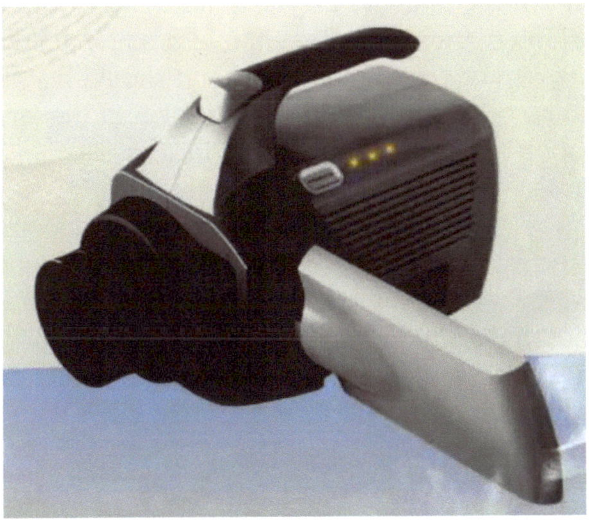

Figure 12.15. A portable X-ray device with a screen, the size of a video camera.

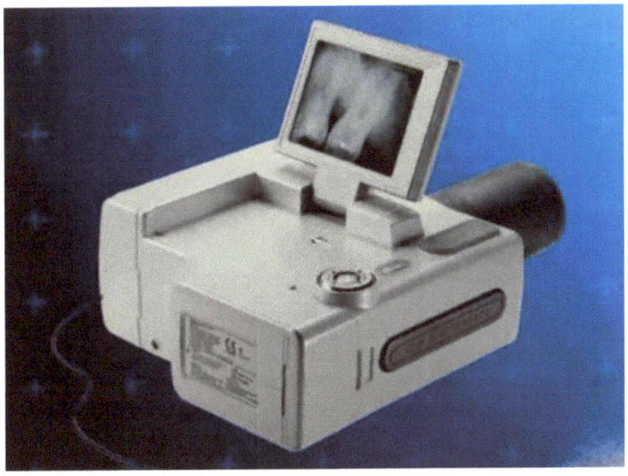

Figure 12.16. Portable x-ray device.

However, the quality of X-ray images with many devices can vary greatly, so the dentist sometimes finds himself in a dilemma as to whether he can realize the planned plan. For this reason, the basic requirement of today's oral implantology in improving diagnostics is supplementing the X-ray image with one more, additional, plane. The need for a three-dimensional display has created, on the market, an ever-increasing offer of digital-volume tomographic devices, which, in addition to the 3- D display, also provide a classic display, an unreconstructed orthopantotomographic image, as with a classic X-ray machine.

The basic goal of radiological diagnostics of preoperative procedures is to establish the morphological and functional prerequisites for ultimate success. A good diagnosis is based on a clear and precise examination of the adjacent anatomical structures, and a clear visibility of the mandibular canal and mental foramen, maxillary sinuses, nasal cavities and the condition and relationship of the present teeth is placed in the foreground.

Three-dimensional planning and navigation using the software allows viewing in three main plane directions (axial, coronary and sagittal). In addition to the panoramic analog view, a view of one segment and an entire view of the jaw is obtained (Figure 12.17).

When planning the installation of implants, attention should be paid at the beginning to visibility in two planes, which enables good spatial visibility. It is important that the corresponding image is one to one, which depends a lot on how the x-ray technician has positioned the patient. Errors and ambiguities in the recording, which can be obtained, often depend on the patient himself - his calmness during the recording. Some patients cannot be placed in the ideal position by the x-ray technician, even with repeated imaging; position of the spine, short neck, in case of large retrusion, patients who are nervously labile and cannot maintain a still position during imaging, etc. All of this greatly affects the precision of details that are extremely important for the dentist when making the implant placement plan.

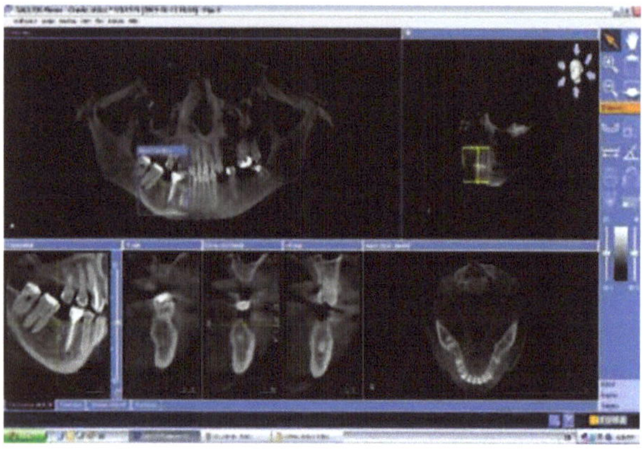

Figure 12.17. Three-dimensional recording (3D).

The connection of 3D X-ray data in the navigation procedure, in the future, will be a field of increasing interest of dentists for the improvement of diagnostics and planning, which will greatly increase the safety of patients during operative procedures. Like this, the X-ray procedure enables us to fulfill two goals: the immediate postoperative relationship of the implant with the adjacent anatomical structures and the control of the postoperative course; observation of resorptive processes in the healing phase, control of the performed procedure. This X-ray image controls the position of the secondary parts and as a reference image, for comparison with later controls. The ability to monitor the main success parameters of oral surgery and implant placement, as well as early observation of bone breakdown, depends on the quality of the X-ray.

As x-ray diagnostic methods, the following are available today: orthopantomography, transverse tomography, intraoral dental imaging, computerized tomography, as well as digital volume tomography.

Panoramic tomography scans

The basic image for planning and treatment is an orthopantomographic image, which provides a useful representation of the bony part of the jaw, maxillary sinuses, as the mesiodistal space in two dimensions. The difficulty that occurs when making a panoramic tomographic image lies in the fact that the focus-object distance and the object-film distance are not constant, which means that the magnification factor changes within the image itself. With modern devices, the path of the focal field follows the jaws, so that distortions in the size and dimension of the bone are avoided, but there remains an error in the mesiodistal measurement, which is not insignificant. When there is a minor change in the positioning of the patient, distortion occurs, that is, deformation, which, of course, makes it difficult to assess the important details of the image.

Transverse tomogram

The advantages of the transverse tomogram are the display of the buccolingual width of the jaw and the possible detection of lingual concavities. Tomographic images showed that the quality of the image, with the use of a program with a fixed projection direction, largely depends on the positioning of the patient. Of decisive importance for the successful outcome of the clarity of the image is the adjustment of the patient's position, matching it with the position of the jaw, so that it is vertical in relation to the given direction of projection. It should be taken into account that the oblique position of the jaw in relation to the central ray results in an unclear image, whose interpretation is not reliable.

The advantage of the transverse tomographic image is that it can be an additional program of the device for panoramic tomography; therefore, it can be useful in situations where the application of digital volume tomography is not available, which provides the implantologist with another plane.

Intraoral shots (retroalveolar)

Classic intraoral images also belong to the scope of x-ray diagnostics (Fig. 12.18). Their advantage is high resolution, which is why they can be used for the detection of the peri-implant space, as well as for the diagnosis of peri-implantitis. However, if the initial bone changes are less than

0.2 mm, they can hardly be registered with this technique. In the case of too vertical or too horizontal adjustment, the consequences are deformations, ie distortions on the recording, which should be taken into account.

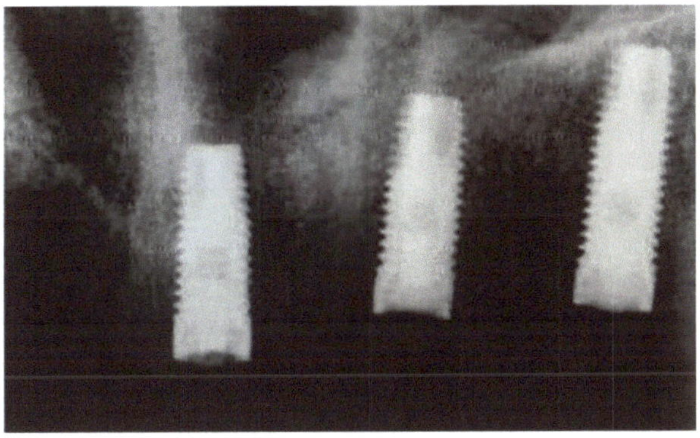

Figure 12.18. Intraoral x-ray of the implant made by portablex-ray device.

Computed tomography

Computed tomography (CT) is one of the newer methods of radiology. It is very useful for planning the installation of implants as a whole, and especially for detecting the existence of unfavorable anatomical conditions. As for the reliability of the image, especially in the stage of planning the installation of the implant and its positioning, it is, for now, the most accurate method, and the magnification is always constant: one to one! By deciphering the data obtained by CT and the corresponding software, in practice, a direct practical application is possible for the planning of implant placement. Transferring data and applying templates for implant positioning is a great relief for the implantologist.

It was much more difficult for the pioneers of oral implantology to plan implant-prosthetic treatment based on the then imperfect orthopanic images. Today, implant placement planned based only on the digital orthopantomographic image represents a big mistake, due to the lack of relevant data for implant positioning.

Computed tomography provides a clear cross-section of the bone of the target site for implant placement. The obtained tomographic image clearly shows the structure of the bone, the size and quality of the lamina, as well as the shape and exact position of the anatomical structures.

By planning and assessment, based only on orthopantomography we do not know the exact position of the anatomical structures in the cross-section, which is very important when it comes to, for example, the exact position of the mandibular canal and the mental openings. From the author's experience, on the orthopantomographic view of the sinus and the floor of the sinus, we see that part only in the orthogonal projection, and in the real state, the bone can exist either above or below the sinus cavity.

It should be emphasized that during the augmentation procedure, an orthopantomogaph scan can be used to determine whether sufficient bone volume has been obtained by augmentation, because there is only an examination of the height of the bone. After augmentation of bone defects with bone substitutes and the creation of new bone, the author's experience shows that by relying only on orthopantomographic images, a false image can be obtained, because there is no insight into what happened to the bone if only an image of the height, but not the bone volume, is obtained. Computerized tomography provides a realistic image of alveolar ridge augmentation. And there is also missing information on bone density after augmentation at the place of planned implant placement. Despite the tremendous advances in radiographic computer technology, reliable bone density determination of segments of interest has not yet been achieved. Computed tomography provides precise measurement results of the cross-section, but the bone density of the cross-section cannot be determined visually. Measuring bone density is not only a problem of oral implantology, it is also a problem of medicine in general. For this reason, there is no relevant data on bone density in the upper and lower jaw. However, during the implementation, when it comes to assessing the quality of the bone, the computed tomography findings can complement the clinician's experience. Only in this way can one assess, or rather assume, whether the bone is porous - type D4 or not.

Practice and experience show that with an unclear orthopan-tomographic image, on which unclear anatomical details are essential for planning the implant procedure, which implies planning of the entire implant-prosthetic treatment, one should not try to start planning with such unclear images. It is necessary to make a 3D recording on the basis of which a plan of the whole is made treatment treatment. Overlooking some details during planning, minor and serious incidents are possible during implant installation. Computed tomography must show clear details; whether it is about the measurement values of the section of undermined bone sites-concavity of the alveolar ridges, bone defects, etc. With computed tomography, it is possible to determine the degree of achieved osseointegration of integration and similar details. Overlooking these details during implant placement, ridge perforation may occur during bone preparation for the implant bed. During the surgical phase of implant placement and implant positioning, monitoring the position of the implant with the surrounding anatomical structures using digital intraoral sensor is great relief for the safe installation of the implant(see Figure 12.12).

Digital volume tomography

Digital volume tomography (DVT) as an X-ray imaging method available to every dentist today. In the literature, it is also defined as CBCT (Cone Beam CT) and this technique was described as early as 1998. More than fifteen years have passed since its introduction into dental practice, and the unique name of this radiological modality is still being debated. So, today in practice we meet different names, which denote the same radiological principle. Synonyms for Cone Beam CT (CBCT) radiography are Cone Beam Volumetric Tomography (CBVT) and Dental Volumetric Tomography (DVT). Knowing the different names eliminates confusion when interpreting different literary materials and professional presentations. Basically, this method belongs to the family of computerized tomographic radiology technique, because the data obtained during radiography, with specially designed computer programs, merge into a three-dimensional radiological record of the radiographed region. The essence of the technique is a source of radiation, which emits a cone-shaped beam of rays, during which with just one circular exposure of the patient, a sufficient amount of radiological data is acquired that enables the reconstruction of a three-dimensional radiological record (Figure 12.19).

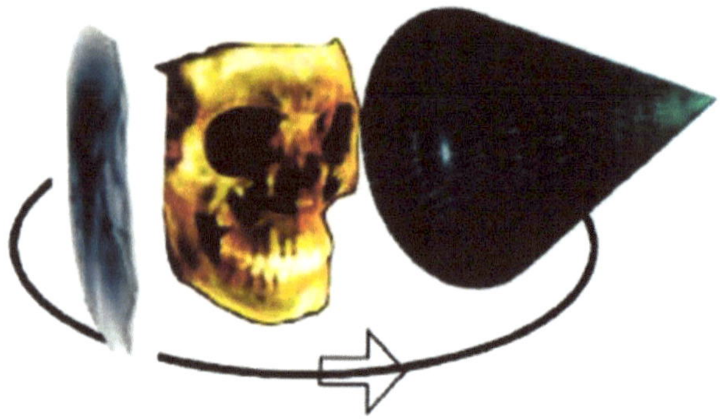

Figure 12.19. Šematski prikaz DVT.

For a proper understanding of the concept, it is extremely important for the dentist to understand that, unlike classic CT records that include a series of layers, by choice, that extend through the entire neck or head (that is, part of them), CBCT records usually have the shape of a cylinder of different dimensions (depending on the choice of device), the inclusion of the desired anatomical details depends on its correct positioning.

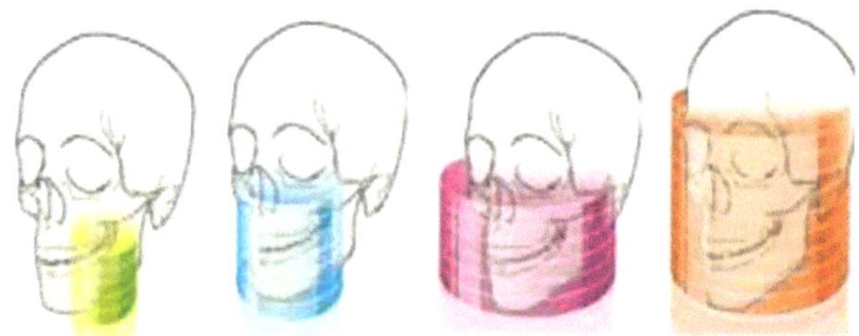

Figure 12.20. An adequate selection of the size of the radiography field significantly reduces the dose of X-ray radiation (it is communicated to the patient).

Only a selection of the largest fields have x-ray emission bands like classic CT devices (Figure 12.20). The idea is to correctly estimate the size of the desired anatomical details, in order to perform the radiography with the smallest required field, which would consequently result in a lower radiation dose delivered to the patient. Also, the larger the size of the radiography field, the "larger" the details we will observe, and the resolution of the image decreases with the growth of the field size. In this way, the patient is protected from unnecessary radiological radiation. The size of the field varies from 6x4cm and even up to 18x20cm. The resolution of the image ranges from 80-330μm, and the dentist with an adequate selection of the size of the imaging field receives an image that will be easier to interpret, i.e. higher recording resolutions. Although three-dimensional radiographic techniques in the form of CT X-ray devices have long been used in dental practice, we can safely say that it was the CBCT technique that introduced the world of three-dimensional radiographic records into everyday dental practice. The benefit of this technique is primarily reflected in the ability to create a three-dimensional radiological image (record) with a radiation dose many times lower than classic CT radiographic techniques. This is a justification for answering relatively "simple" questions by the interpretation of a three-dimensional record. In the second place, the availability of radiography devices has increased with the increase in their supply on the market with the decrease in the price of radiography compared to classic CT devices. In third place, but no less important, is the fact that the method of interpretation of recordings has been significantly improved by the development of software packages in which tools of importance for oral implantology have been designed.

The advantage of using DVT in oral implantology is a three-dimensional representation of a segment or the entire jaw for planning individual implants, but also for extensive treatment in the presence of reduced bone mass and the threat of neighboring anatomical structures or possible augmentation planning (Figure 12.21). Instead of multiple scans of the skull, the dataset in DVT enables, based on its possibilities for reconstruction in additional planes, a complete representation of the jaw region. Magnification, one to one, is independent of patient positioning, which is an advantage of DVT.

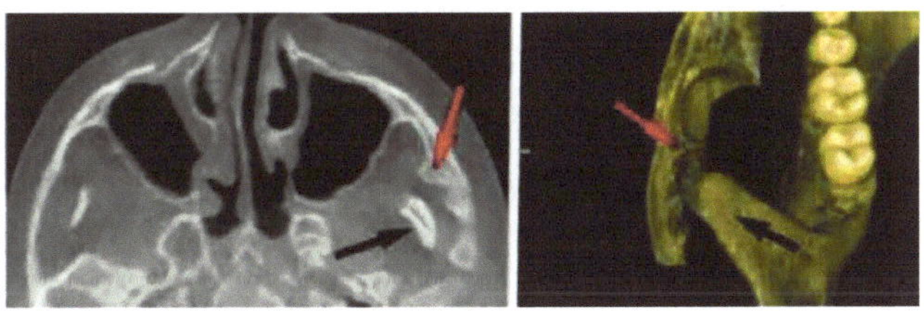

Figure 12.21. Occlusal scan of the sinus. TMJ scan

Limitations within DVT are the absence of soft tissue imaging. In the presence of metalwork in the patient's mouth, DVT recordings are characterized by less sensitivity to artifacts than in the case with computed tomography. DVT, in contrast to a conventional panoramic tomographic scan, represents only a partial view of some regions (several millimeters thick). For X-ray implantology diagnostics, compared to today's techniques, in terms of providing a three-dimensional image, one should expect a view without deformation, with a magnification that is one to one, which is important for increasing the safety of implant installation. Despite all the modernization of X-ray techniques, the most important requirement is still today: **reducing radiation for both the patient and the doctor**.

Although in the framework of modern implantology, as part of "retrograde planning", anatomical risks due to peri-implant augmentative and other surgical procedures can be avoided, anatomical knowledge still belongs to the essential factors of the success of implant placement. Three-dimensional images using CT and DVT techniques as part of the therapeutic plan enable an exact representation of all relevant anatomical structures, both bones and soft tissues, arteries, veins and nerves without deformations, and in this way secure observation of anatomical "traps" is ensured. In any case, even today, and in the future, we should expect even greater progress in terms of facilitating the installation of implants. Planning the entire operation is the foundation of success. Implantology planning will increasingly be based on computer-guided implant placement. The conclusion can be drawn from this that the process of implant planning has gone through many stages, and the most based on visual and routine planning with assistance of radiological two-dimensional (2D) image. The concept of computer-guided implant installation, in addition to detailed visibility of anatomical structures, bone quality and density, also enables the best prosthetic and surgical plan solutions.

The process of computer-guided implant placement begins with the fabrication of the stent. Static computer-guided implant placement uses a surgical stent with an embedded titanium cylinder that serves to determine the direction and depth of planning bone preparations. Dynamic, computer-guided implant placement is a type of navigation technology that enables implant placement based on a virtual plan, following the movement of the implant instrument with an electronic camera, without the use of a surgical stent (Figure 12.22).

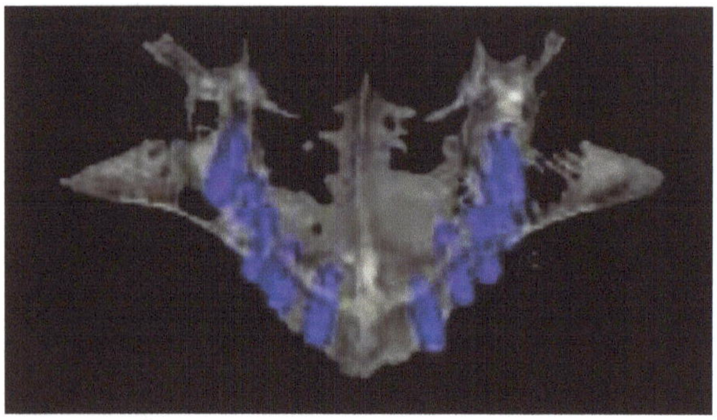

Figure 12.22. Computer-guided implant positioning at basis of virtual planning for the Nobel Biocare implant system.

Until recently, computer-guided implant placement was only available for individual implant systems (Nobel Guides, ImPla). Today there are "open" or "closed" computer systems guided installation of implants, depending on whether the system allows the application of implants from different manufacturers or is intended exclusively for using a certain type of implant. Systems of computer-guided implant placement can be divided into local and global, depending on whether the surgical stent is made in its own laboratory, or electronically sends the virtual plan to another laboratory that makes the stent. The procedure of making a stent involves the creation of a study model on which, using the wax-up or setup procedure, the missing teeth are modeled. After the test in the mouth, the modeled teeth are translated into X-ray contrast teeth using material (barium sulfate). The purpose of this is to determine the exact position for the installation of the implant in the planning process, the distance from the mandibular canal, as well as the position of the future prosthetic work (Figure 12.23).

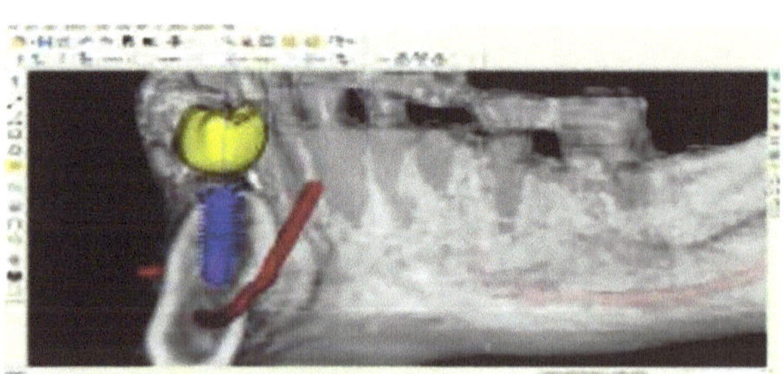

Figure 12.23. Virtual implant positioning.

The exact position of the virtual model is translated into the actual condition in the mouth, and the landmarks are modeled teeth made of X-ray contrast materials, which have a clear morphology and position. An X-ray stent is made on the basis of X-ray-contrast teeth made of acrylic or vacuum-made foil adapted to an toothless or edentulous ridge. After making the image, the data is entered into the software for bone structure analysis and virtual implant placement. Open planning systems enable the virtual placement of implants from all manufacturers of certified implant systems, as well as the creation of models of new implants based on dimensions, if implants are not on the list. The process of virtual implant placement is very complex and requires a good knowledge of prosthetic planning principles, as well as knowledge of anatomical details, which ensures safe surgical implant placement. The translation of virtual planning into the implementation of implant installation begins with the creation of a surgical stent with the exact position for the installation of the implants themselves. The intended position of the implant is made possible by position positioners, which have the ability to adjust and align with the virtual plan with a precision of 0.1 mm. By making a surgical stent, it is possible to check whether the position of the titanium guides on the surgical stent completely matches the position of the virtually planned implants, which represents the final stage of making the surgical stent.

Advantages of computer-guided implant placement

The advantages of computer-guided implant placement, from the dentist's perspective, are numerous compared to other methods:

- achieving safe conditions for greater planning success and precise implant positioning;
- greater safety and comfort during the surgical procedure, especially if it is performed without flap lifting;
- for performing the surgical procedure, this method enables the accurate selection of surgical instruments in advance, which shortens the intervention time, and thus reduces trauma, both to the bone and to the surrounding tissues, and consequently the healing period immediate loading and prosthetic

work can be performed immediately after implant placement;

- better aesthetics are achieved because the entire process of computer-guided implant planning is aimed at achieving the optimal prosthetic solution.
- there is complete visibility of the planned implant position, complete predictability of the course of the surgical procedure stages and control of parallelity of the implants themselves. A significant advantage is that the surgical intervention takes much less time, and the future surgical course and appearance of future prosthetic work can be explained much more clearly to the patient;
- from the point of view of the implantologist, with this method of planning, in addition to observing the position of the implant, the position of the carrier can be clearly observed and at the same time the parallelism of the implants can be checked, which is extremely important for the final outcome.

One of the major disadvantages of computer-guided implant placement is the relatively high dose of radiation to the patient when taking X-rays, which is especially pronounced when taking CT scans. In the future, eliminating this shortcoming will be a priority task in the development of new technologies. Three-dimensional radiological records of the CBCT technique are characterized by exceptional accuracy so that, after a properly performed recording technique, where the patient's "absolute" rest during radiography is primarily considered, images are obtained that realistically depict, without deformation, the necessary anatomical characteristics of the patient (Figure 12.24). A special feature of the program for the interpretation of recordings is that the measurement of the linear dimensions of certain structures on the recording, regardless of the relative enlargement (zooming) of the structure in the program, remains absolutely accurate.

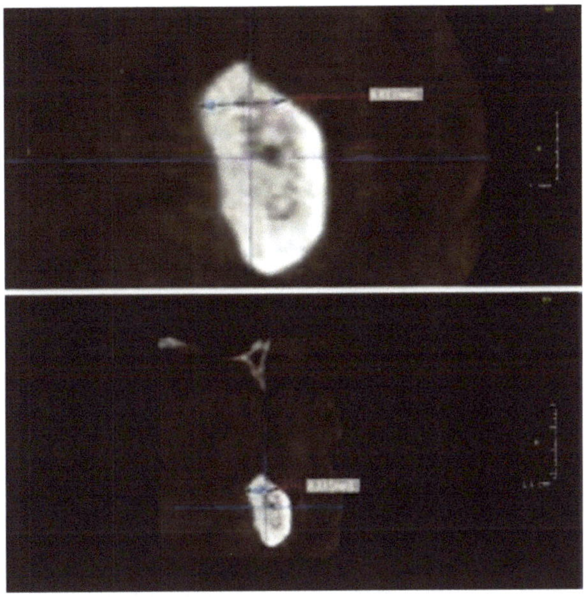

Figure 12. 24. The possibility of enlarging the radiographic display, up to the limit of the resolution of the image, provides security when measuring and evaluating anatomical details, while maintaining the absolute accuracy of the display.

Bone tissue details are reliably observed on CBCT images, and the characteristics of soft tissue structures are registered only in absolute volume, without the possibility of qualitative assessment of their structure. It is important to note that with the CBCT technique, even with a wrongly positioned patient who was not calm during the radiography, the image does not lose its use value because the program allows its reorientation without losing the accuracy of displaying the radiological structures (Figure 12.25).

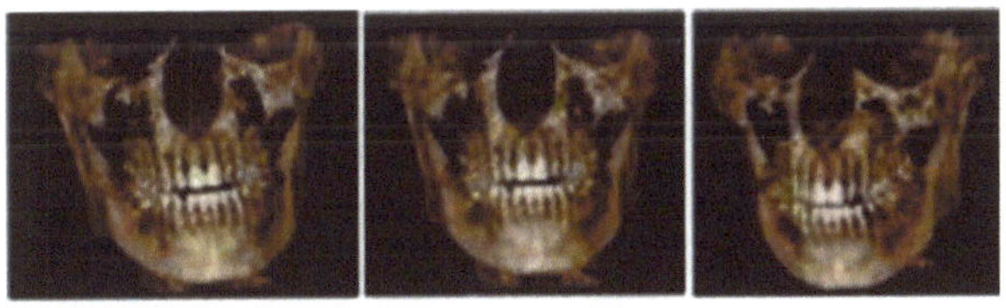

Figure 12.25. The software features of the program allow subsequent "positioning" of the radiographic record, eliminating the need to re-image incorrectly positioned patients during radiography.

For easier interpretation in implantology, the so-called DVR (dental volume reformat) view was developed. This kind of display can be said to have an option that has a similar display for orientation on the recording, which is generated based on an individually drawn tomographic plane (Figure 12.26). This plane corresponds to the shape of the observed jaw, and the tomographic sections show the dimension of the bone in the buco-oral diameter that was inaccessible by "classical" radiological techniques. Three-dimensional reconstruction of anatomical structures greatly facilitates spatial orientation.

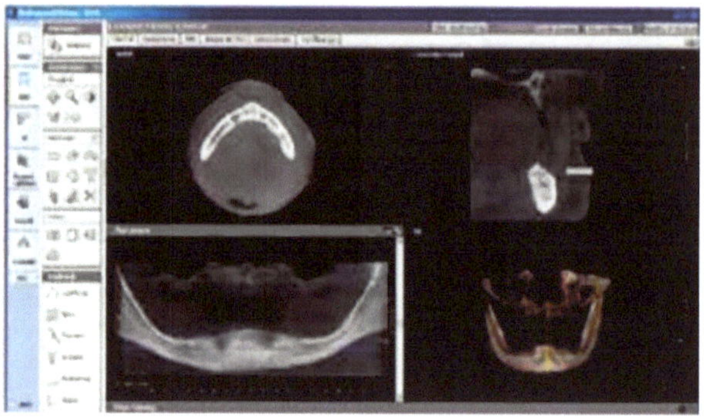

Figure 12.26. DVR or dentally oriented record review offers a comprehensive panoramic view and tomographic sections generated in relation to an individually formed tomographic plane, according to the anatomical characteristics of the jawbone.

Particularly interesting are the tools that enable a reliable pre-implant analysis of the available bone foundation, and the marking - "mapping" - of the bony path of the lower dental nerve canal and the virtual positioning of the graphic implant models stand out. Mapping of the mandibular canal facilitates visualization of the spatial distribution of the nerve, which makes planning easier and more reliable (Figure 12.27).

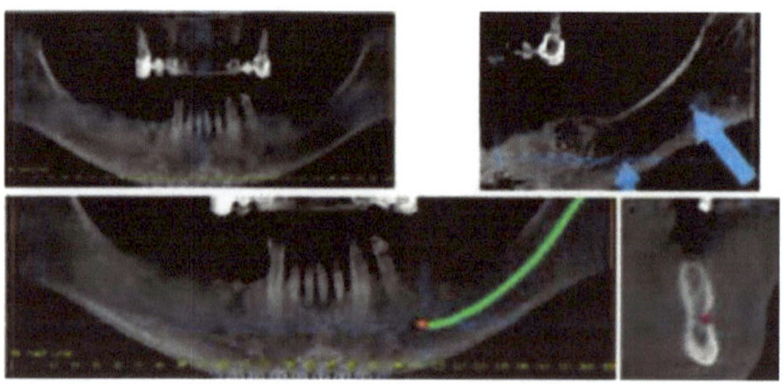

Figure 12.27. The procedure of "mapping" the bony path of the lower dental nerve allows the location of the "mandibular canal" even when identification is difficult during examination of a tomographic section.

Tomographic sections generated from CBCT records have significantly improved characteristics compared to linear tomographic sections, which have been the mainstay of implantology in our country for the past ten years (Figure 12.28):

- no superimposition of layers;
- there is a possibility to choose the resolution of the recording;
- There is no deformation of the recording and they can be reliably recorded
- perform linear measurements;
- software marking of nerve paths is reliable;
- It is possible to determine the amount of bone foundation
- for placement of endosseal implants;
- It is possible to assess the "quality" of the bone.

A reliable assessment of the available bone foundation enables safe planning of implant placement. Software packages offer the possibility of virtual implant positioning, individually, depending on the observed characteristics of the bone foundation on the radiological record (Figure 12.29). The implant software libraries have a wide selection of implant manufacturers and product lines and, most significantly, they are the dimensions of the positioned "virtual" implants within the CBCT images identical to the dimensions of the real implants that would be installed in the same anatomical place. Regardless of the magnification of the image, the relationship between the dimensions of the implant and the radiographic record remains the same. Nevertheless, after the planning performed on the native image (without radiological guides), the surgeon's experience is necessary to identify the estimated anatomical localization on the image and in the mouth. Programs offer the possibility of exact estimation of the distance of certain points by means of millimeter graduation of the distance of the tomographic sections, when the orientation is done in relation to the central line of the jaw, present teeth or a characteristic anatomical detail, according to the number of tomographic sections. Planning and verifying the position of virtual implant models facilitates the assessment of the complex relationship of the implant to the surrounding anatomical structures. The dimensions of the implant, regardless of computer zooming, remain "absolute" and reliable. The programs have wide "libraries" of implant systems and production lines, so they support a wide range of users in their daily work.

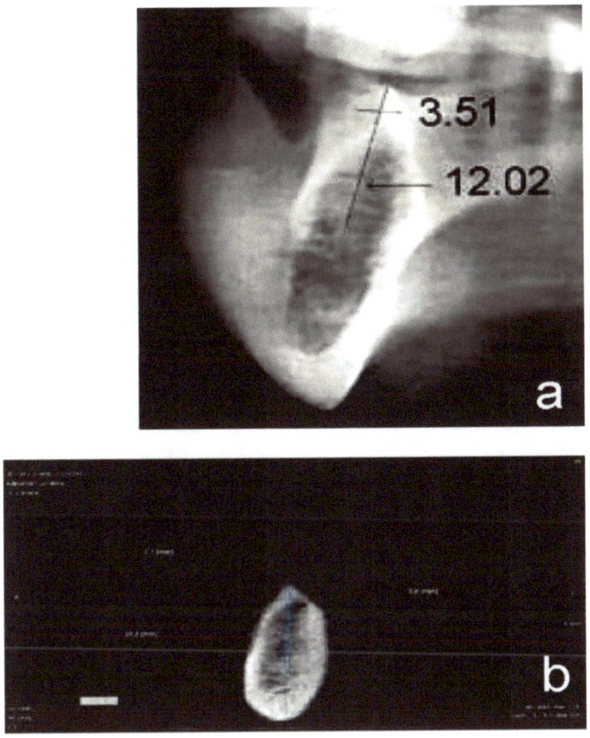

Figure 12.28. Comparison of display clarity: (a) on the left, linear tomography; (b) on the right, a tomographic view generated from CBCT scan.

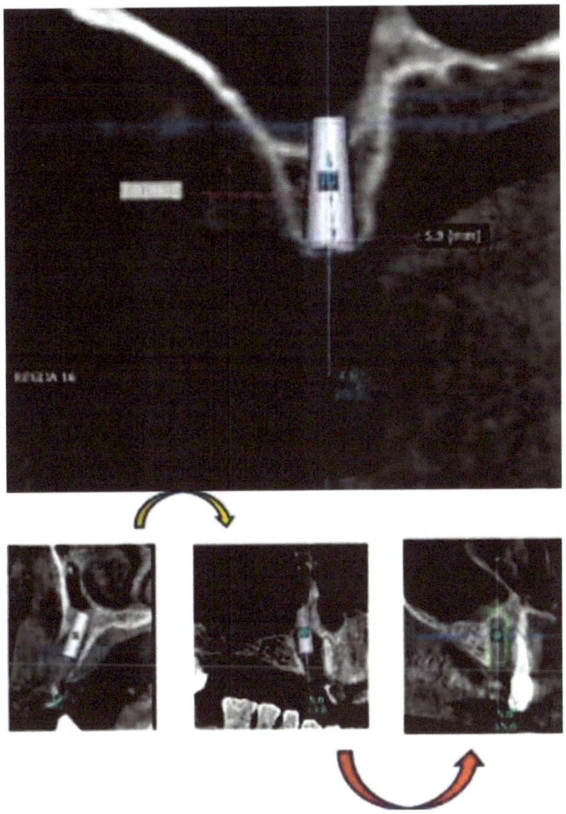

Figure 12.29. (a) Example of a virtually positioned implant; (b) An example of implant position verification shows that in certain cases, planning the position solely on the basis of transverse tomographic images can lead to a planning error; positioning of implants in relation to anatomical structures, as well as in relation to neighboring teeth.

Verification of implant position is also a more important tool because it provides insight into the spatial relationships of implants and anatomical structures 360° circularly in relation to the axis of the implant. Harmonization of the prosthetic reconstruction plan with the surgical plan, i.e. prosthetic formation directed insertion of implants, is one of the significant advances of three-dimensional CBCT technology, which forms the basis for the formation of surgical stent-guided implantation. Defining the prosthetically desired tooth position can be done with the help of radiographic guides or plaster study models on which the desired position of the future restoration is planned (Figure 12.30). Radiographic guides can be used in the form of specially made prostheses or temporary crowns. Radiographically the guides are positioned in a defined position in the patient's mouth and are radiographed together with the patient. Study models are radiographed or scanned with standard extraoral scanners, and the obtained digital ones the data, based on orientation points, are subsequently superimposed with the patient's radiological record.

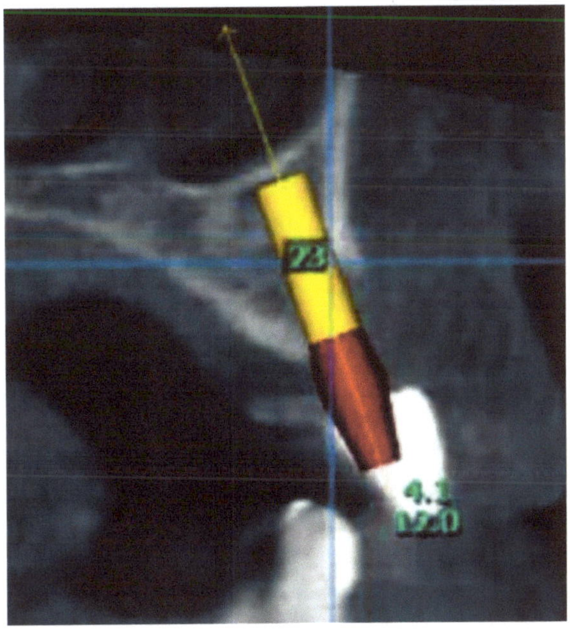

Figure 12.30. Radiological guide and virtual planning of implant installation based on the outline of the tooth crown in the desired position.

Example of implant planning

After accessing the patient's radiological record, an individual tomographic plane is defined that corresponds to the shape of the patient's jaw (Figure 12.31). Individual definition of the tomographic plane is extremely important due to the generation of accurate tomographic sections, which are formed in an orientation at right angles to the tomographic plane. An inadequately formed tomographic plane can create an error in observation section either by the observed width or by the shape of the observed section.

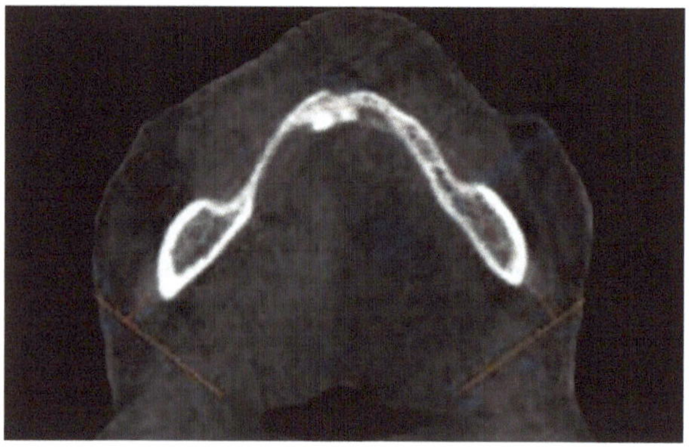

Figure 12.31. Individually formed tomographic plane in accordance with the shape of the jaw.

After the formation of the tomographic plane, detection of the canal of the lower dental nerve is performed if the planning is done in the lower jaw. Detection or mapping of channels is performed with a specially designed software tool, which enables the joining of a series of graphic points registered in successive tomographic sections of the smallest thickness, which move parallel to the previously defined tomographic plane. The minimal thickness of the section, in the orthogonal projection, enables accurate localization of the roof and floor of the mandibular canal and graphic marking of its lumen (Fig. 11.32-11.34). As a final result, a graphical line representation of the mandibular canal path is obtained.

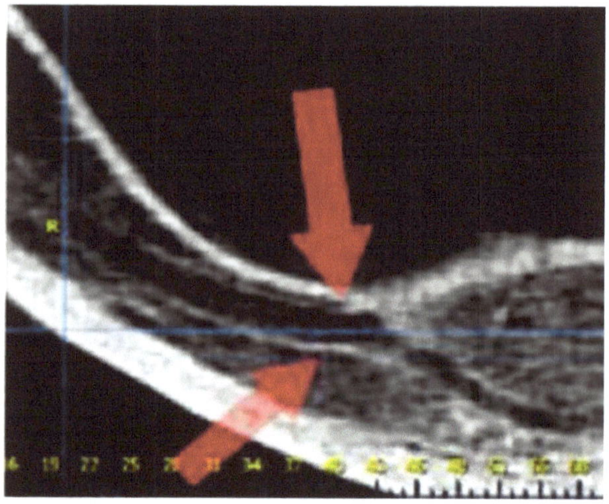

Figure 12.32. Tomographic sections of minimal thickness make it easier to observe the structure of the roof and floor of the mandibular canal. Arrows indicate the borders of the mandibular canal.

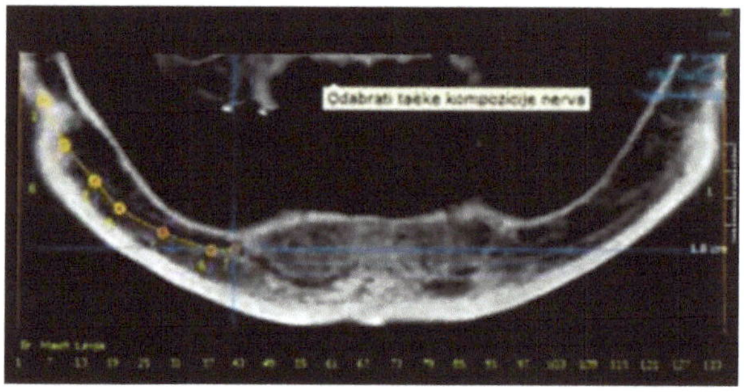

Figure 12.33. Channel "mapping" course.

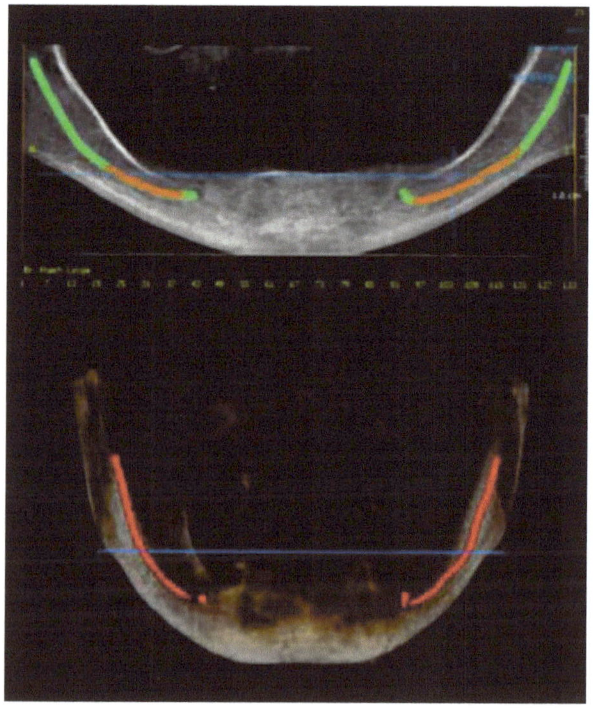

Figure 12.34. Marked ("mapped") mandibular canal.

After the mapping is completed, it is easier to observe the structure of the canal and minimize the possibility of its injury in a subsequent surgical act. Planning the position of the implant is done in relation to the surrounding anatomical structures and universal rules, which define the distance implant-nerve, implant-tooth, implant-implant, in a sufficient width of the alveolar bone. When planning is done in relation to the remaining teeth, orientation is facilitated, both for planning itself and for transferring data within the surgical field. When it comes to planning in the toothless jaw, the situation is complex, both for virtual planning itself and for transferring the plan into the operational framework. Such situations gave rise to the development of a still "exotic" field in oral implantology, the so-called navigational implant placement. However, since this area of oral implantology is not yet widespread in our country use, the experience of the operator is still of crucial importance. The beginning of planning is done by identifying the middle of the jaw, on the basis of which relationships are formed about the necessary implant-implant spacing and their possible positions (Figures 12.35 and 12.36).

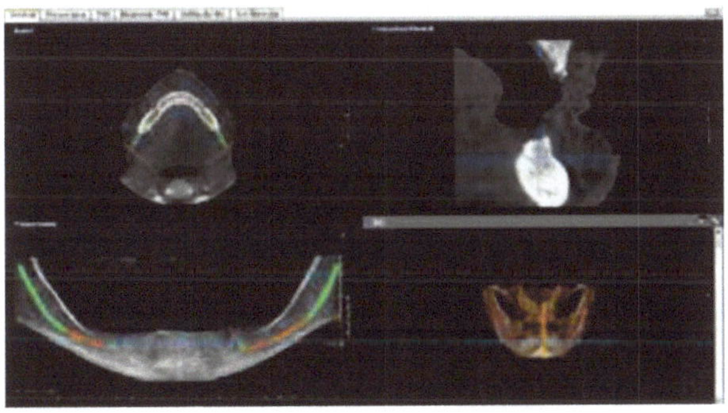

Figure 12.35. Determining the middle of the lower jaw.

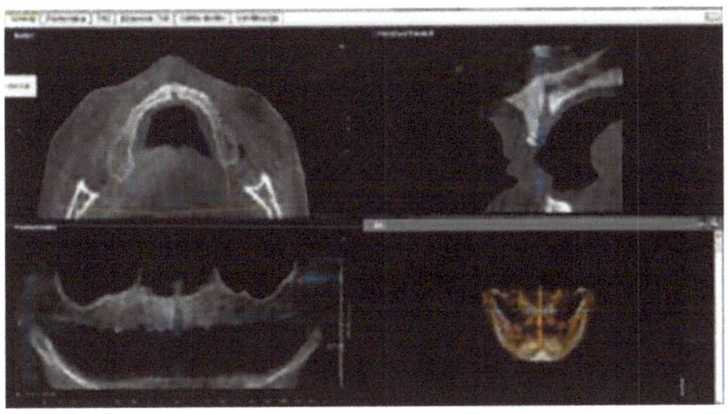

Figure 12.36. Determination of the middle of the upper jaw.

Planning is done separately for the upper and lower jaw due to the different shape of the tooth row (ellipse and parabola), which require the necessity of drawing two tomographic planes in order to achieve accurate transverse tomographic sections. Different shapes of the tomographic plane, in the same patient, can be seen in Figures 12.35 and 12.36. After defining the middle of the jaw, on the basis of the necessary implant-implant distance of 2 mm and on the basis of the desired diameter of the implant, we define places where the analysis of the bone foundation is performed (Figures 12.37 and 12.38). The "millimeter" bar at the bottom of the panoramic view serves to define the distance.

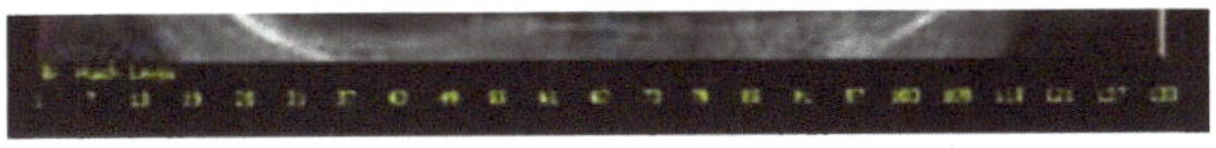

Figure 12.37. The millimeter tape makes it easy to measure the distance of the desired tomographic sections.

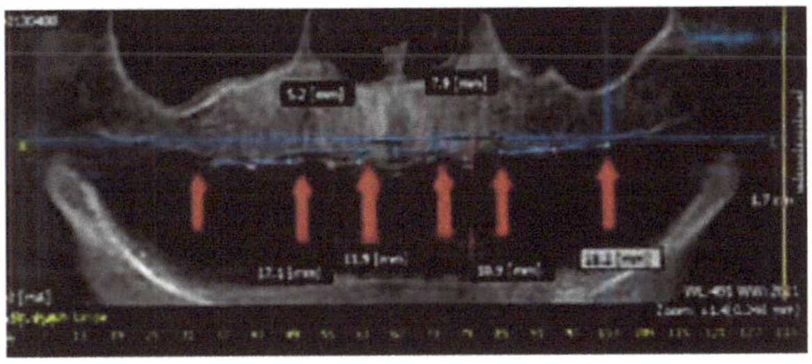

Figure 12.38. Defined preferred sites for bone foundation analysis in the upper jaw.

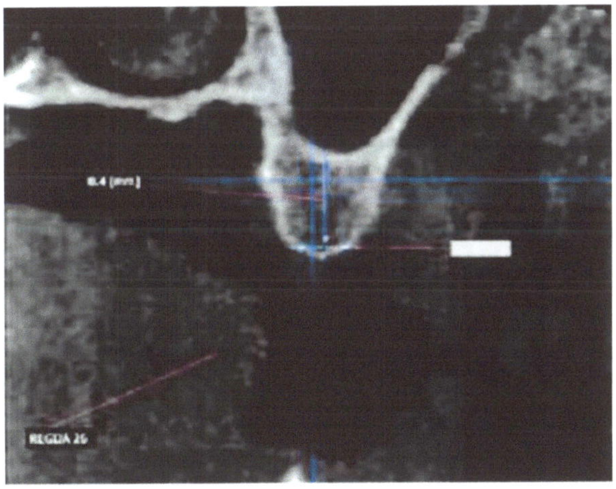

Figure 12.39. Display of one of the regions where the upper jaw was analyzed.

After the analysis of the bone foundation, the virtual planning of the implant position is started, and then the implant position is verified in relation to the available bone and the surrounding anatomical structures (Figures 12.39 and 12.40).

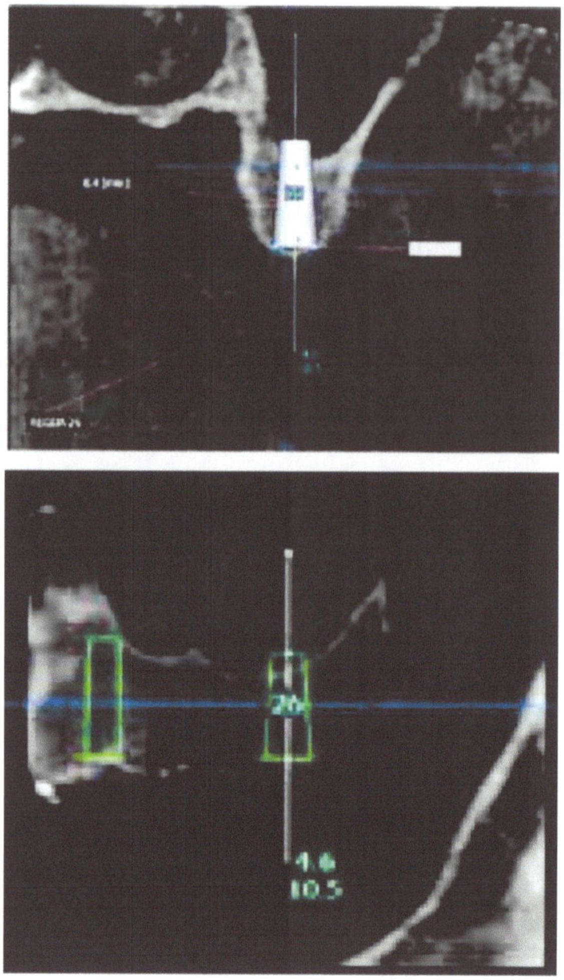

Figure 12.40. Planning and verification of implant position

An example of planning a surgical procedure to definitive prosthetic work

Planning is carried out in the same way for all selected regions, in order to obtain as a final result the possible position of the planned implants in relation to the available bone and in relation to each other. Although revolutionary steps have been made in relation to previous technological principles, primarily with the possibility of exact assessment of the available bone width and height, with the possibility of observing vital anatomical formations (surrounding teeth and nerve pathways), the problem of transferring the findings to the operative field still remains. The solution to this

problem can be found in the application of navigation implant placement, as a well-defined and tried-and-tested principle. However, until the high costs of performing such operations and the organizational and technological limitations of our market are eliminated, this type of operation is still not routinely applied in our country (Figure 12.41). Figures 12.42-12.60 show an example of a complete implant-prosthetic rehabilitation procedure for one patient.

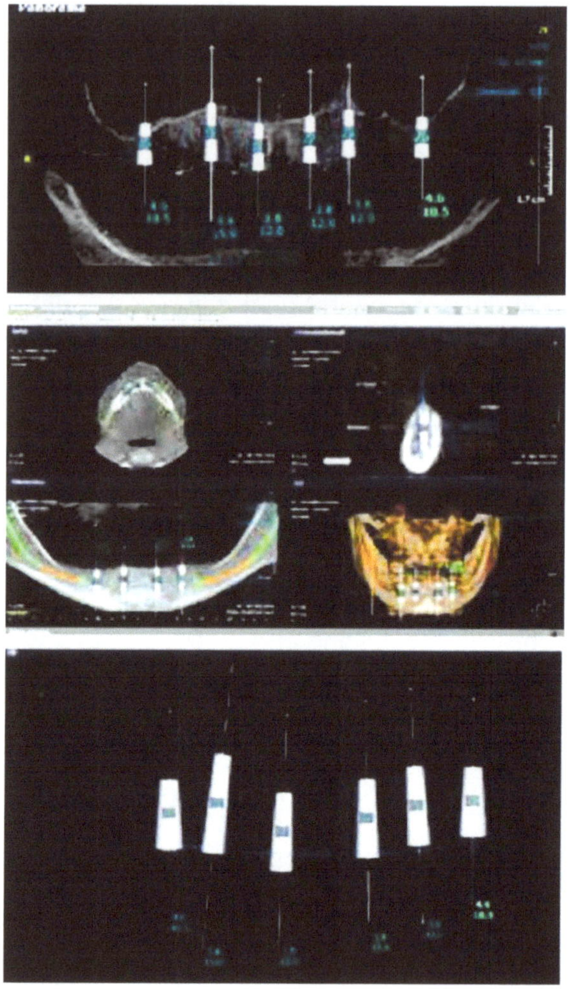

Figure 12.41. Possible interrelationships of implants after planning in two-dimensional and three-dimensional projection.

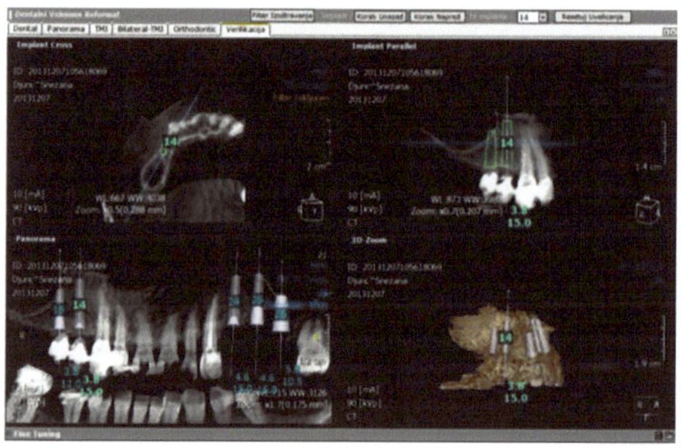

Figure 12.42. Verification of the position of the implant in the premolar region of the upper jaw.

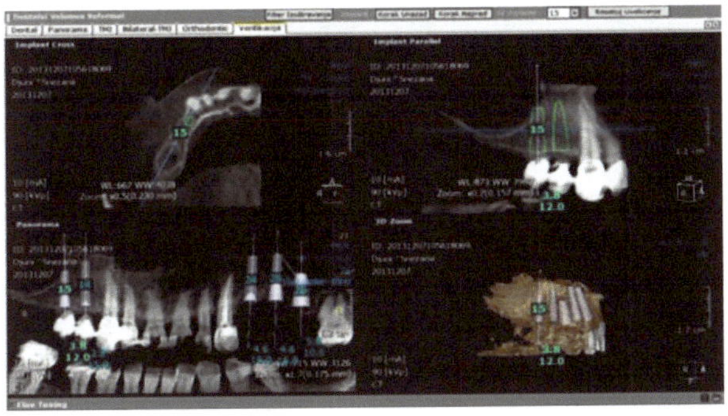

Figure 12.43. Verification of the position of the implant in the premolar region of the upper jaw on the right.

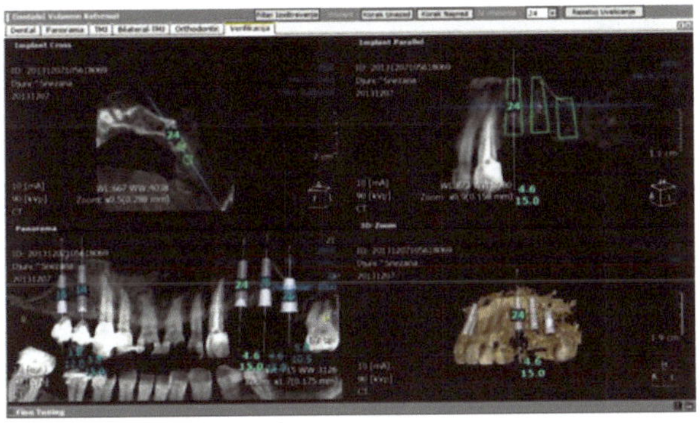

Figure 12.44. Verification of the position of the implant at the site of the upper first left premolar.

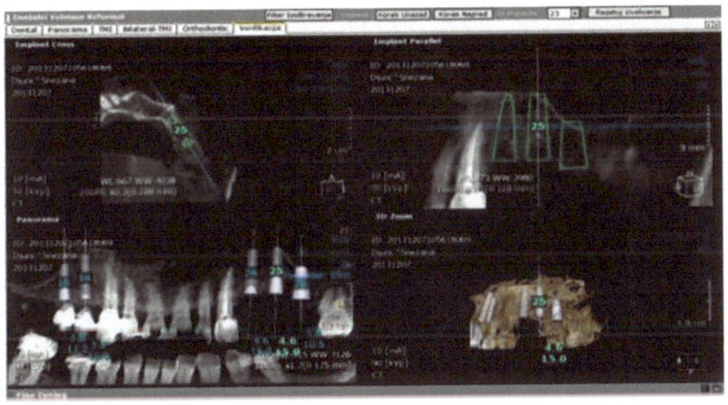

Figure 12.45. Verification of the position of the implant at the site of the upper second left premolar

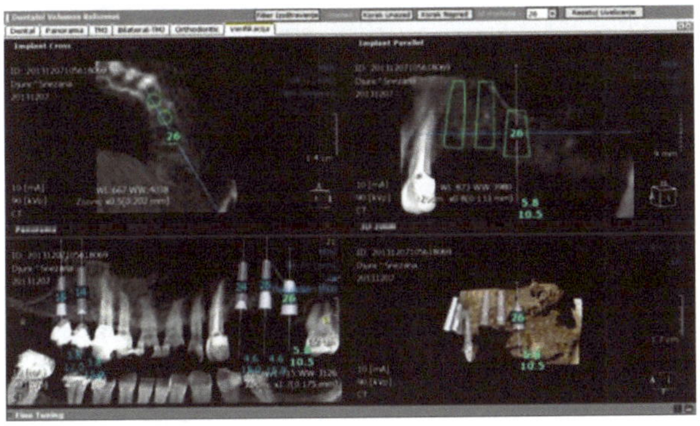

Figure 12.46. Verification of the position of the implant at the site of the upper first left molar

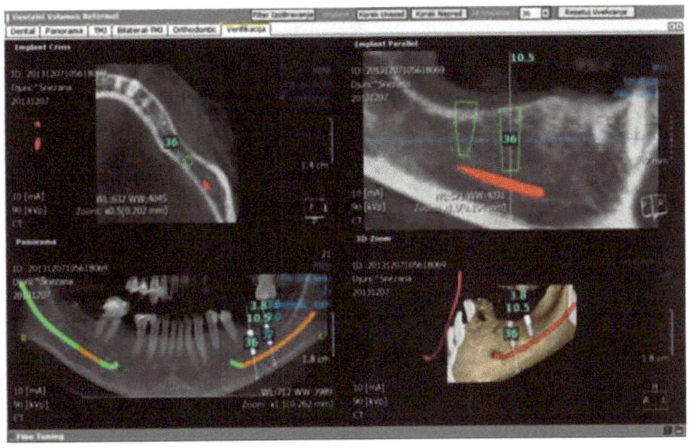

Figure 12.47. Verification of the position of the implant at the site of the lower first left molar

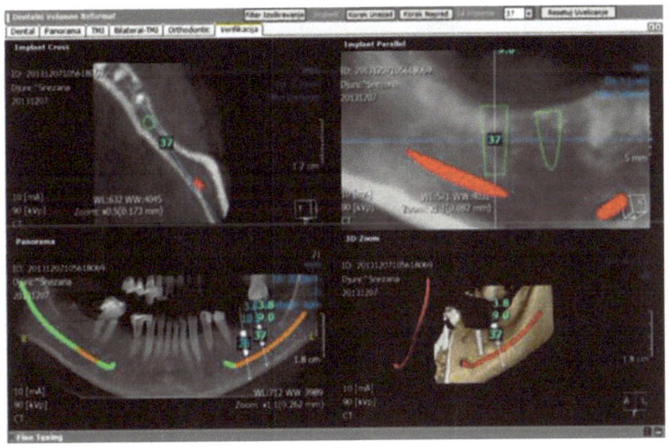

Figure 12.48. Verification of the position of the implant at the site of the lower second left molar

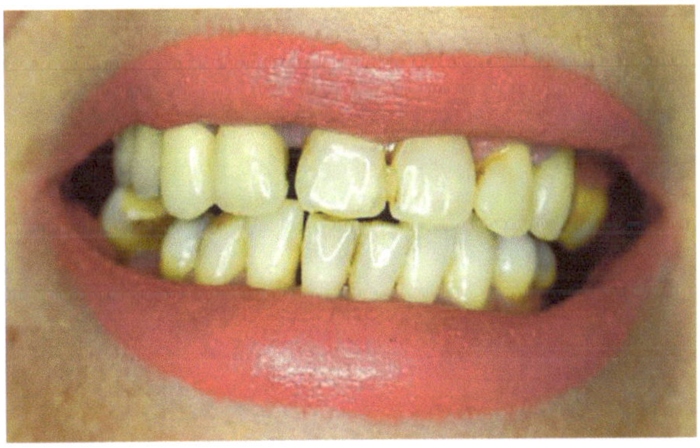

Figure 12.49. Appearance of the initial state with mobile prosthetic work.

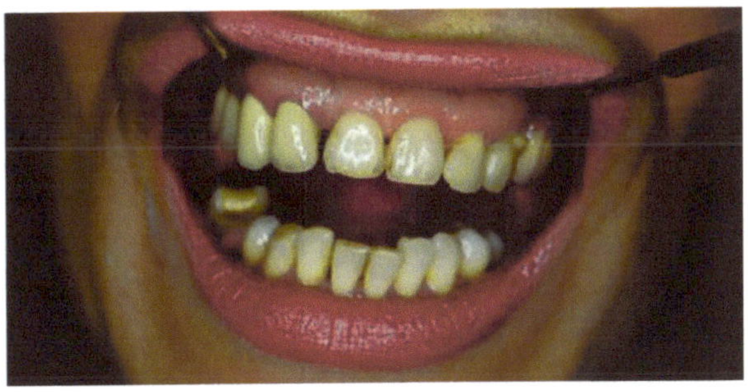

Figure 12.50. Found condition with a skeleton prosthesis in the upper jaw.

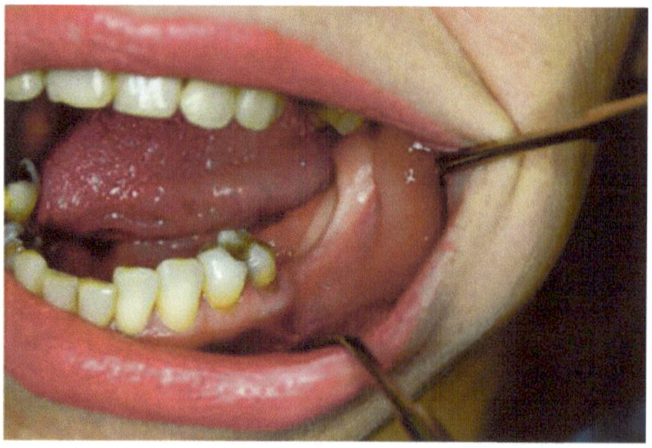

Figure 12.51. Found condition in the lower jaw on the left.

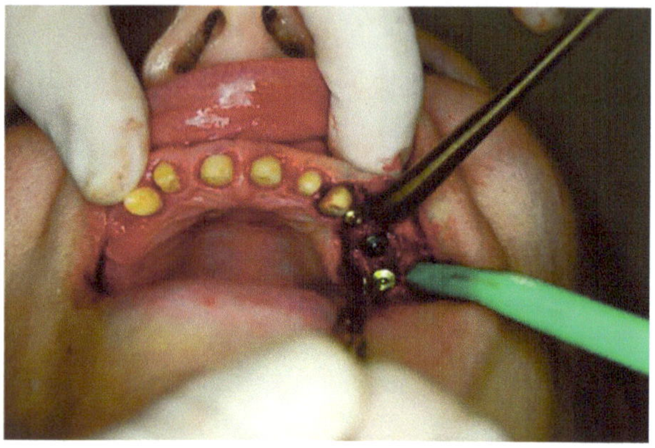

Figure 12.52. Embedded implants (Biohorizons implants) planned in the region 24, 25, 26.

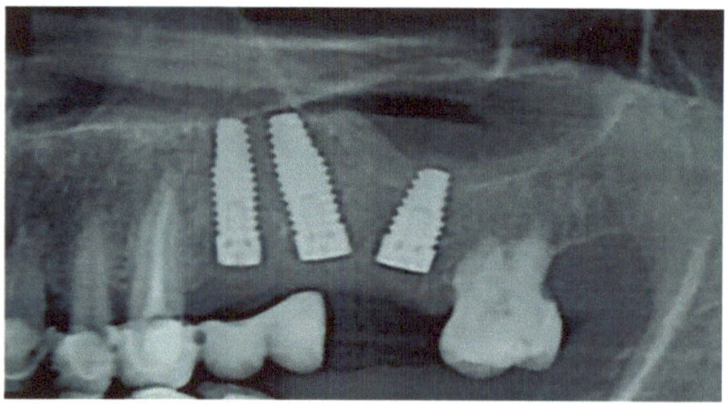

Figure 12.53. Control shot after implant installation region 24, 25, 26

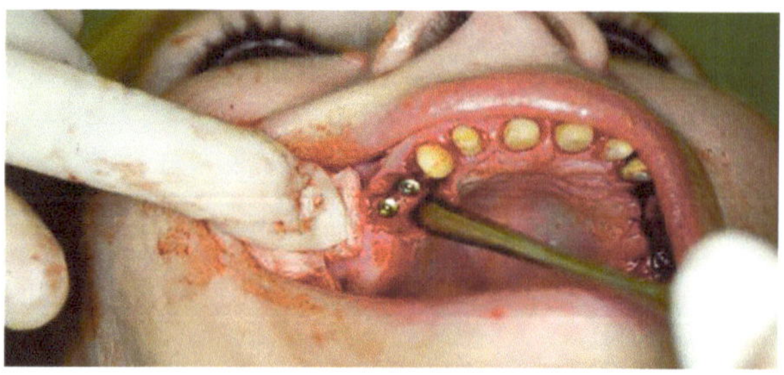

Figure 12.54. Embedded implants (Biohorizons implants) in the region 14 and 15.

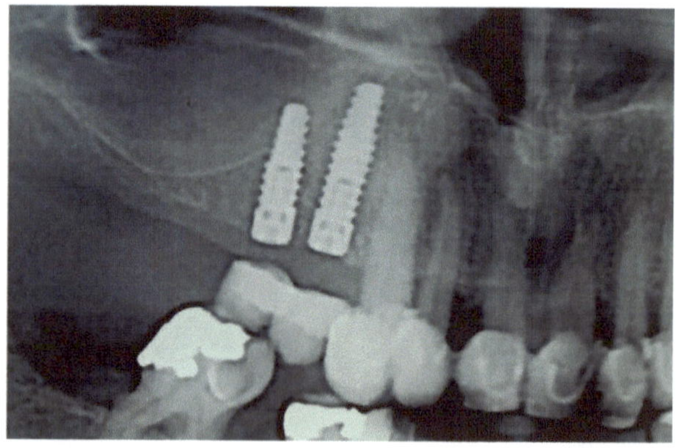

Figure 12.55. Control shot after installation of regional implants 14 and 15 (T. Zlopaša)

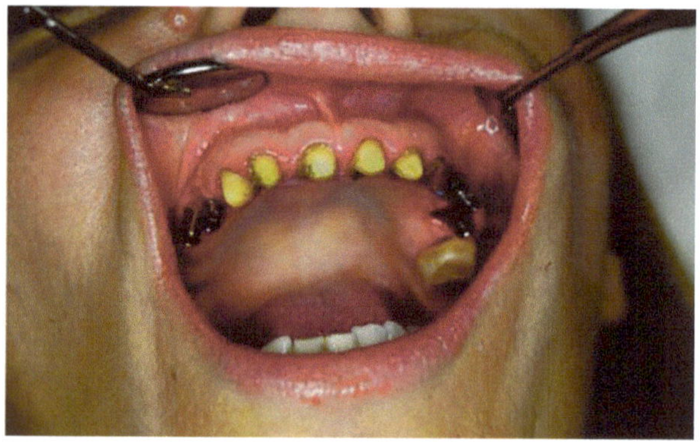

Figure 12.56. Placed definitive supports (abutments) of the prosthetic of work.

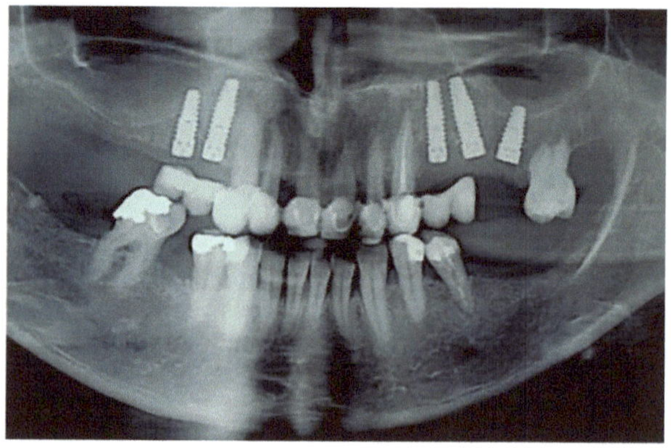

Figure 12.57. Control shot after the installation of implants that are aligned with the created 3D planning (T. Zlopaša).

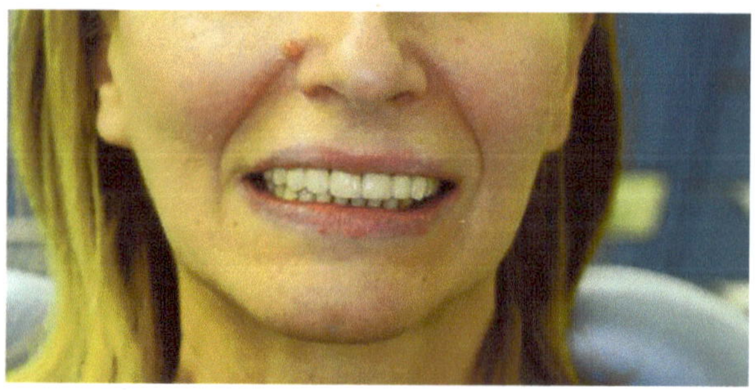

Figure 12.58. Aesthetic appearance of definitive prosthetic

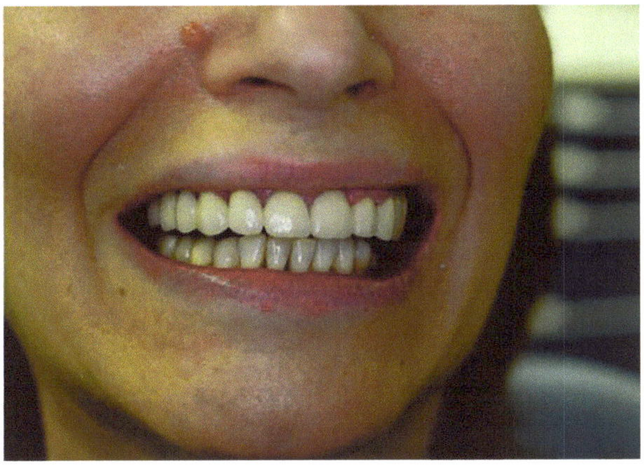

Figure 12.59. Definitive implant prosthetic rehabilitation (T. Zlopaša)..

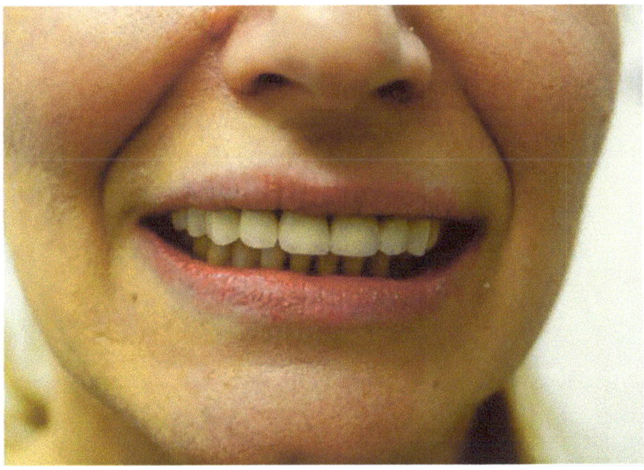

Figure 12.60. Aesthetic requirements and patient comfort met. Compare the initial state of the solution with mobile skeletal prostheses.

Tomographic sections of regions and virtual planning of implant placement

What does a case that would explain the virtual planning of implant placement look like in practice? The first step in computer-guided implant placement is to obtain a profile image and vertical dimension. The following images (Figures 12.61-12.97) show all procedures in the analysis of one patient.

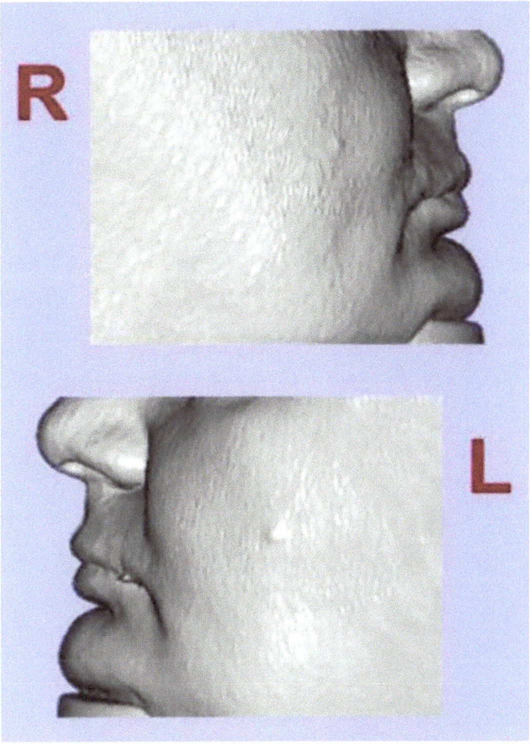

Figure 12.61. Vertical dimension and profile shots of the face (right and left).

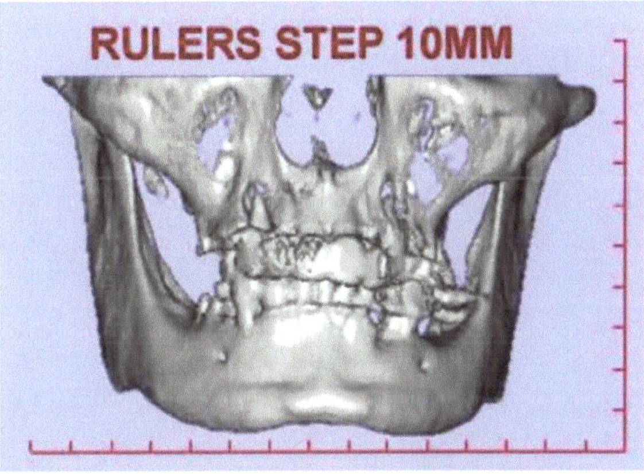

Figure 12.62. Image of bone system reconstruction (AP position) of the same patient.

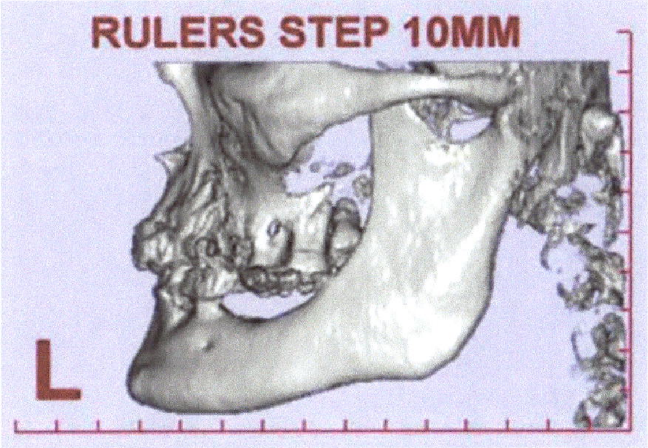

Figure 12.63. Profile shots of the upper and lower jaw.

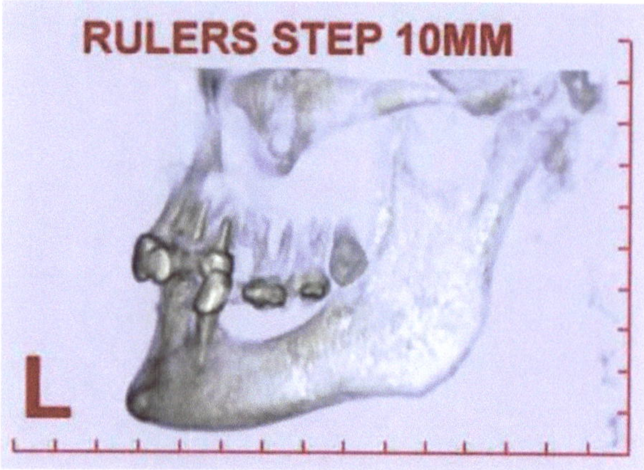

Figure 12.64. Lateral shots.

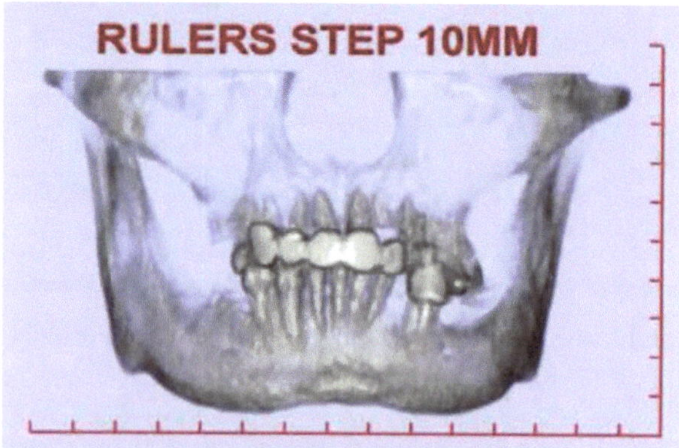

Figure 12.65. AP bone system reconstruction.

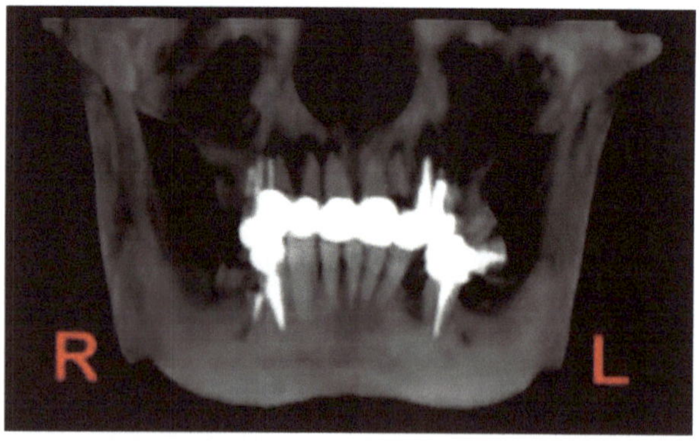

Figure 12.66. X-ray (AP) scan.

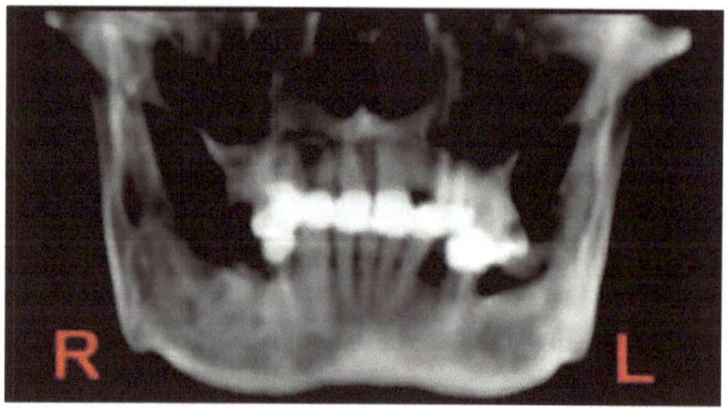

Figure 12.67. AP reconstruction

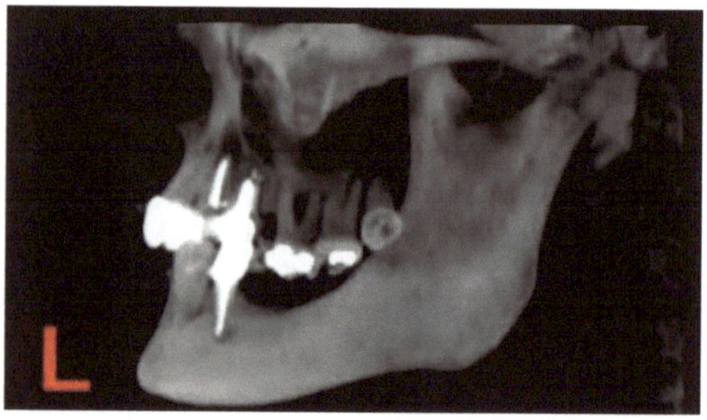

Figure 12.68. Lateral reconstruction of the left side – clarification of mental opening.

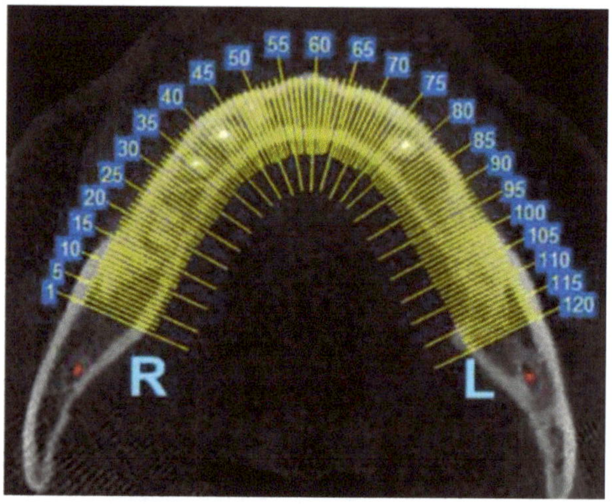

Figure 12.69. 120 sections of the mandible.

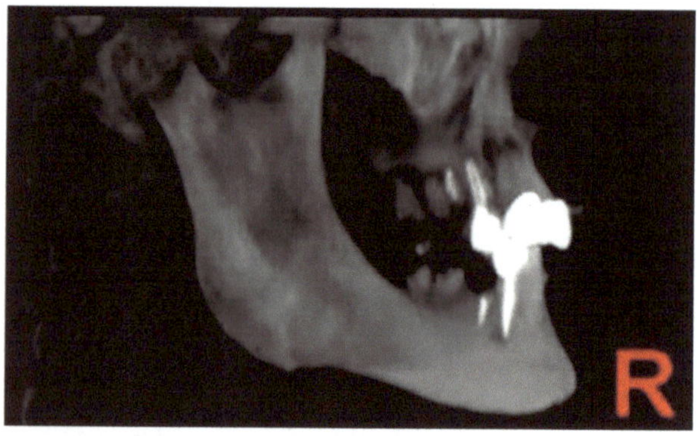

Figure 12.70. Right profile shot.

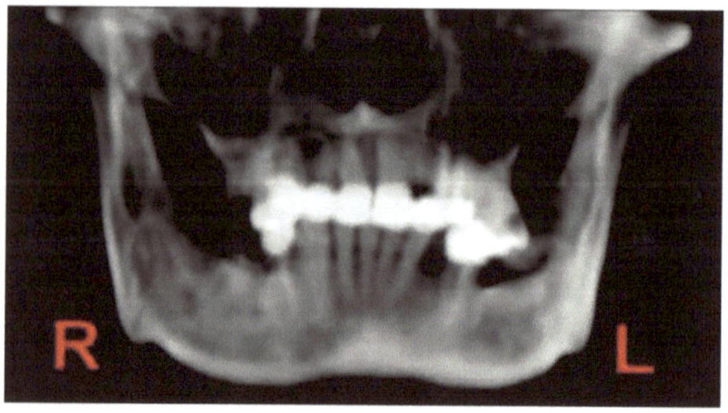

Figure 12.71. Antero-posterior view.

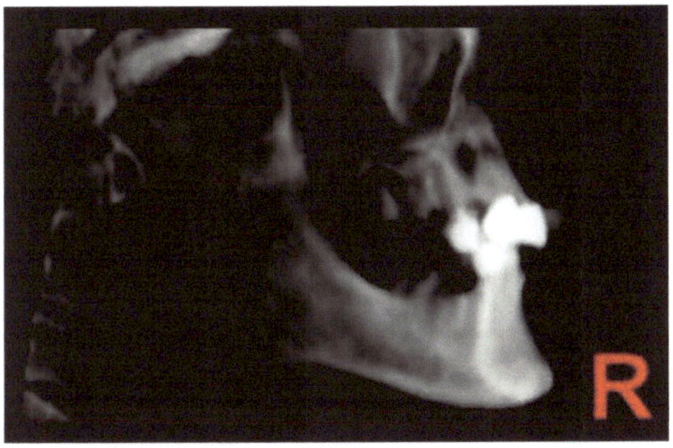

Figure 12.72. Lateral reconstruction of the right side.

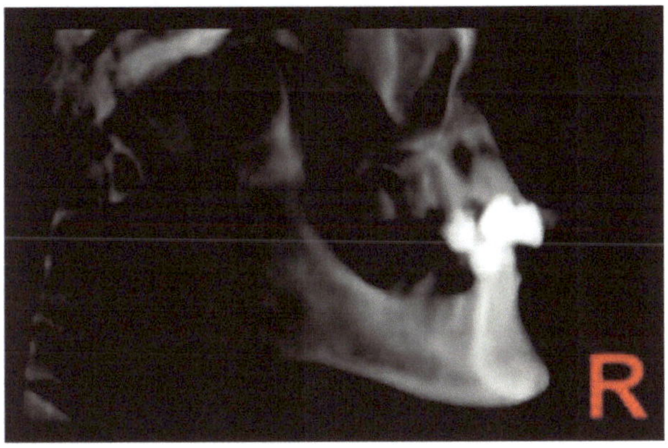

Figure 12.73. Profile view of the right side.

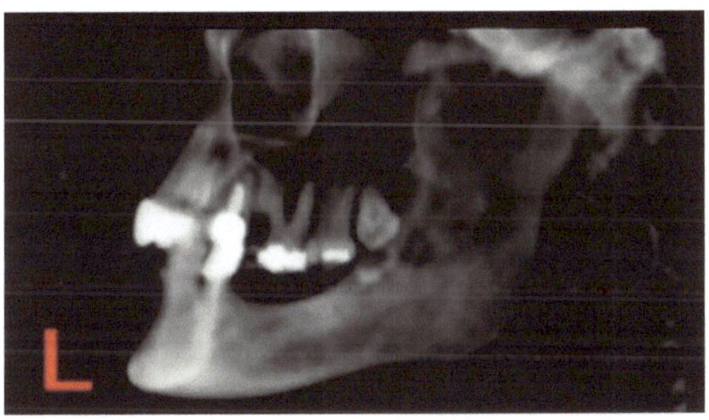

Figure 12.74. Left profile shot of the position of the molar roots and the sinus cavity.

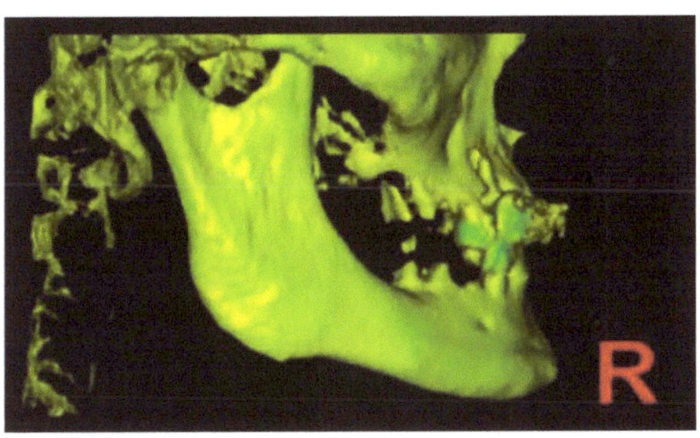

Figure 12.75. Right side profile shot with details of TMZ, the stragglers roots, their position.

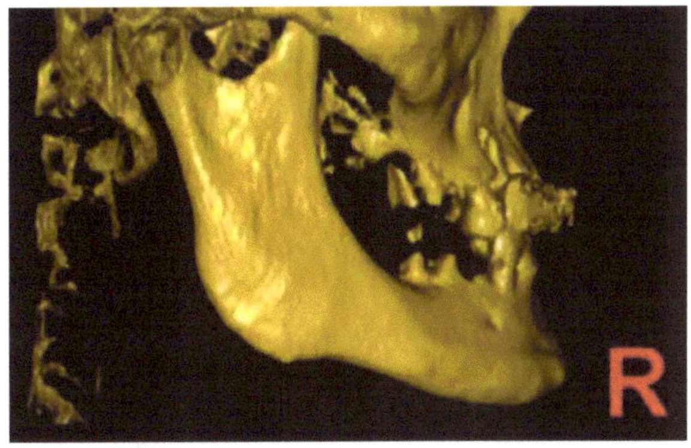

Figure 12.76. Right profile shot.

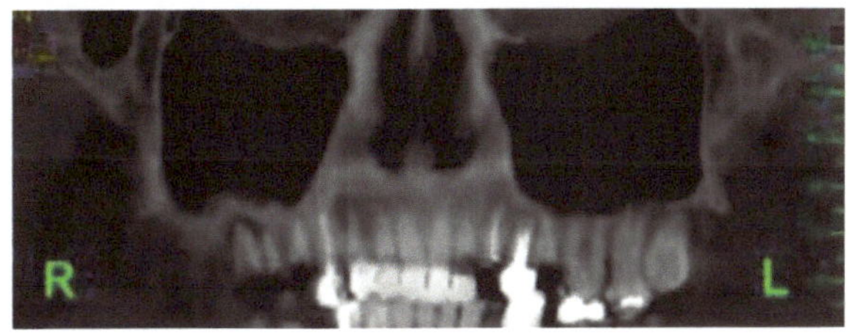

Figure 12.77. Anatomical structures, condition of teeth and roots with all periapical changes. Presentation of maxillary cavities.

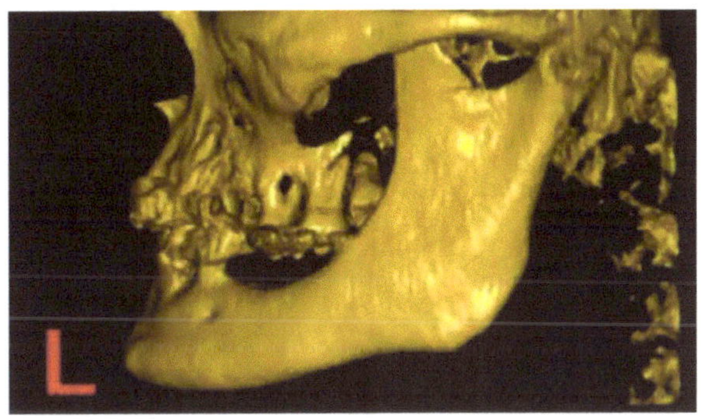

Figure 12.78. Left profile shot - position of molars and wisdom teeth.

Compare the above pictures with the classic orthopantomographic x-ray and pay attention to the relationship of the molars with the maxillary sinus.

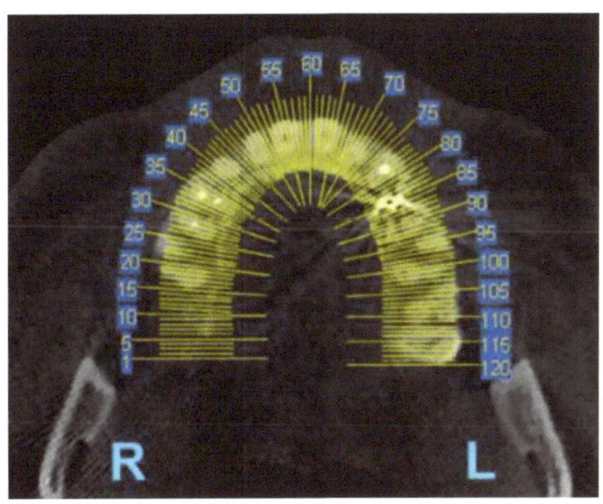

Figure 12.79. 120 crossections in the upper jaw.

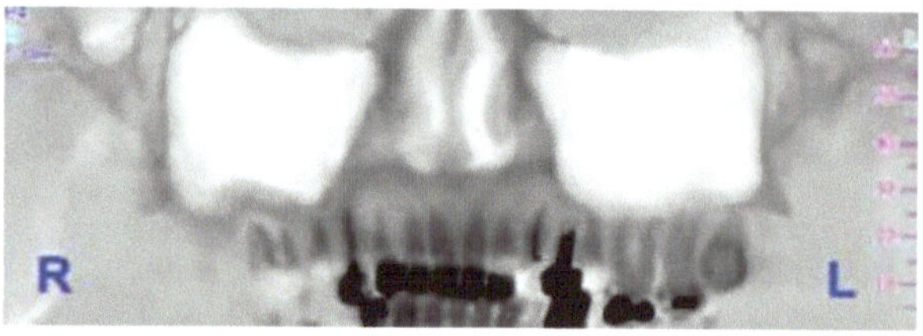

Figure 12.80. Extending the boundary of the pneumatized parts in the upper jaw.

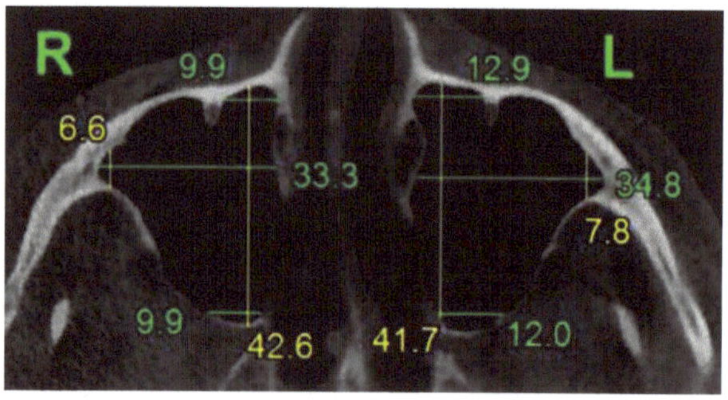

Figure 12.81. Measuring sections of sinus cavities.

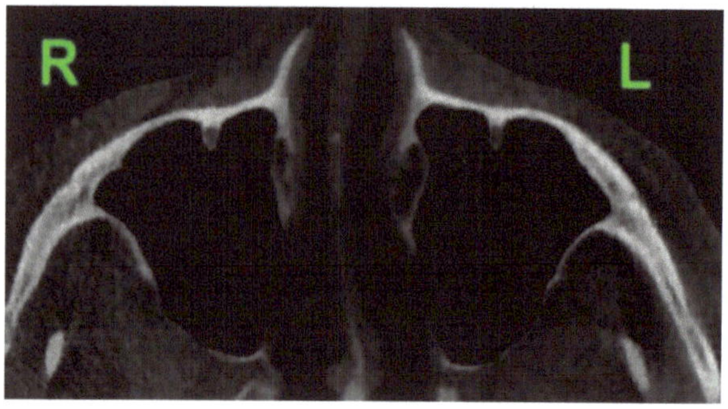

Figure 12.82. Sections of the maxillary cavities.

One of the very important possibilities is to document the found state with a video (pictures 12.83 and 12.84). This is extremely important for the dentist because he can always show the patient what condition he came to the office with.

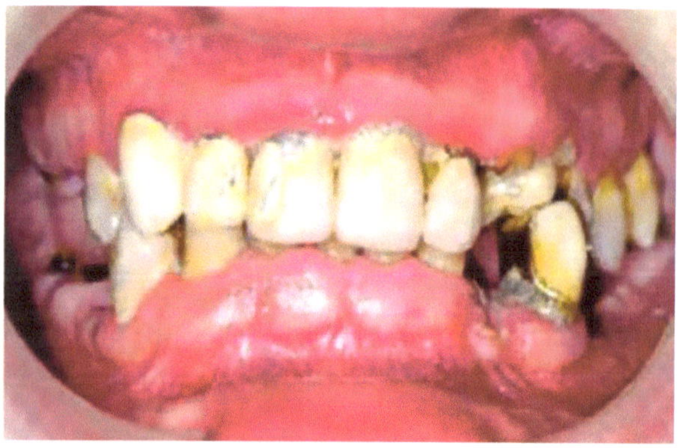

Figure 12.83. Oral cavity status.

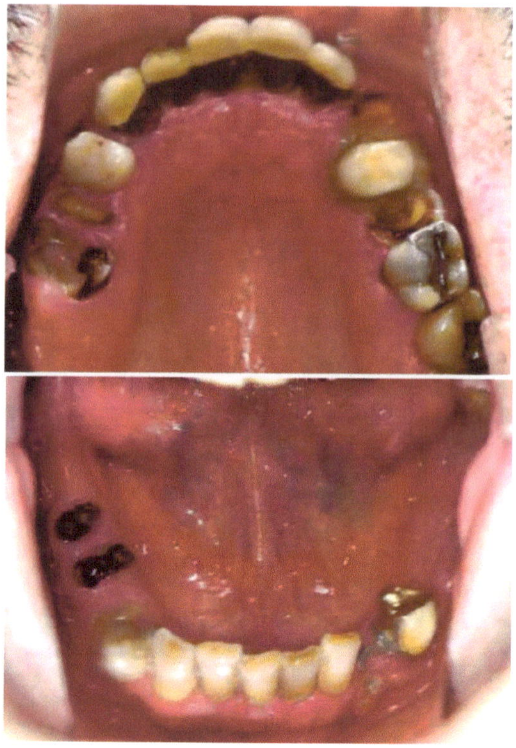

Figure 12.84. Oral cavity state, intraoral.

Of special importance are cross-sectional images of tooth positions in certain regions, with measurements of bone mass by height and width, in the case of planning post-extraction immediate implant placement (Figures 12.85- 12.97).

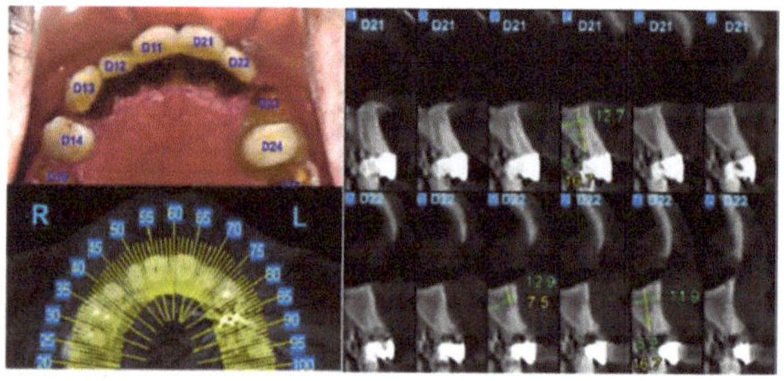

Figure 12.85. A snapshot showing the 64-section position of the central incisors with measurements of bone mass by height and width in in the case of planning post-extraction immediate implant installation.

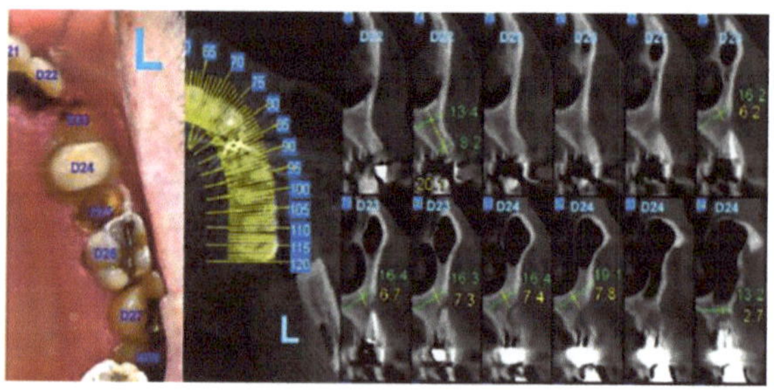

Figure 12.86. Unit of measurement for tooth region 22 - horizontal and vertical diameters of the alveolar bone.

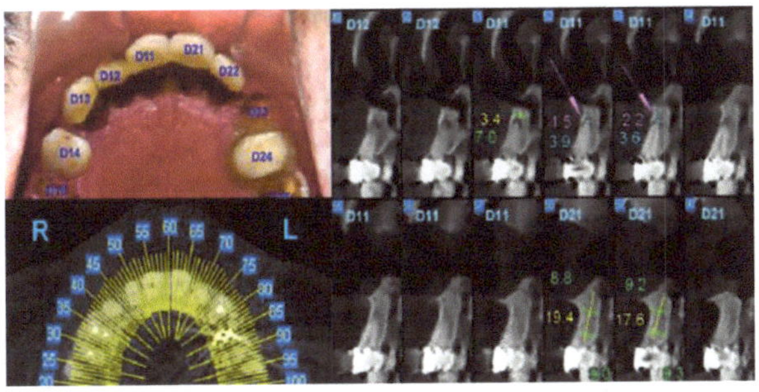

Figure 12.87. The position of the pink arrow indicates the relationship of the periapical lesion to the buccal lamella.

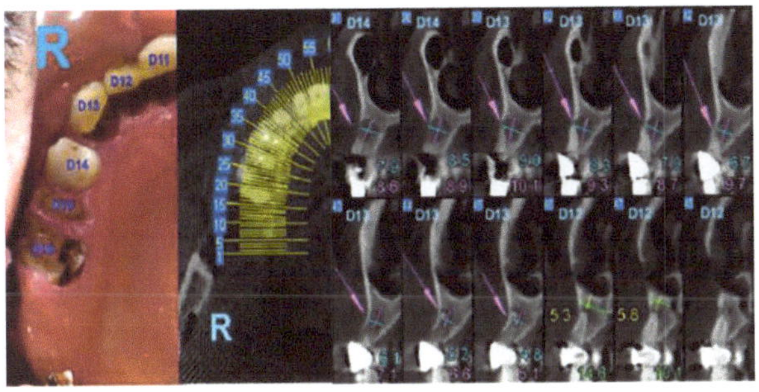

Figure 12.88. The measurement indicated by the pink arrow indicates the craniocaudal diameter of the periapical lesion.

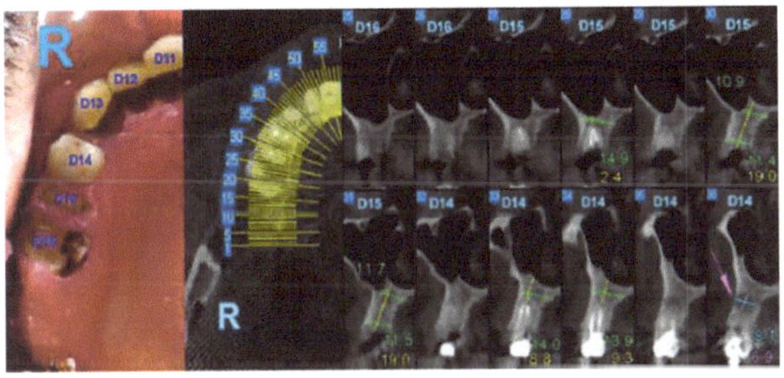

Figure 12.89. The relationship between the floor of the nasal cavity and the maxillary sinus with the measurement sections of the regions of interest.

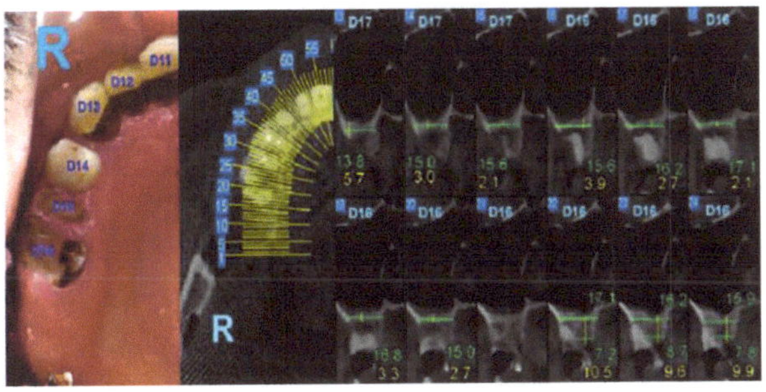

Figure 12.90. Measurement sections of the horizontal and vertical cortical bone of the floor of the maxillary sinus in the region of the first and second molars.

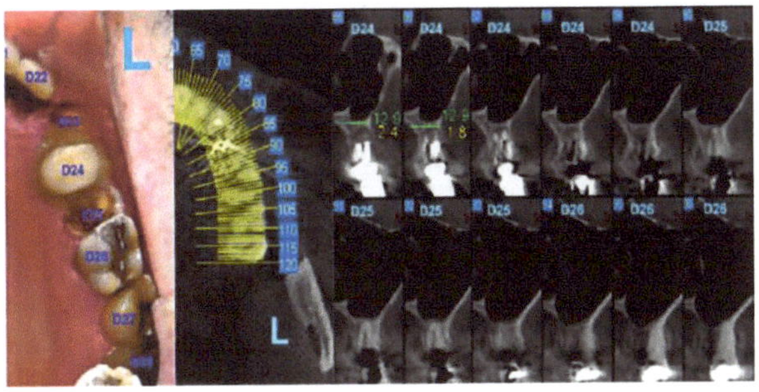

Figure 12.91. Measurement sections of the lower nasal concha and maxillary sinus.

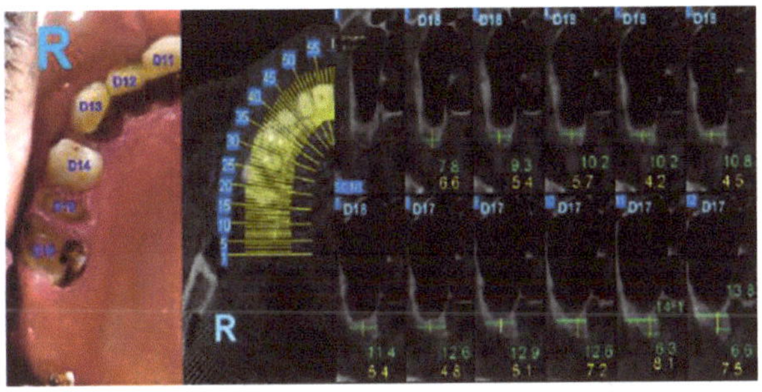

Figure 12.92. Measurement sections of horizontal and vertical bone in the region of teeth 17 and 18.

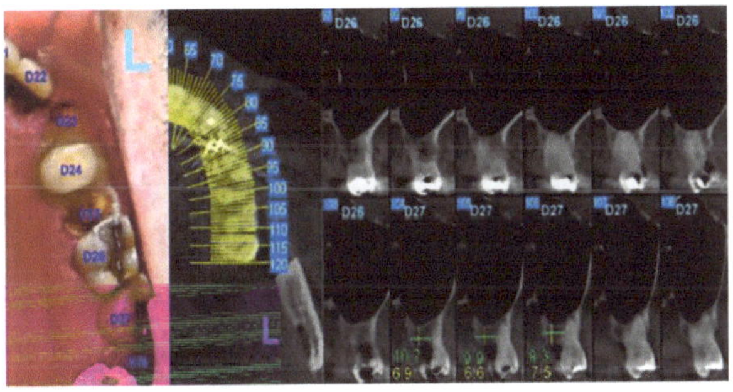

Figure 12.93. Measurement sections of the cortical bone of the floor of the maxillary sinus.

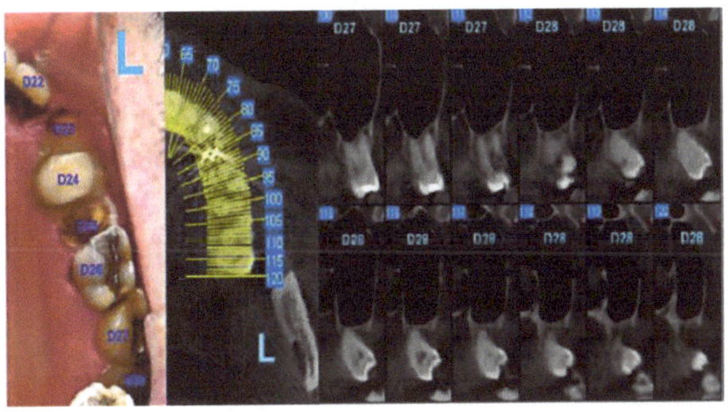

Figure 12.94. The position of the second upper molar - a clear relation of the buccal and palatal roots to the maxillary sinus can be seen.

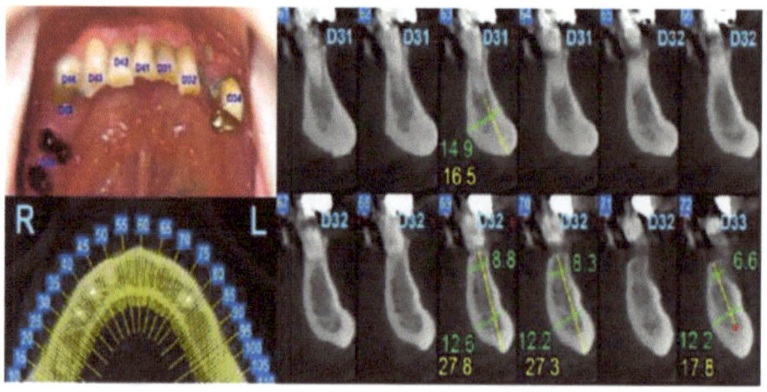

Figure 12.95. Measurement sections of the alveolar bone in the region of teeth 31 and 32.

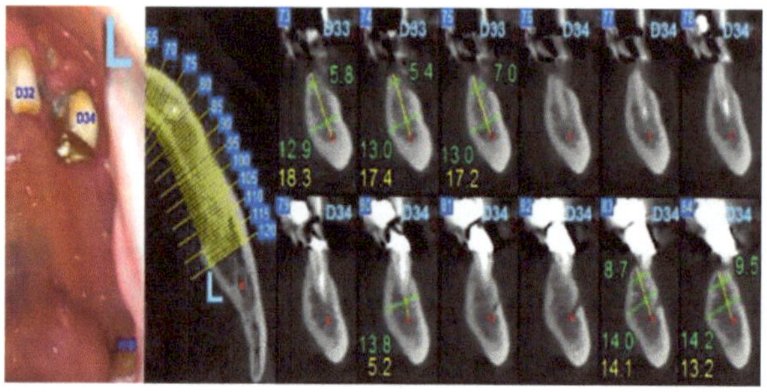

Figure 12.96. Measurement sections in the lower jaw show the relationship between the apex of the lower premolars and the mandibular canal. Measurement sections of the D33 region from the tip and platform to the mandibular canal. Measurement sections of the D34 region from the apex of the tooth to the mandibular canal (yellow line) and a vertical section at the level of the apex (green line).

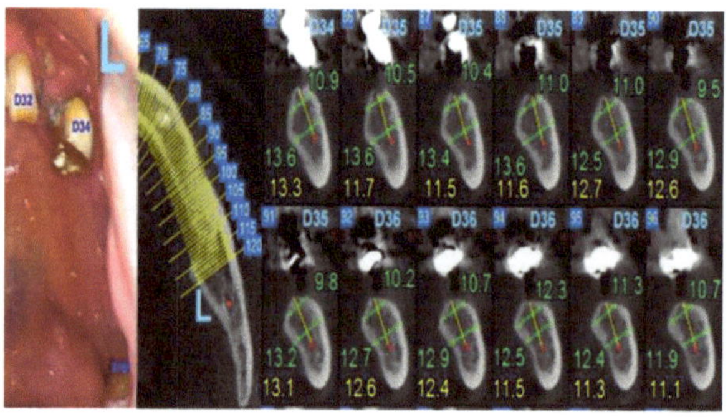

Figure 12.97. Measurement sections of the same - region 34 from the top of the alveolar ridge to the mandibular canal (yellow line), vertical section of the platform and vertical section of the border of the positioned implant (green line).

Virtual positioning of the implant in relation to the n. alveolaris inferior

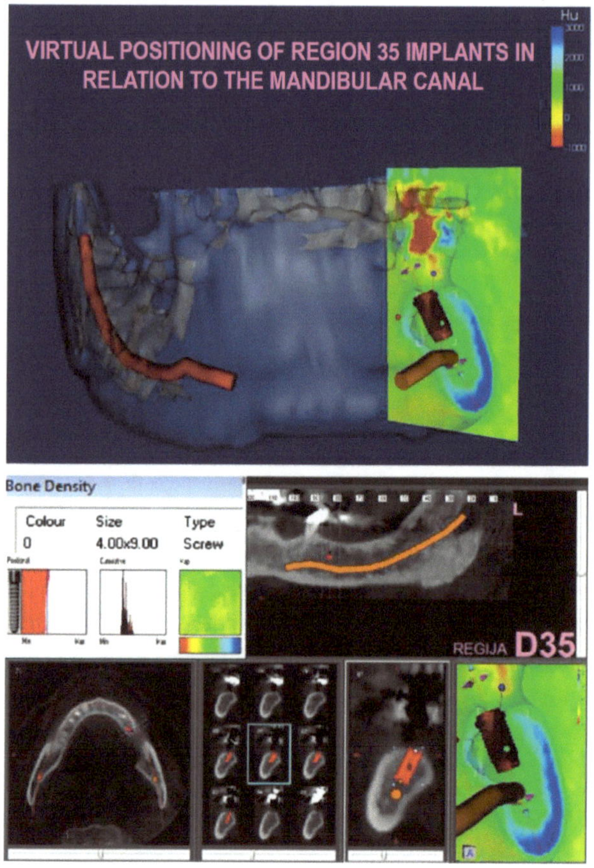

Figure 12.98. Virtual positioning of the implant in the region of the second premolar aligned with the measurement sections of the available alveolar bone and the distance of the implant from the lower dental nerve - marked in red.

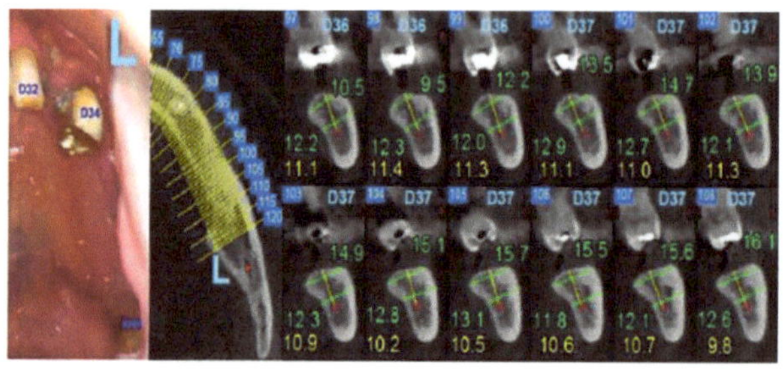

Figure 12.99. Vertical sections in the region of teeth 36 and 37 from the apex and platform to the mandibular canal (yellow line). Horizontal sections of the available bone to select the diameter of the implant (green arrow).

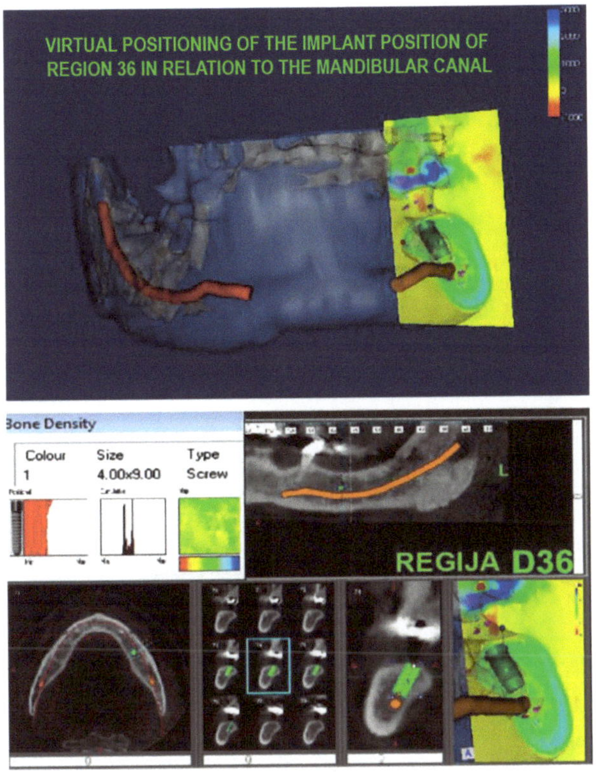

Figure 12.100. Virtual positioning of the implant in the region of tooth 36 aligned with the measurement sections of the available alveolar bone and the distance of the implant from the lower dental nerve. Horizontal section of the position of the mandibular canal with the diameter and length of the implant in relation to the plateau and the lower dental nerve marked in green. The marked square shows the ratio of the diameter of the implant to the available bone.

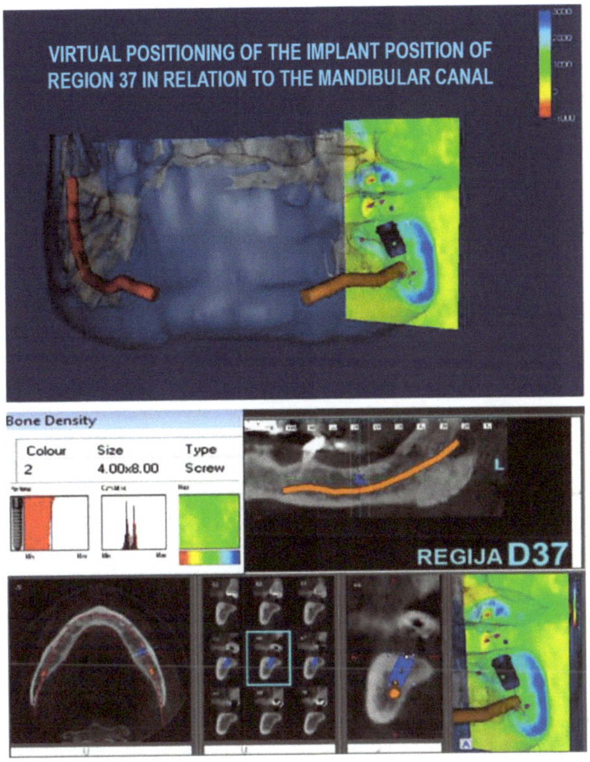

Figure 12.102. Virtually positioned implant in the region of tooth 37 and cross-section of the alveolar ridge. The position of the mandibular canal with sections of the diameter and length of the implant marked in blue in relation to the plateau and the mandibular canal. The ratio between the diameter of the implant and the available bone is shown in the marked square.

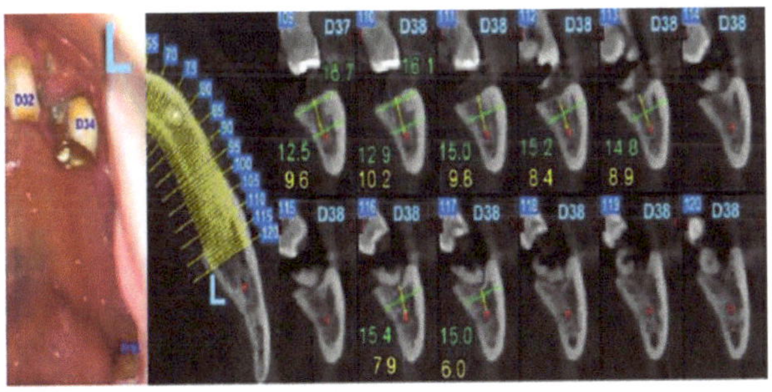

Figure 12.101. Measuring sections from the apex of the residual root to the mandibular canal and the horizontal width of the alveolar ridge.

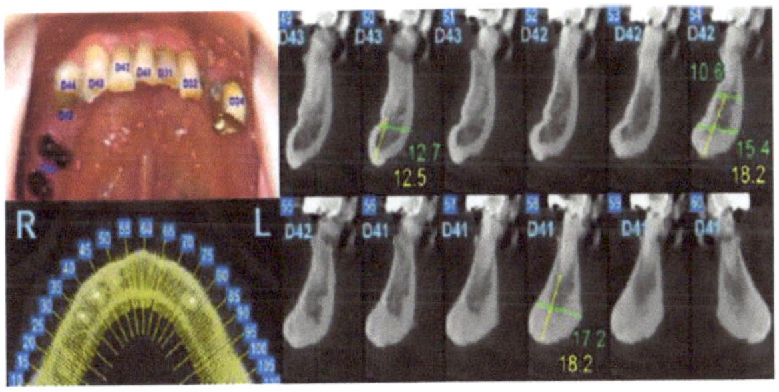

Figure 12.103. Measurement sections in the region of teeth 41 to 43, from the apex to the cortical bone of the mandible. Measuring section D 42 from the apex to the cortical bone of the mandible. Horizontal section D 42 from the top of the apex to the cortical bone.

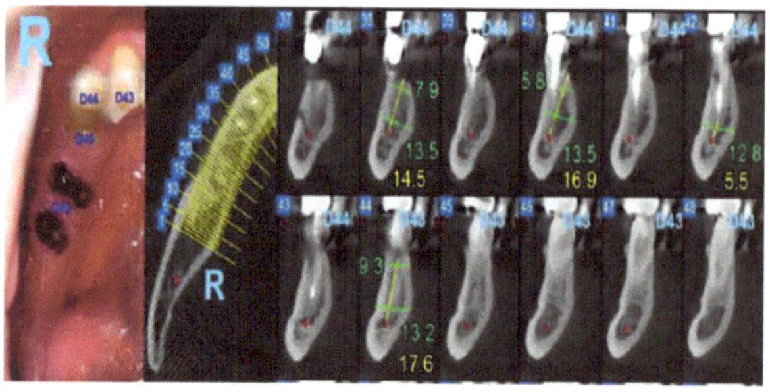

Figure 12.104. Measurement sections in the lower jaw on the right side, from the top of the apex to the mandibular and mental canals.

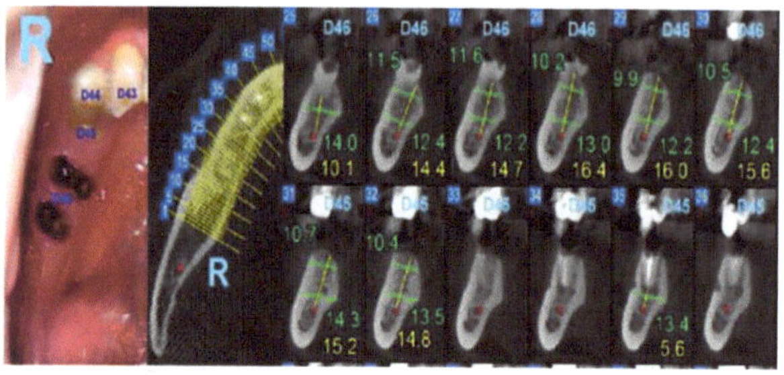

Figure 12.105. Section from the apex of the residual root to the mandibular canal.

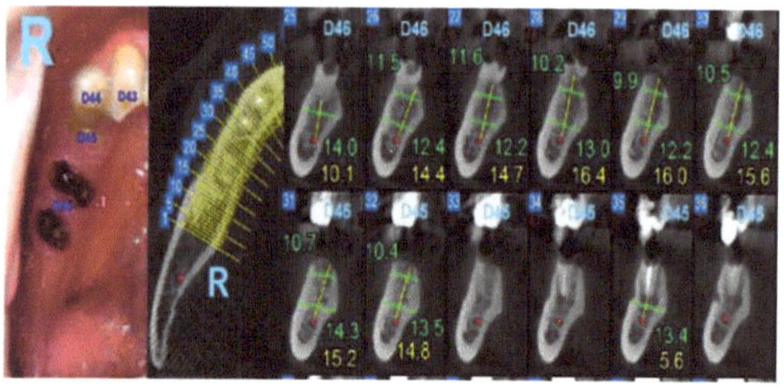

Figure 12.106. Measuring section from the tip of the alveolar bone to the mandibular canal and from the tip of the residual root to the mandibular canal (yellow line) and horizontal sections of the platform and available bone for selecting the diameter of the implant.

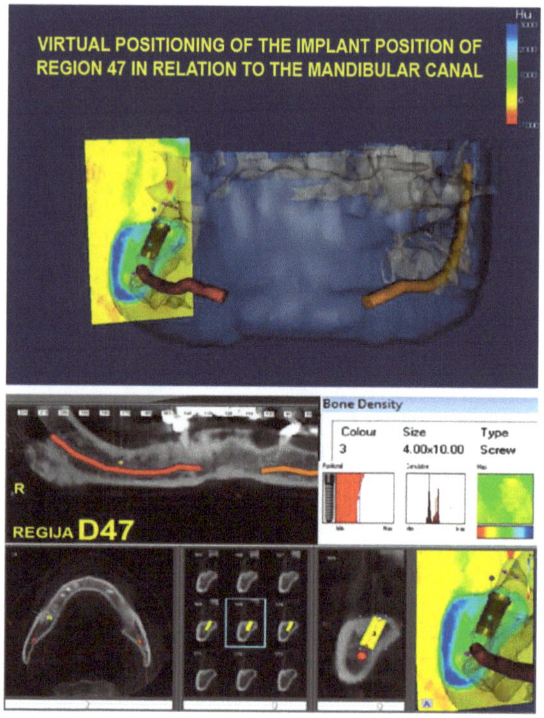

Figure 12.107. Virtual position of the implant in relation to the mandibular canal in the region of the second lower right molar. Cross-section of the position of the mandibular canal marked in red, cross-section of the diameter and length of the implant marked in yellow. The ratio between the diameter of the implant and the available bone is shown in the marked square.

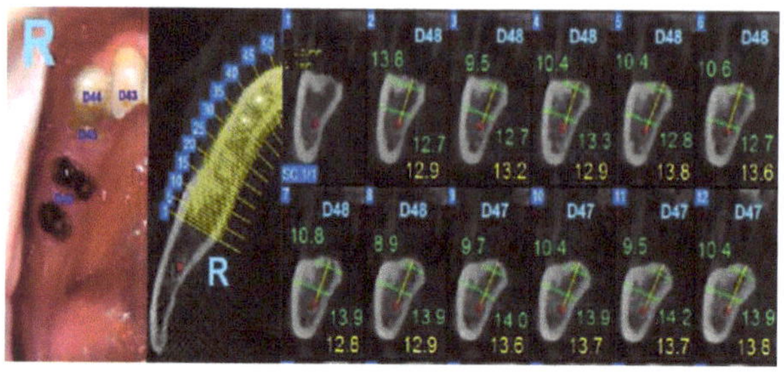

Figure 12.108. Measurement sections of regions 44, 45, 46, 47 and 48 with diameters and length of implants according to available bone.

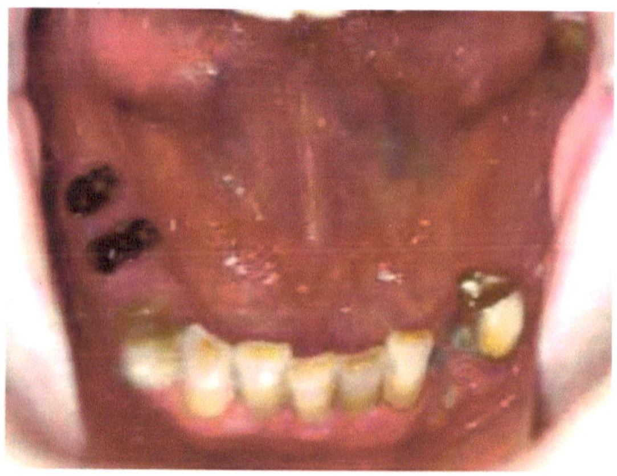

Figure 12.109. A condition in the lower jaw.

13

Risks in Oral Implantology

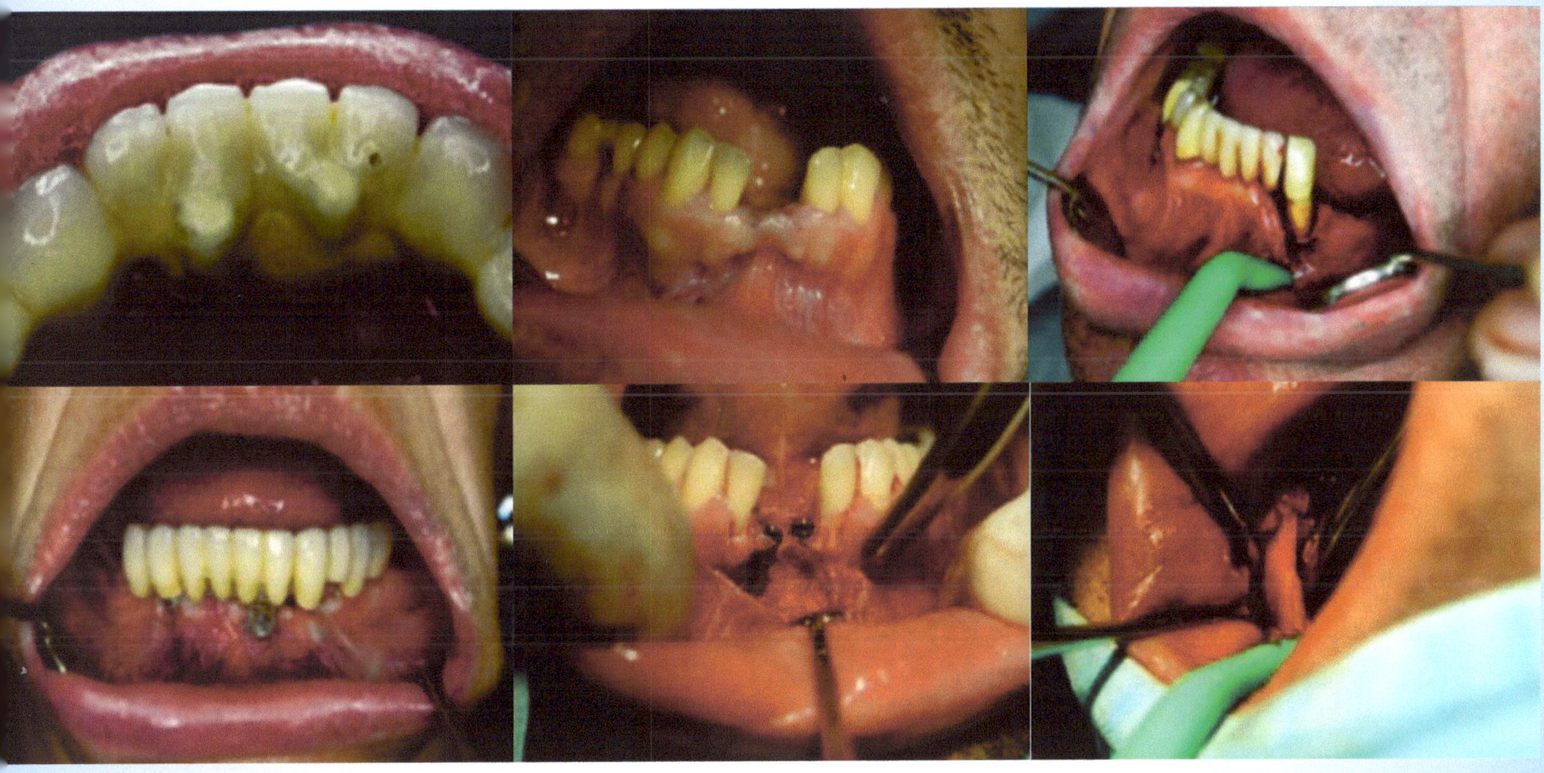

In oral-surgical routine procedures, whether it is tooth extraction or implant placement, sometimes the practitioner is unwittingly faced with injuries or damage to certain anatomical structures. It can be said that tooth extraction is the simplest and cheapest procedure in oral surgery, but it can also be risky with unforeseen and unwanted serious complications!

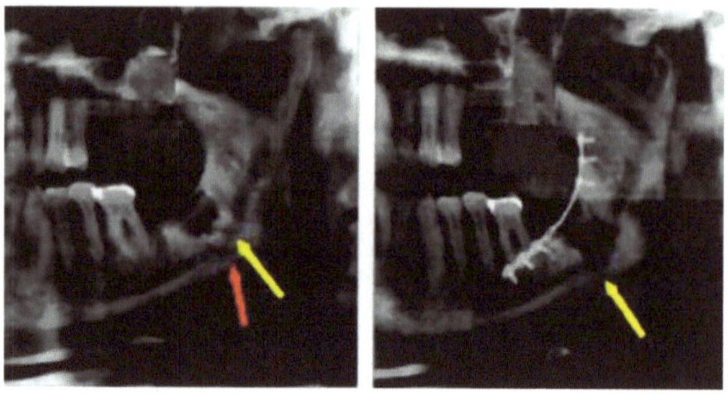

Figure 13.1. Fracture of the lower jaw as a complication of wisdom tooth extraction in the lower jaw.

During the extraction of teeth, especially the surgical extraction of impacted teeth (Figure 13.1), more severe postoperative complications occur more often than during the installation of implants, even the installation of several implants in the same session. It happens that sometimes the removal of an impacted wisdom tooth is a much riskier procedure than the installation of any implant system.

In principle, nerve damage to the inferior alveolar nerve and mental nerve during wisdom tooth extraction can be the result of sharp or blunt trauma, the result of edema and hematoma formation, local anesthesia, as well as wound infection that can develop into more serious complications. For this reason, wound treatment and suturing should be given great attention.

Interruption of the continuity of n.alveolaris inferior and n.lignvalis, is possible through the careless use of rotating instruments in the first row. When a tooth is luxated, the mandibular nerve n.alveolaris inferior can be exposed to blunt trauma, and this manifests itself in a disturbance of sensibility of a transitory nature.

Postoperative complications in oral surgery for implant placement are caused by several factors. Rare and unpleasant incidents can be: postoperative sensitivity disorder of the lower dental nerve, injury to blood vessels, severe infections, etc.

When removing wisdom teeth, incidents can occur that are excluded during the installation of implants, for example, fractures of individual segments of the mandible.

Iatrogenic injuries n. mandibularisa inferior or n. lingualis, are manifested by a disturbance of sensibility, which is a great inconvenience for both the patient and the dentist (for the dentist, an additional inconvenience is a possible court process).

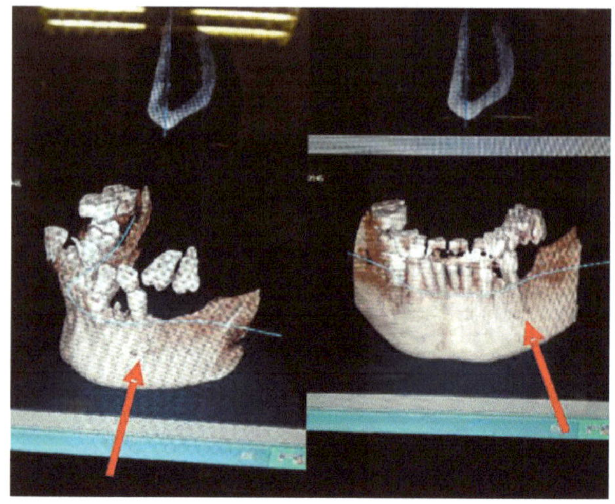

Figure 13.2. Often, on orthopantomography, anatomical variations that can cause injuries to the n. alveolaris inferior and n. mentalis. Anatomical variations are revealed only on a 3D scan, as in the case shown, where there were two openings of the chin nerve (n. mentalis).

These complications can occur during the installation of implants and it is very important to point out the guidelines regarding the procedure, what to do and what to expect after a postoperative sensitivity disorder. These accidents during implant installation can also happen due to an inappropriate number of revolutions of a sharp drill, which can result in entering the mandibular canal and completely cutting the nerve itself. Nerve injuries are also possible due to poor assessment of the dimensions (length) of the selected implant, as well as the length of the bone preparation drill. According to some research, during oral surgery and implant procedures in the lower jaw, the percentage of complications of temporary or permanent damage to the lower dental nerve is about 5%.

Manifestations of sensitivity disorders of the lower dental nerve are reflected on the teeth in the innervation zone, with permanent numbness. Sensibility disorders appear as paresthesia, expressed as hyperesthesia, hypoesthesia, and up to complete anesthesia - numbness.

Damage to the lingual nerve leads to loss of sensitivity in the area of the front two-thirds of the lateral half of the tongue. In addition to the loss of sensory sensitivity, the complication is manifested by a reduction or even loss of the sense of taste.

In oral implantology, there is also a risk of sensibility disorders, in addition to the inferior alveolar nerve, there is also an injury to the n. mentalis. There is a risk of injury to the mental nerve when installing an implant in the premolar area. Before the procedure, you must have a clear overview of the position of the metal openings, and the 3D image provides the clearest and most accurate view (Figure 13.2).

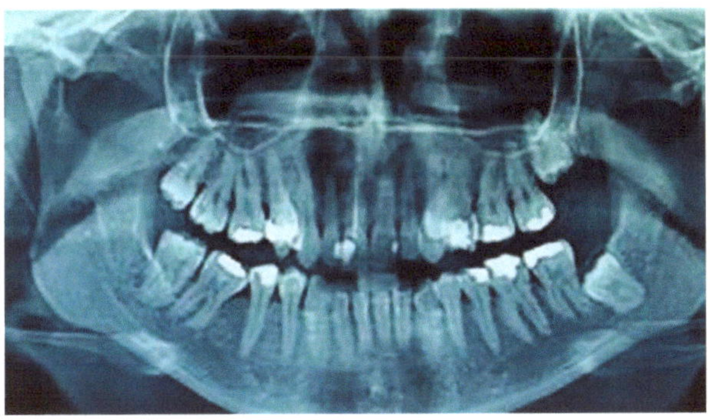

Figure 13.3. Extracting an impacted wisdom tooth is always a traumatic and risky oral surgical procedure.

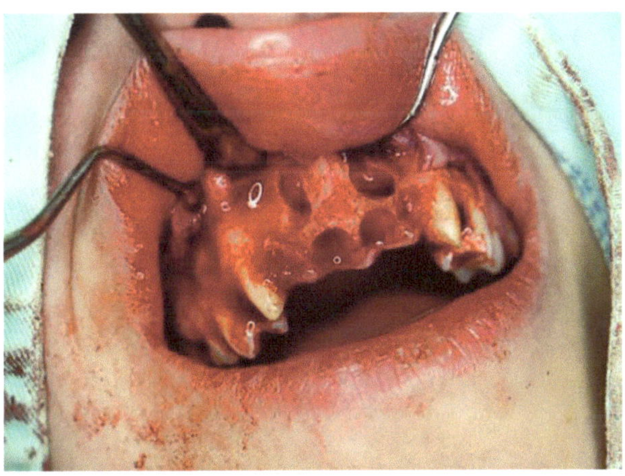

Figure 13.4. Condition after root resection of central incisors. By cutting the root, opening a multitude of infected tubular channels, the homeostasis and regeneration of the apical region and lamellar bone are irreversibly disturbed. Augmentation with a bone substitute is necessary. Omitting the augmentation procedure during implant placement in those regions is a risk factor.

When planning the installation of endosseous implants and in the past, numerous diagnostic procedures were applied to examine the spatial limitation due to the presence of the mandibular canal. Today, as in the past, it is a panoramic tomographic image. Newer generations of X-ray machines have an incomparably lower exposure to X-rays and better visibility. Using appropriate magnification factors and selected measuring templates, the distance from the top of the alveolar ridge to the upper border of the bone is obtained, i.e. roof of the mandibular canal. Clarification of the position of certain anatomical structures in a 3D image can be marked by coloring (Figure 13.2).

It is considered that the safe distance from the implant to the roof of the mandibular canal is 2 mm. In order to minimize the possibility of injury to the mandibular canal, control retroalveolar X-rays should be taken intraoperatively, if necessary, during the bone preparation phase with drills of selected diameters and lengths. Today, it is much easier with the use of intraoral digital sensors (RVG), whereby the parallelism of the implants can be controlled during installation (Figure 13.5 and 13.6).

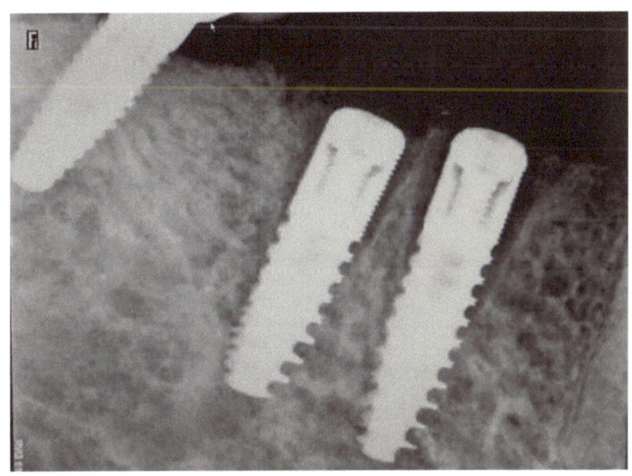

Figure 13.5. The safety of implant installation is significantly increased by the use of the RVG intraoral sensor. With the intraoral sensor as an auxiliary method, it is possible to monitor the parity of the implant position during implementation.

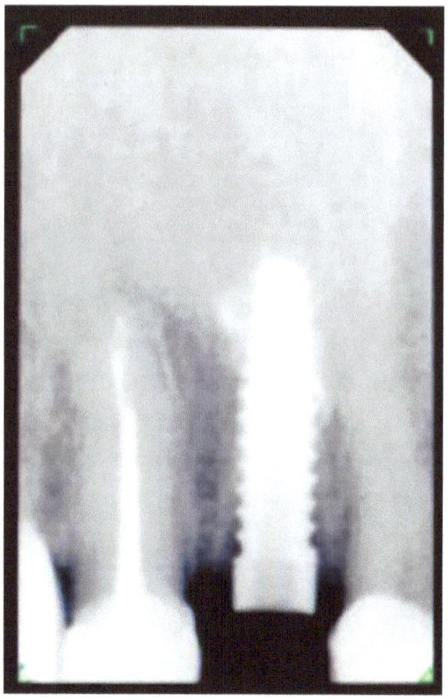

Figure 13.6. Monitoring the position of the implant on the screen with an intraoral sensor (RVG) during installation makes the implantation safe.

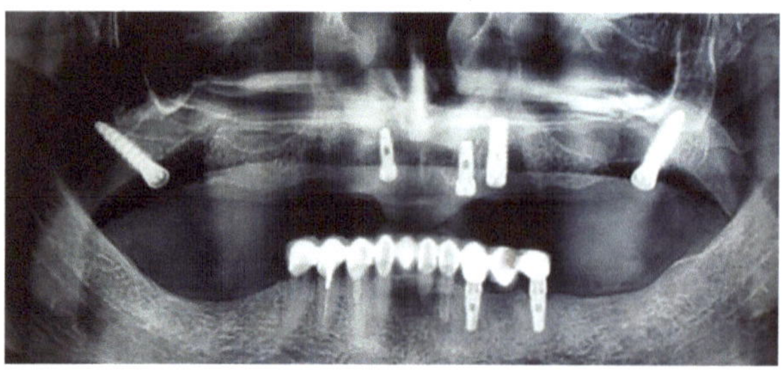

Figure 13.7. The presented implant procedure (in the picture) is a big risk in oral implantology, because it is not in accordance with the implant-prosthetic principles of rehabilitation. "Justification" may be in the express request of the patient and the courage of the implantologist to satisfy the patient's wishes. Experience advises not to engage in similar risky interventions in correcting other people's mistakes.

A group of researchers (Vasquez et al., 2008), in a study that included 2,584 implant procedures, in the lateral region of the lower jaw, in which panoramic tomographic images and measurement templates were used to determine the length of the implant and the relationship with the mandibular canal, observed only two cases of postoperative paresthesias, which is about 0.08%. Both of these cases of paresthesia are related to imprecisely selected measuring templates or template displacement during bone preparation.

It should be emphasized that the position of the chin (n. mentalis), as a landmark, is an extremely important strategic orientation point in implant placement, which is located between the first and second premolars, and shows very wide variations (Figure 13.8. - red arrow).

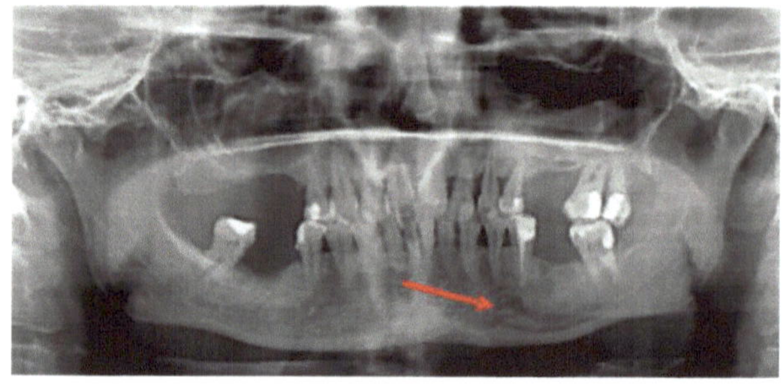

Figure 13.8. Variations n. mandibularis and n. mentalis on the left side of the lower jaw, indicated by a red arrow.

Nerve injuries, in relation to the degree of damage, can be: neuropraxia, axonotmesis or neurotmesis.

Neuropraxia (grade I) is characterized by the lowest degree of damage and is a completely reversible loss of function of a nerve, without anatomical damage.

Axonotmesis (II degree) is a more severe damage to a nerve due to the interruption of the continuity of endoneural structures and axons (nerve fibers) with preservation of the nerve sheath.

Neurotmesis (III degree) is the most severe degree of nerve damage, with complete interruption of nerve fibers and complete loss of nerve conduction, when reinnervation (regeneration) is impossible, with permanent loss of sensitivity.

In principle, all these mentioned degrees of lesions can lead to complete anesthesia in the region of innervation of the corresponding nerve. In the first two terms, neuropraxia, there is a deterioration of the nerve fibers of the surrounding border zone, and axonotmesis is manifested by degenerative changes in the border zone and axons, reestablishment of sensitivity can be expected.

Differentiating different degrees of severity of nerve damage by the usual routine clinical examination, such as the sharp-dull test, is not possible. To determine the degree of sensitivity disorder, specialist neurological examinations and tests are required.

One of the routine methods of examining sensitivity disorders is to inject an anesthetic and wait for the numbness of the lower lip. After that, a slight lesion of the nerve is made with the tip of the needle or probe. The patient's response will show whether the continuity of the nerve is preserved. In cases of nerve injury, it is recommended to wait, with the application of anti-edematous therapy for a period of three to four days, to prevent edema of the nerve itself in the bone canal caused by iatrogenic compression. Steroids should be started, for example, prednisone 5 mg or pronisone 20 mg in doses that are successively reduced daily. You should prescribe a medication that has an anti-inflammatory, anti-exudative, and mucolytic effect, which accelerates the disappearance of swelling - edema, exudate and blood vessels - hematoma, normalizing the locally disturbed circulation of blood and lymph. After the procedure, give one ampoule of dexamethasone (4 ml), and in the postoperative course, continuously use vitamin B-complex tablets for the regeneration of the injured nerve.

If it does not spontaneously recover in 3-4 months, a consultation with a maxillofacial surgeon is recommended. When it comes to nerve regeneration, neurologists are more competent (if they can help, at least in terms of precise diagnosis of the degree of injury). Research by Progel (2006), in 51 patients with pronounced disorders of sensibility, n.alveolaris inferior and n.lingualis, the only recommended choice of therapy would be a microsurgical intervention in an institution where it is possible to perform it. In the aforementioned study, significant improvement was observed in 10 patients, a weaker improvement in 18, and no improvement in 22; in one case, the consequence of the microsurgical intervention was worsening of the condition.

Where to start to avoid risks?

The aim of the preliminary examination is to show any relative or absolute contraindications for implantation at an early stage of the examination. It would be completely useless to perform all the computed tomographic analyses, evaluations and planning of the entire implant procedure if the patient is unable to open his mouth wider than three finger lengths (Figure 13.9).

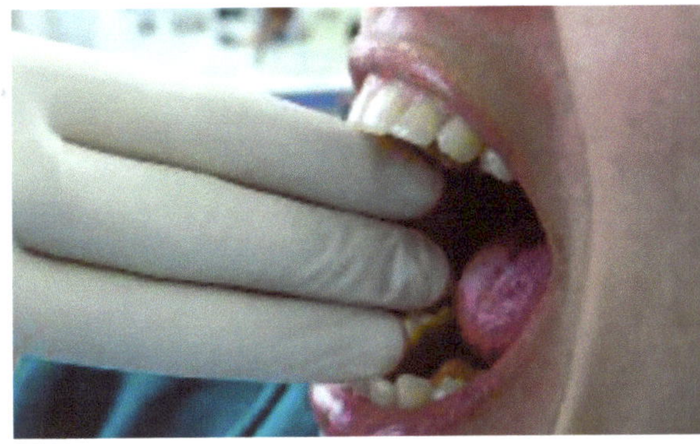

Figure 13.9. The possibility of opening the mouth - if the intraocclusal distance is less than three fingers, it is much more difficult to work during the procedure.

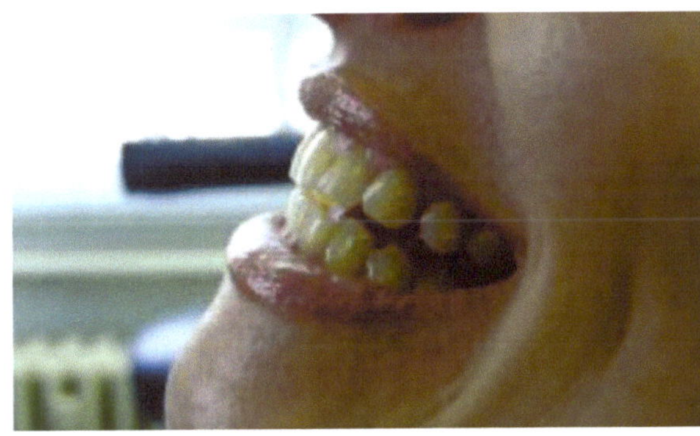

Figure 13.10. Assessment of the condition of interjaw relationships is extremely important before the decision to install implants (whether orthodontic treatment is required).

At the beginning of the examination, the interjaw relationship must be assessed and established, as well as the ideal minimum height in relation to the antagonists, i.e. the minimum height required for mounting the brackets (Figure 13.11).

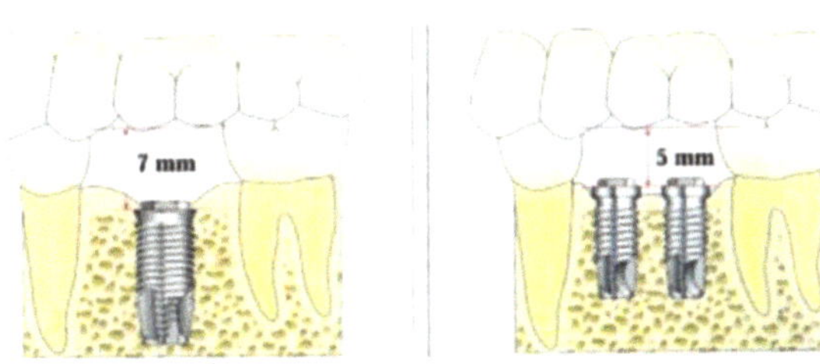

Figure 13.11. Lower height compared to antagonists of 7mm is considered a risk factor.

In the preliminary examination, general risk factors should be excluded:

- General examination - patient's health condition;
- Cause of toothlessness - caries, periodontopathy, trauma; resections...

- Extraoral examination - laugh line, lip shape;
- Oral examination - inspection, palpation, height and width of dental arch, hygiene, condition of gums, smoking;
- Existing functional condition - interjaw relationship, abrasiveness;
- Radiographic examination - orthopantomography, intraoral, near the floor of the sinus in the upper jaw and the position of the mandibular canal in the lower jaw and
- Periodontal examination - pocket depth, bone loss.

Aesthetic risk factor

In the conversation with the patient, such questions should be asked that the patient's wishes and requirements when it comes to aesthetics can be assessed from the answers. If the requirements are unrealistic, there is a risk that such patients belong to an ungrateful group of patients for implant placement. It is one of the risk factors for future dental headaches. In this regard, before installing the implant, it should be established when and in what way the teeth were lost.

The most complicated aesthetic risk factors exist in cases in the frontal region of the upper jaw where the loss occurred due to injuries most often and after root resections. Every such case must be approached with great caution. Even with congenital anodontia of the lateral incisors, the situation must be carefully assessed, because aesthetic risk factors are always present. If the mesiodistal space is less than 6 mm, orthodontic treatment should be performed. In such cases, the width of the crestal bone of the alveolar ridge can be an additional risk factor for achieving a satisfactory aesthetic result.

A few decades ago (when the author began to study and apply implants) it was believed that implantology arose primarily from functional, not aesthetic motives. That position has been advocated for a long time, but modern implantology, in many cases, has set the aesthetic requirement as primary. However, there are cases where aesthetic risk factors are not only not primary, but also negligible, or even non-existent. It depends on the person, case, age and gender, where function is the most important requirement. In those cases, there can only be occlusal risk factors, to which special attention must be paid (Figure 13.12).

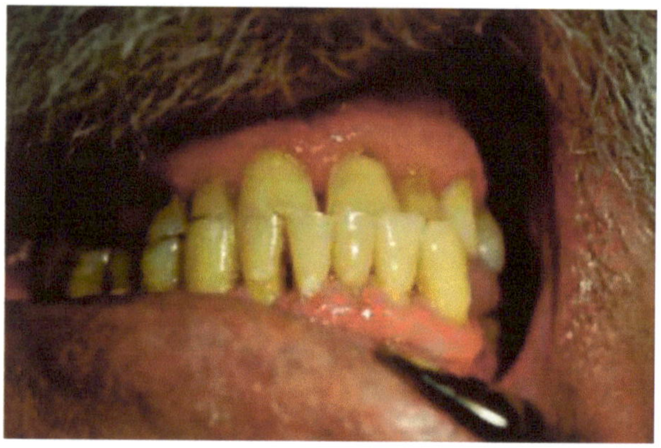

Figure 13.12. The type of patient in whom aesthetics are not primary.

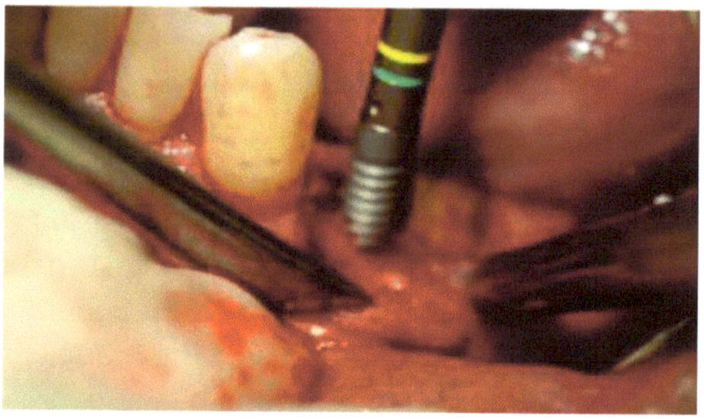

Figure 13.13. The diameter and length of the implant are important to eliminate the risk of masticatory forces acting on the implant and surrounding tissues.

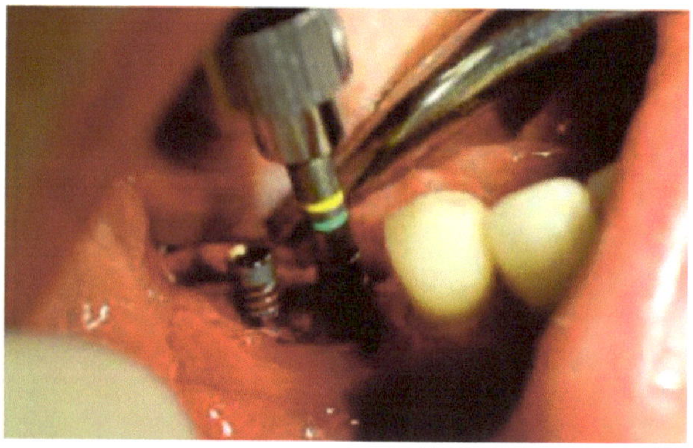

Figure 13.14. Wide diameter, position and number of implants with atraumatic implant placement is the initial step in eliminating occlusal risk factors for failure.

Occlusal Risk Factors

Occlusal risk factors are always present. The basic principle in such cases is the choice of implants (quality, diameter, and length), as well as their number

(Figures 13.13 and 13.14). Achieving good primary stability is one of the most important goals of the implant placement procedure. If these conditions are met, the primary loading of the implant within physiological limits promotes integration processes. The presented implants, at the follow-up examination after two years, showed extremely good stability and successful osseointegration. A significant role in the success of the process after implantation was played by coordinated occlusal contacts, by shaping the biting surfaces, and the inclination of the cusps adapted to gnathological requirements.

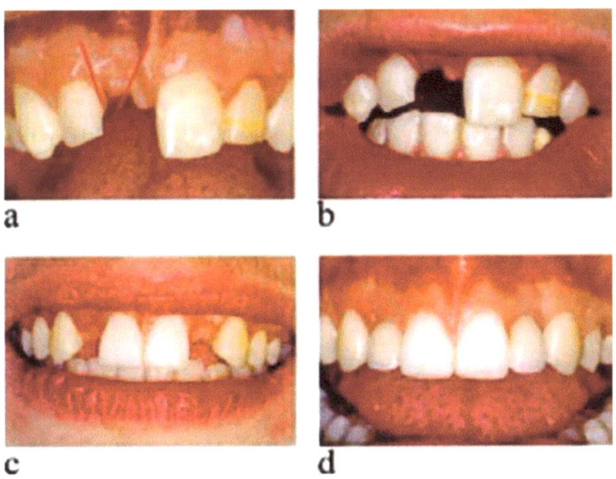

Figure 13.15. Traumatically lost central incisor (a) and the condition after wearing partial dentures with compression created bony and aesthetic risk factors. (b). Hypodontia of lateral incisors (c). By orthodontic movement of the canines, a mesio-distal space was created for the lateral incisors and the installation of reduced-diameter implants.

Figure 13.15. in the top row, shows the loss of a right central incisor as a result of trauma. The lost tooth, in another institution, was replaced with a temporary movable acrylate prosthesis ("frog"). The consequences are visible: quantitative loss of bone and soft tissues, and the papillae are also at risk. Implant therapy requires compensation with bone substitutes, and the waiting period is at least 8 to 12 months. A more justified procedure than a movable acrylate prosthesis was the installation of implants, immediate loading and a provisional acrylate crown. But it should be emphasized that even with the best result of bone defect compensation with bone substitutes, there are always bone and aesthetic risk factors during delayed implant-prosthetic rehabilitation.

Gingival risk factors

A successful aesthetic outcome of implant rehabilitation depends on the condition of the gingiva and interdental papilla. A successful aesthetic result is the harmony of soft tissues (gingiva and papillae) and good prosthetic work.

Important factors for good aesthetics are:

- Laughter line - gingival or dental;
- Gingival quality – thickness (biotype);
- Papilla - relationship with the neighboring tooth.

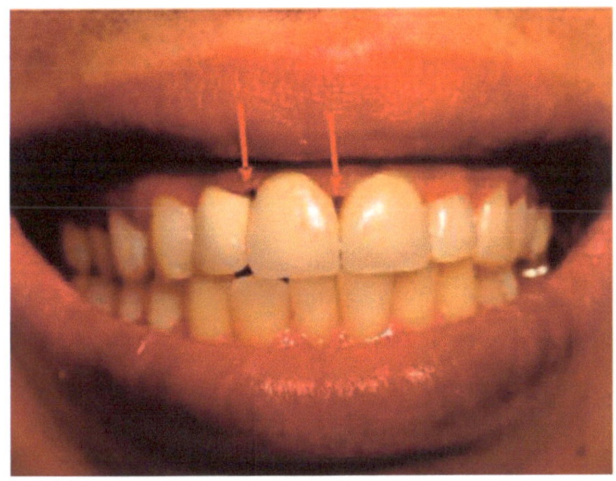

Figure 13.16. The papillae are threatened (red arrows), and the unfavorable smile line makes visible the aesthetic failure caused by imprecise prosthetic work - wide crowns in the neck part of the implant.

Dental risk factors

The visibility of dental risk factors depends on the high smile line: poor prosthetic work, shape and color of teeth, visibility and biotype of gingiva and destroyed interdental papillae. Dental risk factors are numerous and are shown in Figures 13.15, 13.16 and 13.18.

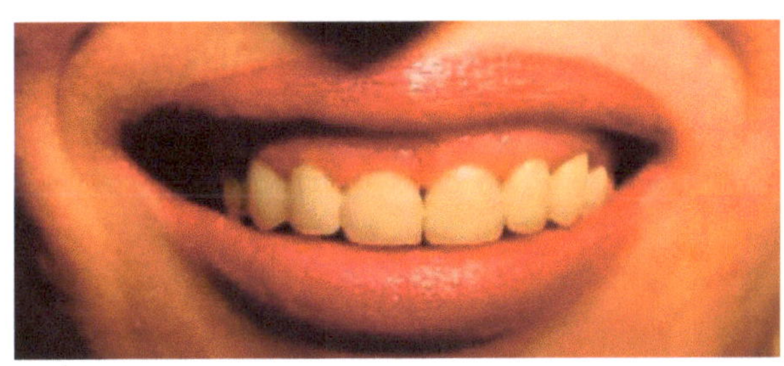

Figure 13.17. With a high smile line, the interdental papilla must be preserved. Prosthetic work on implants risk factor interdental papilla of central incisors.

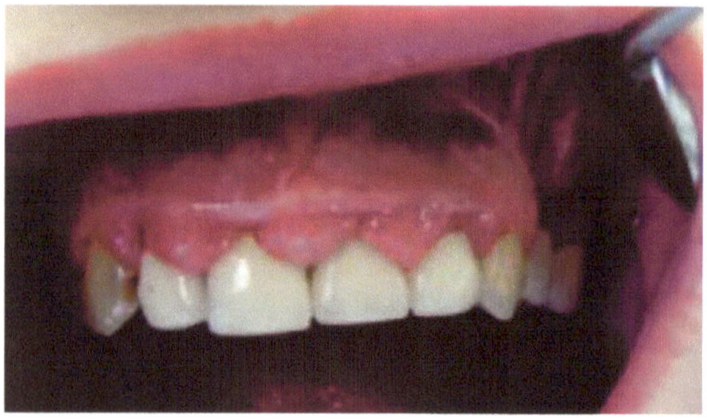

Figure 13.18. Bad condition of the gums represents a high risk factor for the application of implants. The presented condition is a consequence of poor prosthetics and poor oral hygiene.

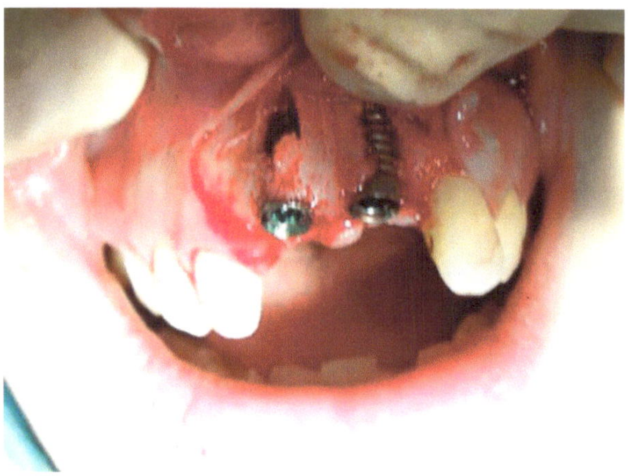

Figure 13.19. Resected roots, destroyed lamellar bone. After extracting the roots of the central incisors, the dentist created an aesthetic risk factor for the patient with a provisional acrylic prosthesis ("frog"), promoting alveolar bone resorption by compression. Augmentation was done with a bone substitute mixed with autologous bone chips.

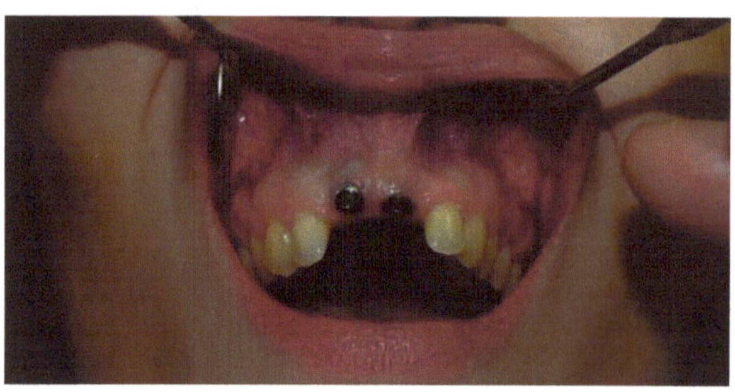

Figure 13.20. The successful outcome of augmentation resulted in good osseointegration and soft tissue healing. There remains an aesthetic risk factor as a consequence of root resection, as well as wearing an acrylate mobile prosthesis after extraction of the resected roots.

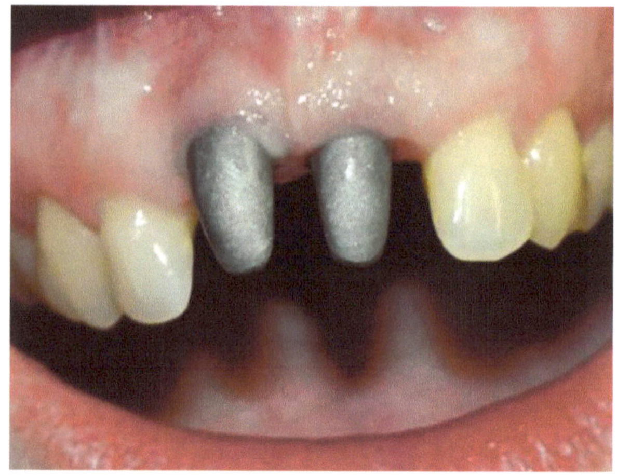

Figure 13.21. Since augmentation of the perforated lamellar bone, immediate implant placement and good bone integration resulted in success, there is an aesthetic risk factor, which partially eliminates the favorable lip shape and laugh line. After extracting the resected roots, the so-called "frog" is also inadmissible as a temporary solution.

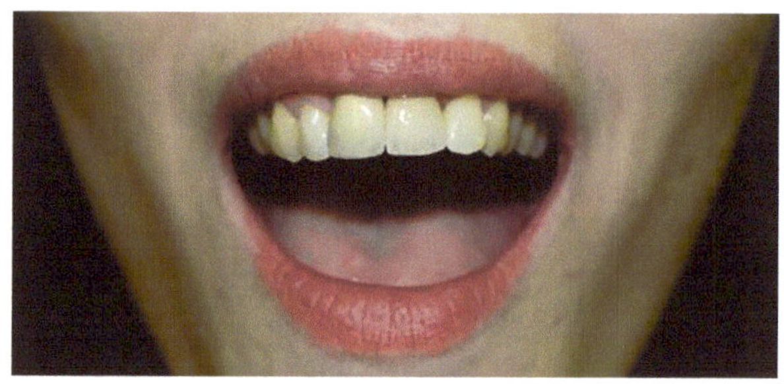

Figure 13.22. The aesthetic risk factor eliminates the favorable position of the upper lip - the favorable laugh line. Figures 13.25 and 13.26.

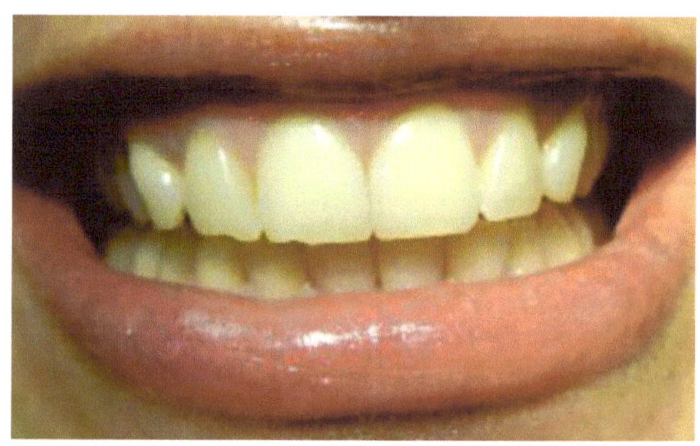

Figure 13.23. Natural ideal appearance of preserved interdental papillae thanks to good bone support and absence of minimal periodontal changes.

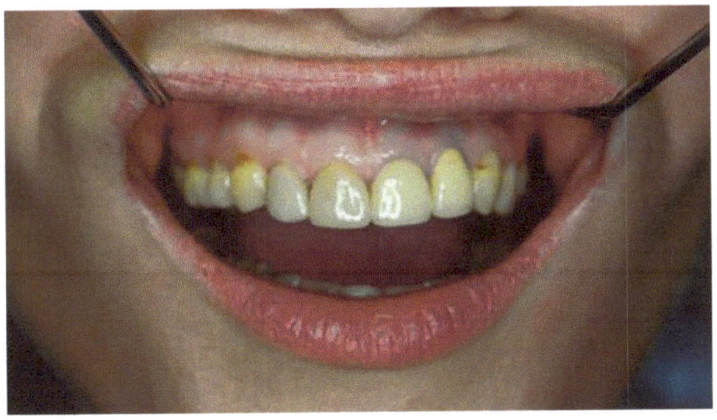

Figure 13.24. Screening of the neck of the implant and the support (abutment) in thin gingival biotype is an aesthetic risk factor.

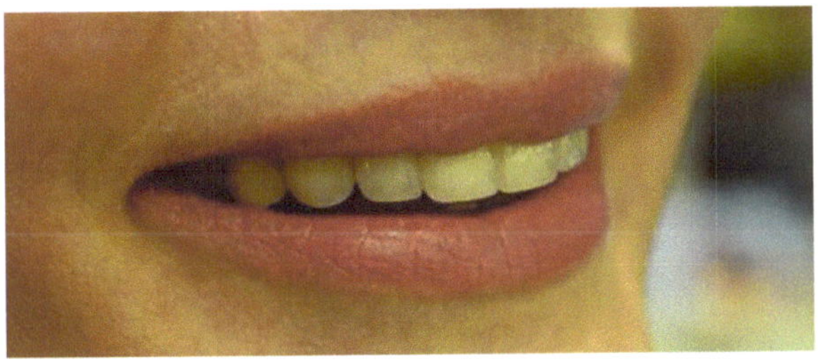

Figure 13.25. Partial toothlessness compensated by implants, the shape and position of the lip is determined by the aesthetic risk factor.

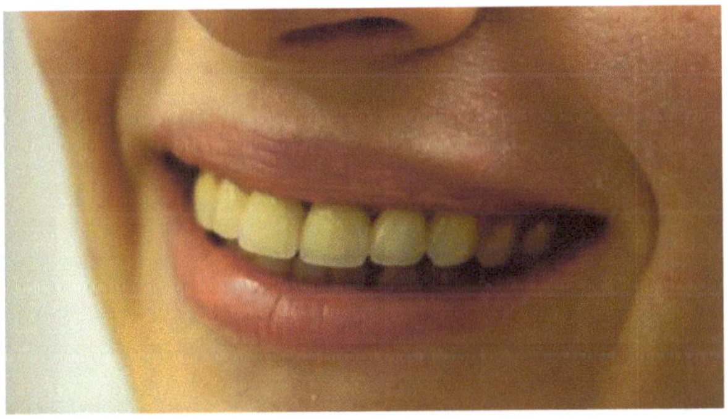

Figure 13.26. After the augmentation of the lamellar wall of region #21 and #22 (see Figure 13.16), the position of the lip and laugh line is favorable for the aesthetic result. The most frequently repeated mistake with routine tooth extraction that needs to be replaced with implants. During extraction, carefully and slowly apply all movements (luxation and rotation) in order to leave as much bone mass as possible in the alveolar wound. Preservation of the alveolus and filling with a bone substitute is a recommended procedure.

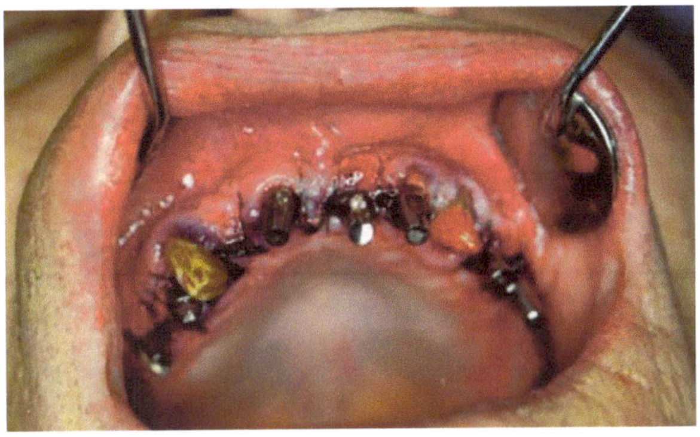

Figure 13.27. Immediate installation of implants with immediate loading. The answer to the question of whether to leave natural teeth depends on the status of the teeth. Canines are good supports for prosthetic work. However, after a long time since implantation, periodontal changes can be a risk factor - experience shows that.

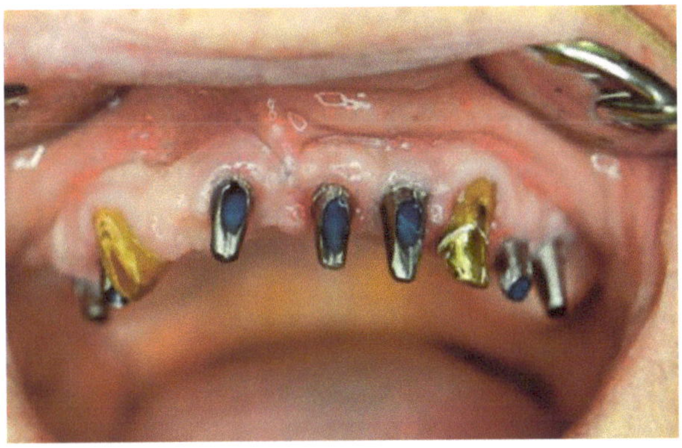

Figure 13.28. Appearance of healed tissues, well-integrated implants, lege artis of healed canine with extension. Status report after eight weeks. Compare with the previous picture (13.27).

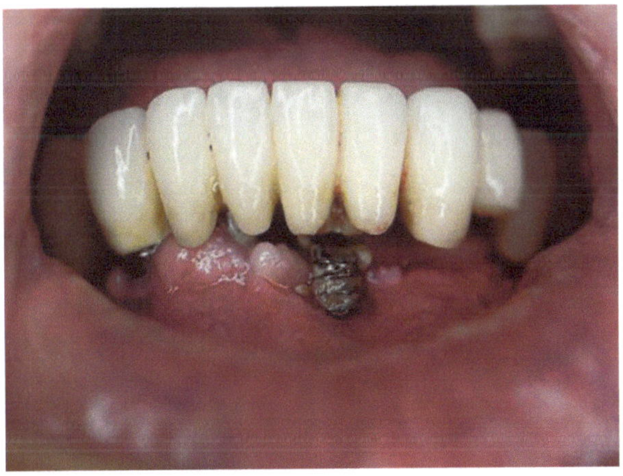

Figure 13.29. The risks in the presented case were created before the start of the implantation: poor planning by choosing low-quality implants of inappropriate diameters in relation to the available horizontal bone. The patient could not correct the dentist's mistakes even if he maintained good oral hygiene. Compare with pictures 13.30. and 13.38. Patient's condition 15 years after implantation, despite heavy smoking and poor oral hygiene.

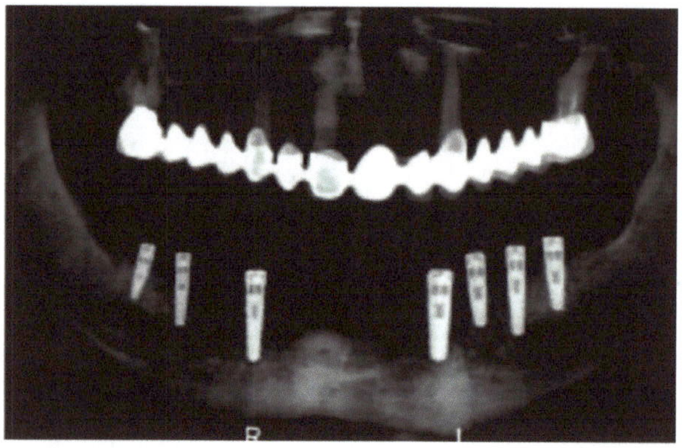

Figure 13.30. Built-in implants of the Nobe-Replace-Biocare type with wider diameters - sufficient width of the horizontal bone. Alveolus preservation after tooth extraction, augmentation of lost bone. The degree of achieved primary fixation of the implant determines the next procedure - primary or delayed loading. The applied procedures are the prevention of failures as shown in Figure 13.29.

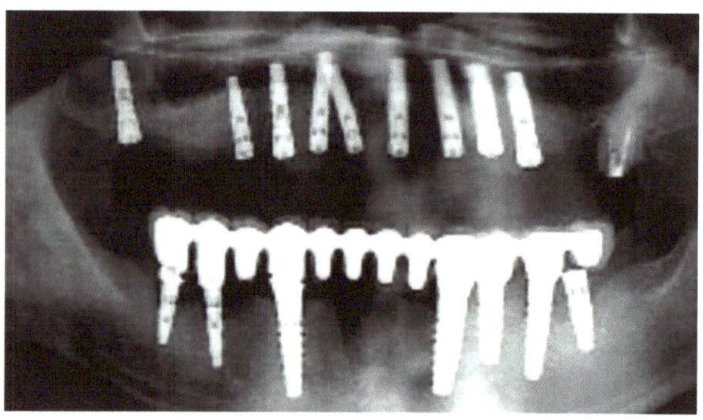

Figure 13.31. Immediate installation of Nobel Replace Biocare implants, immediately loaded except for the implant installed in the tuber of the upper jaw. Control image of the upper jaw after 6 months and the lower jaw after 10 years (see the initial state of the installed implants, Figure 13.28). Fracture of the carrier screw is a complication and a risk factor, and in the presented case it caused the migration of the implant, indicated by the red arrow.

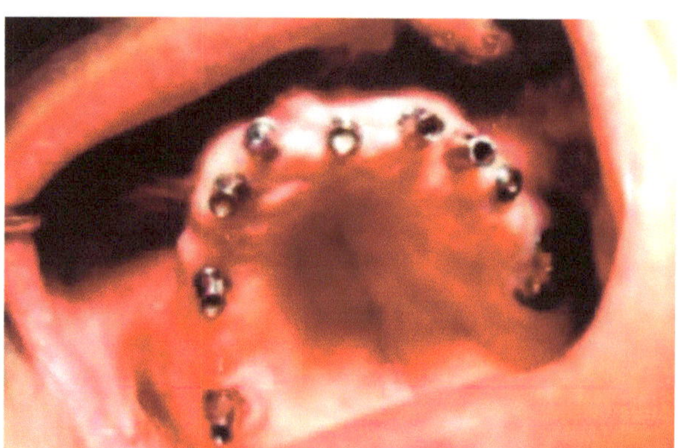

Figure 13.32. Healing after six months. Placed abutment on the implant embedded in the tuber of the upper jaw. Upper left left molar (low sinus floor) which will not be connected to the definitive prosthetic work, and the distal part of the bridge with the occlusal support of the hanging members will reduce the action of occlusal axial forces on the neighboring implants.

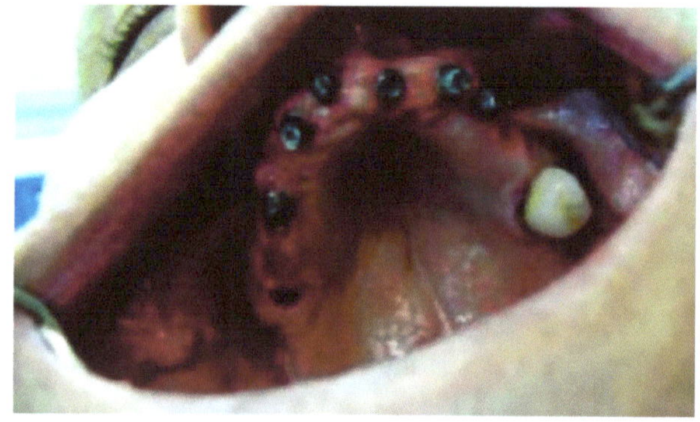

Figure 13.33. Placed implants in the same patient. Implant placed in the tuber of the upper jaw on the right (indicated by the red arrow). A crown was made on the molar (left due to the low floor of the maxillary sinus - see picture 13.30) which will not be attached to the construction of fixed prosthetic work. The toothless region is compensated by a member resting on the crown (Figures 13.31, 13.34 and 13.35).

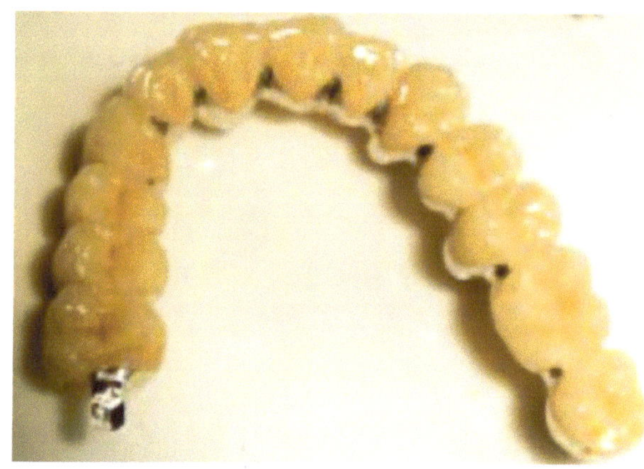

Figure 13.34. Appearance of definitive prosthetic work in metal ceramics, left metal collars and occlusal abutment on the crown. In case of molar loss, the prosthetic work remains intact.

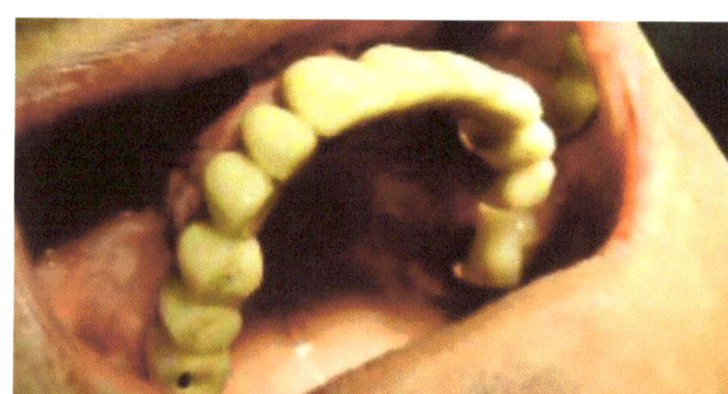

Figure 13.35. Definitive prosthetic work. A left molar left for an occlusal support to cushion the matic forces on the suspended bridge members, shown in Figure 13.34. Tying an unreliable tooth into definitive prosthetic work would be a mistake.

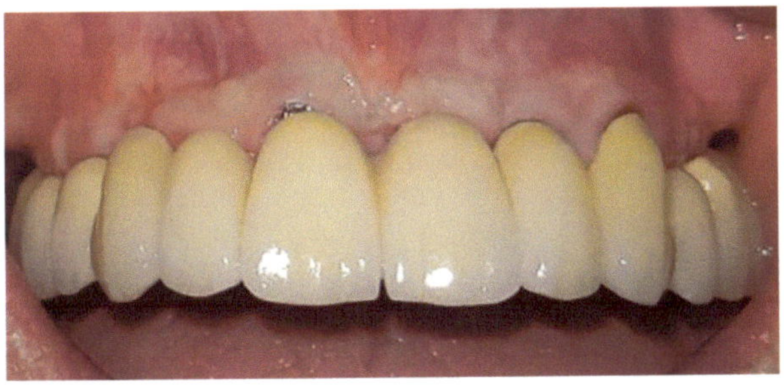

Figure 13.36. Definitive metal-ceramic prosthetic work after 12 years with left occlusal rest on retained molar. With the loss of the remaining molar, the prosthetic work remains unchanged, possibly shortening one hanging member, which depends on the condition of the antagonist.

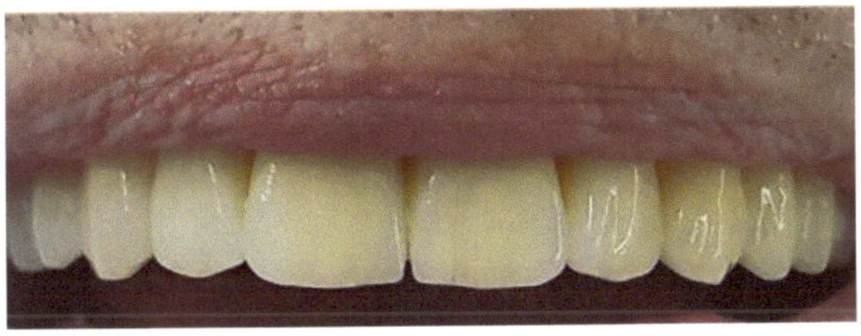

Figure 13.37. The shape and position of the lips, in the presented case, means that aesthetic gingival risk factors in the upper and lower frontal region do not exist.

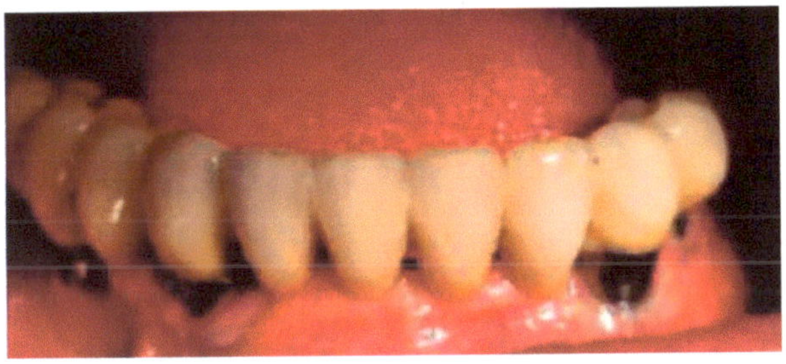

Figure 13.38. By leaving the collar in the neck area, the risk factor for plaque deposition is reduced and the possibility of better cleaning is created. Heavy smokers are always a risk factor for implantation success. Collars in the neck area and hygienic bridges in the lateral regions (the picture shows the condition after 15 years) reduce the risk of failure. Hygienic bridges made in the lateral regions.

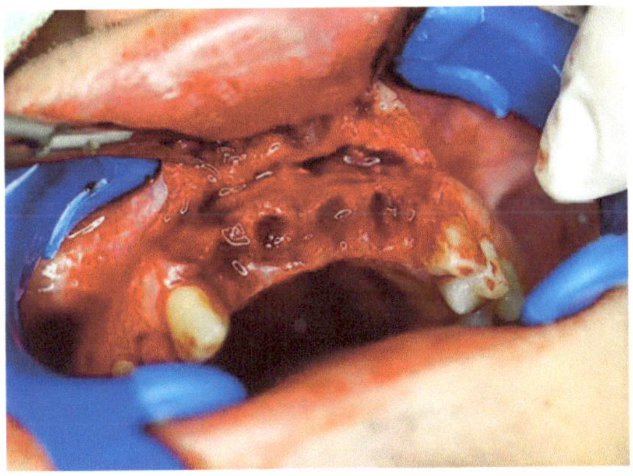

Figure 13.39. Larger bony defects in the frontal region of the upper jaw are a greater aesthetic than functional risk factor. Augmentation avoids the aesthetic risk factor by creating quality bone support for healing and shaping of soft tissues, why a longer waiting time is needed.

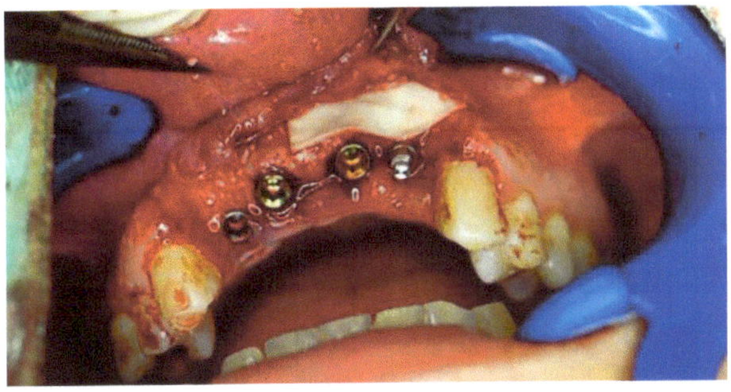

Figure 13.40. With the immediate installation of the implant, achieve good primary fixation, replace bone defects with a bone substitute, covered with a collagen resorptive membrane.

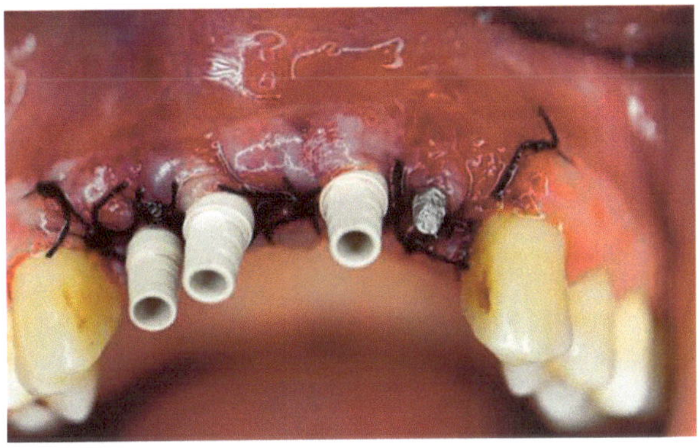

Figure 13.41. Installed temporary supports (abutments) for the construction of a provisional bridge. After 8 months, replace them with definitive brackets, the condition found determines whether it is necessary to perform additional augmentation to shape the alveolar arch and create better bone support, which would create the conditions for the regeneration of the interdental papillae.

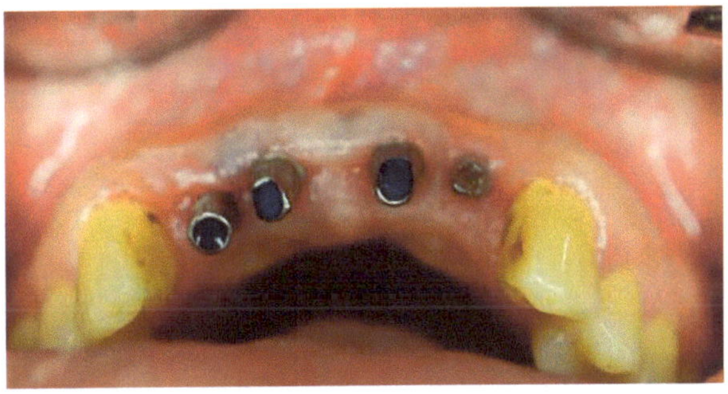

Figure 13.42. By augmentation of bone defects, the arch of the alveolar ridge was shaped, good bone support was created for the formation of stable soft tissues, which eliminated bone and gingival risk factors. Status report after 12 months. Compare with picture 13.39.

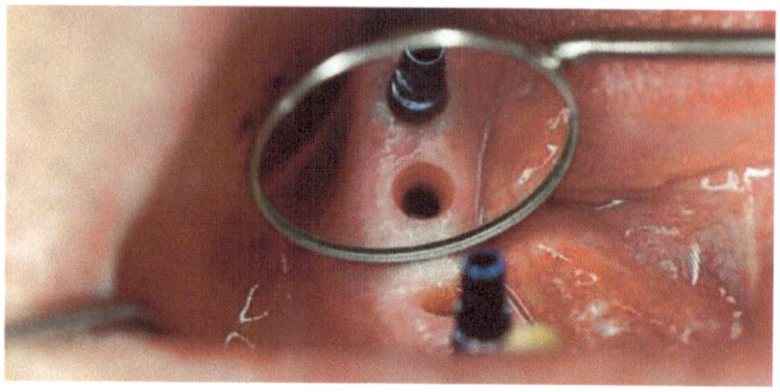

Figure 13.43. Quality keratinized gingiva is a protection against risk occurrence of peri-implantitis

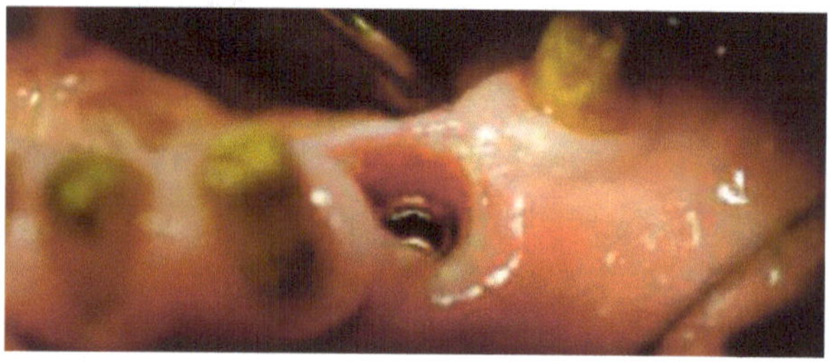

Figure 13.44. A deeply embedded implant is a mistake, and a quality thicker layer of keratinized mucosa can be a factor to eliminate the risk peri-implant changes.

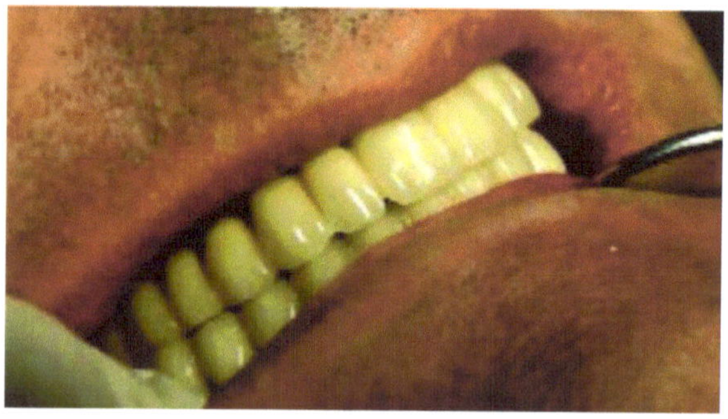

Figure 13.45. Balanced occlusion established, maintenance condition long-term functions of the entire implant-prosthetic treatment long-term survival of the implant in the bone. Controlling established balanced occlusions, elimination of premature and too strong occlusal contacts, biomechanical risk factors are eliminated.

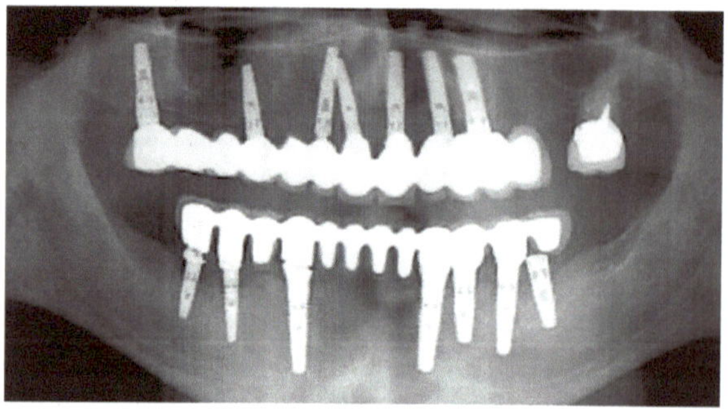

Figure 13.46. Condition of the jaw after 10 years for implants in the upper jaw, and 15 years in the lower jaw (Nobel Repalce Biocare implant system). Fracture of the mounting screw on the left side - red arrow. By loosening the screw, a microcrack (yellow arrow) is created suitable for the deposition of plaque and bacterial content, causing peri-implant infections.

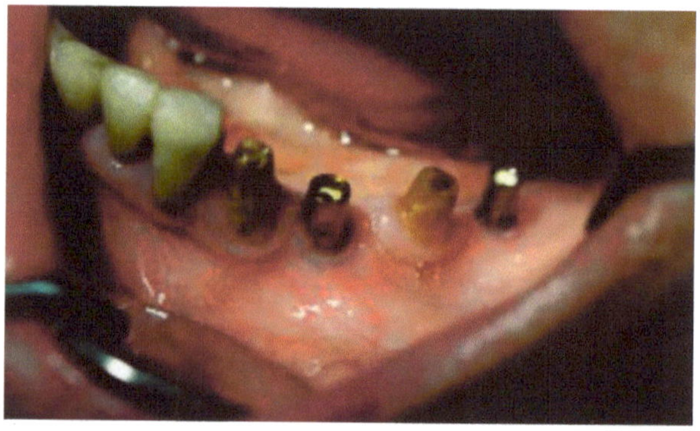

Figure 13.47. Bonding of implants and natural teeth is a greater risk factor than when prosthetic work is placed only on implants. Bad assessment of the condition of natural teeth is a risk factor for implant prosthetics treatment.

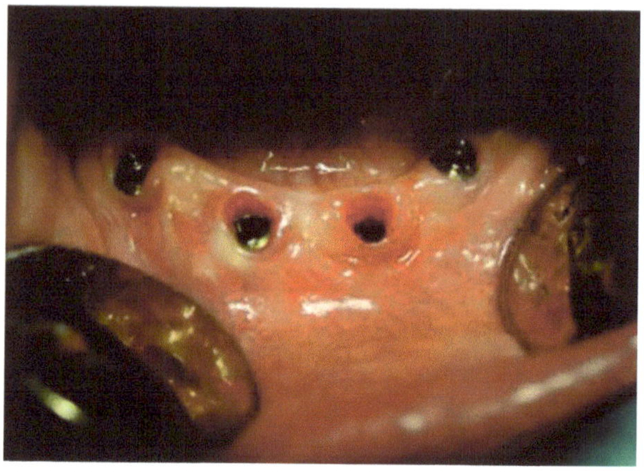

Figure 13.48. Healthy keratinized gingiva is protection against the risk of peri-implantitis. Retention clips on implants. To the patient advise periodic controls to remove accumulated plaque and tartar.

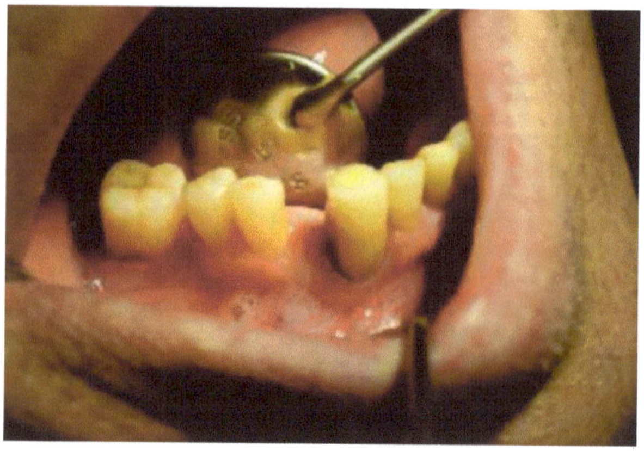

Figure 13.49. Dislodged canine in the lower jaw, loss of lamellar bone, unfavorable interdental space, indicated procedure after extraction of the dislodged tooth, compensation of the bone defect of the lamellar bone with bone substitutes and a waiting period of 6 months. However, the time available and the position of the patient (Australia) required a different procedure.

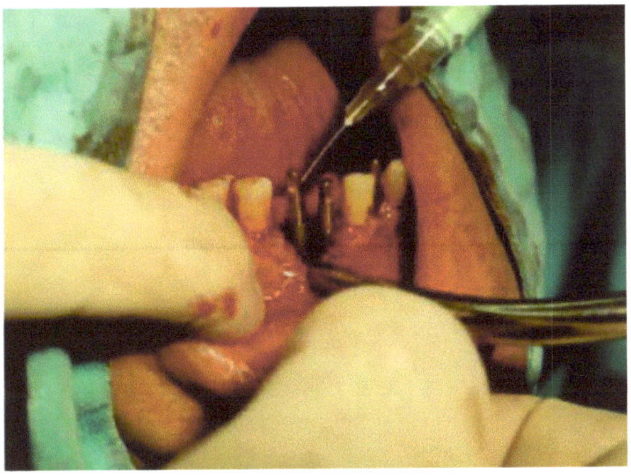

Figure 13.50. The interdistal space determines the diameter of the implant, and the height of the alveolar bone determines its length.

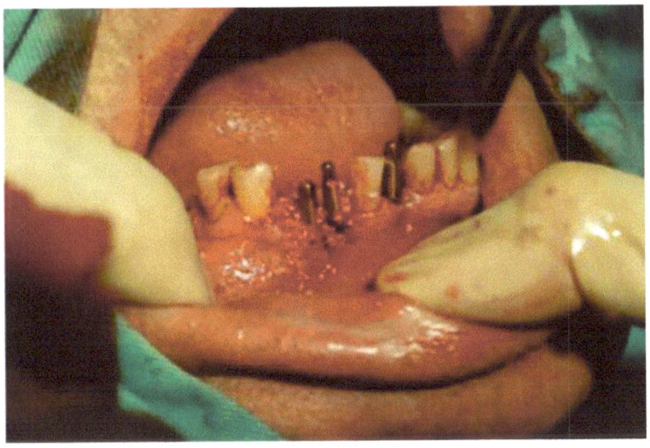

Figure 13.51. Immediately installed one-piece implants (3 mm), replacement of the lost lamellar bone with bone substitutes, which is covered with a collagen resorbable membrane.

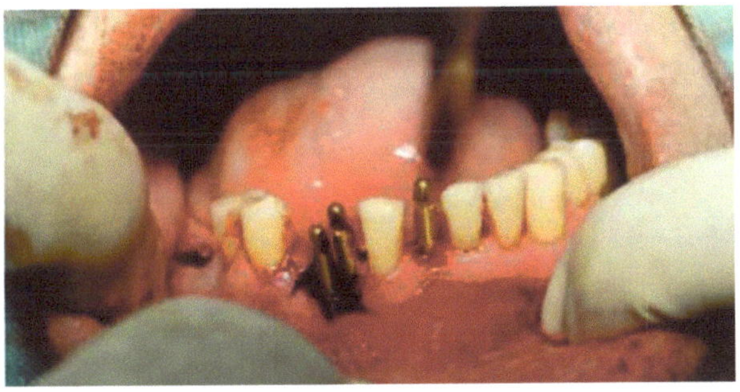

Figure 13.52. Gingival defect - the aesthetic solution of prosthetic reconstruction in the lower jaw is made possible thanks to the favorable shape of the lower lip. Immediate installation of implants with bone defect augmentation.

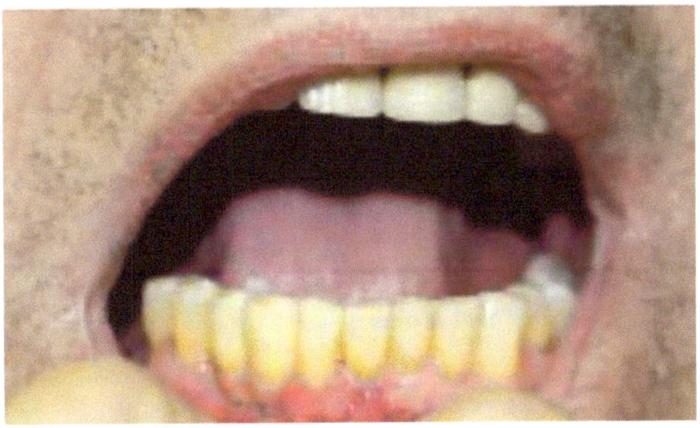

Figure 13.53. The patient shown in the pictures from 13.49. to 13.52, he came for a follow-up examination only after 7 years (he lives in Australia).

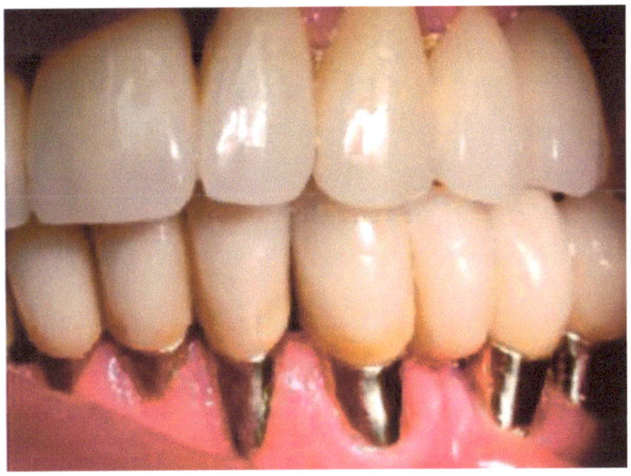

Figure 13.54. Fulfillment of occlusal and hygiene requirements is a prerequisite for the success and longevity of installed implants and the preservation of natural teeth with gingival recession. Good oral hygiene makes the soft tissues stable.

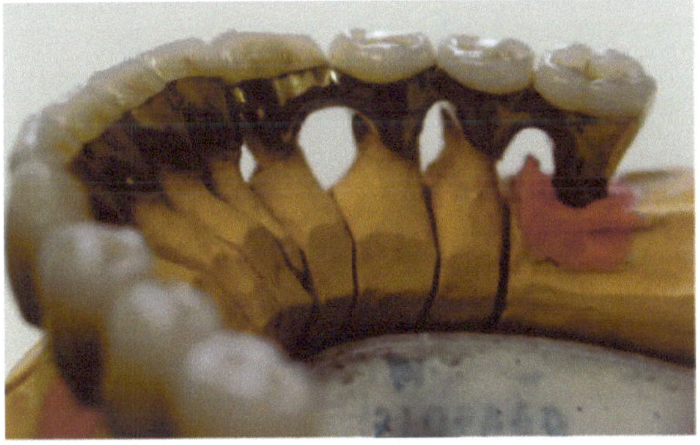

Figure 13.55. Desirable prosthetic reconstruction on implants and natural teeth in the lateral region - shaping of occlusal surfaces (morphology of cusps) in accordance with gnathological principles and the possibility of maintaining oral hygiene. The position of the lips eliminates aesthetic problems in the lateral regions, especially in the lower jaw.

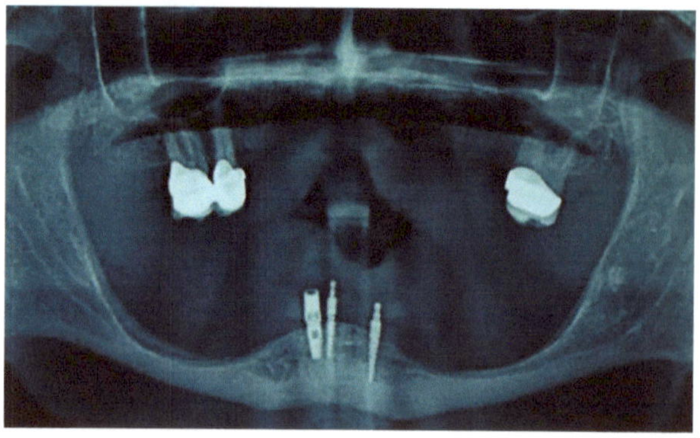

Figure 13.56. In case of extreme alveolar bone resorption, the only possible method of implant-prosthetic rehabilitation is the installation of implants with spherical heads and retention clips. Repeat ridge augmentation performed to obtain possible available bone for installation of implants. Trying to solve it with a different procedure is a risk with foreseeable failure.

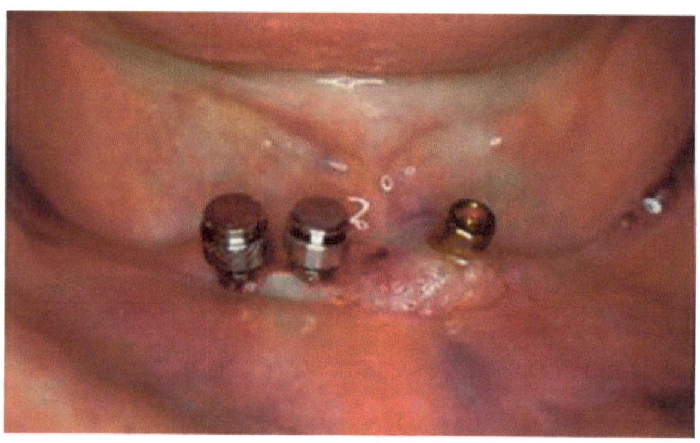

Figure 13.57. The appearance of the retention clips on the spherical heads of the embedded implants after successful augmentation (Figure 13.56).

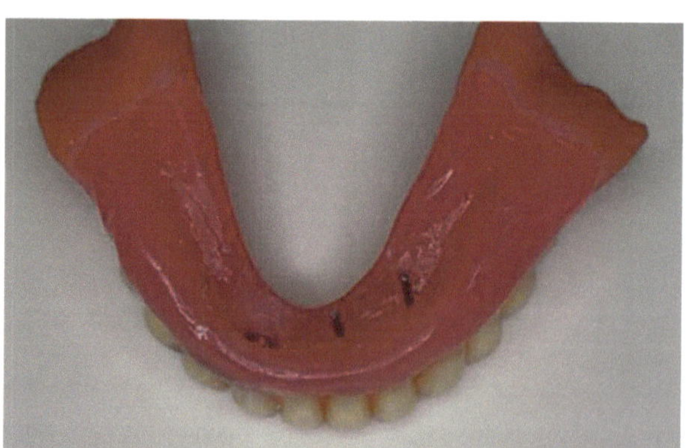

Figure 13.58. Soft acrylate base and built-in retention clips increase the comfort of wearing a mobile lower prosthesis.

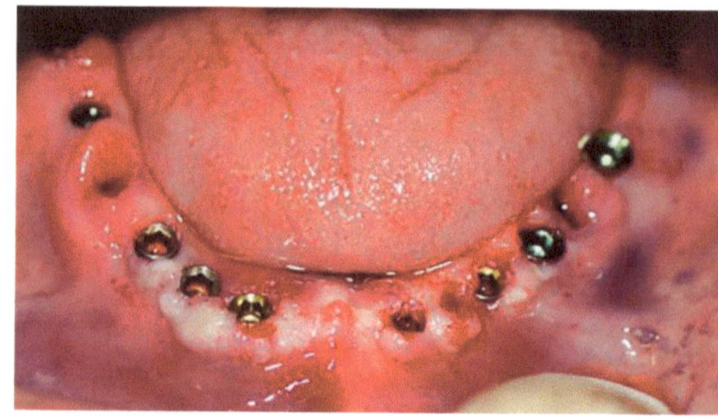

Figure 13.59. Loading multiple implants with prosthetic work in a block is a risk factor, confirms the experience of the author of the book. In the case shown, it is possible to make a prosthetic work in three parts.

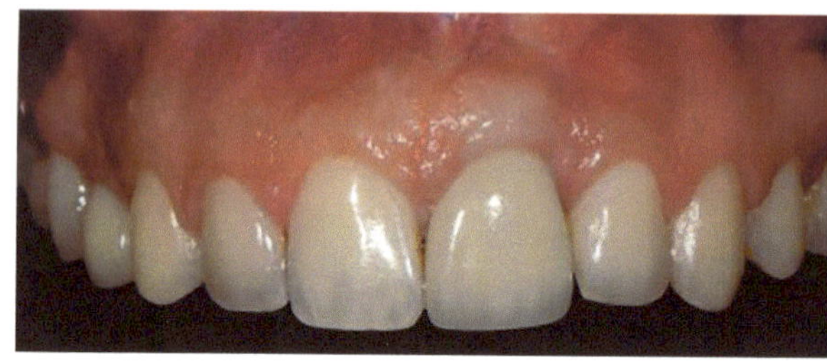

Figure 13.60. Compensation of central incisors with implants. Augmentation increased good bone support and a favorable biotype gingiva of the central incisor (12) resulted in exceptional aesthetics success..

Bone and implant risk factors

There are several types of these risk factors, and the most important is to recognize:

- existence of buccal concavity;
- ratio of neighboring implants

The existence of vertical bone resorption. A very common risk factor is the deceptive surface appearance of the alveolar bone. An experienced practitioner recognizes such cases. A tomographic analysis is mandatory in such cases in order to show the sharp peak of the residual alveolar bone, which is significantly narrower than the plateau, by a few millimeters.

The plateau is the structure of the residual alveolar ridge (RAG) that arises after shaping-flattening the top of the RAG in order to obtain the desired width for installation of an endosseous implant of a selected diameter. Visually, the concavity of such a ridge is emphasized, which represents the risk of perforation of the alveolar ridge during implant placement, which is why special caution is necessary when planning the

diameter and length of the implants and their number (Figure 13.59).

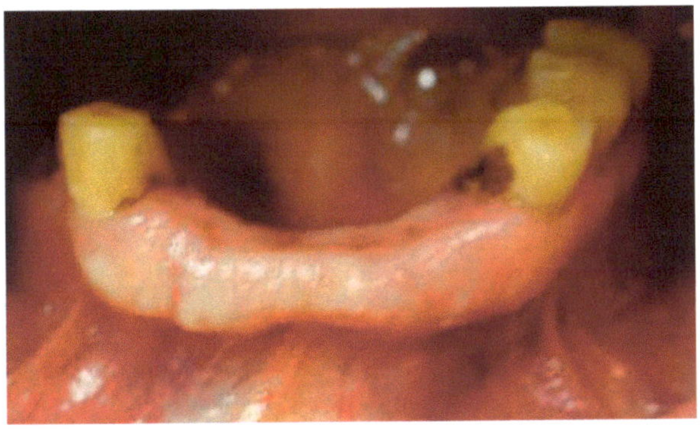

Figure 13.61. Concavity of the alveolar ridge is a major risk factor for perforation on the labial and lingual sides. Adequate selection of the diameter of the implant and caution with the drilled bed are required with the appropriate diameter of the drill bit.

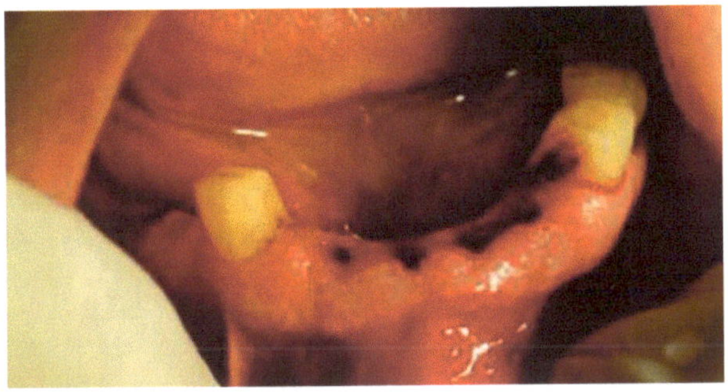

Figure 13.62. A clear position where the implants should be installed, and the selection of the appropriate diameter and length of the implant is important.

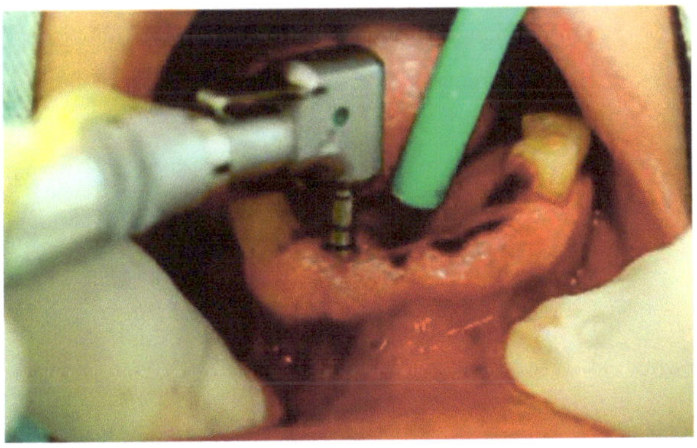

Figure 13.63. The direction of bone preparation is crucial for the success of implant placement.

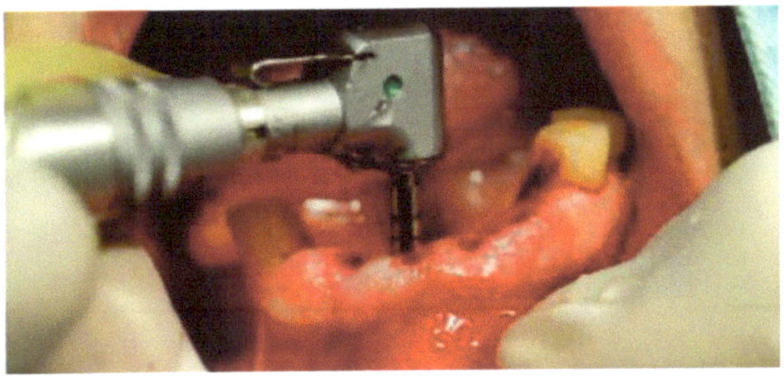

Figure 13.64. The markings on the drill determine the length of drilling the implant bed in the bone.

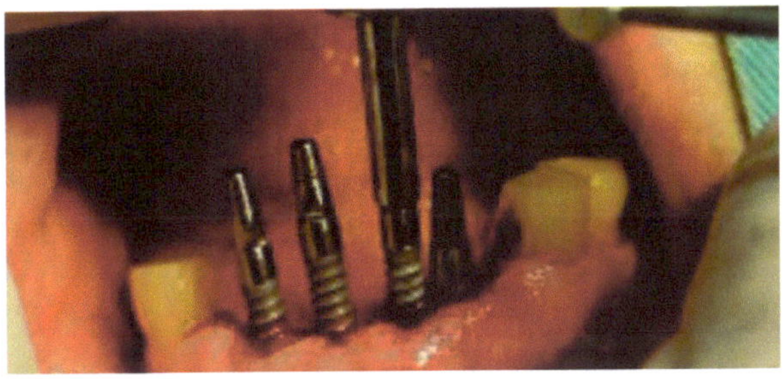

Figure 13.65. Positioning of 3-diameter one-piece implants mm. The insufficient width of the alveolar bone is compensated by the length of the implant.

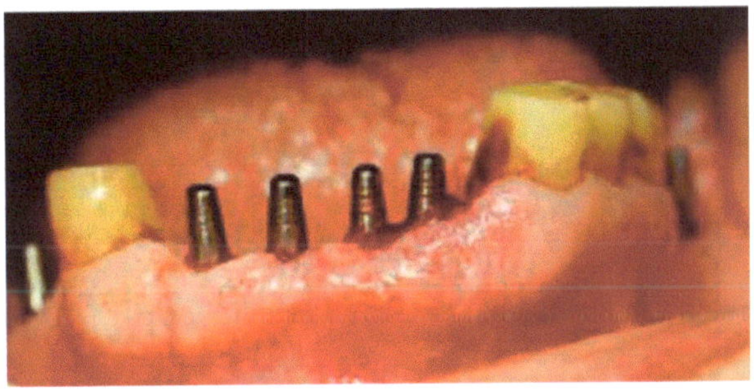

Figure 13.66. Placed implants in the bone without raising the flap, primarily loaded. By choosing the appropriate diameter of the implant, despite the concavity of the alveolar ridge, the risk of perforation was avoided. The success of the procedure depends on the experience of the dentist.

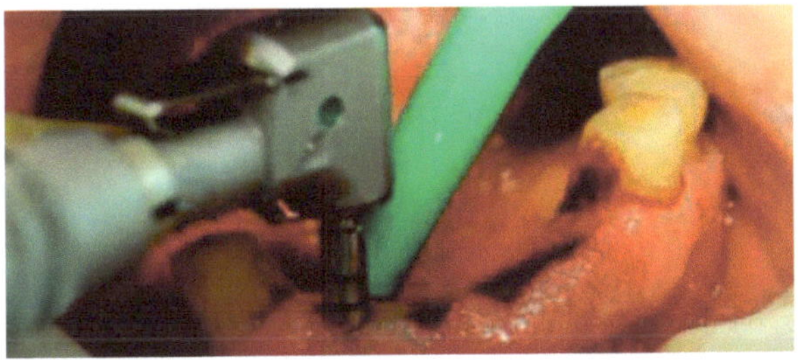

Figure 13.67. The visually deceptive shape of the alveolar ridge (buccal concavity) is a risk factor. The platform of the case shown is narrower than the top of the ridge. At 3 mm from the top of the ridge, the plateau is only 2.5 mm wide. Caution is required due to possible perforation of lips and tounge.

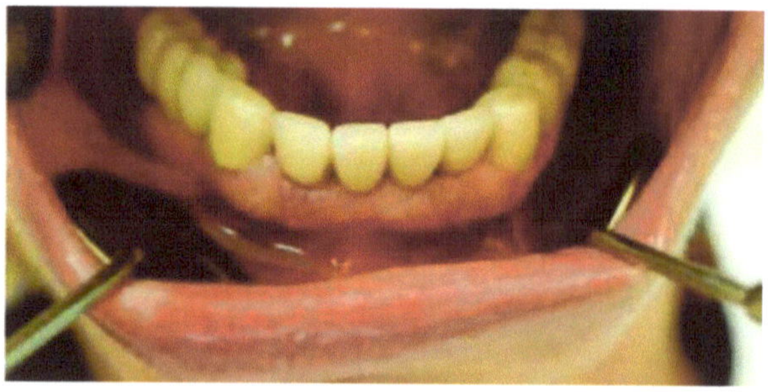

Figure 13.68. Definitive prosthetic work on immediately installed implants without raising the flap. The risk factor of perforation was avoided by installing an implant with a suitable diameter adapted (3 mm) to the dimensions of the horizontal available bone.

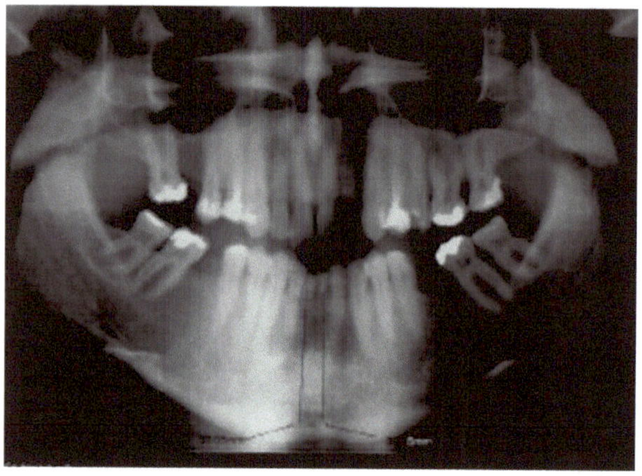

Figure 13.69. Residual milk teeth (in a 34-year-old patient) they caused a decrease in the width of the alveolar bone and the interdental space. Risk factor for labial and lingual bone perforation. The available bone parameters indicate that planning requires extensive augmentation, which should be explained to the patient.

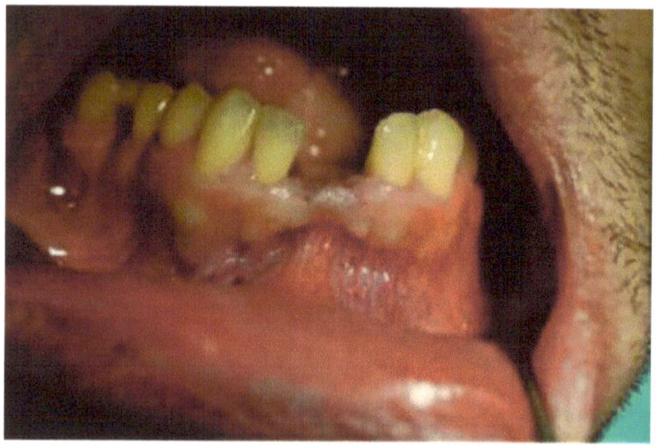

Figure 13.70. Situation after extraction of milk teeth in a patient shown in the previous radiographic image (13.69). Pronounced labial concavity.

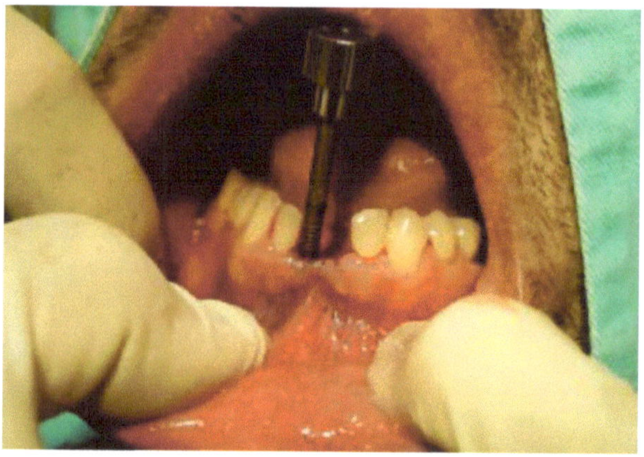

Figure 13.71. Risk for perforation (due to ridge concavity) despite good direction of the drill bit.

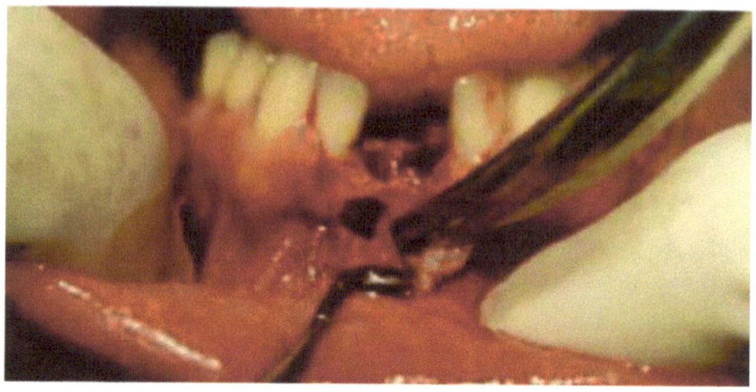

Figure 13.72. Perforation of the labial wall of the bone.

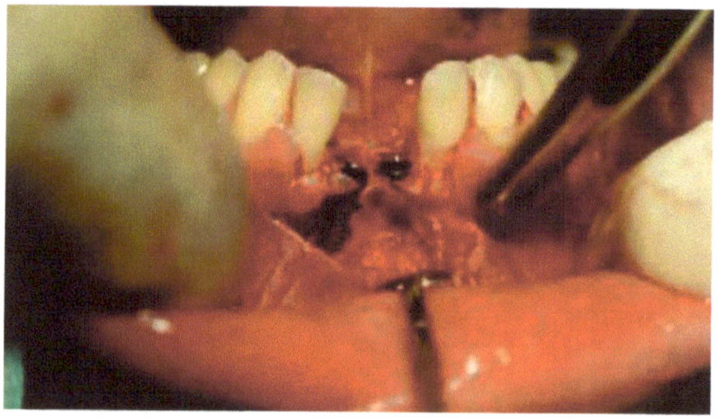

Figure 13.73. Perforation of the labial bone wall. The experience of the author of the book determined the immediate installation of implants and the application of augmentation with a bone substitute with a collagen resorbable membrane.

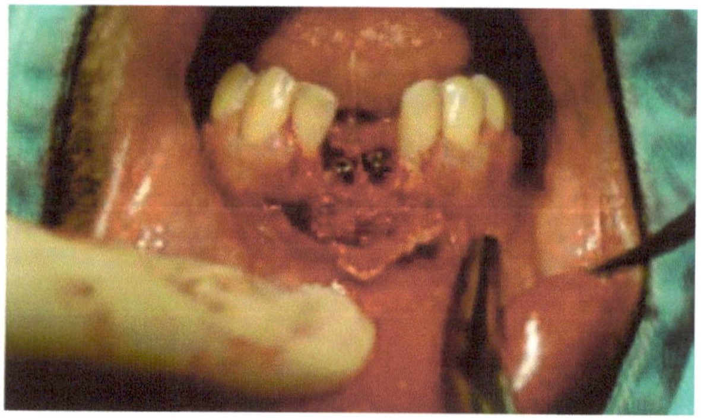

Figure 13.74. Augmentation of the perforation with a bone substitute.

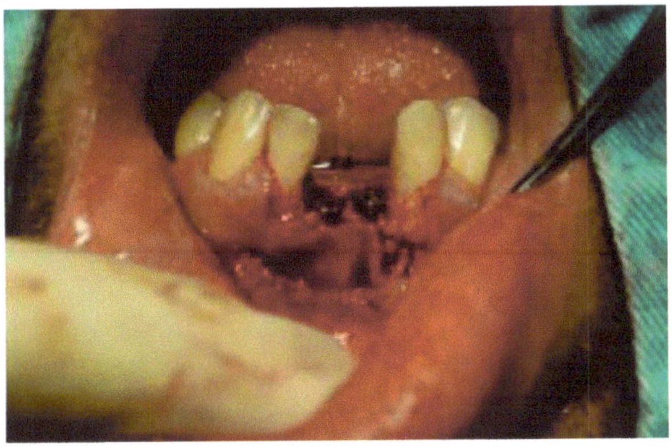

Figure 13.75. Placed collagen resorptive membrane.

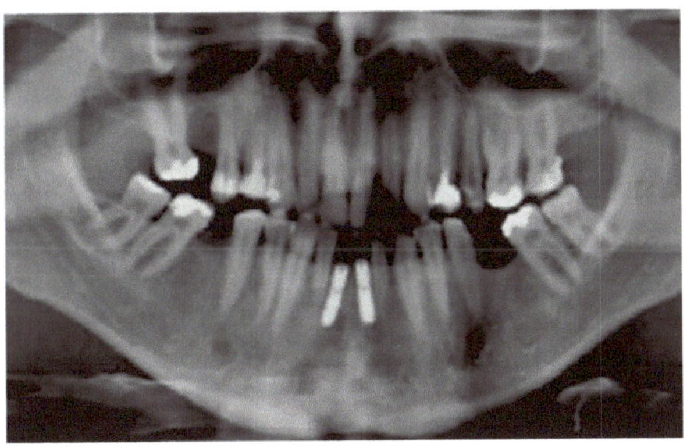

Figure 13.76. The space between the implant and the roots of the adjacent teeth is also a risk factor.

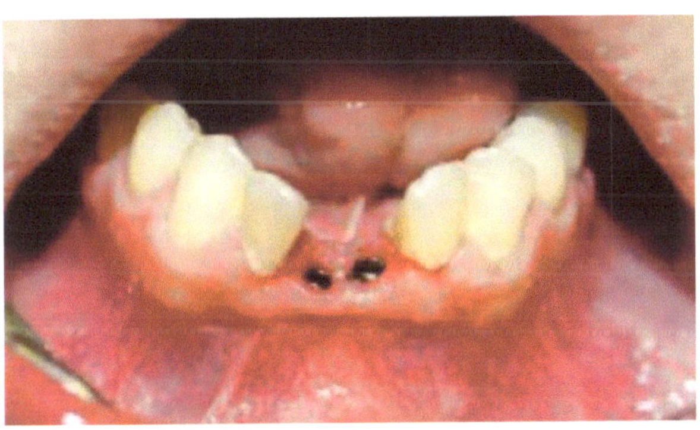

Figure 13.77. Reconstruction of the papilla complicated by retention of milk incisors. Status after 12 months.

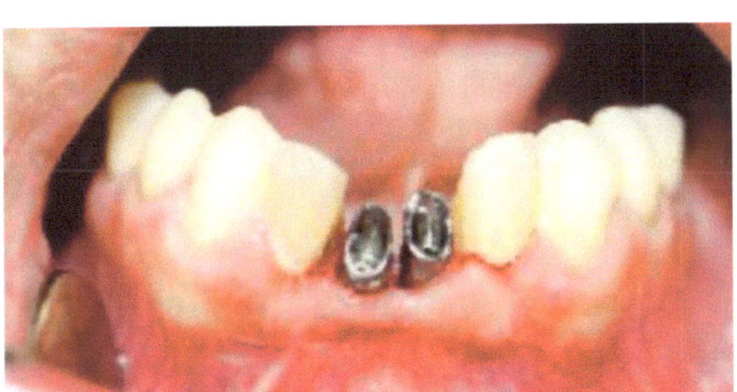

Figure 13.78. Mounted supports after healing formed interdental papilla.

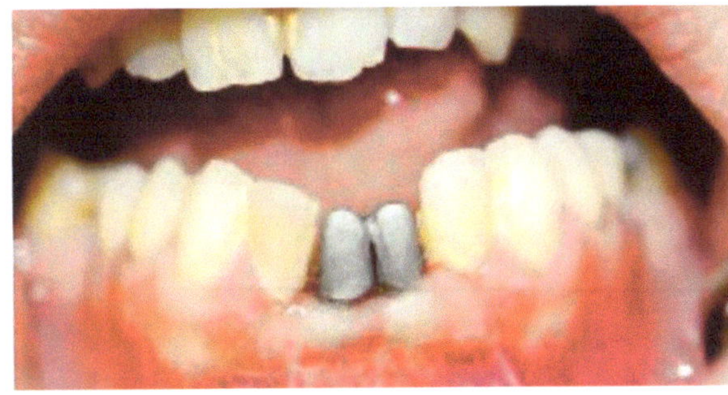

Figure 13.79. Test of metal construction. Need to pay attention to detail of the structure, the space that allows the regeneration of the papilla.

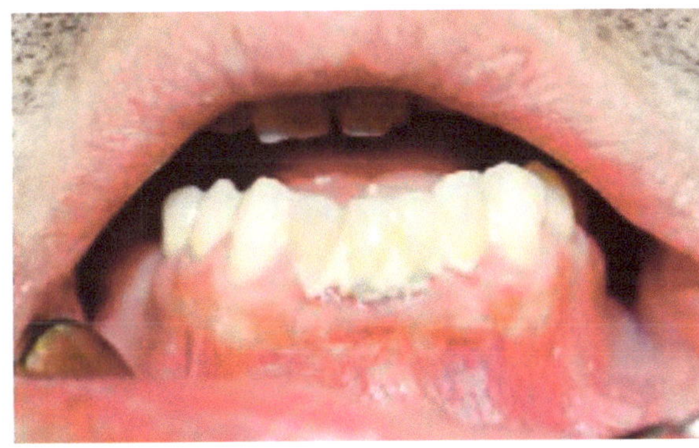

Figure 13.80. Control after 3 years. Poor oral hygiene and accumulation of plaque and calculus - risk factors depending on the patient..

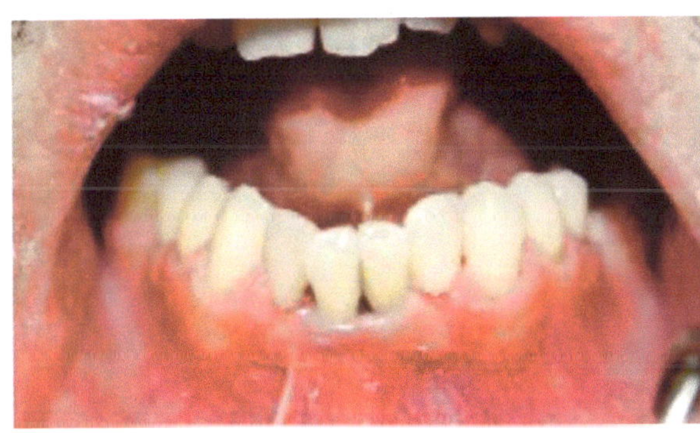

Figure 13.81. Condition after 5 years. Bad oral hygiene is not improved compared to the previous period (Figure 13.80) – abundantly plaque deposition, compromised interdental papilla.

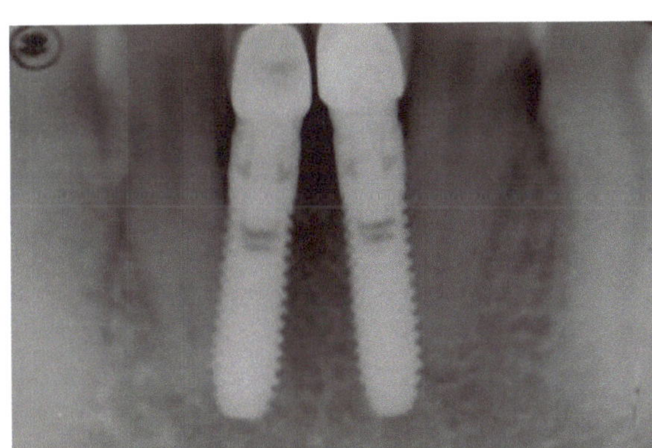

Figure 13.82. X-ray at the control examination after 10 years. The risk of using a standard diameter implant due to the proximity of the root of the

natural tooth. The use of implants smaller than 3 mm in diameter would reduce the risk of failure. The most important factor in eliminating the risk is the arrival of the patient for regular check-ups, which prolongs the time the implant stays in the bone.

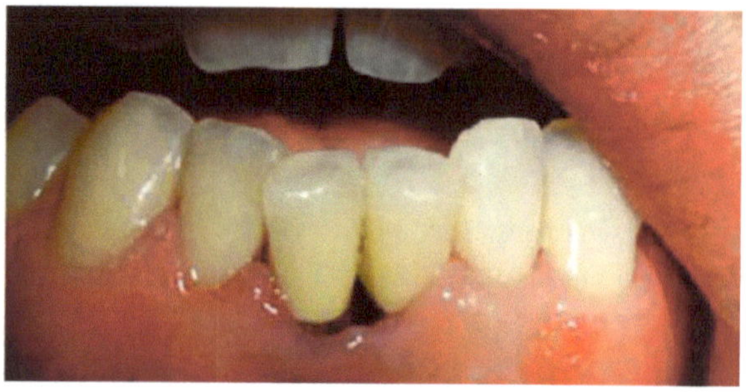

Figure 13.83. Endangered papilla due to plaque deposition - a consequence of irregular attendance at regular check-ups. Condition after 10 years.

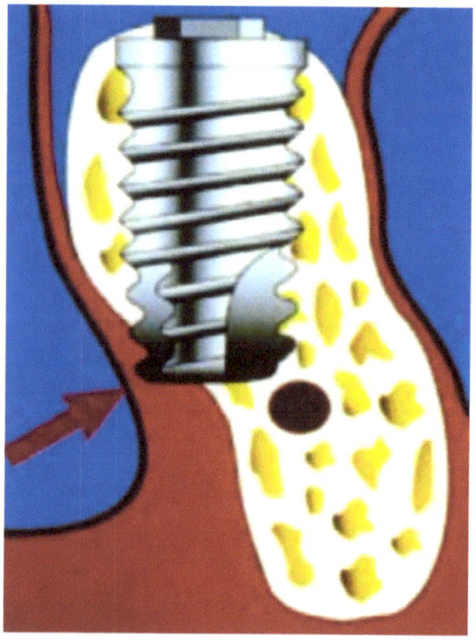

Figure 13.84. Schematic representation of the risk factor of perforation on the lingual side as a result of the installation of implants with standard diameters greater than 3.5 mm in case of insufficient deployable width of the horizontal bone.

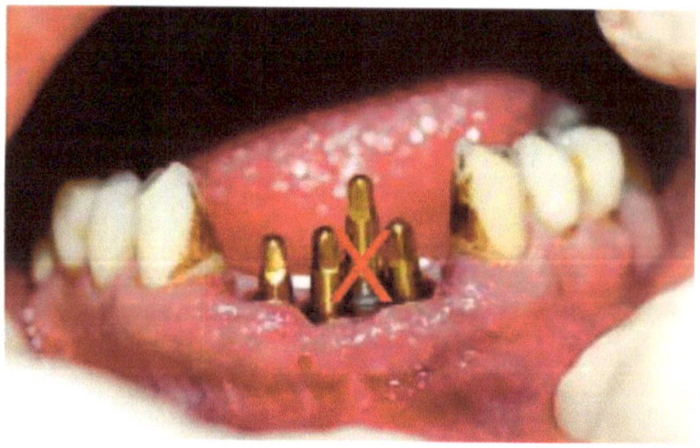

Figure 13.85. The number of lost teeth often cannot compensate for the same number of implants.

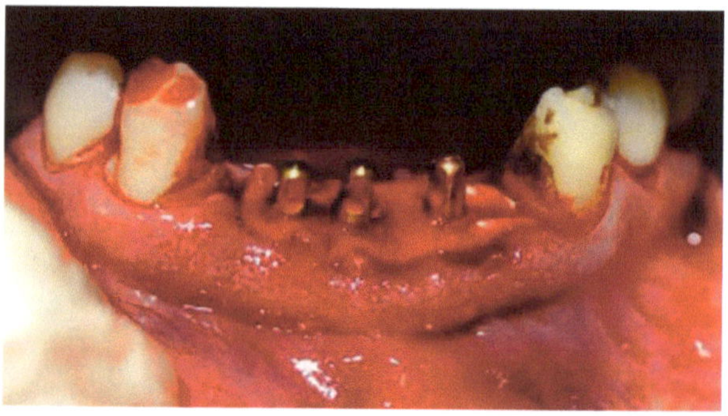

Figure 13.86. Compensation with smaller diameter implants (3 mm), maximum length (18 mm). Such cases can be successfully resolved with two implants of appropriate diameters and lengths.

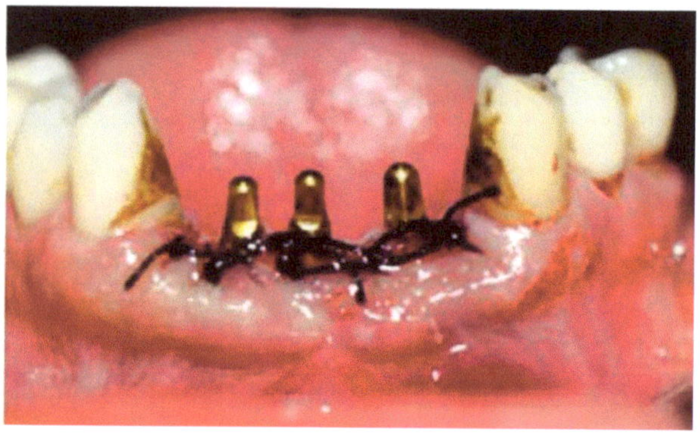

Figure 13.87. Immediate installation of the implant with immediate loading with a provisional bridge. The embedded implant with a diameter of 3 mm and a maximum length of 18 mm allowed by the vertical available bone.

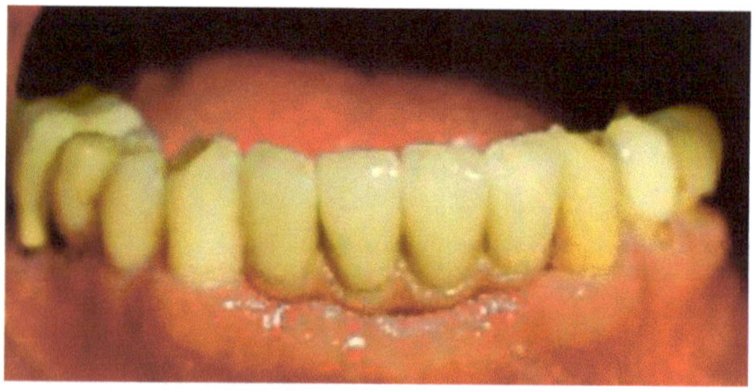

Figure 13.88. Aesthetic appearance after 6 years.

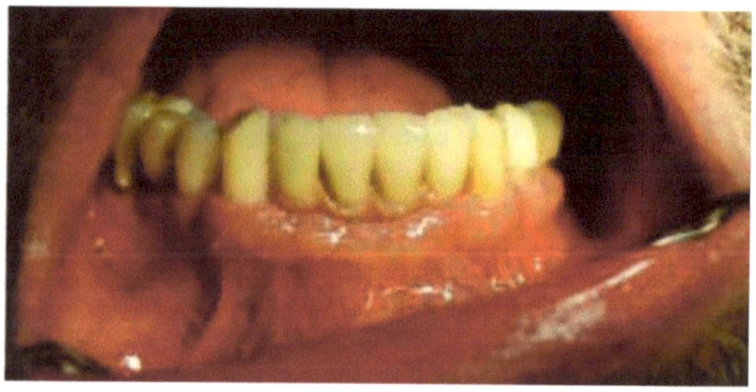

Figure 13.89. Control after 10 years. Good oral maintenance hygiene contributes to an unchanged state.

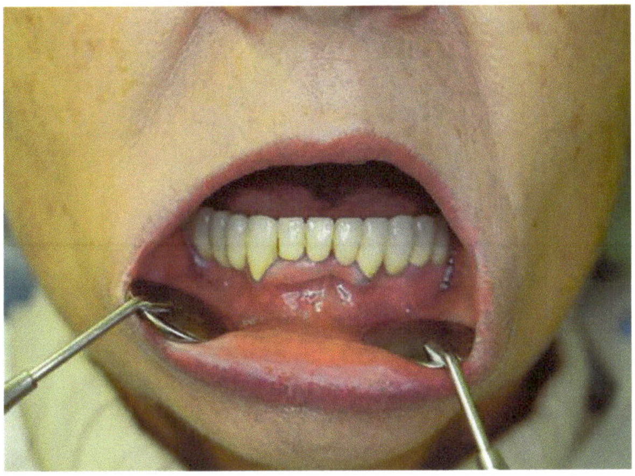

Figure 13.90. Concavity of the alveolar ridge in the frontal region of the mandible is a major bone risk for implant placement.

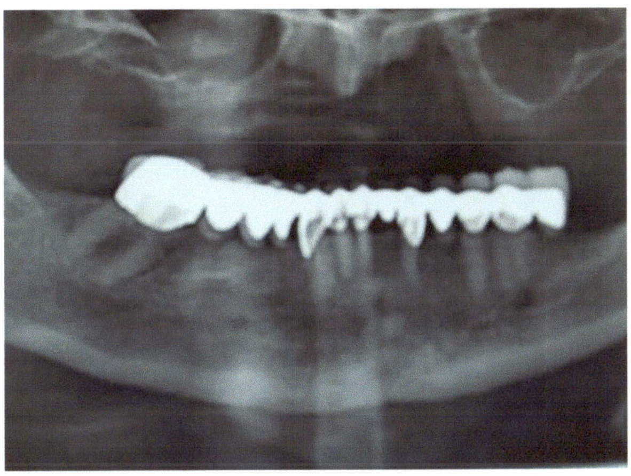

Figure 13.91. The size of the bone defect cannot be established on the orthopantomography.

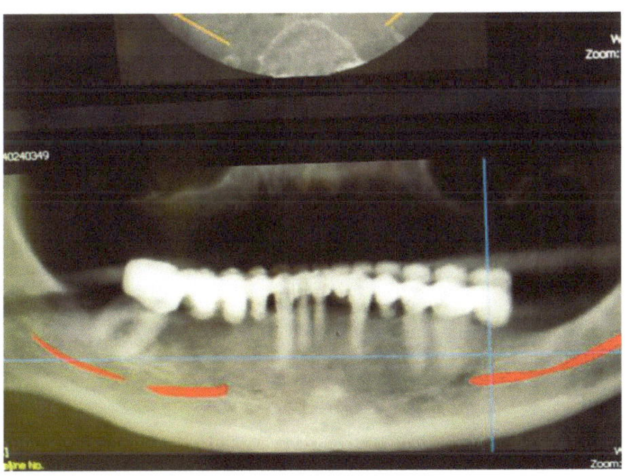

Figure 13.91a. The size of the bone defect cannot be ascertained with a 3D image either. Clear position of the mandibular canal and mental openings.

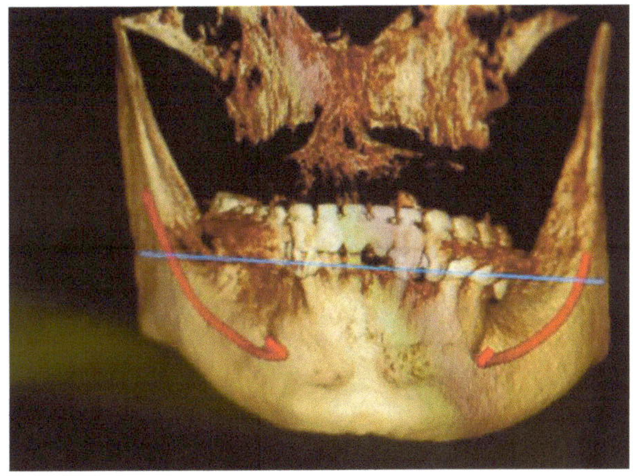

Figure 13.92. 3D imaging clearly shows anatomical structures, but not the true state of the bone defect.

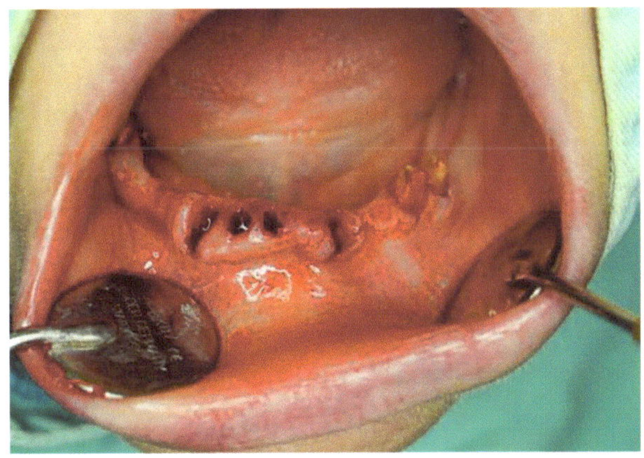

Figure 13.93. After removing the worn-out prosthetic work, the loose teeth were extracted.

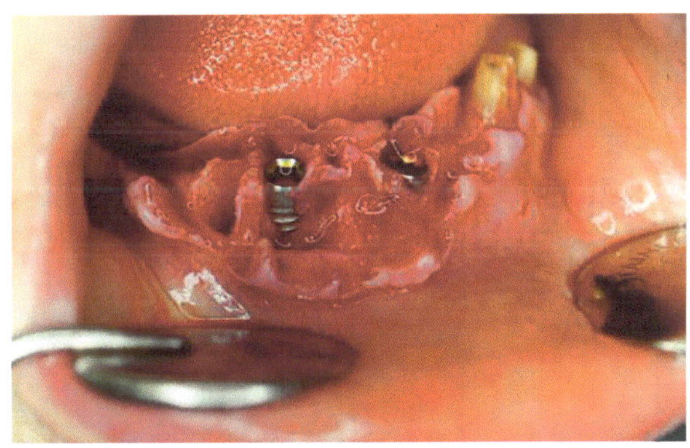

Figure 13.94. Presentation of the condition after lifting the flap - large bone defects are a risk factor of implant-prosthetic rehabilitation. The treatment plan is possible in two ways:

1. Augmentation of bone defects with a bone substitute by covering with a collagen resorbable membrane with a wait of at least 6 months. Provisional compensation - mobile acrylate prosthesis.
2. Immediate installation of the implant with immediate loading by provisional fixed prosthetic work in the composite. This procedure depends on the experience of the dentist.

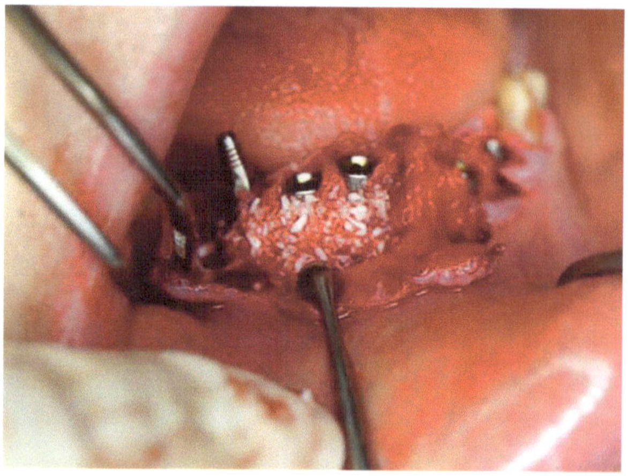

Figure 13.95. Healing and stability of soft tissues depends on the quality of bone support achieved by augmentation.

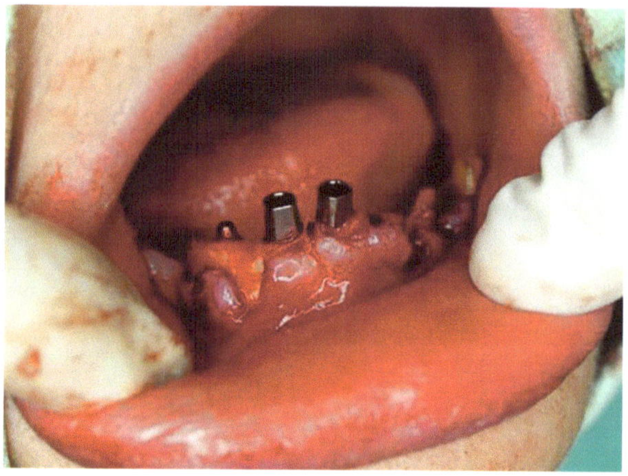

Figure 13.96. With such complex interventions, it is important to assess the predictability of implant-prosthetic rehabilitation success, where the therapist's experience is dominant. The final stage of immediate installation of implants and augmentation sewn with resorbable thread.

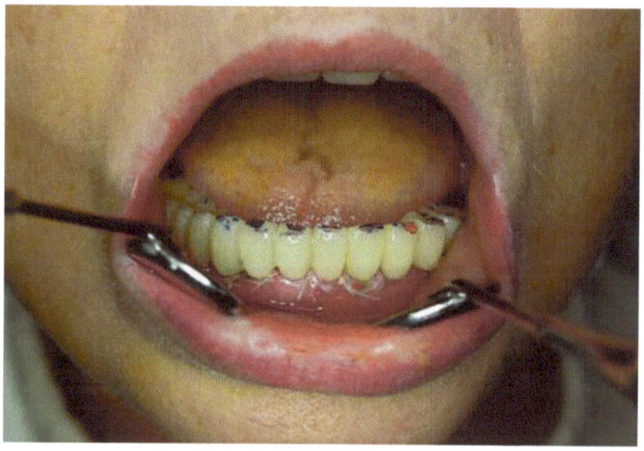

Figure 13.97. After the immediate installation of the implant and augmentation, a provisional fixed composite bridge was made. The use of resorbable thread allows not to tear the provisional bridge to remove the sutures.

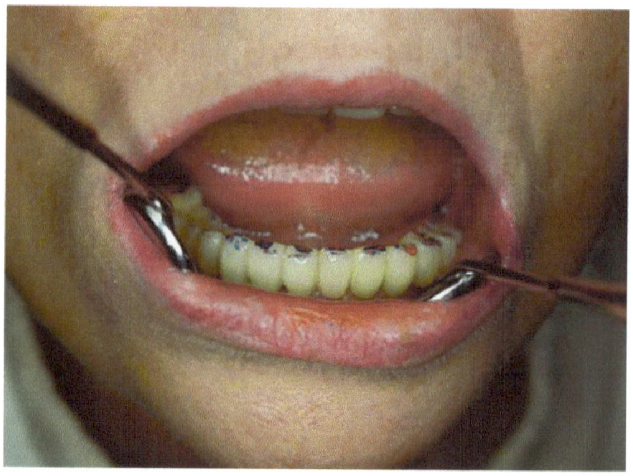

Figure 13.98. Establishing a balanced occlusion on a provisional fixed prosthetic work in composite is an extremely important stage in rehabilitation procedures. The characteristic of this composite material is its resistance to fracture, which enables a longer waiting period until the definitive prosthetic work is made, due to the healing of soft tissues and achieved good bone integration.

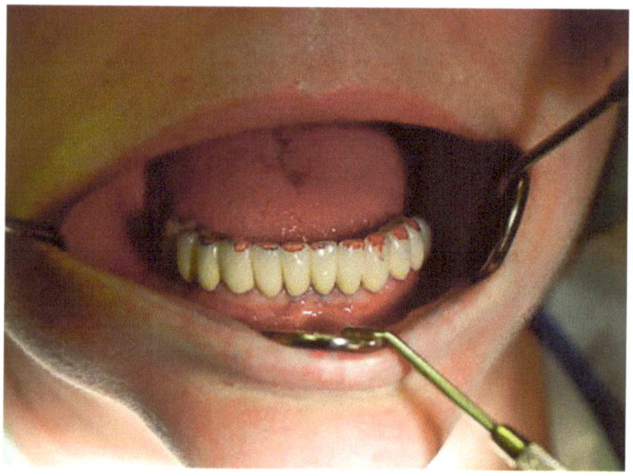

Figure 13.99. Appearance of definitive prosthetic work. Achieved balanced occlusion, removal of premature and too strong occlusal contacts are eliminated risk factors of implant-prosthetic rehabilitation. It is important that the conditions for maintaining oral hygiene are created by making prosthetic work.

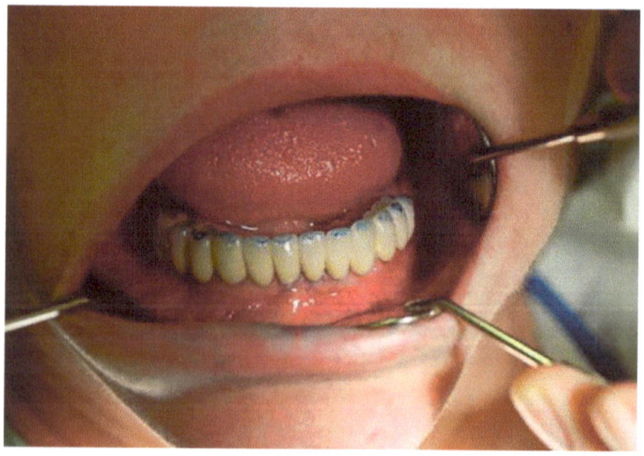

Figure 13.100. Definitive prosthetic work in metal-ceramics. Checking the established occlusion is an important factor in eliminating the risk. See Figures 13.93, 13.95 and 13.96.

Patient-specific risk factors

There are several risk factors that depend on the patient. Some of them have already been mentioned, when it comes to wearing mobile temporary compensations. And possible reasons for toothlessness (especially in the front segments of both jaws) should be revealed in the anamnesis. Otherwise, the main patient-dependent risk factors are:

- Quality of oral hygiene maintenance;
- Aesthetic requirements - realistically achievable or not;
- The presence of harmful habits - avid smokers.

The size of the mesiodistal space can also be a risk factor. If it concerns the frontal region of both jaws, especially in the upper jaw, it is primarily important for achieving aesthetic results (which also depends on other factors, primarily the laugh line). The required minimum or ideal mesiodistal space is shown in Figure 13.101. (a. the minimum interdental space required for implant placement, to fill the gap when the central incisor is missing; b. the minimum mesiodistal space to compensate for one tooth in the frontal region with a small diameter implant; c. the minimum mesiodistal spaces, to rehabilitate partial toothlessness in the lateral region with standard and larger diameter implants). Very often, in practice, one encounters cases that at first glance cause the therapist's concern and the impossibility of predicting the aesthetic demand. Earlier inadequate prosthetic rehabilitation can also make the implant procedure complicated and risky.

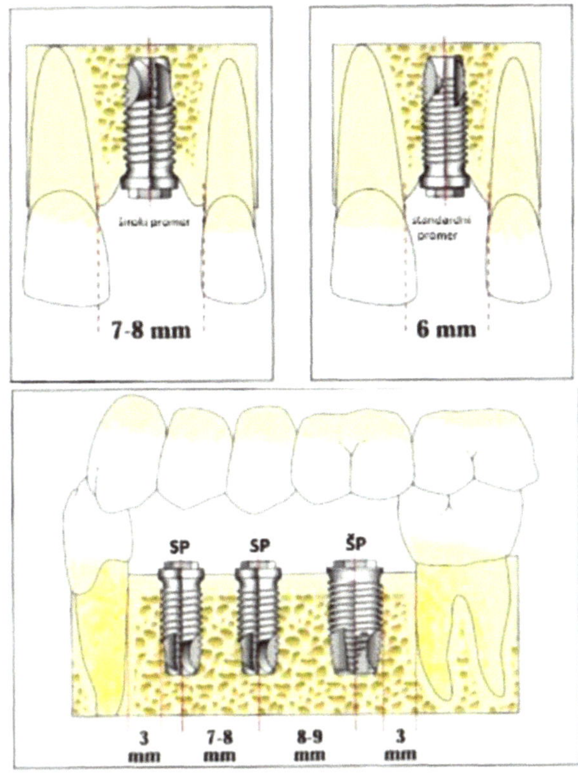

Figure 13.101. A minimum mesiodistal space of 7-8 mm is necessary for replacing one tooth with a standard diameter implant; and a minimum mesiodistal gap of 6 mm is required for a smaller diameter implant. The minimum clearances for standard and larger diameter implants in the lateral region are different.

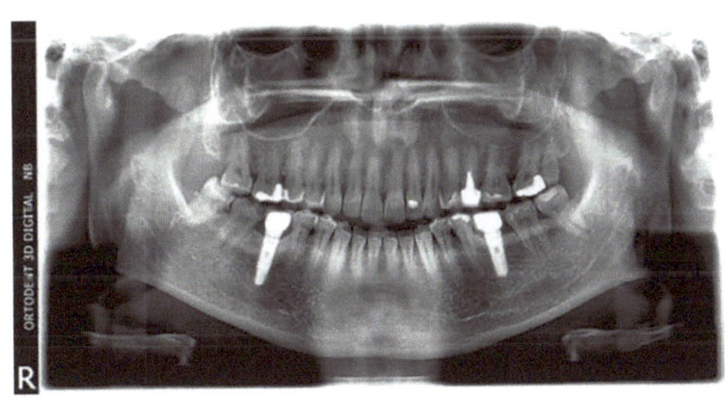

Figure 13.102. In the lateral regions, in place of the molars in both jaws, if the mesiodistal space and sufficient horizontal width of the available bone allows, implant the widest diameter implants, where the forces of action are the strongest. It is important to shape the cusps in accordance with gnathological principles.

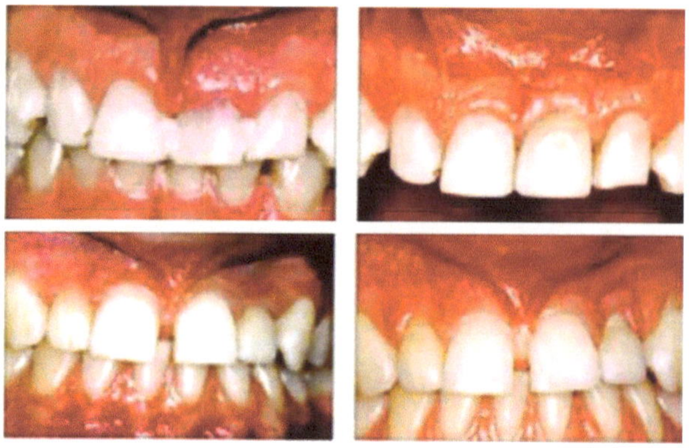

Figure 13.103. Presentation of the compensation of the upper left central incisor with the installation of implants and temporary prosthetic work. In such situations, special attention must be paid to the labial part of the bone lamella, which is thin, and very often it is so thin that a membrane and bone substitutes must be used during implant installation. b) The clinical result can be seen after 4 years, where very good bone integration was achieved. c) View of the compensated right lateral incisor (#12) with an implant in an 18-year-old patient. Previously, the tooth was unsuccessfully restored with composites. On the very thin gingiva, you can see trauma from excessive brushing with a brush when washing. d) An implant was installed at the site of the lateral left incisor, on which a temporary crown was placed. A definitive metal-ceramic crown was placed on the right lateral incisor. In cases where the contacts with the antagonists are quite strong, it is better to leave that contact in the metal.

In cases where the tooth is in supraocclusion ("floated out"), patients most often request the shortening of that tooth. But the final outcome is tooth extraction and implant placement. In such cases, there is a significant portion of healthy and solid apical bone, and the author's experience suggests that immediate loading is one of the preferred solutions. In order to achieve good primary stability, the apical part of the bone should be at least 5-6 mm. The benefit for immediate loading depends on the depth of the alveolus after tooth extraction in the terminal phase of periodontitis. That part of the alveolus is in the shape of a "funnel" and should not be deeper than 3-4 mm. If that part of the alveolus is deeper and wider, a significant part of the implant remains outside the bone and in the alveolar "funnel", and is not in intimate contact with the walls of the alveolar bone, it is recommended to fill that space with some bone substitute.

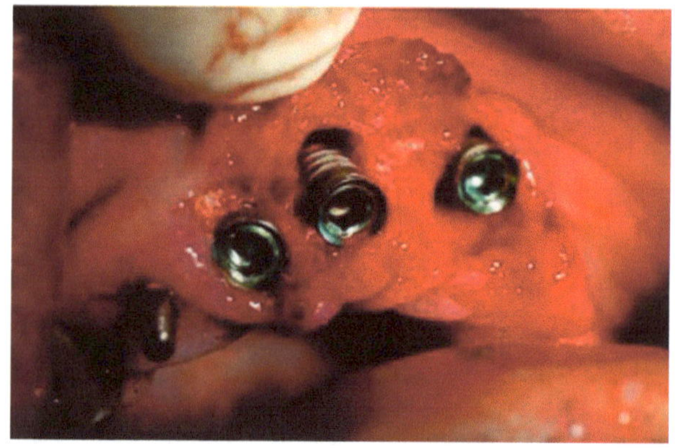

Figure 13.104. After tooth extraction in the frontal region of the posterior jaw, where the thickness of the lamellar bone is below 2 mm, the implant should be positioned more palatally, and the space between the surfaces of the lamellar bone and the implant should be augmented with bone substitutes to avoid the risk factors of metal screening due to resorption of the lamellar bone. Weakening of bone support would cause gingival recession. Shaped collagen resorbable membrane for placement. If there is a possibility, the procedure can be performed using the PRF method.

In any case, it is better to use a wider implant. However, some authors believe that it is better to leave the coagulum to fill the interstices in order to regenerate the bone tissue. In the case of a decision to replace the immediate load with a wait for healing (2-3 months or more), one must think about the need for the patient to wear temporary compensations - mobile prostheses during that time, which endangers the formation of soft tissues and favors greater atrophy of the surrounding alveolar bones. For example, in a patient who has lost a central and lateral incisor, the situation due to untimely treatment becomes more complicated due to the reduction of the mesiodistal space, and the problem is increased by the loss of the papilla, which cannot be regenerated (Fig. 13.81). The advantage of immediate loading is multiple: putting the bone into function, the formation of new bone is faster and stronger, which accelerates the process of osseointegration. Immediate loading with precise fixed prosthetic work also helps to preserve the interdental papilla. The situation becomes much more complicated if implant-prosthetic rehabilitation is delayed. For example, in a patient who has lost a central and lateral incisor, the situation due to untimely treatment becomes more complicated due to the reduced mesio-distal space, and the problem is magnified by the loss of the papilla, which cannot be regenerated.

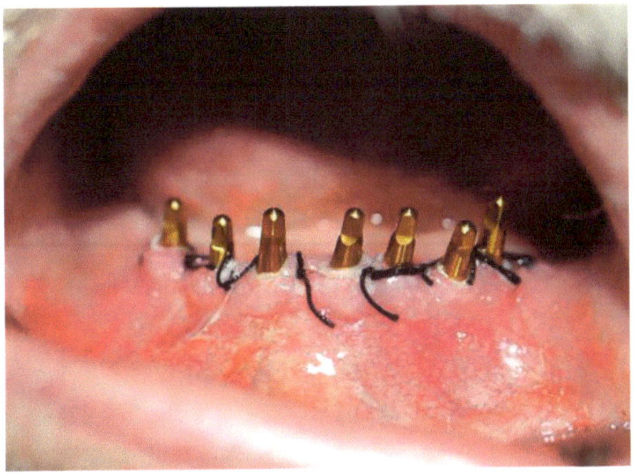

Figure 13.105. Immediately installed one-piece implants (3 mm). The experience of the author of the book shows that the occurrence of peri-implantitis with one-piece implants is much less frequent (under the condition of maintaining good oral hygiene and precise prosthetic work) than with two-piece implants. A possible reason is the absence of a microcrack (the space between the endosseous part of the implant and the support (abutment), which prevents the deposition of plaque, calculus and bacterial content.

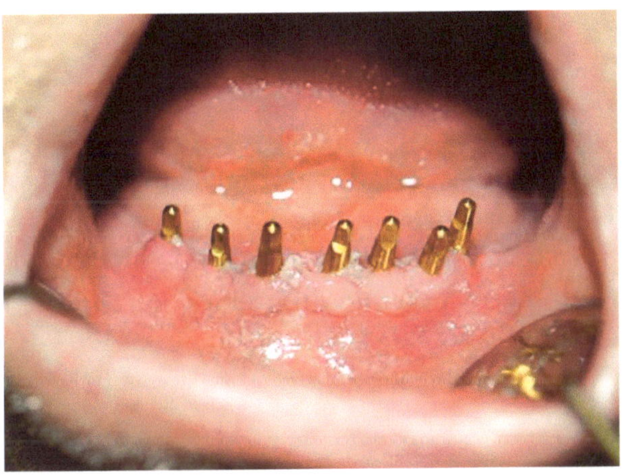

Figure 13.106. Appearance of healed soft tissues after 10 days. The advantage of this one-piece implant system is (3 mm), which is a support for prosthetic work made of a softer material than titanium, and it is possible to adjust the parallelism by grinding without transferring thermal stimuli to the endosseous part of the implant and the surrounding tissues. Good primary fixation allows immediate loading with a fixed temporary acrylate or composite bridges.

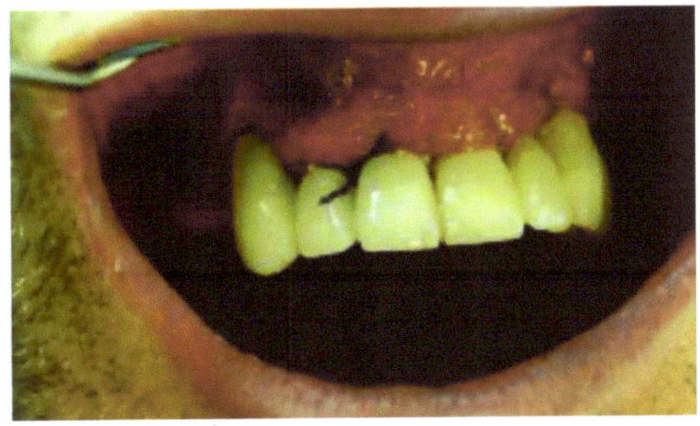

Figure 13.107. A typical example of a patient with risk factors: unfavorable anatomical structures, poor oral hygiene of a heavy smoker. Unfavorable for cooperation. The persuasion that the two remaining teeth should be extracted and replaced with implants failed. He was satisfied with the provisional fixed bridge. He presented after three years with a broken provisional acrylic bridge. Two loose teeth were extracted and replaced with implants (pictures 13.108 and 13.113).

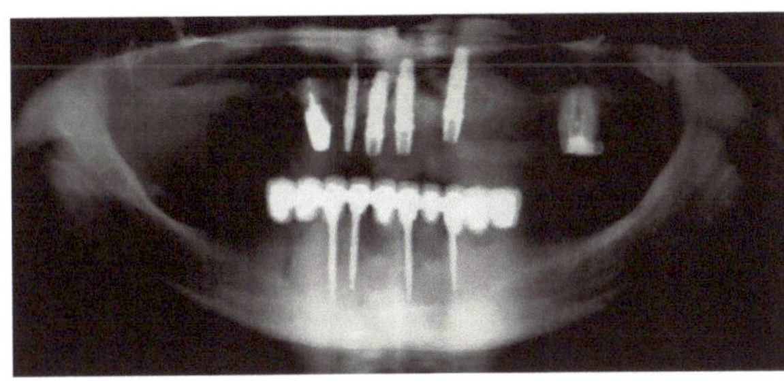

Figure 13.108. Extreme disadvantage of anatomical structures: width razor tip ridge 1 mm, and plateau 1.2 mm; The favorable length enabled the installation of implants with a narrow diameter of a maximum length of 18 mm. Augmentation with bone substitutes was performed. Risk presented to the patient with an emphasis on maintaining oral hygiene and reducing smoking.

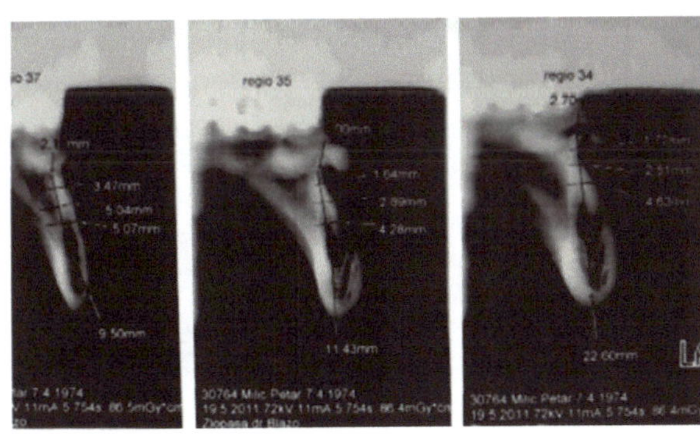

Figure 13.109. A detailed analysis of the parameters determined the therapy plan for the presented patient. The parameters of the horizontal expanded bone precluded the insertion of satisfactory implants with larger diameters. The decision for the procedure was made based on the patient's statement that he will not wear a mobile acrylate prosthesis at any cost.

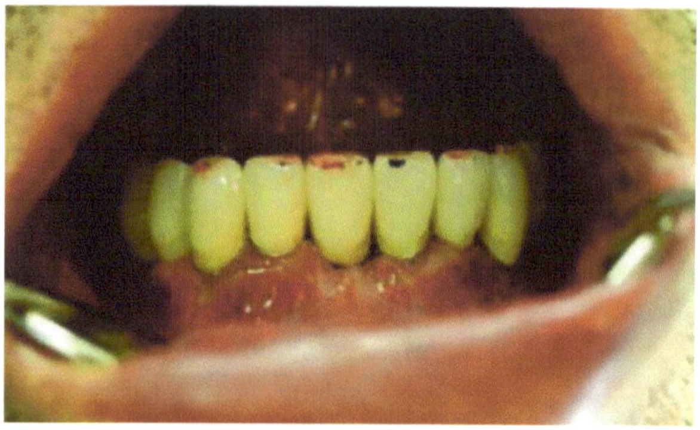

Figure 13.110. Precise temporary restoration of immediately loaded implants of small diameter. Occlusal balance is the most important phase for the success of the therapy. All risk factors are presented to the patient.

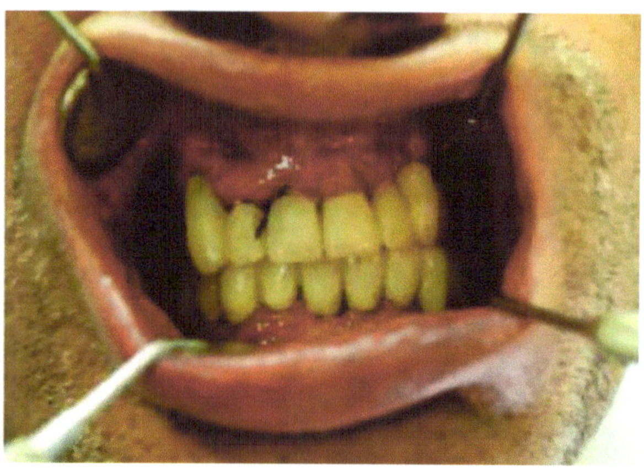

Figure 13.111. Temporary condition after implant installation, temporary fixed prosthetic works in composite. The patient is satisfied that he is free from mobile total acrylate prostheses that he could not tolerate. Extreme urge to vomit and when taking impressions.

In the case of loss of front teeth due to trauma, if the lost tooth is not replaced with an implant immediately after the trauma, the consequences are the same as in the previously described case: destroyed papilla and accelerated material bone loss.

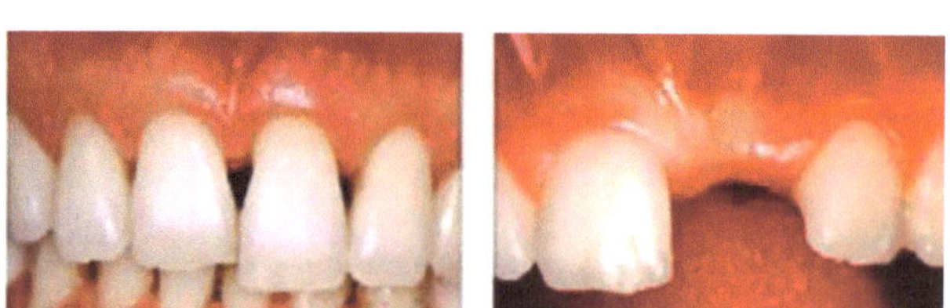

Figure 13.112. The emerging tooth was shortened several times, finally extracted. Replacement with acrylate flipper denture accelerated bone resorption. Augmentation is also indicated, with a long wait. By immediate implantation into a fresh alveolus and using periapical bone for good primary fixation, these problems would be eliminated. However, the application of the flipper denture made the treatment procedure extremely complex!

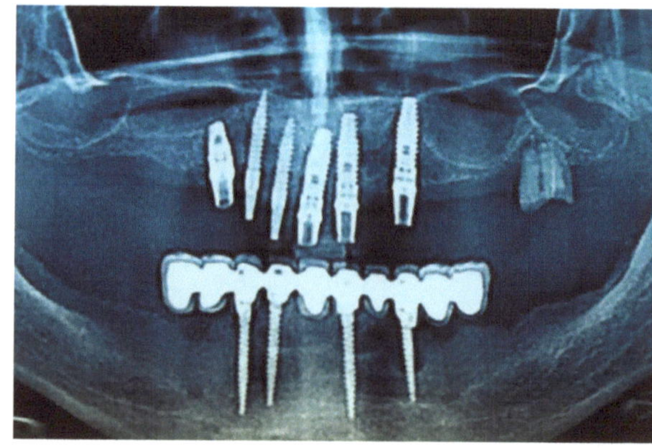

Figure 13.113. Patient with extreme anatomical disadvantages (compare with Figures 13.95-13.100) heavy smoker with extremely poor oral hygiene. The patient did not allow tooth 13 to be extracted (see Figure 13.108). The patient's request was fulfilled, the implants were placed primarily loaded with a provisional acrylate bridge. The patient presented only after 6 years, with broken acrylate temporary bridges, which he used well until then. Residual roots were extracted, which the patient did not allow in the first procedure, and two implants were inserted. The patient did not comply with the given instructions: maintaining oral hygiene and reducing smoking. Condition of narrow-diameter implants in the lower jaw after 6 years with the appearance of peri-implantitis in region 33 (indicated by the red arrow). The causes of peri-implantitis in this patient are: poor oral hygiene, heavy smoking and biomechanical causes. The life of the implant was extended by augmentation (it has already been 7 years of using fixed prosthetic work). A typical example of a patient who creates the risks of implant-prosthetic rehabilitation, despite his unrealistic demands being met.

In such cases, when the central incisors are lost due to trauma, the clinical picture is very favorable for implant placement if it is done immediately after tooth loss.

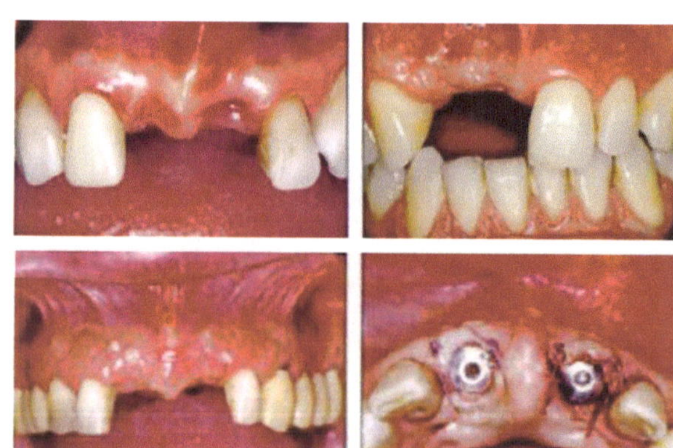

Figure 13.114. Figure a. shows loss of central incisors; b. disturbed interdental space due to untimely therapy Images c. and d. a similar case of lost central incisors that were compensated by immediate implantation of standard diameters. The diastema left behind was caused by untimely removal of a strong frenulum, which fulfilled the patient's aesthetic

request. It is very important to save the papilla during surgery. Risk avoidance should be considered starting from the preliminary examination, and good planning allows predictability of success.

Risk factors caused by poor planning

The next case shows taking a risk with wrong planning, with the consequences of the failure of the entire treatment and discomfort for the patient.

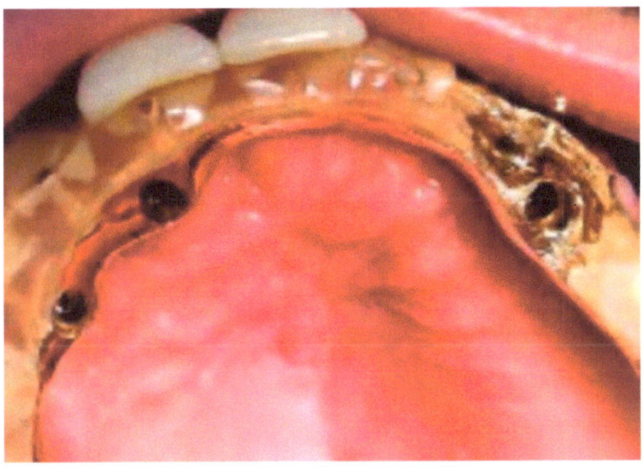

Figure 13.115. When planning the implant-prosthetic restoration, the biomechanical requirements were not taken into account. Sufficient availability of the bone in which the implant is placed is only one of the parameters for the final success of the entire procedure.

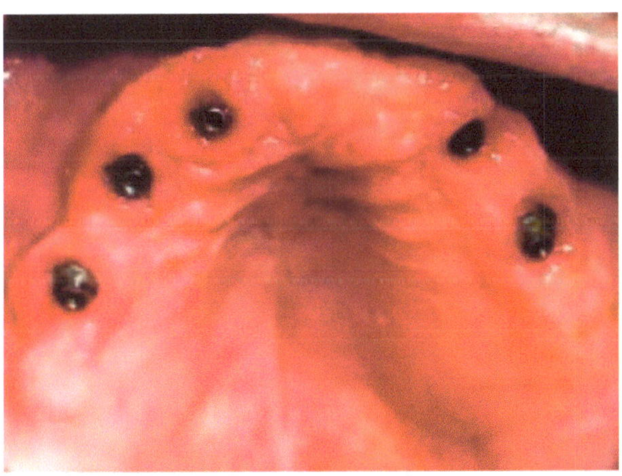

Figure 13.116. Often, at first glance, the sufficient width of the ridge in the upper jaw can be misleading during planning due to the poor quality of the bone (D4), which is why the whole project can be unsuccessful. The patient was treated in Stockholm (Sweden).

Despite the fact that the implant-prosthetic rehabilitation was done abroad and with the highest quality implants (Brenemark), complications followed. The cause of the failure was already in the preliminary examination. A thick layer of mobile mucosal tissue and poor planning (number and placement of implants and prosthetic solution) were the reasons for the failure. The entire conception was not in accordance with the biomechanical requirements. The combined fixed-mobile structure dislocated the remaining implants to a considerable extent with symptoms of peri-implantitis and bone defects. There was inflammation of the soft tissues around the implant, accompanied by pain, so the patient could not use the poor prosthetic work. Such a risk should not have been taken for the following reasons: too thick keratinized and mobile mucosal tissue, unfavorable interjaw relationships and poor occlusion caused excessive forces, primarily horizontal forces on the implants. These risk factors jeopardized the achieved osseous integration. Due to the aforementioned risk factors, there were frequent fractures of the movable part of the prosthesis, which also had consequences on the implants. Planning and thinking in the specific case presented should have been directed in a different direction. Practical experience confirms that the restoration of such cases should not be done with a telescope crown for biomechanical reasons.

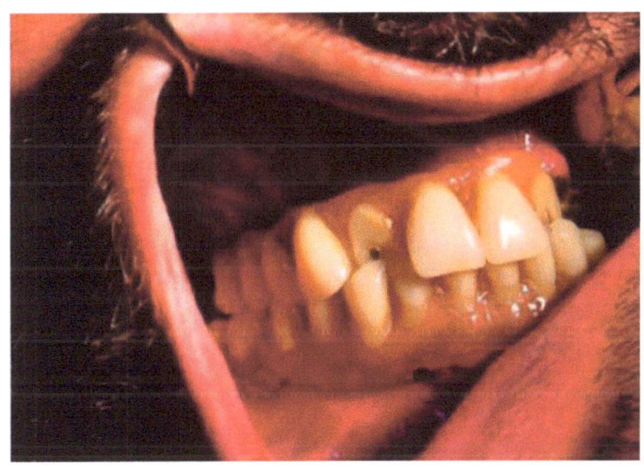

Figure 13.117. In the presented case, interjaw relationships, soft tissue condition, poor bone quality, and poor occlusion were a major risk for implant placement, which resulted in failure.

Next case (Fig. 13.118). First of all, the shape of the arc of the alveolar ridge catches the eye. It can be immediately assumed that the fulfillment of aesthetic requirements will be unpredictable. Fulfilling the patient's wish that the solution is based exclusively on fixed work, a detailed analysis of the situation must be carried out beforehand. Due to the elevation of the sinus floor (two implants on the left and one on the right), a one-year wait was necessary. The decision to fulfill the patient's request with a fixed compensation was made based on the smile line and the shape of the lip that covers the edge of the alveolar ridge, which is therefore not visible.

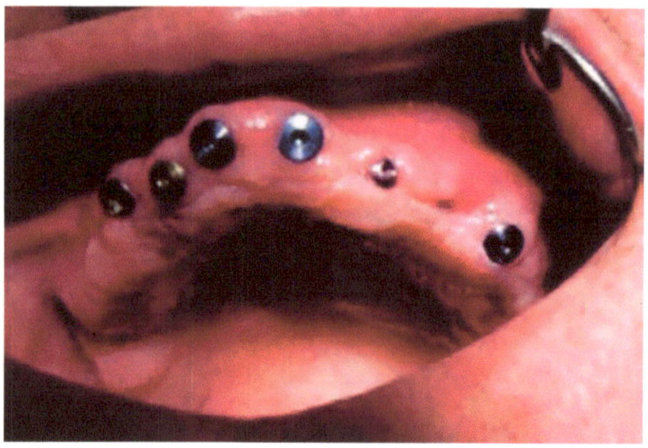

Figure 13.118. Built-in Nobel-Replace implants. Uncritical approach, low sinus floor, failed installation of 2 implants in the lateral region on the left side - low sinus floor, make implant-prosthetic rehabilitation risky. The implantology procedure was performed in another institution. The patient requested the author of the book to perform prosthetic reconstruction, which was not accepted for several reasons. Do not get involved in inheriting other people's failures and make subsequent failures.

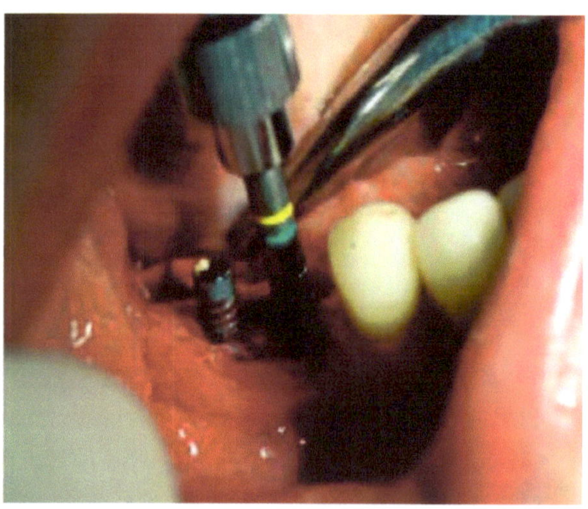

Figure 13.119. When there is enough available bone in the lateral region, it is best to install an implant with a wider diameter because the forces in that area are the strongest during mastication.

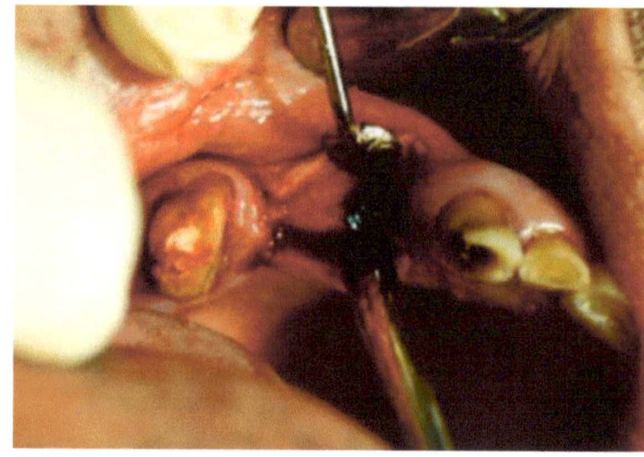

Figure 13.120. If there is sufficient bone available in the lateral region, it is best to place an implant with a wider diameter because the forces in that area during mastication are the strongest.

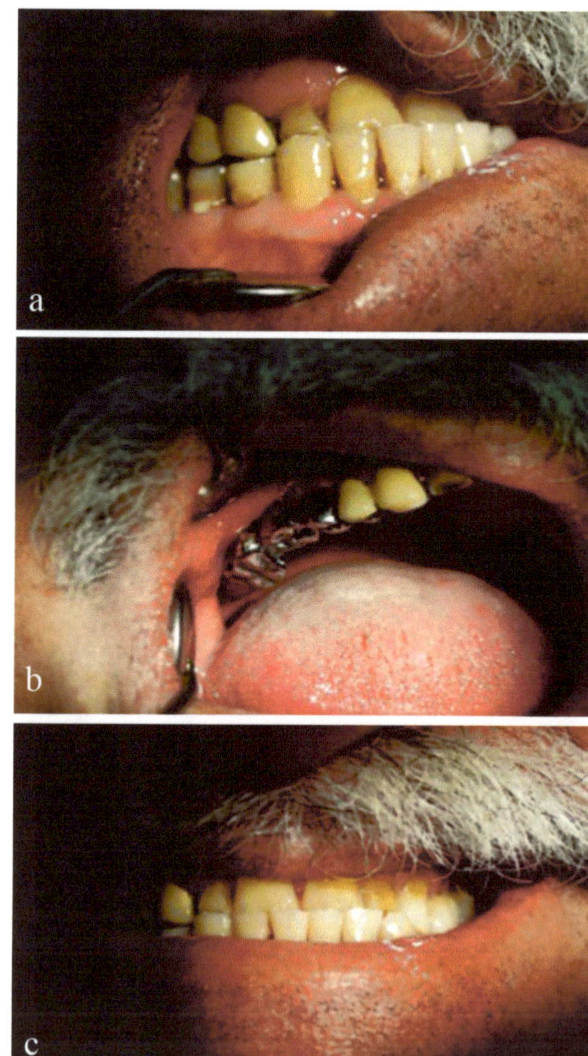

Figure 13.121 (a,b,c) In the patient shown, aesthetic factors were not important, but the establishment of chewing function, which was also the express request of the patient.

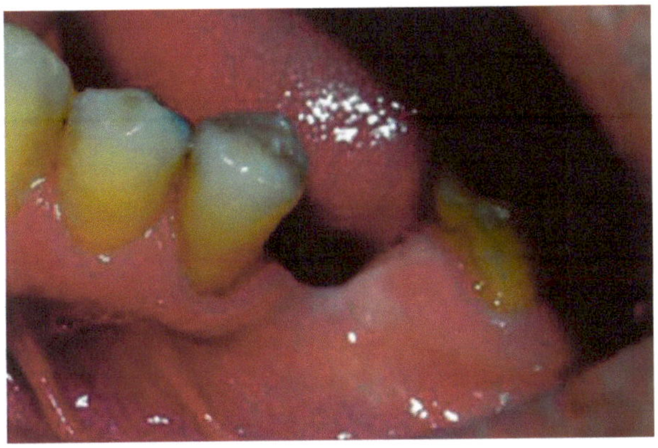

Figure 13.122. In places where there is an excessive mesiodistal space and uneven distribution of the amount of alveolar bone, it is often not possible to fill that space with one implant of a wider diameter. A good functional result can be obtained by installing two implants of standard or narrow diameter (3mm).

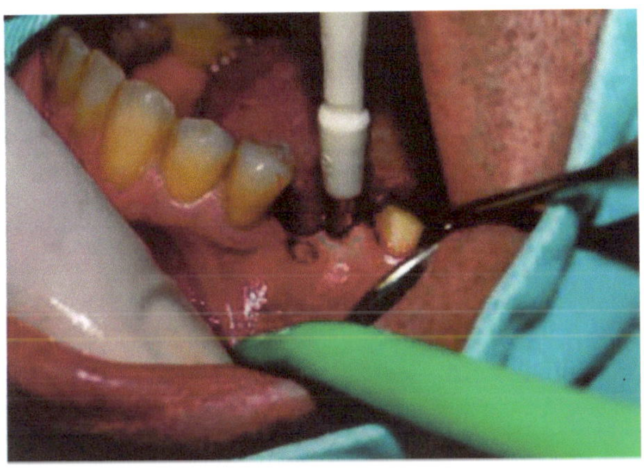

Figure 13.123. Marking the position of the implant - installation using the "Flapless" technique.

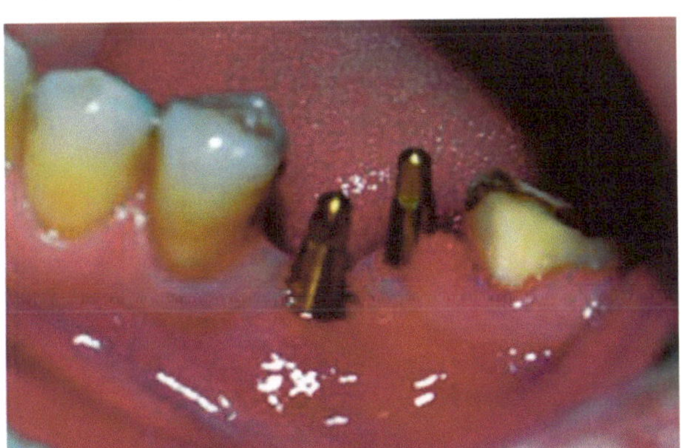

Figure 13.124. Space filling with two 3.2 mm diameter implants. By avoiding flap elevation, soft tissue healing around the implant is faster and of better quality. The condition immediately after implant placement.

Visible principles of implant crown modeling

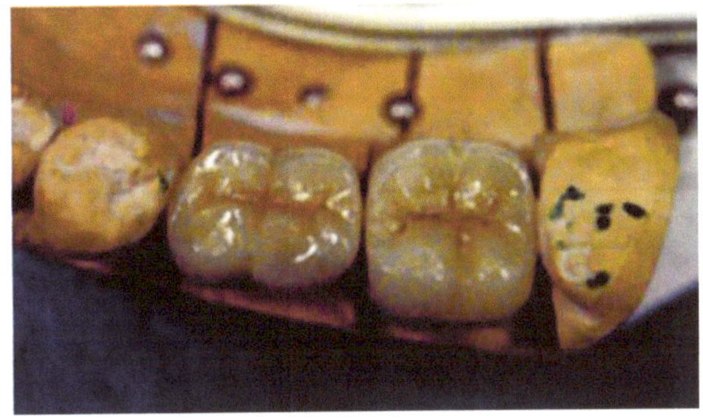

Figure 13.125. Form a definitive crown with an intermediate implant space to allow access to interdental brushes for cleaning. Occlusal appearance of the crown, modeling the morphology of the crowns in accordance with gnathological principles during lateral movements of the lower jaw, on the first molar (#36), which is anchored to two crown implants on the second molar (#37).

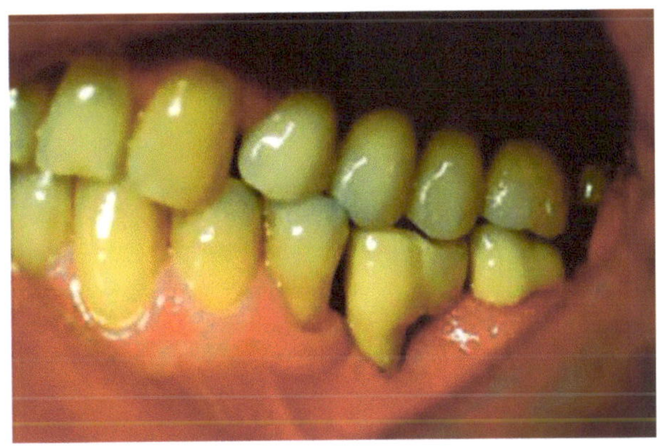

Figure 13.126. Definitive prosthetic work on the first molar (#36) with an inter-implant space accessible for interdental cleaning brushes.

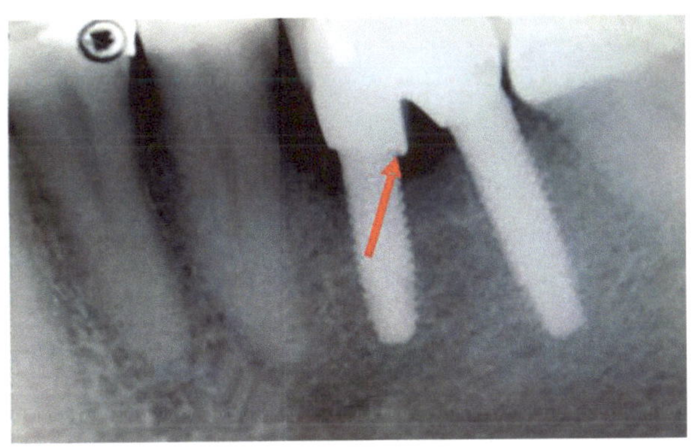

Figure 13.127. Control shot after 5 years. Preserved marginal bone and free inter-implant space for cleaning. Laboratory error: the width of the crown (red arrow) in the neck of the implant caused marginal bone resorption, which was absent on the second implant (yellow arrow). Risk factors with more serious consequences can be secreted in the dental laboratory.

Peri-implantitis risk factor for implant loss

The loss of an implant as a result of a disease of the peri-implant tissue affected by a pathological process is, as a rule, an unpredictable risk. The soft tissue surrounding the transmucosal part of the implant is called the peri-implant mucosa. The dimensions and structure of this tissue are similar to the gingiva of natural teeth. Taking the concept of biological width as the thickness of the soft tissues attached to natural teeth and implants, there are fundamental differences between these two tissues. The root of the tooth is covered with cement that extends from the enamel to the tip of the root, and the collagen fibers that join at the border of hard and soft tissues spread vertically along the length of the root (Fig. 13.128).

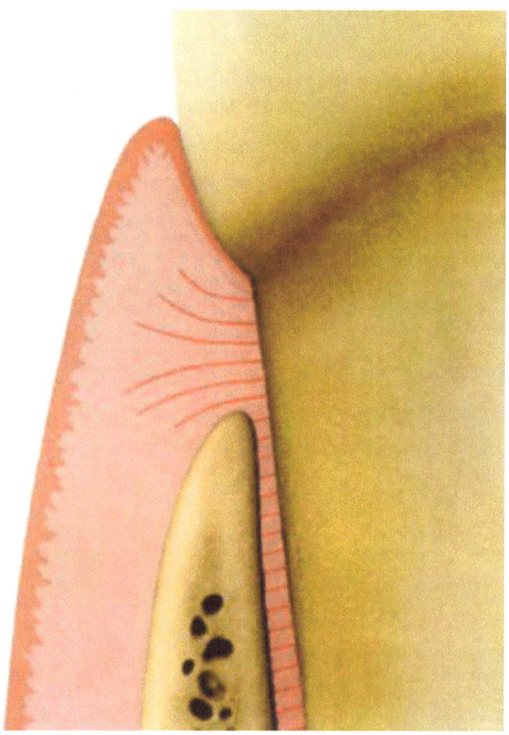

Figure 13.128. Schematic representation of soft tissues and tooth roots.

The periodontium is an integral part of the periodontium, which is located between the root of the tooth and the alveolar bone. Alveolar bone supports the teeth during various functional loads. Bone metabolism takes place in such a way that the bone receives the necessary physiological stimulation through the teeth and periodontium. Pedriodontal fibers transmit the forces that act on the tooth, they are also transmitted to the wall of the alveolar cup, which are then transmitted to the bone beds, which support the alveolus. The tissue that fills the periodontal space consists of many different collagen fibers The tissue that fills the periodontal space consists of numerous collagen fibers, various cells, blood and lymphatic vessels, nerves and nerve endings and basic extracellular substance. The basic role of the periodontium is the attachment of the tooth to the alveolar bone and the support of the tooth in response to various functional events. The periodontium cushions and neutralizes the action of forces during mastication. In the cushioning of masticatory pressure, in addition to collagen fibers, other mechanisms are also involved: vascular, resilience mechanism, hydrodynamic mechanism, and the shape of the alveolus also plays a role in cushioning. The implant does not have all these components (Fig. 13.129). First, the implant has no cement. For this reason, collagen fibers cannot be attached to the implant surface either biologically or mechanically which is the case with natural teeth. In the peri-implant tissues, collagen fibers are distributed in different directions, and in the lateral parts, in relation to the surface of the implant, collagen fibers are organized parallel along the axis of the implant (Fig. 13.129compare with figure 13.128). In addition, the biological attachment formed by the border epithelium and connective tissue of the peri-implant mucosa provides an effective barrier that protects the surrounding milieu of the implant from the contents of the oral environment.

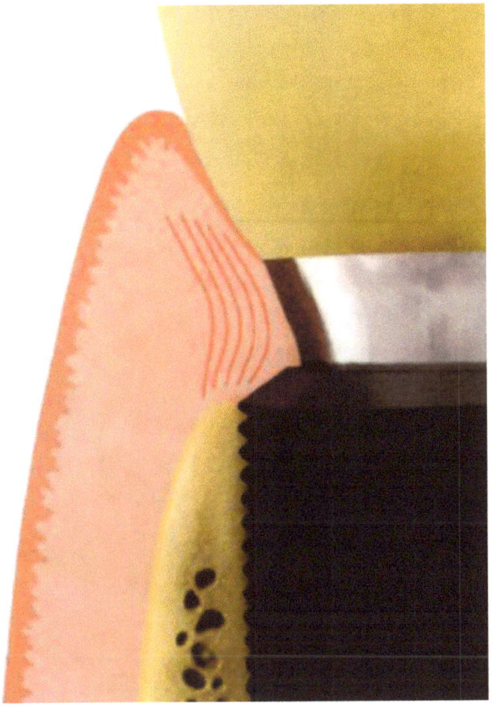

Figure 13.129. Schematic representation of implants and peri-implant tissues.

Implant placement causes damage to soft and hard tissues, which is a temporary and short-term disintegration process. If the procedure is performed with minimal trauma, conditions are created for the process of healing and integration of soft and hard tissues to be fast and complete. The tissue reaction in the healing process at the site of the implant recipient begins with the formation of a coagulum, and within a few days vascular structures and inflammatory cells infiltrate the coagulum, forming early granulation tissue. The healing process continues with the replacement of early granulation tissue with organized connective tissue, ultimately resulting in osseous integration. Through the healing process of the mucosa around the implant, a barrier epithelium is formed, which adheres to the neck of the implant and prevents the penetration of contents from the oral cavity into the peri-implant space. Apical to the formed epithelium, the connective tissue integrates with the titanium surface of the implant, preventing further migration of the epithelium. Barrier epithelium and connective tissue with the implant establish a specific biological width of the peri-implant mucosa. The integration of hard and soft tissues with the implant is a dynamic physiological process that lasts several weeks.

If only the mucosa around the implant is affected by the inflammation, then this process is defined as peri-implant mucositis. It is a reversible inflammatory process that affects only the mucosa, and the therapy is simple and successful. If the inflammatory pathological process also affects the alveolar bone around the implant, then the disease is defined as peri-implantitis. At the beginning, the pathological process begins around the neck of the implant, and most often during osseointegration. If the causes of the pathological process are not noticed and not removed in time, the processes of osseointegration will be stifled, and the implants, which were primarily stable, will become mobile. A detailed examination of the peri-implant tissue is an extremely important procedure for determining therapy if signs of inflammation are observed. Clinical symptoms of peri-implantitis are manifested by signs of acute or chronic inflammation of the peri-implant mucosa. The color of the mucosa is more intensely red or paler than normal, depending on the type of inflammation; the symptoms of inflammation of the exudative type are most often manifested. In this stage of inflammation, alveolar bone resorption does not occur, unless bone resorption has already occurred in the first phase of osseointegration. The expected bone loss at this stage of the inflammatory process depends on the type of implant. With threaded implants, the loss is up to the first notch, and with cylindrical implants, the expected bone loss corresponds to the bone level at the junction of the polished and rough parts of the implant body. In case of peri-implant mucositis, the rule is that treatment does not require systemic administration of antibiotics. If for some reason there are indications of progression of the pathological process, prescribe tetracyclines and metronidazole tablets first, or amoxicillin with the addition of clavulanic acid, augmentin, one tablet every 12 hours. If the prescribed therapy does not calm down the inflammation, due to edema and inflammatory infiltrate, the peri-implant mucosa is enlarged, thereby deepening the peri-implant sulcus. The loss of alveolar bone increases the migration of the attachment epithelium in the apical direction, forming a peri-implant pocket causing alveolar bone destruction. It manifests as infrabony defect around the implant. Horizontal loss of alveolar bone can occur extremely rarely. The most common form of bone loss is characterized by a symmetrical circular type of bone resorption around the implant. If the resorption affects the peri-implant bone in the first two coronary thirds - this is a bad prognosis for successful therapy and the implant should be removed. In order to prevent the occurrence of pathological changes in the peri-implant tissue, periodic mandatory controls of patients with implanted implants are extremely important in order to apply adequate therapy.

Methods of examination of peri-implant tissue are very similar to methods of examination of periodontal tissue (Figures 13.130 and 13.131). The examination of the peri-implant tissue starts with examining the depth of the pocket with a periodontal probe, in the same way as when probing the periodontium. (In the literature, the English term PPD-probing pocket depth is used). The depth of the pocket around the implant can vary, and, for this reason, bleeding is the primary diagnosis, and the depth of the pocket is secondary. But, if the depth of the pocket around the implant is greater than 6 mm, a thorough examination of the pathology of the process is required. The assessment of peri-implantitis is based on the determination of marginal bone loss, which is proven by an intraoral X-ray and comparison with the image taken immediately after implant placement. Then, the extent of gingival bleeding is examined by probing. Probing is a reliable and similar method of examining peri-implant as well as periodontal tissue. In healthy tissue, the probe encounters resistance from the peri-implant mucosa as well as in healthy gingiva around the natural tooth, while in peri-implantitis and periodontitis the probe penetrates without resistance to the apical position of the epithelium, depending on the degree of inflammation. Several scientists have looked at the frequency of peri-implantitis. Their research showed that in patients with one or two implants, the percentage of peri-implantitis ranged from 28% to 56%. The severity and causes of the disease were different. In 10% to 15% of patients, more severe complications with greater bone loss around the implant have been proven. Most of the patients who were included in these studies had the same implant system. Their conclusion is that peri-implantitis does not depend on the implant system. The etiology of peri-implantitis is multicausal, but two factors stand out as primary causes: bacterial infection and biomechanical factors. In conditions of inadequate maintenance of oral hygiene, the deposition of plaque around the neck of the implant causes inflammation of the peri-implant mucosa. Cell infiltration and destruction of connective tissue is manifested subepithelially. The pathological process spreads, affecting the peri-implant epithelium, which gradually separates from the transmucosal part of the implant. With the loss of alveolar bone and the migration of the attachment epithelium in the apical direction around the implant, a space similar to a periodontal pocket is formed. Scientists who researched the frequency of peri-implantitis found that the destruction of soft and bone tissues is significantly more pronounced around the implant than around the natural tooth. The reasons are weaker vascularization peri-implant mucosa, as well as differences in the ratio of collagen and fibroblasts in the peri-implant tissue in relation to the gingiva in a natural tooth. This affects the reduced biological potential of the peri-implant mucosa, and the easier and faster development of the pathological process. Figure 13.130. Schematic representation of diagnosing periodontal changes by probing.

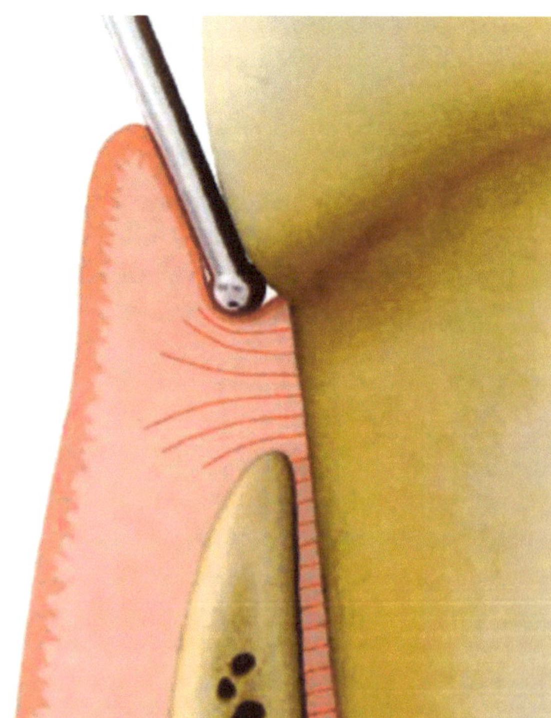

Figure 13.130. Schematic representation of periodontal diagnosis change by probing.

As for the bacterial content, it is similar in periodontitis and peri-implantitis. The composition of the subgingival bacterial flora around the implant is very similar to that around the natural tooth. This applies to both healthy and pathologically altered tissue. Experience shows that the number of pathogenic micro-organisms of subgingival dental plaque is significantly reduced around implants in patients with total edentulism who have had implants.

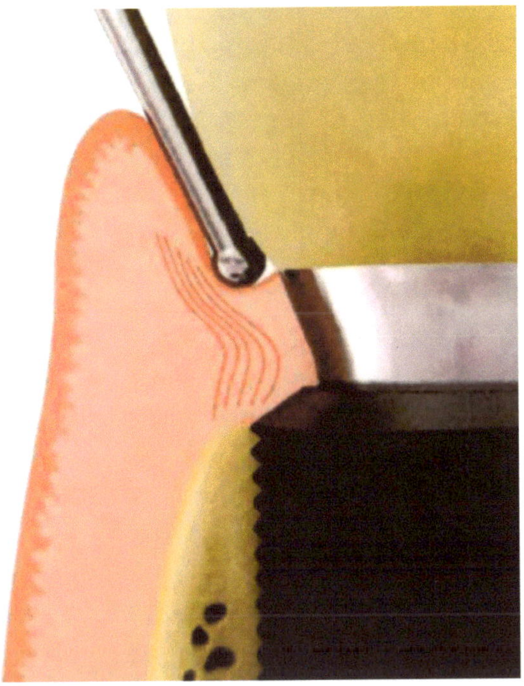

Figure 13.131. Schematic representation of peri-implant diagnostics change by probing.

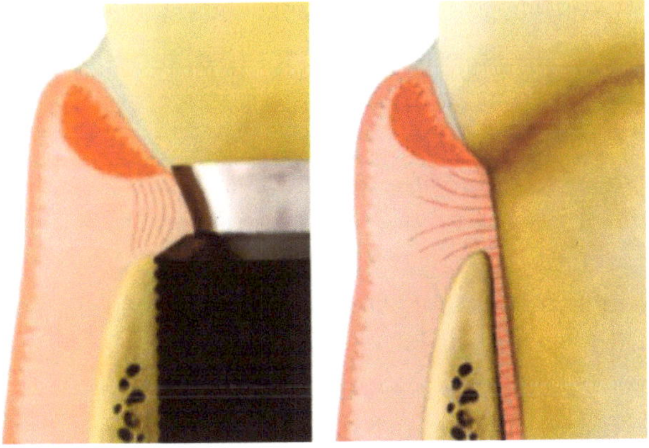

Figure 13.132. Schematic representation of peri-implant mucositis in compared to a natural tooth.

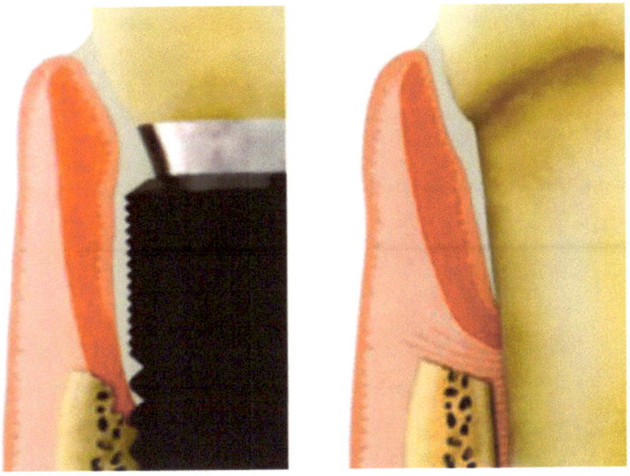

Figure 13.133. Schematic representation of peri-implantitis - compare with picture 13.132.

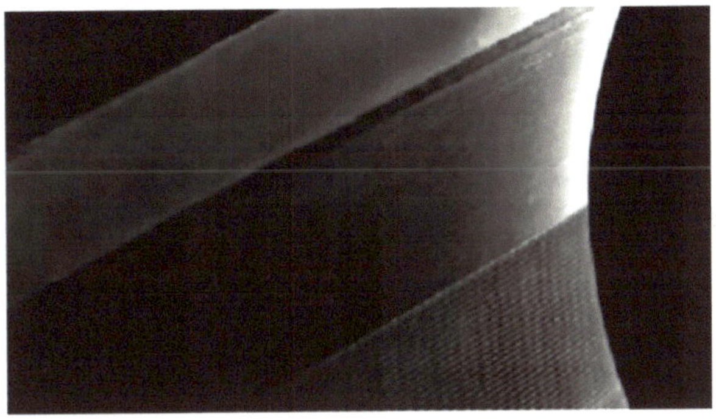

Figure 13.134. The design of the implant neck processed with Laser-lock technology; the conditions of mucosal attachment to the surface of the neck of the implant are significantly improved.

The biggest problem and dilemma in professional circles, as well as in research centers in the field of dental implantology, is the design of the implant and the processing of its neck, as well as the connection of the implant with the support (Fig. 122), which can be conical, hexagonal, triangular, friction or a combination of some of these ways. In the connection between the implant and the support, for reasons of prevention of preserving the integrity of the mucosal attachment around the neck of the implant, there must not be an intermediate space, defined by a microcrack. If there is a microcrack between the implant and the support, a dead space will be created as a predilection place for the deposition of plaque and the development of microorganisms that can cause inflammatory reactions of the peri-implant tissue. An additional risk factor for the occurrence of peri-implant changes is the trauma created by masticatory forces, which are transmitted to the implant itself via the implant carrier, and it is known that the greatest tension of forces is at the neck of the implant (unlike a natural tooth, where the forces are strongest in the apical third of the root teeth). These are the factors that can influence the creation of inflammatory processes around the neck of the implant, with a tendency to descend towards its apical part. If treatment is not started after diagnosing inflammatory processes, the process will progress to peri-implantitis, with possible loss of the implant. To prevent this, the creators of implant systems are racing to design a more "receptive" surface the neck of the implant, around which newly formed collagen fibers (similar to Sharpay fibers) will be placed faster and continuously, perpendicularly, with the aim of imitating the epithelial attachment and preserving the crestal bone, which supports the soft tissue and the papilla, which gives successful aesthetic results that will be constant for throughout the survival of the implant in the bone.

Treatment of the surface of the implant neck is done in several ways: Laser-lock technology ("Biohorizons"), microchannel treatment with a channel size of about 200 microns ("Astra") and "platform-switch". It is important that the technological treatment of the implant neck enables the speed of migration of osteoblasts and fibroblasts towards the implant neck, which will form new bone. For this reason, the aim is to treat the surface of the implant for which osteoblasts have a greater affinity, which achieves a faster and better attachment of osteoblasts, which affects the stimulation of osseointegration processes, which of course results in greater stability of the implant. Another risk factor, in addition to the bacterial one, are biomechanical factors. The author's experience is that biomechanical risk factors are formed in the dental laboratory due to non-respect, and often ignorance, of gnathological principles during the fabrication of prosthetic work. It is not without reason that Professor Dr. Mr. Graber from Basel (Switzerland, 1981) wrote a book on gnathology exclusively for dental technicians ("Gnatologie-Die Zahntechnik L'odontotecnica la technique dentarie", Einsiedeln, 1981). Inadequate, oversized shaping of occlusal surfaces, slopes and shapes of cusps that are not adapted to lateral movements of the lower jaw, and to all movements in general, especially the existence of premature contacts, can be factors in the cause of peri-implantitis with the consequence of implant loss. The author's experience is; that the majority of failed implant placements are more related to occlusal-articulation problems than to the surgical protocols of implant placement. If the occlusal-articulation relations between the compensation worn on the implants and the antagonist are not established, changes occur that are characteristic of occlusal trauma on natural teeth, and are manifested in a similar way by peri-implant bone trauma. Occlusal trauma is manifested by the loss of marginal bone around the implant. But this process should be distinguished from normal physiological loss of alveolar bone that occurs around the implant (it is the highest in the first year after implant placement, and it decreases significantly later). In the first year of functioning implants, where good bone integration has been achieved, the normal physiological loss of the marginal bone amounts to 1 to 1.5 mm, and then this annual loss decreases significantly and ranges from 0.1 to 0.2 mm. Unlike the changes in the peri-implant tissue caused by the pathological process, the normal annual physiological loss in the range of 0.1 to 0.2 mm ensures a favorable transfer of pressure to the implant and bone. Bone loss can be increased if there are parafunctions (bruxism, bruxomania, nail biting, pipes, unilateral chewing, etc.). The risk of increased bone loss caused by the biomechanical factor, as already emphasized. In cases where both risk factors (bacteriological and biomechanical) are combined, the causes of peri-implant changes must be precisely identified in order to determine therapy in a timely manner and for it to be successful. Who are the patients at high risk for developing peri-implantitis? These are primarily smokers and patients who did not follow the doctor's instructions for maintaining oral hygiene. This group also includes those who never came for check-ups after implant placement, or did not come for regular annual check-ups. The quality of the treatment of the implant surface and the quality of the material (titanium from type 1 to 4) from which the implant is made and how the neck of the implant is coated cannot be ruled out as the etiology of peri-implantitis. Laser technology for processing the neck part of the implant is a big advance in the prevention of peri-implantitis. In terms of bacterial content, animal experiments and analysis of human biopsies have found that the inflammatory lesions of peri-implant mucositis and gingivitis are similar. It has also been proven that inflammatory processes caused by infection in the marginal part of the gingiva and the peri-implant part of the mucosa are similar. Both processes are reversible and amenable to successful therapy. It is very important to recognize the clinical symptoms of initial peri-implant mucositis, which is characterized by discrete soft tissue inflammation. The symptoms of inflammation of the exudative type are most often manifested. This type of inflammation is the result of plaque accumulated due to inadequate oral hygiene. Accumulations of dental plaque are present in the region of the peri-implant mucosa and peri-implant sulcus. Clinical symptoms are manifested by discoloration and swelling of the peri-implant mucosa, as well as bleeding when touched with a probe. In this initial stage of the disease, alveolar bone resorption is absent, unless it occurred during the period of osseointegration. In patients with peri-implant mucositis, it is necessary to develop motivation for good maintenance of oral hygiene. It should be explained to them that the treatment is exclusively domain and their action, aimed at the rehabilitation of gingival diseases around implants. If there are deposited hard deposits and plaque, they need to be carefully removed with special plastic instruments and ultrasonic devices with plastic attachments. Recommend to the patient the mandatory purchase of the device (Waterpick), as well as other means for maintaining hygiene around the implant (pictures 13.125 - 13.136).

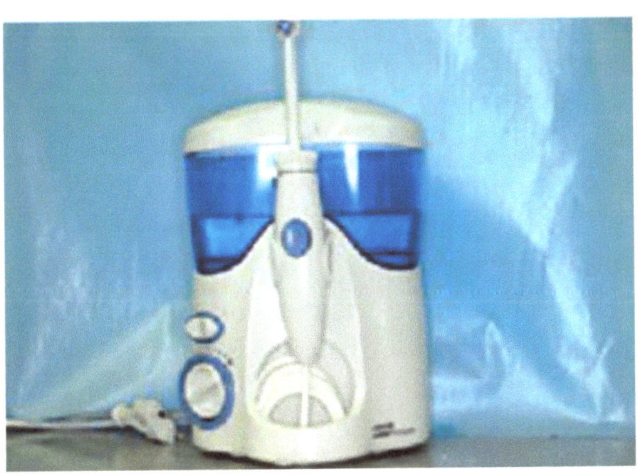

Figure 13.135. Device for maintaining oral hygiene.

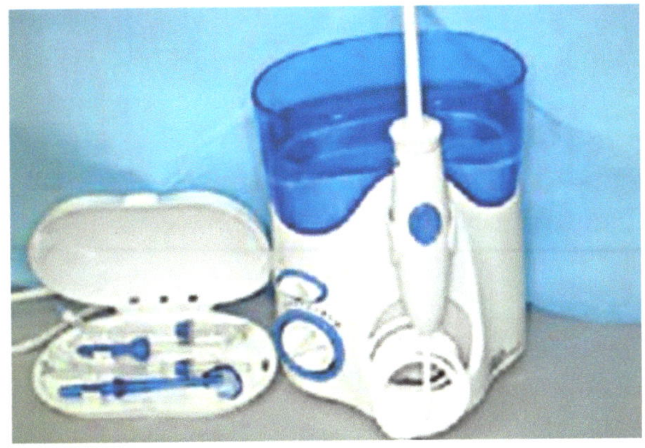

Figure 13.136. Additions for family members.

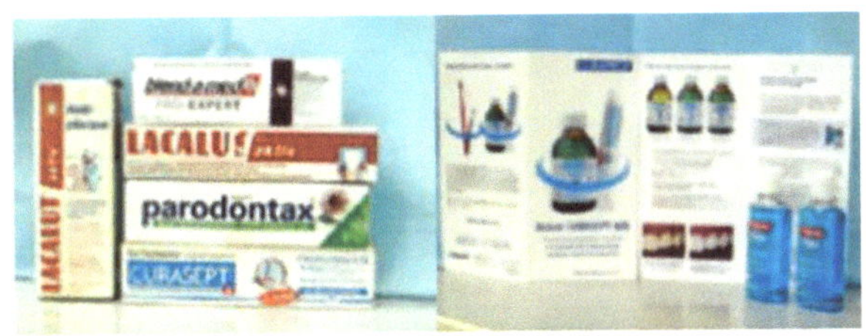

Figure 13.137. Additional means for maintaining oral hygiene, which needs to be recommended to the patient.

Since inflammation of the peri-implant mucosa and peri-implant tissue is caused by infection, the goal of therapy for these diseases is to eliminate the cause of peri-implantitis. The first step is to eliminate the peri-implant pocket and stop bleeding on probing (Figures 13.130 and 13.131). Successful treatment should prevent the loss of tissue around the implant, and in order to achieve this, it is necessary to control the course of the infection. Part of the therapy is a detailed explanation to the patient of what caused the disease, and the cause of the disease can be the patient himself, which needs to be emphasized and explained. If serious complications have developed, establish the causes. First of all, determine whether the only cause of the disease is poor maintenance of oral hygiene. Experience shows that peri-implant changes are caused by a lack of motivation to maintain oral health hygiene by the patient, the therapy is much simpler and more successful than the disease of peri-implantitis which is "created" by a dental technician or dentist. Peri-implantitis caused by a doctor's mistake during implant placement has more serious consequences than peri-implant mucositis caused by failure to maintain oral hygiene. Mistakes that are in the domain of dentists - poor planning, overheating bones during implant installation, errors in assessing the quality and quantity of available bone, installation of implants of inappropriate diameter, poor prosthetic reconstruction, from occlusion to the impossibility of using interdental proximal brushes (Fig. 13.138 and 13.140) to maintain oral hygiene around the implant - it is much more difficult to correct and rehabilitate.

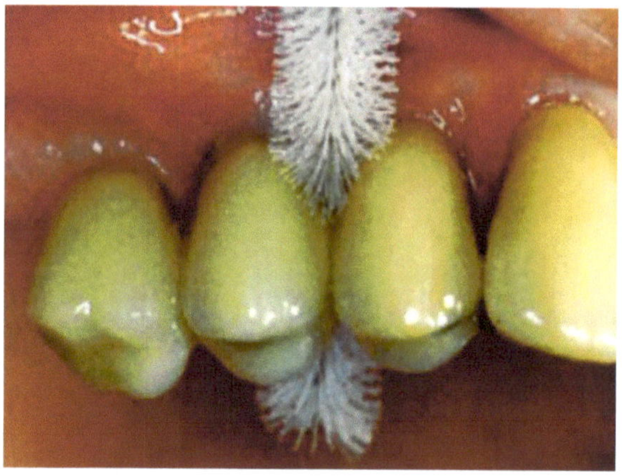

Figure 13.138. Application of interdental, approximal brushes for maintenance of oral hygiene should provide adequate prosthetic reconstruction.

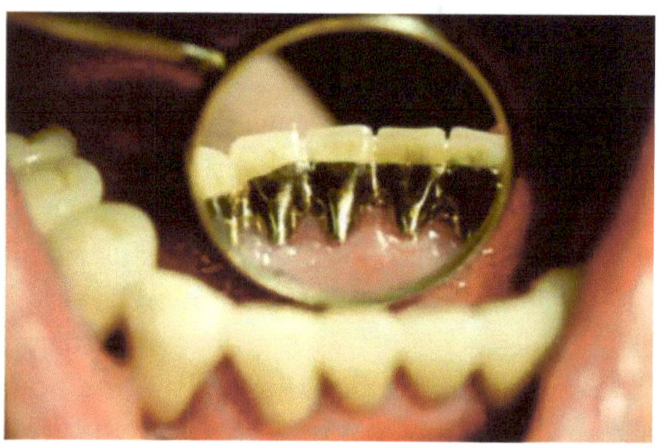

Figure 13.139. Appearance of healthy periodontal tissue around metal-ceramic crowns on gold.

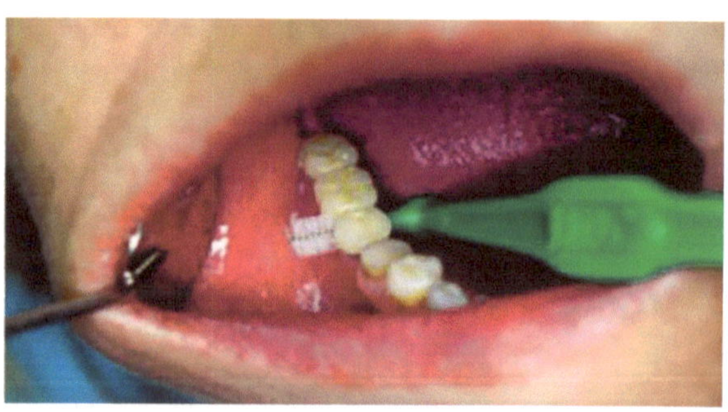

Figure 13.140. The use of interdental brushes is a condition for maintaining healthy peri-implant tissue.

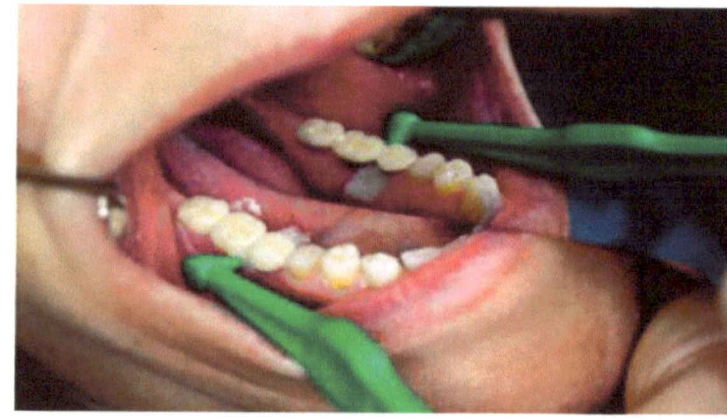

Figure 13.141. Maintaining oral hygiene in a patient with three implants is made possible by precise prosthetic work.

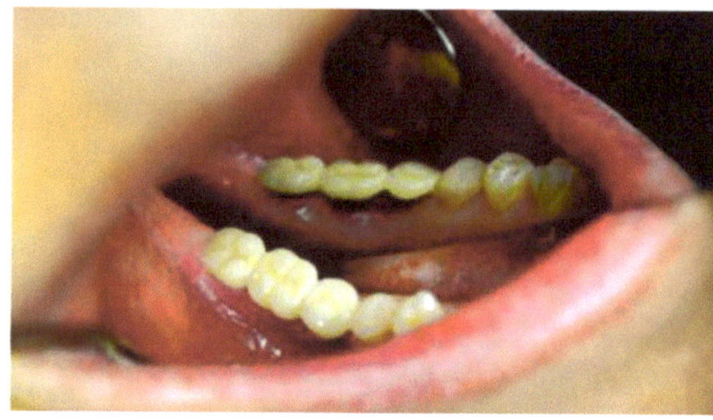

Figure 13.142. "Lege-artis" performed prosthetic work on implants. Oversized occlusal surfaces with exaggerated cusps, which can be a biomechanical risk factor.

Prosthetic work should enable, as much as possible, easy maintenance of oral hygiene, accessibility with interdental-proximal brushes (Fig. 13.139, 13,140 and 13.13.141). In many cases, in patients with signs of peri-implant tissue disease, it is not possible to maintain oral hygiene due to poor prosthetic work. In successfully performed prosthetic works, after many years, the gingiva around the implant is still healthy (pictures 13.139, 13.152 and 13.153 and 13.155).

To maintain oral hygiene around the implant, patients should be advised to use the "Water pick" device, which has several types of brushes and attachments, with which, by irrigation under the pressure of a liquid stream, it is possible to thoroughly clean the peri-implant space. With interdental brushes in the inter-implant spaces, fine vibrations and under a stream of liquid, it is possible to thoroughly clean the peri-implant space. There are various types of solutions with deodorant and disinfecting effects on the market (Figure 13.137). Also, there are many types of toothpaste that are specifically designed to maintain the health of the gums. An educated hygienist or dental nurse should explain to the patient in detail the use of the recommended means for maintaining oral hygiene, not only when it comes to implant problems. If the patient with peri-implant mucositis followed the instructions for oral hygiene, regardless of the successful therapy of peri-implant mucositis, it is necessary to precisely check the occlusal-articulation relations. In this regard, possible excessive occlusal load should be eliminated, and it is of particular importance to register premature contacts that can cause gingival recession and bone resorption around the implant, identically to gingival recession in natural teeth. The procedure of registering occlusal contacts with a traumatic effect on the peri-implant tissue should be performed patiently and meticulously. Control the contacts of the occlusal surfaces in all positions and movements. Too strong occlusal contacts on prosthetic work carried by implants should be reduced to a minimum, even placed in minimal subocclusion, especially at the beginning, in order to achieve the best possible osseointegration over time. If the symptoms of parafunctions are present, it is necessary to establish the causes, and, if possible, remove the traumatic effect on the implants by wearing protective corrosive bulwarks, especially at night, when parafunctional movements are most manifested.

If a detailed clinical examination reveals that a peri-implant pocket has been formed by a pathological process in the peri-implant tissue, surgical therapy is necessary - removal of the altered peri-implant tissue. Thus, the resulting bone defects in the bone around the implant are removed, and mucogingival defects should be corrected. Bone defects around implants are eliminated by methods of resective or regenerative surgery, which aims to eliminate peri-implant pocket.

With resective therapy, a full-thickness flap is moved apically (see chapter 10 on augmentation) and the implant and alveolar bone damaged by the pathological process are exposed. By raising the flap, a clear overview of the affected region is obtained and it is necessary to remove the pathologically changed tissues - chronically inflamed granulation tissue, with special curettes to the healthy bone. After the surgical treatment of the affected area, the implantoplasty procedure follows, which involves mechanical treatment of the implant surface coronal to the alveolar bone. This procedure is performed for smaller destructions, when regenerative therapy is not required. How the procedure will be applied depends on the design of the implant neck - whether the surface of the implant neck is rough or smooth. If the surface of the implant neck is rough, sometimes it is necessary to radically process it with a diamond bur of a finer structure and then polish it, with copious pouring of cold sterile physiological solution, so that heating the implant does not endanger the achieved osseointegration in the part that is not threatened by the pathological process. Finally, the processed surface should be detoxified with some chemical agents, such as chlorhexidine solutions 0.12% to 0.2%, Curasepta which is a chlorhexidine solution 0.20%, lacalut solution, etc. Care should be taken that chemical detoxifying liquids do not get into contact with the peri-implant bone, so that its necrosis does not occur. This procedure can be performed for smaller destructions, where regenerative therapy using the augmentation method is not required, because the metal filings left behind during processing the surface of the implant with a diamond burr would remain and jeopardize the regeneration and healing of the wound.

Treatment of larger bone defects resulting from peri-implantitis requires the use of resective surgical therapy. Preoperatively, the symptoms of inflammation in the peri-implant soft tissues should be calmed down. It is necessary to prescribe antibiotics depending on the degree of inflammation (amoxicillin or augmentin with the addition of metronidazole 400 mg). Before applying resective surgical therapy of peri-implantitis, prosthetic work should be completed so that access to the surgical field is fully inspected and accessible for placement of replacement material, whether it is an autologous bone block or a bone substitute. The filling of the defect must be performed in such a way as to allow unhindered repositioning of the flap or its coronary movement, so that after the placement of surgical sutures, the treated region was completely covered.

Reductive surgical procedures correct unfavorable soft tissue relationships and bone defects around implants. The procedure for tissue resection and regenerative therapy depends on the size of the bone defect. If the bone defect is extensive, regenerative therapy based on the principle of "moderate bone tissue regeneration (GBR)" is necessary. The GBR method involves the application of collagen bone substitutes (Bio-Oss), and if the size of the defect requires a more extensive augmentation procedure, Bio-Oss can be mixed with autologous bone, covered with a collagen resorbable membrane. In larger bone defects, the bone defect must be compensated for with a bone block of autologous bone, taken from the chin or retromolar region. The bone block should be fixed with titanium screws that are removed after 6-8 weeks. If the peri-implant bone defect is large, and the block is not sufficient, the augmented block should be covered with collagen bone substitute (BioOss). It is mandatory to cover it with a resorbable or non-resorbable titanium membrane, which must be removed after 3 months. Postoperatively, the patient is prescribed antibiotics and analgesics, and intramuscular dexomethasone is given as a preventive measure against the occurrence of major postoperative swelling. The patient is given additional instructions for maintaining hygiene, with mandatory rinsing the mouth with chlorhexidine solutions or similar solutions. Advise the patient to rinse with sage or chamomile tea. After rinsing with these liquids, teach the patient how to apply additional agents to accelerate wound healing, such as Fibrolan (USA), Solcoseryl (Switzerland) or Placentinex (Italy). The stitches are removed after 8-10 days.

It happens that the membrane, due to suture dehiscence, is exposed before the scheduled deadline. In this case, it is necessary to continue rinsing with chlorhexidine solutions (0.12% or Curasept 0.20%) to prevent the occurrence of infection, which would jeopardize the success of the treatment. If there are no signs of infection, the exposed membrane can remain for 6 to 8 weeks, in order to continue the osseointegration process. In the postoperative period of healing of the peri-implant soft tissues, it should be emphasized to patients who are passionate smokers that they absolutely must quit smoking. The goal of regenerative therapy of a bone defect in the peri-implant space is not only to stop the development of pathological processes around the peri-implant tissue, but to achieve its complete healing (restitutio ad integrum).

Peri-implantitis caused by dentist's mistake

The most severe forms of peri-implantitis can be caused, first of all, by the mistakes of the dentist, and then by the dental technician during the fabrication of the implant-supported superstructure. A dental technician must know how important it is to maintain oral hygiene and, by creating prosthetic work (construction), enable easy maintenance of oral hygiene in the inter-implant spaces. A very common occurrence in our laboratories is that the dental technician, at the place of the dental bridge between the implants, "erases" a depression on the plaster model, so that the dental bridge rested more closely on the alveolar ridge, considering that it achieves better aesthetics. This is a big mistake, because "arbitrary" erasure compresses the soft peri-implant tissues around the implant, creating chronic decubitus, which can cause inflammation of the peri-implant tissues. An additional problem is the non-respect of bio-mechanical fasteners by creating occlusal surfaces contrary to gnathological requirements. The problem can also be aggravated by the patient's poor oral hygiene. The consequences of such errors are peri-implantitis with larger bone defects around the implant. The dentist is responsible for the consequences. The following images show obvious errors, solely to the detriment of the patient.

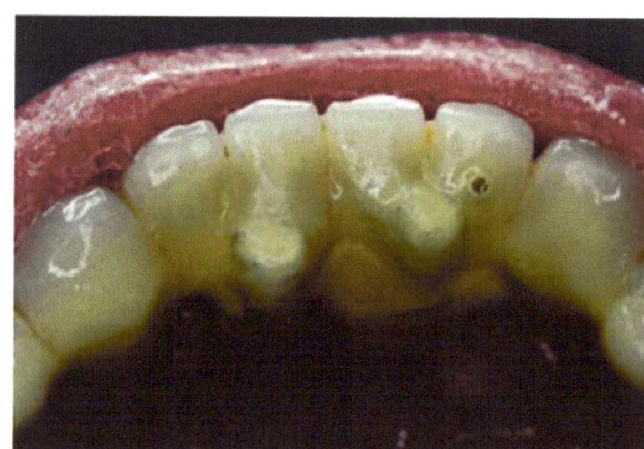

Figure 13.143. Frequent mutual mistakes: dentist, dental technician and patient. Dentist's mistake: positioning of an implant of inappropriate diameter, clearly visible from both the lingual and vestibular side. The laboratory's error is the lack of a "collar" that prevents the accumulation of plaque and the compression of wide crowns in the neck area on the papillae, due to which the passage of approximal brushes is not possible. Patient error: failure to maintain oral hygiene.

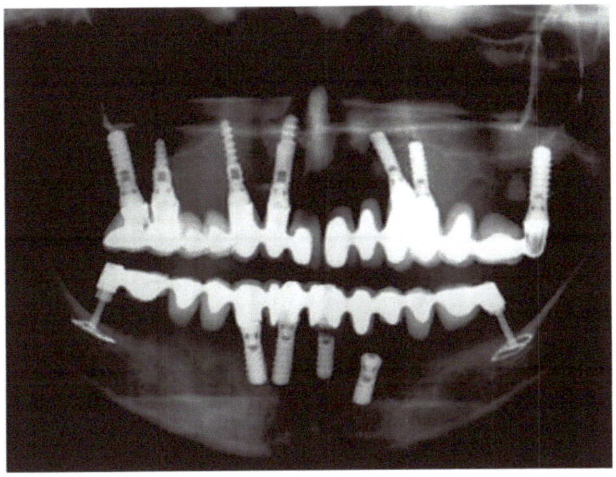

Figure 13.144. The radiographic view only confirms the dentist's mistakes. In the upper jaw, the arrangement of implants of different diameters. The positions of the implants in sites #23 and #24 preclude the creation of prosthetic work to meet esthetic and functional requirements. Perforation of the sinus floor with a narrow-diameter implant, where mastication forces are strongest. In the lower jaw, the installation of the so-called The "disk" of the implant with a long support arm is in danger of breaking due to the tension of masticatory forces, which experience confirms. Due to the length of the span between the "disk" implant and the attachment of the bridge, the arms of both "disk" implants broke in the symphysis. (fig. 13.146 and 13.148). Four implants in the frontal region, with inadequate diameters, caused recession of the peri-implant soft tissues and resorption of the vestibular bone wall. The consequences of the risk shown in the following figures.

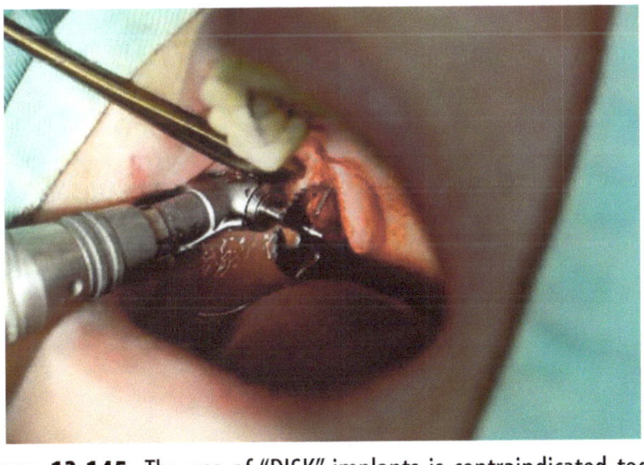

Figure 13.145. The use of "DISK" implants is contraindicated today, when modern oral implantology surpassed the past with new designs, copying nature, it is not only a risk in the design of the implant (breakage of the support), it is also a risk during implantation from serious injuries to the patient with circular cutters. The patient is exposed to morbidity during implantation and even stronger and more complicated removal of the broken endosseus part of the implant. Applying similar procedures today (installation of "DISC" implants) is a huge step backwards. The picture shows a detail from the practice of the author of the book. Reviews of experienced implantologists confirm the superiority of these implants of the past.

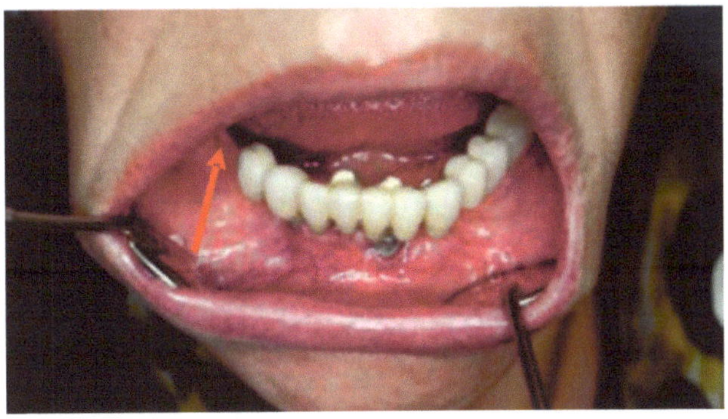

Figure 13.146. Situation with broken "disk" implant arms (red arrow) - increased biomechanical risks with remaining hanging bridge members.

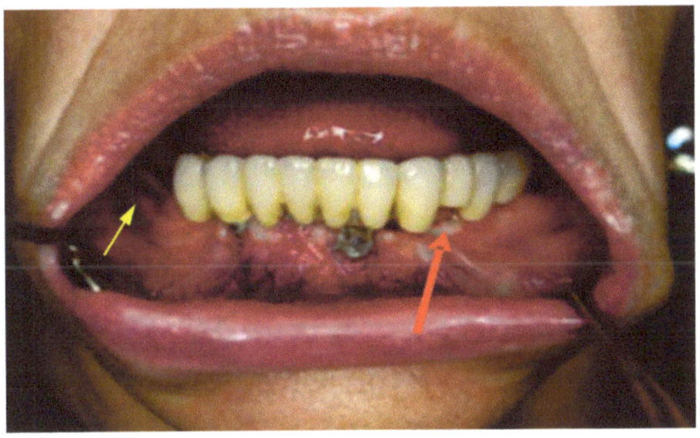

Figure 13.147. Recession of the peri-implant gingiva and resorbed vestibular bone lamella are the consequences of an inadequate diameter of the implant in proportion to the available bone. Pay attention to the lower left premolar (red arrow). Shortening into definitive prosthetic constructions is evidence of wandering, without a set plan and the application of outdated "disk" implants with a long arm of the support prone to breakage (yellow arrow). Done in an educational institution. See Figure 13.146

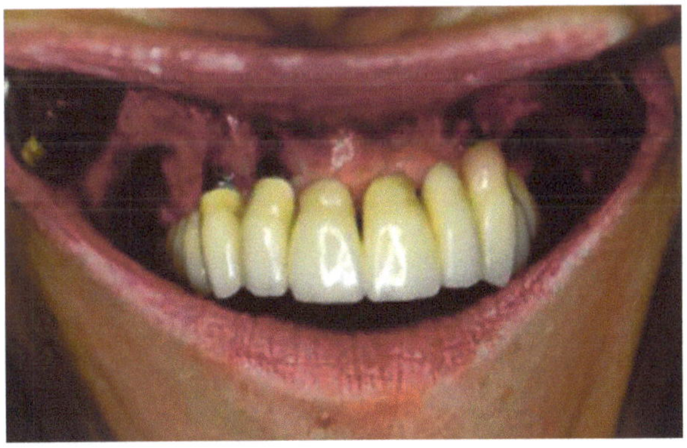

Figure 13.148. Consequences of bad planning. The selection of inappropriate implant diameters in proportion to the available bone, positioning and installation of the implant creates a risk of not being able to create a precise prosthetic work. See picture 13.144.

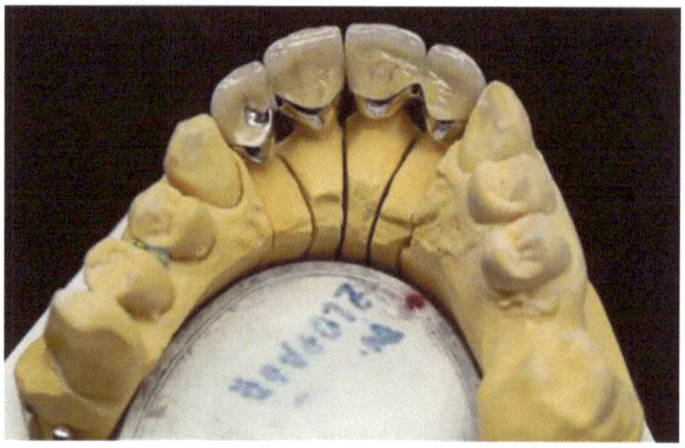

Figure 13.149. It is very important that the dentist has knowledge of prosthetics as well as oral surgical knowledge, in order to explain to the dental technician how to create prosthetic work on implants. Appearance of prosthetic work on implants in the frontal part of the upper jaw. High palatal collar, space for a regenerated papilla and the possibility of maintaining good oral hygiene.

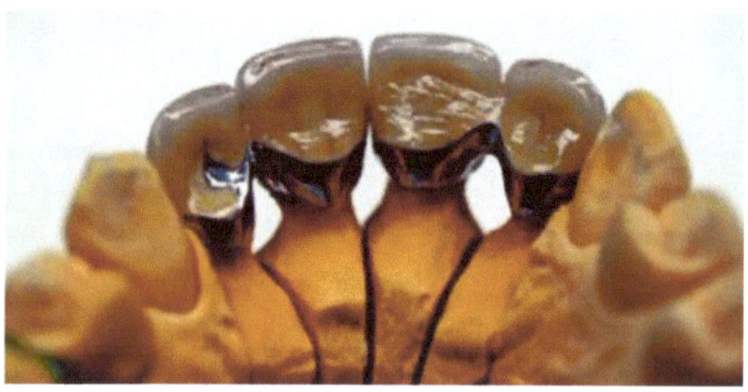

Figure 13.150. The interdental papilla must not be compressed, and with the prosthetic design, the retention of food residues and the deposition of plaque in the periodontal and peri-implant tissues cannot be prevented. Precise prosthetic works do not jeopardize the integrity of surrounding tissues, their health is maintained.

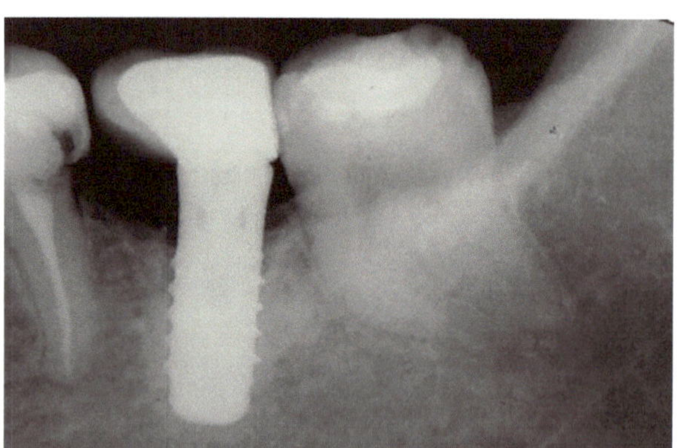

Figure 13.151. Faults: Design and dimensions of the implant - a wider diameter is indicated due to the reception of masticatory forces, which are strongest in the lateral region. The implant had to be placed at the level of the cortical bone, which would enable a different design of the crown. By making the crown, biomechanical risk factors were created - lever action, food residues and plaque deposition for the rough part of the implant surface.

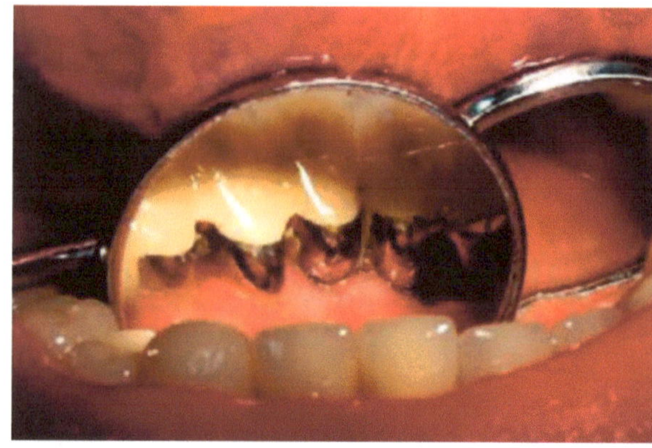

Figure 13.152. A high collar on the lingual side has no effect on aesthetics and enables the health of the surrounding tissues. Avoiding this prosthetic detail and covering it with ceramic (three layers: opaque, dentin, glaze layer), narrows the interdental and inter-implant space, which causes compression on the surrounding gingiva, especially on the papilla. Difficulty in cleaning, especially the impossibility of using approximal brushes, is a risk factor for plaque deposition and inflammation of periodontal and peri-implant tissues.

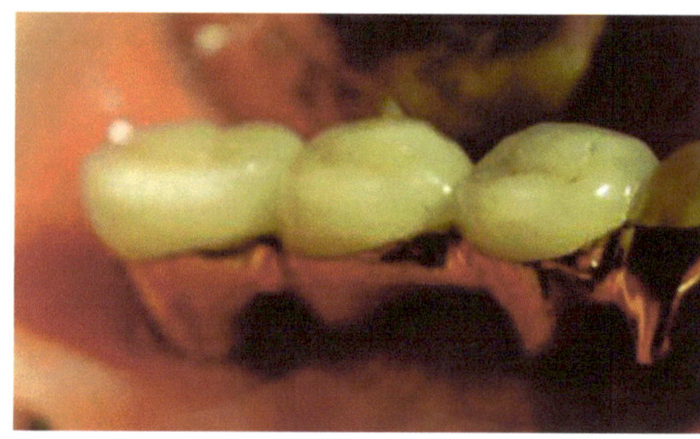

Figure 13.153. View of the bridge from the lingual side on the implants, which is surrounded by healthy peri-implant tissues. Biomechanical requirements are met by shaping the cusps, according to gnathological principles.

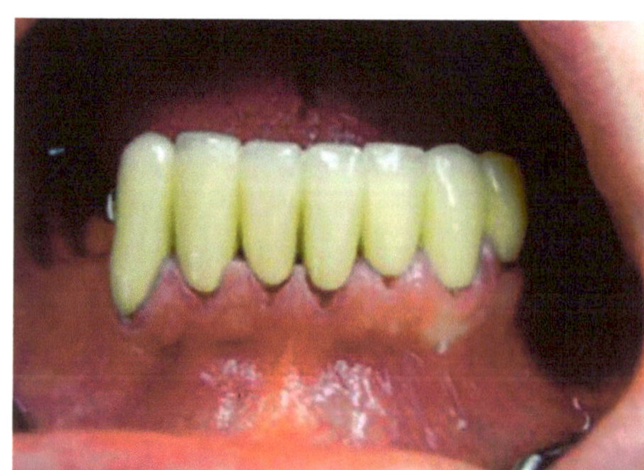

Figure 13.154. Presentation of a case where bad prosthetics created periodontal problems, which resulted in tooth loss.

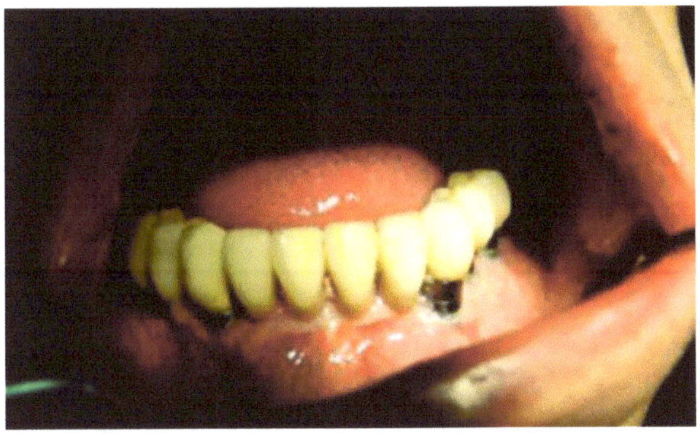

Figure 13.155. Case report in a patient who is an avid smoker, with poor oral hygiene and prosthetic construction and details of the prosthetic construction that prevent the deposition of plaque and dental calculus, which enables long-lasting implants in the bone. Presentation of the condition 15 years after the installation of the Nobel Replace Biokare implant. Complete osseointegration was achieved, and the peri-implant tissues showed no signs of inflammation, despite poorly maintained oral hygiene. The author's experience shows that plaque deposition is much less in cases of total toothlessness rehabilitated with implants, than in cases where there is a combination with natural teeth. When planning an implant-prosthetic replacement, take into account the shape of the lip due to the harmonization of function and aesthetics and, based on that, plan the performance of prosthetic work in the lateral regions.

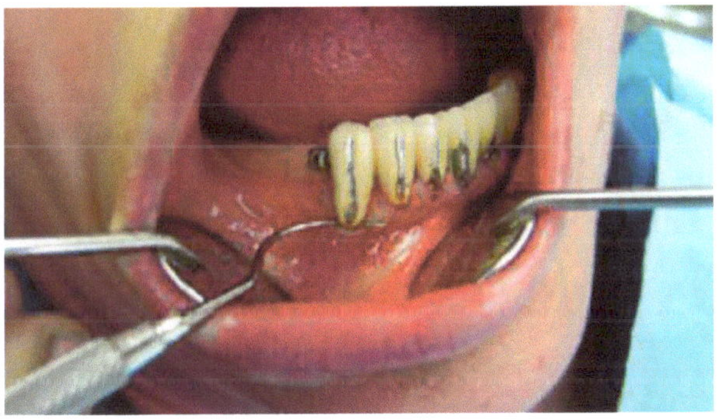

Figure 13.156. In this case, the responsibility lies with the doctor who fixed the imprecise prosthetic work. If the impression is imprecise, the dental technician must not start work on such an impression. The biggest mistake dentists make is taking an impression immediately after tooth preparation, without waiting for the traumatized gingiva to heal after grinding with diamond burs. The author's experience recommends that you should wait at least 7-8 days, and in some cases even longer.

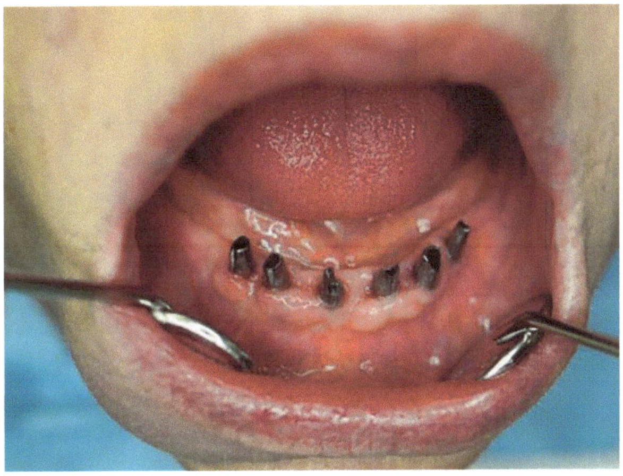

Figure 13.157. Immediate implants. Condition after 3 months: good implant stability and soft tissue healing. The success of the implant procedure can be compromised in the dental laboratory.

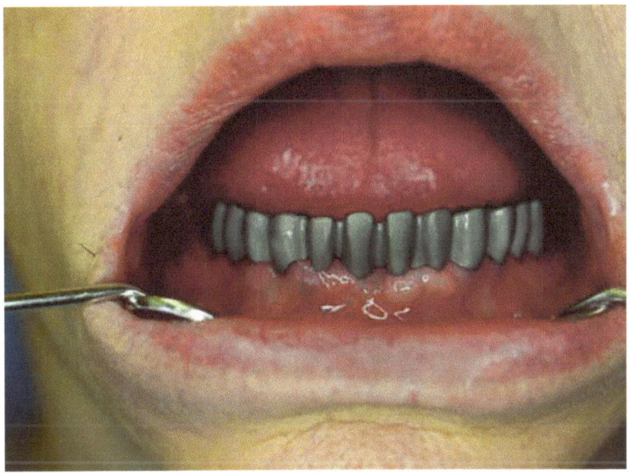

Figure 13.158. Risk factors are created in the dental laboratory. This construction is a risk factor for successful implantation, because it is impossible to maintain oral hygiene, the impossibility of using interdental brushes.

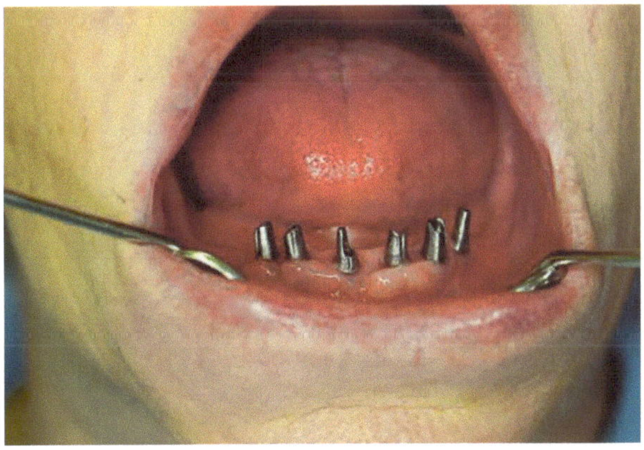

Figure 13.159. Augmentation and implantation successfully performed. Quality osseointegration and soft tissue healing achieved. The success of the entire implant-prosthetic treatment depends on the quality of the prosthetic work.

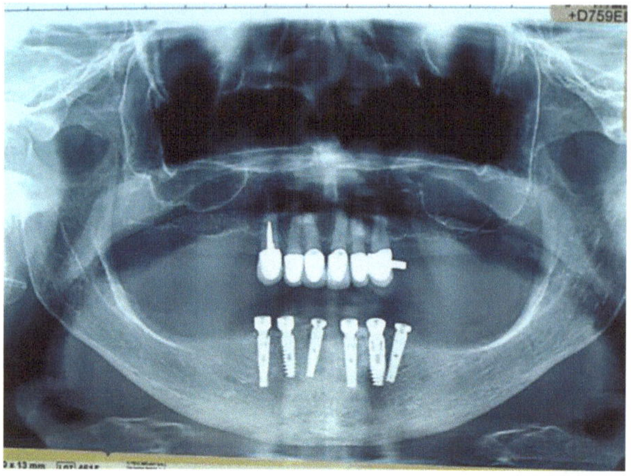

Figure 13.160. Radiographic representation of immediate implantation (Figures 13.157 and 13.159) and augmentation in the frontal region of the lower jaw with an immediate fixed provisional bridge.

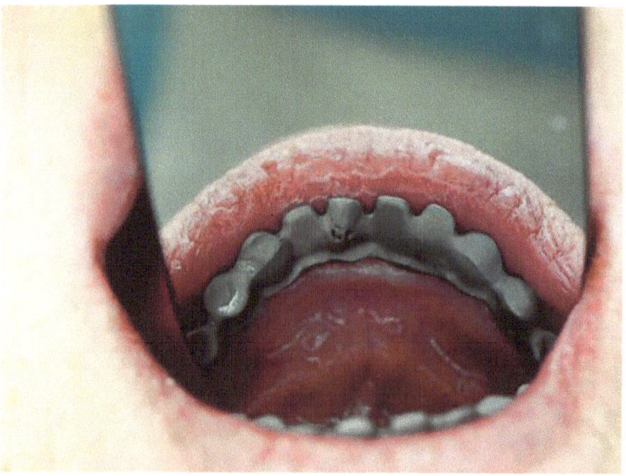

Figure 13.161. Making such a construction in the laboratory is proof that the dental technician does not know the problems in oral implantology. If the dentist in implant-prosthetic rehabilitation accepts such solutions, the consequences are risks with serious complications.

Allergic reactions as a risk factor

During implant-prosthetic treatment, as well as during any other treatment, the occurrence of allergic reactions to the applied agents and medicines is also possible. Such reactions can cause a mutual panic reaction, both of the patient and the dentist, which is often unnecessary. Generally speaking, an allergic reaction can be to everything that is used in dental practice. People are more and more allergic to food, probably due to genetically modified food products.

The time of onset of an allergic reaction varies from a few minutes to several hours, and the changes caused by an allergy can vary in appearance and intensity. An allergic reaction can be manifested by fever and a rash on the skin, which is considered moderate urticaria or bronchoconstriction, and a reaction with hemodynamic collapse can occur. An allergic reaction can be early, which occurs in the first few minutes to half an hour, or late, which occurs after one or two hours, or manifests itself during the day. Early allergic reactions to the drug are more serious, violent, and require immediate intervention, because they can be life-threatening. The patient should be observed for the first fifteen minutes. Late allergic reactions are milder and often appear only as a rash on the skin, but still require attention. Allergic reactions due to oral administration of drugs are less severe due to slower absorption of the drug. Local reactions at the site of drug administration or systemic allergic reactions may occur. In the case of systemic allergic reactions, the clinical picture is mostly manifested by urticaria with occasional swelling of soft tissues (most often eyelids or lips). Skin changes may be accompanied by itching. In addition to this, attacks of suffocation may occur, with or without chest pain, with cardiovascular system complaints, drop in blood pressure, weakness and dizziness. If the digestive tract is affected, vomiting, nausea and diarrhea occur.

The most common allergic reactions are to penicillin, and the most severe form of allergic reaction to penicillin preparations is manifested by anaphylactic shock, and if not intervened within a few minutes, it can end tragically. Also, violent allergic reactions can be to non-steroidal anti-inflammatory drugs.

Previously, Gelastipt was used in dental practice - a preparation in the form of a spongy cube, which served as a tampon to stop bleeding after tooth extraction and prevent alveolitis. This preparation contained a penicillin component. On one occasion with a female patient (in Switzerland), the author, after tooth extraction, put a Gelastit tampon in an alveolar wound after which a major allergic reaction happened followed by fever, face redness, breathing difficulties, and symptoms of suffocation, difficult swallowing. The patient fell on the floor. Adrenalin and antihistaminic were administered, stopping that unexpected and difficult life-threatening incident.

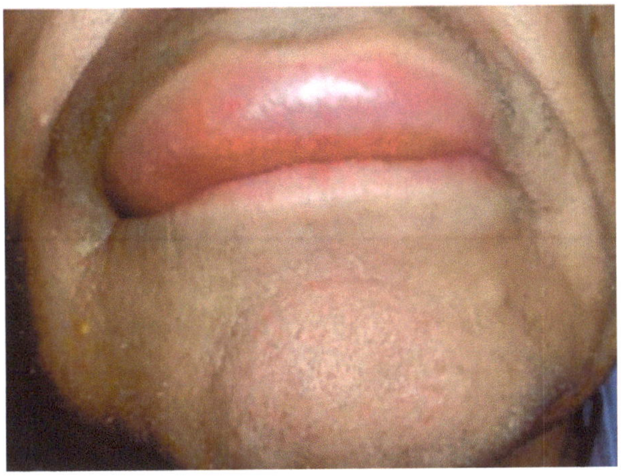

Figure 13.162. Turbulent course of late allergic reaction.

Once an allergic reaction begins, the use of drugs that suppress the effects of histamine on the cardiovascular and respiratory systems is indicated. It is a fact that after every oral surgery, dexamethasone is prescribed intramuscularly, which has anti-inflammatory and immunosuppressive effects, which is why its effect is manifested not only by reducing postoperative edema, but also by suppressing any allergic reaction. Otherwise, it is a legal obligation for every dental practice to have a kit for emergency treatment of anaphylactic shock, with strict control of the date by which the medicine can be used. The precaution must be maximum and the dentist must be well aware of how to react in case of sudden violent allergic reactions.

Despite the fact that there are many available today antihistamines, however, progress is slow when it comes to diagnosing allergens, and the number of allergy sufferers is skyrocketing. A scientific and philosophical question arises: does man pay a price to evolution for discovering soap, hot water and many chemical preparations that he uses, and those violent allergic reactions do not exist in animals. A person becomes increasingly sensitive from the use of chemical means for hygiene, to some parts of textiles and to many types of food, as well as to many medicines, analgesics, cosmetics and similar preparations.

In violent allergic reactions, the dentist should recognize whether it is Quincke's edema. Quincke's edema is an acute violent and painful swelling in the form of hives (urticaria) due to skin edema.

Quincke's edema occurs suddenly, most often on the swollen face. Swelling of the eyelids closes the eyes, facial features disappear, and the itching is severe. A few hours after the onset of the reaction, edema can affect the mucous membranes of the throat and block the upper airways, causing laryngeal dyspnea. Quincke's edema responds to the same causes as urticaria. Most often after the use of antihistamines withdraws in a few hours. If the reaction is violent and may threaten life, give corticosteroids intravenously immediately. Some bloating after treatment can last up to 24 hours. In order to prevent unwanted and life-threatening incidents, the patient should be referred to the Emergency Clinical Center immediately. If there is no such possibility, apply the intravenous corticosteroid LEMODSOLU (methylprednisolone). LEMOD-SOLU is a preparation in the form of powder and solvent for intravenous administration, and the strength of the medicine is 20 mg, 40 mg, 125 mg and 500 mg. The dosage of the drug depends on the symptoms and severity of the manifestation of the allergic reaction. This medicine contains the active ingredient methylprednisone, which belongs to a group of medicines known as corticosteroids. Corticosteroids are hormones produced in the body by the adrenal gland. Corticosteroids are important for the body's defense against inflammation, allergic reactions and some other stress conditions. The preparation Lemod-Solu contains a synthetic corticosteroid, which acts in the same way as corticosteroids that are naturally synthesized in the body. At the same time, PRONISON tablets of 20 mg are prescribed. A dose of this drug depends on the disease and response to therapy. Starting doses vary from 5 mg (a quarter of a tablet) to 60 mg. The medicine is dosed once a day, usually in the morning. This medication must be discontinued gradually. With this medicine, at the same time, the drug XYZAL of 5 mg is prescribed (one film tablet per day), which is an antiallergen-antihistamine for systemic use in allergic reactions, and the third drug to be prescribed is CONTROLOC of 20 mg.

The number of allergens is constantly increasing, considering the complexity of their detection and the fact that there are more and more allergens, knowledge of this problem is extremely important for the dentist.

With the introduction of new chemical preparations, as well as the application of new substances that have not been used so far in dentistry, allergic reactions of greater or lesser intensity can be expected. In oral implantology, cases of extremely violent allergic reactions have been recorded in the literature for augmentations using xenogeneic or synthetic-alloplastic bone substitutes (Figure 13.162). 100 years ago, the word "allergy" did not exist. Manifestation of the severity of the allergic reaction depends on the way the allergen enters the body.

Reactions with typical allergy symptoms after the application of xenogeneic materials, be it bovine, porcine or materials derived from algae, as well as synthetic alloplastic materials (hydroxyapatite, tricalcium phosphate, bioglass, polymer and others), have not been described and there are no valid statistical data.

But after augmentation, whether autologous or blocks of xenogeneic origin and other materials of xenogeneic and synthetic origin were applied, there were violent reactions not only in the augmented areas, but they spread, involving the entire mucous membrane in the oral cavity, spreading with large hematomas all over the body. face, affecting the neck as well, which can lead to the complete failure of the entire treatment (Chapter 10).

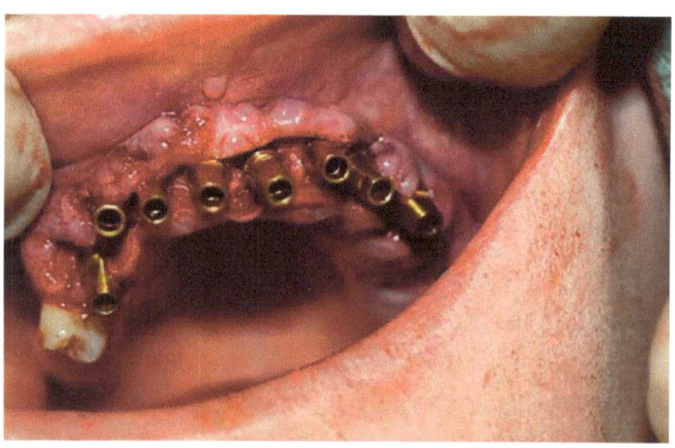

Figure 13.163. If at the end, after extremely complex treatment of disability in the oral cavity with implant-prosthetic procedures, with the result of high-quality bony integration and stable soft tissues, then it can be said that the implant-prosthetic rehabilitation was completely successful, shown in Figure 13.164.

Why such reactions occurred in the subcutaneous tissue is not clear, especially since the hematogenous changes occurred outside the interventional region. Such changes are possible in older patients due to the fragility of the capillaries. The affected parts of the face and neck are immobile and very painful under pressure. It is basically an interstitial blood deposition. Prophylaxis with antibiotics and the use of Heparin-Gel (6000 I.E.) are advised to accelerate the establishment of disturbed homeostasis and prevent soft tissue necrosis. Diagnosing the cause of allergic reactions primarily depends on a well-taken history. It is desirable that the patient has medical documentation, from which previous conditions and reactions can be determined, whether it is about the food taken; the use of various analgesic ointments or the medicine taken. If the allergic reaction occurred immediately after taking the medicine, it is necessary to find out the generic name of the medicine taken, followed by a laboratory test. Unfortunately, there are no reliable methods for detecting many allergens. In any case, at the beginning of an allergic reaction, if there are home conditions, you should take histamine, and the patient should be urgently referred to an institution for emergency interventions. When it comes to the occurrence of allergic reactions during dental treatment, the dentist must know to react calmly and professionally and to know what risk and unwanted outcome can occur.

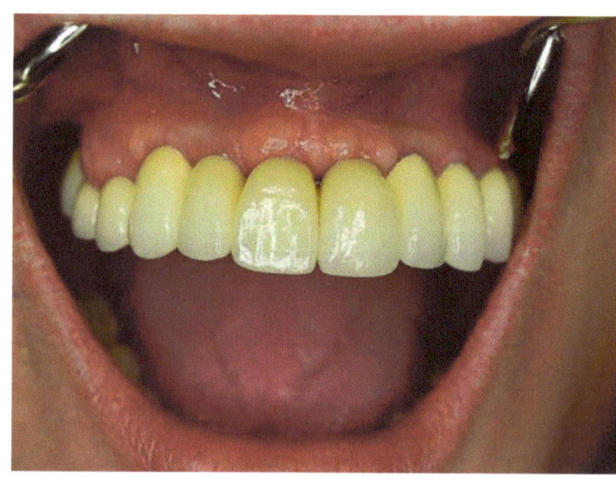

Figure 13.164. The end crowns the work!

14
Indications And Contraindications For Implant Placement

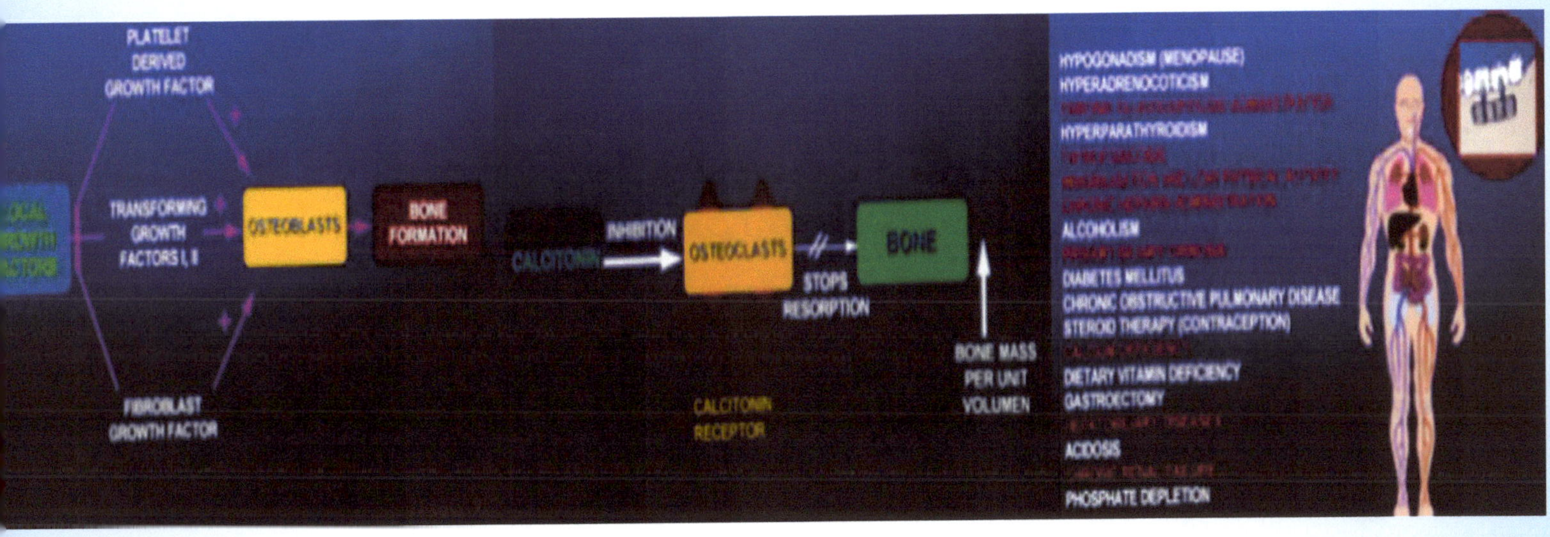

In most textbooks, the indications and contraindications for the application of a procedure are discussed, as a rule, at the beginning of the text, immediately after the definition of the procedure itself. However, it seems that in a book like this it is more appropriate to talk about indications and contraindications for the application of implant-prosthetic rehabilitation after considering all aspects related to the procedure itself, all dilemmas that need to be resolved and ways to avoid possible risks of failure. Therefore, I decided to talk about the indications and possible contraindications for the installation of dental implants, for a procedure that today, after many years of distrust of the scientific public, has gained universal approval and acceptance, almost at the very end of the book, after considering the most important practical aspects related to the procedure itself.

Indications

At today's level of development of oral implantology, when the possibilities of diagnostics are almost brought to perfection and when implants made of materials that are not only absolutely biocompatible, i.e. harmless, but also have the properties of bioadhesiveness, i.e. the induction of specific reactions between bone and the material that is implanted, it could be concluded that dental implants can be used in all situations where one, more or all teeth are missing.

1. **Lack of one tooth.** The lack of one tooth, especially if the neighboring teeth are healthy, is an ideal indication for the installation of endosseous implants and the restoration of a lost tooth, especially in the frontal region. (Fig. 14.1)

In such situations, the best possible rehabilitation is achieved, because adjacent, healthy teeth are preserved, and an ideal aesthetic result can be achieved. (Fig. 14.2)

Whether, along with implantation, there will also be a need for augmentation of bone tissue if the tooth was lost a long time ago and there is significant bone resorption or a lack of buccal cortical lamella, depends on the case by case and specific assessment of an experienced implantologist, which was about enough talk in previous chapters. (Fig. 14.3)

By replacing one molar, grinding of two adjacent healthy teeth is avoided. (Figure 14.4)

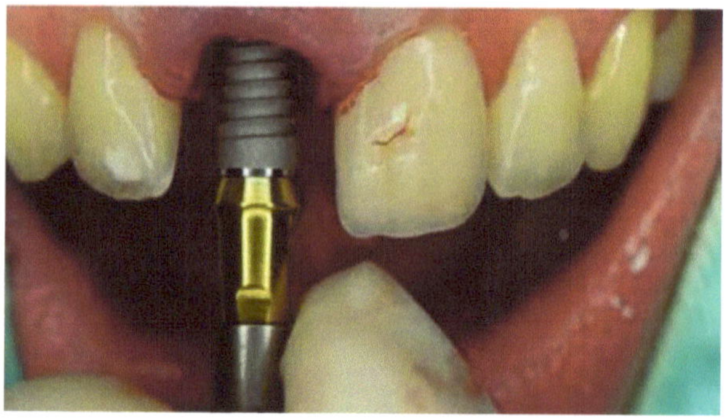

Figure 14.1. Replacement of one tooth by implanting an endosseous implants.

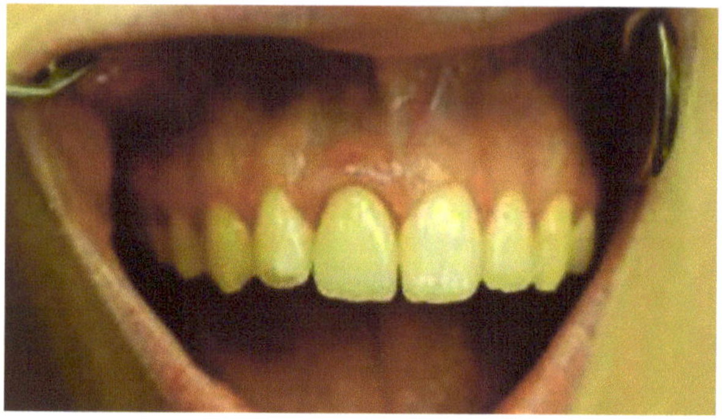

Figure 14.2. Ideal aesthetic result on endosseous implant images 14.1.

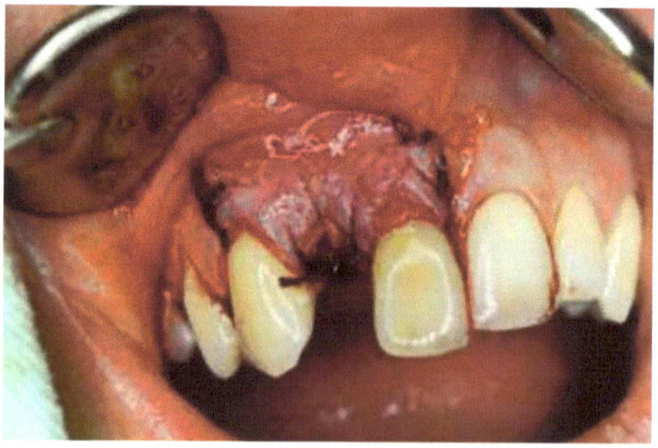

Figure 14.3. Buccal cortical lamella augmentation.

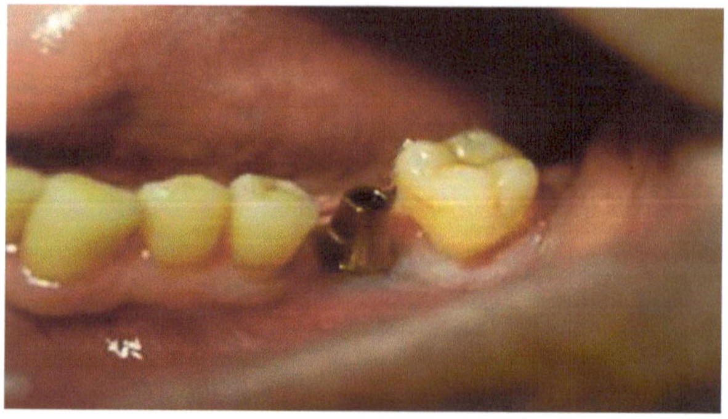

Figure 14.4. Molar replacement with an endosseous implant avoids grinding of two healthy adjacent teeth.

2. **Lack of multiple teeth.** When multiple teeth are missing, toothlessness can be inserted or free, when the dental array is actually shortened.

The installation of endosteal implants is an ideal solution for the care of free, distal toothless ridges, because classic prosthetic therapy with removable dentures is a very ungrateful solution since such partial dentures are, as a rule, uncomfortable and less stable. (Figures 14.5-14.7)

When it comes to inserted toothlessness, it can be successfully solved with classic bridges, provided that the gap between the teeth is not excessively large. However, if the gap between the teeth is greater than two or three (lost) teeth, then that situation, as a rule, should not be solved with classic bridges, especially when the teeth bordering the toothlessness are healthy (so they need to be ground to install the bridge supports). The installation of two or three implants, at the ends of the toothless saddle, in such a situation is the ideal solution, because the prosthetic work is fixed only on the implants. In certain situations, depending on the assessment of an experienced implantologist, it is possible to install only one implant that is attached to natural teeth (the conditions for such a decision are commented on in earlier chapters of this book). The installation of endosseous Implants In the case of edentulIsm is especially indicated if in this way the creation of mobile prosthetic work (partial dentures) is avoided, because the comfort achieved for the patient is incomparably better.

The scope of today's oral implatology in the rehabilitation of distal edentulous alveolar ridges with implant-prosthetic treatment is confirmed by the case of a patient who, four decades ago (1976), with the insertion of endo-osseous leaf implants connected to a natural tooth, I preserved comfort in the oral cavity with fixed prosthetic work instead of an unpleasant partial acrylic prosthesis (Figure 14.8). The patient then had all her teeth and did not want to wear an uncomfortable partial denture. Recently (November 2016) a practicing doctor from another city and state called me for advice, the patient has pain due to a dislodged canine on which a fixed prosthetic work connected to Linkov's "First generation" endosseous implant is anchored (Fig. 14.8). In the meantime, the patient lost all her teeth, she was retained by prosthetics work done four decades ago. A dentist in another institution, after extracting all the teeth, used the residual fixed prosthetic work to retain a partial acrylate prosthesis with a wire hook. It is important to emphasize that alveolar bone resorption is much less on the edentulous distal alveolar ridge where the implant was installed, (because all the time the bone was functioning as a support for the implant) from resorption of the alveolar bone on the opposite side (indicated by the red arrow). Since implant retention clips were unknown at the time, the embedded endosseous leaf implant, which is still strong after four decades, can still be used to stabilize the lower acrylate prosthesis. The patient's complaints were caused by the loosening of the natural tooth, not the implant. On the contrary, the bone is more preserved than on the opposite side, where the compression of the acrylate plate has enhanced bone resorption. The tightly integrated implant can further be used to retain the total acrylic prosthesis in two ways; by creating a crown on the implant support of the edentulous saddle, continue the retention of the mobile acrylic prosthesis with a wire hook or drill a recess in the acrylic part of the prosthesis into which the fixed implant support can enter. Fill the widened recess with soft acrylate, which will approximately replace the role of the retentIon clIp. The comfort of the patient, considering the advanced life age, can be extended.

The extent of today's oral implantology in the rehabilitation of distal edentulous alveoral ridges by implant-prosthetic treatment is confirmed by the case of a patient who, four decades ago (1976), by implanting endosseus leaf implants connected to a natural tooth, preserved comfort in the oral cavity with fixed prosthetic work instead of an unpleasant partial denture. Recently (November 2016), the attending physician from another city and country called me for advice, the patient has pain due to a loose canine on which the fixed prosthetic work is connected to the Linkov's endosteal implant of the "First Generation" (Fig. 14.8). In the meantime, the patient lost all her teeth, and the prosthetic work done four decades ago was retained. The dentist in another institution, after removing all the teeth, used the remaining fixed prosthetic work to retinate the partial acrylic prosthesis with a wire hook. It is important to emphasize that the resorption of the alveolar bone is much lower on the toothless distal alveolar ridge

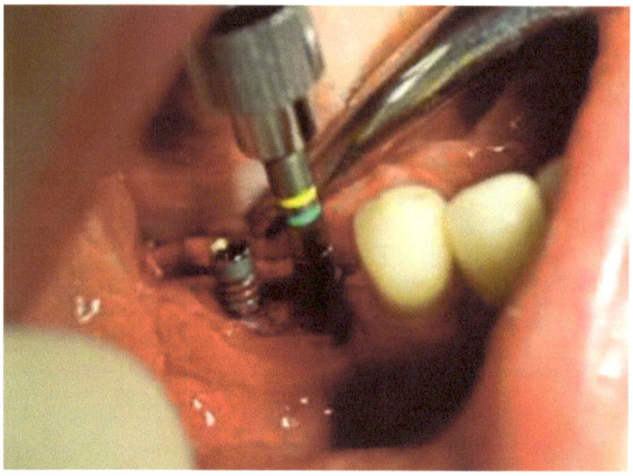

Figure 14.5. Distal toothless alveolar ridge. Installation of two endosteal implants.

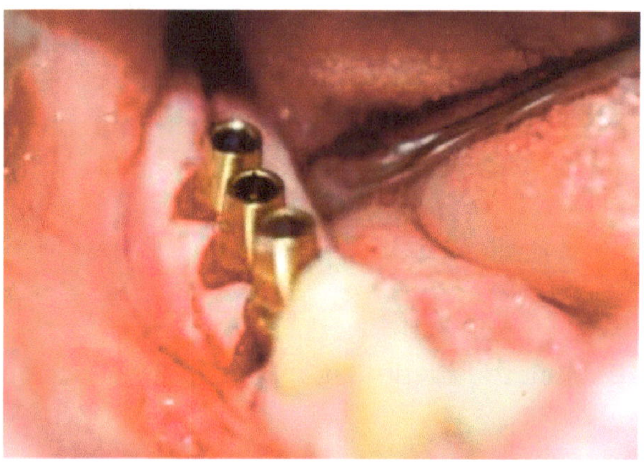

Figure 14.6. Endosteal implants in the distal toothless ridge.

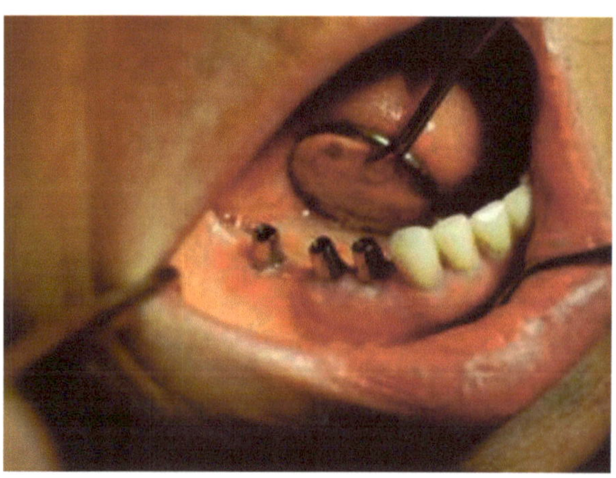

Figure 14.7. Implanted endosteal implants in the distal toothless alveolar ridge.

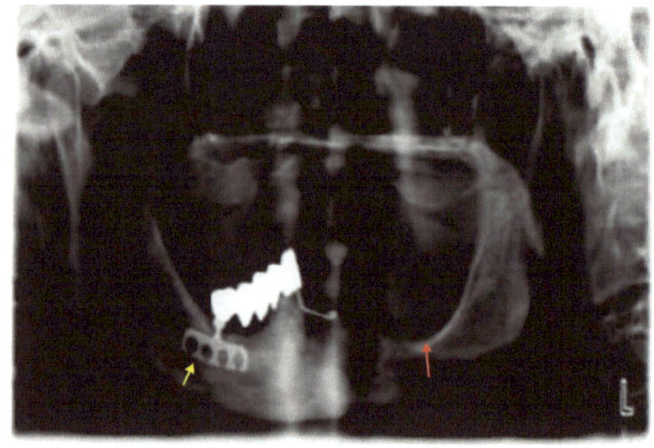

Figure 14.8. Implant-prosthetic rehabilitation of the distal toothless alveolar ridge with a leafed Linkov endosteal implant four decades ago, when the patient was replaced with a one-sided partial acrylic prosthesis with fixed prosthetic work, anchored on the endosteal leaf implant and a natural tooth. (To compare, the resorption of the alveolar bone caused by the compression of the partial acrylic prosthesis (red arrow) is higher than the bone of the implanted implant region (yellow arrow). The work of the book's author (1976.). At the time of placement of the first-generation leaf-shaped open Link implant, the patient had all teeth, except for regions 44.45, 46 and 47.

where the implant was implanted, (because for the entire time the bone was in function as a support for the implant) from the resorption of the alveoral bone on the opposite side (indicated by a red arrow). Since retention clips on implants were not known at the time, the implanted endosteal leaf implant, which is still solid after four decades, can still be used to stabilize the lower acrylic denture. The patient's problems were caused by disentangling the natural tooth, not the implant. On the contrary, the bone is more preserved than on the opposite side and where the compression of the acrylate plate promotes bone resorption. The tightly integrated implant can be further used to retinate the total acrylate prosthesis in two ways; by making a crown on the implant bracket of the toothless saddle, the retinating of the mobile acrylate prosthesis can continue with a wire hook or drill a recess into the acrylate part of the prosthesis into which the fixed implant bracket can enter. Fill the expanded recess with soft acrylate, which will approximately replace the role of the retention clip. The comfort of the patient, given the advanced age, can be extended.

3. **Lack of all teeth.** In the case of complete edentulousness, by installing an appropriate number of endosseus implants, the patient can be rehabili-

tated with fixed prosthetic work instead of a total denture, which is an incomparably more comfortable solution (Fig. 14.11). As pointed out earlier, even if there are no conditions for the placement of the appropriate number of implants to perform fixed prosthetic work, the placement of at least two implants can significantly improve the retention of total dentures (Fig. 14.9 and 14. 10) which is much more comfortable for the patient, especially when it comes to the care of edentulousness in the lower jaw. In extreme toothless atrophied alveoral ridges in the lower jaw, where there is no possibility of implant placement for fixed prosthetic work, total acrylic dentures can be stabilized with retention clips on the implants. (Figures 14.9 and 14.10.)

The solution in the edentulous lower and upper jaw with fixed prosthetic work on implants is incomparably more comfortable than a mobile acrylic prosthesis. (Fig. 14.11 and 14.12).

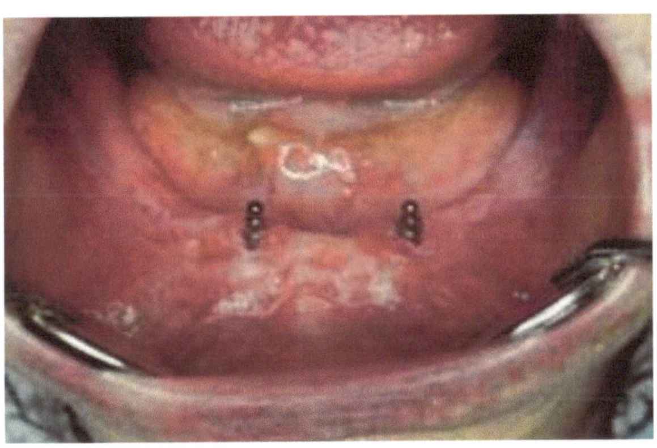

Figure 14.9. Endosseus implants, implanted and loaded to stabilize the lower total denture.

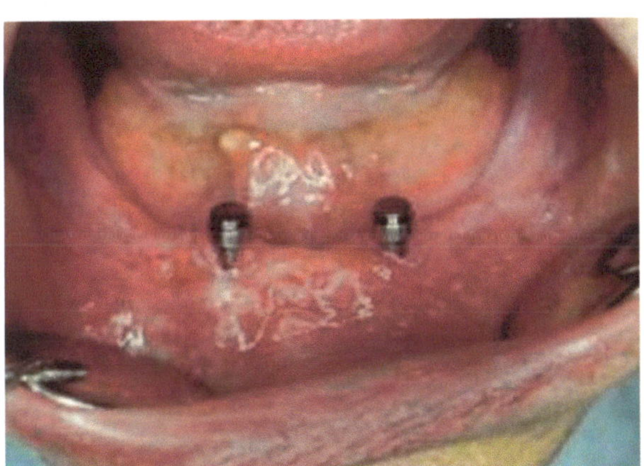

Figure 14.10. Retention clips on implants that remain in the acrylic part of the denture.

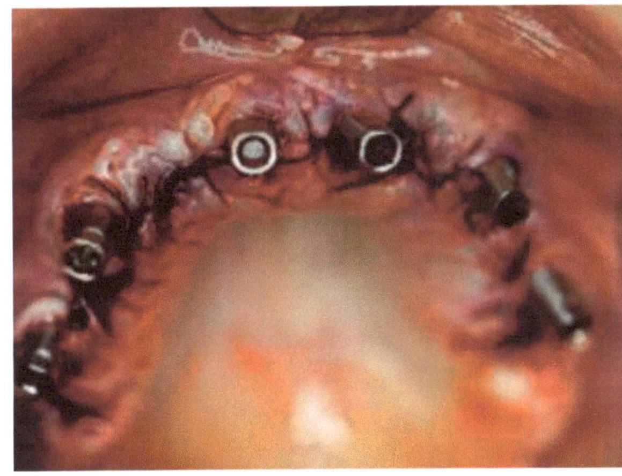

Figure 14.11. Immediately implanted endosteal implants and immediately loaded with fixed tentative work in the edentulous upper jaw. By restoring bone function, its resorption is slowed down, as opposed to an acrylic prosthesis that is promoted.

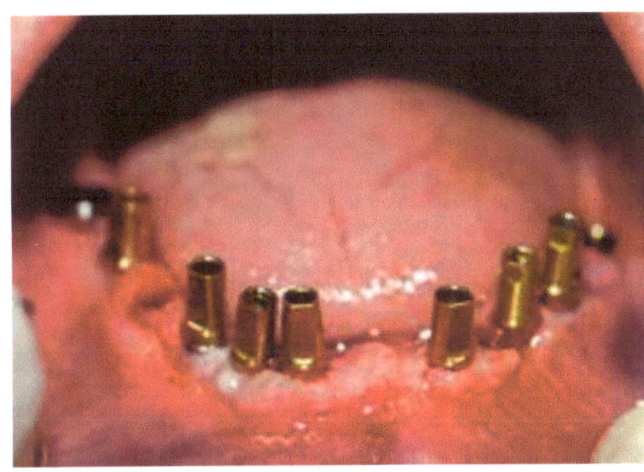

Figure 14.12. Immediately implanted endosteal implants in the edentulous lower jaw with definite abutments.

Contraindications

As is generally the "rule", the development of the profession also reduces the number of contraindications to the use of a procedure. When it comes to oral implantology, whose development has reached unprecedented proportions in recent decades, it is not surprising that the number of contraindications to the use of endosteal implantation has drastically decreased since the time of its inception, which the author witnessed. It could be freely said that absolute contraindications for the placement of dental implants essentially do not exist in everyday dental practice - there are numerous cases, which will be listed below, when it is not advisable to immediately start the implantation, but to postpone it until the situation changes. This means that all contraindications, which will be listed, are in fact restrictions of a temporary nature until the conditions are met for the implantation to be performed subsequently in the interested patient. It is not disputed that there are situations when it is not advisable to perform the implantation at the moment when the interested patient comes forward; in other words, there are situations when the implantation should be postponed until favorable conditions are created. All those contraindications, essentially relative, may exist due to unfavorable local or general conditions, and sometimes the age of the patient can be a factor in giving up prosthetic rehabilitation of the patient by implanting implants on which the planned prosthetic work would be fixed.

1. Local contraindications. Local contraindications are probably more common than others and relate to the situation in the mouth. Most often, it is about poorly maintained oral hygiene and the lack of motivation of the patient to adequately maintain it. Indeed, if a patient comes forward with a desire to have implants placed in the area of missing teeth, and with evidently poor oral hygiene, such a patient is definitely not a candidate for endosseus implants, at least not at that moment. However, the reasons why it is not indicative to approach the implantation should be discussed and explained with such a patient. But this does not mean that such patient should be definitely rejected. The recommended procedure would be, in a few visits, to completely remedy the situation in the oral cavity and to explain to him how the situation thus remedied should be maintained. In particular, it should be explained in detail that the maintenance of oral hygiene should be carried out even more in detail if implants are installed and that, in these conditions, the maintenance of oral hygiene is much more complicated and requires much greater effort. If, in the coming weeks, the dentist concludes that the patient has fundamentally changed his behavioral attitude when it comes to maintaining oral hygiene, the initial contraindication to the placement of oral implants will no longer apply. Thus, the initial contraindication was not absolute, but relative in nature.

It has already been pointed out that the presence of parafunctions creates biomechanical circumstances that can have a very negative impact on the success of implant-prosthetic therapy. Such circumstances should be recognized in a timely manner and their negative effect should be commented in detail with the patient. It is not disputed that the presence of parafunctions represents a definite risk to the success of implantation, which has already been discussed in the early chapters, but this is not in the true sense of the word a contraindication to implantation - no, the patient should be informed about this risk, and the final decision is made jointly by the implantologist and the patient. A similar negative effect on the end outcome of implantation may also have unfavorable intervicular relations, as well as unfavorable anatomical circumstances (lowered under the maxillary sinus in the lower jaw or high position of the mandibular canal in the lower). However, these are not contraindications in the true sense of the word, although they require detailed consideration of ways to overcome their adverse effect. And these are circumstances that should be discussed with the patient, but an experienced implantologist can always find a way to overcome them, either by choosing implants or additional surgical interventions (augmentation, sinus-lift) or by the method of modeling that will be worn with implants.

2. Age of the patient. The patient's age is sometimes classified as a possible contraindication, both due to the likely presence of some general diseases and due to the potentially weaker mental activity of older people. However, the "calendar age" of the patient, especially nowadays, does not provide any even remotely valid data on his "biological age". At one time, it was believed that people in advanced age (it was never known what exactly this meant) were not always able to responsibly perform the necessary activities to ensure the success of implant rehabilitation. This may be true for individuals, but it has nothing to do with the age of the patient. An experienced implantologist should, in a conversation with the patient, carefully consider all the circumstances important for the successful maintenance of the implant in each individual case, and the definitive decision is not based on the age of the patient, but on the conclusion of his motivation and willingness to follow instructions, both in terms of maintaining oral hygiene and all aspects of treatment and postoperative and postimplantation course.

3. General contraindications. General contraindications for the placement of oral implants, mainly, refer to the presence of general diseases that could pose a risk for any oral surgical intervention, starting with routine tooth extraction. However, even in the case of such potential contraindications, it should be in mind that they are, as a rule, temporary and not absolute in nature. In doing so, it seems even more important to point out that people with impaired health also have a basic right to function better and look more beautiful; if this can be achieved by implant-prosthetic rehabilitation, what would be the justification for avoiding such a thing with the excuse that there is a risk? After all, by gaining the patient's trust and adequately suppressing the pain during the intervention, it is understood by both professional and careful work, the stress that the patient experiences during the implant placement is lower than during most other oral surgical interventions.

According to the generally accepted classification of diseases given by the American Association of Anesthesiologists (ASA), the so-called ASA classification, healthy patients were classified in the first, and patients with discrete systemic changes in the second group. Patients of these 2 groups are by far the most common candidates for dental endosteal implants. It is almost unbelievable that patients with severe systemic diseases or complications of these diseases would come forward with the desire to undergo implant-prosthetic rehabilitation in such a situation. In the vast majority of cases, there are no general complications for dental implants because patients who would have such contraindications do not come with such desires. If data on the existence of such disease were to be obtained in the medical history, the procedure is the same as for any other oral surgical intervention - consultation with the appropriate specialist who treats the underlying disease and possible preparation of the patient before the procedure.

And, one should never lose sight of the fact that the patient will benefit very significantly from implant-prosthetic rehabilitation: better chewing function and a more beautiful appearance. Only an apparent dilemma remains: should such benefits be denied to people who are not healthy? The question remains: is it humane? Each therapist should answer such questions independently in accordance with their conscience!

At a time when oral implantology was not developed and applicable at today's level, the general contraindications that were considered and as absolute were systematized in the following order:

Heart disease and other cardiac weaknesses were considered in the first place as the most common absolute contraindications for implant placement.

The order of general contraindications includes: systemic diseases, kidney diseases, uncontrolled diabetes mellitus, diseases of the immune system, hyperparathyroidism, diseases of coagulation disorders, diseases of the bone system and osteomalacia.

The list of general absolute contraindications also includes acute leukemia and malignancies. These diseases are an absolute contraindication to the placement of implants, but it is certain that patients with such severe diseases do not think about the placement of dental implants given the short survival period.

However, it happens that such patients seek help from a dentist due to pain in the oral cavity of different origins. The dentist must also know about the manifestations of these diseases in the oral cavity. For example, symptoms of general anemia, neutropenia and thrombocytopenia are also clearly manifested in the oral cavity through discoloration of the mucous tissue. Neutropenia can cause reactivation of chronic focal infection, periodontitis, herpes labialis accompanied by ulcero-necrotic lesions. Mucous hemorrhages (echimoses) are often seen in the oral cavity. Thrombocytopenia may increase bleeding gums as well as major petechial mucosal hemorrhages. Lymph nodules may also appear in the parathyroid gland.

Also, a decline in the immune system can be a temporary general contraindication to implant placement. The decline of the body's immune system can significantly impair homeostasis and must be taken into account in patients who want implant-prosthetic treatment. The decline of the immune system is caused by viruses and can be an absolute contraindication to implantation, one of the most dangerous viruses is the HIV virus, which was discovered and isolated only in 1983.

The characteristic changes caused by this virus are often also clearly manifested in the oral cavity as Kapovši's sarcoma, clearly expressed as angiomatous pink or purple plaque with uneven nodules of irregular shape. Ulcerations are also pronounced, most often localized on the hard part of the palate: with candidal changes, the golden color gives the image of pseudo-membranous plaque. The occurrence of hemorrhagic lesions, leukoplakia, cervical microadenopathy, which is an expression of systemic polyodentopathy. When it comes to kidney diseases, primarily diabetes mellitus as a complex disease, it can also manifest itself on oral health, firstly on the paradontium. A diabetic who maintains strict glycemic control is not contraindicated for the placement of implants. Nevertheless, the implantologist must be familiar with the basic symptoms of these diseases, and in the anamnestic approach to examine what type of diabetes it is., one must have insight into the severity of cardiovascular and renal disease, arterial hypertension as well as neuropathic problems.

Diabetic patients who are not insulin-dependent, and who are compensated and regularly controlled by the attending urologist, show proper glycemic control with anamnestic data and the absence of diabetic complications, implant placement is indicated. In diabetic patients, special attention must be paid, first of all, to periodontal procedures during the healing period, in order to avoid the occurrence of infections, especially in the first week of the epithelialization phase.

In patients who are dependent on insulin therapy, and if they are still with cardiovascular and renal complications, the decision to use implant-prosthetic treatment must be approached very carefully. In any case, the decision on implanting the implant should be made by consulting an appropriate specialist, primarily an endocrinologist.

The above indicates that the implantologist should know the basic symptoms of this disease. This disease, or syndrome, is also characterized by chronic hyperglycemia. From today's point of view, diabetes diseases are classified on the basis of clinical and therapeutic aspects;

Clinical aspect:

- skinny and obese people, children and adults exposed to diabetes

Therapeutic aspect:

- insulin-dependent and insulin-independent diabetes.

The current classification of diabetes is based on physio-pathological criteria:

- type 1: insulin-dependent
- type 2: does not show an immunogenic aspect, and this form of diabetes is not dependent on insulin administration.

In younger patients under 40 years of age, the clinical picture is manifested by the following symptoms:

- sudden weight loss;
- nocturnal polyuria;
- feeling thirsty
- asthenia and
- gingival and periodontal inflammation.

A urine analysis can be used to determine whether or not such patients are dependent on insulin, and the clinical picture can often change. Diagnosing diabetes can be through pathophysiological complications; manifested in the eyes, neurological disorders, cardiovascular and renal diseases, and also manifestations in the oral cavity.

Patients with diagnosed hyperparathyroidism must be approached with caution and can be considered one of the general contraindications. In general, hyperthyroidism is caused by a disturbed homeostasis in the metabolism of calcium and phosphorus, followed by pronounced hypersecretion of parathyroid hormone with symptoms of the disease: diffuse pain in the bones; spontaneous bone fractures, especially on the femur and other bones, in Paget's disease and cancer. All this can have an impact, if implants are installed, on the osseointegration processes.

Patients with coronary disease

When considering a patient with coronary disease during a phase when there is a temporary contraindication for the placement of implants, it's important for the patient to be familiar with not only implantologists but also all dental specialties. In cases involving implant procedures, awareness of the symptoms of coronary disease is crucial primarily for safety reasons rather than as a strict contraindication, as incidents related to such diseases can occur at any time.

Patients with coronary disease often experience changes in their blood vessels, which result in a reduced supply of oxygen to the heart. A lack of oxygen at the cellular level within the myocardium causes the heart to work harder to fulfill its functions.

Patients with angina pectoris can typically be identified through thorough questioning about their medical history. The most common symptoms in these patients include the onset of pain in the chest area and the left shoulder when engaging in activities such as walking briskly, climbing stairs, or exerting themselves in other ways. These symptoms may also occur in cold conditions, often leading them to stop and rest to compensate for the lack of oxygen required by the heart muscle (myocardium).

Extreme caution is necessary for patients who have experienced a previous heart attack, as the heart muscle may be permanently damaged, and their blood vessels are often weakened.

The clinical signs that indicate a pre-infarction state and may lead to an actual heart attack include:

- Anxiety and a fear of death
- Chest pain, which is often the first symptom of a heart attack
- A feeling of strong pressure or heaviness in the chest
- Cough, fatigue, nausea, and loss of appetite.

Pain starting in the chest spreads to other body parts; on the shoulders, arms, elbows, back, and neck, especially in the lower jaw and part of the abdomen. There is no rule for the spread of pain because the pain in the chest can stop and continue to manifest strongly on the left or right arm. It does not stop even after the application of nitrates.

The mentioned manifestations are accompanied by a rapid and irregular pulse. Sweating and the urge to vomit are also symptoms of a heart attack. Rapid swelling of the feet, ankles, legs, and abdomen is also possible. All these symptoms are accompanied by a feeling of strong weakness and fatigue.

What is the implantologist's procedure in patients with previous infarction?

It is necessary to delay implant intervention for at least six months to a year after pectoral angina attacks and previous heart attacks. Even after that, the author of the book advises that the written consent of the cardiologist is also necessary.

When deciding on oral surgical implant procedures, it is desirable to fulfill the following conditions:

- Request a written report and opinion from the cardiologist confirming that oral surgical intervention is possible.
- Address the factors that lead to emotional stress (such as fear of intervention), which can increase adrenaline secretion and subsequently raise the myocardium's oxygen demand.
- If necessary, which is often the case, prescribe anxiolytics or sedatives.
- Use a surface anesthetic and a thin needle to ensure a painless puncture and anesthetic injection.
- Be familiar with the characteristics of different anesthetics.
- Monitor the prothrombin level and temporarily discontinue anticoagulants to prevent bleeding during oral surgery.
- Prepare all conditions to carry out the surgical intervention with precision, minimizing aggression and duration, which largely depends on the experience of the implantologist.
- Do not prescribe drugs containing acetylsalicylate (aspirin) or drugs from the phenyl-butazone group and their derivatives, which can act as anticoagulants.
- Coronary disease, changes in the heart valves, are classified as serious contraindications for implant placement.
- Changes in the heart valves (Cardiopathia valvularis) today belong to temporary contraindications for implantological procedures. Today, the treatment of this disease is possible in more ways. A dentist plays a crucial role in dental therapy, which includes prophylaxis—the removal of all sources of focal infection. In cases of bacterial endocarditis, this approach is fundamental for the rehabilitation and treatment of valvulopathies.
- For patients with diseased heart valves, it is essential to eliminate all sources of infection, particularly waste bacteria originating from dental issues. The treatment principle for these patients involves the following steps:

   1. Radically removing all diseased teeth, including those with infected roots, granulomas, and any devitalized teeth.
   2. Rehabilitating the supporting structures of the teeth, known as the periodontium, to thoroughly eliminate harmful bacteria, especially oral streptococci.

- Acute rheumatic joint inflammation, primarily triggered by streptococcal infection, is a more serious systemic condition. Acute rheumatism can lead to significant changes in the pericardium, myocardium, and endocardium. Endocarditis can have severe consequences, resulting in heart murmurs as the valves lose their elasticity. This may lead to permanent damage to the mitral and aortic valves, significantly increasing the risk of bacterial endocarditis.
- Patients suffering from endocarditis belong to the risk group of all dental interventions, and in the case of implantological interventions, they must be protected with antibiotics, because thrombus can form on the valves. If you want to install implants in such patients, you must approach with great caution.

Conclusion

However, coronary insufficiency, with the development of oral implantology, no longer represents an absolute contraindication for implant surgery, but requires caution and cooperation with a cardiologist and his support.

Psychogenic pain and other unpleasant sensations in oral implantology

The decision to focus this chapter on the study of psychogenic pain and other unexpected unpleasant sensations stems from decades of clinical experience. My dedication to exploring this issue within oral implantology arises from my own encounters with psychogenic pain. Despite my long experience and the belief that I had successfully performed an implant-prosthetic procedure, I once mistakenly miscommunicated with a patient. I suggested that they consult a neurologist and psychiatrist, as objective evaluations indicated no pathological changes in the mouth. Unfortunately, this well-intentioned advice was taken as an insult by the patient.

Another reason for my focus on this topic is the lack of literature addressing the treatment of psychogenic pain and other unpleasant sensations following successful implant-prosthetic interventions. This important issue is notably absent from dental and implantology textbooks. A logical question arises: where should psychogenic pain and unpleasant sensations be classified after a successfully completed implant-prosthetic treatment plan? They do not fit neatly into either contraindications or complications of implant treatment. Psychogenic pain exists as a phenomenon that has not yet found its place in implantology literature. While textbooks may overlook such topics, the scientific community has produced numerous works that delve into the study of psychogenic pain.

The decision to focus this chapter on the study of psychogenic pain and other unexpected unpleasant sensations stems from decades of clinical experience. My dedication to exploring this issue within oral implantology arises from my own encounters with psychogenic pain. Despite my long experience and the belief that I had successfully performed an implant-prosthetic procedure, I once mistakenly miscommunicated with a patient. I suggested that they consult a neurologist and psychiatrist, as objective evaluations indicated no pathological changes in the mouth. Unfortunately, this well-intentioned advice was taken as an insult by the patient.

Another reason for my focus on this topic is the lack of literature addressing the treatment of psychogenic pain and other unpleasant sensations following successful implant-prosthetic interventions. This important issue is notably absent from dental and implantology textbooks. A logical question arises: where should psychogenic pain and unpleasant sensations be classified after a successfully completed implant-prosthetic treatment plan? They do not fit neatly into either contraindications or complications of implant treatment. Psychogenic pain exists as a phenomenon that has not yet found its place in implantology literature. While textbooks may overlook such topics, the scientific community has produced numerous works that delve into the study of psychogenic pain.

In everyday dental practice, we occasionally encounter patients who, despite the exceptional efforts of the dental professional, remain unsatisfied with the outcomes of their treatment. This dissatisfaction may pertain to either the function or aesthetics of prosthetic work and can surface as vague complaints that arise after the treatment is completed. One particular issue is pain, which may differ in duration and nature from the expected postoperative pain.

Persistent idiopathic facial pain (PIFP) is recognized as one of the most challenging and distressing pain syndromes faced by medical and dental practitioners. This type of pain was first identified in 1947 by McElhin and Horton, who referred to it as atypical facial pain. Although such cases are not uncommon in clinical settings, there is still no consensus on the causes, terminology, classification, and diagnostic criteria related to this condition. Furthermore, these painful conditions are often under-researched and frequently overlooked by practitioners.

Terminology

Several names are used for this type of pain, such as: Persistent idiopathic facial pain (PIFP), atypical facial pain, orofacial pain, and psychogenic pain. This type of pain is not etiologically explained and represents a differential diagnostic challenge. Similar syndromes described are "burning mouth syndrome" and "temporomandibular joint pain", "atypical odontalgia" and "phantom tooth syndrome". Several terms are used in the literature without a general consensus, so often the same pain can be called by different terms, and the same term can be used for two different types of pain.

Characteristics

Persistent idiopathic pain after implant placement occurs immediately after an oral surgical procedure or later, without a clear, known and confirmed reason. According to the International Pain Association, a duration of more than 6 months is necessary for the pain to meet the criteria of chronicity. Complaints can refer to pain as well as other sensations: burning, stinging, stabbing, throbbing, tingling, and a whole series of graphic descriptions that the patient uses to describe the sensations that torment and preoccupy him. The pain does not have a typical quality corresponding to the anatomy of the transmission of sensory signals and does not correspond to any of the known pain syndromes (trigeminal neuralgia, headaches, sinusitis, etc.). There is no objective loss in sensitivity and it is most often localized maxillary and unilateral. A psychogenic component is often suspected, which may or may not be confirmed.

Frequency

Chronic orofacial pain accounts for 20-25% of chronic pain conditions. The prevalence for a duration of 6 months is between 1-3% of the population. According to Locker & assoc. slightly less than 10% of the population had some unpleasant sensations in the oral region for a measured month. Bonica in 1980. finds that 5-7 million Americans suffer from some type of chronic pain in the oral and facial regions, and that 25-45% have experienced some type of pain in this region in their lifetime. According to most studies, pain occurs in the female sex, according to some studies more often in the late sixties and fifties, and according to some studies, the age distribution is insignificant. The frequency of persistent idiopathic pain after implant placement is not statistically measured, while PIFP pain after other dental procedures is between 3-6%. This is also important to point out that the incidence of trigeminal neuropathic syndrome after implant intervention in the upper jaw is extremely high around 0.9% and is rarely described in the literature. In these cases, it is a confirmed violation of the trigeminal branch. Likewise, neuropathic orofacial pain after implant placement and other dental interventions (endodontic root canal treatment, apicotomy, tooth extraction, cystectomy) is stated to be idiopathic pain. Mueller and Cavo in 2001. Have through an extensive review of the literature on the topic of pain and implant placement, found that the professional literature on this topic is scarce, and by examining sensory experiences in the postoperative period, they have come to the conclusion that there is no significant statistical correlation between implant placement and chronic pain, which speaks in favor of other etiological factors, including the psychogenic factor. The necessary differential diagnosis should exclude medical and dental causes, it is indicated to do X-ray and MRI of the head, consult a neurologist, maxillofacial surgeon and anesthesiologist specialist in painful conditions, psychiatrist and internist. Conditions that must be differentially diagnostically excluded are: eye diseases, ear diseases, sinusitis, nasal disorders, periodontal diseases, odontalgia, glossodynia, headaches, cranial neuralgia, central origin of pain. Then psychogenic type pain, pain in delusional, hallucinatory and other psychotic disorders, somatoform pain, hypochondrial preoccupation, pain related to depression and anxiety states.

Clinical course

When the pain in the orofacial region persists even after the acute postoperative phase and in addition to classic conservative methods, the first suspicion of chronic type pain without a clear cause appears. There is also a possibility that pain or other sensations were expressed to a lesser extent and preoperatively, and that this was not recorded anamnestically or the symptoms were understood as a result of a bad overall oral situation. If dissatisfaction with the results of implant-prosthetic treatment cannot be objectively explained through a critical analysis of all aspects of the work, from the installation and quality of implants, prosthetic work, periodontal surgery, application of augments and other materials, the search for the cause of the painful syndrome begins. However, sometimes the understanding of the origin of complaints cannot be explained by an objective finding. The patient continues to persistently complain even after support, reassurance and minor interventions. The implantologist is then at a crossroads; when he either rejects the patient and refers him to another specialist, or works on correcting his work in the hope of removing the patient's dissatisfaction and complaints. If it really was a mistake, the complaints should disappear, and the patient is satisfied with his new appearance and function of the teeth, which also improves his quality of life. However, if this does not happen, the spiral of repeated attempts and dissatisfaction continues. Then it is recommended to pay attention in detail to the nature of the complaints that the patient is complaining about. The patient uses a series of comparisons to which he associates the pain. It is necessary to pay attention to the fluctuation of these sensations, when they intensify, whether they depend on the time of day, at what intervals they occur, what increases them and what decreases them, how they respond to analgesics and whether there is any psychological connection with the pain. The doctor gradually begins to suspect that there is some psychogenic factor in the etiology of the pain. In the beginning, it is difficult to prove it. The patient often seeks the help of another implantologist on his own initiative or turns to another specialist. Given that the tests he performs are not coordinated, each doctor looks at the patient's situation partially from his own perspective, and some of them think that they can solve a complicated case, and out of omnipotence or profit motive, they take further steps in reparation of the found condition - iatrogenization is inevitable. What has been shown to be a feature of this type of pain in some cases is a temporary improvement after an intervention that tries to eliminate the pain, this improvement is often short-lived and the patient soon complains of old complaints. Thus, in one case, the author of the book referred a patient who suspected psychogenic pain to a maxillofacial surgeon who, believing that it was atypical maxillofacial pain, decided on anesthetic block therapy. However, after completing the therapy with anesthetic blocks lasting several weeks, the patient continued to complain even more about the old complaints. Such cases of short-term improvement after the introduction of a new therapy are also found in other branches of medicine, which speaks in favor of becoming a factor of psychological suggestion. Of course, we are talking here about cases when all objective diagnostic and therapeutic methods have been exhausted and when the suspicion of a psychogenic factor becomes more and more real. In practice, such patients wander from "door to door" on their own, ie. from doctor's office to doctor's office, and case integration is missing, which further worsens the patient's condition. It happens that the implantologist, whether he worked with superficial knowledge or medical vanity, with a non-collegial approach, contrary to the Hippocratic Oath, instead of helping the patient, leads him into even bigger problems. In this case, a multidisciplinary approach and high-quality, open, written medical and oral communication between colleagues is necessary.

If all factors as the cause of pain or other unpleasant sensations are excluded, we can suspect that it is psychogenic pain. Psychogenic pain is a condition in which pain is caused, intensified or prolonged by psychological factors and causes a significant degree of suffering and reduced quality of life. A person with this type of pain syndrome spends a significant amount of time thinking about and trying to relieve the pain. In addition to pain, as stated, there is a whole series of sensations such as burning, stinging, stabbing, throbbing, which similarly occupy the patient's attention. The characteristics of this pain are: chronic course, imprecise and deep localization, variable intensity from mild to intense and other accompanying unpleasant sensations. Sometimes it is possible to clearly connect certain psycho-social stresses as provoking factors, and sometimes it is done with unconscious and interpersonal factors that cannot be recognized, named and verbalized. Comorbidity of psychogenic pain with depression or anxiety is common, and it can also be "masked depression" that manifests itself through various somatizations. This disorder is located in the "gray, transition zone" of diagnosis between the specialties of psychiatry, neurology and dentistry, and within psychiatry it can be classified under several disorders.

Classification of persistent facial atypical pain

The International Classification of Headaches compiled by the International Headache Society places persistent idiopathic facial pain (PIPF) in subgroup 13-18: "Central causes of facial pain", along with other entities, such as anesthesia dolorosis, central pain after stroke, pain as a consequence multiple sclerosis and burning mouth syndrome. PIPF is included in the group "Cranial neuralgias and central causes of facial pain," under diagnostic number 13,14.4. PIPF is diagnosed when all possible systemic and local causes have been ruled out. The international classification of diseases in the chapter of complications of surgical treatment not specified elsewhere (T 80-T88) includes pain due to the installation of orthopedic prosthetic bodies (knees and hips), dental implants and grafts can also be classified here, which is not a consequence of other known recorded complications (T84). This diagnosis is closest to what is described as pain caused by a complication of surgical procedures in oral implantology. Undoubtedly, these diagnosis often include those patients who have a psychogenic influence on pain.

Classification of psychogenic pain

It is necessary to emphasize that every idiopathic pain is not psychogenic, and when existing doubts are considered after exhaustive treatment and confirmation, then it is useful to consult psychiatric diagnostic criteria. According to the international classification of mental disorders ICD-10 (somatoform disorder) represents "frequent presentation of physical symptoms and constant requests for medical tests despite repeated negative results and reassurance from the implantologist that the symptoms have no physical basis." If there is a somatic illness, it does not explain the nature and existence of the symptoms or the exhaustion and preoccupation of the patient. The patient usually rejects any attempt to discuss the possibility of psychological causes, this may also be the case in the presence of obvious depressive or anxiety states." How problematic this group of disorders is for psychiatry itself, is shown by the fact that even in the classification of somatoform disorders (ICD 10), difficulties and even contradictions in defining this disorder can be observed. The characteristic of this group of disorders is that they are not mediated through the autonomic nervous system and are not limited to specific systems or parts of the body, which separates them from multiple and undifferentiated somatizing disorders. The American Classification of Mental Disorders (DSM V) places such conditions within a large group of somatoform disorders in which somatization and conversion disorders with hypochondriasis, dysmorphobia, and pain disorder are separated as subtypes. In these disorders, according to ICD-10, "there is usually a certain degree of attracting attention, especially in patients who are offended by the failure to convince the doctor of the physical nature of their illness and the need for further research and testing."

Characteristic in this case is the variability of symptoms, ie. a sensation for which an adequate medical, physical cause cannot be found, persistent non-acceptance of the implantologist's opinion that there is no physical explanation for the symptoms, and a certain degree of impaired social and family behavior. Somatization disorder can also take on elements of hypochondria, which is characterized by the development of fear of a certain disease and a certain bad outcome of treatment, a pessimistic attitude with accompanying anxiety-depressive symptoms, and in more extreme cases, consequent suicidal ideas. An implantologist who engages in giving superficial evaluations to a patient who visits several offices must also keep this in mind. In the case of chronicity, and if complaints of persistent, severe and debilitating pain persist that cannot be fully explained by physiological processes or somatic disorders and usually occur in circumstances that indicate that the pain is related to conflicts or problems, then according to the international classification of diseases (ICD-10) calls this phenomenon "Persistent somatoform pain disorder". According to the same classification, it is stated that "It is usually the result of increased support and attention, whether personal or medical". Respecting the subjective psychological reality of pain and other unpleasant sensations for the patient, another diagnostic category from ICD 10 is taken into account - "Elaboration of somatic symptoms due to psychological reasons" when symptoms that are due to a disease or some medical treatment (in this case implantology) "become overemphasized and prolonged due to the patient's psychological condition. A behavioral syndrome of attracting attention (histrionic syndrome) develops, which may also include additional (usually non-specific) complaints that are not of somatic origin. The patient is usually uncomfortable with physical pain or disability and is often preoccupied with concerns, which may be justified, about the possibility of prolonged or progressive disability or pain. , can also be motivational factors. Some cases are clearly motivated by the possibility of financial compensation for an accident or injury (in this case implantological intervention), but this syndrome does not have to be resolved even when such demands are satisfied".

Building on this disorder, ICD 10 also recognizes the diagnosis: "Deliberately causing symptoms or simulating symptoms or disabilities, somatic or psychological (artificial disorder)". These individuals with no proven medical disorder persistently simulate symptoms. A sensitive, difficult, and sometimes impossible understanding of the motivation for this behavior is essential, with the basic question whether it is a conscious search for profit and material compensation (the high cost of implant-prosthetic treatment) or an unconscious motivation to divert attention.

Psychodynamic aspects of pain

The reaction of the patient and the doctor is frustrating; the physician may react with feelings of irritability, anger, powerlessness, guilt, and incompetence. The patient also develops feelings; from dissatisfaction and suspicion, all the way to accusing the implantologist of the damage caused. What is important to emphasize is the subjective dimension of the symptoms, which is superimposed on the previous oral intervention. Certain people develop a subjective, unconscious intolerance towards new bodies in the mouth, which is expressed in implanted implants. Descriptions of pain and other sensations that change the quality of life and fluctuate in intensity cannot be explained by an objective finding. It is also possible that the factor of excessive expectations exists in the sense that the implant-prosthetic intervention will change the patient's life in all aspects of functioning, and that the suppressed dissatisfaction in other aspects of functioning will pass after the implantological intervention. If the patient had some form of anxiety or depressive disorder before the implant intervention, or met the criteria for one of the personality disorders, in those cases there is an unconscious emotional hyperinvestment in implant-prosthetic intervention, which is expected to solve all problems. Further unrecognized psychological conflicts that can lead to psychogenic sensations are those related to difficulties with accepting changes related to aging, loneliness, "empty nest syndrome", unsatisfied need for attention and closeness, fear of physical weakness and finally fear of death. Various unresolved family and interpersonal conflicts and dissatisfactions can be the source of somatic manifestations that some medical, in this case, implant-prosthetic intervention can trigger. The implantologist should be careful about potential interpretations and connection of psychological facts with pain, because patients generally perceive it as an insult and unjustified psychiatry, which further increases resistance in further cooperation, complicates finding a solution. It takes enormous patience and tact of the implantologist, and acceptance of the fact that pain and other unpleasant sensations, regardless of the fact that they are not medically explainable, represent a subjective psychological fact and the patient's reality.

The terms essential for understanding these phenomena are alexithymia and somatization. Alexithymia (blindness to emotions) which means a person's inability to express, recognize and communicate their feelings with others. Somatization refers to the process of turning unacceptable emotional conflicts into physical symptoms, signs and doubts. Thus, these patients cannot express their depression and anxiety in words and connect them with certain facts from their inner psychic and external life, connect them with events from the past and present, or express concern for the future, but through the mechanism of conversion - converting conflicting emotions, and they express all this through bodily sensations. Such persons may have more pronounced obsessive personality traits with a pronounced need for control, meticulousness and efficiency, and if something fails in the realization of those mechanisms, it becomes unbearable for them and they unconsciously resort to escaping into the somatic - "it is easier for them to be hurt by the body than the soul"- , "it is easier for the implantologist or implant-prosthetic therapy to be blamed for their misfortune, than they themselves or life itself with all its unpredictability". Such questions, of course, enter the field of psychosomatics and are the subject of psychiatry and psychotherapy, not oral implantology and maxillofacial surgery.

Treatment

Treatment of idiopathic and psychogenic pain is a real challenge and there are no reliable guidelines for it. Cases of idiopathic facial pain that occurred after the installation of implants and extremely successfully performed prosthetic work were presented, which were successfully treated with tricyclic antidepressants (amitriptyline, nortriptyline), benzodiazepines (lorazepam, clonazepam and relaxation techniques). There are data on the use of anticonvulsants (lamotrigine, pregabalin, carbamazepine), but no data on significant success. This group of psychopharmaceuticals cannot be exempted from application in these cases. We find works on the local application of 0.025% capsaicin and opiate analgesics (tramadol, codeine) with satisfactory results in some cases.

Conclusion

Pain syndromes of unknown origin in the oral and facial region are often unrecognized or are recognized late, and further education and research in this field is needed. It was my challenge to pay attention to this still unknown in oral implantology. As prevention of such unwanted events, which can never be predicted with certainty, nor prevented, it is recommended: good psychological preoperative preparation for implant-prosthetic procedures, consideration of patient expectations, which may be unrealistic. Work on fears of implantological surgical intervention, subjective feeling related to the fact that the implant as a "foreign body" will become an integral part of the patient's body and will not behave in the organism as a "foreign body". Using anamnestic data to find out about experiences of pain tolerance, preoperative and postoperative pain therapy and anamnestic data on mental disorders. Good differential diagnosis and an early multidisciplinary consultative approach prevent further complication of the clinical situation and interpersonal relations between the implantologist, the medical team and the patient.

Clinical example 1.

A patient in her forties enters the psychiatric office holding gauze in her mouth, evidently after some dental intervention. She just got her last tooth out. She states that for many years she complained of pain, burning, stinging in her mouth, and because of this, she tried several interventions at several dentists that did not bear fruit. She had never seen a psychiatrist before. When asked how she explains the fact that the pains occurred even after various interventions, she answers that this is exactly why she had her teeth extracted. This is, of course, an extreme case, which raises the question of the expertise and ethics of dentists and implantologists who did not recognize what kind of disorder it was, with the fact that such people, upon mentioning that their complaints could be of a psychological nature, quickly change doctors and wander away from the office. to the doctor's office.

Clinical example 2.

A patient in her sixties came forward to solve her case exclusively with implant placement, due to constant pain that she could not determine. After the initial satisfaction after the installation of several implants and the aesthetically successful prosthetic work, after three years, he started to complain of vague pain and other strange sensations in the upper jaw. After re-imaging, examination, treatment, several interventions, the doctor decides to replace the implant, suspecting (3D image) that a barely noticeable periapical shadow on one implant could be the cause of pain that the patient could not determine and localize. After the operation and satisfaction for a while, the patient again does not complain about pain and other sensations, however for a short time. During several repeated examinations, the finding is: complete absence of inflammatory symptoms of soft tissues and peri-implant changes, complaints of undetermined pain continue. The pain is characterized by fluctuations in intensity, intensification in the evening hours, short-term improvements after minor implatological interventions. However, she did not get a satisfactory answer and solution from all the dentists and implantologists she approached.

In the end, after visiting many surgeries, she stopped complaining of vague pain and new requests began. She is dissatisfied with the color of her teeth. It required a lighter color than A2, which is among the lightest. Not recognizing a patient with psychogenic pain, treating with anesthetic blocks is a big mistake.

The experience of the author of the book confirms that psychogenic pain is most often caused by an "aesthetic defect", which "everyone sees", especially those who should not see it, which leads the patient to psychological suffering. In fact, psychogenic pain is suffering, which can end up going from depression to suicide.

The loss of frontal teeth is described as a special psychological pain, and it depends on many factors: age, gender, social status, education, occupation, the rest of the life perspective in longing and suffering to compensate for the lost part of one's body...

A person constantly looks in the mirror that the scheme of aesthetic disorder of her body burdens her more and more, burdening her closest family-closer with pain that she cannot localize and explain. It is extremely important to recognize psychogenic pain for appropriate therapy.

15

Peri-implant Infections

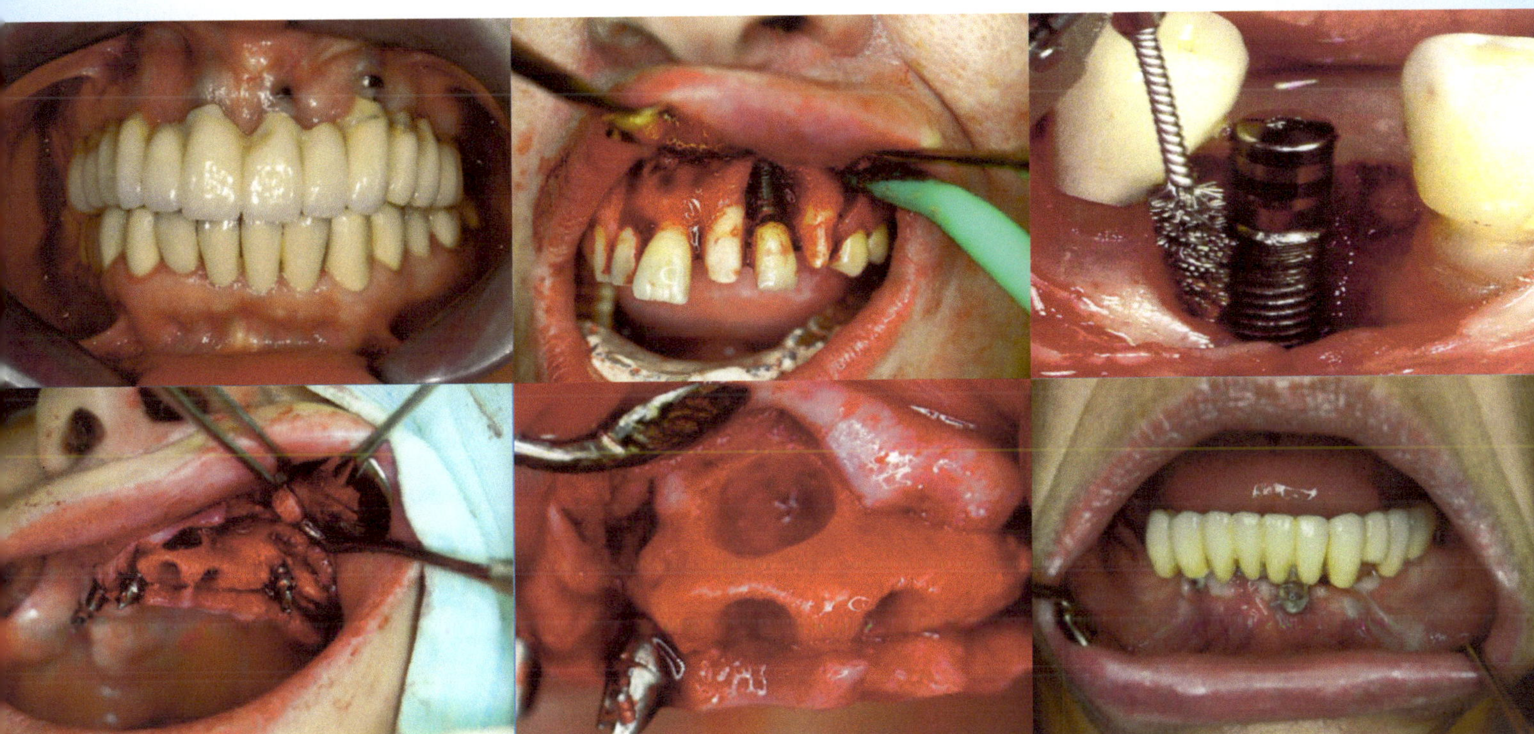

Oral implantology in the last two decades, it can be said, experienced a rapid development, both in the scientific and technological sense. This branch of medicine has become a fusion of art and science. The art of oral implantology is how to plan and predict the final harmony of the patient's face, while at the same time ensuring the successful restoration of bone structures, soft tissues and teeth on the implant. High aesthetic requirements must be accompanied by the stability of all tissues and the perfect function of all these structures over a long period of time. Bone integration is no longer discussed, because it is no longer a priority, although recently it is insisted that implants be made of a combination of titanium and zirconium materials to accelerate bone integration and soft tissue healing. Today, there is more and more talk about a successful aesthetic result. The art of tissue reconstruction is the ability to apply all new information and scientific knowledge from literature, biology, and technology in everyday practice.

The philosophy of implant-prosthetic treatment should be: choose an effective and least invasive procedure and technique for living tissues, and achieve a successful aesthetic and functional result.

The author of the book, as a witness of the time when oral implantology was stagnating, and there were no beaten paths to follow, remembers that the percentage of failures was not negligible. Experience, therefore, points to caution. Despite the fact that this issue has already been discussed in the previous chapter, new findings clarify peri-implant infections in more detail. Many implant systems have been created today. Progress is in the design and processing of the implant surface, especially the design of the structure of the part that is in contact with soft tissues. But, on the other hand, we also have the abuse of the basic goal of progress, because the interest of every industrial production is profit, including the implant industry. Numerous manufacturers of the implant industry offer "new" systems on the market, mostly copies of proven implant systems, but also of different quality. Marketing praise from manufacturers about the advantages of their implant system over others should be taken with a grain of salt until it is verified and confirmed in practice. Many plagiarisms are without a certificate and with a significantly lower price than the copied implant system. The large offer and competition on the market of implant systems caused the price to drop. Such a supply trend, mainly for profitable reasons, also enabled a more massive application. On the other hand, the number of serious complications in the tissues that are in direct contact with the implant has also increased. The percentage of peri-implant diseases ranges from 1-20%, but valid statistical data are still lacking.

The role of the implant is to replace the diseased root of the natural tooth, if it is lost (Figure 15.2). Root disease of a natural tooth can be caused by inflammatory processes in the root itself (pulpitis, gangrene with periapical bone lesions) and periodontal changes around the root. The inflammatory process in the root of a natural tooth is manifested by the symptom of pain. However, the disease of its substitute (implant) has a completely different course; from symptom manifestation, diagnosis, to treatment. Natural root disease is easier and faster to diagnose. Also, treatment with endodontic access is easier, faster and more successful. The implant as its direct substitute, which takes over all the roles of a natural tooth, from function to aesthetics, due to the biologically inert material from which it is made, does not get sick in the same way, and the symptoms of the disease at the beginning are very different.

Implant disease means the cancellation of the role that the implant assumed as the successor of the root. Comparing the gingiva and mucosa around the implant and the natural tooth is also different. The surrounding soft tissues around the implant react to the colonization of the bacterial content with faster inflammatory lesions, i.e. by infiltration of leukocytes in the connective tissue. Inflammatory lesions around the implant spread faster, progressing apically, than around the natural tooth, because the mucous membrane around the implant contains fewer fibroblasts. For this reason, the mucous membrane around the implant is a weak barrier for the penetration of microorganisms from the accumulated plaque. The paucity of fibroblasts in the mucous membrane is manifested by the insufficient content of collagen fibers and matrix, and during the reparative phase, it promotes the progress and spread of the inflammatory infiltrate in the mucosa around the implant.

Illness around the embedded implant is diagnosed as peri-implantitis, because the inflamma-

tory process affects the tissues around the integrated implant that is in operation. At the same time, with the progression of peri-implant mucositis, there is a loss of supporting bone.

Inflammation of the peri-implant mucosa is a reversible process, limited to the soft tissue around the implant. It manifests itself without symptoms and without loss of supporting bone, and is most often the result of poor oral hygiene and accumulated plaque.

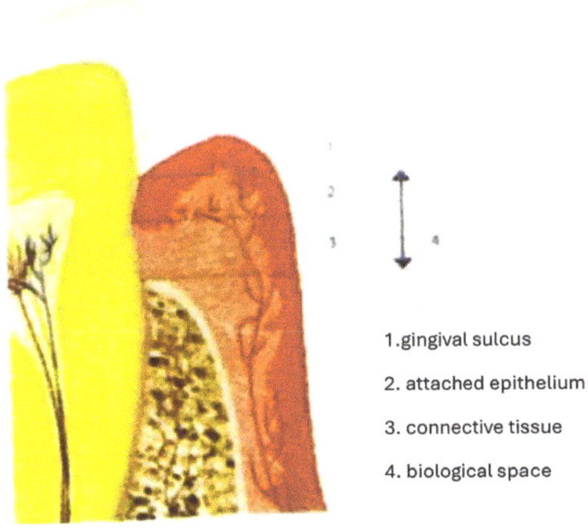

Figure 15.1. An overview of the composition of the biological space around the natural tooth. Biological space consists of attached epithelials and connective tissue of the dento-gingival complex. These anatomical structures fill the space between the gingival sulcus and the alveolar bone. The anatomy of the peri-implant tissue cannot be described in detail, but as with a natural tooth, the implant body in a well-integrated implant must be surrounded by biological space. The formation of the anatomy of the peri-implant tissue depends on the position of the implant.

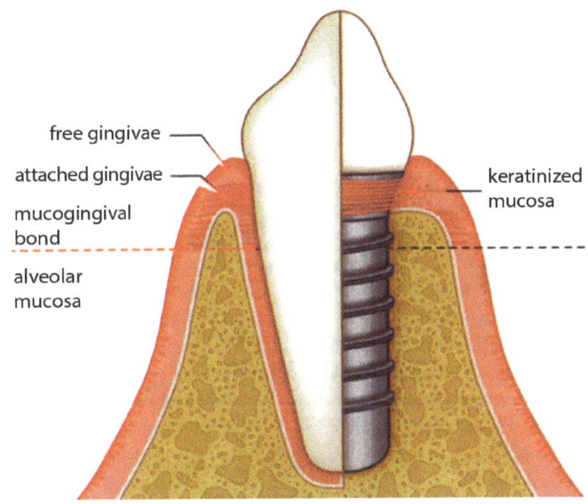

Figure 15.2. Schematic representation of the tissues surrounding the root of the natural tooth and the tissues surrounding the implant.

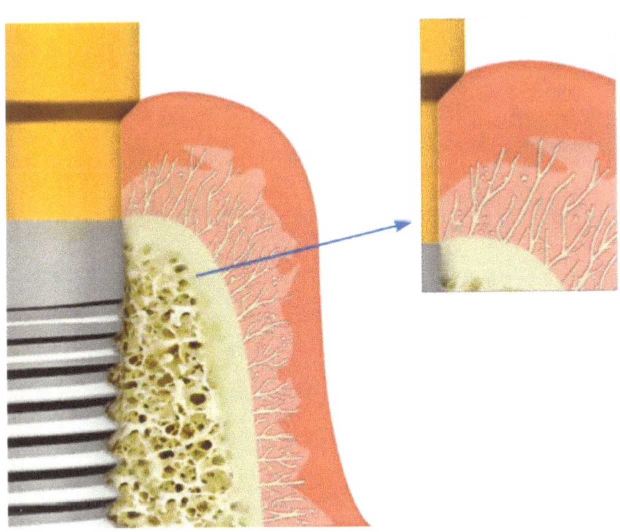

Figure 15.3. The connective epithelium of the integrated implant followed the axis of the implant body, which makes the gingival edge less resistant. The connective fibers surrounding the implant and its abatement (prosthetic abutment) are provided parallel to the implant surface. The gingival sulcus around the implant is more rounded than the gingival sulcus of a natural tooth and passively adheres to the surface of the implant. The deposition of plaque and bacterial content causes the formation of inflammatory lesions that progress apically faster than in a natural tooth.

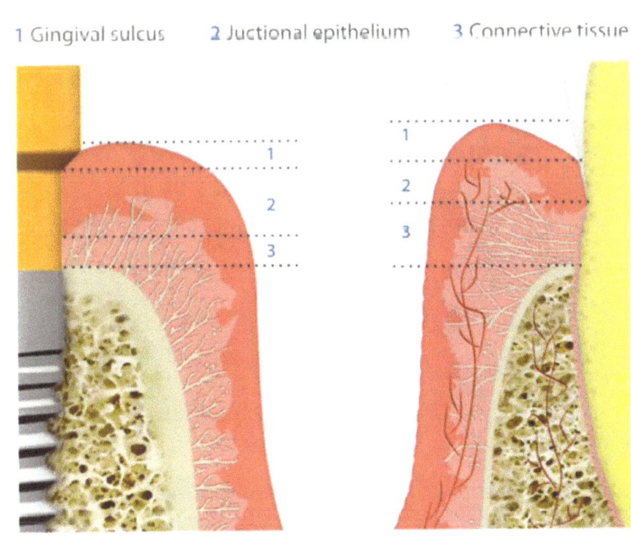

Figure 15.4. Comparison of the soft tissue ratio of the implant and the natural tooth: 1. gingival sulcus, 2. Attached epithelium, 3. conjunctival membrane The macular tissue around the natural tooth consists of a solid attached gingivae and a movable alveolar mucosa. Periodontal fibers around the natural tooth extend vertically to the root surface and grasp the root cement.

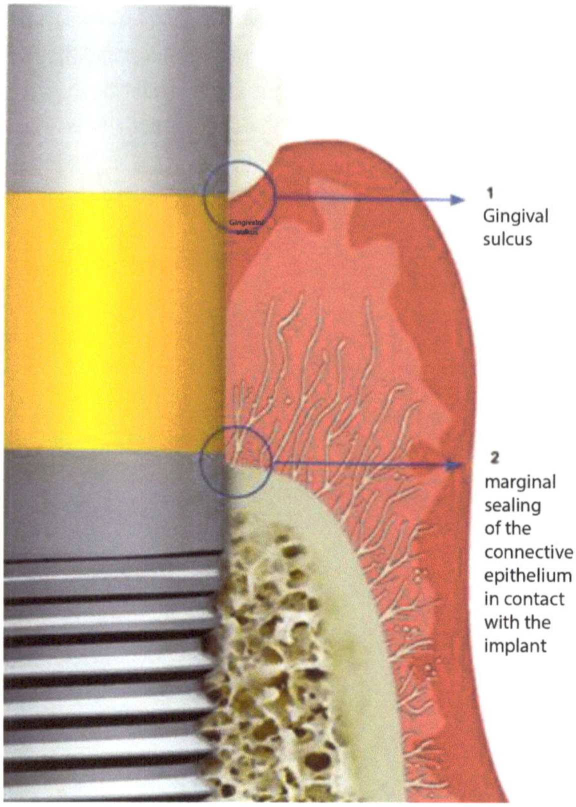

Figure 15.5. The gingival sulcus around the implant differs from the gingival sulcus in the nature of the new tooth due to its passive adhesion to the abatement surface. The deposition of plaque and bacterial content in the gingival sulcus causes faster and inflammatory processes around the implant than around the natural tooth.

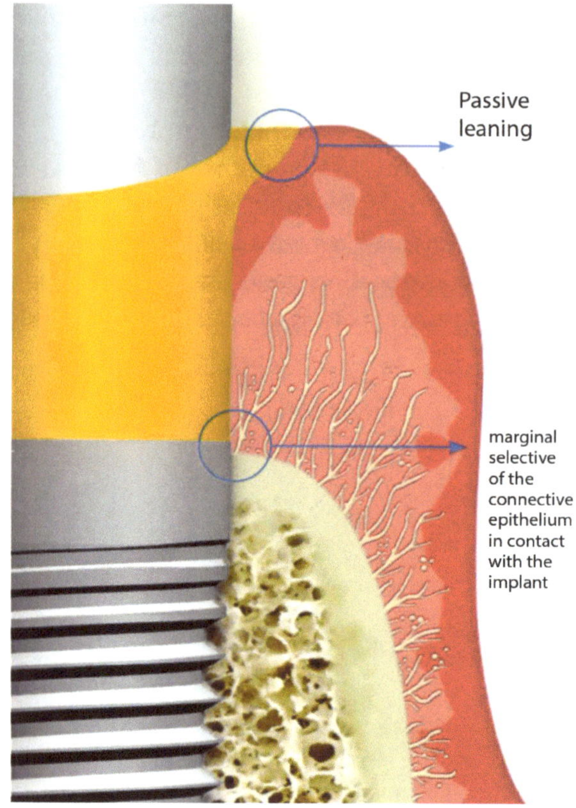

Figure 15.6. Schematic representation of the passive fit of the gingival sulcus around the implant.

Peri-implant mucositis (Figures 15.7. and 15.8) is manifested by minor bleeding when probing, and peri-implantitis is also manifested by marginal bone changes. Peri-implantitis is a complication of serious character, as it is the most common cause of implant loss (Figures 15.9. and 15.10.)

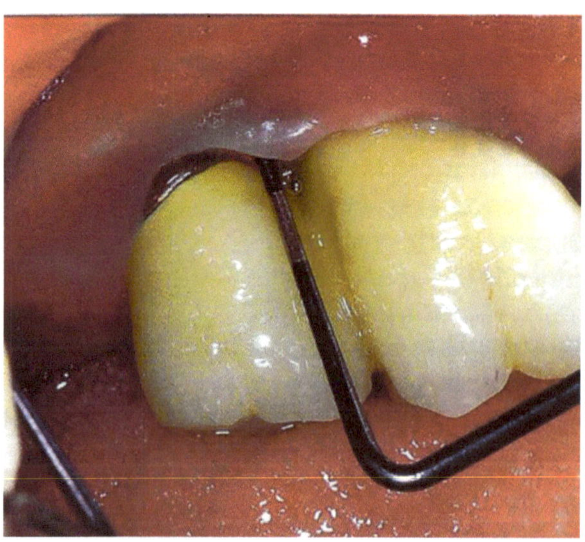

Figure 15.7. Sounding with light pressure at the beginning is the most important diagnostic sign for peri-implant inflammation.

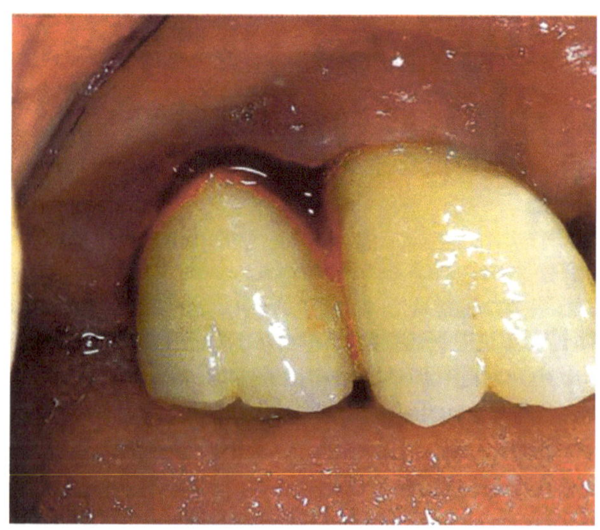

Figure 15.8. Bleeding during probing is evidence of peri-implant mucositis.

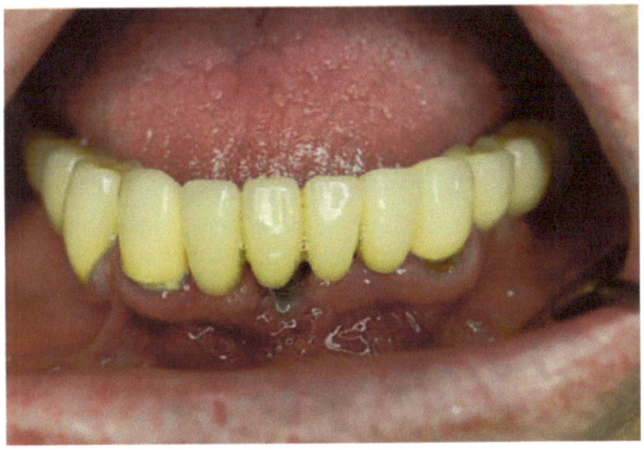

Figure 15.9. Peri-implantitis – advanced phase.

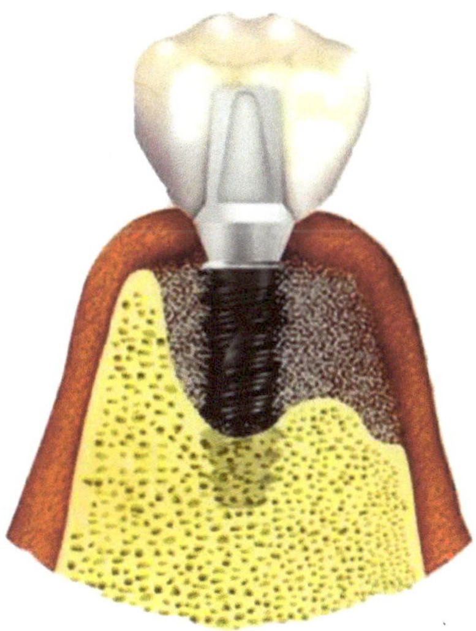

Figure 15.10. Schematic representation of peri-implantitis.

Peri-implantitis is a destructive inflammatory process that affects soft and hard tissues immediately surrounding the implant. Peri-implantitis is one of the unwanted and unforeseen reactions that can result in impaired function and loss of the implant.

Inflammation in the region around the implant involves more complex pathohistological, biochemical, physiological, microbiological and immunological processes. Research has proven that the biofilm that is created around the implant represents a group of microorganisms that inhabit the immediate environment of the implant and can cause a defensive reaction of the organism – inflammation.

The findings of the contents around the lost implant are very similar to the contents found in various forms of inflammatory periodontal diseases.

In recent years, the accumulation of knowledge from clinical practices and animal experimental studies has enabled a better understanding of these processes. Of utmost importance were, of course, studies that study the zone of direct contact between the titanium surface of the implant and the surrounding tissue. At the beginning, when the author of this book also began to deal with problems in oral implantology, the main interest was focused on the nature of the relationship between bone and implants. Today, the focus has been extended more to soft tissues with the aim of better integration of the implant with the mucous part. Based on the collected facts from practical knowledge, a practical application in the treatment of this serious complication is also based. Paradoxically, the design of the implants and the increase in the surface roughness of the implants have improved the bone integration processes with the implant, and on the other hand, the roughness of the surface of the implants in the neck area with marginal bone loss increases the possibility of penetration and accumulation of bacterial content, which is still a completely unexplained topic.

Peri-implantitis is preceded by a milder form of inflammation peri-implant mucositis, which is easily treated with better oral hygiene. As soon as peri-implant mucositis is diagnosed, this is a first warning and the patient should be emphasized the obligation to increase the number of medical controls, which is the basis for the treatment of peri-implant changes. It is the obligation of the dentist to reanalyze the possible causes of the appearance and pathological changes around the implant.

Periodic mandatory controls are invaluable for maintaining the health of the peri-implant milieu, i.e. homeostasis, after the completion of the implant prosthetic treatment. This must be emphasized to the patient! The explanation of the dentist must be shaped into a story that will interest the patient to understand the importance of the advice. The dentist and the patient must be clear about the origin of peri-implantation changes, which can result in serious consequences. The patient easily remembers the possible causes of implant disease: poor hygiene and passionate smoking.

However, the dentist has a more complex obligation in discovering the cause of peri-implantitis. He must initially find out what intensity the marginal bone loss was and what factors caused the bone loss. Loss of marginal bone increases the possibility of peri-implantitis. The underlying reason may be biomechanical in nature, and the combination with the bacteriological factor leads to more severe peri-implant changes with the consequences of implant loss. An experienced physician applies the prevention of peri-implantitis from the very beginning of the implant prosthetic procedure: starting from a history of good planning, the number and position of implants, the absence of traumatic damage to soft tissue and bone during implant placement. The market also offers expensive lasers for the treatment of peri-implantitis, and practical experience confirms that all this is not as successful as the marketing advertisement recommends, which will be explained in the part of this chapter where the treatment of peri-implantitis is discussed. When it comes to serious complications, in order to understand the problems of the onset and development of peri-implantitis, the dentist must follow new scientific findings that have recently been significantly expanded.

Where should we start in order to take preventive action in practice to prevent the onset of peri-implantitis of serious inconvenience for both the patient and the doctor? When placing implants, care should be taken that there is sufficient distance between the implants, as well as the distance from the implant to the adjacent tooth. The quality of bone integration also depends on the interim implant distance. If the distance between the implants is less than 3 mm, it may in the presence of other factors, favor the occurrence of peri-implant changes. If, due to insufficient interim implant space, there is a loss of marginal bone, it should be expected that this will adversely affect the surrounding soft tissues, in 1 row, the preservation of the papillae. If it is planned to connect the implant with the natural tooth, care must be taken that the gap between the root of the natural tooth and the implant is at least 1.5 to 2 mm. Very often, in order to maintain favorable interim implant spaces, smaller diameter implants are indicated. Statistics confirm that the survival rate of implants after 10 years is higher when the prosthetic work is anchored only on implants. (99.2%), than when the prosthetic work is anchored at the connection of the implant with the natural tooth (82.2%). Practical experience confirms that the success of the entire treatment largely depends on the stability of soft tissues. Stable and healthy soft tissue, keratinized mucosa around the implant, is not only an aesthetic advantage, but also a prevention of peri-implantitis. From practical experience, the author of the book believes that keratinized mucosa is one of the very important conditions for maintaining the stability of soft tissues around the implant, as well as for the long-term survival of bone implants, unlike mobile mucosa. Appearances of stable keratinized mucosa in Figures 15.11. to 15.17) demonstrate the success of implant rehabilitation and the predictability of implant survival.

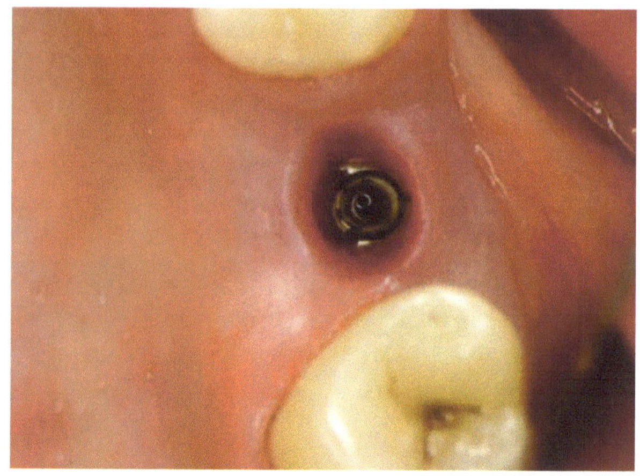

Figure 15.11. The practical experiences of the author of the book confirm that keratinized mucosa as a stable healthy soft tissue is not only essential for the realization of aesthetics but also for the long survival of implants.

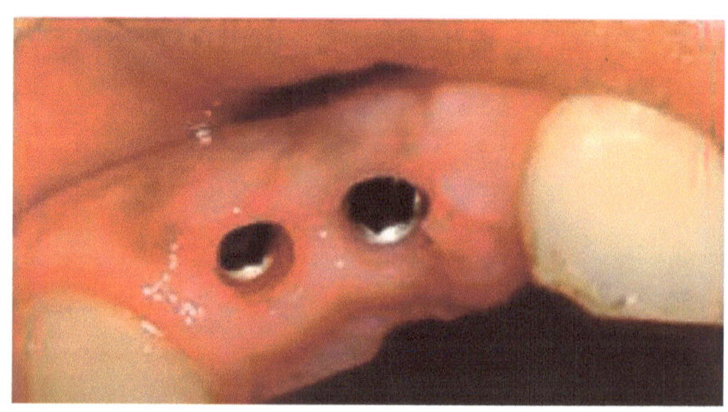

Figure 15.12. Appearance of healthy keratinized mucosa (region #11 and #12) after immediate implantation and immediate loading of the implant. Balance after 8 months.

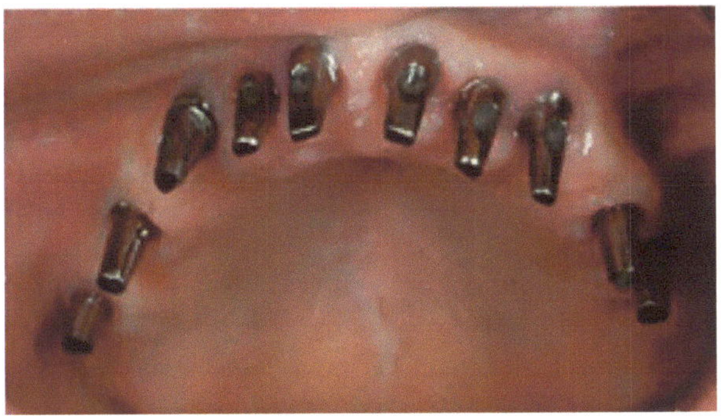

Figure 15.13. Healing and formation of keratinized mucosa is the best prevention against peri-implant changes, which is supported by precise prosthetic work and oral hygiene by the patient. The experience of the author of the book confirms that this is best achieved by placing definitive abutments immediately upon implant placement. The less trauma to the soft tissues by removing and placing the supports, the faster and better the healing of the mucous gingiva.

The following recordings show complex cases and procedures of the procedure. Despite the complexity of the presented cases, 5 years after the implant prosthetic treatment, control examinations and radiographic analysis, it was found that no peri-implant changes occurred in any patient. Performance results depend on many factors - good work planning, good oral hygiene and regular mandatory controls.

Movable mucosa around the implant is a weak barrier to the penetration of microorganisms into the peri-implant space, which also favors the deposition of plaque, as well as the difficulty of maintaining oral hygiene.

The formation of peri-implantitis can be promoted by microcracks, i.e. distance between the abatment and the implant body. The amount of deposited plaque and microorganisms in the area also depends on the size and distance. For this reason, the occurrence of peri-implantitis in one-piece implants is significantly less frequent.

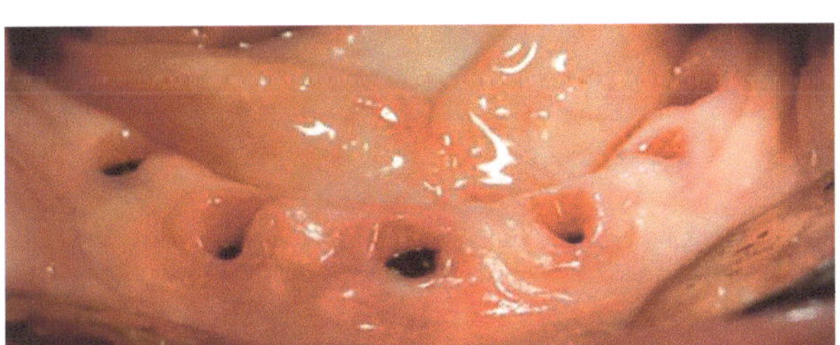

Figure 15.14. Stable keratinized mucosa in the lower jaw after 12 months.

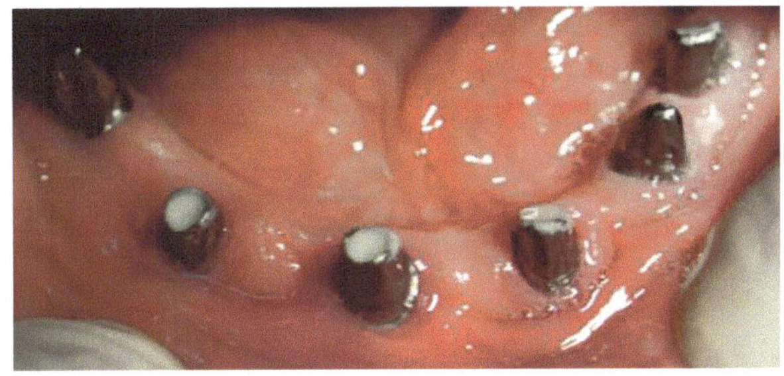

Figure 15.15. Appearance of healthy and good target tissue around the Brenemark implant system support after 12 months.

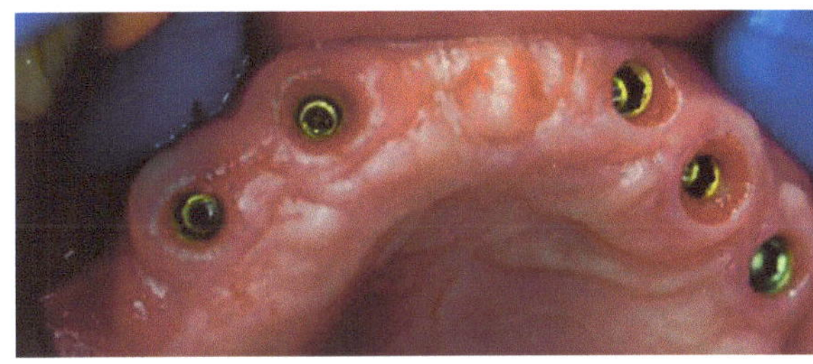

Figure 15.16. It appears well healed keratinized mucosa after one year of immediate implantation and immediate loading.

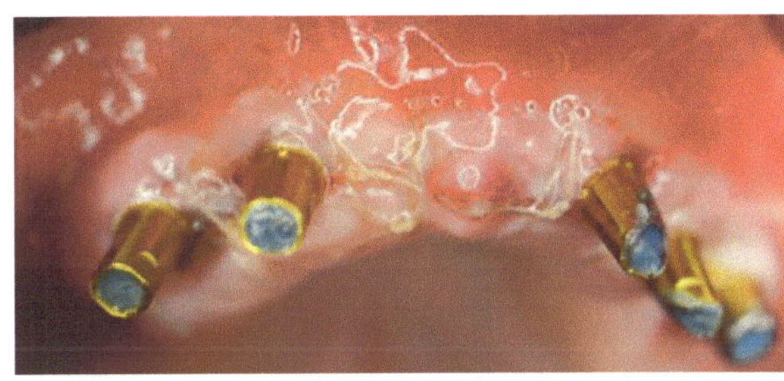

Figure 15.17. The appearance of healed soft tissues around the definite supports that are placed simultaneously with the implanted and loaded implants, which is evidence of a justified procedure. Displayed condition after 8 weeks, and definitive prosthetic work is not recommended after 6 months.

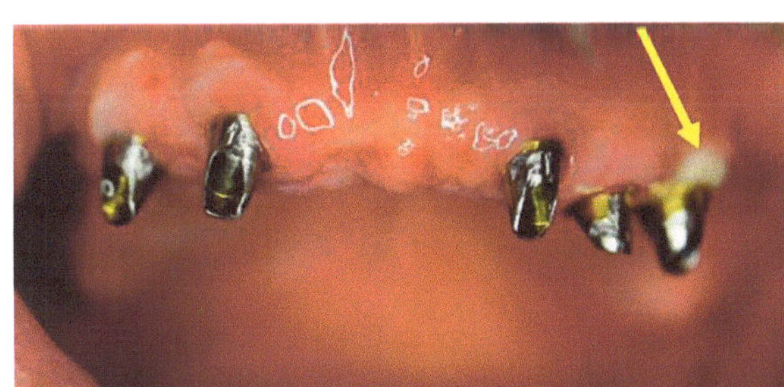

Figure 15.18. Experience confirms that definite supports should be placed immediately upon implantation, thus achieving both faster and better healing and shaping of soft tissues. Appearance of an ideally restored alveolar ridge arch and healed keratinized mucosa. The abutment on the implant in region #15 had to be removed for paralysis processing. When reapplying, mild compression was performed on the healed soft tissues. If this procedure were repeated several times, it would be possible to introduce a microorganism into the space between

the abutment and the implant body. All supports are placed at the same time as the immediate implant placement and tightened with a dynamometer up to 35 Ncm.

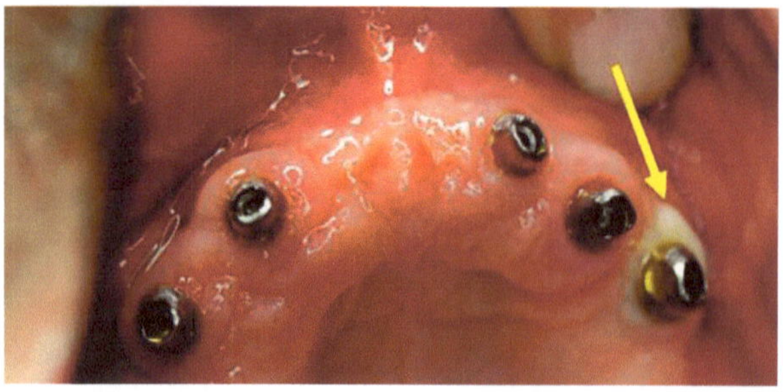

Figure 15.19. Appearance of healing of peri-implant soft tissues on the palatal side. Around the support of the region #14, compression on soft tissues (marked with a red line) is visible. This is due to reinforcing the support in the laboratory (the traumatization of soft tissues should be avoided by placing and removing the gingiva-former, but by placing definite supports when installing implants).

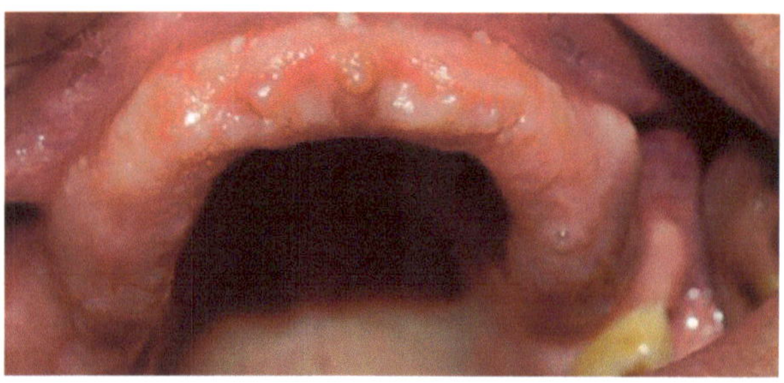

Figure 15.20. The patient is a perennial user of upper partial acrylic dentures. The appearance of the alveolar ridge; stable soft tissues, and by radiological assessment of the condition of the available bone, the placement of implants of standard diameters without raising the lobe is indicated, which accelerates healing and treatment.

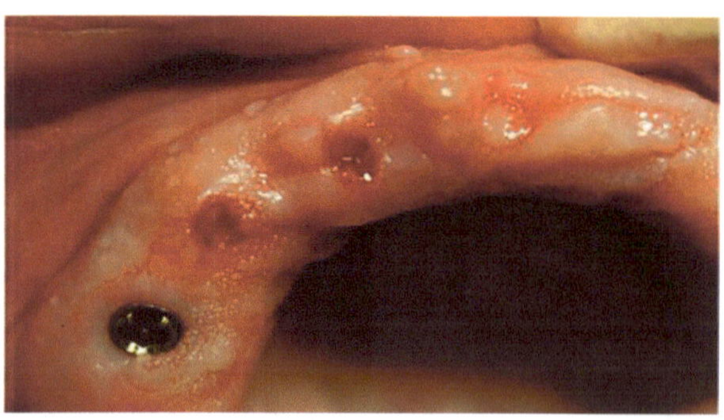

Figure 15.21. Quality keratinized mucosa facilitates implant placement without raising the lobe, thus accelerating tissue healing and shortening the time of the entire implant-prosthetic rehabilitation. Marking the position of the implant by removing the "plugs" of the keratinized mucosa.

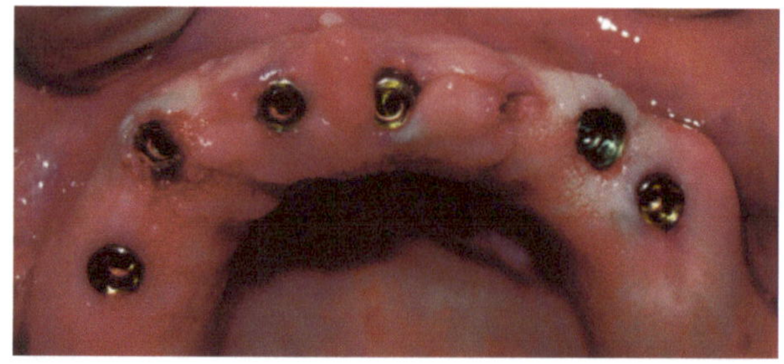

Figure 15.22. Successful implant placement without a lobe lift, with a predictable outcome, depends on the experience of the dentist and good judgment. Stable soft tissues promised a successful result of implanted prosthetic treatment.

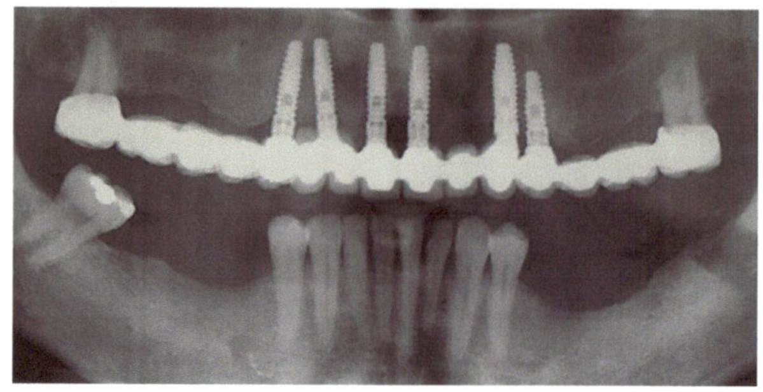

Figure 15.23. Radiographic representation of implanted implants without lobe lift. Control image after 6 years - stable soft tissue barrier is from peri-implantitis (Figures 15.21. and 15.22.)

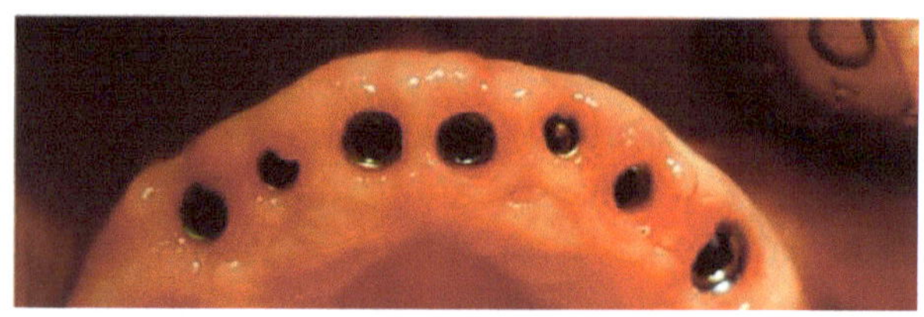

Figure 15.24. Appearance of the remodeled alveolar arch and healing of the keratinized mucosa in well-integrated implants. The formation of a healthy peri-implant gingiva is a solid barrier to the formation of peri-implantitis.

Fundamentals Of Morphology And Histology

In order to better understand the processes related to the occurrence of peri-implantitis, it is necessary to consider the basic morphology and histology of the periodontal milieu (Figure 15.1.).

The peri-implant tissue is composed of the following epithelial and connective tissue structures:

1. gingival epithelium-turned towards the oral cavity.
2. sulcus epithelium - facing the surface of the implant but without contact with it
3. connective epithelium in contact with the implant.
4. biological space

The mucosa immediately surrounding the visible part of the implant opening is a healthy tissue of light pink color and a typical slightly darkened keratinized part. Connective undifferentiated epithelium that is not keratinized and surrounds the neck of the tooth in a width of about 2 mm. This connective epithelium after tooth growth serves as the epithelial sheath of the oral cavity. The connective epithelium is physiologically important, as it enables the two-way exchange of metabolites, immune cells, biochemical compounds and microbiological products and mucus as a barrier against the oral microbiological flora. So far, there is no reliable data that the binding epithelium can be created in contact with non-biological materials such as titanium and take on the same histo-physiological characteristics as in contact with natural teeth. Recently, there have been announcements that this bond is being promoted by a combination of titanium and zirconium materials, which has not yet been proven, and practice has confirmed.

Histological differences should also be considered for a better understanding of peri-implant processes.

The soft tissue around the natural tooth is different from the soft tissue that forms around the implant and abutment. The soft tissue around the natural tooth forms on the solid narrative gingiva and movable alveolar mucosa. The width of the attachment gingiva is different and varies from 1 to 9 millimeters. In contrast, the terminology referring to soft tissues around implants is not uniform in the literature. The differences between the soft tissues surrounding the implant and the artificial tooth support from the soft tissues around the natural tooth are:

a) Periodontal fibers around the natural tooth extend vertically to the root surface and grasp the root cement. The connective fibers of the tissues surrounding the implant and its abutment are provided parallel to the surface of the implant and abutment.
b) Peri-implant connective tissue contains fewer fibroblasts and more collagen fibers and its structure is more similar to the structure that also characterizes scar tissue;
c) The attached epithelium around the implant is more pliable, and therefore represents a weaker protective barrier than the attached epithelium around the natural tooth;
d) The gingivae around the natural tooth is more vascular. It is assumed that inelastic collagen connective tissue fibers are responsible for the existence of keratinized tissues, with most periodontal ligament fibers being inelastic. For this reason, in a natural tooth and after complete surgical excision, a narrow belt of attached gingiva is regenerated in most cases. Unlike natural teeth, implants can be surrounded by keratinized or mobile alveolar mucosa.

The important fact is that the loss of some tissue around the implant progresses much faster than around a natural tooth.

Tooth extraction is accompanied by horizontal and vertical bone resorption due to loss of function. This process in the bone is accompanied by the process of moving the attached mucogingival tissue towards the coronary. Implant placement is often associated with recuperation of the resorbed bone, so displacement of mucogingival displacement may occur. For this reason, uniform attitudes regarding soft tissue augmentation are missing in order to obtain the width of the keratinized mucosa in the area of the implant and abutment. Therefore, different soft tissue augmentation protocols are proposed:

- as a separate preparatory procedure before implant placement;
- as part of the surgical procedure for implant placement;
- as part of a two-stage implant placement procedure
- subsequently when the implant has already been opened or is already under load.

It is assumed that the first three procedures are more justified to predict the outcome, than after a certain time when the implants are damaged. The author of the book applied 12 procedures in most cases in fixed prosthetic works. In cases where peri-implant changes have occurred, aesthetic problems are also present, which is why patients predominantly appear with a delay, without knowing that biological complications are also present.

In case of decision and need for soft tissue augmentation, two methods can be applied:

- Enlargement of keratinized mucous membrane with apically displaced lobe-vestibuloplasty in combination with free gingival graft and
- Increase in soft tissue volume by subepithelial connective tissue graft or free gingival graft to increase the width of the keratinized gingiva.

Connective Tissue

There are cross-sectional studies related to the characteristics of the connective tissue surrounding the implant. According to some, only endosteal integration occurs without the formation of the periodontal ligament, while animal studies have shown that the formation of desmodontal structures are possible. Also controversial are findings on collagen structures in the peri-implant region, their type and direction of provision in relation to the surface of implants with some common characteristics, but also differences in collagen type and vascularization in relation to natural teeth.

Titanium oxides are assumed to react with collagen fibers and affect their arrangement. Thus, in animal studies, implant designs that differ in the transmucosal part were investigated. However, there are also no reliable animal studies related to this problem that have been confirmed in human research. It has been shown that hydrophilicity has no impact, while microtopography of the implant surface has an impact on the formation of biofilm deposits, but still these data are not differentiated to find application in practice. The implant systems "ICX-Templant" and "Roxolid-Straumann" (a combination of titanium and zirconium materials), point out contrary to scientific research that the hydrophilicity of the surfaces of the implants of these implant systems affects the faster integration of tissues around the implants.

Transmucosal Part Of The Implant

More and more research supports the fact that the integration of soft tissue in the transmucosal part of the implant is a prerequisite for protecting the alveolar bone from potentially harmful factors from the oral cavity milieu. Thus, due to the suspicion that the rough surfaces of the implants are suitable for settlement of bacterial colonies, the implant manufacturers applied the finest techniques and polishing of the transmucosal part of the implant. In contrast, some research again suggests that the somewhat rougher surfaces of implants are stimulating for adhesion of epithelial and fibroblast cells. From future research, we expect a response to this controversy regarding the surface of the transmucosal part of the implant. Recent findings confirm the importance of implant surface treatment and that the immune response to inflammatory processes depends on the physical and chemical composition of the implant surface. The physical and chemical composition of the implant surface can affect the local metabolism of the peri-implant tissues and is considered an important element of the reaction between the implant as an inert material and the living tissues surrounding the implant. For this reason, it is important to choose the highest quality implant systems.

Peri-implantant Oxide Titanium Layer

Under the influence of water, air and other compounds from the oral environment, titanium creates oxides that are organized into stable mineral structures that serve as a protective layer of the titanium body of the implant itself. The characteristics of this oxide layer, depending on the type of chemical bonds and the very composition of titanium in which various compounds can be installed, affect its protective function and bio compatibility.

From the very beginning of the contact of the implant with the blood and proteins that make it up, oxidative processes begin. Peri-implant tissue healing is faster in implants with a porous surface compared to a smooth surface. It is assumed that the healing process is facilitated by stimulation of osteo-areal cells. Thus, implants that have undergone technological treatment with pure gas and the release of anode currents acquire stronger osteophilic properties. All this points to the importance of applying the highest quality implants with a certificate from renowned manufacturers.

Etiological Factors of Peri-implantitis

In addition to bone necrosis caused by the taxidermy of the implant bed and the formation of a layer of microbiological biofilm, additional etiological factors that may result in inflammatory processes in the immediate tissue structure around the implant are also listed. Early complications are most often caused by inadequate preparation of the implant bed, and it is necessary to pay attention to the following precautions during preparation and bone: reduction of the rotation speed of the drill bit and sufficient cooling with saline solution. The preparation of the implant tray should be conducted intermittently, which allows the bone to "rest". With this procedure at the same time sudden stress on the bone itself is also reduced. Minor trauma to the bone allows the use of a sharp drill bit. The main cause of peri-implant infections is the formation of bacterial biofilm, while possible additional factors are listed as:

1. periodontitis;
2. excessive smoking;
3. systemic diseases;
4. use of alcohol;
5. genetic factors;
6. implant overload;
7. pathological processes In the mucosa;
8. prosthetic works;
9. wound dehiscence;
10. positioning of implants;
11. use of bio-phosphates, etc.

Microbiological Factors

The set of deposited microorganisms, primarily bacteria, creates a layer or biofilm that surrounds the implant, has a specific organization and structure by which it can become resistant to bacteriocine influences and the immune response of the organism.

Initial Stages of Osteointegration

Establishing direct contact between the bone and the implant without creating connective tissue is the basis of successful osteointegration. Brenemark was the first to explain the concept of osteointegration; as the ability of bone to coalesce to the surface of the implant under certain conditions without soft tissue interposition.

In recent years, many animal studies have been performed that have attempted to shed light on the dynamics in the immediate zone surrounding the implant through a variety of complex histometric methods. However, the conclusions obtained in these studies can only be partially applied to human bone. Despite the latest findings, the histochemical processes that begin osteointegration have not been fully discovered. It is assumed that the very beginning of these processes begins the binding of plasma proteins to the titanium surface, which triggers further into the biochemical cascade that allows cell adhesion. Increased activity of progenitor bone cells, undifferentiated mesenchymal cells, preosteoblasts and osteoblasts, results in osteointegration at best.

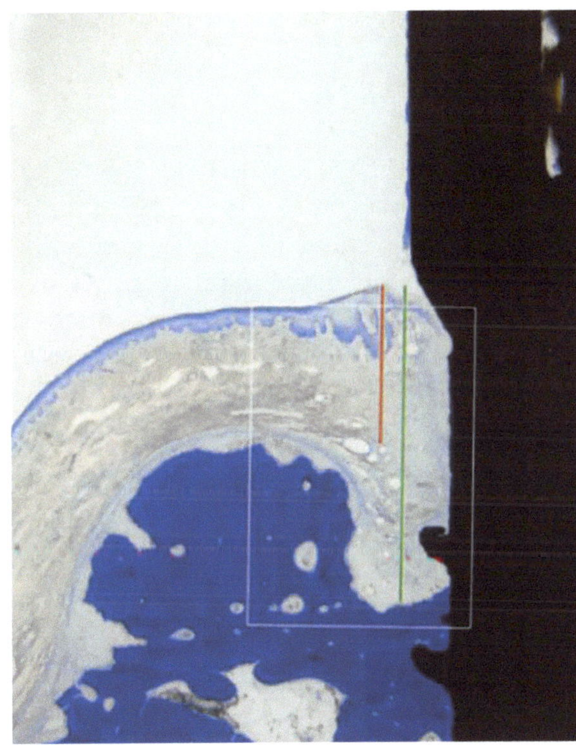

Figure 15.25. Resorption of the crestal part of the alveolar bone due to insufficient initial biological width. In the square, the red line indicates a resorption of 1.3 mm, and the green line indicates a loss of crystalline bones of 2.7 millimeters. In animal studies, it has been proven that for the development of a more stable biological width, the supracrestal surface of implants with apical coronary expansion should be at least 3 millimeters (source of histological images Frank Schwarz, Jurgen Becker)

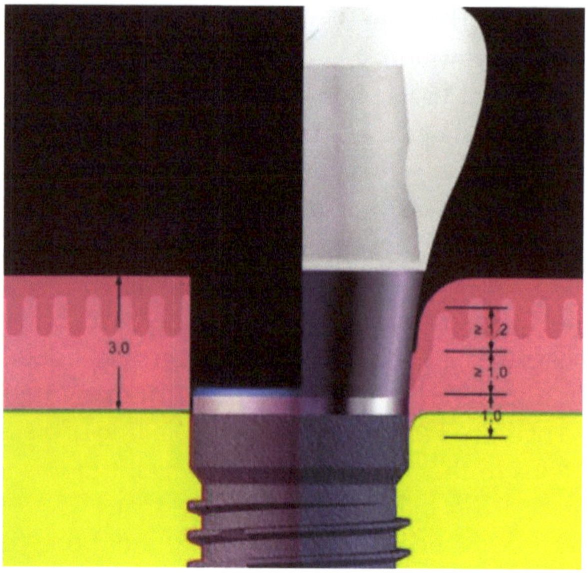

Figure 15.26. Implant with reduced hat of machined neck over 0.4 millimeters, and the treated part of the bone does not enter below the ridge.

Biological Latitude (Biological Space) And Dentogingival Complex

Biological width is defined as the distance between the highest coronary extension to the alveolar bone, i.e. Biological width is the structure around the implant. The biological width consists of the epithelial attachment, the sulcus of the epithelium of the sulcus base and the connective tissue (see Figures 15.1.15.4).

It averages up to 3 millimeters. When the tissue has a height and thickness of 3 mm, this structure will be built and the vestibular wall will remain at the same level. In other words, the biological width contains an epithelium of about 1 mm and a connective tissue junction of 1 mm. The dentogingival complex also contains parts of the gingival sulcus of about 1 mm. Below this level, resorption of the peri-implant bone can be expected. If the initial tissue is of a thin biotype, the biological width will be built at the expense of bone loss. It is concluded that tissue biotype is decisive for soft tissue stability. Some research proves that the soft tissue biotype is essential for the aesthetic and functional stability of the peri-implant tissue. Any loss greater than 1mm in height-thickness of the tissue leads to its visual discoloration.

Based on the studies and available data from the literature, it can be concluded that for the stability of soft tissues around the implant, it is necessary to:

- 3 mm tissue height;
- 3 mm tissue thickness and
- 3 mm attached gingiva around the implant.

It can be concluded that in order to achieve perfect aesthetics, when the peri-implant tissue is reconstructed, the following should be provided:

1. The thickness of the buccal new wall and the level of the interdental bone. The buccal wall bone is attached to the tooth and will be resorbed horizontally and vertically as soon as it is removed. The resorption process should be stopped by augmentation with bone substitutes;
2. formation of biological width; thus preventing bone resorption
3. ideal position of the implant, which provides a satisfactory aesthetic result, i.e. a distance of 2 mm from the buccal level of the tissue. Augmentation with bone replacers between the surface of the implant and the buccal bone wall will create good bone support for soft tissue, which will prevent tissue loss and maintain its maximum volume stability.

Further, the relationship between the treated and coarse surface of the implant that is most likely to affect bone resorption. The optimal ratio of these surfaces is still unknown. The results of the research of these relationships are presented in subsequent histological studies (Figure 15.25. to 15.31)

The conclusion of these studies is that the polished or treated surface of the implant leads to marginal bone resorption and results in a peri-implant infection.

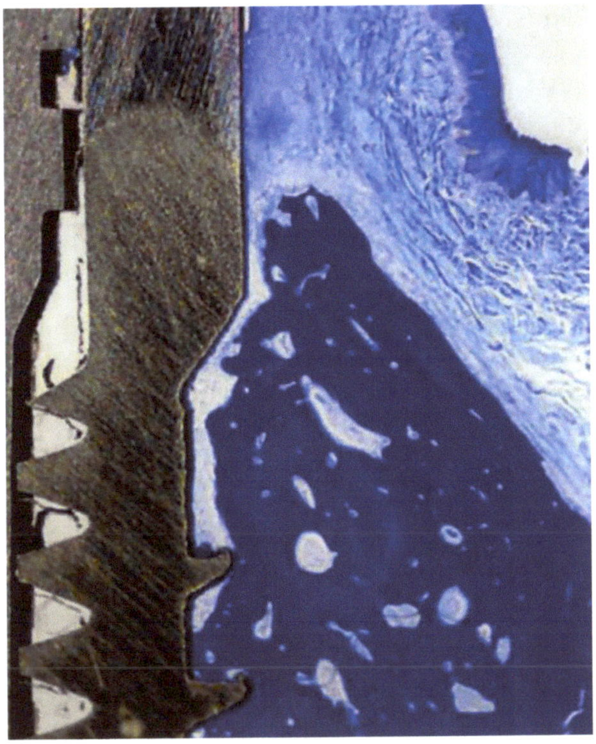

Figure 15.27. Healing of the wound even after 4 weeks in standard diameter implants, with the formation of connective tissue in the gap between the bone part and polishing of the treated part of the implant.

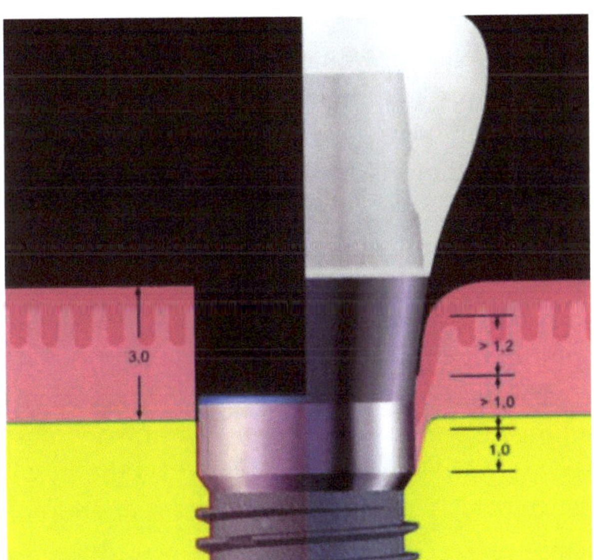

Figure 15.28. An implant with a treated neck 1.5 millimeters wide that is implanted about 0.4 millimeters above the ridge according to the standard protocol.

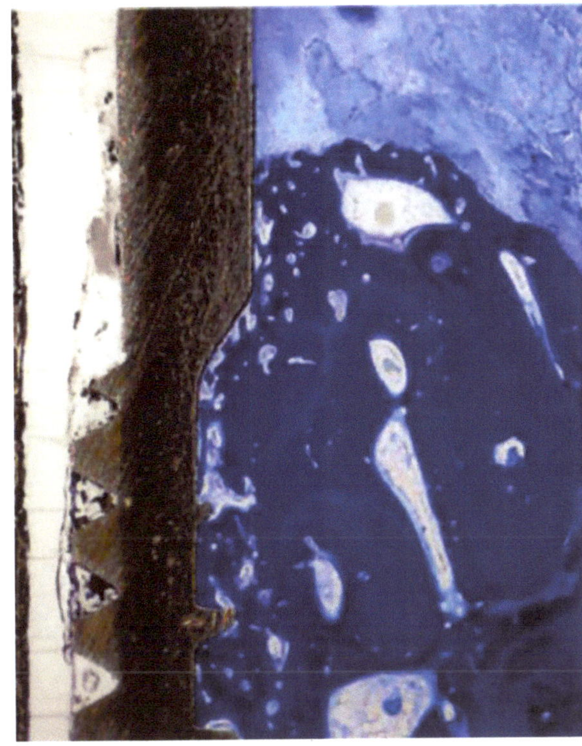

Figure 15.29. Wound healing after 4 weeks - animal model. Direct contact of bone and implant at insertion and depth levels.

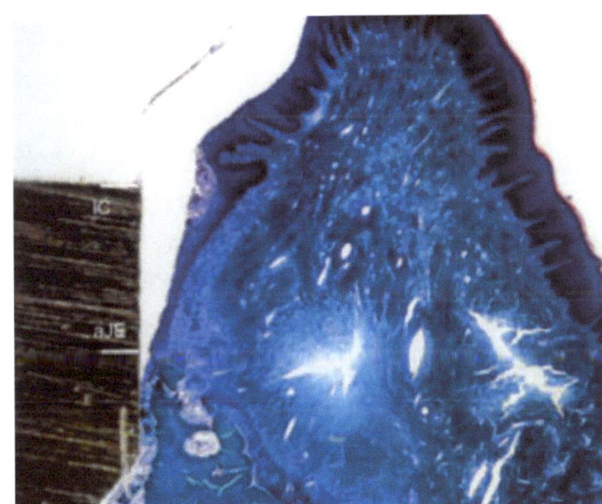

Figure 15.30. A binding appeal that usually proliferates with the treated implant surface with appropriate implant attachments.

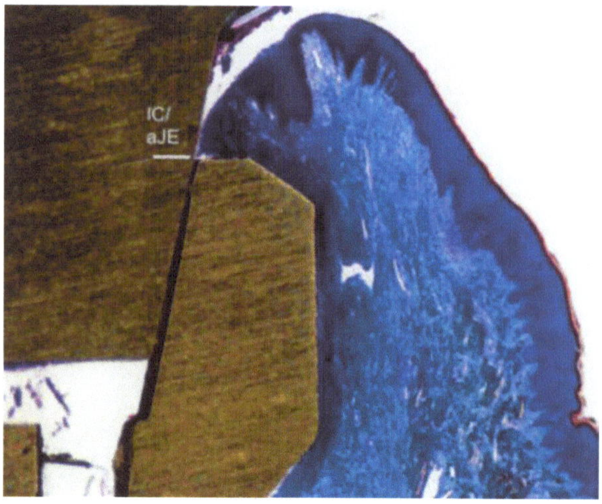

Figure 15.31. A 5-millimeter circumferential horizontal mismatch was sufficient to prevent the borderline epithelium from receding in the direction to the apex.

Pathogenesis Of Peri-Implant Infection

A number of inflammatory and immune reactions may also occur in the implant environment that have not been fully investigated. The classic division into acute and chronic inflammation in this case cannot be applied. At the very beginning, there is an inflammatory reaction of an acute type with the accumulation of numerous information cells, and later this process takes place through T lymphocytes and antibodies that are produced. In 1 phase, bacteria can cause a peri-implant infection. The passage of antibodies depends on the permeability of blood vessels. The reaction of the immune system in a peri-implant infection can be: nonspecific, non-adaptive or specific and adaptive, i.e. functional.

Histopathological Phases Of Persistent Infection

Early peri-implant mucositis is the first stage when supragingvinal plaque changes dominate and bacterial-induced changes in the junctional epithelium occur upon activation of non-specific immune response mechanisms. Bacteria stimulate the secretion of cytokines IL-8, and T8 lymphocytes who secrete both pro-inflammatory and anti-inflammatory cytokines. By increasing the value of inflammatory cytokines, the degree of inflammation of the tissues around the implant increases. Cytokines are important mediators of physiological and pathological processes in the peri-implant environment. Scientific findings indicate that cytokines as an important mediator of pathophysiological processes also affect the metabolic processes of peri-implant tissues. In the peri-implant fluid of the peri-implant sulcus, there is a multitude of cytokines, and they are directly influential on the immune response and the occurrence of inflammation of the peri-implant tissue process.

Recently, the importance of genetic susceptibility to the onset and development of peri-implantitis has been given so that the GD14 gene plays an important role in explaining genetic influences on peri-implantitis, because genes that control inflammatory processes also play an important role in the modulation of the stage of peri-implantitis. It has been proven that the development of peri-implant changes is influenced by a very complex interplay of genetic factors and factors from the external environment. Local inflammatory cytokines increase local secretion and metalloprocess activity by damaging the structure of peri-implant tissues by stimulating resorption mechanisms. The production of anti-inflammatory cytokines reduces inflammatory processes that damage tissues. With the progression of peri-implant inflammation, the concentration of cytokines in the peri-implant fluid increases. It should be emphasized that there is an individual difference in the degree of production of inflammatory mediators, which indicates the genetic presence in these processes.

One of them is the cytokine IL-8 that secretes monocytes, macrophages and fibroblasts endothelial cells, hepatocytes and chondrocytes. Cytokine IL-8, is present in peri-implant processes, and differs from other cytokines in its ability to activate neutrophil granulocytes, releasing leukines from granules. T4 lymphocytes are the main regulators of the immune response. For example, the human immune response to infections is regulated by the cytokine balance, which can have an impact on peri-implant infections, because neutrophil granulocytes, macrophages, T lymphocytes, plasma cells, etc. accumulate. This pathophysiological process causes the loss of collagen structures in the internal and external space of the subepithelial collagen tissue. The apical tip of the connective epithelium is unchanged at this stage.

Developed Peri-implant mucositis. This phase leads to the formation of a gingival pocket and the structure of the typical epithelium that lines it. The immune response involves more and more antibodies in response to bacterial colonization. Monokines at this stage can stimulate new osteoclasts. At this stage, resorptive processes in the peri-implant area are not yet recorded.

Advanced Peri-implant mucositis. The formation of a pocket with a biogingival film represents the transition to an advanced stage of inflammation in the implant environment. This phase is dominated by the spread of cellular infarction to the apical, pocket ulceration and degeneration of sub-epithelial tissue. All this promotes the spread of microorganisms and the formation of microabscesses. The migration of nuclear granulocytes weakens the dominance of plasma cells. Cellular immunity is characterized by the presence of T cells.

Macrophases are stimulated by either saccharides and gram-negative bacteria. Cellular immunity is characterized by the presence of T cells. Macrophases are stimulated by orposaccharides of gram-negative bacteria. By stimulating the osteoclasts, the initial resorption of the peri-implant alveolar ridge begins.

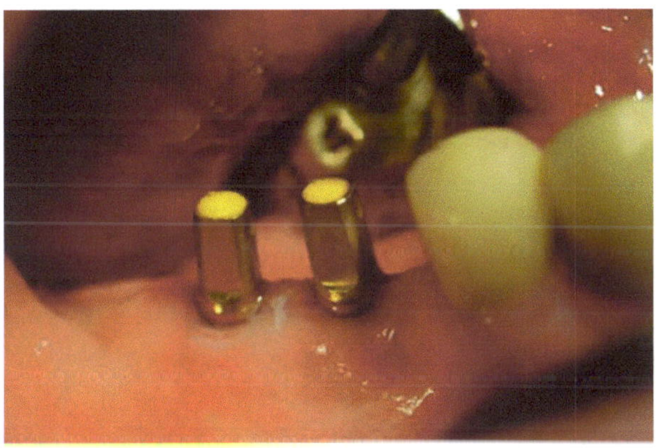

Figure 15.32. Display of implanted implants, immediately loaded; at the same time, definite abutments are placed instead of healing caps. It looks like well formed and healthier keratinized mucous membranes after 6 months. This is a preventive defense against peri-implant diseases with precise prosthetic work.

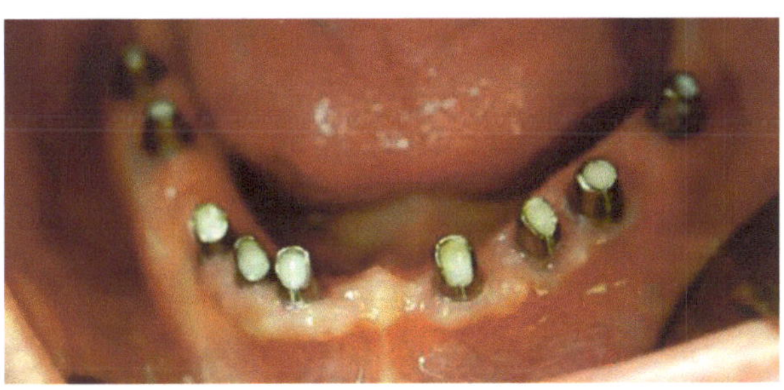

Figure 15.33. The appearance of a stably formed keratinized gingiva after immediately implanted implants of standard and wider diameters. Simultaneously installed definite supports instead of healing caps. Immediately loaded implants with temporary fixed acrylic prosthetic work. Balance after 12 months.

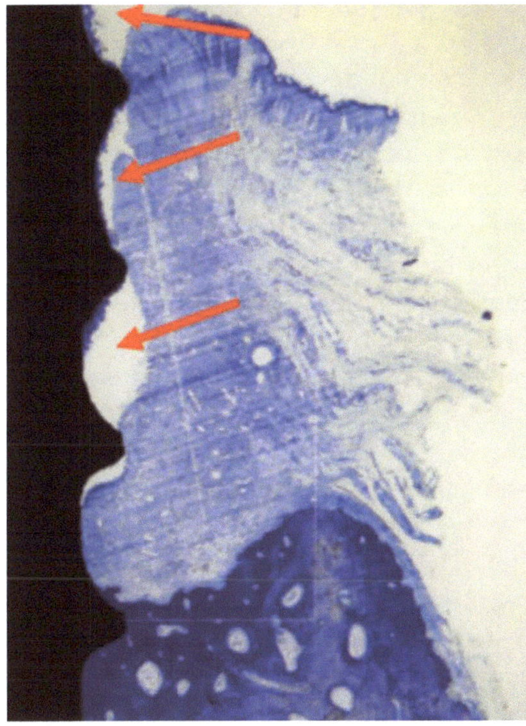

Figure 15.34. The histological finding of persistence of the peri-implant pocket (red arrow), continues to be thickening and proliferation of inflammatory cell infiltrate. Alveolar bone resorption, pocket epithelium. Plasma cell dominance, osteoclast activation with alveolar bone resorption.

Peri-implantitis

Processes started at earlier stages continue. Osteoclasts are multicore cells that are formed through the fusion of mononuclear progenitor cells of the bone marrow. Osteoclasts release proteolytic enzymes that break down the bone collagen matrix, and fragments of collagen are phagocyticized. Osteoclasts are specifically controlled through the osteoprotegrin system (OPG). The OPG-ligand-osteoprotegrin system is a TNF (tumor necrosis factor) protein and is produced in osteoblasts, T-lymphocytes and bone marrow cells. The interreaction between OPG-L and the other clasts leads to the fusion of the initial forms of osteoclasts, increasing their activity and reducing the apoptosis of mature osteoclasts, which all results in an increase in bone resorption. OPG is synthesized in many cells such as in bone marrow cells and fibroblasts of the periodontal ligament.

In addition to the known etiological factors of peri-implant diseases, bacterial infection and biomechanical problems, the latest research also points to a genetic predisposition to peri-implantitis, which was previously emphasized. It is assumed that the complexity of genetic processes with factors influencing from the external environment plays an important role in the emergence of inflammatory processes in the stages of peri-implantitis. The main factors of damage to the implant tissues are the secretion of aggressive enzymes, metalloproteinases, whose activity in the peri-implant milieu is regulated by cytokines. Information cytokines increase secretion and metalloproteinase activity, which is manifested by stimulation of bone resorption and destruction of peri-implant tissues.

Defense against peri-implantitis begins at the very beginning of implant-prosthetic rehabilitation, with the Preventive Plan and Preventive Procedures (Figures 15.15. to 15.24), in order to smoothly enable the prevention of peri-implantitis.

The views that one should wait at least 24 weeks or longer for the implants to be loaded were completely rejected by the author. Practical experience confirms that the implants should be loaded immediately after implantation with a precise acrylate bridge, thus manifesting patient comfort in terms of function and aesthetics. Also, the author's experiences have confirmed that for the formation of soft tissues it is better to immediately place definite abutments on the implanted implants (Figures 15.32. and 15.33).

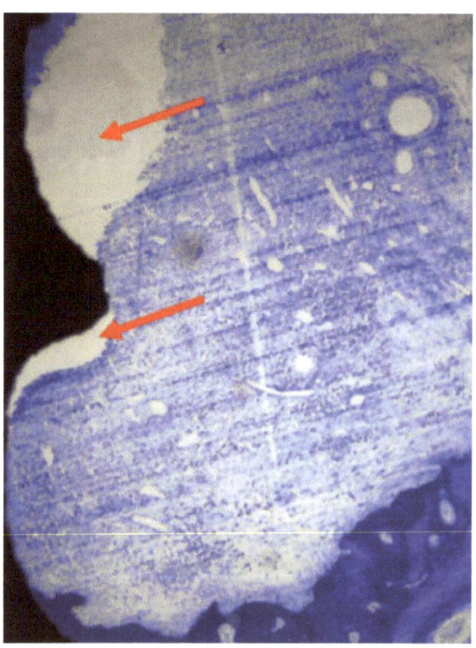

Figure 15.35. Combined marrow and bone defect (red arrows).

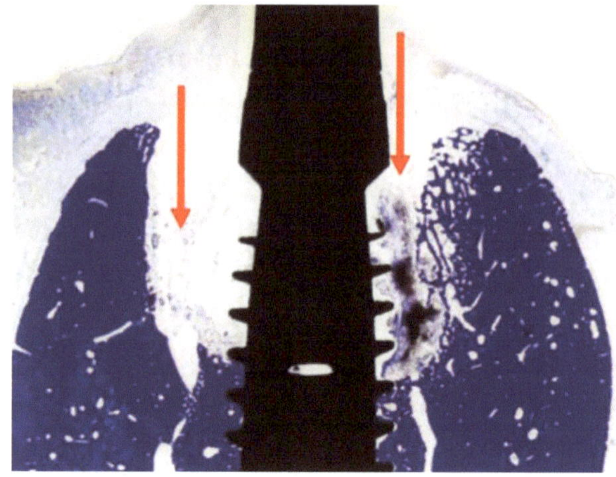

Figure 15.36. Typical circular intraskeletal defect (red arrows).

Diagnosis

The main cause of mucositis and peri-implantitis is bacterial contamination, and the author's experience confirms that the occlusal load of the implant leads to a process complicated by infection of the pathogenic microorganisms of the oral cavity. Clinical and laboratory tests are very important for proper diagnosis of peri-implantitis. The most important step for the successful treatment of peri-implant changes is the early recognition of signs of inflammation of the peri-implant tissues (mucositis, which in most cases is reversible), whether it is a clinical, radiological or microbiological study. This first step in the treatment of peri-implant infection is crucial to establish a diagnosis. The experience of physicians is one of the essential factors for early recognition of signs of changes in the peri-implant environment. There are numerous diagnostic procedures for early diagnosis of peri-implant infections, starting from traditional clinical parameters, to radiological testing of marginal bone levels, and even to microbiological and genetic tests. These procedures are very important to make an accurate diagnosis.

To prevent the occurrence of peri-implant infections, the necessary steps should be taken even before the start of implant-prosthetic rehabilitation; starting with history, good planning, avoiding tissue trauma during implantation and making precise prosthetic work.

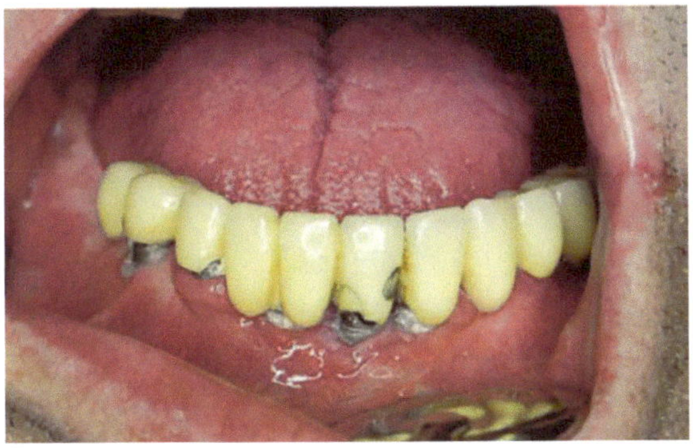

Figure 15.37. Prosthetic work on implants - a typical example of a predisposition to these diseases; poor oral hygiene; smoking; poorly designed prosthetic work on implants. Genetic and other factors of emerging peri-implantitis in this patient cannot be excluded. The patient came forward for examination and advice. When he was presented with a diagnosis based on a clinical trial and advised on further procedures, he did not show up again. The treatment was done at an educational institution.

Peri-implant Changes Indicators

1. radiologically proven loss of surrounding alveolar bone;
2. implant mobility;
3. formation of a peri-implant pocket;
4. bleeding during periodontal probing.

Abscess formation (Figure 15.38) It can be considered a rare complication since drainage of secretions can easily take place. If an abscess is formed, an urgent procedure is carried out that allows the evacuation of purulent content, with systemic antibiotic treatment. There are atypical indicators of peri-Implantitis that are not characteristic of this process itself. The swelling and redness of the surrounding soft tissue cannot be sure indicators of the process in the bone bed of the implant. Pain in itself is not an indicator of the development of peri-implantitis.

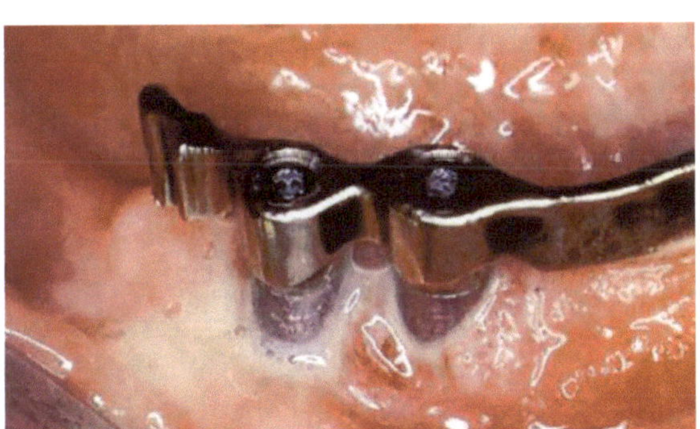

Figure 15.38. Diagnosis: submucosal abscess and peri-implantitis of region #44 and #45.

Clinical Trials

In addition to diagnostic procedures, a clinical trial is the most important factor in considering possible complications. Clinical parameters imply the use of appropriate indices that enable quantitative and qualitative analysis of the appropriate criterion. Clinical parameters should be the main factor in diagnosing peri-implant events.

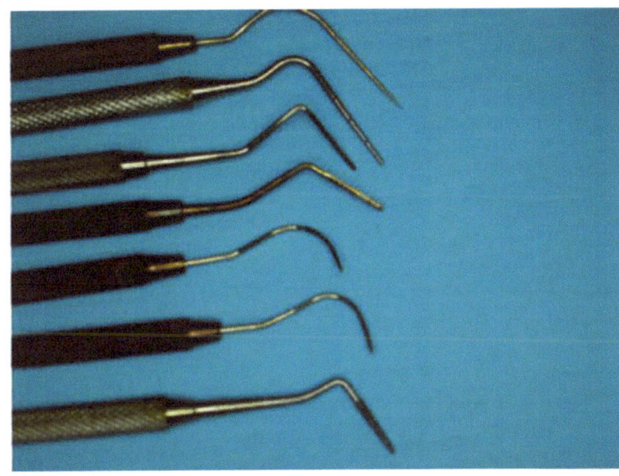

Figure 15.39. Periodontal probes to diagnose peri-implant changes.

In determining clinical parameters in practice, the first step is the procedure of using periodontal probes (Figures 15.7, 15.40, 15.43, 15.48). In this way, analogous to periodontal diagnostics, the following clinical trial parameters represent its basis:

a) plaque index;
b) gingival index;
c) bleeding secretions when provoked by a probe;
d) the quality of the exudate;
e) probing depth;
f) gingival recessions;
g) hyperplasia and epithelial attachment level.

Plaque Index

Silness-Loe studies this index represents the initial amount of non-mineralized plaque along the gingival edge. The pressure index is determined using the following formula:

$$\text{Plaque Index} = \frac{\text{collection plaque index}}{\text{the collection of tooth surfaces on which it is determined}}$$

The plaque index represents the sum of the index values of plaque deposited on the surfaces around the implant. Already, the value of the plaque index speaks of poor oral hygiene.

The Sines-Lou Plaque Index uses the numbers:

0 - no plaque;

1 - dental plaque at the edge of the gingiva;

2 - a larger amount of plaque visible to the naked eye;

3 - the abundance of dental plaque, and the interdental spaces are filled with plaque.

This index has been modified by Mombelli and adapted to only one implant system (ITI implant):

0-No plaque;

1-plaque visible after probing - probe passage in the polished part of the implant;

2-plaque visible to the naked eye.

The calculation of the plaque index is performed at 6 points per implant, if possible, i.e. as far as prostetic work allows: mesio-buccal, medio-buccal, dysto-buccal, mesio-oral, medio-oral and dysto-oral.

Peri-Implant Mucosal Detachment Index

The gingival index by Lou and Sinles determines the degree of inflammation of the gingiva within 4 degrees and is represented by the following formula:

$$\text{Gingival index} = \frac{\text{collection of gingival indices}}{\text{collection of tooth surfaces on which the index is determined}}$$

The higher values obtained by this formula indicate a higher degree of inflammation of the gingiva.

The Gingival Index by Silens and Lou uses the numbers:

0 - healthy gingiva without signs of inflammation, traffic color and bleeding;

1 - existence of inflammation, redness, swelling, bleeding caused by probing and pressure;

3 - severe inflammation, severe redness and swelling, tendency to spontaneous bleeding and ulceration.

The gingival index has been modified by Mombeli to be adapted to the ITI implant system. When studying and determining the condition of the peri-implant mucosa on only one and the implant system, the obtained results may differ on other implant systems, because each system has its own characteristics in the design and technological processing of parts that are in contact with bone and soft tissues, according to the author of the book. For example, a new implant system, Roxsolis (Roxsolid), which is a combination of titanium and zirconium, has been applied recently. It is stated that this combination of materials from which the implant is built accelerates bone integration, i.e. To shorten the time of osteointegration physiological processes from 6-8 weeks to 3-4 weeks. This characteristic is important for patients with diabetes, for example, and passionate smokers because faster healing of bone soft tissues is a defense against peri-implant infections. It is certain that the technological treatment of the implant surface affects the metabolism of tissues that are in contact with its surface, but nevertheless, these processes are scientifically clarified.

Mombelli Gingvinal Index:

0 - There is no curling of the perimortem mucosa when probing;

1 - Isolated SPOTTED BLEEDING,

2 - Linear bleeding along the marginal edge of the mucosa;

3 - Deep bleeding

Determination of the gingvinal index is performed with 6 points per implant, if possible, i.e. as far as prosthetic work allows: mesio-buccal, medio-buccal, dysto-buccal, mesio-oral, medio-oral and dysto-oral.

During longitudinal studies, a large correlation between gingvinal mucosal index and peri-implatal bone loss was not demonstrated.

Bleeding After Probing

Bleeding after probing indicates the state of inflammation of the peri-implant tissues. If possible, as far as prosthetic work allows, the probe is applied to the peri-implant pockets in six points: mesio-buccal, medio-buccal, dysto-buccal, mesio-oral, medio-oral and dysto-oral. The probing determines whether bleeding occurs after a period of 15 seconds. The bleeding index after probing is calculated using the following formula:

$$\text{Bleeding on probing (\%)} = \frac{\text{a collection of cities that bled}}{\text{zbir surface of the tooth on which the probe is made}}$$

A high bleeding index is associated with severe peri-implant inflammation. Although a negative bleeding index at probing is associated with healthy periodontal disease, this cannot be said with certainty when it comes to the implant. Leckholm was unable to determine a relationship between a positive bleeding index and histological, microbiological, or radiological deterioration around the implant. The authors believe that bleeding can also be caused by traumatization of the peri-implant tissue.

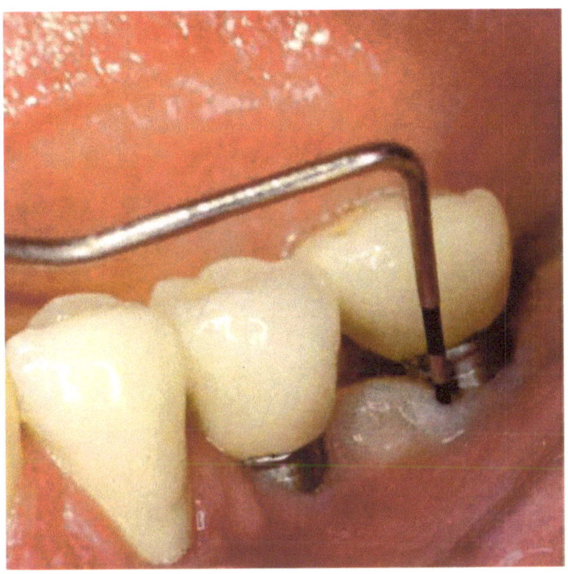

Figure 15.40. The depth of probing next to the implant is 5mm; gingival recession 1mm; attachment epithelium level 6mm; no bleeding, no separation.

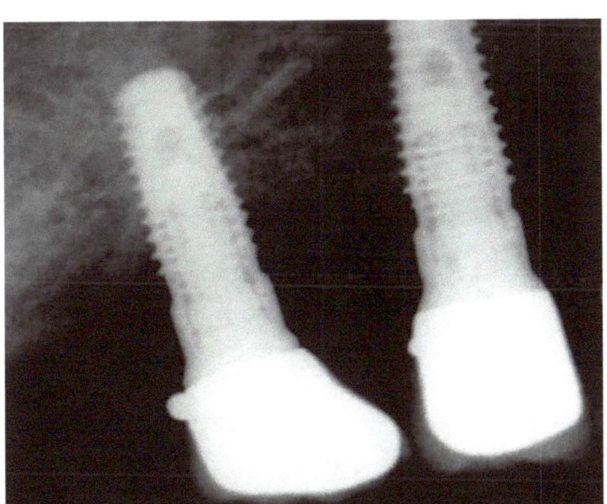

Figure 15.41. Radiographic representation of peri-implatitis bone defect type regions #24 and #25. 12 months after implant insertion.

Probing Depth, Gingival Recession, Epithelial Absorption Level

In a healthy peri-implant milieu, the physiological probing depth does not exceed 3mm. In the literature, we find that these strains were performed on animals, so the apical spread of the attachment epithelium cannot be accurately determined. Research has shown that the probe passes deeper in the direction of the marginal bone around the inflamed peri-implant mucosa than around the healthy tissue around the implant. This is explained by the decompression of collagen fibers in the presence of inflammation. The pressure of probing should not exceed 0.25 Ncm, which is considered standard in periodology. Also, it is recommended to probe around the mini-implants. The penetration of the probe tip can be influenced by a multitude of factors-angulation and diameter of the probe, micro and macro design of the implant and suprastructure, as well as the consistency of the peri-implant mucosa.

Some of the results of probing are shown in figures (15.40, 15.43, 15.46, and 15.48).

The depth of probing can be associated with peri-implant inflammation, but it is not possible to draw conclusions about the degree of bone resorption. Increased values of the probing depth must always be compared with the values of the probing before prosthetic work. In this way, all factors that can affect the increase in the depth of probing and create unfavorable conditions for the occurrence of mucositis and peri-implantitis can be considered.

Experience from practice indicates that the doctor examines the future prosthetic work modeled in wax and suggests to the dental technician to eliminate all factors that could favor peri-implant changes. When testing the metal supraconstruction on implants, it is necessary to remove all the details that perform compression on the surrounding soft tissues. Prosthetic work should be performed in such a way as to allow the circulation of the spit and accessed brush in all parts around the implant, in order to maintain good oral hygiene.

Probing is performed at 6 points per implant if possible, when prosthetic work has already been set: mesio-buccal, medio-buccal, dysto-buccal, mesio-oral, medio-oral and dysto-oral.

Probing is essentially the main method in the diagnosis of peri-implant infections. Bleeding to provocation after probing and fubina probing determine the degree of inflammation.

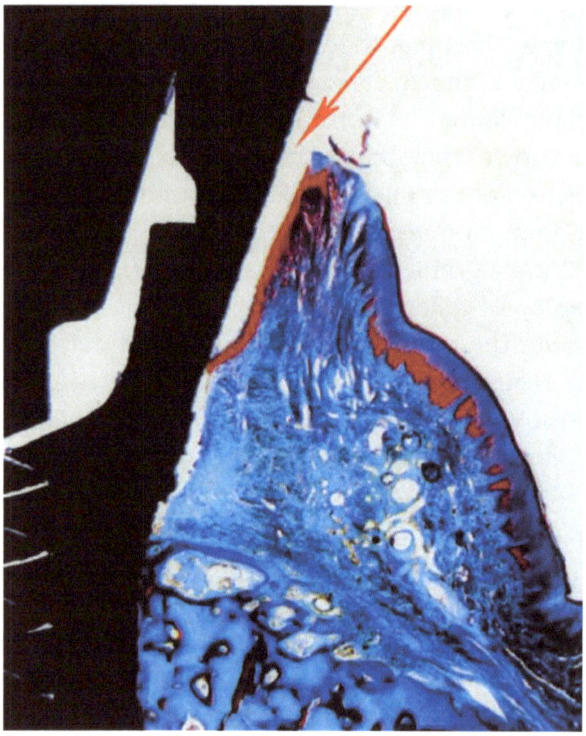

Figure 15.42. Histological sample showing peri-implant tissue 6 weeks after transmucosal healing. The connective eepithelium and subepithelial tissue are clearly separated from the implant surface by a crack (indicated by a red arrow).

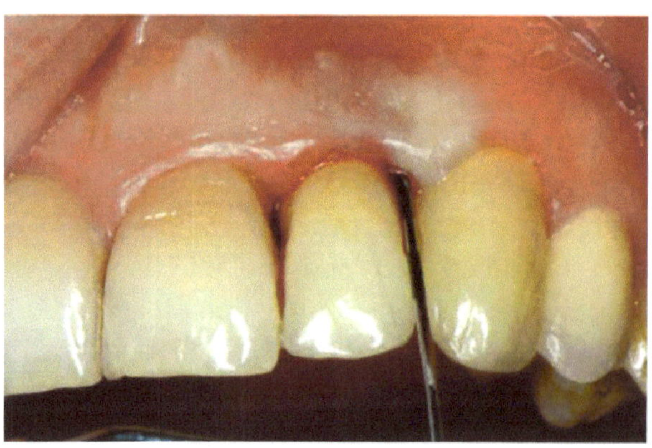

Figure 15.43. Probing of a bone defect in the form of a tunnel on the distal side. The diagnosis is peri-implantitis.

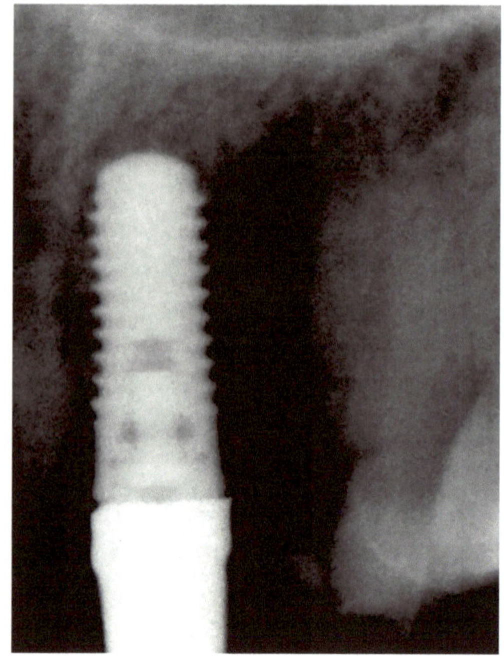

Figure 15.44. Radiological presentation of a bone defect in the form of a tunnel of a region with peri-implantitis.

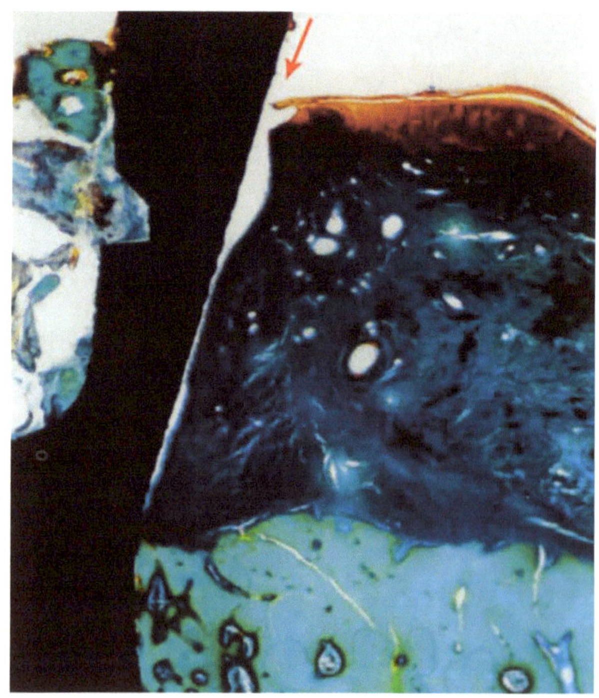

Figure 15.45. Hisotological findings 2 weeks after probing. The soft and hard tissue surrounding the implant does not show any changes. A mild inflammatory herbal infiltrate was observed in the subepithelial connective tissue of the adjacent junctional epithelium along its entire length.

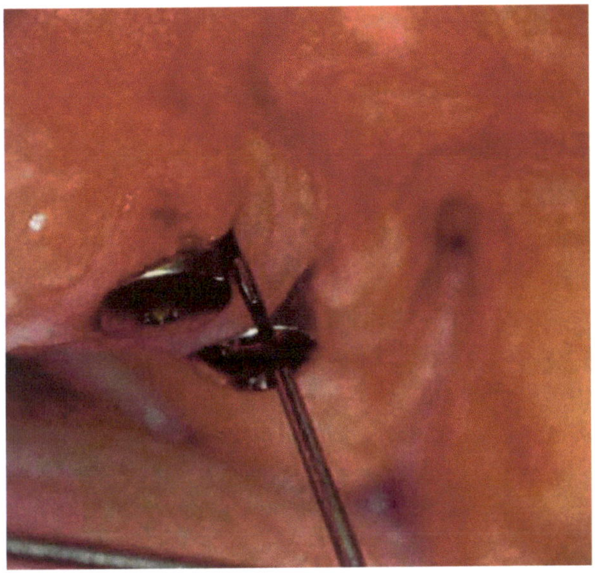

Figure 15.46. Depth of union 3-4mm, recession 0,level of attached epithelium 3-4mm, presence of bleeding and suppuration

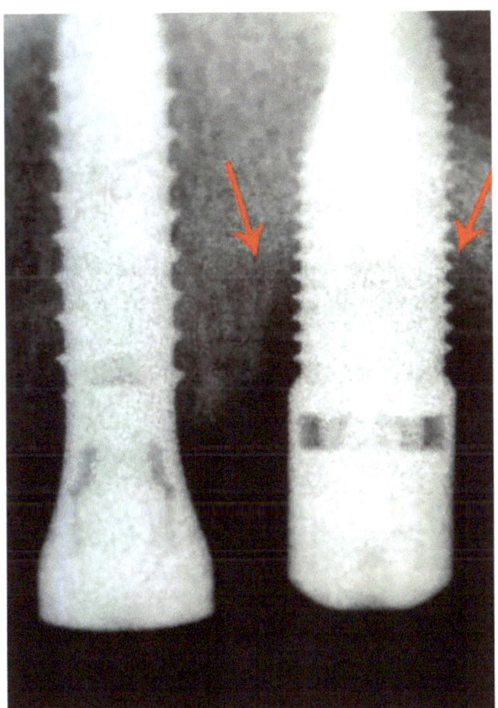

Figure 15.47. Radiographic representation of the previous image - Pateliform defect - cup shape (Class II),horizontal defect (Class I). Diagnosis: peri-implantitis.

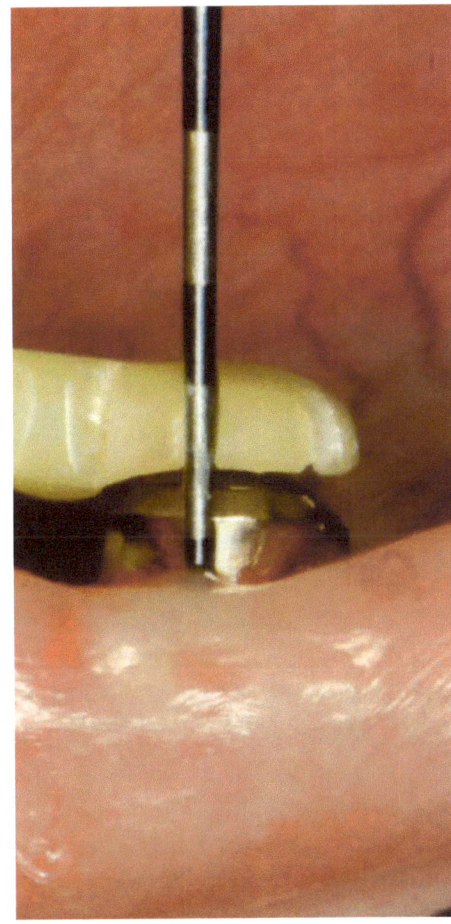

Figure 15.48. Clinical probing using periodontal probes to diagnose peri-implant infection.

Determination Of The Content Of Peri-implantate Sullucid Liquid (Peri-implant sulcus fluid)

Several studies show a correlation between peri-implatal infection and an increase in inflammation mediated values (proinfalamic cytokines) in the sulcus fluid in peri-implatitis. The fluid composition approximates that of blood serum. The succulent fluid has a larger immunological reactiveness than saliva. In inflammation of peri-implant tissues, the volume of sulcus fluid is significantly increased by the presence of deposited plaque. The pulsating fluid contains proteases, collagenases, glycosamine, glycan, pro-inflammatory mediators such as Il1-beta and prostaglandin E2. Benk (Behenk) with a three-year longitudinal study demonstrated a positive correlation between increased volume of peri-implant sulcus fluid and loss of peri-implant bone.

Supuration And Manure Content

Manure is a pathological inflammatory exudate consisting of neutrophils, polymorphonuclear granulocytes, decomposed tissue, microorganisms and serum. Advanced peri-implant infections are clinically manifested by the appearance of manure and suppuration.

Clinical Determination Of Implant Mobility

From a practical point of view, even when there is a pronounced bone loss around the implant, the applicative part of the implant that is still osteintegrated can be used for further survival of the implant in the bone, with thoroughly performed augmentation. The result of augmentation depends on the size and configuration of the bone defect. In the event that after the period required for healing and remodeling of the new bone it is found that the level of bone compensation is insufficient, additional augmentation should be performed. If, after some time, minimal mobility of the implant is also found, it is considered that there has been a complete loss of osteointegration.

The mobility of the implant can be determined manually or using instruments. By manual movement of the implant, the finding of mobility in the horizontal and vertical direction, with the appearance of pain, is a sign of peri-implant inflammation. By instrument percussion, a clear, hypersonic sound can be heard over the osteointegrated implant, while a blunt, hypersonorous sound is obtained in an implant encapsulated with connective tissue.

Today, laser electronic methods are used to measure implant mobility. With this method, the implant is percutaneous 16 times for 4 seconds. The device then reads the result of implant mobility on a special mathematical scale.

The values obtained indicate the degree of mobility of the implant:
-8 to +9- physiological mobility = zero degree
+10 to +19- mobility by palpation = first degree
+20 to +29- visible mobility = second degree
+30 to +50- third degree

The values of osteointegrated implants cannot be fully confirmed by this method. Higher values are obtained in the upper than in the lower jaw. With this method, different results are obtained in implants of different lengths.

Using resonant frequency analysis, more accurate results are obtained. This apparatus, at the base of the piezoelectric effect, shows frequencies from 3500 to 8500 Hz, while the second element measures the reaction of the implant and directly shows the solidity of the bond between the implant and the bone. Resonant frequency analysis values increase during osteointegration, and decline if integration is unsuccessful. The coefficient of implant stability is the unit of measurement of this method and ranges from 1 to 100 Hz. Many studies have shown that the coefficient of implant stability increases over time in osteointegrated implants.

Clinical Manifestations

By consensus at the Sixth European Round Table in Periodontology, peri-implantitis was defined as an infectious disorder. Peri-implant mucositis involves an inflammatory reversible lesion of the mucosa, while peri-implantitis also affects the surrounding bone. Peri-implant mucositis is limited to the mucosa, while peri-implantitis also applies to the bone. Peri-implantitis should be distinguished from reversible soft tissue inflammation and early complications following implant placement, such as necrosis and dehiscence.

Peri-implant infections are clinically manifested in three different forms: peri-implant mucosal hyperplasia, mucosal hyperplasia and peri-implantitis (Figures 15.48 and 15.49). Differential diagnosis of peri-implantitis requires differentiation of reversible inflammation and peri-implant soft tissues without involvement of alveolar bone (peri-implant mucositis and peri-implant mucosal hyperplasia), then early complications within the healing period of the implant, as well as cases where there is no primary inflammatory component (for example, bone necrosis due to overheating due to inadequate permeation of the implant bed with blunt drills, with the absence of abundant saline cooling, dehiscence defects).

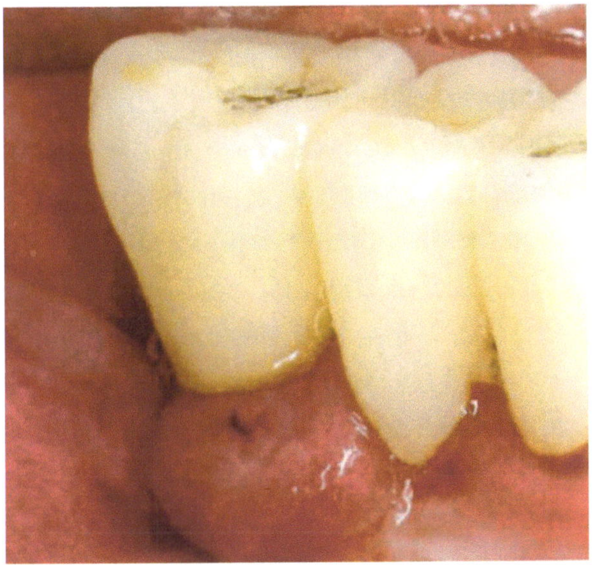

Figure 15.49 Diagnosis: peri-implantitis with mucosal hyperplasia

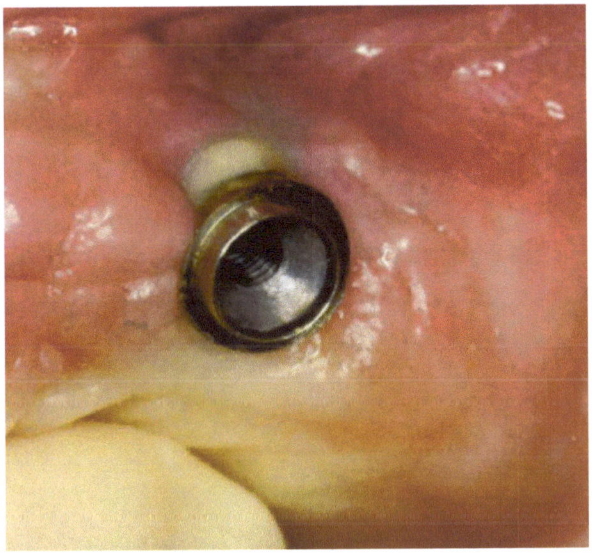

Figure 15.50 Diagnosis: Peri-implantitis

The following parameters can be used as safe diagnostic signs of peri-implantitis:

1. **Radiologically proven intraskeletal or supracrestal loss of the supportive alveolar bone.**
2. **Implant mobility.** Implant mobility is a sign of insufficiently achieved or completely unfulfilled osteointegration
3. **Formation of peri-implant pockets.** Intraskeletal and vertical bone loss is the cause of the formation of peri-implant pockets.
4. **Bleeding after probing.** Bleeding after careful probing with a periodontal probe may be associated with suppuration and pus expression.

Intraskeletal loss may have: patella-form, tunnel-form and fissure-form. There is currently no known correlation between forms of bone loss and etiological factors. The remaining amount of the osteointegrated implant can be used as a prognostic factor (less or more than 1/3 of the implant length). The physiological process of peri-implant resorption must be considered. In two-part implants with submerged bone healing, the average crestal bone loss was 0.9-1.6 mm in the first year and 0.02-0.15 mm in subsequent years. In contrast, implants with transmucosal healing, show an average crestal bone resorption of 0.09mm per year in the lower jaw and 0.01 mm in the upper jaw. The actual amount of residual bone around the implant can only be reliably determined histologically.

The formation of a peri-implant abscess is very rare and is perceived by an unusual progressive form, as pus usually appears from the sulcus when the connection between the soft tissue and the implant surface is poorly formed. Depending on the localization of the infection, as well as on the histological value of the loss of the peri-implant bone, the abscess can nevertheless survive from the peri-implant abscess to the submucosal abscess, which must be treated as an emergency. This procedure is based on the basic principle that pus should always be removed when it appears. In addition to the incision of the abscess, it is necessary to remove the causes of infection ("Secanta causa-Secante effectus"). Antibiotics should be administered to accelerate therapy, as the possibility of neurosurgical treatment of inflammatory processes around the implant surface is greatly narrowed.

The following examples are not characteristic of the diagnosis of peri-implantitis:

Swelling and redness of the peri-implant soft tissue do not have to be signs of peri-implantitis. Hyperplasia does not also speak of the condition of bone tissue. Hyperplasia most commonly occurs around the implant that lacks a keratinized gingiva or manifests itself during prosthetic therapy (Figure 15.50).

Pain occurs at the initial stage of peri-implant mucositis.

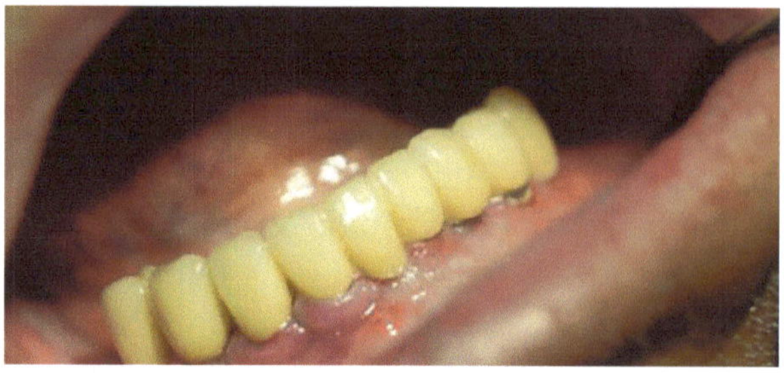

Figure 15.51 Peri-implant changes in mucosal tissues without change in bone tissue condition. Cause poor oral hygiene.

Classification Of Peri-Implant Bone Defects

Based on clinical trials of peri-implant bone defects, a division can be made according to bone involvement by inflammation. These peri-implant defects can be intraosseous (Type 1) and supra-alveolar (Type II), as shown in Figures 15.51 and 15.52.

Intraskeletal defects can be clinically divided into 5 types (Figures 15.54-15.58):

- Type 1a. Manifested as a mild buccal or oral skeletal defect, V-shaped dehiscence as the mildest degree of bone resorption (Figure 15.52);
- Type 1b. Buccal or oral bone defect with semicircular bone resorption towards the middle of the implant;
- Type 1c. Circular bone defect spreading vestibularly, with the preserved part of the lamella vestibularly (Figure 15.55);

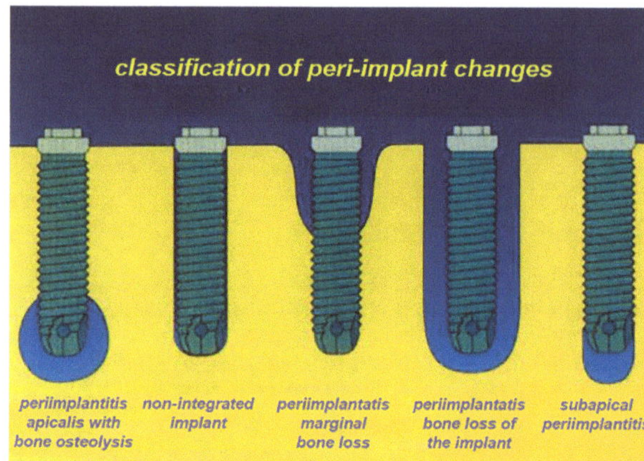

Figure 15.52. Schematic representation of peri-implant changes in bone defects

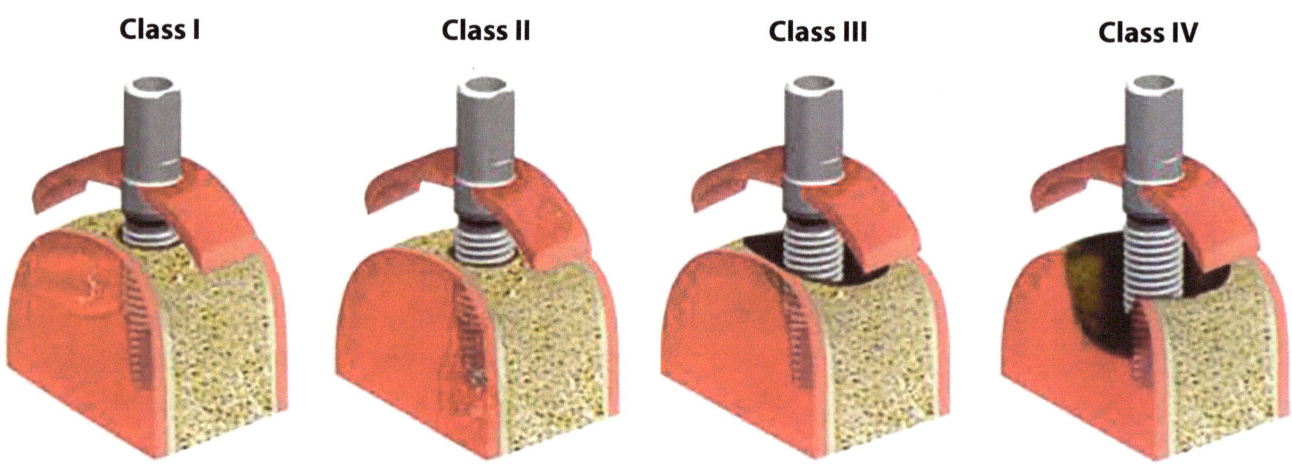

Figure 15.53. Schematic representation of the classification of peri-implantitis and bone damage by Jovanković and Spikerman

Classification Of Peri-implantitis Based On The Degree Of Bone Damage By Jovanović And Spikerman

In order to determine the degree of disease and the choice of therapy Jovanović and Spikerman (1995) published a classification of peri-implantitis based on the degree of bone damage (Figure 15.53).

Based on this classification, the following classes are distinguished:

- Class 1: moderate horizontal bone loss with minimal bone component;
- Class 2: moderate to advanced horizontal bone loss with minimal bone component;
- Class 3: minimal to moderate horizontal bone loss with co-ordered peripheral bone lesion;
- Class 4: bone damage with moderate horizontal bone loss and advanced peripheral bone lesion with loss of vestibular and/or lingual lamella.

Types of peri-implantitis from 1a to 1e start from the crestal part of the alveolar ridge, progressing towards the floor of the intraskeletal defect and can be biri measured in four locations marked with a blue circle: mesial, distal, buccal and oral. Horizontal defects determine the distance between the mesial and dostal, as well as the buccal and oral bone walls. The spread of the dehiscence defect can extend from the crestal part of the alveolar bone in height and width. (Figure 15.61).

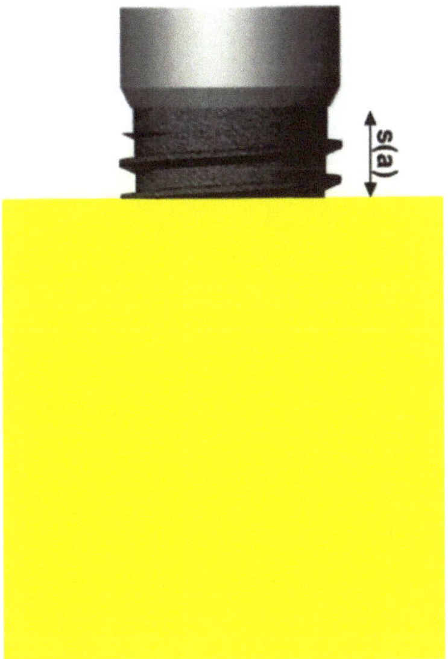

Figure 15.54. Classification of bone defects caused by peri-implantitis supracrestal bone defect.

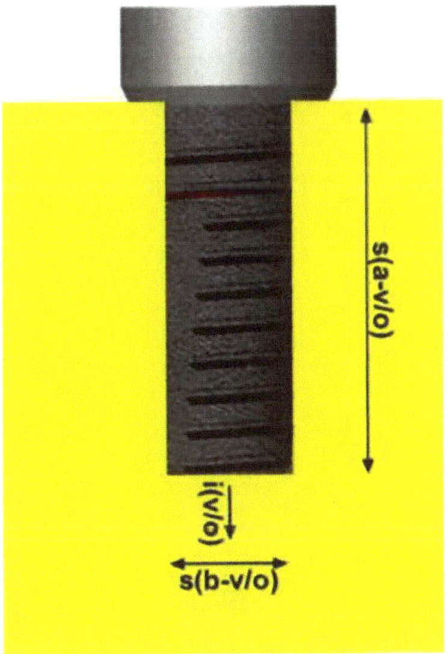

Figure 15.55. Frontal cross-section of the dehiscence defect

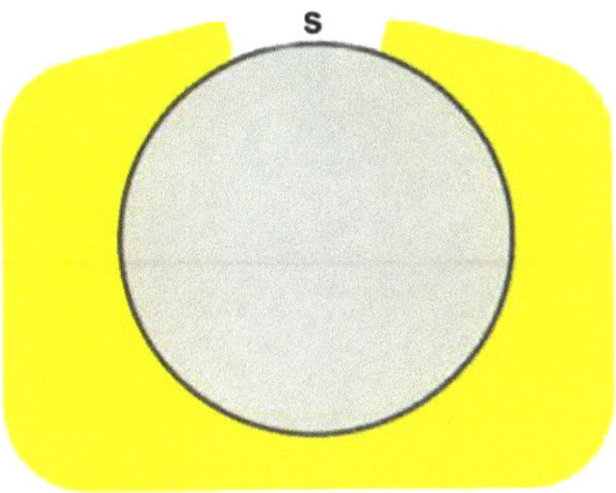

Figure 15.56. Mildest degree (type) of buccal intraosseous bone defect-vestibular dehiscence (class 1a)

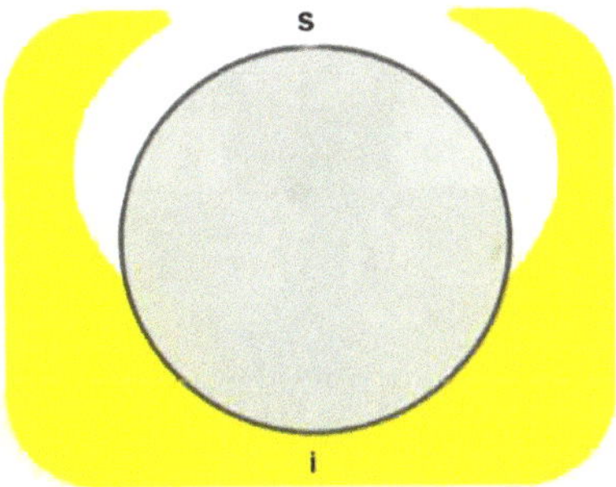

Figure 15.57. Semicircular bone resorption up to half of the implant body, intraosseous bone defect (class 1b): vestibular dehiscence with semicircular defect.

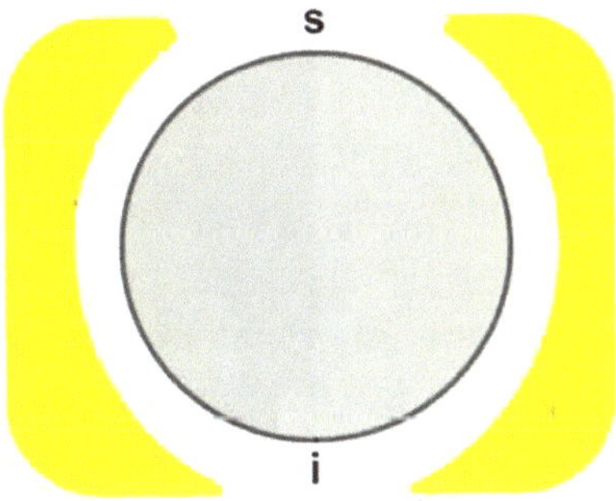

Figure 15.58 Intraosseous defect (class 1c), vestibular dehiscence with semicircular defect

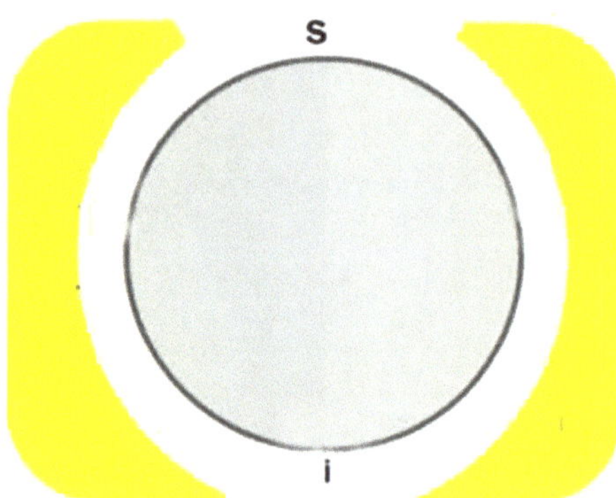

Figure 15.59. The circular bone defect of the lamella is a defect that spreads vestibularly, and part of the bone lamella is not preserved (class 1d)

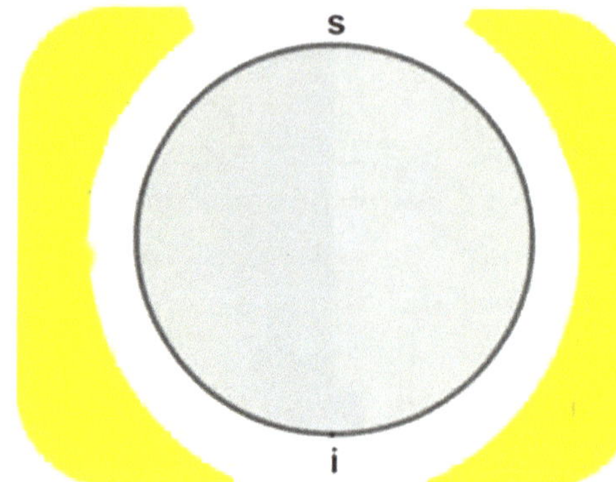

Figure 15.60. Intraosseous circular defect with dehiscence and circular bone resorption (class 1e).

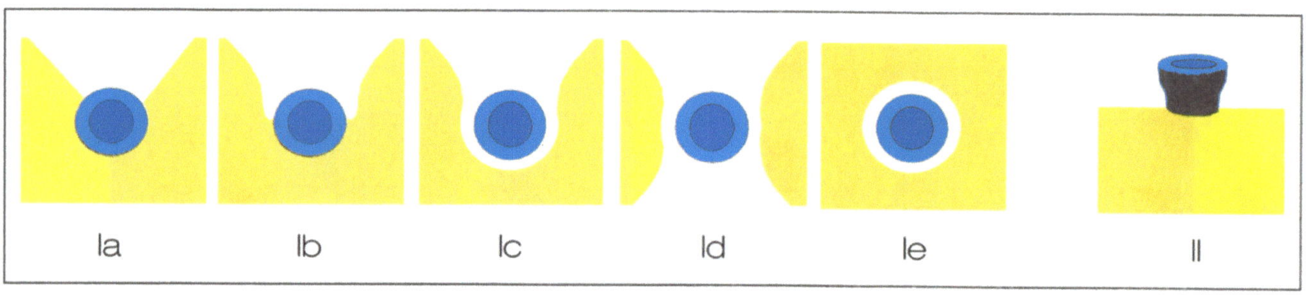

Figure 15.61. Schematic representation of subdivisions of peri-implant bone defects by the same author (Schwarz). Class 1 describes the appearance of intraosseous bone defects and class 2 describes supra-alveolar defects. Point marked with a blue circle and determines the interosal components of the defect (s) the height of the bone defect (class 2) (i) or the width of the defect (class 1).

Radiographic Classification

The radiographic classification allows a quick examination of the marginal bone and serves as the basic method for examining peri-implantitis. Generally, the current bone level should be compared to the bone level immediately after implant placement.

Radiographically detected peri-implantitis may not necessarily be accompanied by bone loss due to inflammation. This must also take into account the physiological atrophy of the bone and the assessment of the peri-implant part. It must be taken into account that the radiological assessment cannot determine with certainty the state of the buccal and oral compact structure-only a possible reassessment of the supra-alveolar defect is possible.

When making decisions on the treatment plan for cases indicating the existence of peri-implantitis, it should be known that the clinical and radiographic findings do not coincide (Figures 15.71 and 15.72). Also, it should be known that there is a possibility that appropriate procedures (primarily bone augmentation) can significantly extend the life of the implant that was affected by peri-implantitis (Figures 17.73, 15.74, 5.75, 15.76 and 15.77).

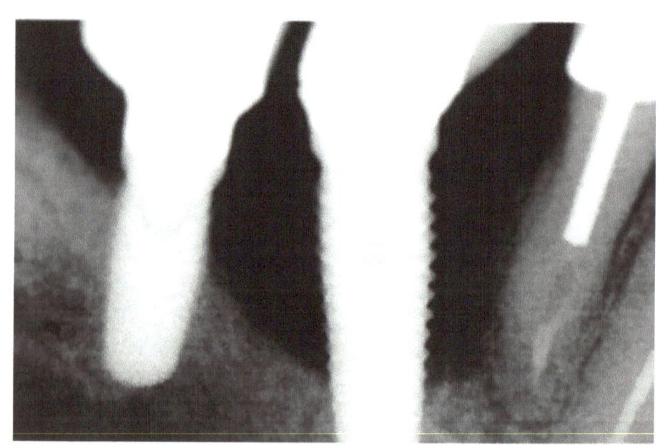

Figure 15.62 Horizontal bone defect

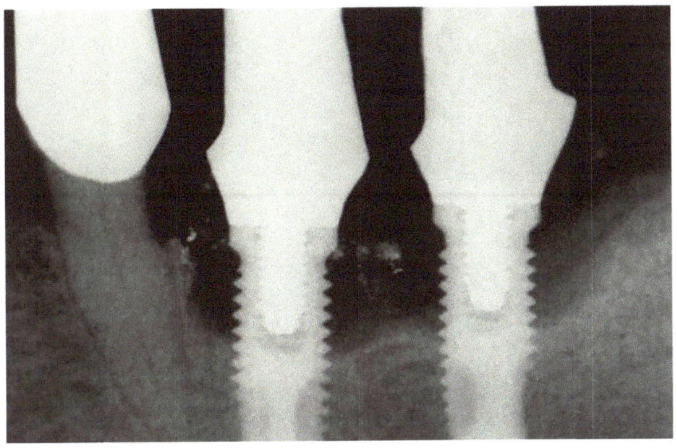

Figure 15.63 Bone defect tunnel shape

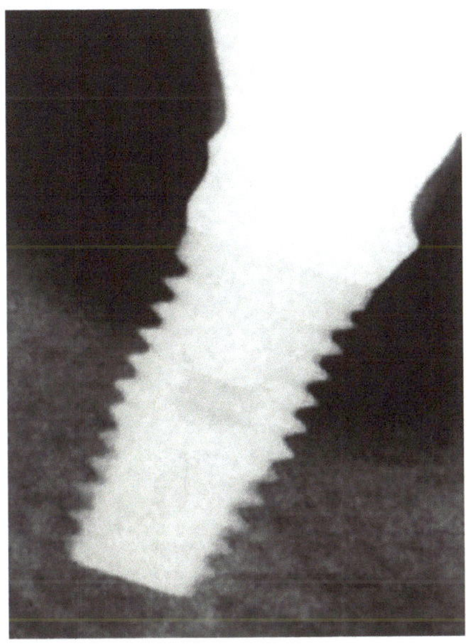

Figure 15.64 Horizontal bone loss

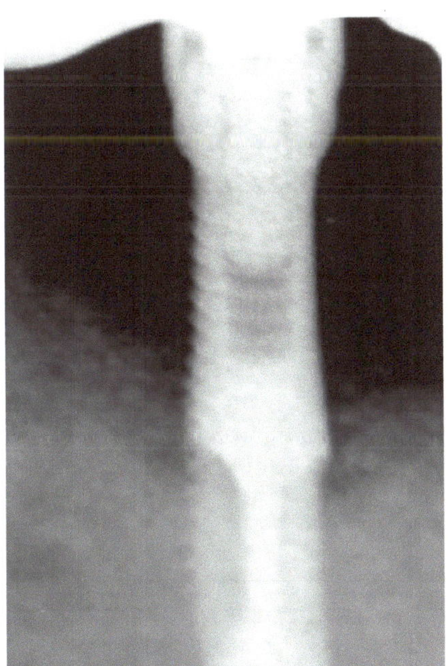

Figure 15.65 Patellar defect type

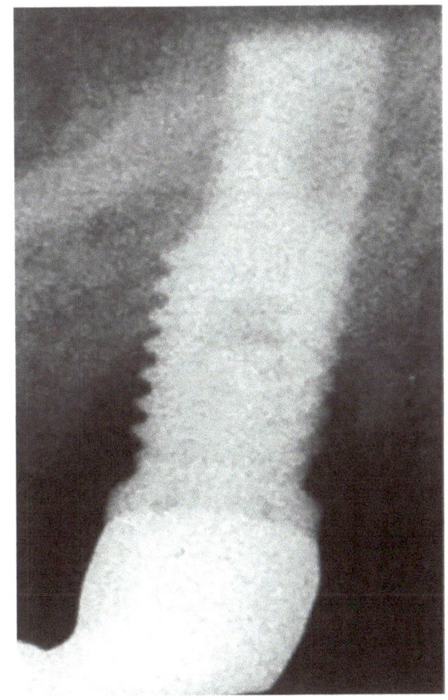

Figure 15.66 Gap bone defect

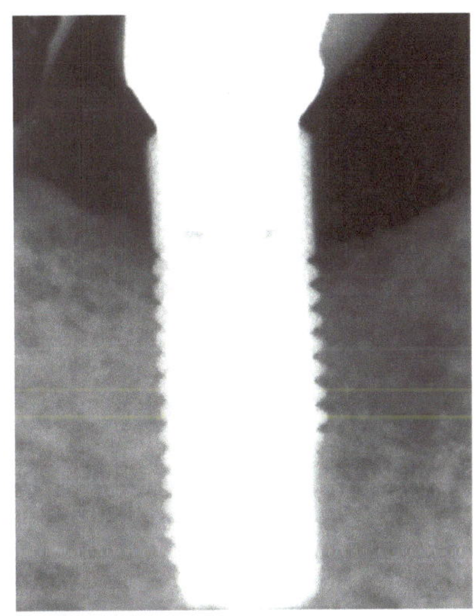

Figure 15.67 Patelliform and horizontal bone resorption type

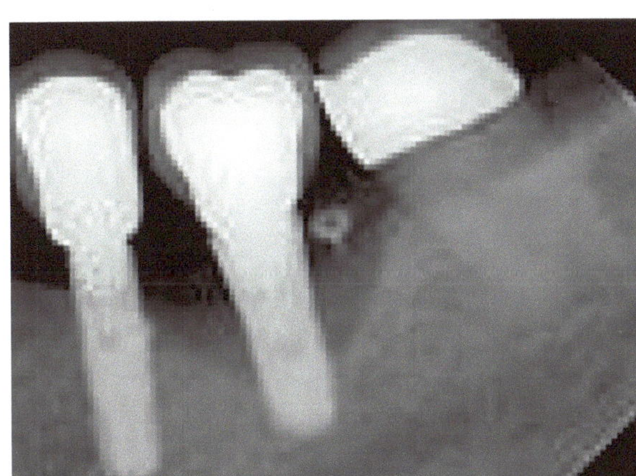

Figure 15.68 Bone defect in the shape of the pelvis. Augmentation with autologous bone block

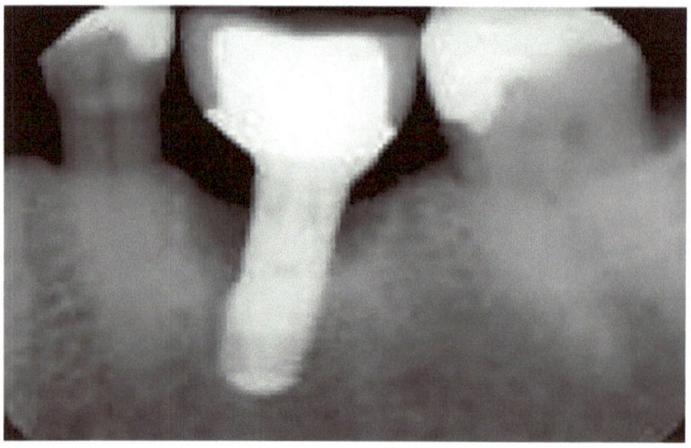

Figure 15.69 Bone defect in the shape of the pelvis. Augmentation with xenogenic bone substitutes.

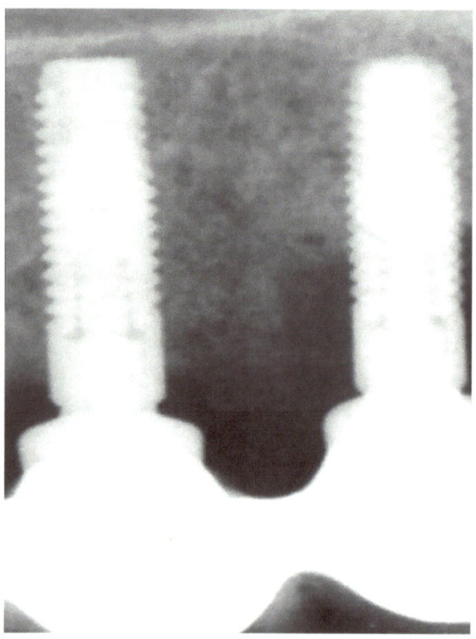

Figure 15.70 Horizontal tunnel bone resorption type

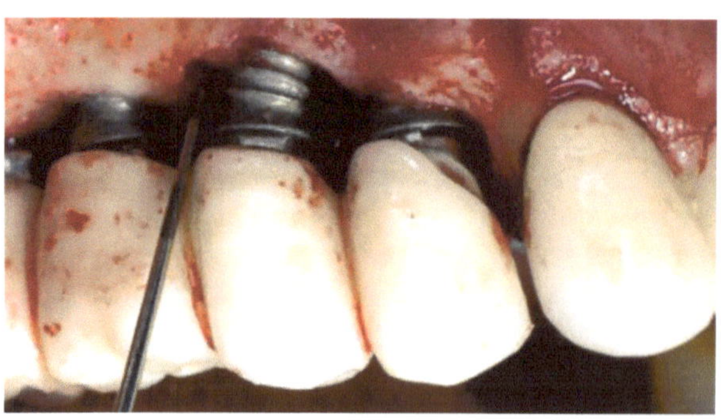

Figure 15.71 Clinical finding of the implant in the lateral region of the upper jaw that is not in accordance with the radiographic finding shown in the following figure

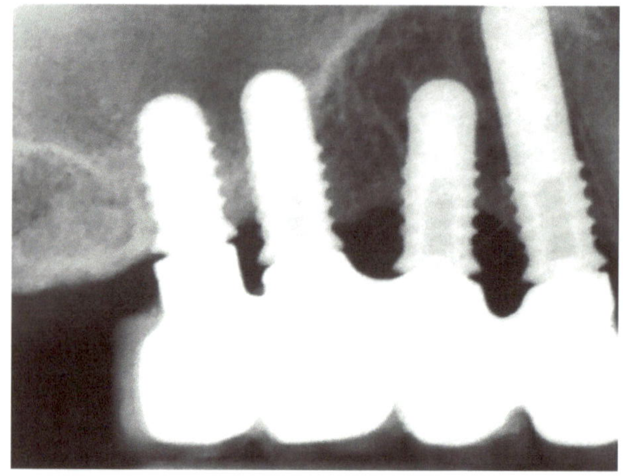

Figure 15.72 Radiographic finding of the same region, which completely deviates from the clinical finding. Compare with Figure 15.71.

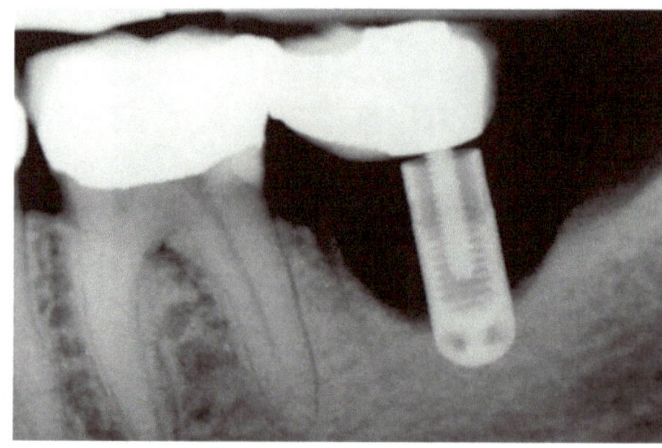

Figure 15.73 Terminal bone resorption phase around the cylindrical implant. Augmentation with bone replacers prolongs the survival time of the implant (see Figures 15.68, 15.69, 15.74, 15.76 and 15.77)

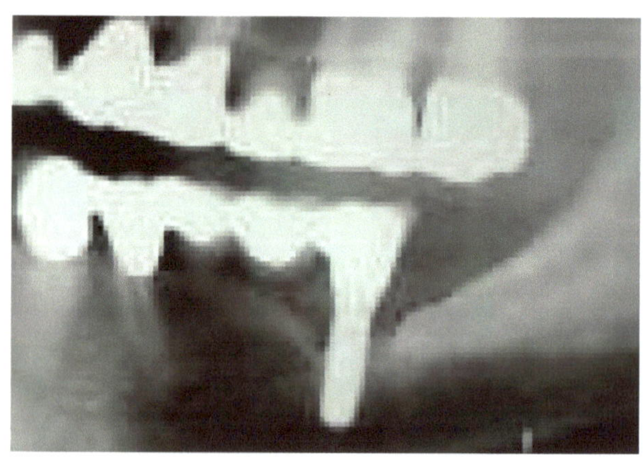

Figure 15.74 Treatment of peri-implantitis by defect augmentation also prolongs the time of implant function. Considering the period when these systems were applied, this implant has been in operation for at least two decades. One of the reasons for the occurrence of a bone defect is the bonding of the implant with a natural tooth (instead of having two individual implants immediately installed without bonding).

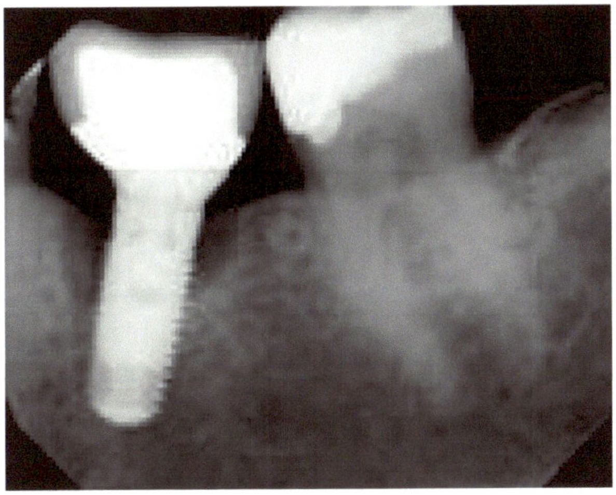

Figure 15.75 Peri-implantitis of the region #36

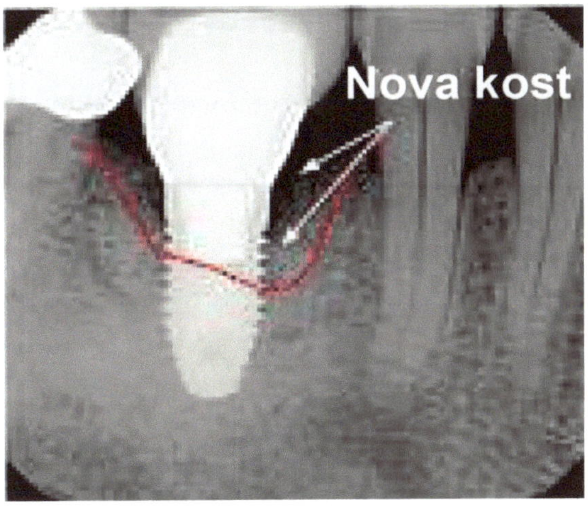

Figure 15.76 Creating new bone after augmentation of a bone defect around the implant.

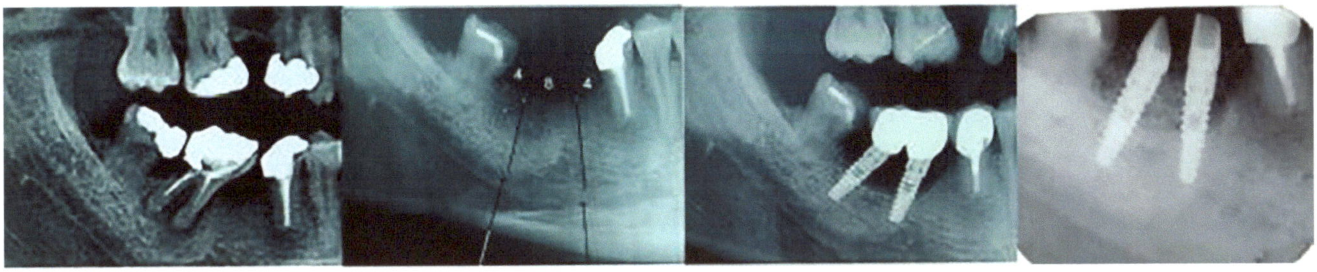

Figure 15.77 a) After molar screening (#46), alveolar preservation was performed; b) appearance of augmented region after 8 months; c) patellar form peri-implantitis after 4 years, the cause of the peri-implant infection was residual cement that was not seen on the radiographic scan. After removing the prosthetic work and augmentation, the implantats are firmly integrated.

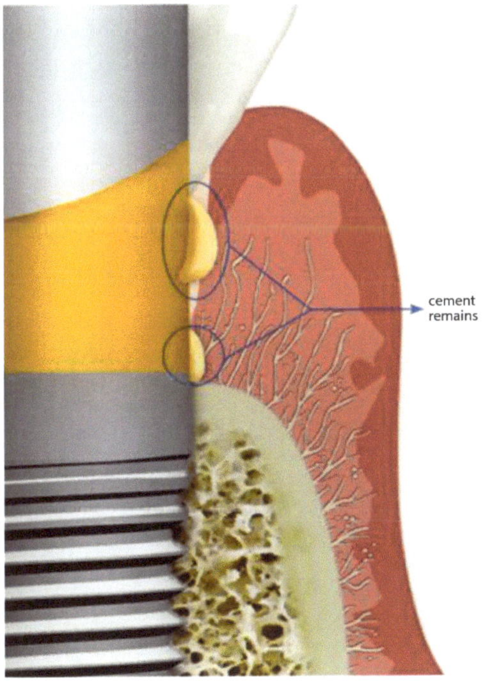

Figure 15.78 Cement residues can cause serious complications of peri-implantitis and implant loss

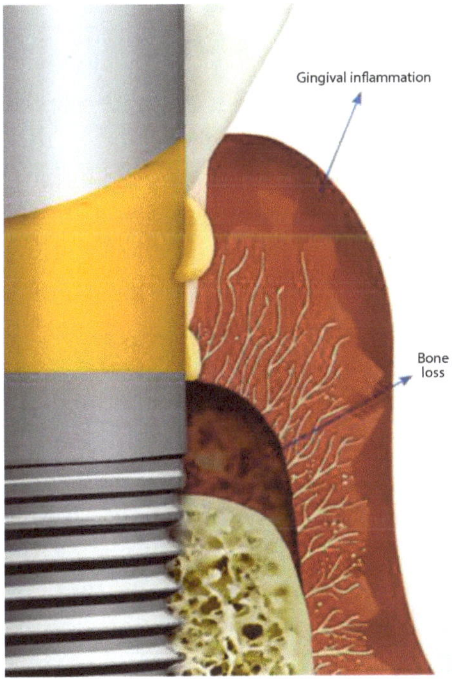

Figure 15.79 An overview of the consequences of residual cement causing soft tissue inflammation with consequences of peri-implantitis.

Treatment of Peri-implantitis

When it comes to the treatment of peri-implantitis, it should be emphasized that peri-implantitis is one of the most serious complications of implant-prosthetic rehabilitation of the oral cavity. It is important to emphasize that the treatment of peri-implantitis is very difficult and with an uncertain outcome. Considering the multifactorial causes of peri-implantitis, the treatment protocol will depend on diagnosing the cause of the peri-implant disease, not masking the problem (Figure 15.80). -"Secante causa-secante effectus" - "Remove the causes - the consequences will not exist" - with the help of adequate treatment.

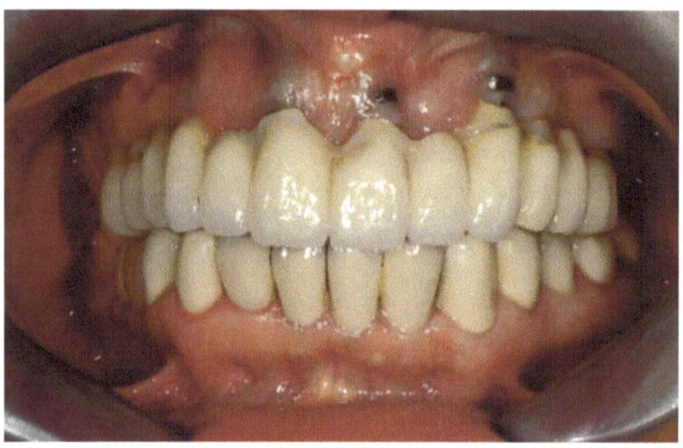

Figure 15.80. Wrong approach to solving the problem of peri-implantitis. Masking with composites hides the problem and exposes patients to all sorts of troubles.

There are many theories about the occurrence of peri-implantitis based on reinfection of the peri-implant tissue, because between the implant and the suprastructure there is an intermediate space that can be reduced, but not completely removed. Some studies state that this marginal space is from 14 to 160 microns and that it cannot completely resist the penetration of bacteria from the oral cavity, because pathogenic microorganisms are several times smaller than the existing crack between the surface of the implant and the superstructure. The colonization of bacteria may occur immediately after fixation of the support (abutment) and prosthetic work, because in such an environment, warmth and humidity create favorable conditions that allow the growth of bacteria. Their settlement in the intermediate space between the carrier and the body of the implant depends on the diameter of that gap, which also depends on the implant system and technological processing. During chewing, due to the creation of capillary forces and micro-movements, there is an exchange of tissue fluid from the surface of the implant and peri-implant tissue. This mechanism enables the creation of permanent reinfection, which is explained as the most common cause of peri-implantitis. Theoretical explanations go further, speculating that even the highest precision and the best technological treatment of the implant surface cannot eliminate the need to insert some materials into the peri-implant space to compensate for the surface roughness of the implant and the superstructure as a replacement for the lost tooth. Preparations have already appeared on the market to prevent peri-implant diseases. The author believes that for now these considerations are only at the level of theory, and practice is the one that can accept and confirm them.

Treatment of peri-implantitis was based on procedures and experiences from periodontitis therapy. However, practical experience confirms that the method of treating peri-implantitis is much more complex.

The first procedure in the treatment of peri-implantitis is the removal of the biofilm that caused the infection on the surface of the implant. How and in what way to remove the infection from the surface of the implant depends on the dentist, that is, the method he will apply. The laser method of removing infection from the implant surface has already been widely proposed and applied. One such laser device is "BIOLASE" (picture 15.81), which also has an anti-infective, i.e. bactericidal, effect.

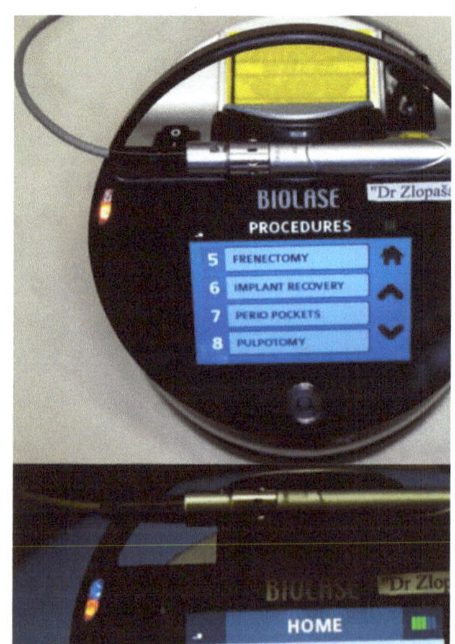

Figure 15.81. BIOLASE laser devices (Biolase, Inc. USA, 4 Cromwell, Irvine).

The therapy of peri-implantitis with this BIOLASE-type laser (Fig. 15.81) is based partly on the disinfection of the surrounding soft tissue and on the sterilization of the implant surface after the removal of the granulation tissue. Since the energy of the diode laser is absorbed in the dark spectrum (thus heating everything that is dark in color), the surface of the implant is heated. In the instructions for use, caution is emphasized during application, so as not to overheat the surface of the implant, which is fatal for the surrounding bone. This laser has a heating power of 0.6-1 w for 30 seconds, and it can't remove deposits from the surface of the implant, but only has a bactericidal effect. When asked by the manufacturer: how can the heating of the implant surface be controlled, the received explanation warns of caution and doubt. Namely, the temperature is controlled by touching the diode with a finger. Regardless of the manufacturer's claims that the success rate of treatment with this method is up to 65%, the conclusion is that its application is an unnecessary risk taking because heating the surface of the implant can do more harm than good. Arbitrary determination of the heating of the diode with the finger, which heats the surface of the implant, can be individually different, and therefore an introduction to risk. The marketing characteristics of such expensive devices described by the manufacturer should be taken with a grain of salt. Previous experiences and many evidences from the literature confirm that in many cases where laser technology was used, the results were similar to cases treated with conventional methods.

The treatment of peri-implant mucositis is non-surgical, mechanical processing removes deposited plaque and concretions in the sulcus of the mucosa. Treatment of mucositis is carried out by agreement with the patient, because the outcome of the treatment depends on the cooperation of the patient. The inflammatory process cannot be stopped without the cooperation of patients - by stopping smoking and improving oral hygiene. If there is no improvement, a surgical approach is necessary. Since each patient is individual, the results of the treatment may be variable. The surgical procedure must also provide a wide access to the treatment of the implant surface. After removing the granulation tissue, it is necessary to mechanically clean the surface of the implant with rotating titanium brushes (Figures 15.82 to 15.84).

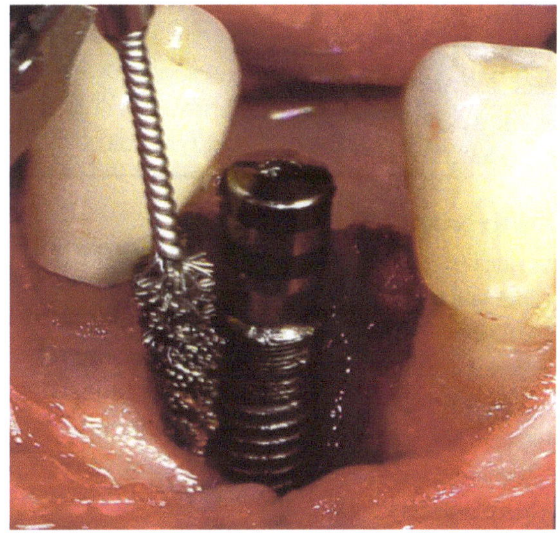

Figure 15.82. Mechanical cleaning of the implant surface with a rotating titanium brush.

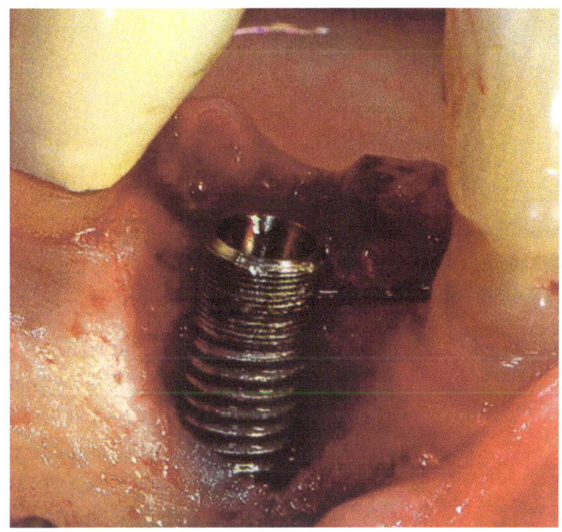

Figure 15.83. Appearance of the implant surface after removal of peri-implant granulation tissue with a titanium curette.

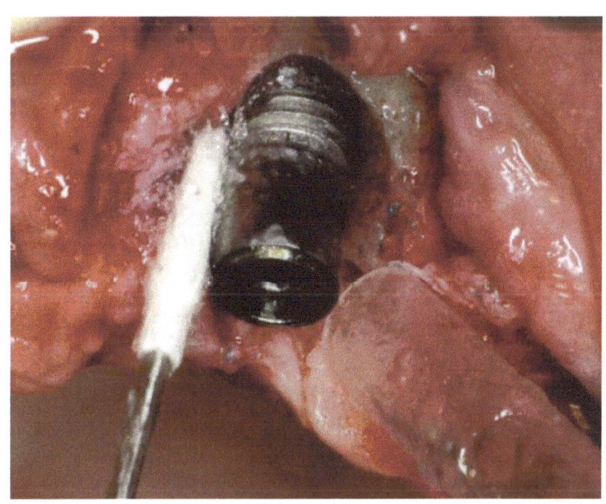

Figure 15.84. Disinfection of the surface of the implant can be done with rotating brushes soaked in a chemical solution for disinfection.

After thorough removal of the altered peri-implant tissue, the surface of the implant is cleaned with rotating titanium brushes and its surface is decontaminated. How to decontaminate the surface of the implant and surrounding tissues, various procedures and various devices are mentioned in the literature: ultrasonic, laser, sandblasting, as well as the application of chemical agents. All these procedures are still more on a theoretical level than on a practical level. It is contraindicated to treat the implant surface with steel instruments. In practice, a cotton ball soaked in solution with a thorough saline rinse is used to decontaminate the implant surface and surrounding tissues for cleaning.

The procedures described above are followed by the procedure of augmentation of the bone defect, i.e. compensating for the absorbed delicacy by covering the surface of the implant (Figure 18.85.). The amount of bone replacements depends on the defect configuration. Augmentation of bone defects is still with an uncertain outcome and risk, because the causes are multifactorial and individual.

Despite the tremendous progress of oral implantology, when it comes to replacing resorbed peri-implant bone with bone replacements, much remains unresolved. The results of augmentation are not always the same for bone defects of different configurations. All this shows how serious complication peri-implantitis is. For example, a group of authors (Aghazadeh & assoc.) found that (after 12 months, the second study after 24 months) the resorption of the covered bone defect with xenogenic material was lower than when autologous bone was used. Also , when asked whether the combination of bone graft, which was obtained by mixing shavings of autologous bone with xenogenic materials with bone substitutes, has an advantage, there is still no definitive answer from science.

However, practical experience confirms that the results of resorbed bone replacement were better in some patients with a xenogenic bone substitute, covered with a resorptive membrane, than with an autologous bone. Also, augmentation with xenogenic materials has a certain advantage due to reduced patient morbidity. It was also shown that filling the bone defect with shavings of the autologous bone above the level of the crestal bone did not give much better results.

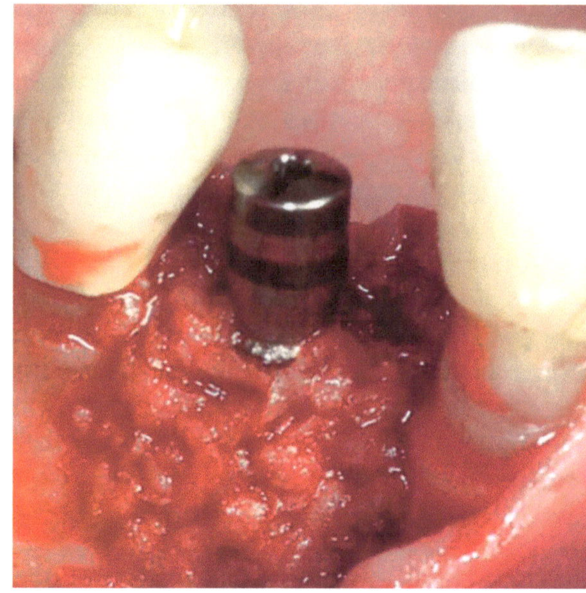

Figure 15.85 After mechanical cleaning and disinfection, the bone defect was filled with autologous bone shavings taken from the retromolar region of the mandible.

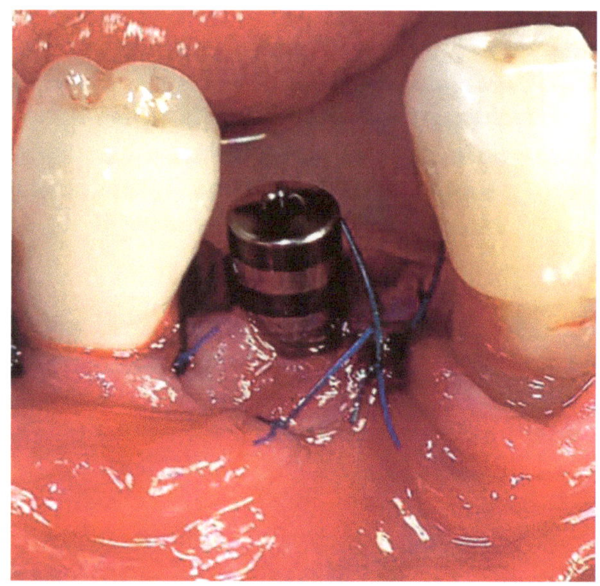

Figure 15.86 Formation of surrounding tissues by suturing.

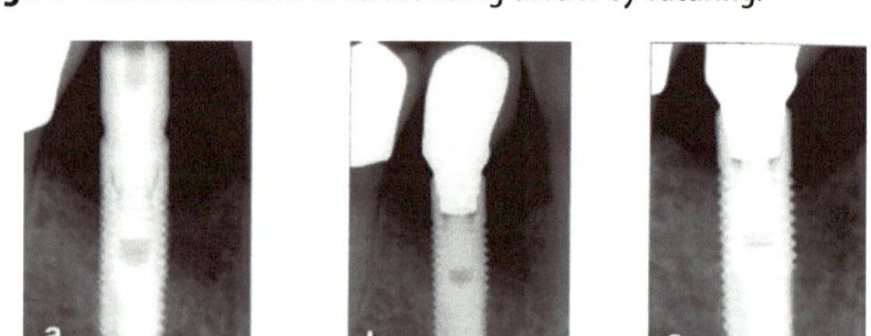

Figure 15.87 Peri-implantitis. Typical pelvic bone defect. a. formation of surrounding tissues by suturing, b. condition three months after augmentation, c. condition after 10 months

The observation of the author of the book, derived from the experiences of compensating bone defects with bone substitutes, the application of collagen resorptive membranes or titanium, according to the protocol is mandatory, the results of augmentation were approximately the same. However, obtaining different healing results of bone peri-implant defects, after surgical procedures performed according to the same protocol, lead to the interpretation that other factors are present in the pathophysiology of the peri-implant milieu that are not easy to detect. If the membrane is a barrier from the growth of connective tissue into the augment, there is no valid data that collagen membrane resorption takes place at the same time in all patients? That is, is its barrier role timely equal in all patients? Of course, this question does not arise when a titanium membrane is applied. Since the etiology of peri-implantitis is multifactorial, the question arises whether this multifactoriality can also affect the course of the time duration of the role of the collagen membrane as a barrier against the penetration of connective tissue after covering the bone substitute in the same way as in all patients? The answer to this question is not yet known.

This is supported by the fact that various types of collagen membranes from different manufacturers are offered on the market. However, the prospects do not provide adequate explanations that would clarify these dilemmas.

The most important factor for the speed and quality of augmentation remodeling into new bone, whether of autologous or xenogenic origin, is vascularization. This leads to thinking, can covering with collagen mebrane, given the multifactoriality of the cause of the disease, be a hindrance to faster blood circulation of the placed augment and faster formation of the coagulum? The author of the book on several cases of the aforementioned thinking checked in practice and came to the conclusion that the speed of remodeling of the new bone depends largely on the way of lifting the lobe, its processing and the immunity of the organism. Is it not logical that the coagulum will infiltrate into the placed material rather than when a precursor such as an membrane is placed on it in the initial phase? To the answer to this dilemma multifactorial facts must be added that science has not yet fully clarified. In many cases, this dilemma was tested in practice by the author of the book - in some patients, the result was better without the use of a collagen resorptive membrane, than in some where it was used.

Report of cases that confirm the complication of diagnosing and treatment of peri-implantitis

The presentation of three cases will show the seriousness of peri-implantitis as a complication and the importance of timely diagnosis and treatment. It is interesting that the arrival of the patients for the control examination was also motivated by different symptoms. In the first case, the patient presented due to a disturbance that caused profuse bleeding, not only by touching the brush, without pain symptoms, but with easily visible inflammation of the peri-implant tissues. In the second case, the patient (case II) came in because of pain disturbances, the localization of which she did not know how to determine. There were no signs of inflammation of the surrounding tissues, and the keratinized gingiva was firm and stable. In the third case, the patient (Case III) contacted the dentist who installed her implants due to the problem of bad breath and dissatisfaction with the aesthetics of prosthetic work. The answer of the dentist who performed the implant-prosthetic treatment was that everything is fine and without changes. However, the patient went to see another dentist, who after the examination advised her that her case required urgent treatment. The patient (case - 1), treated in Moscow, presented due to profuse bleeding of region #22, without the presence of pain (Fig. 15.88). Light probing without pressure revealed a deep pocket, and a minimal touch with the periodontal probe on the inflamed tissues manifested itself in profuse bleeding. By raising the flap, it was observed that the vestibular lamellar bone was completely destroyed, with an abundance of granulation tissue present (Figures 15.89 and 15.90). The implant was firmly integrated palatally from the middle third to the apex of the implant. The clinical condition was much worse than the x-ray showed! The radiographic view shows slight periapical changes above the implant; however, on the removed implant, there was an abundance of granulation tissue (Figure 15.89). Extraction of the implant was extremely difficult and complicated (Figures 15.91 and 15.92) despite the fact that the vestibular lamellar bone was completely destroyed. For the most part, the implant was well integrated palatally, which could not be ascertained on the radiograph. There was a danger when the implant was removed from the fracture of the palatal bone. After the detailed treatment of the alveolar wound, the bone defect is filled with bone substitutes, covered with a resorptive membrane. A temporary prosthetic work was made (Figure 15.93), and the patient was explained that he should wait at least 6 months to see the result of the augmentation. It was emphasized to him that the repetition of augmentation may happen, given the size of the bone defect. Similar cases must be approached with maximum caution, and the outcome is always uncertain, which should be presented to the patient. The question arises, what is the etiology of peri-implantitis in region #22 despite the good condition of the other 9 implants? Periapical lesions on the implant affecting the function of the implant are reported in the literature. It can be assumed that the etiology is multifactorial: vascular disorder, ischemia, overheating during implantation, contamination of the implant surface and the quality of the implant system. The further course of patient care and the final result are shown in Figures 15.94 to 15.103.

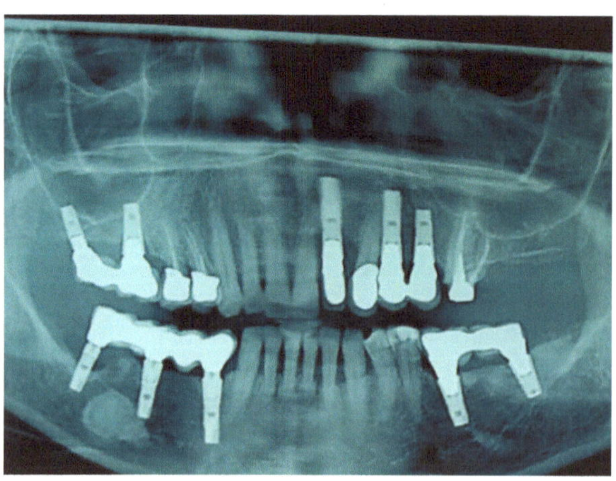

Figure 15.88 Found state. The radiographic representation deviates from the objective state in the mouth.

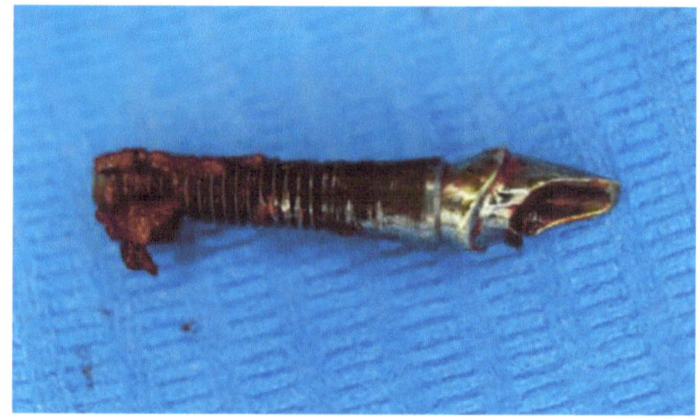

Figure 15.89. Extracted implant with an abundance of granulation tissue.

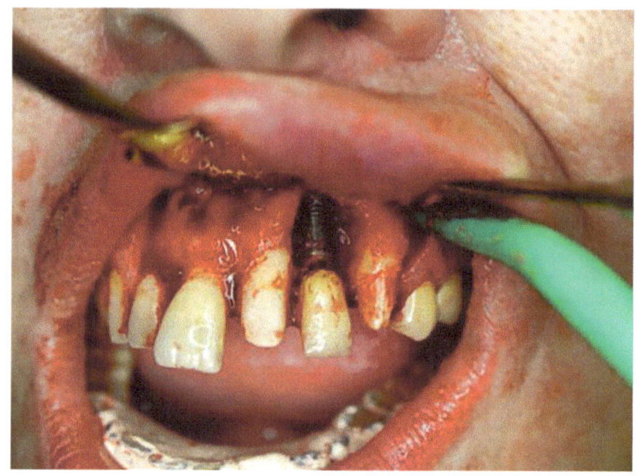

Figure 15.90. Appearance of initial state after lobe lift. Destroyed vestibular bone lamella.

It was explained to the patient that he should wait at least 6 months to see the result of the augmentation. It was emphasized to him that recurrence of augmentation may occur due to the size of the bone defect. Similar cases must be approached with the utmost caution, and the outcome is always uncertain as to what should be presented to the patient.

The question arises what is the etiology of peri-implantitis in region #22 despite the good condition of the other 9 implants? The literature lists periapical lesions on the implant that affect the function of the implant. It can be assumed that the etiology is multifactorial: vascular disorder, ischemia, overheating during implantation, contamination of the implant surface and the quality of the implant system.

The further course of patient care and the end result are shown in Figures 15.94 to 15.103.

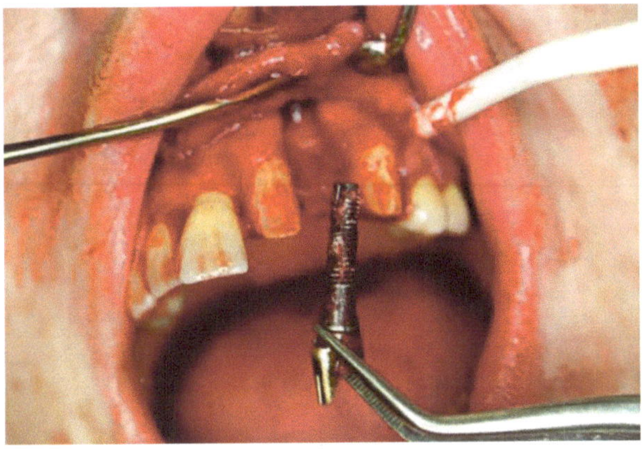

Figure 15.91 An implant of an unknown quality system was removed.

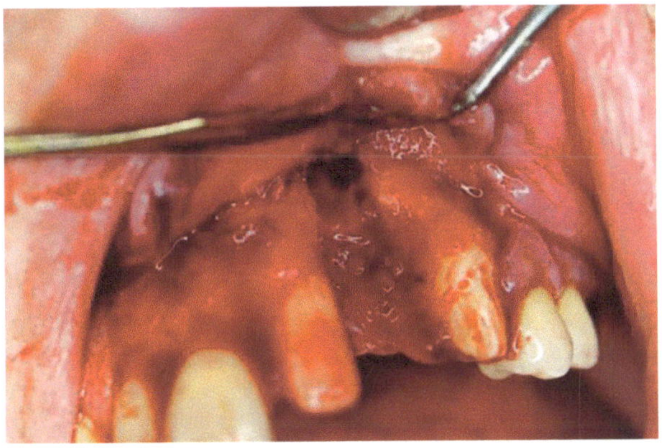

Figure 15.92 Major bone defect. Wound thoroughly treated. Augmentation was performed, and the bone substitute was covered with a resorptive membrane.

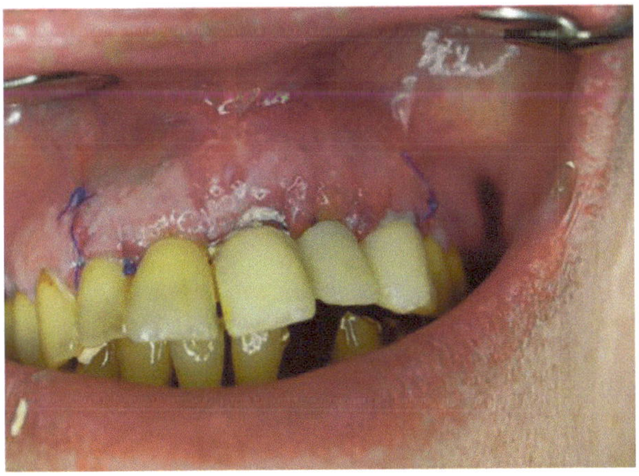

Figure 15.93 Bone defect augmentation of region 22 and temporary bridge installed.

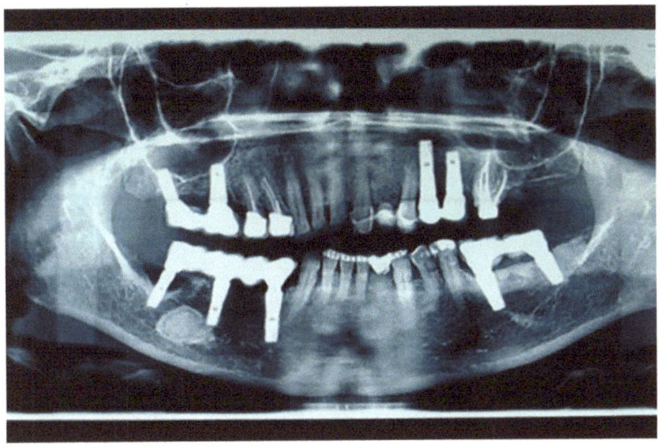

Figure 15.94 Radiographic view after implant removal and bone defect filling with bone substitutes and application of a resorbable collagen membrane.

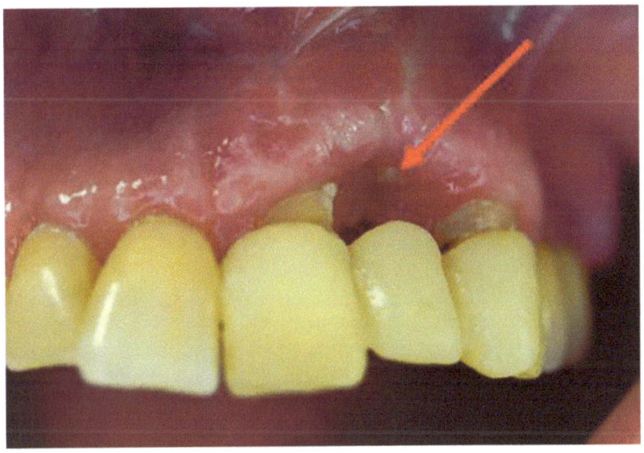

Figure 15.95 Balance after 6 months. The success of augmentation of major bone defects can be expected by applying appropriate autologous bone blocks. This option did not exist in the patient shown.

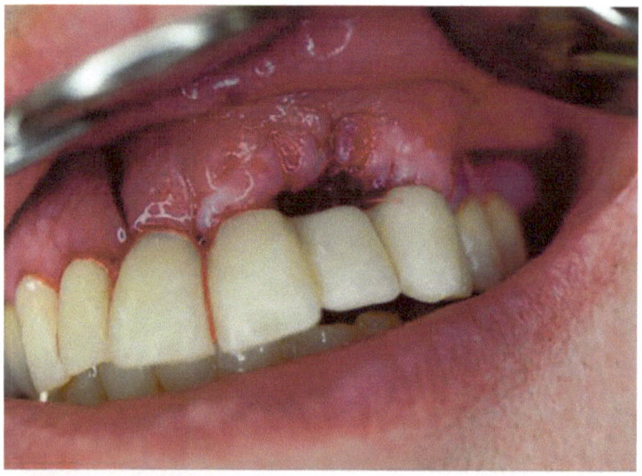

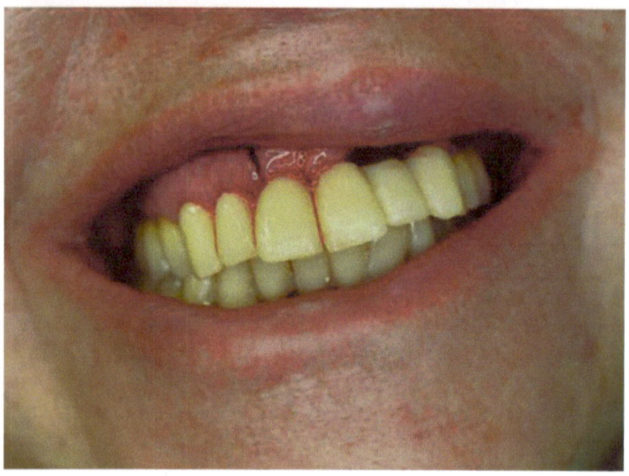

Figure 15.96 Additional augmentation and tentative compensation was made including tooth #21. Given the size of the defect, the solution should have been sought in restoration in a classic prosthetic manner, without implant placement in the augmented region #22.

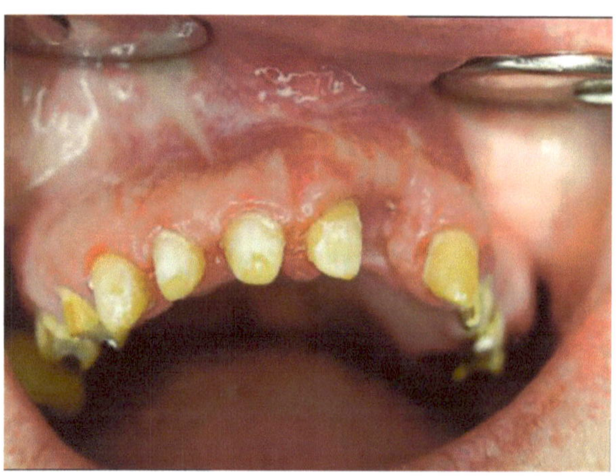

Figure 15.97. Given the condition of the existing teeth in the frontal region (color and rotation of the central incisor #11), it is a more justified solution to continue the treatment with classical prosthetic work in metal-ceramics.

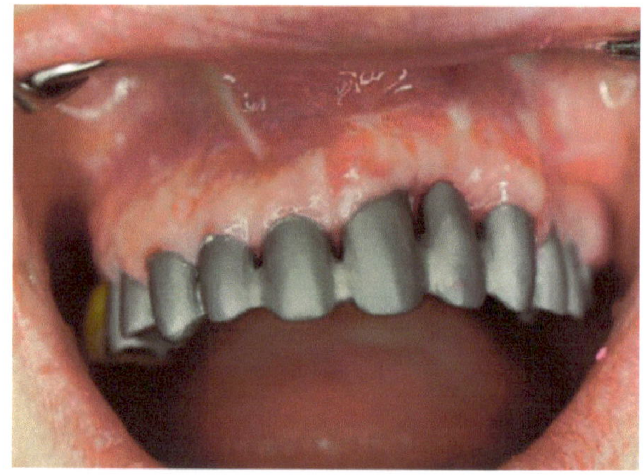

Figure 15.98. Precise prosthetic work from both an aesthetic and functional point of view is a more justified solution in the presented patient than reimplantation of implants in region #12, where repeated small mentation of hard and soft tissues did not achieve the desired result.

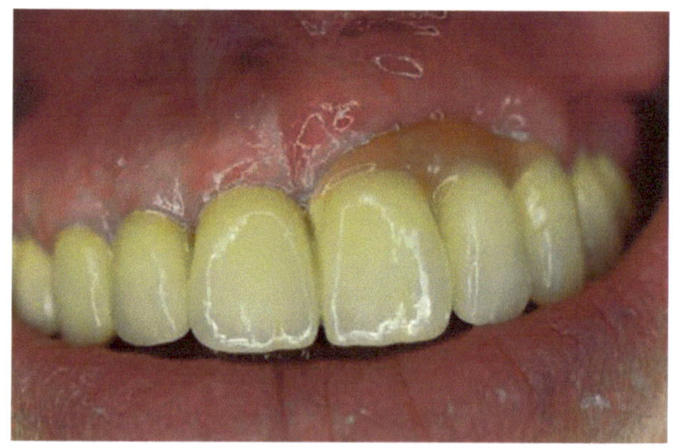

Figure 15.99. Soft tissue augmentation is a surgically complex procedure in oral surgery often alone due to the unpredictability of treatment outcomes, depending on the size and bone defect. Replacement of resected soft tissue with prosthetic work is one of the solutions that meets aesthetic requirements. If the line of laughter, the shape and position of the lip allows for solutions without this detail, it should not be insisted on because compression on the papillae of adjacent teeth is avoided and oral hygiene is easier to maintain.

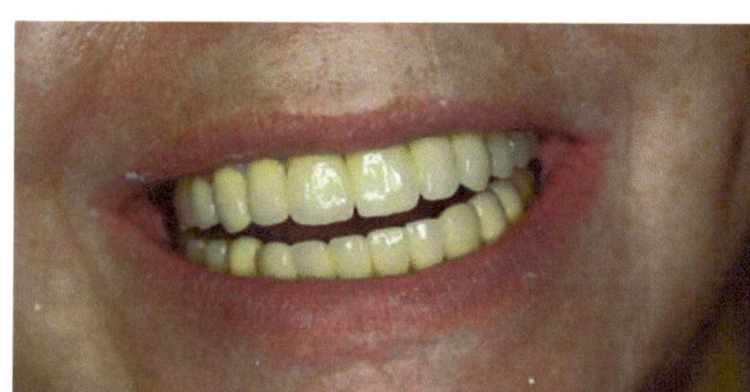

Figure 15.100. The treatment of the presented complex case confirms the view that the successful result of treatment requires the experience of a dentist and knowledge of prosthetics, to explain to the dental technician the essential details during the preparation of prosthetic work (work by T. Zlopaša)

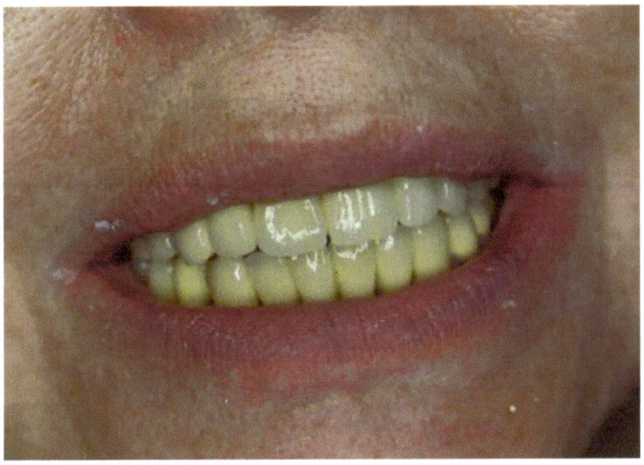

Figure 15.101. The final outcome of the treatment confirms the justification of the adopted treatment plan without entering into the adventure of implant placement in the augmented region.

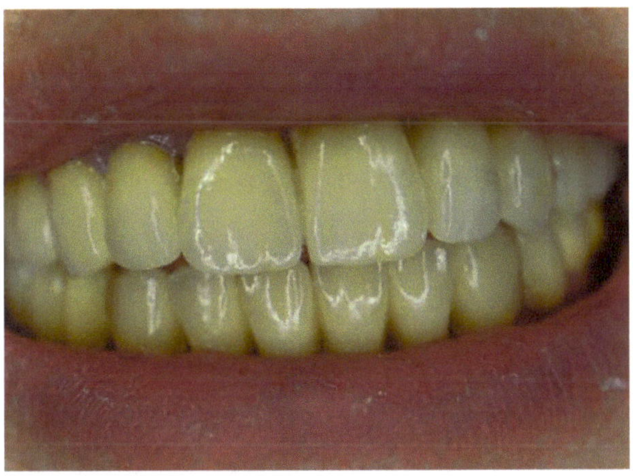

Figure 15.102. Achieved aesthetic and functional result. Established balanced missing occlusion, which is extremely important for the long-term survival of bone implants.

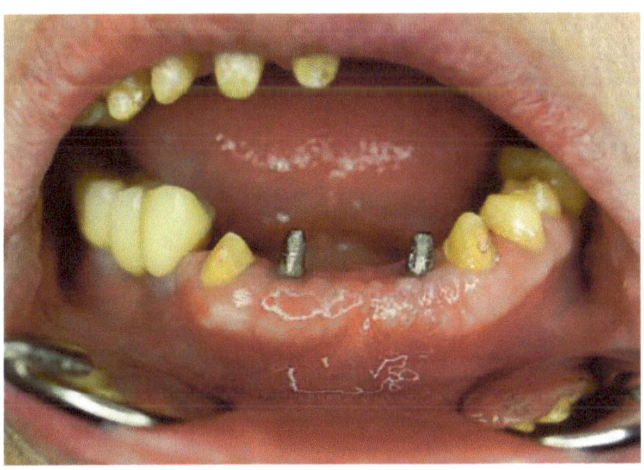

Figure 15.103. Implant-prosthetic rehabilitation in the lower jaw required the following stages: extraction of detached incisors in the frontal region (#31, #32, #41, #42) implant placement in regions #32 and #42, fabrication of metal-ceramic crowns on the remaining teeth and alteration of prosthetic works in the lateral regions (done in Moscow) for 2 reasons: establishment of balanced occlusion and compliance of the color of the ceramics with the new prosthetic work (work by T. Zlopaša and B. Zlopaša).

The following example is a patient (Figure 15.104) with pain sensations in the frontal region of the upper jaw. The patient was unable to localize the pain, emphasizing that it makes her anxious in the first place due to sleep loss. The clinical finding did not show any signs of inflammation of the surrounding tissues, and percutaneously and while applying pressure, present teeth were not sensitive. Otherwise, the patient was not satisfied with the previous prosthetic work done in another office. She was advised to undergo an endodontic revision, perform upgrades and repeat prosthetic work. Time was left for her to reflect on the advice she was presented with. The patient always came with an escort from one of the family members. After a few days of reflection, the patient returned with a strong request to remove all teeth and install implants. This request was also made by the family. Chances are that this "pain" also tired the family. Once again, the family and the patient were persuaded by explaining to them in detail that her case can be solved without implants with less morbidity and financial costs. A period of 10 days was left for them to think carefully about our proposal. Persuasion was futile. We tried to find a reason to give the patient and family a longer period of 2 months to think about our proposal. The pressure from the family and the patient forced us to accept their demands. The patient was suggested to keep premolar (15) to avoid sinus lifting. An explicit request was also the extraction of that tooth. After the immediate installation of 5 implants and sinus lifting, a good primary fixation was achieved, a tentative prosthetic work in acrylate was set. The implanted implant is not primarily loaded by sinus-lifting. The patient and the family were extremely satisfied with the temporary bridge, because all interference with the "headache" from the tooth she complained about ceased. After a long waiting period (8 months) post implant placement, fixed prosthetic work was performed in metal ceramics. Patient and family satisfaction was achieved with aesthetics (Figures 15.106 and 15.110) manifested itself with enthusiasm because the patient stopped bothering them with "headaches" on a daily basis. The patient's satisfaction with the cessation of "pain" was in anticipation of a new prosthetic work: a nicer lighter color, a nicer tooth shape, a nicer appearance, probably the expected return of a youthful appearance. However, after 3 years of satisfaction, everything returned to the beginning. Repeated "headache" in the area around the implant that cannot be determined. A 3D scan was taken again.

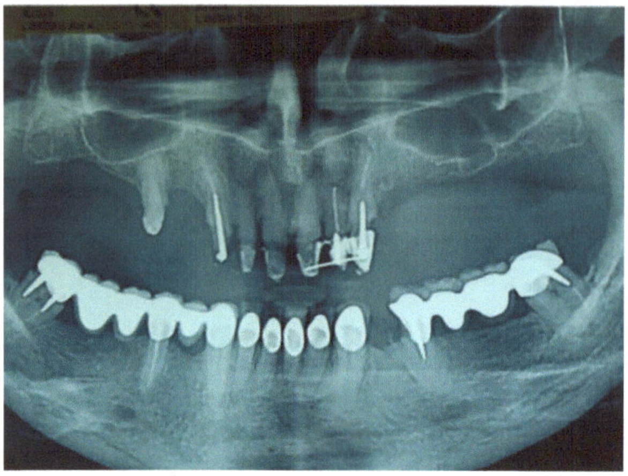

Figure 15.104. X-ray of a patient with pain of unclear localization and dissatisfaction with the existing prosthetic work performed in another institution. Proposed endodontic therapy, root canal revision, cast upgrades and classical prosthetic work in metal-ceramics.

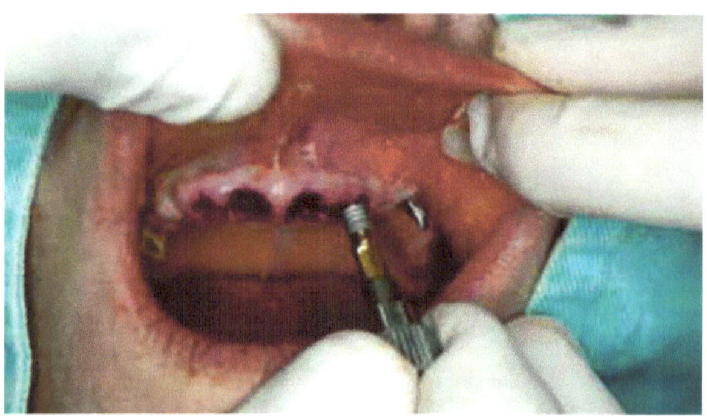

Figure 15.105. Immediate installation after extraction of existing teeth.

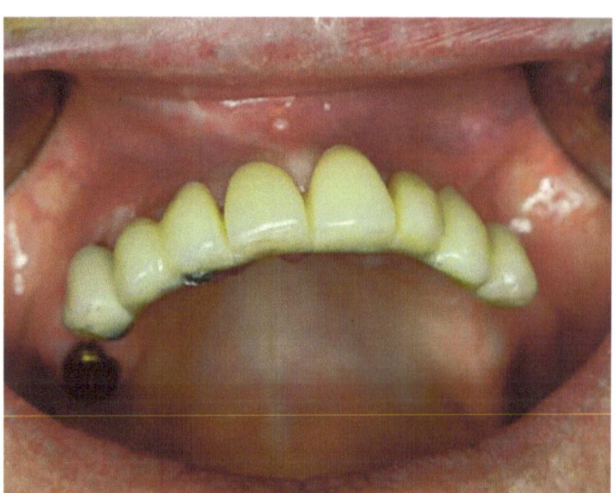

Figure 15.106. The implant in region #15 is primarily loaded due to the performed sinus lifting. The patient was extremely satisfied with the next 6 months, because all the disturbances she complained about in anticipation of a new prosthetic work and a better appearance were gone. After 3 years, the patient appears with the same problems she had with her teeth and unsuccessful prosthetic work.

We suspected that there was a barely noticeable periapical shadow on 1 implant, the assumption that this could be the cause of pain sensations. The implant was removed (it was firmly integrated) and a new implant was placed (Figures 15.115 and 15.116.) and the prosthetic work was repeated with the request of the patient of the brightest color. After a while, the same story was repeated.

It will turn out to be a typical psychogenic pain from the domain of psychiatry, not oral implantology. Experience confirms that such patient is difficult to reckognize. Find out as much as possible about the patient's requirements and expectations in the history and conversation with the patient. Such patients are typical as contraindicated for implant-prosthetic treatment, and as already emphasized, they are difficult to reckognize at the beginning. It would be logical if the implantologist suspected the patient to refer him to a psychiatrist-psychoanalyst for an interview, which the patient would perceive as an insult. The conclusion is that a patient with psychogenic pain is impossible to initially recognize despite decades of experience. (See Chapter on "Indications And Contraindications For Implant Placement")

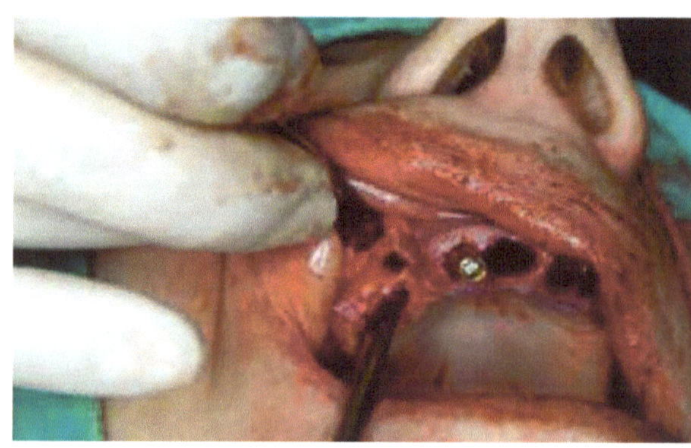

Figure 15.107. Immediately implanted in regions #15 by sinus lifting.

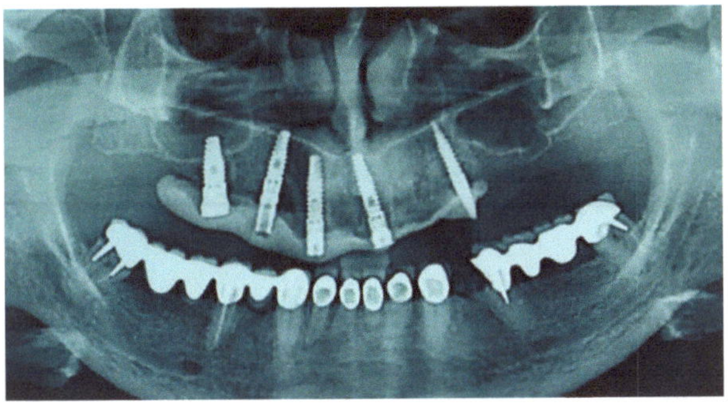

Figure 15.108. Radiological presentation of implanted implants, performed by sinus lifting of region #15 with implanted prosthetic work in the composite

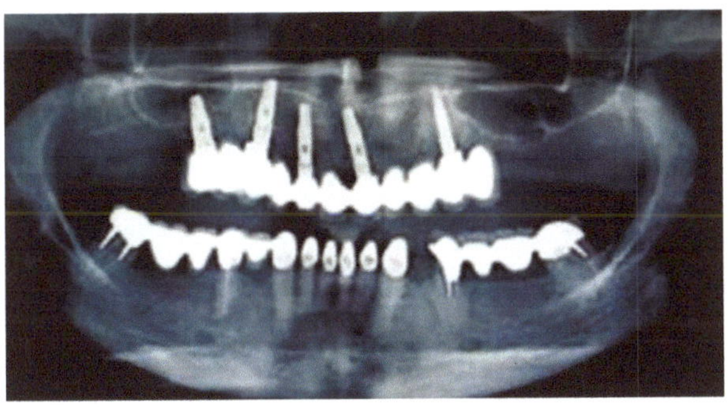

Figure 15.109. Control radiographic display after one year, successful installation and successful outcome of sinus lifting.

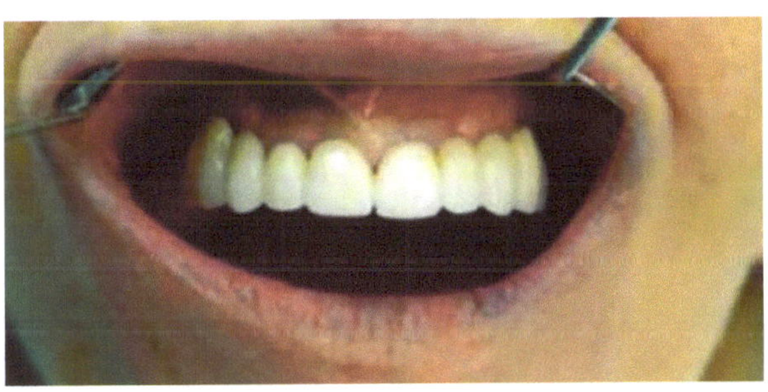

Figure 15.110. Patient satisfaction lasted 3 years. Appearance of keratinized mucosa with vestibular side and no signs of inflammation.

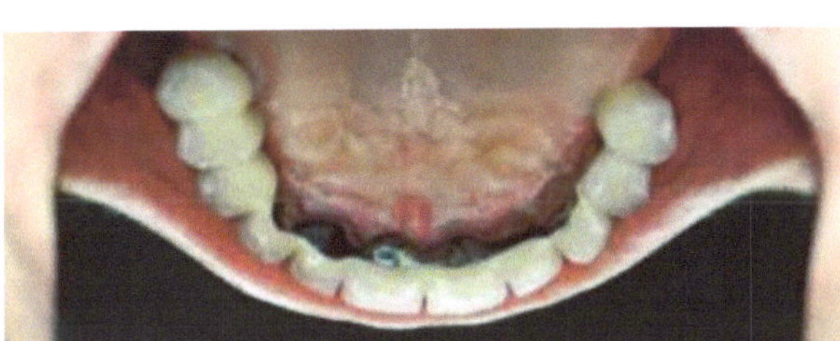

Figure 15.111. Appearance of soft tissues on the palatal side without signs of inflammation. Left high collar for easier maintenance of oral hygiene.

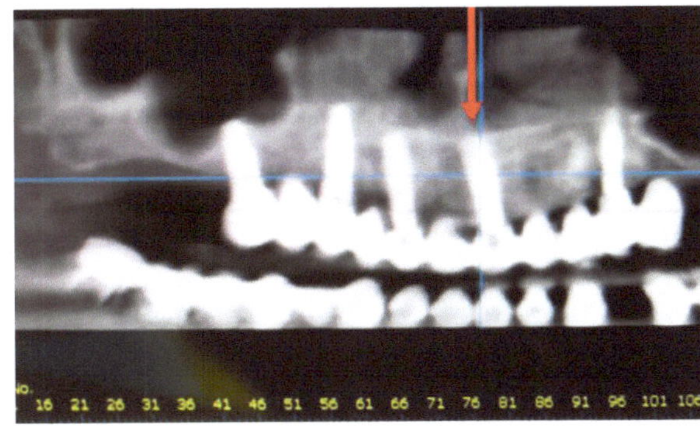

Figure 15.112. After 3 years, the patient reappeared with the same sensations of "headaches" around the implants that they did not know how to determine. The 3D scan shows a stable condition around the implant and the success of sinus lifting region #15. A barely visible shadow in the apical part of the implant is marked with a red arrow. Refer to the following figure.

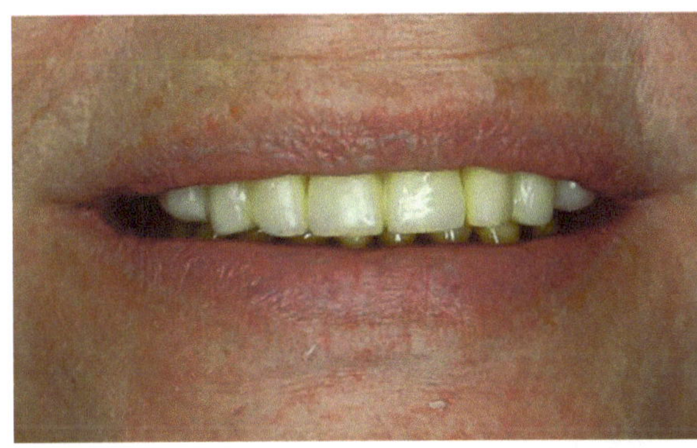

Figure 15.113. The patient was satisfied with the achieved aesthetics and function for 3 years.

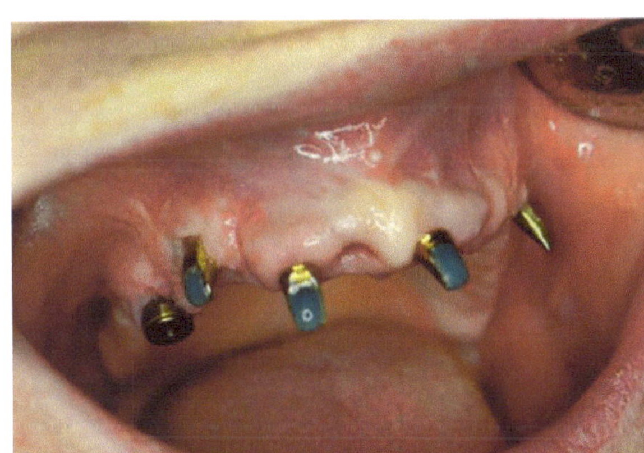

Figure 15.114. Appearance after 3 months of reimplantation. Region #11 of the removed implant is visible.

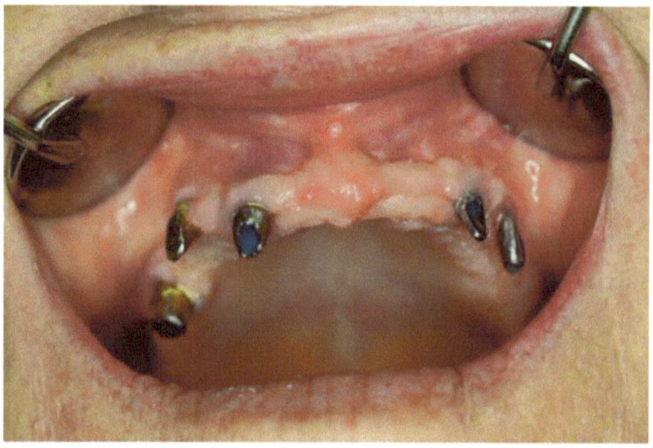

Figure 15.115. After 6 months, the implants showed the maximum degree of integration and stably formed soft tissues. At the express request of the patient, the prosthetic work was repeated, requiring a lighter color. The patient again complains of pain that he cannot define. By fulfilling all the unrealistic demands of the patient and his dissatisfaction, the correct diagnosis was made: Typical psychogenic pain. (Described in Chapter 17).

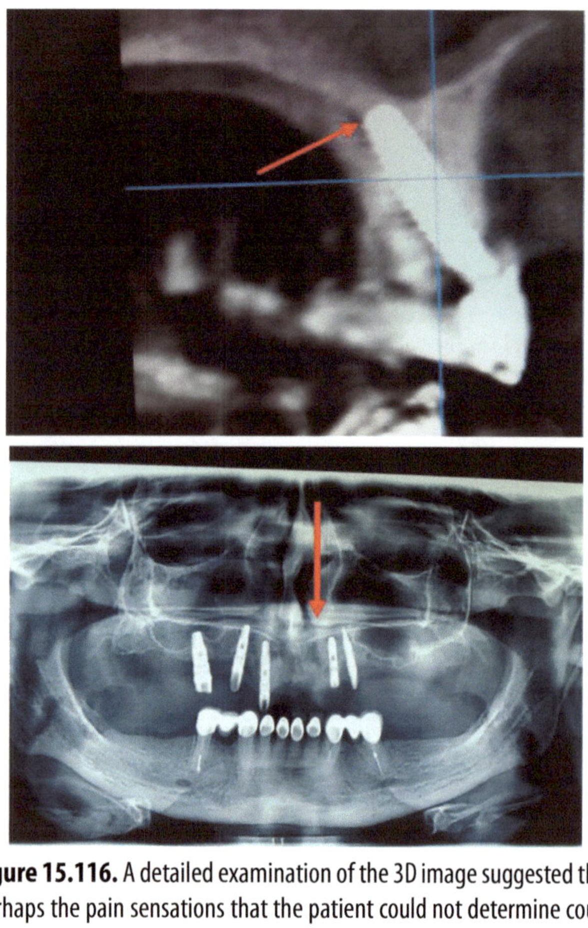

Figure 15.116. A detailed examination of the 3D image suggested that perhaps the pain sensations that the patient could not determine could be caused by peri-implant changes on the apical part of the implant from the palatal side? The prosthetic work was successful. Percussionally, all the implants, including the one that was suspected to be the cause of the pain, produced a clear hypersonic sound. The region #11 implant was removed and a new one was placed in region #22.

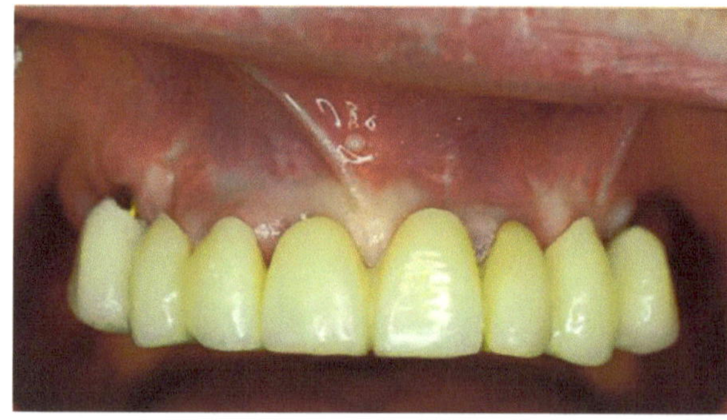

Figure 15.117. Appearance of definitive prosthetic work after 12 months, without pain sensations. A metal polished collar was left on the tooth of region #14 due to easier maintenance of oral hygiene and reduced plaque deposition, which allows the shape of the lip.

After three years, the patient (case III) returned to the dentist who performed the implant-prosthetic rehabilitation, reporting discomfort and bad breath. The dentist assessed her condition and explained that her oral health was stable with no pathological changes. However, the patient was skeptical of this conclusion and sought a second opinion from another dentist.

To her surprise, the new diagnosis revealed a chaotic condition that required urgent attention due to a very serious and complex problem (see images 15.118, 15.119, and 15.120). The initial diagnosis was accurate, and the advice given by the second dentist was warranted.

The subsequent treatment procedures for this patient are illustrated in images 15.118 to 15.133.

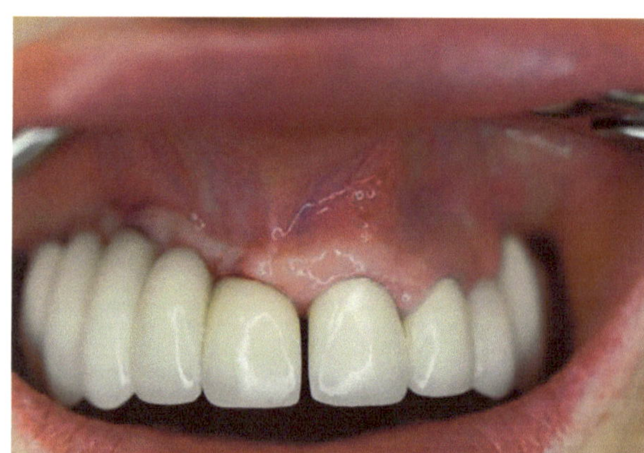

Figure 15.118. The appearance of incorrectly performed prosthetic work that is anchored on implants and diseased teeth.

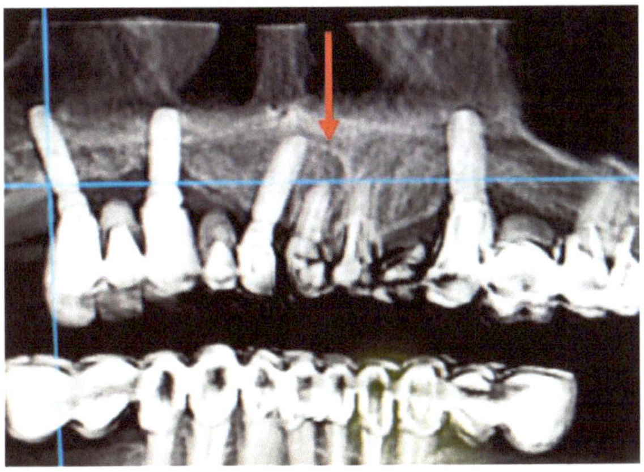

Figure 15.119. Orthopantomography clearly showed bony defects in regions #12, #16, #17 and #24, clearly visible cyst (red arrow).

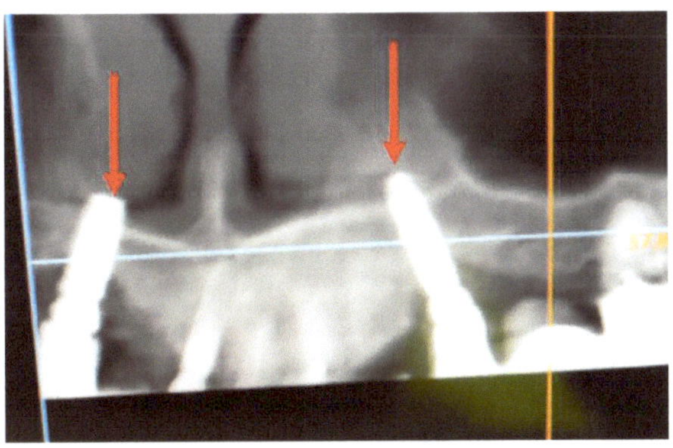

Figure 15.120. Pierced cortical bone of the floor of the nasal cavity (indicated by red arrows).

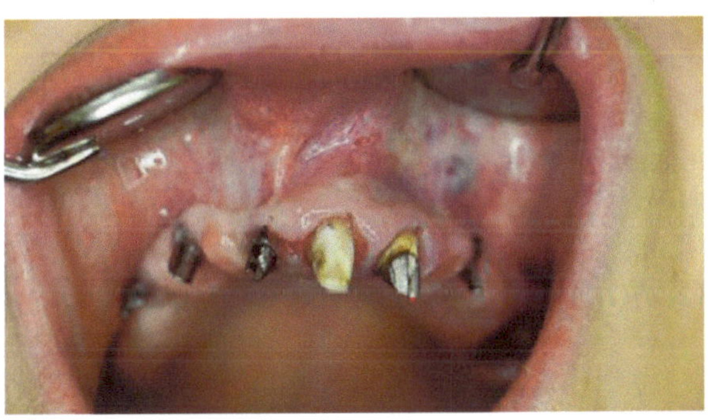

Figure 15.121. Pierced cortical bone of the floor of the nasal cavity (indicated by red arrows).

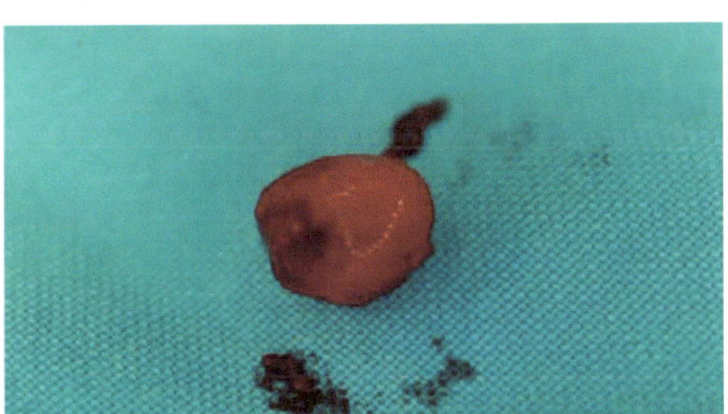

Figure 15.122. Appearance of the extracted cyst.

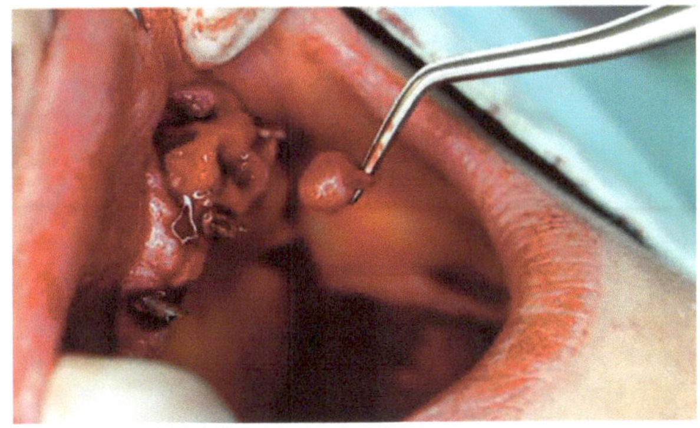

Figure 15.123. Region #11 cyst completely removed.

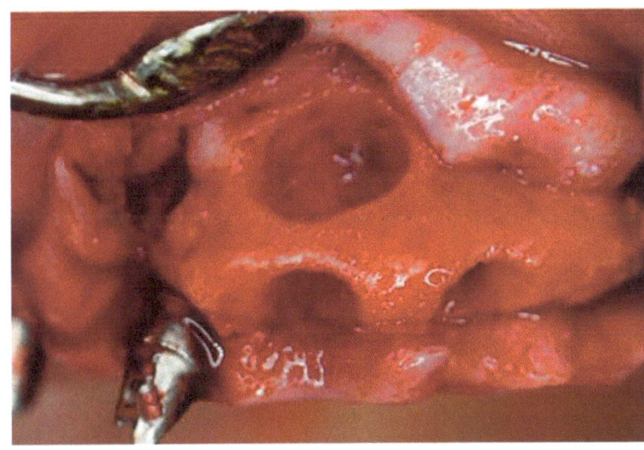

Figure 15.124. A large bony defect after cystectomy, with visible per-implatitis around the adjacent region #10 implant.

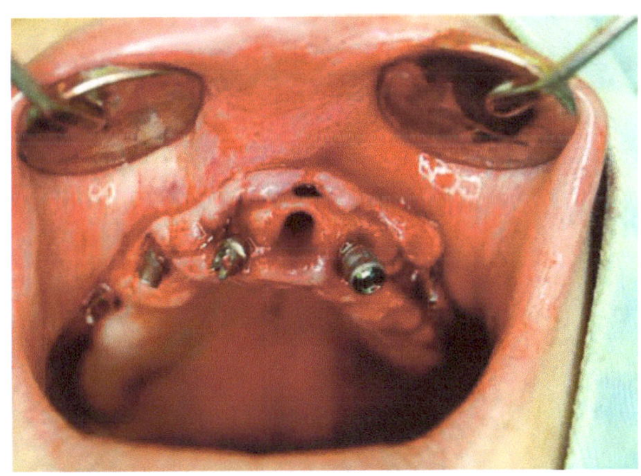

Figure 15.125. After removing the cyst, an implant was placed in region #21. At the same time, the bone defect was filled.

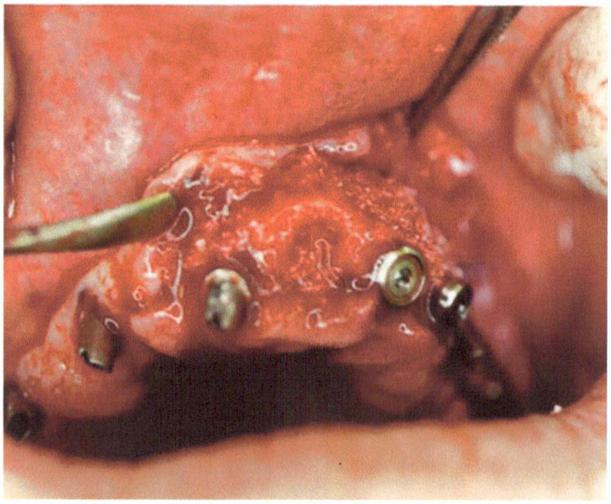

Figure 15.126. Augmentation of the bone defect due to cystic destruction and bone resorption in the peri-implant space of the existing implant.

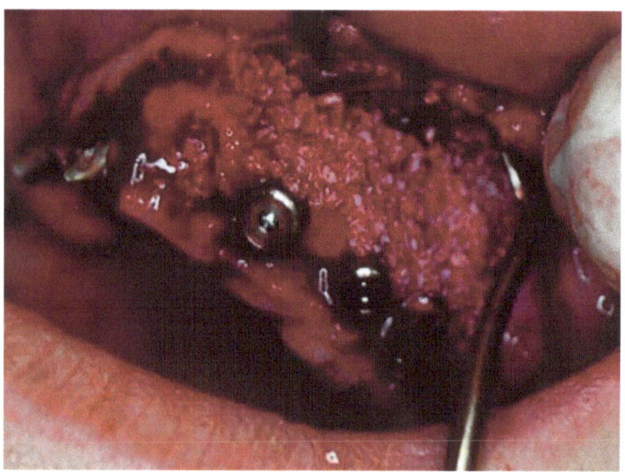

Figure 15.127. Filling bone defects in other regions with bone substitutes.

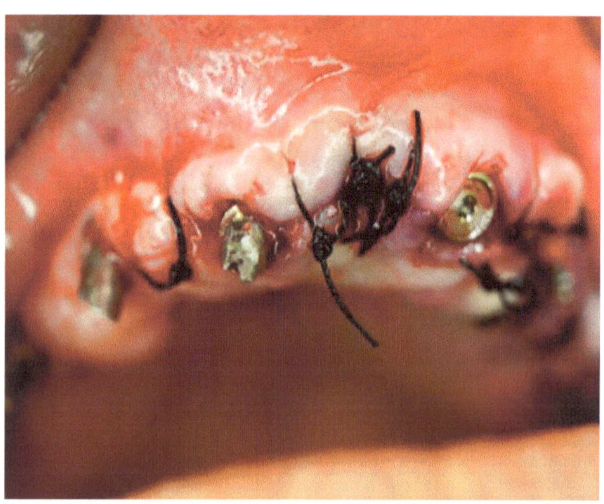

Figure 15.128. Stitched augmented region.

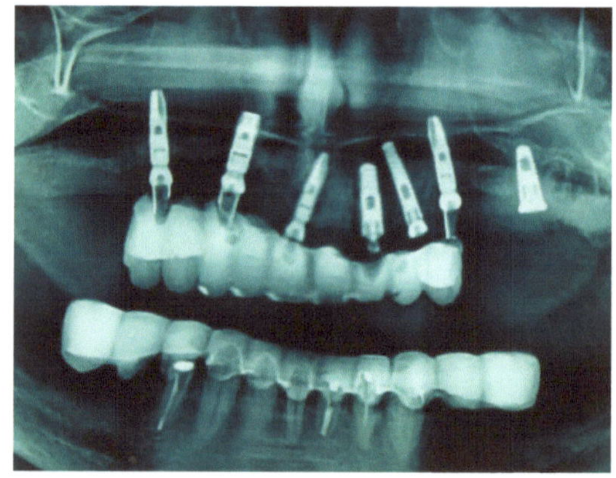

Figure 15.129. Radiographic view on orthopantomography of installed implants and augmentation of bone defects.

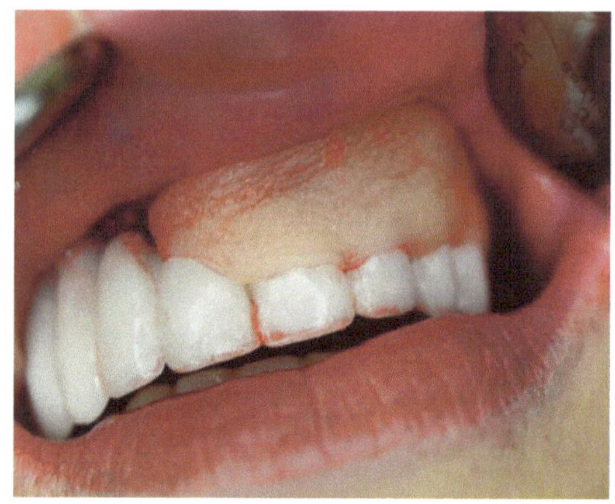

Figure 15.130. On the immediately installed implants, after the augmentation of bone defects caused by peri-implantitis, Reso-pack was placed (the characteristics of Reso-pack are that it is very easy to handle, it is hydrophilic and ready to be placed on soft tissue with very good adhesion. The pack remains elastic all the time , so that ulcers cannot occur by compressing the package.In addition to containing a cellulose matrix as a base, Resopack also has disinfectant, astringent and At the same time, it has a pleasant taste, and Reso-pack is not removed after 2-3 days is necessary, and it depends on the doctor's assessment, the packing can be repeated several times.

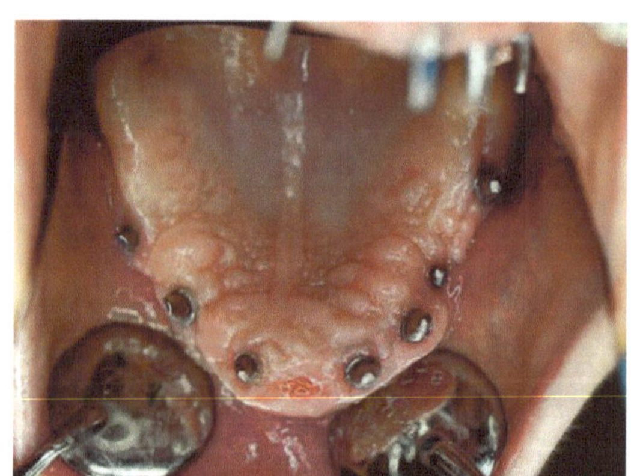

Figure 15.131. Presentation of healed tissues after cystectomy, augmentation of bone defects, immediately installed and integrated

implants, primarily loaded with temporary fixed prosthetic work. (work by Tamara Zlopaša).

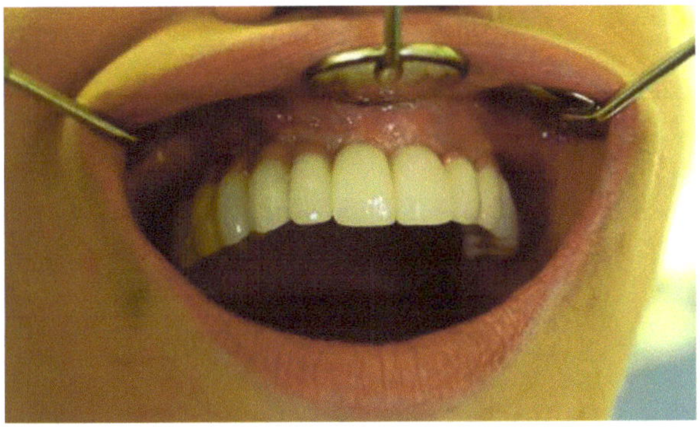

Figure 15.132. The definitive result of the entire implant-prosthetic rehabilitation (see pictures 15.18 and 15.130). (work by Tamara Zlopaša).

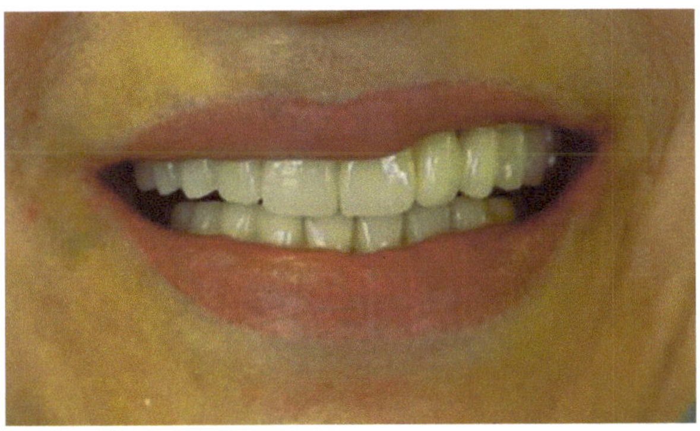

Figure 15.133. A successful outcome to the mutual satisfaction of the patient and the doctor.

Examples Of The Treatment Of Peri-implant Infections

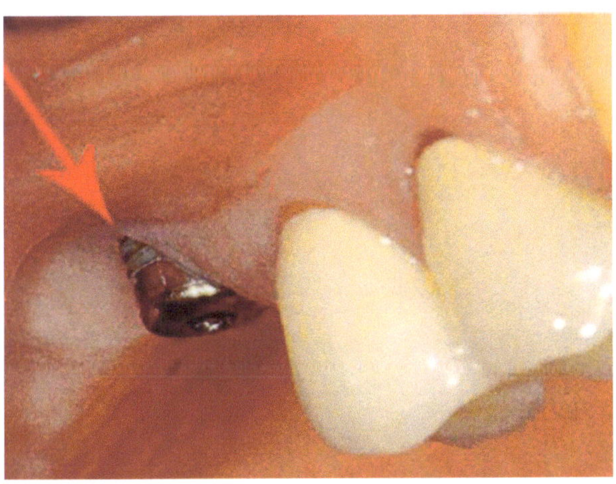

Figure 15.134. Recession of the gingiva around the implant followed by bone resorption. It is necessary to create visibility of the defect by raising the mucoperiosteal flap (region #16). (picture 15.135).

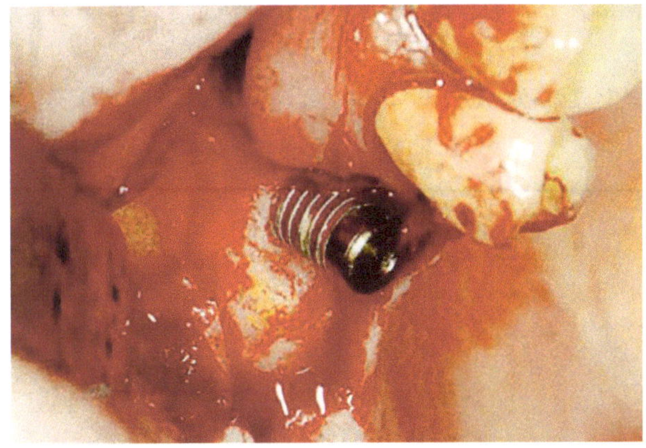

Figure 15.135. Recession of soft tissue in region #16 about 4mm buccally, which is accompanied by appropriate bone resorption, and a small part of the implant is surrounded by keratinized mucous gingiva. It is necessary to take a connective tissue graft from the palate with preserved full thickness, shape and size of the defect.

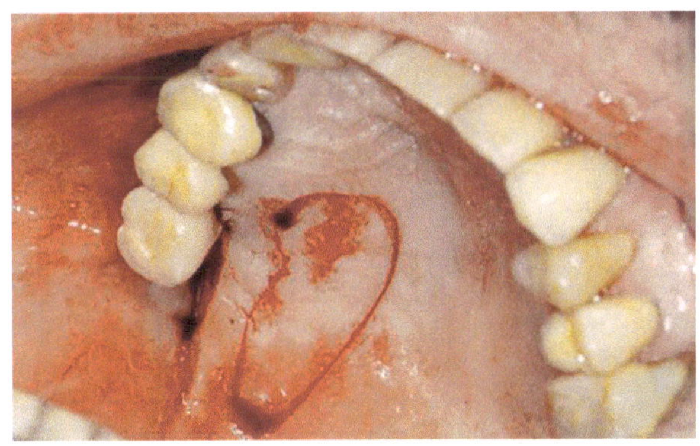

Figure 15.136. A connective tissue graft of the shape and size of the prepared region was taken from the palate.

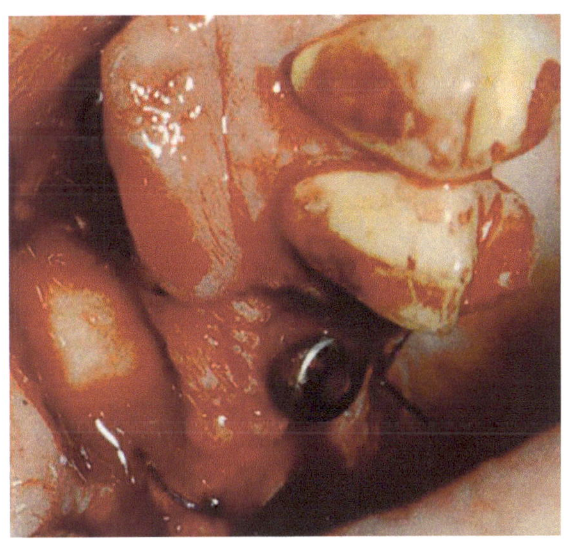

Figure 15.137. The placed bone substitutes are covered with a subepithelial graft from the palate, which is sutured buccally (Fig. 15.138). Previously, the rough surface of the implant was polished with a diamond bur and polished with titanium polishers. Disinfection with Curasept ads 212 solution or 0.2% chlorhexidine solution.

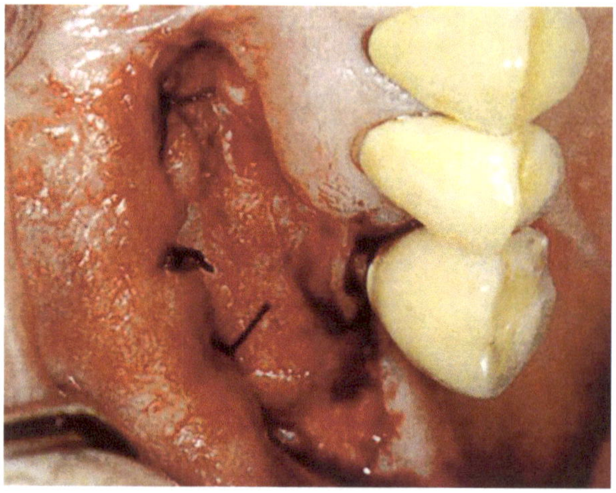

Figure 15.138. Subepithelial connective tissue graft.

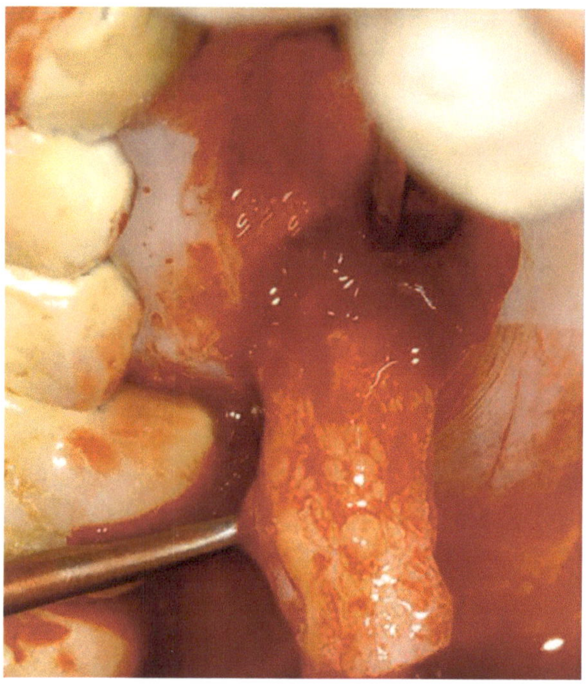

Figure 15.139. After three months, the surgical intervention was repeated and vestibuloplasty was performed in combination with a free gingival connective graft, performing a marginal incision along the mucogingival connection with two vestibular relaxing incisions in the region #16 and #15. After that, the mucosal flap in the vestibulum was prepared, and the coronal edge was sutured apically to the underlying periosteum.

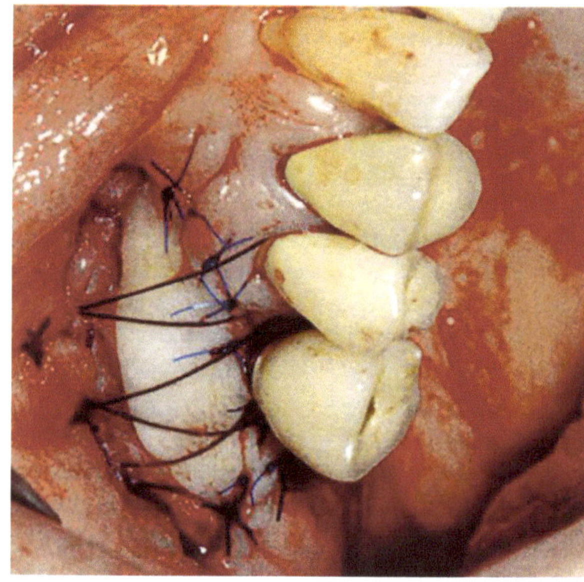

Figure 15.140. Appearance of a sutured free gingival graft, with its cranial edge only pressed against the periosteum mattress with sutures. Sutures must be kept for at least 10 days after surgery.

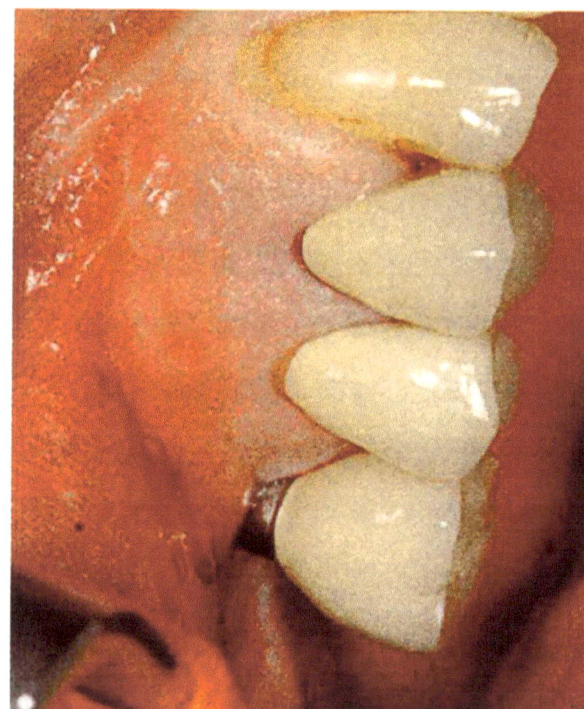

Figure 15.141. Condition after three months. The part of the implant that was affected by soft tissue recession was covered by a subepithelial connective tissue transplant taken from the palate, the soft tissue was thickened, but the buccal mucosa was not keratinized. Possible repetition of another operation. This shows that the result of soft tissue augmentation is not always predictable.

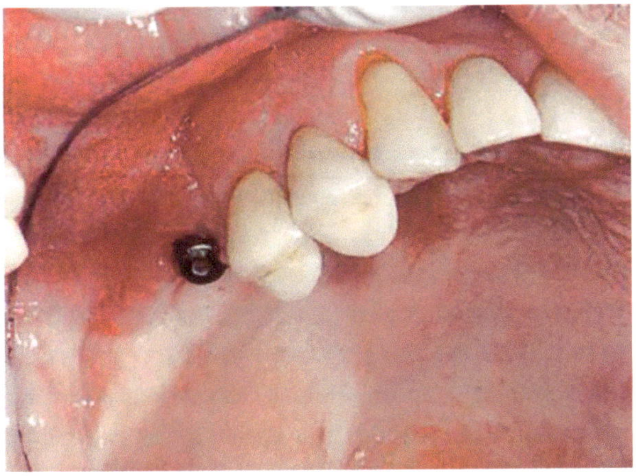

Figure 15.142. After a horizontal periosteal incision, the flap was advanced coronally and sutured. Condition after two weeks.

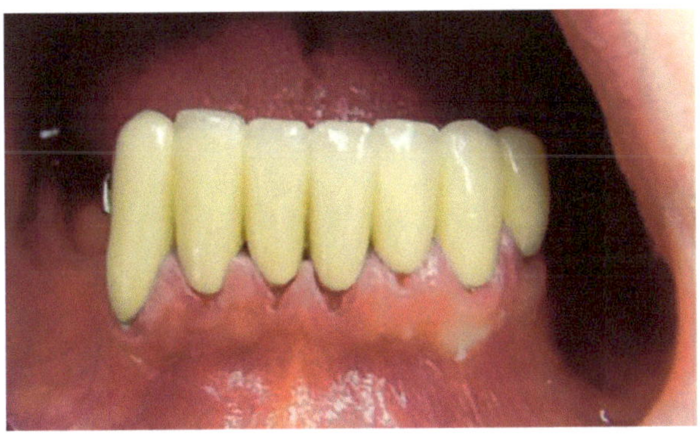

Figure 15.143. The causes of peri-implantitis in this case are: unfavorable anatomical structure - concavity of the alveolar ridge (narrow ridge of the alveolar bone). The selection of the diameter of the implant must be coordinated with the dimensions of the available bone. In addition, the patient is a heavy smoker.

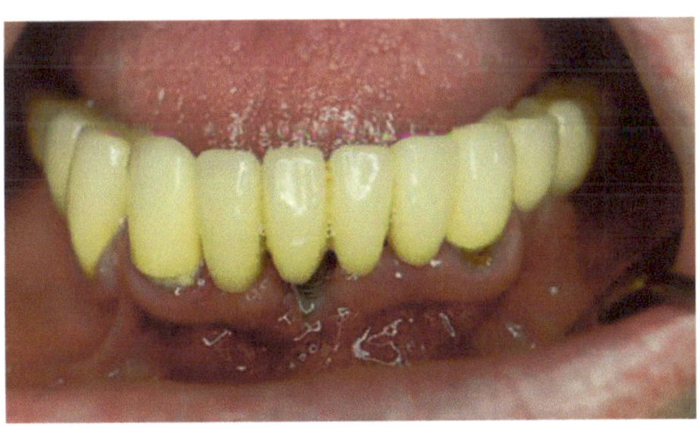

Figure 15.144. Peri-implantitis. After 6 years, the patient presented with bleeding gums. Causes: poor oral hygiene, accumulated abundant plaque lingual partially vestibular, heavy smoker, unfavorable anatomical structure - concavity of the alveolar ridge.

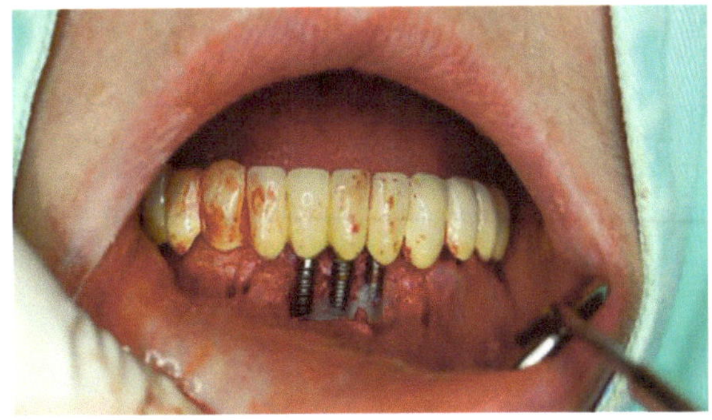

Figure 15.145. Peri-implantitis with extreme bone resorption. For five years, the patient did not feel any changes or complaints. Embedded implants of reduced diameter (diameter).

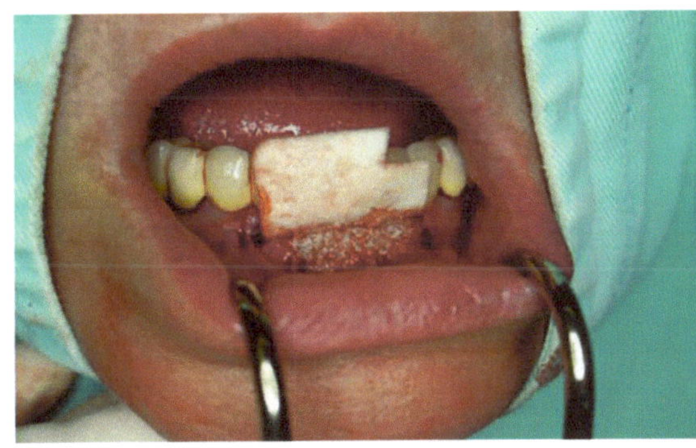

Figure 15.146. Covering the bone defect with bone substitutes and a collagen resorbable membrane.

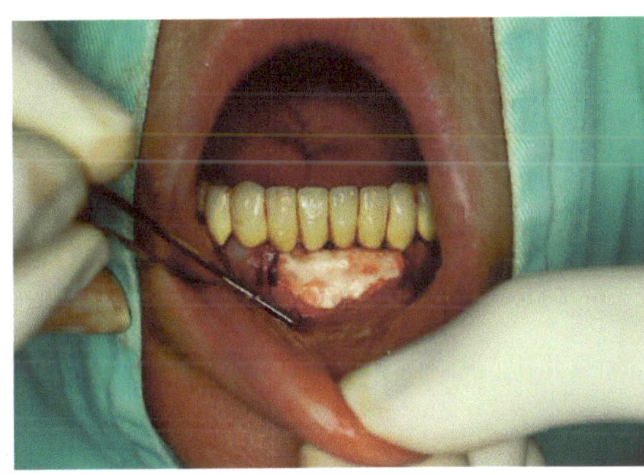

Figure 15.147. After the augmatation of the defect, the result of the treatment is unpredictable.

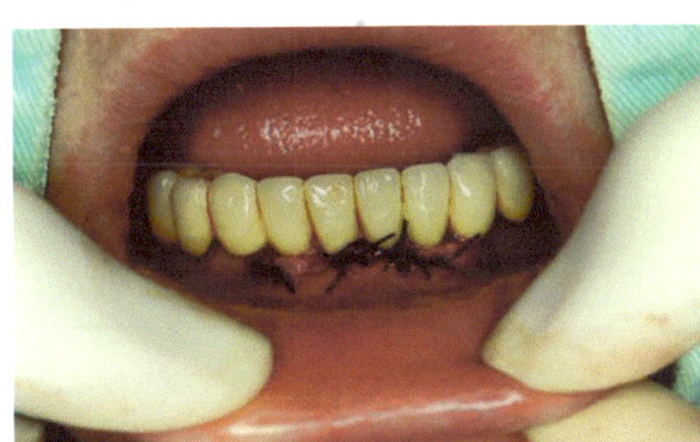

Figure 15.148. Placed sutures after the augmentation.

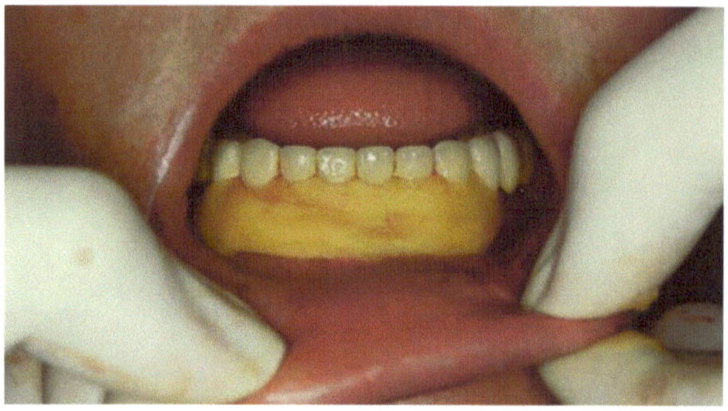

Figure 15.149. Reso-pack promotes and accelerates the healing of soft tissues.

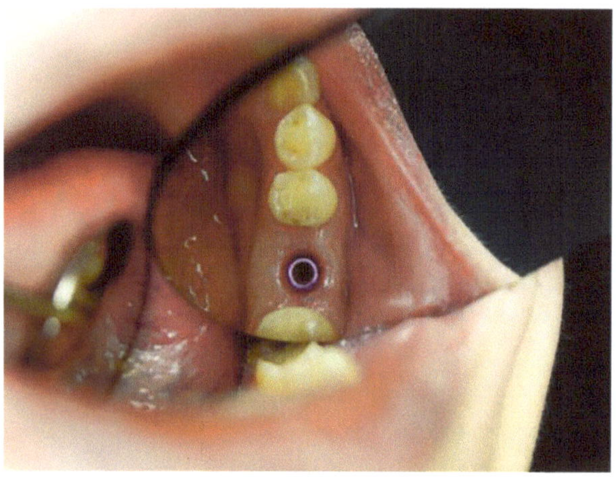

Figure 15.150. The appearance of a well-keratinized mucosa around the immediately implanted implant.

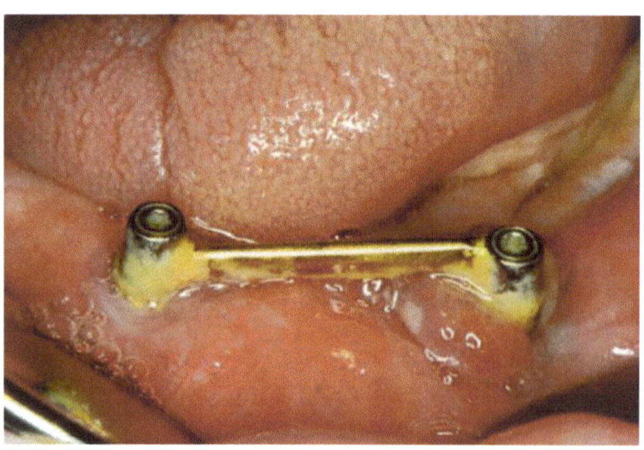

Figure 15.151. Peri-implantitis of the Dolder's crossbar support implant for stabilization of the lower total prosthesis. Poor oral hygiene and abundantly deposited plaque caused peri-implant infections. The outcome was a loss of stability of the lower total prosthesis.

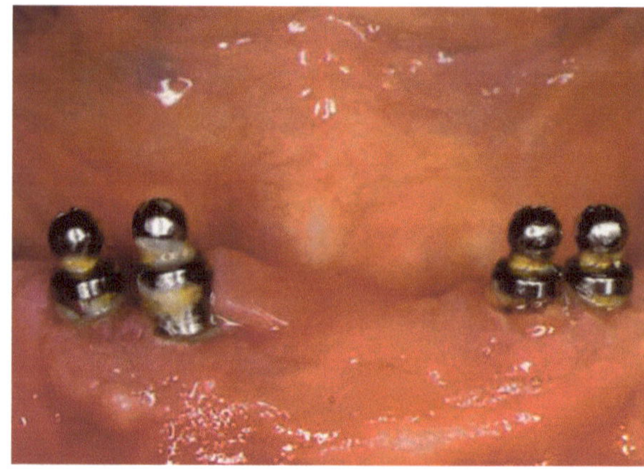

Figure 15.152. Plaque build-up on round-head retention clips weakens their ability to retain clips, and thus the stability of the lower total denture.

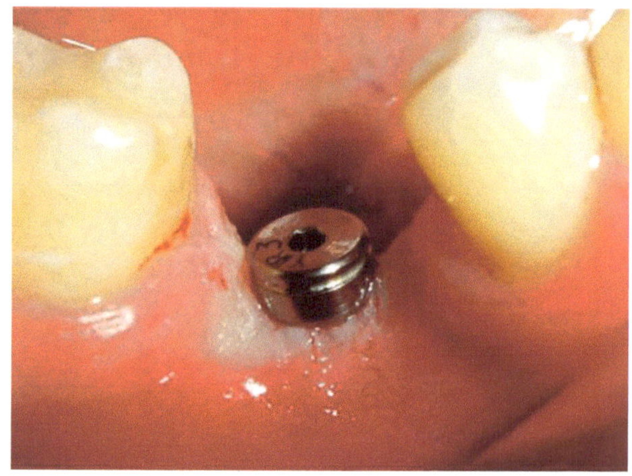

Figure 15.153. Healing caps should be used temporarily while the carrier is processed in the laboratory and the crown is made. Gingiva-former can only be used for delayed implant loading, if the bone is of poor quality and primary fixation of the implant has not been achieved.

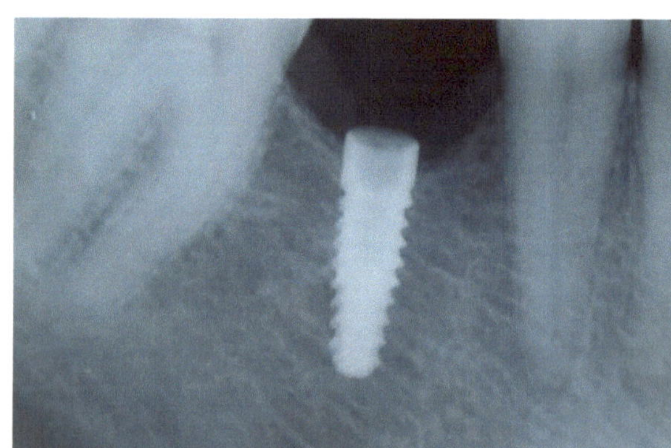

Figure 15.154. The quality of the formation of soft tissues in the neck part of the implant depends on the processing and design of the thread structure of the embedded implant at the level of the bone and on the biological width, which is the prevention of peri-implant changes.

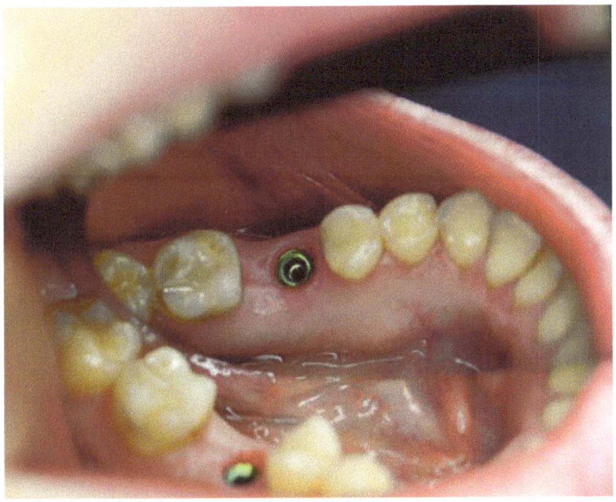

Figure 15.155. The appearance of well-formed keratinized gingiva in molar replacement is a protection against pei-implant infections.

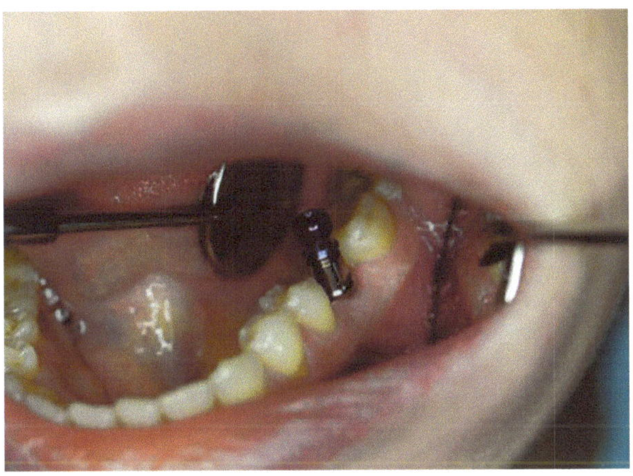

Figure 15.156. Implant position transmitter.

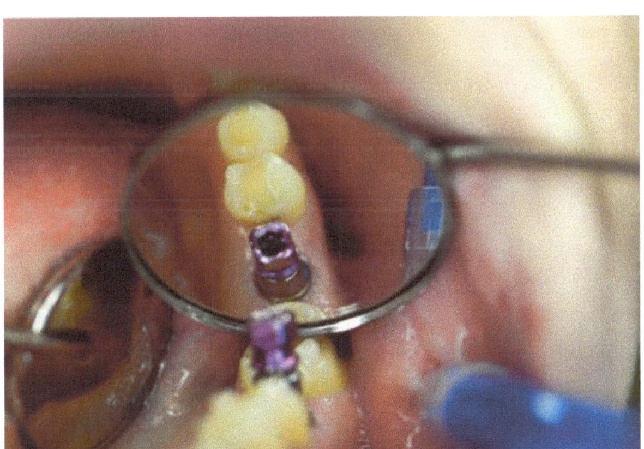

Figure 15.157. Stable keratinized gingiva is a factor for the long-term stay of the implant in the bone.

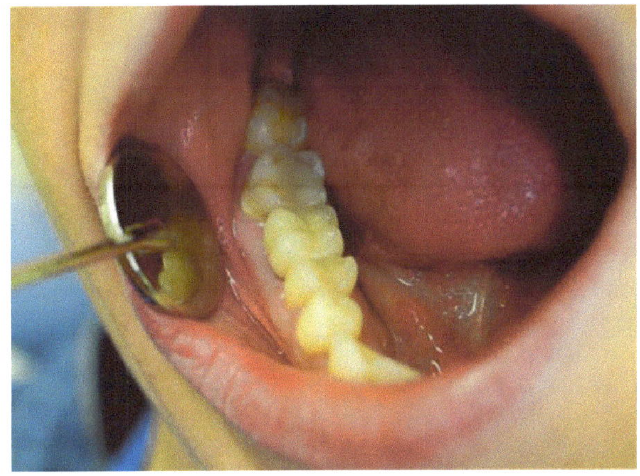

Figure 15.158. The occlusal surface must be in accordance with gnathological biomechanical principles. The appearance of the compensated molar on the wide-diameter implant, which is important for the uniform reception of the given forces during mastication, reducing them to the physiological limits of action, thus protecting the peri-implant environment.

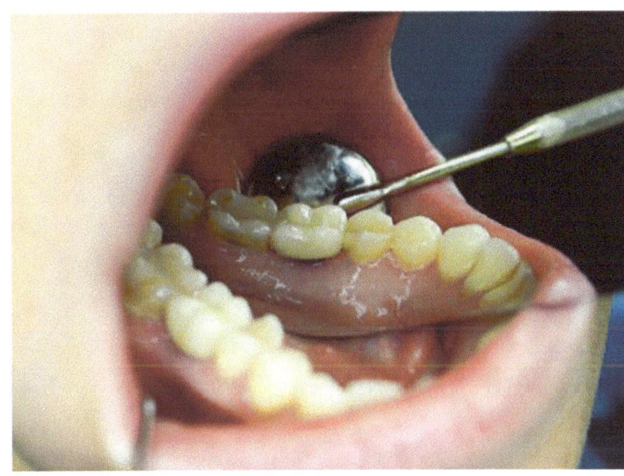

Figure 15.159. Condition 8 years after makinq definitive crowns. In the molar regions, lingually and palatally, and very often in the premolar regions, a high collar should be left, which prevents the easy deposition of plaque, and allows for better and easier maintenance of oral hygiene, protection against peri-implant infections.

At the end of this chapter, the presentation of this case illustrates the seriousness of peri-implantitis as a complication with an unpredictable treatment outcome. The patient's medical history outlines the sequence of procedures involved in the entire treatment process. Seven years ago, the patient underwent implant prosthetic rehabilitation. Although this procedure was carried out correctly, adhering to all the principles of oral surgical-prosthetic protocol and utilizing high-quality implants at the time (Brenemark's implant system), the case demonstrates that the patient encountered a more significant problem than the one they faced at the beginning of the treatment.

The treatment procedure was performed in the following sequence: first, diseased teeth were extracted, followed by the augmentation of bone defects in both the upper and lower jaw. The patient was fitted with an immediate temporary acrylic prosthesis, which he wore for six months. After this period, a two-phase implantation with delayed loading was carried out. Six months later, definitive prosthetic work was completed for both jaws, beginning with the installation of the implants.

Four years after the completion of the implant-prosthetic treatment, the patient returned to the attending physician due to issues in both jaws (see pictures 15.160 to 15.162). Re-augmentation was conducted around the installed implants using xenogeneic bone substitutes (Fig. 15.130).

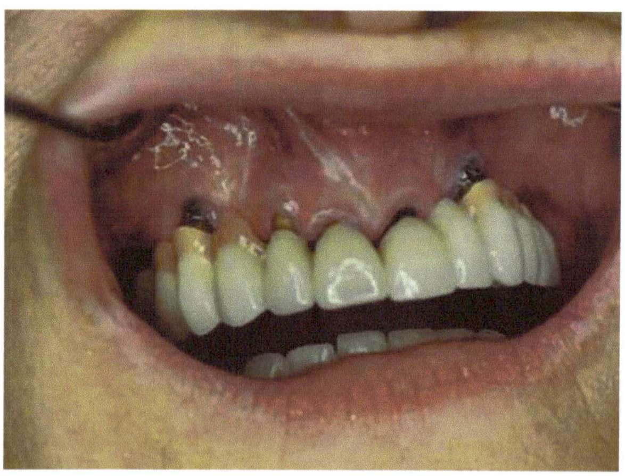

Figure 15.160. Presentation of the situation after 7 years. The case was handled abroad.

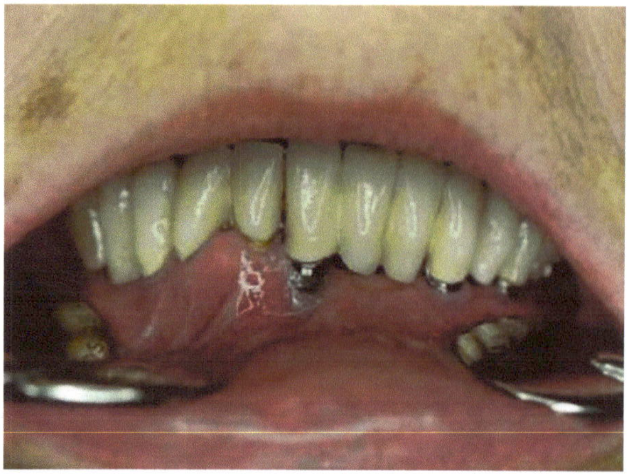

Figure 15.161. Condition in the lower jaw; despite the recession of the gingiva around the implants, the integrated implants are stable, as is the prosthetic work. The case was treated at a university clinic.

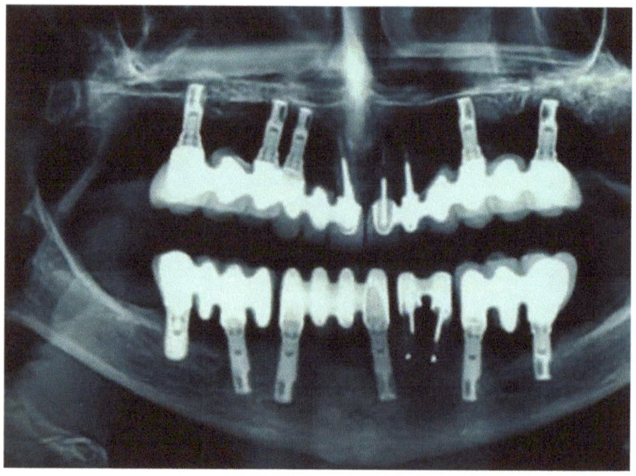

Figure 15.162. Radiographic view of the condition (April 16, 2016) 7 years after the start of implant-prosthetic rehabilitation and subsequent repeated augmentation of bone resorption around the implant.

Conclusion

Throughout decades of work and during the writing of this book, the author adapted his views to align with advancements in the profession, scientific evidence, and practical requirements. In analyzing the case presented, it is evident that the surgical procedure was conducted according to the established protocol for implant prosthetic rehabilitation. The highest quality and most expensive Brånemark implants were used, indicating that the entire treatment was executed correctly.

However, the patient encountered more significant issues than at the start of the treatment, raising the question of which procedures should be applied to achieve a successful treatment outcome (see pictures 15.160, 15.161, and 15.162).

After four years, the peri-implant changes were addressed with repeated augmentation around the implant. However, the treatment resulted in the same condition, as shown in the orthopantomographic image. This raises the question: what should be the first step in treating this extremely complicated case, and what actions should be taken next?

The patient should be referred back to the dentist who performed the initial treatment. It is important to explain that the installation of the implant and the overall treatment were conducted conscientiously and professionally. A collaborative approach is recommended—reach out to the colleague to discuss and agree on the next steps to ensure the best outcome for the patient.

Discussion

Branemark's implant system is still regarded as very high quality today. However, in the context of modern developments in oral implantology, the design of Branemark and similar implant systems is considered superior to newer systems that feature modified design details. This superiority is evident in the technological processing of the implant surface and in specific design elements that are essential for osseointegration and the formation of stable soft tissues around the neck of the implant.

Branemark was the pioneer of osseointegration, though at that time, there was less emphasis on the integration of soft tissues with the implant surface. Additionally, the design of Branemark implants, particularly at the apical part, does not mimic the anatomy of a natural root, which reflects a deviation from nature.

Most of the latest implant systems feature a rounded design at the apical end of the implant, which mimics the apex of a natural tooth root. Significant advancements have been made in the design of the section of the implant that comes into contact with the cortical bone and soft tissues. Recent research confirms that the arrangement and shape of the threads— particularly the double-bend design and the angle of inclination—are crucial for several reasons. These design elements facilitate better self-threading into the bone, thereby reducing stress on the surrounding bone during the implant installation process. Additionally, the thread designs in the neck of the implant promote the integration of both hard and soft tissues. This allows the implant to effectively withstand the strongest chewing forces.

When addressing larger bone defects, particularly when augmentation has been carried out using only xenogeneic bone substitutes instead of autologous bone blocks, it's important to consider the implications of using a temporary mobile acrylate prosthesis. Compressing the augmented material with such a prosthesis may lead to unfavorable outcomes, promoting bone resorption.

For larger bone defects (as discussed in Chapter 18), a more effective approach involves simultaneous implantation and augmentation by using bone blocks or autologous bone chips mixed with xenogeneic bone substitutes, which should be covered with resorbable collagen membranes. Regardless of the source of bone substitutes, it is advisable to avoid the use of a mobile acrylate prosthesis as a temporary solution.

A more effective solution involves the use of a fixed provisional acrylate bridge, or newer materials made from composite blocks, which is placed outside the area of occlusion. This is immediately followed by the implantation of reduced-diameter implants (2.8 mm). After 12 months, these mini-implants can be replaced with standard or wider diameter implants, depending on the success of the augmentation procedure and the amount of available bone in both horizontal and vertical dimensions.

Immediate implant installation, followed by immediate loading, is a well-documented procedure with a high success rate when certain conditions and parameters are met. The dentist's experience, skill, and knowledge are crucial for the effective application of these techniques. If a dentist lacks sufficient experience and dexterity, opting for a two-phase implant installation with delayed loading may be a more appropriate choice.

When it comes to immediate installation of implants and immediate loading, it is a very successful procedure with predictability of outcome, verified and documented by successful outcomes of implant-prosthetic rehabilitation in practical application. Such treatment procedures stimulate osseointegration, remodeling, and new bone formation, and avoid trauma to soft tissues. In contrast to that principle, mobile acrylate prostheses (as a temporary solution) exert compression on the augmented bone ridge, which achieves the opposite effect.

16

Application Of Implants In Developing Individuals - Children And Youth

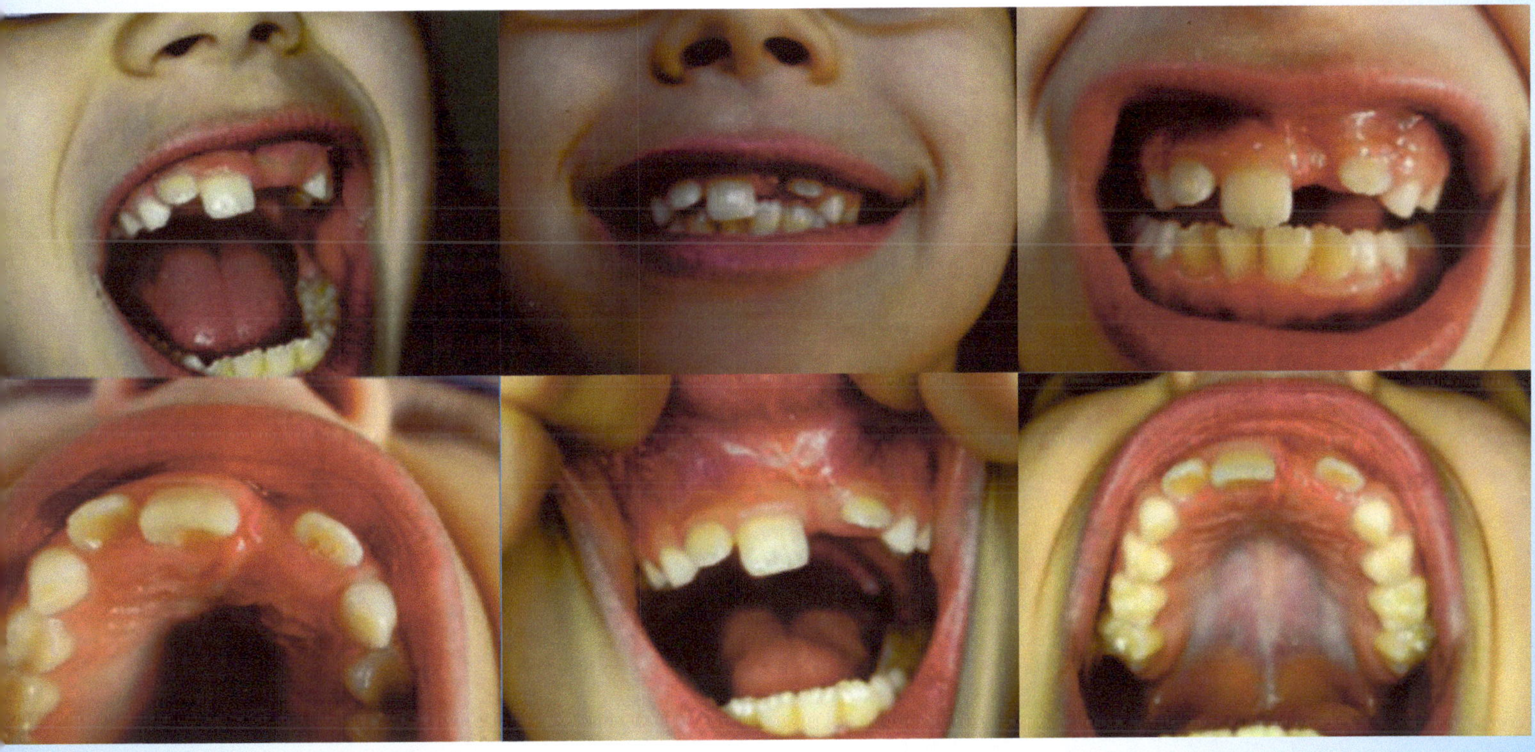

With the rapid advancement of oral implantology, the indications for using dental implants are continually expanding. Until recently, the use of implants in growing individuals—such as children and adolescents— was not widely considered. However, there has been a growing application of implantology for children and teenagers who experience oligodontia (the condition of having fewer than the normal number of teeth) or anodontia (the absence of teeth) as well as in cases of premature tooth loss. At a stage when the entire body is still developing, the use of implants for oral rehabilitation necessitates a continuous updating of our knowledge regarding anatomy and physiology. Specifically, it is essential to have a detailed understanding of the physiological changes related to growth and development in the jaws and facial structures.

Currently, there is a limited amount of literature that publishes the results of implanted dental devices during this developmental period, covering aspects of both functionality and aesthetics, as well as the effects on bone growth and surrounding tissues. Congenital partial or total anodontia, as well as tooth loss due to trauma, is often observed in patients who are still growing. Traditionally, it has not been common to perform prosthetic oral rehabilitation for these patients after implant placement. Instead, they were typically fitted with removable prostheses that children could take out at will. Fortunately, children adapt to this type of care quite quickly and can effectively use these prostheses, especially when they understand the importance of wearing them.

The main reason for using removable prostheses during this growth period is related to the child's mental and emotional development. Children can be unkind to their peers when they notice any physical differences, which can lead to harsh experiences for those with dental issues. There have been instances when prostheses have fallen out or broken during play, causing children to feel embarrassed and even reluctant to attend school. Such experiences can significantly affect their mental well-being.

The use of mobile acrylate prostheses can lead to side effects that may result in more severe oral disabilities in individuals still in their growth phase. Firstly, the pressure exerted by the acrylic prosthesis on the bone can cause increased and accelerated resorption of the alveolar ridge, which has not yet fully developed. Secondly, there is a risk that the prosthesis, often referred to as a "frog," may be swallowed or aspirated by the child. The risk increases significantly when wire hooks are involved.

The atrophy of the bone in this area can become so pronounced that, once growth is complete, it becomes very challenging to implement any fixed prosthetic solution that meets modern aesthetic standards. Additionally, the presence of mobile acrylate prostheses in growing individuals can result in soft tissue deformations and accompanying periodontal complications. These severe consequences highlight the importance of careful consideration when using such prostheses during the growth phase.

The use of dental implants in developing children raises two important questions: first, are there any potential complications associated with the use of implants in children and adolescents whose jaw growth is not yet complete? Second, can we predict the success of such procedures?

Placing implants during this stage of life requires specialized knowledge that is not necessary when working with adult patients. The issues related to the growth and development of the skeletal and dental structures, and their impact on the predictability of success, necessitate a thorough evaluation by specialists in pediatric and preventive dentistry. These specialists should refer patients to an implantologist with expertise in oligo- and anodontics for further consultation.

Despite existing uncertainties, there is increasing pressure on dentists, presenting both challenges and opportunities in utilizing implants to address pediatric prosthetic needs.

Oral implantology is gaining increasing confidence, with a success rate of up to 98% for adults. As a result, there is a growing consideration for applying implantology as an optimal solution for younger patients. Based on my experience, I have successfully performed several implants in adolescents aged 16 to 18. However, I have hesitated to do the same for younger children due to various uncertainties. This concern prompted me to enhance my understanding of bone physiology and the development of the skeleton and facial bones.

Today, more information is emerging about the advantages of dental implants compared to traditional prosthetic treatments. Parents are becoming increasingly aware of these benefits and are more frequently inquiring about rehabilitation options for their children. This growing interest has drawn my attention to the challenges of oral implantology, particularly when it comes to using implants in children and developing individuals. This remains an area of uncertainty and a significant dilemma for practitioners, especially since many assumptions lack validation from scientific research, experience, or clinical practice.

For example, the partial lack of teeth in people with oligodontia or in patients who have ectodermal dysplasia can lead to facial distortion, which, especially in the early years of adolescence, can have negative consequences in the social sphere.

From a physiological perspective, preserving alveolar bone is a primary and valid reason for applying dental implants in patients who are still growing. When a tooth is lost due to trauma, accelerated resorption of the alveolar ridge can occur during this growth phase. Additionally, using a prosthesis as a temporary replacement for the lost tooth can further contribute to bone resorption. In contrast, implant therapy alters the loading mechanism on the bone and slows down its resorption.

Starting early rehabilitation for patients with oligodontia is essential for several reasons. Traditionally, treatment for oligodontia and the absence of teeth has involved classical methods such as adhesive bridges, skeletal metal structures, and often acrylic prostheses. While these approaches can serve as solutions, they present various aesthetic and functional issues. In some individual cases, orthodontic movement of nearby teeth or transplantation may offer alternatives for prosthetic care.

The optimal age for tooth transplantation, from a morphological perspective, is between nine and ten years. This procedure is based on natural principles: much like there is a limited timeframe for transplanting plants to ensure their successful growth, tooth transplantation in children outside this age range carries a higher risk of unfavorable outcomes.

For instance, consider a scenario where a ten-year-old girl loses her central incisors in a traffic accident. In this case, the second premolars (#35 and #45) from her lower jaw can be transplanted into the spaces where the central incisors used to be. Initially, these transplanted teeth can be reshaped into incisors using composite material. Eventually, a more permanent solution, such as metal-free aesthetic crowns, can be pursued for a better appearance.

The convenience of this method in that period of growth lies in the fact that the teeth that are transplanted, at that moment, have intact dental follicles that can induce the formation of new bone in the alveoli. Particularly difficult cases to treat are patients with multiple aplasia or anodontia.

Two decades ago, in Sweden (Gothenburg, 1996), the "Consensus Conference on Oral Implants in Young Patients" was held. Then conclusions were drawn about the terminology that will be used in the diagnosis, i.e. definitions:

- Hypodontia exists when one to five teeth are missing.
- Oligodontia is when six or more teeth are missing.
- Anodontia is characterized by the absence of all teeth.

Based on the growing experience with oral implants and additional augmentative operative techniques, new possibilities for prosthetic rehabilitation of young patients with oligo and anodontia are opening up.

The installation of implants performed too early can lead to unpredictable negative consequences, making future prosthetic care unsatisfactory. To avoid such mistakes, implantologists must consider the potential impact of the implant on the growth process. Evaluating the suitability of implants in a growing child requires an assessment of the child's growth, which includes determining the skeletal age and the growth phase they are in. It's crucial to predict how growth will continue and the effects that the implant procedure may have on this process. Unfortunately, there are currently only a few studies on the long-term use of implants in children. Therefore, it is important to monitor and anticipate the behavior of endosseous implants during growth, particularly in cases of ankylosed primary teeth, especially in the canine area, where hypodontia may be present, whether affecting one or more teeth.

Similar to ankylosed teeth, embedded dental implants do not adapt to the growth and development of the jaw; they remain in their original position. Consequently, in a localized area of the jaw, implants can lead to malocclusion, lose their bony connections, and either fall out or become completely embedded in the growing bone. Unlike natural teeth, implants do not undergo compensatory eruptions or respond to other physiological changes. These critical considerations, mentioned by the author, are supported by practical experience and case studies involving hypodontia and teeth lost due to trauma.

Growth concerning implant placement should be understood from two perspectives: as a dynamic process and a potentially problematic one.

The growth of the maxilla and mandible, including the skeleton and teeth, is a dynamic process that results in significant changes in all three dimensions during the active growth phase. According to Emlow's detailed descriptions, this growth occurs multilocally, meaning that certain growth tendencies hold varying degrees of importance for implantologists.

For improved understanding and transparency, growth is discussed in terms of its main manifestations: transverse, anteroposterior (sagittal), and vertical dimensions, which are significant for potential implant therapy. In both the upper and lower jaws, growth occurs first in the transverse direction, then longitudinally, and finally vertically. Although the growth in the width of the anterior segment of the upper jaw concludes before the adolescent growth spurt, the posterior width of the jaw is directly influenced by the increasing longitudinal growth.

The distance between the canines changes only slightly after the twelfth year of life, while the width in the area of the second and third molars continues to increase until these teeth are fully formed. The central suture, which coordinates transverse growth with the base of the skull, remains open until adolescence and expands by about 2 mm during the puberty growth spurt. This central suture is a critical growth zone that needs to develop undisturbed.

From the fourth year of life to adulthood, the increase in width at the back of the jaw is three times greater than the increase in width at the front.

If a middle incisor is replaced with an implant immediately after eruption, there may be a larger gap between the implant and the adjacent natural tooth. During the period of transverse growth, implants placed in the anterior region of the upper jaw can get displaced as growth occurs. If these implants are connected across the central suture, they could hinder the growth process of the front segment of the jaw.

Once transverse growth is completed, sagittal growth continues. As both upper jaws increase in size, they move away from each other, which occurs at the base of the skull. This creates a space where growth takes place. Simultaneously, the bone undergoes remodeling through a process of apposition and resorption, known as "primary translation." This means that the central part of the face generally moves forward and downward, resulting from a combination of passive lengthening and enlargement.

After the growth of the jaws, this area continues to shift its position as neighboring structures grow in sync. This latter process is referred to as secondary translation, which can occur up to the age of 20 and slightly beyond. However, this secondary translation does not have significant implications for the timing or method of implant placement.

The anterior surface of the upper jaw experiences more resorption compared to the posterior segments, which are stacked or apposed. The growth period of the lower jaw is similar to that of the upper jaw; however, lower jaw growth is more tied to physical development. In contrast, upper jaw growth occurs during adolescence, resulting in a more pronounced sagittal increase. This change transforms the predominantly convex profile of a child's face into a flatter profile seen in adults.

In girls, sagittal growth typically concludes between the ages of 14 and 15, occurring two to three years after the onset of menstruation. For boys, this growth continues until around the age of 18. Young adults may experience growth in this dimension over a much longer period, often reaching adult values only by the ages of 20 to 22.

For implantologists, vertical growth is particularly important and is the last to conclude. Unlike the upper jaw, implants placed in the lower jaw do not interfere with transverse growth, as they cross over the midline.

During the growth process, the upper jaw moves downward in relation to the base of the skull. The most significant change during this stage is the increase in the height of the upper jaw. Concurrently, there is a resorptive lowering of the floor of the nasal cavity and sinuses, which typically occurs more forward than backward. Resorption is about one third less compared to the vertical growth of the upper jaw. This aspect is crucial for the positioning of dental implants. An endosseous implant placed in a person during the active phase of growth can potentially penetrate the sinus or nasal area at its apex. Additionally, due to appositional growth, the implant may later become impacted at the occlusal level.

In a simulated case, it was observed that an early implant placed in the frontal region was lost due to resorption of the anterior part of the maxilla. While the anterior segment of the upper jaw is generally considered suitable for implant placement, the long-term prognosis is unfavorable. Similarly, the posterior part of the upper jaw does not offer a significantly better prognosis. The resorptive activity of the sinus floor, coupled with tooth eruption, greatly promotes alveolar growth. It has been estimated that the vertical growth of the maxilla can exceed 1 cm between the ages of 9 and 25 with the eruption of molars. As a result, a bony crater may develop around the implant, with the apical end situated in the maxillary sinus. Therefore, the key question is not whether the installation of an implant to replace a single tooth is feasible, but rather what the long-term outcomes of such an intervention will be.

There are valid reasons for considering implants to replace individual teeth in children, particularly following the loss of a central incisor. Thanks to favorable extravascularization, a positive immune response, and an uncomplicated healing process, implantology can also be beneficial for children. The insertion of an implant can help preserve alveolar bone that might otherwise become atrophic.

However, long-term follow-up has revealed significant deficits in the development of the alveolar process around the implant. There can also be aesthetic concerns when comparing the implanted tooth to neighboring natural teeth. In some cases, these drawbacks may outweigh the previously mentioned benefits.

Nasal and anterior resorption of the upper jaw poses a significant challenge for early implant placement, even in children with anodontia. Inserting implants in the upper jaw is generally contraindicated until adulthood. Even in cases of children with anodontia, early implant placement is not advisable due to the resorption in the upper jaw.

It is important to note that the growth rate of the lower jaw is similar to that of the upper jaw; however, this growth is associated with overall body development, whereas the upper jaw growth is linked to the development of cranial sutures. Consequently, during adolescence, there is a noticeable increase in the upper jaw's sagittal dimension, which typically concludes a few years later in boys than in girls.

When examining the transverse growth of the lower jaw, we find that the growth in width in the frontal area ceases by around the age of twelve. Unlike the upper jaw, implants placed in the lower jaw do not hinder transverse growth. In children with partial anodontia, it appears that early implantation of the lower jaw, away from the natural teeth, can be successful. The placement of an implant offers the child stable prosthetic support in the lower jaw, which is not achievable through other methods.

For implant procedures in the frontal region of the upper jaw, it is recommended that girls be at least 15 years old and boys at least 17 years old to increase the likelihood of a successful outcome. The same criteria apply to the posterior area of the upper jaw. It is important to note that when the implant is located close to natural teeth, the prognosis is much poorer due to the risk of progressive infraocclusion of the implant, which can lead to long-term complications for both the implant and the adjacent teeth.

The recommendation in this case is to place implants only after growth has completely finished. In children with anodontia, the anterior region of the lower jaw is the only area where implant placement is appropriate. Although this region also experiences a dynamic growth pattern, the alveolar growth remains relatively minor. One advantage is that most of the transverse and sagittal growth occurs early on.

Significant anterior-posterior growth primarily takes place at the posterior edge of the lower jaw, while growth changes in the distal area of the lower jaw are noted only later. There are substantial changes in the transverse, sagittal, and vertical dimensions, which also include rotational growth affecting both the alveolar process and the lower jaw edge. Even in edentulous jaws, growth changes continue to occur in this region.

For this reason, implants should not be placed in the lower jaw until skeletal growth is entirely complete.

What You Need To Know

- If you want to think about installing implants in young people, you must know the laws of jaw growth.
- In children, there is always a high risk for the installation of implants, due to changes in the jaws caused by growth.
- The upper jaw continues to grow even in the second decade of life. In the first years of life, jaw growth is most active. From the age of 5, the face reaches approximately 80% of its final size.
- Consideration of implant placement in children is possible where there is no tooth germ or natural disorders, etc.
- In the pre-puberty phase, development stops until the age of 17, when a new shift in growth begins.
- During puberty, growth lasts the same length of time and does not depend on gender. Females reach their full body height 18 to 24 months before males due to an overall faster and longer puberty phase; men develop stronger jaw arches. In the case of females, by the age of 15, growth is almost complete and therefore they are more suitable for early application of implants.
- The long-term prognosis and predictability of the success of implantation in children is very uncertain because, due to the ankylosing connection of the implant with the bone in the active phase of growth, there may be damage and displacement of natural teeth.

Based on the data presented, it can be concluded that placing implants in developing individuals is more contraindicated than justified. This conclusion was supported by a group of dentists from the University of Mainz in 1996, who noted that the growth of the upper and lower jaws is not limited by dental and skeletal maturity and can extend into early adulthood. Therefore, placing implants in adolescents and young individuals may carry certain risks.

The growth of alveolar bone surrounding an implanted tooth ceases in a manner similar to that of an ankylosed tooth. Vertical bone reduction around an ankylosed tooth is inhibited by processes of active bone apposition and resorption, as well as by the vertical growth of the alveolar bone. Consequently, in patients who are still experiencing residual growth, the installation of dental implants may lead to the prosthetic restoration sitting lower than adjacent teeth, causing infraocclusion. However, combining implant placement with orthodontic therapy can significantly enhance the aesthetic result.

A 17-year-old patient with traumatic loss of the central incisors in the upper jaw was treated at the University of Mainz. In addition to the loss of teeth, a fracture of the alveolar ridge in the anterior upper region was also observed. After emergency treatment, a healing period was necessary for the bone to recover. Two self-tapping implants from Nobel Biocare, with a diameter of 3.75 mm and a length of 13 mm, were then inserted into the healed bone. Bone augmentation was also performed. Following the delayed healing of both the bone and soft tissues, a second surgical procedure took place. This involved raising a flap and placing a support for prosthetic work, which consisted of two metal-ceramic crowns.

After seven years, a significant vertical discrepancy was noted between the prosthetic work on the implants and the adjacent teeth. Three years later, which means ten years after the implant placement, both the implants and the adjacent lateral incisors were positioned extremely low in relation to the other teeth, creating a disharmony with the lip. To address this aesthetic and functional deficiency, an attempt was made to lengthen the incisal edge of the crowns on the implants. However, the position of the incisors in the lower jaw limited the effectiveness of this solution.

At the age of 28, the patient was referred for orthodontic treatment, which proved to be complicated. The treatment plan involved extracting all premolars, closing the resulting spaces, reducing the arch of the upper jaw, and consequently moving the upper lip. Additionally, the lateral incisors were extruded to align them with the lip line. It was necessary to replace the crowns on the implants as part of the treatment.

The case described indicates that using implants in growing individuals is a highly complex and challenging procedure that carries inherent risks. Alongside aesthetic and functional considerations, such as speech, there are also concerns related to chewing ability. When implants are placed in individuals who are still expecting residual growth, adjustments may be necessary over time due to changes in the positioning of the prosthetic work relative to neighboring teeth.

The growth of the upper and lower jaw continues beyond dental and skeletal maturity and can extend into early adulthood. Therefore, placing implants in adolescents and young adults can be quite risky. This is primarily because alveolar bone growth is inhibited near the embedded implant, similar to the effects seen around an ankylosed tooth. Vertical bone retraction around an ankylosed tooth is restricted due to active processes of bone apposition and resorption, as well as through vertical growth of the alveolar bone.

Consequently, in patients who may still experience growth, the premature placement of an implant can result in the superstructure of the implant moving into infraocclusion relative to the rest of the teeth. In such situations, prosthetic-orthodontic therapy may be necessary, which can significantly affect both functional and aesthetic outcomes.

Taking all these factors into consideration, we conclude that implant placement should ideally be postponed until the period when residual craniofacial growth is no longer expected.

The decision about what kind of compensation should be done in that period is individual, depending on the experience of the therapist and his knowledge of the process of growth and development of the skeleton. There are many combinations for applying temporary allowances. Which combination to choose depends on many factors. Already at the beginning of this chapter, it was said that autotransplantation of premolars can be attempted in younger patients. However, this possibility should also be used with great caution, since there are no statistical data for the long-term success from which a valid conclusion could be drawn. From the author's experience, partial mobile prostheses are usually not comfortable both functionally and aesthetically. The author of the book treated one case of a 16- year-old patient with loss of central incisors and one lateral incisor due to a traffic injury. He applied the following procedure: the bone defect was augmented with xenogeneic bone substitutes, the concavity formed by the augment was covered with a collagen resorptive membrane. After 6 months of waiting for the bone healing process to end, an implant-prosthetic procedure followed with the aim of preserving the mesiodistal space during growth.

Two implants with the narrowest diameter (1.8 mm) were used to place a precise temporary prosthetic work consisting of three members. This decision was made for several reasons. After the healing of the alveolar ridge, placing a removable partial prosthesis in the visible aesthetic region of the upper jaw would undermine the results of bone augmentation and cause ongoing trauma to the soft tissues.

After some time, specifically once craniofacial growth is complete, replacing the narrow-diameter implants with standard-diameter implants will be a relatively simple and atraumatic procedure for both the bone and soft tissues. Since the treatment for this patient is still ongoing, the final result remains to be seen.

Based on the available knowledge and examples, we can conclude that patience, allowing for a waiting period, and delaying implant placement in developing individuals, as long as possible, are essential for ensuring successful outcomes.

17

Return of Smile, Security and Self-Confidence by Implant Installation

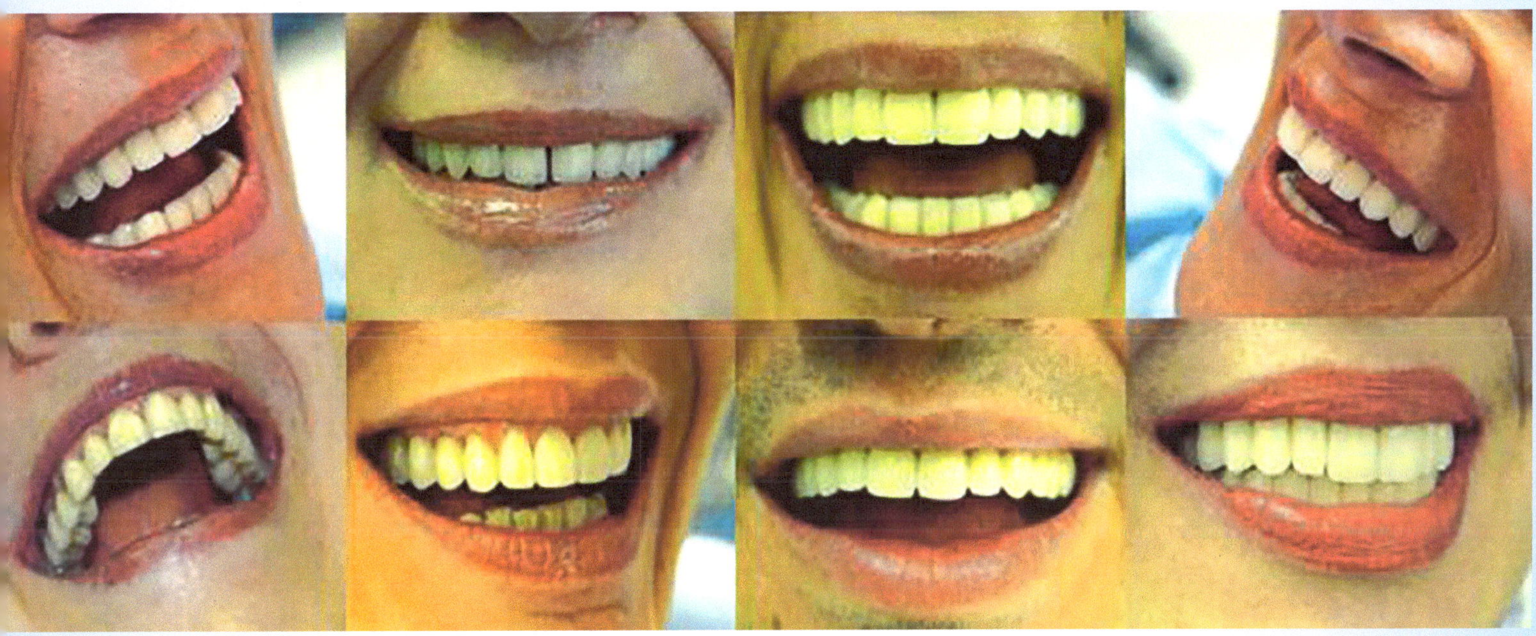

A small number of people recognize the significance and wide range of functions associated with something as commonplace and seemingly ordinary as laughter. Among all species, only humans have been gifted with this ability. Homo sapiens is the only living creature that laughs. Studies show that smiling in response to social stimuli typically begins around the eighth week of life, while loud, expressive laughter can be observed by the twelfth week.

The primary purpose of laughter—expressing an emotional state—grows and evolves in intensity between the second and fifth years of life, transforming into a crucial form of communication with the environment. It's important to note that laughter and the act of laughing change through learning, enriching our experiences and developing alongside us, ultimately becoming a true indicator of our "inner state."

While laughter is a form of emotional and subjective expression, its roots are fundamentally social. As we mature, the social aspect of this mode of communication becomes more pronounced.

The depiction of laughter as merely showing teeth is misleading. A true smile engages the whole face, as 19 facial muscles are involved in laughter. It's important to note that a smile is perceived not just through the teeth and face, but primarily through the eyes.

The reason the author chose to include a chapter on this topic in a book about oral implantology is quite justified. Observations of society reveal that toothless individuals or those wearing loose acrylic prostheses often cover their mouths when laughing, trying to conceal their oral disabilities. This behavior is also seen among people with uncomfortable, ill-fitting, or unstable complete dentures, who fear that their dentures might dislodge while they laugh.

This scenario actually happened to the famous actor Clark Gable during the filming of "Gone with the Wind" when he leaned in to kiss Vivien Leigh, and his prosthesis unexpectedly flew out of his mouth. Similarly, Josip Broz experienced an awkward moment in Washington during a conversation with U.S. President Jimmy Carter when his upper denture ended up under the table.

If oral implantology had advanced to its current level at that time, such embarrassing situations could have been avoided for both of these individuals. In these uncomfortable circumstances, people often feel self-conscious and uneasy.

Laughing and feeling funny is always a pleasant feeling caused by an unusual, unexpected, and creative association. That creative association must not threaten the value system of the person we want to make laugh. Some people are witty and their laughter will provoke a sense of funniness and pleasantness in the interlocutor, in the popular saying, "Don't worry, be happy". Laughter without teeth reveals the "psychological and social tragedy of the personality". Not having teeth is a civilizational failure, not only for the individual, but also for society. Young people without teeth are a tragic image of the individual and society. "There is no laughter in a sad man" - said Njegoševski.

Laughing enhances our wit, transforming it from a subjective trait into a genuine social skill. Individuals who excel in humor experience significant social benefits; they create an enjoyable atmosphere in their interactions, which makes them popular and often perceived as more intelligent. This perception arises from their ability to freely and creatively connect ideas. Consequently, they become more attractive to others.

A warm smile is a universal symbol of kindness. It is often said that smiles inspire smiles: if you encounter a friend without a smile, share one with them. A smile may last just a moment, but the impression it leaves can endure for a long time. Additionally, laughter and humor can serve as a defense mechanism, helping to steer communication in a more pleasant direction.

The previous text highlights the widespread belief that a smile primarily serves to showcase "beautiful white teeth," whether they are natural or artificial, and represents one's emotional state. However, a smile is one of the fundamental and crucial means of communication among humans and encompasses much more than these aspects.

The loss of teeth disrupts the harmony of the face and the functional balance of the masticatory system, which also affects one's smile. This disruption can lead to insecurity in human communication and a loss of self-confidence.

When teeth are lost, restoring the natural harmony of the oral cavity is essential and can often be achieved through prosthetic work. This process is generally simpler in cases of partial tooth loss, where remaining natural teeth can serve as anchors. In contrast, total edentulism requires a more complex rehabilitation procedure.

Moreover, the functional and aesthetic harmony can be only partially restored with mobile, unstable, and poorly fitting acrylic prostheses. This restoration is limited in terms of aesthetic, functional, and particularly psychological aspects.

The treatment of dental disabilities with total and uncomfortable prostheses can significantly impair communication. When prostheses move around in the mouth, individuals may lose the ability to smile and laugh freely, which is one of the most beautiful gifts of being human. The installation of dental implants prompts us to consider the vital role of restoring a lost smile. A smile transformed by implants is distinctly different from one affected by missing teeth or removable prosthetic devices.

The significance of laughter for a person's mental and physical health has been emphasized by American doctor Henry Robinstein in his book "Psychosomatics of Laughter." His research on laughter was conducted with individuals who had healthy teeth, highlighting how essential it is to restore a person's smile and enhance both function and aesthetics through implants. Doing so can truly rejuvenate a person, enhancing their quality of life and helping them regain confidence and joy in their daily interactions!

According to Rubistein, laughter serves as both an excellent muscle workout and a beneficial breathing exercise. It positively impacts the brain by encouraging the production of hormones that can help improve pain tolerance. Laughter also supports better digestion and can aid in treating insomnia, stress, and depression, contributing to a longer and more fulfilling life, as claimed by Henry Rubenstein. This perspective aligns with the popular saying: "Smile sweetly so you don't live short."

In the book "Psychosomatics of Laughter," the author demonstrates that laughter helps cleanse and open the upper respiratory tract, much like coughing, which facilitates easier and more effective breathing. During laughter, respiratory functions significantly improve: exhalation becomes deeper, the pauses that follow are longer, and inhalation becomes deeper after prolonged exhalations. This process helps cleanse the lungs more effectively.

Since laughing enhances breathing by three to four times, it is particularly recommended for individuals with asthma. Studies have shown that a loud laugh can even halt an asthma attack.

Laughter helps to bear pain more easily by acting through three basic mechanisms: distracts attention, weakens muscle tension and causes general relaxation of the body. And it is precisely from this tension that many pains originate, or that tension sustains them. Gelentologists, scientists who study the healing effect of laughter on human health, have found that cheerful people live longer. Gelotology is the science of laughter, derived from the Greek word "helos" - laughter. It has been known since time immemorial that laughter has a beneficial effect on health, and in the sixties of the last century scientists proved it. It all started with an American journalist, Norman Cousins, who was diagnosed with an incurable spinal disease. He refused to take painkillers, left the clinic, locked himself in a hotel room and decided to laugh. He read jokes and watched comedy movies, and he reacted to all of it by laughing uproariously. Laughing relaxed his muscles, moved his vertebrae, and eventually the pain disappeared completely.

Norman was completely cured by therapy which he himself chose - by laughing. Scientists have begun to investigate the beneficial effect of laughter on humans health. And why do we laugh, say scientists, Gelentologists - specialists in this field: Medicinal effect laughter can only be used if stimuli are detected that cause it. Associations were founded in Germany of German laughter therapy specialists. German scientist Mihaela Šefer claims that therapy laughter consists of three groups: the first includes emotional ones stimuli, which directly depend on our mood, in the second, cognitive, which occur when one hears some good joke, comedy shows on television or in the theater, and in the third, motoric, which is conditioned by the physical by contact, eg by tickling. In cognitive and code the decisive importance of motor stimuli is the effect surprises, which can be used most often when watching comedies or hidden cameras on television. Then laughter massages the whole body, claims Professor Karsten Nimic, director of the Institute for Human Biology and Anthropology in Berlin.

When certain information reaches the brain, it activates is a center for laughter, more than a hundred are engaged muscles, from those on the face to the respiratory musculature organs. The supply of cells with oxygen increases, lung ventilation, metabolic processes improve are accelerated, muscles relax, at the same time harmonizes work of the heart and circulation.

Rubenstein, among other things, claims that our laughter allows us to oppose the pain, encouraging the production of hormones called endorphins, that is substances like natural morphine they have a pain-relieving effect. Laughter encourages the process self-medication, because the brain shuts down when laughing production of adrenaline and cortisone, stress hormones, thus the body releases tension. When when we laugh, the hormone serotonin, known as happiness hormone, because those who laugh more often feel get better. Often times when we feel bad, naturally is that we are not laughing, but an effort must be made which, no doubt, will be rewarded. It can be some comedy movie, good joke or joke, hidden camera on television, a telephone conversation with friends who will able to entertain us. All this will be more efficient than medicines. For example, one wittily written the text can cause loud laughter, which is the most effective massage of the entire musculature.

Reading witty articles will be more effective than watching movies with depressing content. Everything is this is much more effective than taking sedatives for calmness in the thinness of excitement.

Laughter is also a medicine for better digestion, because it provokes stomach gymnastics, deep digestive massage tract, affecting the liver and pancreas. Laughter stimulates gall bladder and liver, eliminating excess cholesterol through the bile ducts, which is again reflected favorably and on the pancreas.

The more and deeper a person laughs, the more solid his sleep. And sound sleep is the foundation of human health. How much laughter can affect sound sleep, the author of the book found out for himself, watching a hidden camera on television. The reactions of different types of people to the suddenly set traps that cause laughter to the point of tears, seems relaxing. With the "hidden camera" there is a surprise effect achieved by the motor stimulation of laughter. The author of the book concludes: the deeper the roar of laughter, the stronger the sleep. Robinstein is really right when he claims in his book: when we laugh well, we sleep well. Because laughing is a way to get rid of internal tensions, muscle spasms, so it relaxes the nervous system. And the state of relaxation favors indulging in healthy and sound sleep. Sound sleep is the best prevention of dangerous conditions in the body, primarily prevention of heart attack, hypertension and brain hemorrhage. The great anti-stress effect of laughter is based on the same effect. Relieving tension is the best anti-stress sedative for the entire body.

A new study conducted by scientists from Michigan (USA) showed that employees who work in contact with people and have a fake smile on their face every day are in a bad mood and less productive at work. While those who genuinely smile are significantly more positive and happier. Laughter is also a good medicine for relieving tension in difficult situations. As already emphasized, laughing reduces stress, and psychologists call this the facial feedback hypothesis. Even if a person laughs forcefully and when he doesn't feel like laughing, he can improve his mood and break away from depression and bad feelings.

Laughter is a very complex reflex mechanism whose effector system involves over twenty muscles, (Professor Nimitz concludes that more than a hundred are engaged), and of these, 15 facial muscles are innervated by the seventh cranial nerve. (CNVII-facialis). Neck muscles and abdominal muscles also participate in laughter.

Laughter is a pleasant sensation and an expression of emotional impressions of varying intensity and quality. Laughter is a subjective and strictly individual experience, so its intensity can hardly be measured objectively. It is most often a manifestation of optimism, positive energy, satisfaction and happiness. If laughter is a gift from God, and it is, then a good implant is a gift from a good and experienced dentist.

Since laughter is a very complex reflex mechanism, the return of a lost smile with the installation of an implant is an attribute, an optimistic smile. However, laughter has at least ten attributes: optimistic, sincere, fake, cheerful, giggling, sly, sneer, toothless, shy, painful smile and ... Missing teeth is one of the most visible signs of old age. Science is increasingly trying to figure out why we age, how we age and what aging brings with it. That biological process is unstoppable, but it can certainly be slowed down, i.e. postpone for a certain time. All human beings do not age equally, some slower, some faster. Aging brings with it more and more troubles: "... because there is no worse shame than old age" (Njegoš).

With the loss of teeth, the interjaw relationships also change, which contributes the most to the appearance of old people, because the lower jaw tends more towards a proclined position. The prognathic position of the lower jaw emphasizes the elderly appearance and expression (Figures 17.1 and 17.2). All this affects the psychological and physical function of the entire organism.

Many are concerned with eliminating, or rather, reducing the signs of aging, but charlatans have not helped in the development of the science of aging. Several times during 1953, the sick Pope Pius XII received injections of the tissue of male gonads or monkey glands, as they were called. They were prescribed by doctor Dr. Paul Nyhans, who became famous for it, creating a successful career by "rejuvenating" celebrities. Among those whom Paul Nyhans "rejuvenated" were Winston Churchill, Konrad Adenauer, Bernard Baruch, Duke and Duchess of Windsor and others. Towards the end of his life, Pope John II was also "rejuvenated" in a similar way with various elixirs. All those elixirs that Dr. Nyhans used didn't work, nor did he scientifically explain how they should work. The charlatanism of Dr. Nyhans has never been stopped, and today it has reached its zenith in another way in the pharmaceutical industry, because many manufactured drugs benefit only those who produce them. Unlike Dr. Nyhans, another physician, scientist, Dr. Godsten Roger, specialist in reproductive biology and author of "Digestive Time: Science, Sex, and Aging," for all such "rejuvenation," which Dr. Nyhans and other doctors who engaged in "smearing", Dr. Godsten especially points out Dr. Nyhans, that "he left behind the same thing that he gave to his patients - NOTHING".

But, Dr. Godsten points out, the search for eternal youth and rejuvenation was not only pursued by fraudsters and charlatans, but by serious and respected scientists, in an attempt to stop the deterioration of the body and mind. Their research is not in vain. All those celebrities who were "rejuvenated" by Dr. Nyhans did not solve the most visible sign of old age: total toothlessness - because they were "smudging" unstable total prostheses in their mouths.

Dr. Nyhans really offered his patients "nothing", in contrast to dentist-implantologists, who offer patients "something", specifically for their rejuvenation: better appearance, establishment of chewing function and better communication.

By placing the implant, the patient is rejuvenated, and thus, a younger appearance, a safe and bright smile is restored. His interjaw relations are returned to the previous physiological position, placing the condyles in the maximum physiological distal position, which also changes the facial expression to a large extent. But, that "something" that is achieved in patients from the aspect of function and aesthetics, is accompanied by the more important one: in this "rejuvenation", of the patient, it was achieved from the aspect of physiology, histology and molecular biology that the tissues surrounding the implant are put back into function which they lost by losing their teeth. The loss of natural teeth disrupts the homeostasis of the jaw bone and soft tissues, accelerating their decay, and thus making aging more visible. That is why Dr. Godsten's strongest message is that the average life expectancy of a person has been extended thanks to the influence of many factors, first of all the progress of medicine. Oral implantology is certainly one of the factors in the progress of medicine. By studying the mechanism of aging, biologists are investigating how to slow down these unstoppable processes! One of the manifestations of the aging process after tooth loss is alveolar bone resorption. By installing an implant in the jawbone, that process is slowed down, because the lost function is restored to the bone.

Scientific research is focused on how to preserve fertility as long as possible, how to slow down some degenerative processes, or even eliminate them at the beginning, delaying degenerative processes and diseases. When it comes to degenerative processes in the oral cavity, they begin immediately after birth, and accelerate over the years. After tooth loss, jaw bone loss is an accelerated degenerative process. The bone loses the function that nature has determined for it. All of this causes the smile to lose its brilliance.

Observing the historical development of oral implantology, it seems that until recently not much thought was given to the extent to which the installation of implants enables the return of a safe and bright smile and how much this factor affects the psychophysical health of a person due to the absence of fear that wobbly prostheses will fall out of the mouth when smiling. How much the denial of laughter, and especially the loss of security of expression by laughing loudly, has an effect on the aging process, there are several scientific confirmations. The science of aging may not have matured enough yet, but it can be said that it has passed childhood illnesses and is well on its way to bringing new knowledge that was once thought of in the realm of science fiction. In truth, oral implantology has not thought about restoring a smile through implantation for a long time. But her step forward can be said to have been "Himalayan leaps" when she started thinking about aesthetics. And today, the question can already be asked: does implanting rejuvenate the tissues surrounding it?

It can certainly be argued that some of the interrupted physiological processes of the jaw bone are established by implantation, and by installing the implant in the alveolar bone slows down its material loss, i.e. the resorption of the alveolar ridges. By restoring the function of bone cells, osteoblasts and osteoclasts, as well as cells of soft tissues that lost their function when the natural tooth left them, the degenerative processes of all the mentioned tissues were significantly slowed down. The bone is again under physiological stress which stimulates it on all levels. With the installation of implants, it can be said that the patient is rejuvenated and offered "something", among other things, the return of a safe and bright smile. The bone is again subjected to physiological stress, but the patient is freed from the other, pathological stress, which leads him to old age faster and deeper. Stress is, after all, a disease of our age, which brings with it increased blood pressure, heart problems, ulcers on the stomach and duodenum, restlessness and insomnia, and all of this threatens human health.

Eminent American scientist, professor Dr. Dušan Kosović, psychiatrist and psychoanalyst, wrote the most books in the world about stress that have been translated into several languages - even Japanese and Chinese. In his works, he emphasizes the importance of laughter and laughing as an anti-stress therapy. In his research, he followed patients who did not want to laugh out loud due to missing teeth and found that they fell into depression more easily. Also, he points out that the manner and quality of the smile can be used to determine the condition of the patient and his troubles. Observing patients who were toothless, he concluded that they exhibited more pronounced symptoms of depression. He concluded that patients who replaced wobbly and incongruous prostheses with stable fixed prosthetic works on implants had a significantly changed smile compared to the previous one and that the course of recovery of psycholabile persons was much faster. Likewise, groups of patients who were allowed to laugh again had far less stress symptoms, which significantly improved their quality of life.

And Dr. Rubinstein in his book "Psychosomatics of Laughter" concludes that laughter, without question, improves the quality of life, which is both important and beneficial. Even in psychotherapy, the multiple benefits and desirability of laughter are emphasized. Laughter is used in individual and group therapy, and even several therapeutic techniques are based on laughter. The emphasis is on the patient's more creative, free and spontaneous expression through laughter.

Studying this problem, the author of these lines, in order to maintain good health, advises patients to laugh as often and as much as possible, alone, in society, in almost all places and in almost all situations. Laughter causes pleasant feelings, we get the impression that we are having fun, forget our current worries, brighten up our everyday life at least for a moment, focus on that moment and feel more beautiful and pleasant. Healthy and unrestrained laughter always conveys pleasant feelings to the interlocutor and the environment. It should be emphasized that laughter cannot be separated from personality; laughter grows and changes along with personality. Laughter is one of the most sought after, valued and most important human expressions. Smiling, cheerful people are always liked and desired in society. They are more beautiful and attractive, and they seem more intelligent, precisely because healthy laughter is one of the good indicators of a higher intellectual level through the rapid creation of metaphors for the purpose of wit. Laughter is a true mental therapy that relieves a person, as well as his environment, of stress, protects and develops personality, heals, improves thinking, communicates, and liberates in the most beautiful way. The author of these lines, during his six-month training in Tokyo, noticed that the Japanese learn the art of laughing, which is used as a desirable form of communication. All this shows how much the installation of implants in a narrow region of the human body improves the quality of life, manifested by safe and unrestrained laughter. A smile when getting acquainted opens many doors, a smile that reflects discomfort due to a mistake made reduces its severity, while an apologetic smile contributes to and resolves misunderstandings.

Hence the popular saying: "Honey and smiling mouth, and iron doors open!" Finally, a Chinese proverb reads: "A day without laughing is a wasted day!"

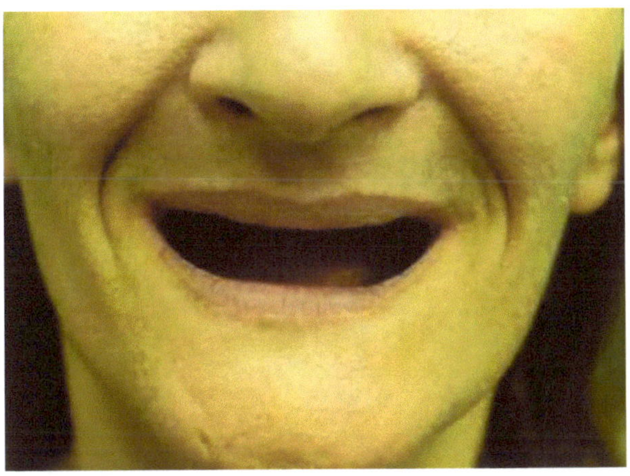

Figure 17.1. A person's emotions color his entire life, internal and psychological, which give tone and meaning to behavior. A person without teeth manifests the sources of emotions in a different way. See the following pictures of the same person who had their lost smile restored.

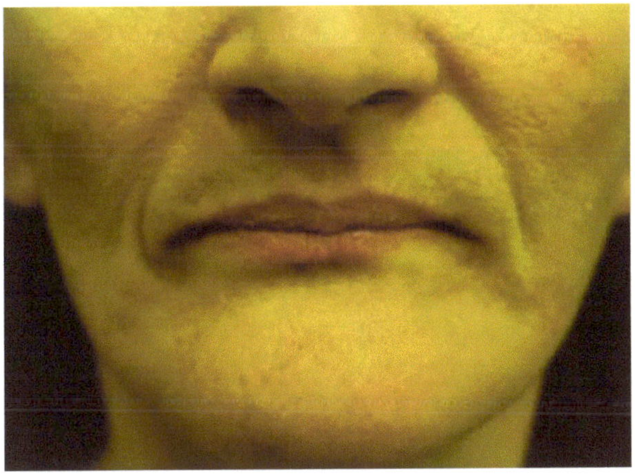

Figure 17.2. The state of mind is expressed on the face. Basic emotions, joy and love, cannot be expressed with the disability of edentulism.

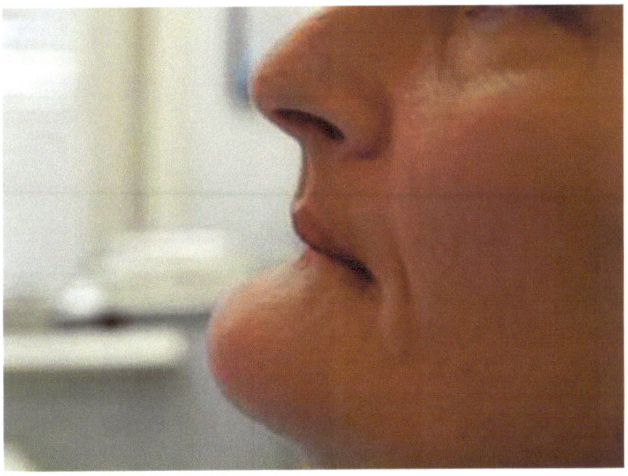

Figure 17.3. Tooth loss changes the interjaw relationships and accentuates the aged appearance of the face. A man is tired if he cannot smile.

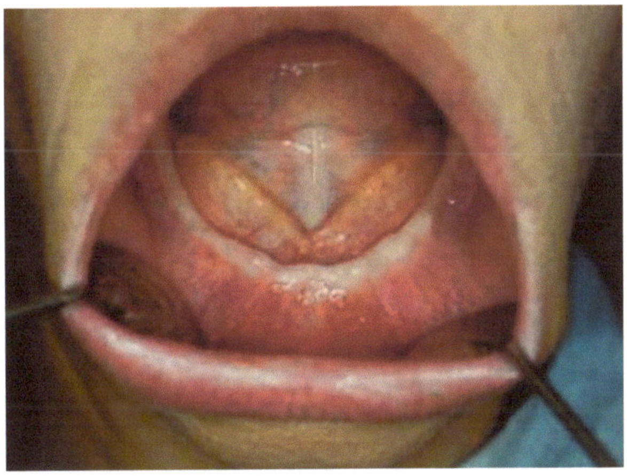

Figure 17.4. A smile starts on the lips, spreads in the eyes. A chuckle comes from the stomach, but a burst of smiles starts from the soul, overflows and makes waves throughout the body. Oral implantology has returned this benefit to toothless people.

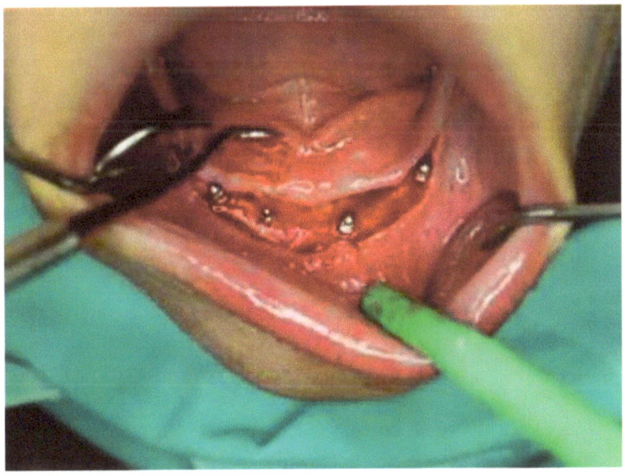

Figure 17.5. Oral implantology made it possible for dentures to be stable in the treatment of total edentulism, increasing the patient's comfort and his safety of function and communication.

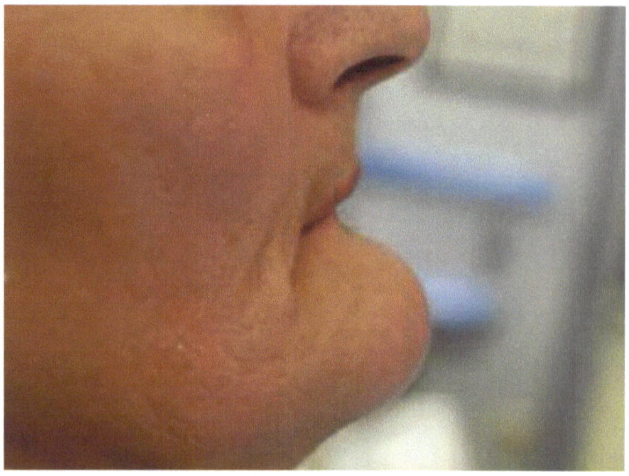

Figure 17.6. A smile increases the face value. A smile makes a person think better of themselves and even if they don't feel like it, it always makes others think better of a beaming face with a smile.

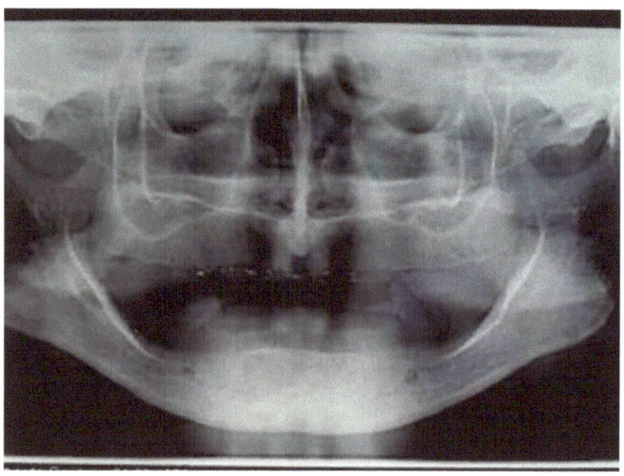

Figure 17.7. "If you have a friend without a smile, give him one." This gift used to not be able to be delivered, because dentists were powerless with such patients.

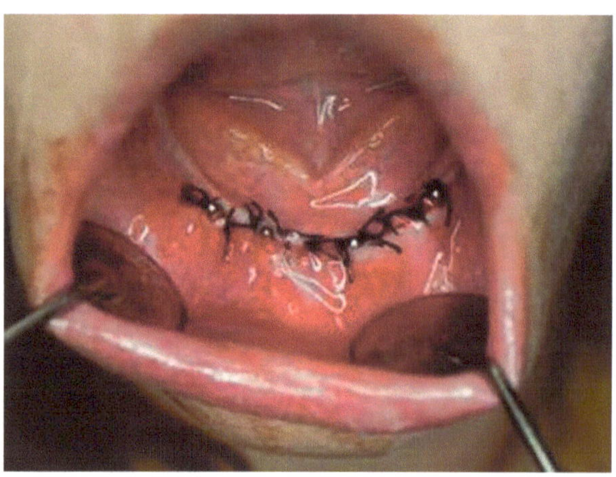

Figure 17.8. Oral implantology restores comfort, confidence and security of communication and the joy of a restored unrestrained smile. Nothing reveals a person's character so powerfully, so powerfully, as laughter. The progress of oral implantology has ensured that the blessing, which among all living beings, is possessed only by man, will not be denied.

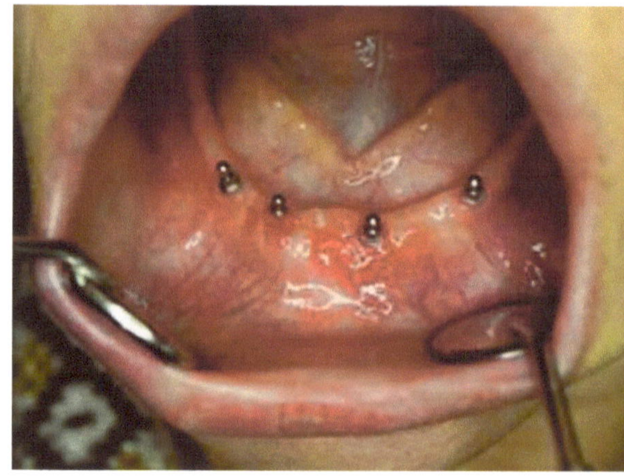

Figure 17.9. Healed soft tissues after 4 weeks

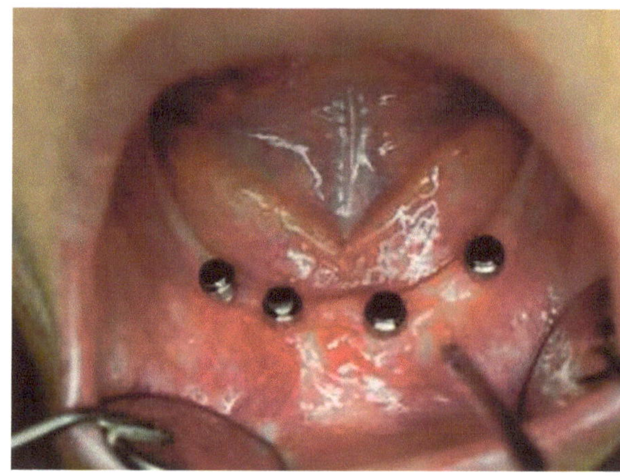

Figure 17.10. Retention swellings on implants enable the functional stability of prostheses in the mouth, and it manifests itself in facial radiance.

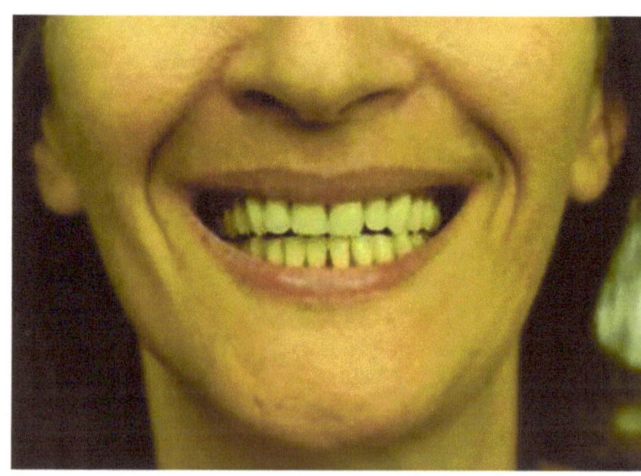

Figure 17.11. A dentist's advice to a patient: "Never stop smiling, because someone may fall in love with your smile."

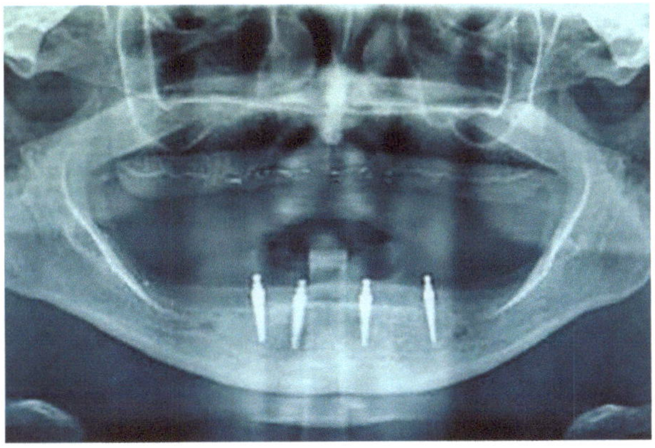

Figure 17.12. Achieved osseous integration of embedded implants that, with retention clips, stabilize the lower total denture, restoring confidence that the denture will not play in the mouth and allowing unrestrained smiling.

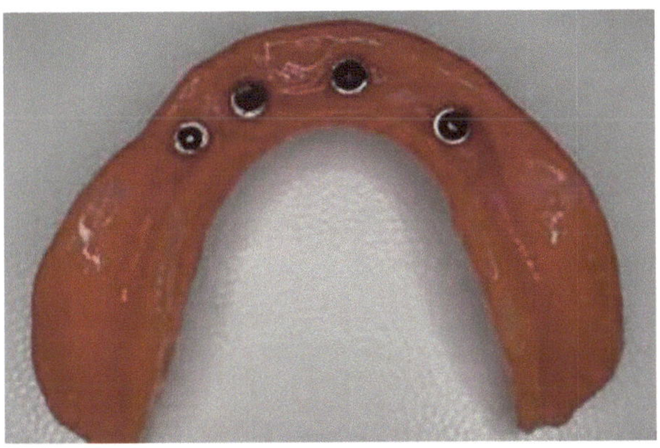

Figure 17.13. Man is a biological being, i.e. a biopsychosocial being, composed of various organs with different structures and different functions. All organs form a structurally functional system. Losing the function of any part of that system violates a person's integrity. Human integrity means an inviolable state of wholeness, ie. the totality of the function. Losing a function like in the oral cavity, man is damaged as a biological being. Oral implantology makes the prosthetic work that replaces the lost organ stable, the damage was compensated by oral implantology.

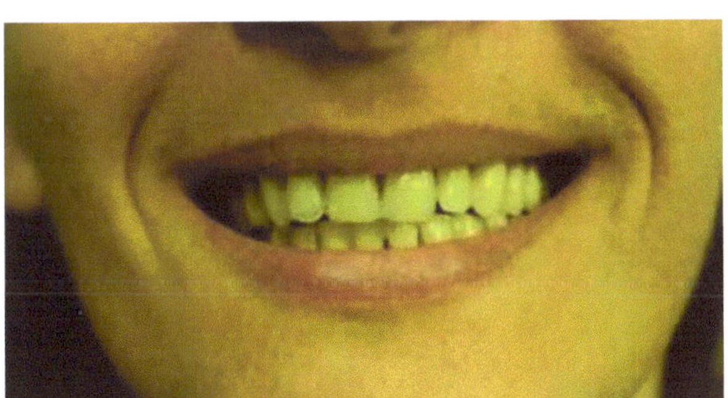

Figure 17.14. A smile costs nothing, but gives a lot. A smile increases the value of every face.

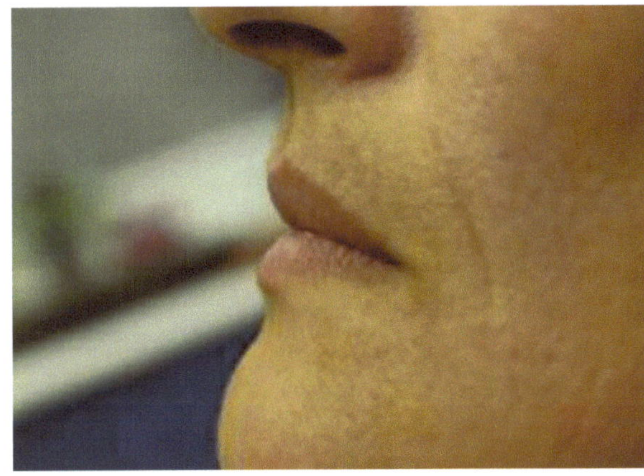

Figure 17.15. A symmetrical face is always a beautiful figure. Restoring the broken harmony of the face is a pleasant feeling. By restoring the function in the oral cavity, the harmony of the face is established. That harmonious relationship is the feeling of a state of objective health.

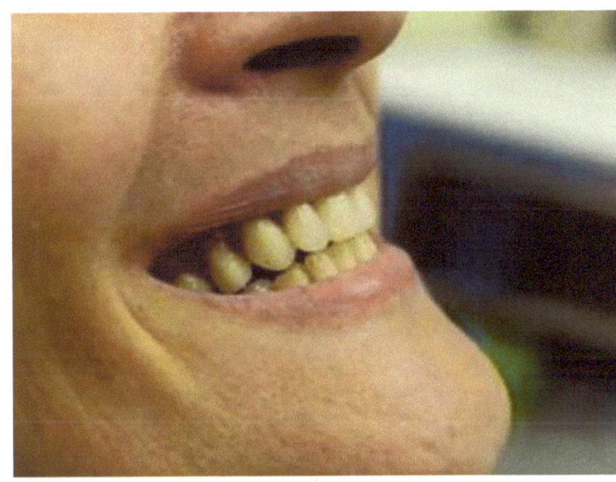

Figure 17.16. A smile enriches those who receive it, not impoverishes those who give it. He who is unable to give smiles is impoverished.

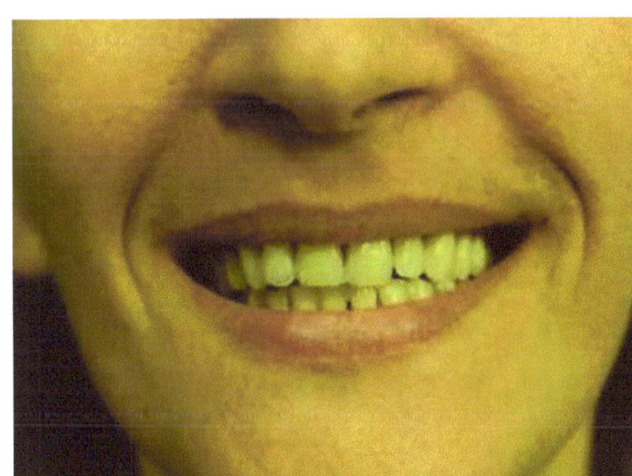

Figure 17.17. Nothing is as powerful and reveals a person's character as powerfully as a smile.

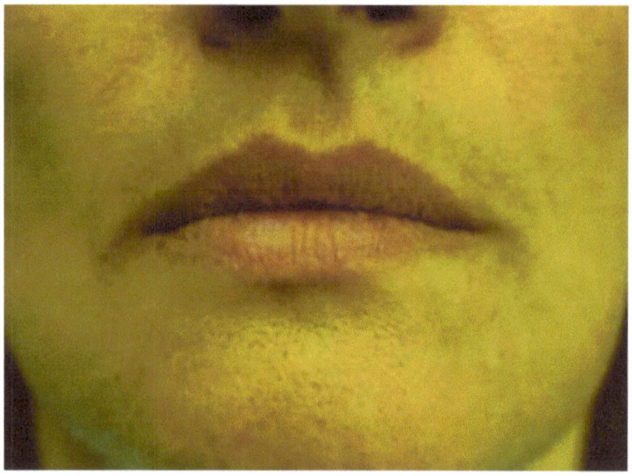

Figure 17.18. There is nothing more beautiful than perfect lips. The perfect harmony of the face, as gifted by nature, is established by prosthetics, and, contrary to nature, by lifting.

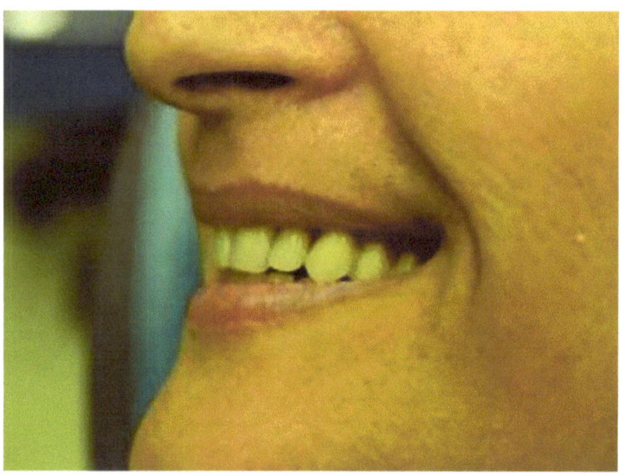

Figure 17.19. Laughter is the only medicine to calm down without negative effects. The state of mind is expressed on the face through a smile.

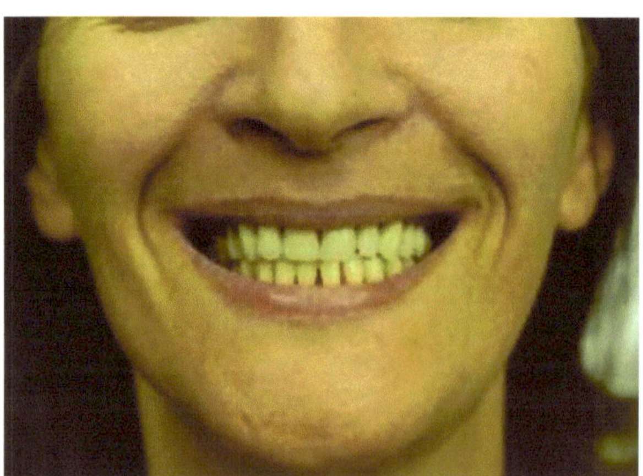

Figure 17.20. There are hundreds of languages in the world, but a smile speaks them all. A warm smile is the universal language of love and a strong bond between people.

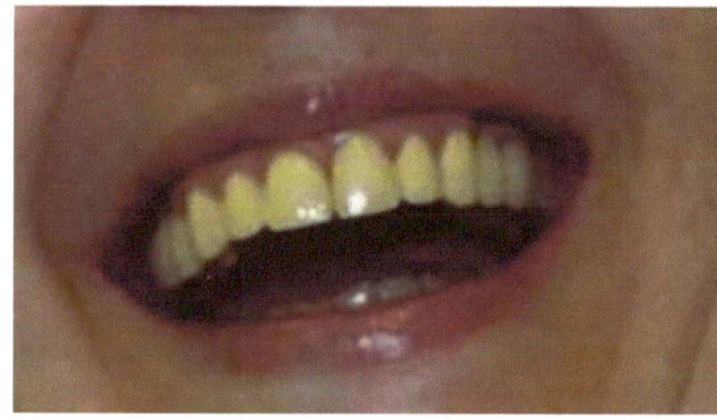

Figure 17.21. The one who knows how to laugh is always stronger than the one who gets angry. A smile only takes a moment, but the memories of it sometimes last forever.

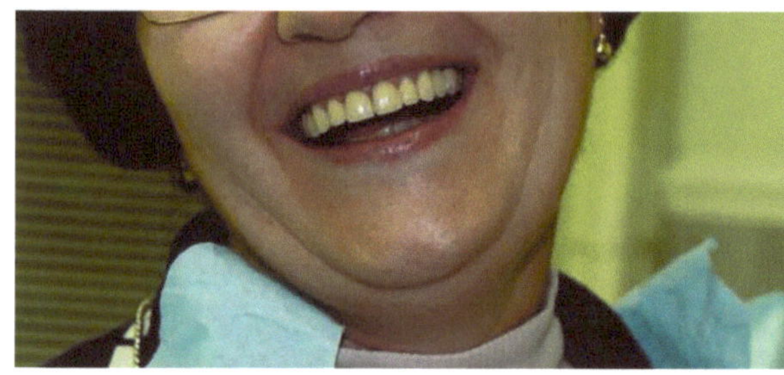

Figure 17.22. There is no face with a smile that is not beautiful. The one who wakes up with a smile, shows the environment all the love of his heart.

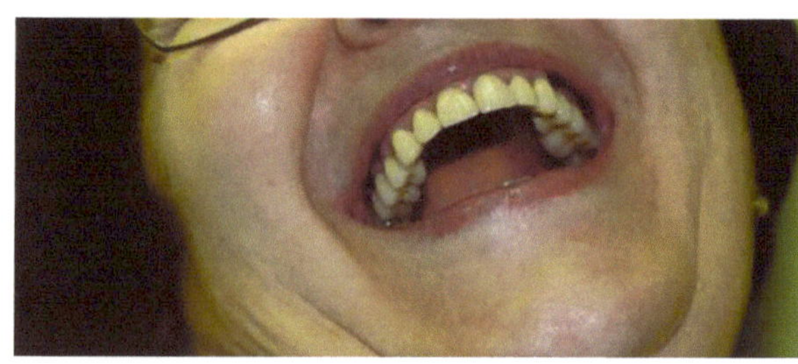

Figure 17.23. The power of modern oral implantology is told in the patient's joyful and witty answer: "I thought I had lost my smile forever. Here it is right under your nose. I forgot it was there!"

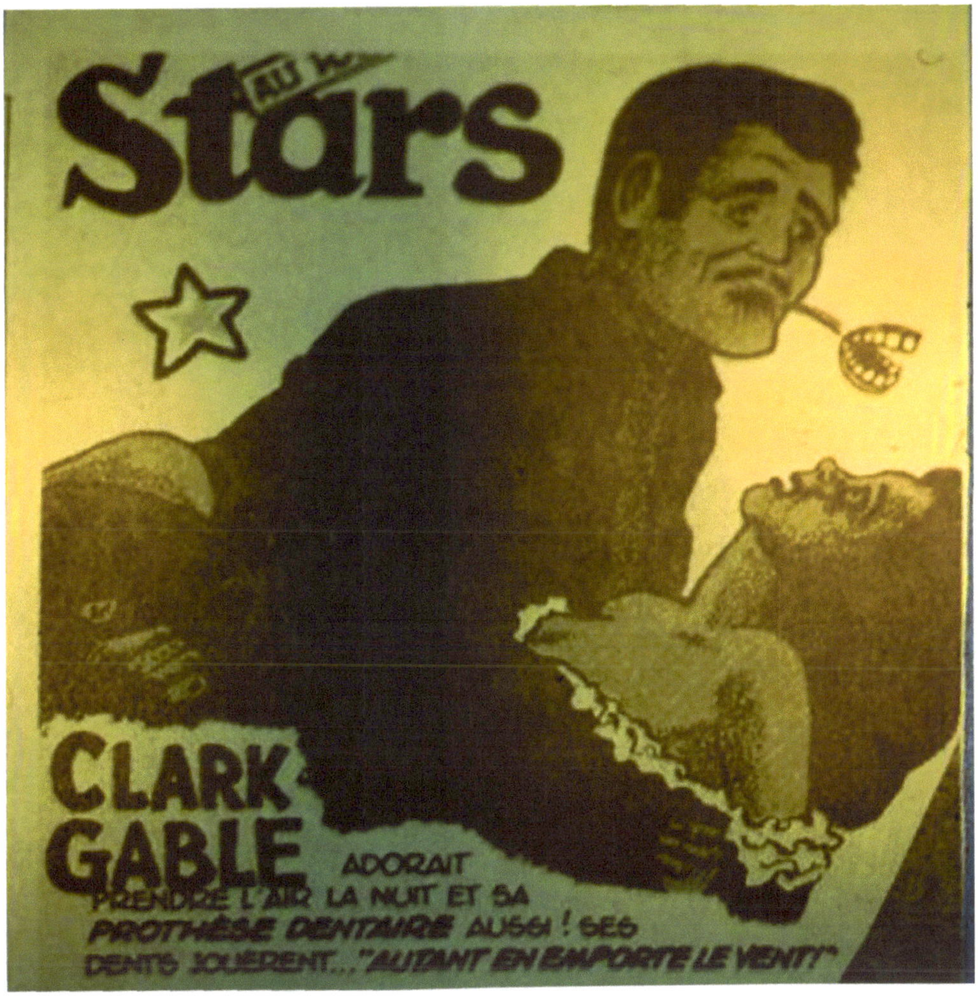
Stars
CLARK GABLE
ADORAIT
PRENDRE L'AIR LA NUIT ET SA
PROTHÈSE DENTAIRE AUSSI ! SES
DENTS JOUÈRENT... "AUTANT EN EMPORTE LE VENT!"

Figure 17.24. Clark Gable liked to wander at midnight, and that wandering was followed by his total prosthesis, it would fly out of his mouth. On the filming of the movie "Gone with the Wind" when he was supposed to kiss Vivian Leigh in one scene, his prosthesis flew out of his mouth and flew away. with a whirlwind. If oral implantology was at today's level, the famous actor would not experience stress.

P.S. WHO MANAGES TO REPLACE A LOST ORGAN TO A MAN AND MAKE LIFE MORE BEAUTIFUL IS DOING A DIVINE WORK.

18

Conversation With A Colleague

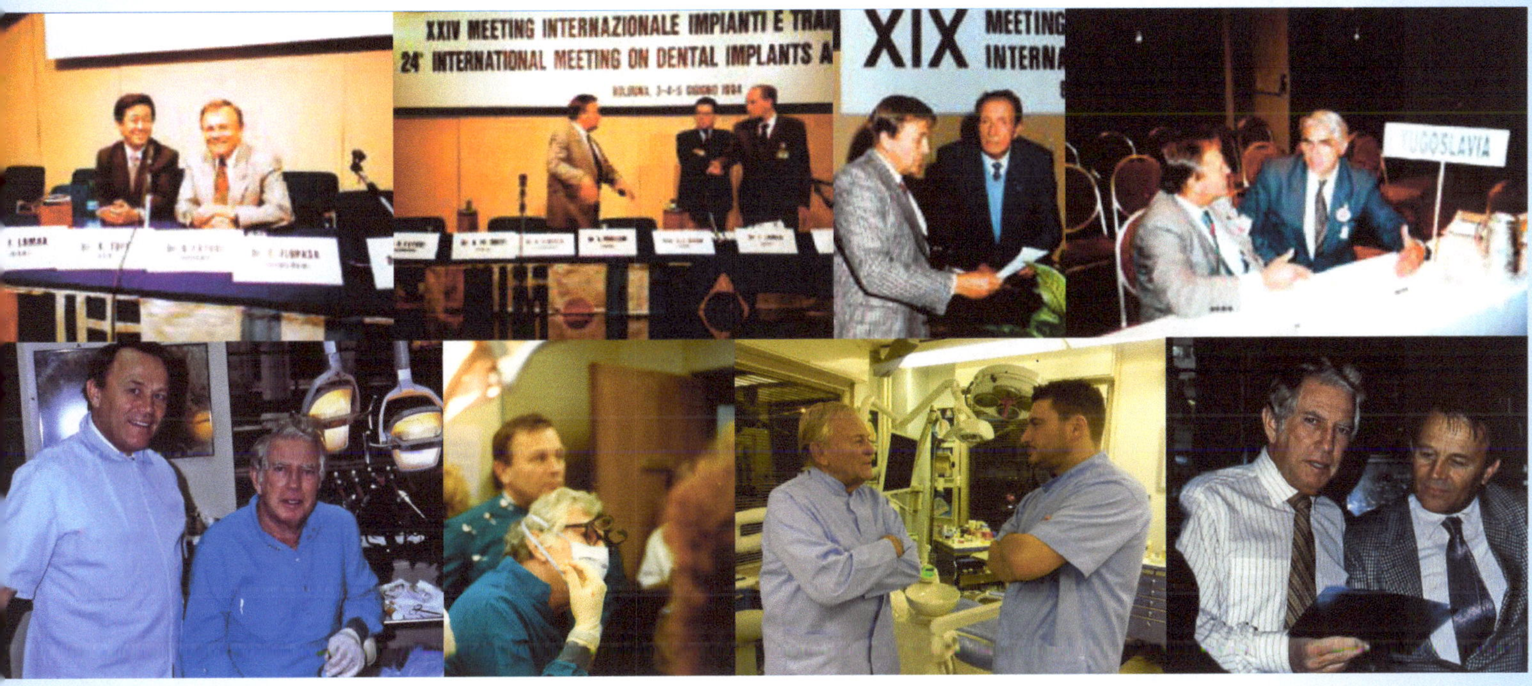

I have designed this chapter to capture the reader's attention without adhering strictly to the order of the questions. It can be seen as the author's inner monologue, set up as a virtual conversation with a colleague who is eager to deepen their understanding of oral implantology. The answers provided stem from my many decades of practice and experience. While many of these answers represent my personal views, I acknowledge that differing opinions are valid. I have aimed to base my responses on scientific evidence. This chapter serves as a recap of content found in other parts of the book. As the Latin saying goes, "Repetitio est mater studiorum" (Repetition is the mother of learning). Many of my answers aim to fill in knowledge gaps, supplemented by more recent findings. It's important to remember that this book is written by a practitioner who shares insights from years of work, moving beyond routine experiences. I have continually refreshed my knowledge, especially in oral implantology. The writing style of this chapter allows the reader to engage with the text in a non-linear manner. Much like the approach taken by Milorad Pavić in "Dictionary of the Khazars," readers can start from the beginning, the end, or anywhere in between—it's all part of a cohesive life-practical whole. I intended for the writing to feel spontaneous, reflective of life itself, with practice being an integral component of that life. I have not shied away from acknowledging my mistakes and have highlighted these admissions in certain answers.

Having dedicated a significant part of my professional life to this matter, I faced a unique challenge in pursuing a path that was uncharted for many at the time. Few understood what this path entailed or even if it truly existed. I encountered intense criticism suggesting that this path was wrong, uncertain, and merely a wandering journey. Now, with the benefit of hindsight, I realize that this path was indeed fraught with unknowns, but rather than succumbing to defeat, I chose to persevere. Courage was the guiding principle that propelled me forward, and this journey continues even today. I acknowledge that, due to many uncertainties, I made mistakes along the way. Truthfully, I wouldn't dare to undertake the same actions today, especially when oral implantology has advanced so significantly. This realization is part of the cost of progress. It's crucial to recognize mistakes and learn from them. Acknowledging errors is vital, as concealing them can be detrimental not only to oneself but also to the patient and the profession as a whole. In your professional journey, it is essential to prioritize understanding your own mistakes to avoid repeating them. Thankfully, thanks to the pioneers of implantology, current generations have a well-established path to follow. However, as in any field of science, a definitive truth is still yet to be reached.

For this chapter, the conclusion would be:
possible questions of the practitioner and answers of the author of the book.

Oral implantology has made great progress. Despite this enormous progress, is implantology still facing great challenges? If so, before whom?

The future has one great quality: it always differs from what we could have predicted (Milorad Pavić). During the writing of this book, I have just completed one chapter, innovations in implantology and new findings, which I did not foresee, confirm the previously stated thought of the Serbian writer. Often, innovation moved at an unexpected speed. New implant systems and new surgical techniques were developed, and widely used implant systems were abandoned, and many of them were placed in the implantological past. The design of the implants changed significantly, the treatment of the implant surface improved, and the knowledge about bone integration deepened more and more. More and more primacy is given to the behavior of soft tissues: preservation and reconstruction of the papilla. Today, function and aesthetics are put on the same level.

I repeatedly revised the content of several chapters because of the continuous advancements in oral implantology. Most books and their new editions are updated regularly to include the latest knowledge. Given the rapid pace of development in this field, I believe that this approach to clarification will be more engaging and relevant for practitioners.

How different is oral implantology today from a few decades ago?

The difference is significant. Implantology is currently the fastest-growing field in dentistry. As a result, it is essential to make considerable efforts to stay updated on new developments. This is particularly important for those seeking to gain adequate knowledge about innovations related to their education or those pursuing further training in the field. It is also crucial for those who aim to organize such education to effectively transfer that knowledge to others, especially students.

The breadth of knowledge in oral implantology has expanded tremendously compared to just a few decades ago. There are two main paths for acquiring knowledge in this area: training and education. Training represents only the first step in understanding the basic technical procedures involved in implantation. Today, various individuals and practices offer training, but many of them lack proper licenses or sufficient experience in oral implantation and complete restoration.

Unfortunately, this situation often arises not from a genuine enthusiasm for the profession, but rather from a focus on profit and the commercialization of the field.

The development of oral implatology requires permanent deepening of knowledge through necessary education, even for those with decades of experience. Education is organized by individuals, often incompetent, but also class associations. It does not matter whether the education will be carried out sporadically and with almost anonymous lecturers or whether this permanent education will be carried out, for example, at Columbia University in New York. At that, one of the most prestigious universities in the world, there is an education program: two-week educations are held three times a year with different programs that follow the latest achievements in oral implantology. In order for the participant to receive a certificate from this University, he must attend all six weeks spread over three times. But it costs money.

In the time, when only individuals began to deal with implantation, how and in what way was knowledge acquired?

When I installed the first implants and started to publish the first results, not a single textbook in the field of oral implantology had been written. There were reports by individuals, and enthusiasts, in magazines or short brochures, mostly about the application of leaf implants. They visited many well-known practitioners, exchanging experiences, attending symposiums and other meetings, and presenting their experiences. It was all about sharing experiences. Literature in the domain of oral implantology was very scarce, and in our country, at that time, no one wrote a single word about implantation.

Today, I can proudly say that back in 1977, at the Dental Week in Petrovac na Moru, I gave the first lecture on the installation of endosseous implants, showing the first patients to whom I installed them. I gave the same lecture a year earlier in Liège (Belgium) at a scientific symposium on transplantation and application of endosseous implants organized by Professor Strel from Liege. At all those meetings dedicated to oral implantology, the lecturers were enthusiastic. Only one name jumped out of the list of almost anonymous people at the time, and that was Leonard Linkov from New York, at that time synonymous with oral implantology in the world. His lectures were always at the end, they would last several hours. The halls were always filled. It was a great honor and pleasure for me that even at that time my name was often included among those lecturers.

How was it accepted on both sides?

In our country, the ferocity of the attack on the idea of implantation, and its challenges, could not have been greater and more frequent. However, in Liège (scientific symposium in 1976) after the same reflective lecture, the atmosphere was completely different. Since then, I regularly received invitations for many foreign symposia and congresses. With us, the situation was the opposite, I had to impose myself.

Is this book also written in an unusual way?

It can be seen from the attached that it is. My intention in this book was to approach the material from oral implantology in a way that is not common in textbooks, to have experience as a guide in thinking about problems, questions, and answers. To some questions in oral implantology, we still do not have definitive answers and clear positions. At least the kind that practice expects from science. The methodology of writing textbooks is special, because books, as a rule, are full of theory and assertions, while there are no questions, dilemmas, and thoughts of the author based on his own experience. For example, whether a problem could have been solved in one way or another. Proven facts are confirmed in textbooks. Similar considerations will not be missing in this book either, but expressed in a way that will be useful to the practitioner. A smart person not only learns from his own experience but also uses the experience of others and draws conclusions based on that. Probably, those who write university textbooks in oral surgery, and who consider the material in oral implantology, will say that some chapters do not belong in this field. However, experience and practice, for example, have shown that prosthetic restoration is an integral part of implant placement. Based on this belief, I treated those chapters with special attention. My approach to that area is multidisciplinary because it is a professional necessity today. After all, I find encouragement in the thought expressed long ago that no book is so bad that it would not be useful at least partially!

Is good theoretical knowledge the foundation of practice?

True, theoretical knowledge is extremely important for a practitioner to be successful in everyday practice. But you should know that theory is easy to learn by reading, and practice and routine are much harder and longer to acquire through work, and experience is the longest, most difficult, most expensive, and often the most painful. But good theory comes only from good practice, and oral implantology is a concrete and practical science.

The experience expressed in the written word must come from proven practical knowledge, which confirms the fact that the best is the knowledge gained by working alongside good teachers and great masters. Real knowledge is not only in the knowledge of theoretical facts, but in the art of using them, that is. with the possibility to perform and realize them yourself.

How did the author's thoughts and attitudes differ from the attitudes of many dentists in the early seventies of the last century who were persistent in challenging the methods of application and justification of implantation?

The attempts, thoughts, attitudes, and courage of the enthusiasts, the pioneers of implantology, were attacked and contested from the very beginning. And to take a new step, to say a new word, that is something that people are most afraid of, wrote the Russian classic Dostoyevsky.

Following this thought, that new step more than four decades ago, was oral implantology, and the new word - "foreign body" in healthy and living bone, which dentists were most afraid of, and they transferred their attitudes to patients, fearing and even more of them. Knowledge is true knowledge only when it is acquired through the effort of one's own thought and verified and confirmed by practice. The profession teaches only those who are constantly tested through practice. I often knew how to spice up my approach to the profession with philosophical thoughts. Life is short, and one's profession is even shorter. But the trace of a person's life and what he did can last a long time

What answers did those who challenged you give to patients interested in implantation?

When asked the questions: "Doctor, what do you think about 'tooth implants' and who can do it and where can I do it?", they would get scary answers:

"By no means! do not allow them to insert a foreign body into your jawbone, which can cause cancer!" Even some authorities from the profession published their ignorance about implantation in newspapers, and weekly and monthly reviews. It was not easy to challenge the majority opinion.

In what way could such attitudes, fierce attacks and challenges be countered?

Lessons can still be drawn from the responses at the time. Back then, I spoke more at foreign gatherings and showed what others kept silent about. Presentations were accepted with understanding. The same lectures in our country are followed by fierce attacks and disputes. I considered it my duty, and I still consider it today, that showing failures did not diminish the contribution to the development of implantology and the professional reputation of those who did not keep their failures silent. On the contrary.

We should not forget the fact that many scientists have invested a lot of effort experimenting on animals, but when it comes to oral implantology, the most "fruits have been harvested" with interventions on humans.

Colleagues remember your confrontation and defense. How did you do it?

The resistance arose because most dentists, at that time, did not know the basic concepts of installing implants and their current scope. On the other hand, they did not even have a vision of the profession. Resistances stemmed from routine complacency and complacency with daily practice. The stagnation of the individual and the profession is caused by the desire to maintain routine, outmoded understandings and stubborn beliefs, contrary to progress.

It should be remembered that Plato (427-347 BC) wrote about the problem of the world's inability to accept that new knowledge that can shake the entrenched conviction of the majority. The reluctance and exclusivity of the majority to significantly expand their horizons is the main brake on the progress of the profession. Not only a brake on the development of the profession, but also of humanity.

The absolute exclusivity in the understanding of what oral implantology offers resulted from the wrong and at the time unacceptable attitude for the majority that it is a "foreign body" in the body, i.e. in living bone.

Human history is full of examples where the majority disagreed with some of the scientific truths, and those who stood for the scientific truth paid dearly for it (Giordano Bruno). Therefore, the polemic at the professional level could not be conducted at the professional level due to the misunderstanding of the majority, but I tried to let the majority know, with witty jokes, that what I advocate has a future.

Humorously, I cited examples that indicated to the dentists present a misunderstanding of progress. For example, when the first railway appeared in France, the first to warn of the dangers of using this means of transport were French gynecologists, they announced a public proclamation and a warning: that pregnant women should be prohibited from using this new technique, because at "fantastic" speeds of 30 km. mass abortions per hour. Today we laugh at such remarks. Then it wasn't like that.

The Serbian doctors did not go any further either. The first electrical switchboard and lamps in Belgrade were made by one Joca Šapčanin. The Belgrade ophthalmologists, professors of the University of Belgrade, were the first to speak out with a public warning to the citizens of Belgrade: that if they use this monstrous light for more than one hour, they will experience massive damage to their eyesight. And we laugh at this remark of the ophthalmologists of the time. But now, not then!

Following the then understanding, sexologists, also professors of the University of Belgrade, spoke out, claiming that such light would change the romance and sexual life of the citizens of Belgrade.

I responded in the same way to the cruelty that happened at the Congress of Dentists of Yugoslavia in Vrnjačka Banja, when I had to interrupt the lecture by turning off the lights in the hall: "The coachman needs to see well, because even with blind horses and oxen he will reach the goal !"

What has had the greatest impact on changing the understanding of the pioneers of oral implantology that the sole goal of implant placement is to establish function?

Time and the development of science caused changes in the understanding that chewing function can be significantly improved by installing implants and that this is the primary requirement of oral implantology. The dynamics of development also influenced the change of attitudes, which the author himself once advocated, that oral implantology primarily stemmed from the functional requirements for a person to be able to chew food. I would support such an understanding by the fact that tooth extraction is not the motivation of science, but the motivation of removing pain: "Sedare dolorum, divinum opus est!" "Relieving pain is a divine work! (Hippocrates).

Based on that logic, at that time, the opinion was advocated that the establishment of the chewing function justified the installation of the implant.

It is an undeniable truth that the laws of nature are the strongest. Oral implantology emerged from this legality. Man sought to compensate for the lost gift of nature to the teeth and to restore the masticatory harmony he had with the natural teeth. That law, the requirement of life, was first recognized and accepted by enthusiasts, not by science. The movement of enthusiasts, pioneers of oral implantology, started from the periphery, not from large scientific centers. Enthusiasts from large centers, everywhere in the world, were on the margins of the university and scientific institutions, because their doors were then closed to them. A high-raised head makes it impossible for a person to see where he is going.

Is the situation reversed today regarding the support and acceptance of oral implantology by science?

The door to modern oral implantology is wide open at all universities in the world. This is its greatness and power because the places where pioneers and enthusiasts performed implantations could not provide scientific support. The vision of the development of the profession cannot be disputed by the pioneers of oral implantology. Scientific centers had to accept it as a logic derived from the laws and requirements of life. Those demands of life were first imposed on science by enthusiasts. To start and finish something, you always need a bit of enthusiasm, wrote Walter.

In which direction will oral implantology move further?

Oral implantology continues to move in the direction of innovation, whereby, as was the case in the recent past, two directions of development dominate:

The first will be aimed at improving the integration of hard and soft tissues, assisted by implant-supported prosthetic work. We should expect constant improvements in the processing of the implant surface, and as for the improvement of the implant design, we should not expect much, but in the improvement of the design details, yes.

Also, there is a constant effort to search for a new generation of materials that will result in better and faster bone regeneration. In this context, zircon is being considered as an alternative material for titanium, both from an aesthetic point of view and in terms of the durability of the embedded implant in the bone. Considerations of zirconium are gaining importance due to its positive impact on periointegration. From the available literature, one gets the impression that all well-known implant manufacturers and research teams, in their future product programs, are looking for metal-free implant design solutions.

However, the fact that the search for such solutions is largely motivated by marketing interests must also be taken into account. For example, zirconium as a material in implantology has not yet met all the high requirements.

The second direction of development, namely, contains the idea of connecting surgery and prosthetics from the finalization-technological aspect, to offer complete dental solutions within which the implant is, in the last case, only one segment on the way to achieving overall harmony of the face, in other words, a beautiful smile with beautiful teeth.

Who should take the central role?

The central role in these concepts is played by navigation systems of the latest generation, which enable the dentist to plan and precisely position the implants, so that the prosthetic treatment and the surgical procedure can be performed in one act.

In which direction will new technological innovations and opportunities lead oral implantology?

The question posed also opens certain dilemmas. Do newly created and offered clinical and technological possibilities have to be encouraged to such a great extent until time confirms it, that is, until practice puts it in its place? Oral implantology is not immune from the goals created by large multinational pharmaceutical corporations, which put the primacy of profitability before science. In many novelties, there are a lot of such phenomena that the profit of the company is more primary and faster than the latest scientific knowledge. For example, the bone substitute market expands its offerings, and it happens that, after a certain time, that bone substitute turns out to be a failure. The offer extends the indications for the application of the manufacturer's product, even when there is no justification for it.

Also, significant questions and dilemmas arise as to which is better: to experiment with marketing offers or to work as experience directs.

In case of extreme atrophy, what solution is possible? Should augmentation be performed and in what way, if it is not possible to install implants, what is the best solution, especially from a functional point of view?

It is likely that, despite the innovations of many implant systems, there will not be an "optimal solution" for all indications in the future, and that there will still be many individual factors that determine the optimal solution, especially for each individual patient.

What conditions should be met in order to recognize the optimal solution at the beginning?

To find the optimal solution, the existence of many limiting factors must be taken into account, first of all anatomical, but also other, equally important limiting factors from the patient himself, such as: time, special requirements, unrealistic expectations, physical load possibilities and psychological aspects, as well as financial resources. All limiting factors should be constantly in the focus of the dentist's attention.

For example, in the case shown in Figure 18.1, where there is extensive bone loss, the question arises, even for the most experienced clinician, what is the optimal solution!? In the past, in the case of almost insurmountable restrictions in the lower jaw, the use of subperiosteal implants was resorted to. Even today, despite the development of science in the wide range of bone substitute materials and the application of the PRF method (Platelet-Rich-Fibrin-fibrin rich in platelets), it represents an insurmountable obstacle for the installation of implants, even those as carriers of retention clips for stabilizing a total acrylic prosthesis. Sometimes you can resort to augmentation, which is a long-term procedure and always with the risk of failure, and in some cases, it is absolutely not possible.

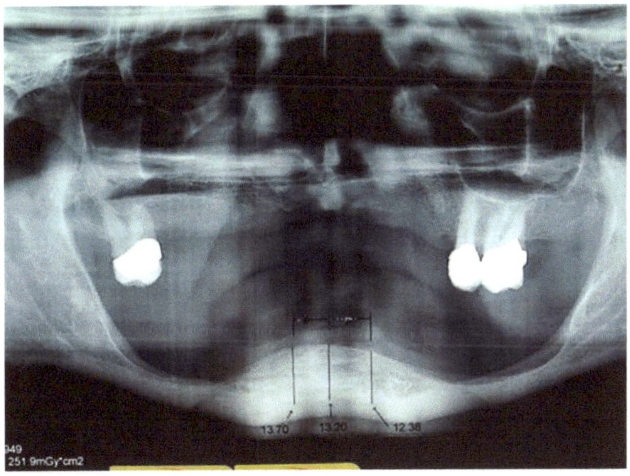

Figure 18.1. Extreme atrophy of the jaw bone in both jaws, often an insurmountable obstacle for implant placement. Augmentation created the conditions for the installation of implants and the application of retention clips. (see fig. 18.5)

What is the basis of success in oral implantation and what principles must be followed in order to achieve success?

For the prediction of success, we can thank the accelerated and great scientific progress of oral implantology. Thinking about the time when the pioneers of implantology, forty or more years ago, were installing implants (to which the author of the book belongs), success could not be predicted. However, the works of the pioneer enthusiasts were not in vain. They forced science to take oral implantology seriously, recognizing its future.

Today, the success of implantation can be predicted. That success is 97-98%, but only with strict adherence to certain principles. The failure rate has been reduced to between 2-4%.

Which principles?

Anamnesis: Anamnesis is the basis and the most important part of the diagnostic procedure. Based on a good anamnesis, an accurate diagnosis can be made and appropriate predictions can be made. First, the causes of disability in the oral cavity caused by tooth loss should be examined in detail.

Bone assessment: assess the quantity and quality of bone in the upper and lower jaw. After that, decide whether there are conditions for successful implantation. Correct assessment of bone quantity and quality is of great importance for the long-term survival of bone implants. Good primary implant stability can only be achieved in good bone.

Intraoral examination and general evaluation of the condition of the mouth: to determine whether there is any soft tissue disease caused by immune or other disorders or poor oral hygiene, excessive mobility of the soft tissue in the upper jaw on the alveolar ridges caused by long-term wearing of a total prosthesis, the so-called fibrous ridge, and Fig. (number and arrangement of remaining teeth, periodontal status).

Radiological assessment: Perform detailed X-ray and tomographic analyses of the bone quality and quantity, possible anatomical limitations, and present pathological changes (residual roots, cysts, etc.). Computer tomography made it easier to determine the position for implant placement. Computed tomography, in contrast to standard radiographic orthopantomography images, provides an accurate and clear examination of the residual bone in all three planes.

Surgery: the surgical procedure must be performed according to all operating procedures (surgeon, assistant, instruments, the environment in which the procedure is performed, etc.). It must be minimally invasive for all tissues, strictly following the protocol prescribed by science. New techniques increasingly simplify the implantation phase and significantly reduce trauma to the bone.

Materials: implants of high standard and quality, which have a guarantee of safety of titanium quality, as confirmed by scientific research and official certificates.

Prosthetic rehabilitation: type of prosthetic works, materials from which they are made, etc.

Control examinations: persistently invite the patient to periodic control examinations. Most often, the patient's failure to report after the treatment is a big problem for many implantologists, because patients who are satisfied (which can be apparent, because the patient does not notice any changes in time) usually do not come for periodic check-ups.

Experience of the dentist: the dentist's experience is one of the conditions for success. The greater the experience, the closer we are to a positive outcome. Only a dentist with extensive experience can predict the outcome, and even that is not always the case!

What is the total percentage of lost implants today and are there any statistical data?

Modern implantology has significantly reduced the number of failed implants. For example, according to data from the literature, more than 100,000 implants are installed annually in Germany alone. Failures happen, but that's the definition of risk! The most common causes of failure are unfavorable anatomical factors: lack of a sufficient amount of bone where the primary stability of the implant was not and could not be achieved. Primary stability can be compromised in cases where there is enough bone, but it is of poor quality (D4). There are no official valid statistical data, but that percentage probably ranges between 2-4%.

Where to look for the causes of implant loss?

The causes of implant loss can be found in: surgical error, poor and unprofessional planning, poor prosthetic work with poorly established occlusion, as well as poor oral hygiene, the negative effect of which is enhanced by excessive smoking. Due to excessive smoking, the healing process of soft tissues is slowed down and of poor quality. It should be emphasized to the patient that excessive smoking is a major risk factor when it comes to overall health, and excessive smoking with poor oral hygiene will result in peri-implant complications and compromise the entire implant-prosthetic treatment.

Why do many dentists, rightly, avoid placing implants in heavy smokers?

Such smokers are often called chronic smokers. Experienced implantologists not only avoid avid smokers from implanting implants, but even refuse such patients because they do not want to accept risk. The healing of soft tissues in heavy smokers is very slow, and most often, it is also compromised. However, today it is considered that after the period of healing and formation of soft tissues, it is allowed to smoke up to ten cigarettes a day.

To avoid risk, what is the first step?

The team must be a well-coordinated team that knows in which order a part of the available instrumentation should be applied, and the instrument technician must adjust the number of revolutions of the drill for bone preparation as required by the doctor. Cooling with physiological solution must be permanent and plentiful. If the principles from the previous answer are followed, the percentage of failure is negligible, ranging between 2-4%.

What should be done to reduce that percentage to a minimum?

To reduce the percentage of failure to a minimum, when the protocol procedures are followed, only the highest quality implants should be applied, which are made with the highest quality technology according to all world standards, backed by scientific research with a certificate confirmed by science.

Should the implant be moistened with saline before insertion?

No! When removing from the original packaging, the part of the implant that enters the bone must not be touched even with sterile surgical gloves. The first contact of the implant surface should be with blood, and a coagulum will form around it (Figures 18.2 and 18.3).

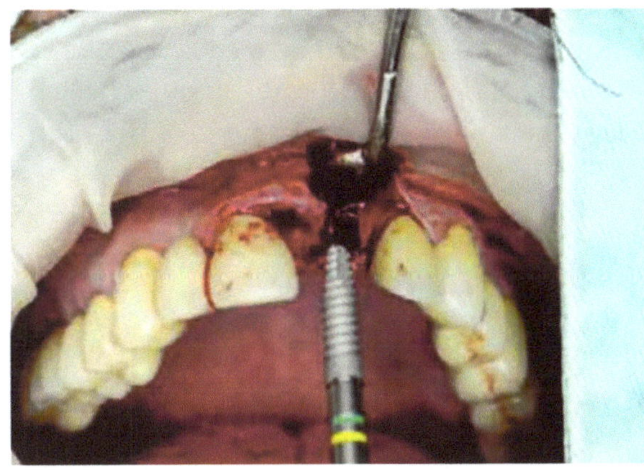

Figure 18.2. Installation after tooth extraction. The diameter of the implant must be wider than the diameter of the root and preservation of the alveolus.

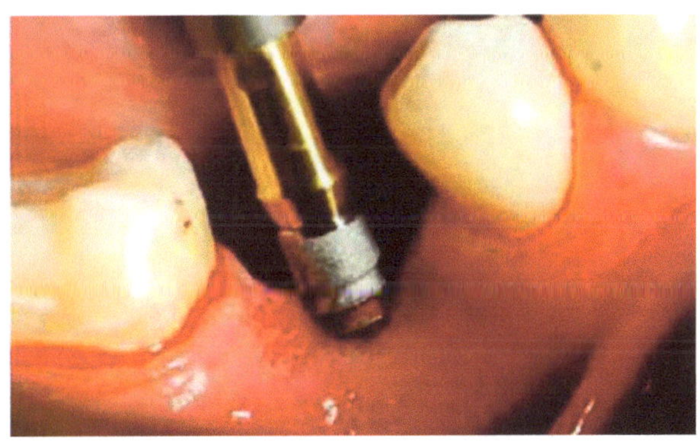

Figure 18.3. The surface of the implant must not be touched with gloves and wetted with saline solution. The first contact must be with blood.

How much does price affect the type of procedure?

Unfortunately, money sometimes determines the type of procedure. Due to the financial situation, we often reach the limit of what is possible. The patient's ability to pay often makes it impossible to realize the planned plan in the best way. However, this does not mean that the implant procedure should be abandoned, which can be achieved with another solution; by choosing the number of implants and a more appropriate prosthetic solution that is adapted to the financial power of the patient (Figure 18.4). The therapist must also anticipate that the chosen solution will justify the effort invested.

The biggest and most useful guarantee of success for the patient is when the implantologist knows what not to do in a specific case, especially if he has the support of the patient as a financier on the one hand and as a collaborator during treatment on the other hand.

Embarking on an "adventure" with unforeseen success is a big risk. However, we should not forget that non-compliance with the agreement by the patient can also be one of the causes of risk.

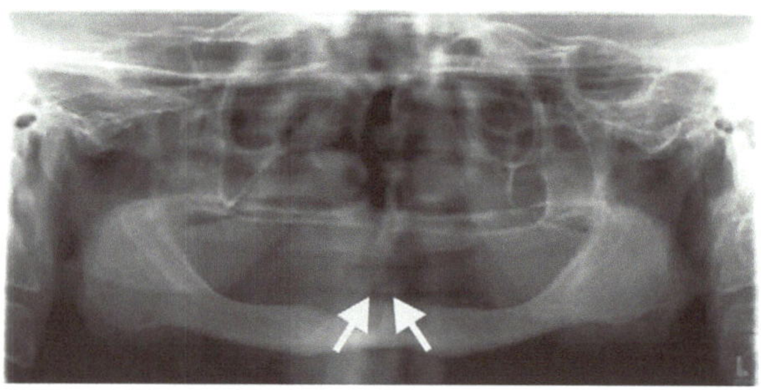

Figure 18.4. Example of a problem case. The solution is reduced to an attempt to increase the volume (indicated by arrows) of the bone by augmentation with an autologous bone block, bone substitutes and the PRF method for the installation of two implants with retention clips.

How much can age and money affect the possibility of implantation?

Today, age is no longer a contraindication. Healing in late life can only be slowed down. What healing will be and for how long, depends on the immunobiological status and the reparable power of organisms. Old age can carry a risk due to the general condition of the organism and contraindications due to some diseases.

When it comes to money and the patient's financial situation, the limit of what is possible is often reached. The question of money is not a shame, nor does it condition the abandonment of the implantology request. In a conversation with the patient, you should find out what his available funds are and, accordingly, plan the method of implantology-prosthetic rehabilitation. Implantation costs depend on the price of the implant itself and its secondary parts. Costs can also be affected by the need for bone and soft tissue augmentation. Therefore, the role of money in the indication of implantological-prosthetic treatment cannot be avoided.

Does it often happen that the limiting factors are so pronounced that they are insurmountable even for a more experienced implantologist, especially with classic prosthetics?

Yes. The following pictures (pictures 18.5-18.7) show the failures of attempts (in the past) to solve total edentulism by inserting subperiosteal implants.

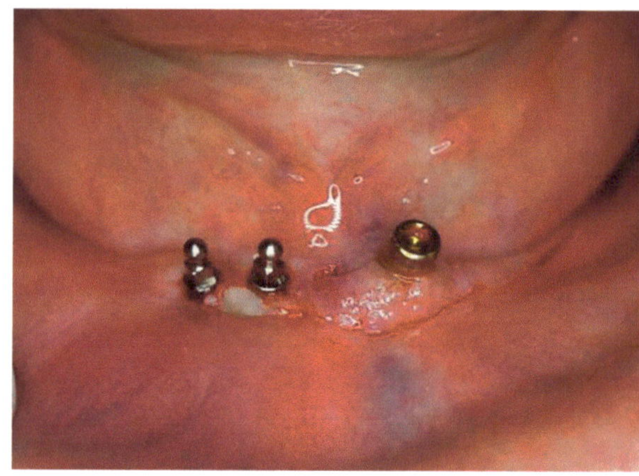

Figure 18.5. Installation of the implant in the augmented region (see Figure 18.1).

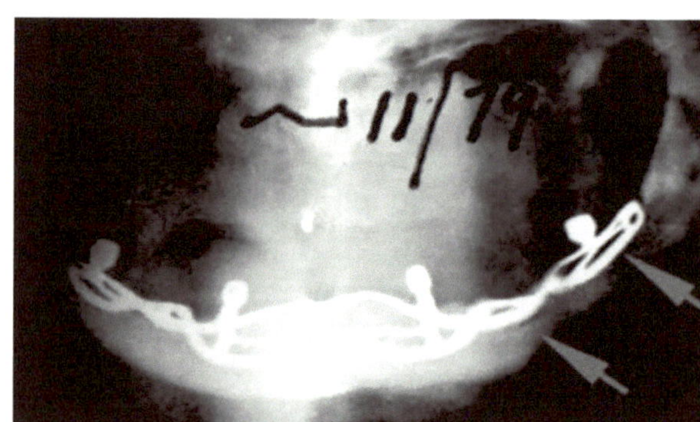

Figure 18.6. An attempt to solve extreme atrophy of the mandible. Bone destruction on the left side caused by the uneven fit of the structure.

Today, a case like this (Figure 18.6) would probably be solved by endosseous implantation in the frontal part of the lower jaw and retention clips, but still with a risk and an uncertain outcome. In the cases shown, it can be stated how scarce radiographic analysis was in the precise marking of anatomical structures.

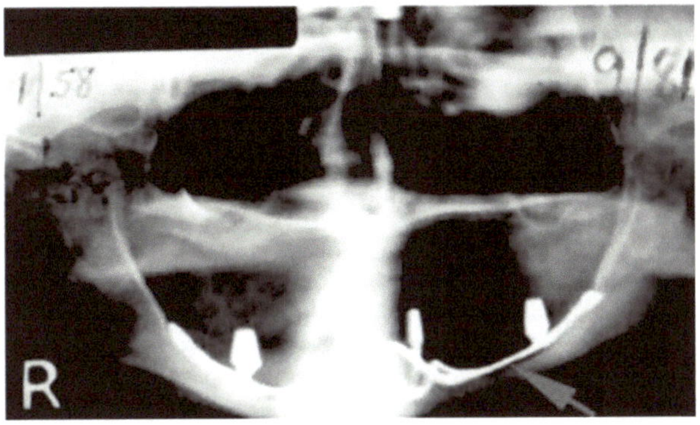

Figure 18.7. What solution could be sought for the presented case even today? Oral implantology still has limits of power then and now!

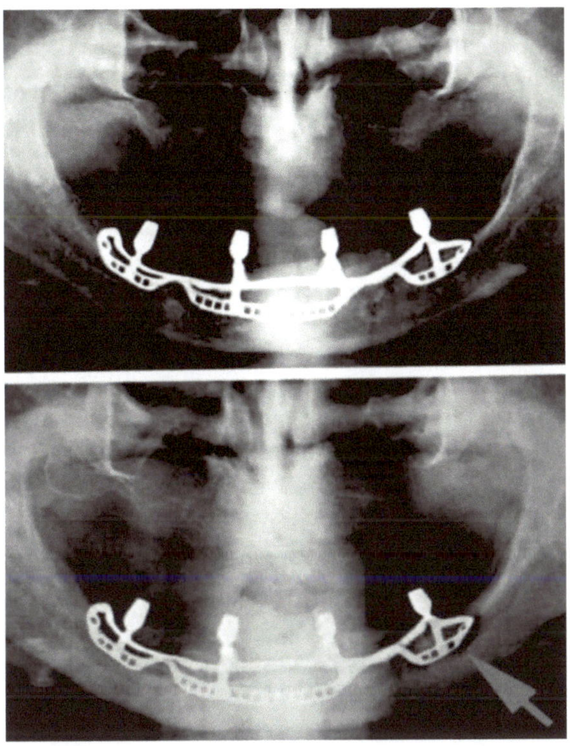

Figure 18.8. Bone destruction by a subperiosteal implant in the lower jaw on X-rays indicated by red arrows.

True, even with the implants we have today, many cases would be solved far more successfully, but not all. However, there are limits to our power. The presented cases are attempts to solve complicated situations when oral implantology did not have today's reach.

Are there any intractable cases for implantation today, and have you recently had a case that could not be treated implantologically?

Despite the great and accelerated progress of oral implantology, there are limits to its power. This is exactly the case of the patient shown in Figure 18.8, with extreme alveolar bone atrophy. Such cases for the dentist represent a special challenge for the lower total prosthesis. Thinking about trying augmentation to increase the horizontal and vertical dimensions of the alveolar bone would probably result in just trying. The loss of alveolar bone in the upper jaw was also extreme, so taking a local autologous bone graft was impossible. The application of extensive surgical interventions, bone removal (from the hip, skull, ribs), for several reasons, was also unfeasible.

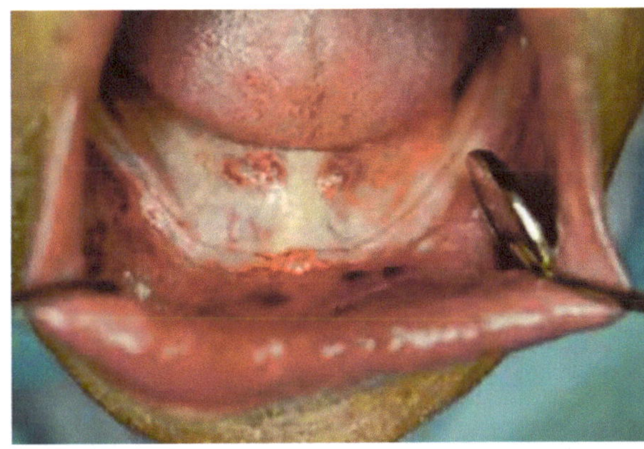

Figure 18.9. A typical example of high risk for implant placement: narrow alveolar ridge, proximity to unfavorable anatomical structures (mandibular canal). Special caution in the position of a sublingualis. Solving a similar case as in Figure 18.4 (work of the author).

After increasing the horizontal and vertical dimensions of the alveolar bone in the front region of the lower jaw, two implants with wider diameters were implanted, and in the distal region it was possible to implant an implant with the narrowest diameter, which was done, but ended in failure (Figure 18.12.)

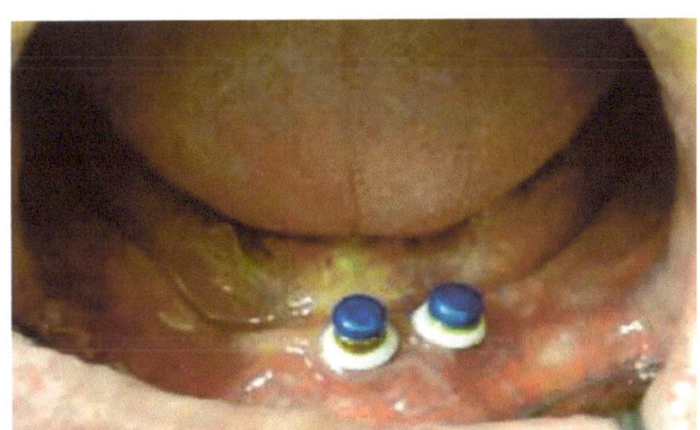

Figure 18.10. The augmentation created the conditions for the installation of two implants with wide diameters, which compensates for the insufficient vertical dimension of the bone. This type of retention clips is less retentive than clips with screw heads (O-ball abutments implant). It is necessary to change Teflon rings (white color) more often.

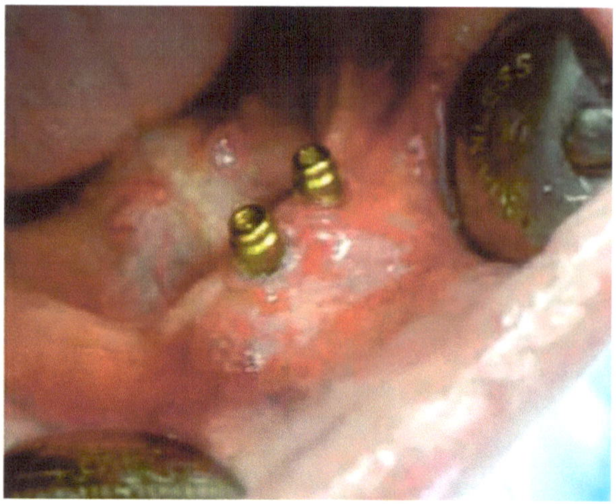

Figure 18.11. The location of the available bone increased by augmentation allowed the installation of two implants with larger diameters. Presentation of the situation after 3 years.

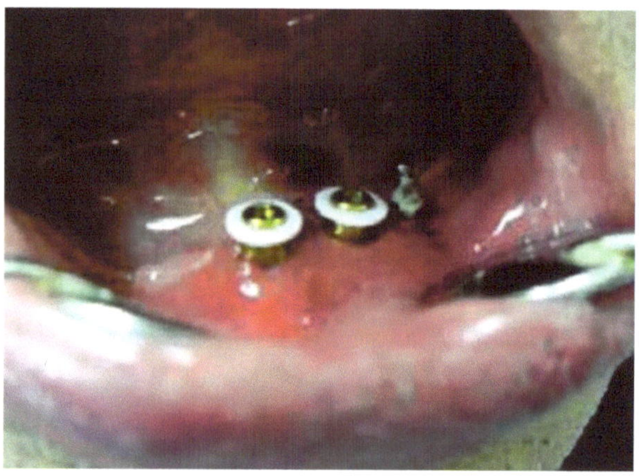

Figure 18.12. Due to weakened retention, one implant of a narrow diameter with a spherical head was added. Teflon retention rings (white in color) worn out over time must be replaced. After 4 years from the installation of two implants with larger diameters, a narrow-diameter implant with a spherical head was installed. Due to plaque deposition and peri-implant inflammation, it was removed.

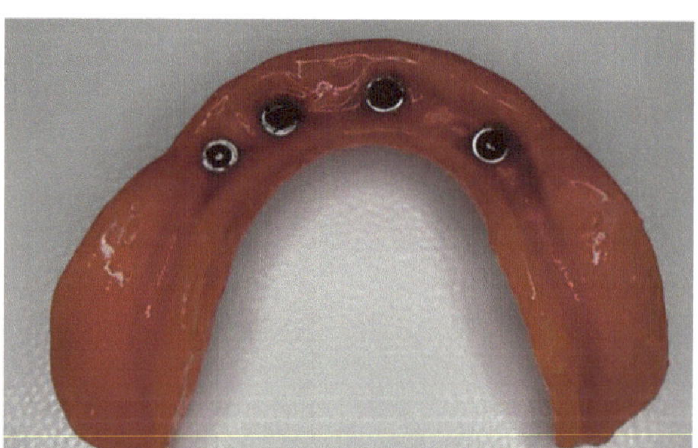

Figure 18.13. The installation of retention caps can be performed in the existing total prosthesis, with an exchangeable base in soft acrylate, which significantly increases the comfort for the patient.

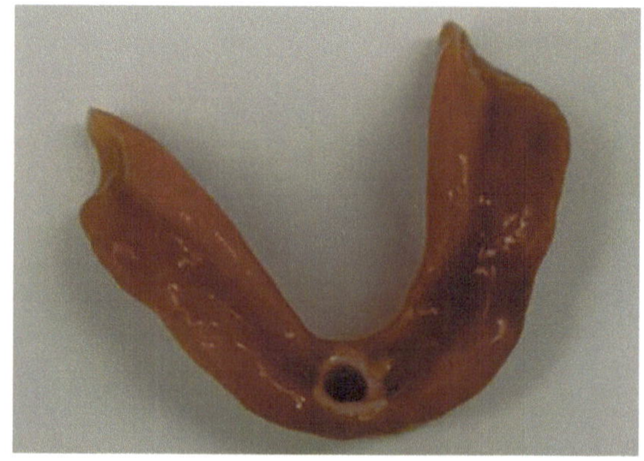

Figure 18.14. Functional satisfaction of the patient can often be met by the installation of a single implant with a spherical head and a retention clip, using the existing prosthesis with a modified base in soft acrylic.

How is the era of leaf implants evaluated?

That period is considered the beginning of more successful implantation because such forms of implants remained in the bone for a long time (sometimes several decades) (Figure 18.15). There are many patients for whom leaf implants have survived for two and three decades. Despite today's scope of oral implantology, I have encountered cases where implantologists in distal edentulous alveolar ridges preferred to install sheet implants rather than the so-called "disk" of the implant. With both systems, implant insertion is very aggressive.

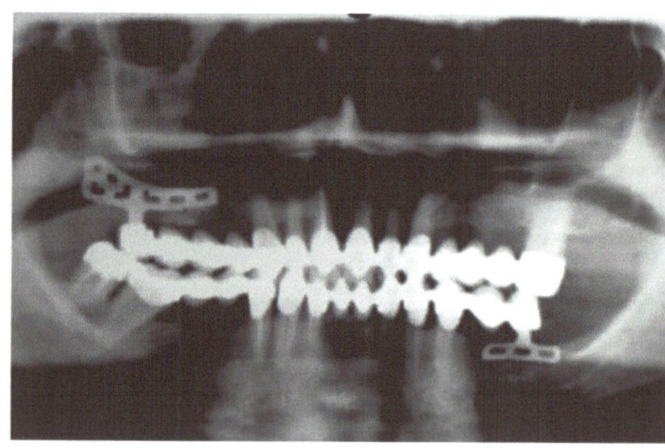

Figure 18.15. Two Linkov-leaf implants in the upper and lower jaw. In the upper jaw, a leaf implant V generation was designed, the endosseous part coated with "titanium plasma" to bypass the floor of the sinus that extends from the tuber of the maxilla. In the lower jaw, due to the insufficient width of the alveolar ridge and the proximity of the mandibular canal, a shorter leaf-shaped implant was installed. Today, such solutions have been overcome. (Author's paper 1977)

Considering the implants that were applied in the past, and in the last decade of the last century, it was considered that the arch endosseous implant is a certain progress in oral rehabilitation in the frontal regions of both jaws. Was the arch leaf implant four decades ago an advancement in implantation?

Half a century ago the installation of implants of such designs was extremely complicated for both the patient and the clinician. The progress was that before similar cases were solved with subperiosteal implants. However, the use of arched leaf implants was applicable only if a sufficient amount of available bone allowed it. It took a lot of courage and routine to hammer such an implant into the bone with great trauma. If today the question is raised whether it was a step forward in the progress of oral implantology, the only fact that supports such a conclusion is that the implants designed in this way persisted in the bone for a long time, and even for several decades.

What was the aggressiveness of the implantation of arch leaf implants in the frontal region of the lower jaw?

The placement of arch implants was performed by experienced implantologists, and the routine experience was accompanied by courage. Cutting the arch implant into the bone with a fissure drill was performed arbitrarily and imprecisely. Routinely, imprecisely without accurate guidance, the incision of the arch of the implant bed into the bone often did not coincide with the arch of the implant. To create an arched implant bed, the surgical procedure must be performed without trauma to the bone, and for an arched implant, it was extremely aggressive to drive the implant aggressively into the bone. Aggressive implantation achieved primary stability, and despite all the shortcomings, the implants remained in the bone for a long time. Two types of arch leaf implants were used: one-piece, where the carrier and the end-osseus part are from one part, the other later form of arch leaf implants from two parts could also be primarily loaded. With this form, there were two possibilities as far as the carrier was concerned; a bracket with spherical extensions that served as retention clips for stabilizing the lower total prosthesis or as a bracket for fixed prosthetic restorations.

The downside of arch-leaf implants in addition to aggressive implantation is; that if the implant gave way in any part, the removal of the implant was very complicated with the consequences of large bone defects. Due to the listed disadvantages, the method of arch leaf implants is among those that have been overcome.

Has the method of arch leaf implants been applied in our country and is there any valid data on success or failure?

I don't think anyone except me in our region has implanted that type of leaf implant produced by "Oraltroniks" from Bremen (Germany). Thanks to the acquired routine with Professor Leonard Linkow in New York and the selection of patients in whom there was a sufficient amount of available bone both vertically and horizontally, in the frontal part of the lower jaw, the arch implants firmly remained in the bone. Since they were from one part, they were burdened immediately. I managed to get only a few patients to "favor" periodic check-ups, and many never showed up again. I guess they were satisfied with the result of the implantation.

At the VMA in Belgrade, an arch implant was created for the length of the entire lower jaw, cast from a chrome-nickel-cobalt alloy. Cutting the implant bed along the entire length of the alveolar bone (the use of stents in oral implantology was unknown at the time) required great manual dexterity from the surgeon. The arch prepared in the bone with a fissure drill hardly matched the arch of the cast implant. The alloy used (chromium-cobalt-molybdenum) from which such implants were made confirms that osseous integration was not thought about at all. Based on the design of the arch implant, a one-piece endosseous implant was designed at the VMA in Belgrade for the rehabilitation of distal edentulous seats in the lower jaw, authored by Professor A. Škundrić. This type of implant has been created in several designs. I had the opportunity to see such an implant installed 27 years ago.

When does osseointegration appear as a term?

Osseointegration as an important term appears in 1981 (Adell et al.), and a large number of implants were already installed in 1980. Although sheet implants were applied, this was the Branemark era when osseointegration processes are increasingly discussed.

What solution should be sought in "hopeless" cases? What then is the optimal solution that experience recommends for a patient when there are no mandibular conditions for fixed work?

Considering all the limiting factors, for many edentulous patients, especially in the lower jaw, despite the enormous progress of oral implantology, the optimal solution will still be: a total prosthesis, with retention clasps of spherical heads, if even possible. It very often happens that due to excessive atrophy, especially in the lateral regions of the lower jaw, there are insurmountable obstacles. If augmentation is attempted, i.e. creation of favorable conditions for implantation, then there are limitations: great pain for the patient, increase in volume and vertical height of the bone with autologous blocks, and a complete, otherwise complicated procedure has an uncertain outcome. The time of treatment would range from 12 to even 24 months. And all this requires high financial expenses.

In the case of severely atrophied alveolar ridges, the installation of implants with spherical heads of retention clips is the optimal and most correct solution. Today, there are several implant systems with spherical heads for the stabilization of prostheses: of various lengths and diameters. The great advantage of installing such implants is the use of an existing prosthesis to which the patient has become accustomed, and the result of the implantation is immediately visible (Figures 18.13-18.14). The implants are put into operation immediately. The most important condition is that there is sufficient bone height to be able to apply implants with narrower diameters. Regardless of the fragility of such implants (diameter of 1.8 mm), good and long-term stability is achieved thanks to their length (from 12 to even 18 mm). Recently, two-part implants with a narrow diameter of 3 mm and a length of 10 to 15 mm have been used for such cases.

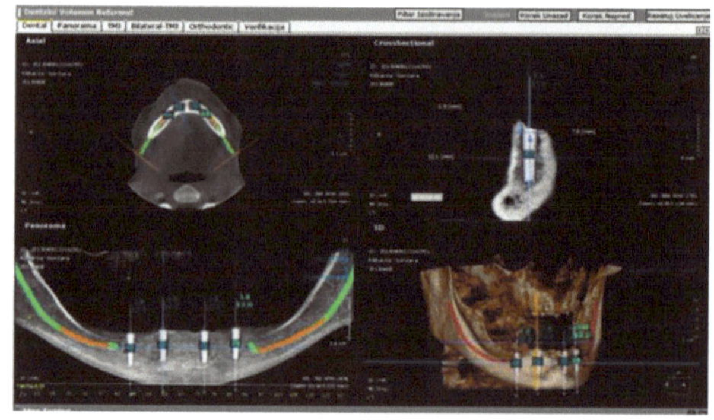

Figure 18.16. The implant installation plan of the presented case. It happens that by lifting the flap, the actual condition deviates from the 3D findings, that is, it is necessary to change the plan. Only by lifting the flap can the visibility of the real situation be obtained.

What is the role of the patient in extremely complicated cases?

Very often, the role of the patient can be decisive. Experience shows that the most complicated patients are those with a neglected condition in the mouth. These are usually patients with poor financial capabilities.

Otherwise, the optimal solution is prosthetic work performed to perfection, from an aesthetic and functional point of view. The entire execution, of the most modern type: firmly fixed or fixed-mobile prosthetic works, requires a longer time and higher financial expenses, especially if augmentation and remodeling of the gingiva with the installation of a larger number of implants is also required. However, even in the case of a patient with good financial possibilities, even after the application of the highest quality implant systems, it is sometimes difficult to fulfill the wishes of the patient despite the professional knowledge and experience of the doctor.

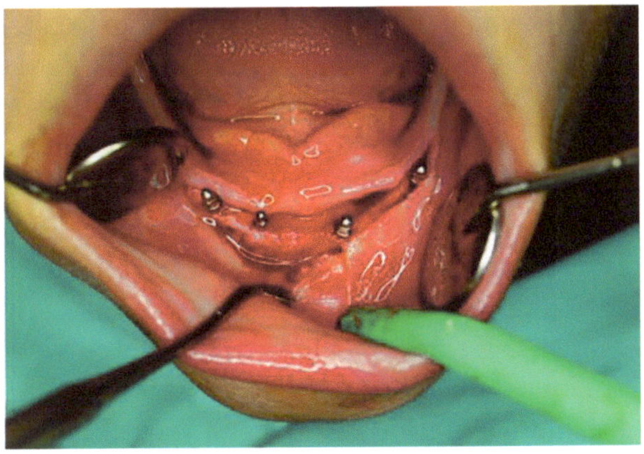

Figure 18.17. In case of extreme atrophy of the alveolar bone, the installation of mini-implants with retention clips is most often performed without raising the flap. However, there is a need to raise the flap due to better visibility of the available bone.

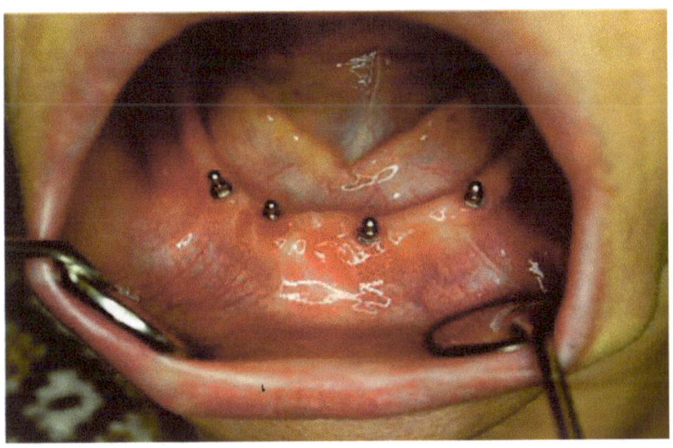

Figure 18.18. When extreme atrophy of the alveolar bone of the lower jaw is present, the best solution is the installation of implants with retention clips to which a mobile prosthesis is fixed. In view of the extreme atrophy (Fig. 18.17), in order to ensure the durability of the installed implants by augmenting the alveolar ridge with bone substitutes, the alveolar ridge was reconstructed in width, which improved the bed of the total prosthesis.

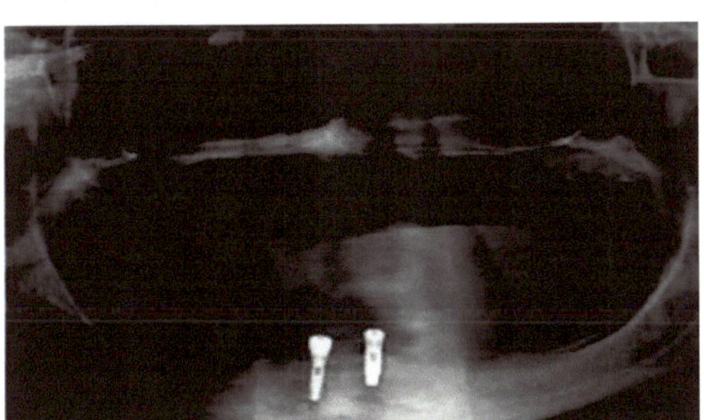

Figure 18.19. Built-in two-part implants of standard and wider diameter in the augmented part of the bone to stabilize the total acrylate prosthesis in the lower jaw. Control shot after 6 years (picture 18.11).

What does personal experience confirm about the above?

It depends on the case. In addition to theoretical knowledge, the most important thing is how many similar situations the doctor has checked through practice and how much, based on such checks, he can predict the outcome, whether it is success or failure. Success depends to a large extent on the availability of computed tomography (3D) data. Relying only on orthopantomography is not enough.

Persistence, without experience and realistic critical perception, leads to failure. In cases where something cannot be done, the patient must be resolutely presented with a very clear position that his case requires a different treatment and that he must accept reality. Even in cases where a solution could be found by installing an implant, one of the important limiting factors is often the impossibility of financing the planned project. If this condition is met, all possible eventual risks must be emphasized and explained. If the clinician is in a quandary about which procedure to use and is not very sure of a successful outcome, the lure of profit can be very dangerous.

The correctness of this conclusion that one should not engage in risky adventures is confirmed by all experienced doctors. The patients I refused for the aforementioned reasons were accepted by other colleagues, accepting the patient's conditions. The colleagues' motive for accepting such patients was probably also a professional challenge, a desire for prestige, and most often, money. In the end, many of those cases would end in failure and mutual disappointment. It happened that a bad assessment ended in appeals or a court case. The implantologist will have the greatest success if he rejects such a patient. This means that he should be analytical and careful in every case!

And what is most important for success to be achievable?

Predictable success in oral implantology requires good knowledge. The best is the one that comes from experience. Risk can best be understood only when failure occurs in practice. This happens even to the most experienced doctors, because the risk usually appears in cases where it was not expected.

First, you need to identify the patient: will he be a suitable collaborator during the treatment. Experience confirms that a thorough medical history is an important first step. Each case should be analyzed in detail. It is important to find out what the patient expects and see if his expectations are in line with realistic possibilities. In other words, a good psychoanalytic assessment of the patient should be made.

On orthopantomographic X-rays study every detail several times, and the use of 3D imaging increases the quality of the examination. Computed tomography provides reliable parameters. If necessary, you should also consult a colleague who deals with this issue.

In which cases is there a risk most often and can it be differentiated?

Risk exists permanently in all procedures. It is important to recognize the case where the risk of failure is closer than success. Such a situation should be avoided or reduced to a minimum.

What should be thought about to avoid the risk, or at least to minimize it?

The risk can occur on two levels: the doctor's mistake, due to a superficial approach in the specific case, or if a patient does not follow the doctor's instructions and does not come for regular periodic check-ups; it is the patient's responsibility, to recognize and prevent an unwanted outcome in time. This should be emphasized to the patient at the very beginning of any implant work.

Is there a belief that for the pioneers of implantology more than five decades ago, when they started dealing with implantation, it was much more difficult than it is today and that the installation of implants was a complicated procedure then?

True, it used to be much more difficult, but only at one stage in the very act of implantation, because today's techniques have far surpassed those of the past. It is also a relief that science has answered many questions that once troubled enthusiasts. The pioneers of implantology could not find answers to the questions posed by their practice in the scarce literature at the time, because oral implantology did not have the scientific support it has today. Therefore, the risk existed even then, but to a much greater extent. It still exists today, and not only when the procedure is performed near anatomical structures that should not be harmed; but after augmentation with bone substitutes in the case of larger bone destructions near the maxillary cavities, the installation of implants in that place is always somewhat uncertain. Despite the new technologies, the risks caused by prosthetic work, and bad planning - occur today, as in the past.

Figure 18.11 shows a case with an emphasized risk. The defect was filled with a bone substitute and covered with a collagen resorptive membrane, which reconstructed the arch of the alveolar ridge in width, which significantly improved the position of the total prosthesis, and reduced the forces acting on the implants (Fig. 18.18).

In the case of larger cystic destructions, what is the procedure for installing endosseous implants?

After radical removal of the cyst, augmentation of the cystic bone defect was performed by filling it with xenogeneic bone substitutes and covering the augmented material with a resorptive membrane. Today, a more expedient procedure is to fill the cystic cavity with a fibrin clot (Advanced PRF) rich in platelets and leukocytes termed "concentrated tissue growth factors". The required waiting time is at least 12 months, and the doctor checks the quality of bone healing with radiographs. There is often no need to rush, because waiting even a few months longer, the installation of implants will result in a better prognosis.

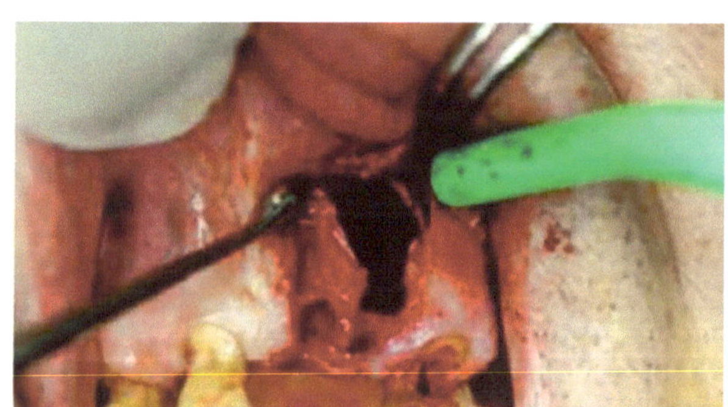

Figure 18.20. The region of cystic destruction requires a long period of bone defect recovery and is a great risk for oral implantation.

What obstacles and surprises can be encountered when installing implants in the place of central incisors in the upper jaw, whether it is an immediate or delayed implantation?

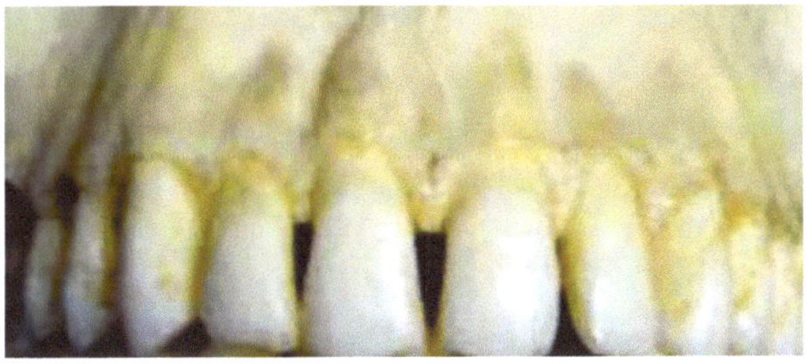

Figure 18.21. Knowledge of the anatomical appearance of the relief of the alveolar bone wall is extremely important for the successful installation of implants in the frontal region. The practitioner should always keep in mind this detail of the anatomical structure of the lamellar bone when making an implant-prosthetic treatment plan.

The lamellar bone of the central upper incisors is usually thin (Fig. 18.21). After the loss of the frontal teeth, with the installation of implants, it is necessary to fulfill not only the functional but, more important, the aesthetic requirements. In most patients, the relief of the labial lamella is obliterated by tooth loss, and this wall of the alveolus is thinner than 1 mm. For a successful functional and aesthetic result of implantological treatment, the buccal bone wall above the surface of the implant should have a thickness of 2 mm. Even with the most careful tooth extraction, with minimal trauma and careful use of rotational movements, in the first year after extraction, the thickness of the buccal wall decreases by over 50%, and 2 to 4 mm is lost at the height of the ridge, which is especially pronounced in the first three months. Although satisfactory bone height remains, there is a risk of fenestration of the implant on the labial side. The choice of implant is very important, first of all, the choice of implant diameter due to aesthetic requirements. An implant of the appropriate diameter should be oriented palatally as much as possible. The risk is all the greater if the periapical process grew larger on the extracted incisors in the upper jaw, which was treated by root resection. In many years of practice, I rarely encountered cases where after root resection the bone at the site of the resected part of the root was histologically compactly organized. For this reason, during my stay in Switzerland, I gave up resection procedures and treated chronic periapical lesions primarily endodontically. Experiences from practice confirm that after each extraction of a resected tooth when it comes to the installation of implants, it was necessary to perform extensive augmentation using xenogeneic bone substitutes covered with a collagen-resorbable membrane. It should be concluded that by resecting the root using the classic surgical method, the favorable conditions for the installation of the implant are not only significantly reduced, but even destroyed. Even trying endodontic treatment and opening an artificial fistula is a far more justified procedure than resecting the root. If we cannot replace the patient's diseased tooth with an implant (mostly for financial reasons), root resection is not justified for the following reasons: root shortening creates biomechanical disturbances (lever action), and local biological disorders of bone healing are caused by disruption of homeostasis at the point of destruction of the lamellar bone wall and artificially shortened roots. By shortening the roots, bundles of infected tubular canals remain open, which disrupts the homeostatic biological balance. Experience confirms that the bone has never been histologically compactly restored in that place, and it is always a diseased place where granulation tissue is formed rather than restored bone. In many years of practice, I have not come across a case treated by root resection where a lamellar bone wall existed. The root resection procedure is more complicated for the patient (pain, swelling, often hematoma) than the implantation procedure.

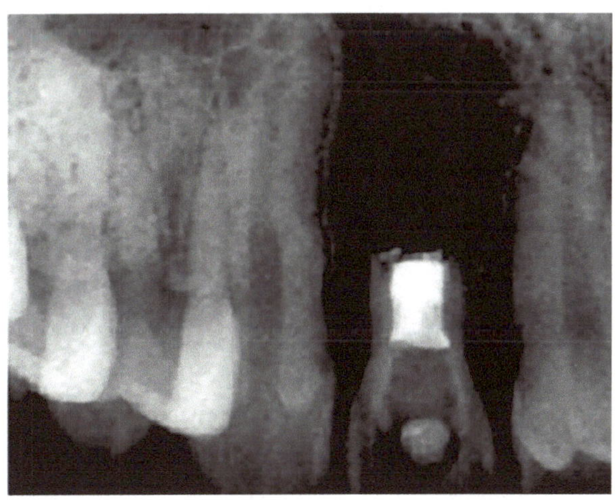

Figure 18.22. Experience shows that the condition after each root resection weakens the labial lamella. It remains a diseased place forever if the tooth is not extracted and repaired with augmentation. The bone structure is significantly weakened, and the decision for implantation also requires

augmentation after tooth extraction. Treatment of periapical changes by root resection in this way is disastrous, even if it is a novice dentist.

What should be done when a complication of lamellar bone fenestration occurs during implant placement?

One should strive to achieve at least minimal primary stability. The maximum possible location of the implant towards the palatal, using as much as possible the cortical part of the palatal bone (Figures 18.18-18.23. To perform augmentation, it is best to cover with an autologous graft combined with a bone substitute, cover with a membrane, and wait at least 6-12 months when the stability of the implant must be checked and checking the thickness of the soft peri-implant tissueThe quality of the soft tissue papilla between the natural tooth and the implant neck, that is, between the implants, will depend on the height of the crestal bone which must support the soft tissues. If the gingiva is insufficiently thick, it is necessary to correct the soft tissues with a free mucosal graft taken from the tuber or the palate, or a substitute such as alloderm. The problem of insufficient attachment and keratinized gingiva is solved by the introduction of free mucosal graft techniques (Nabers, 1966, Sullivan and Atkins 1968). These techniques are today the basis of mucogingival zone enlargement surgery attachment and keratinized gingiva. Regeneration of the attached gingiva is achieved with a free graft taken from the region belonging to the masticatory mucosa, most often from the palate. The graft has squamous layered epithelium with armature, which ensures that the transplanted attachment gingiva after the healing of the surgical wound has the characteristics of a keratinized mucosa.

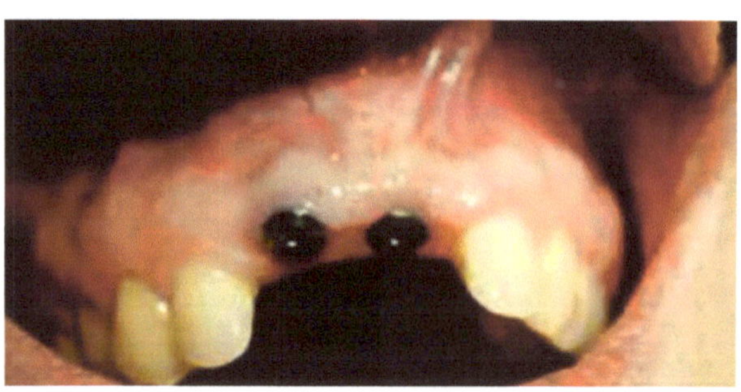

Figure 18.23. The bone defect did not allow locating the implant more palatally. Aesthetic risk factors can hardly be corrected with subepithelial connective tissue grafts. Resection of the roots of the central incisors in the upper jaw destroyed the lamellar bone walls. Due to the destruction of the labial lamella (the central incisors were once resected), it was perforated, and the positioning of the implant was limited.

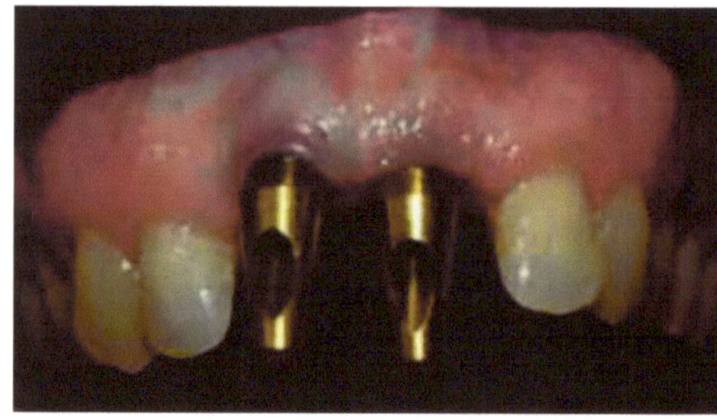

Figure 18.24. Brackets installed after 12 months. High gingival recession on tooth #11 is an exceptional esthetic risk factor.

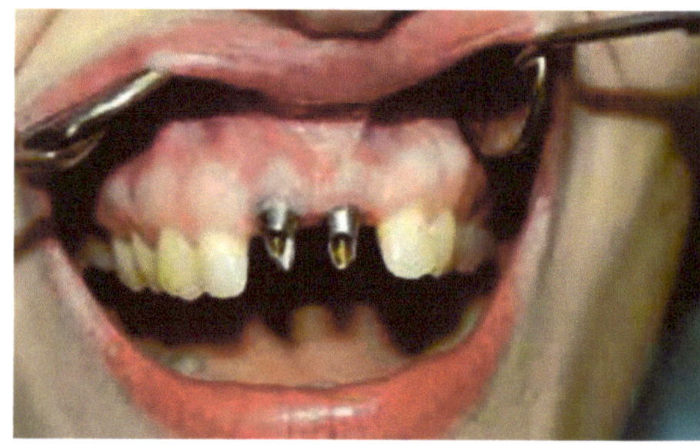

Figure 18.25. Adjusted brackets in the laboratory for prosthetic work after 8 months of augmentation.

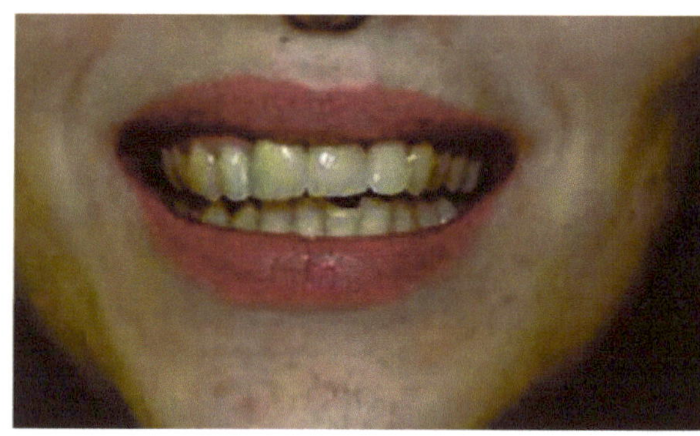

Figure 18.26. The aesthetic defect somewhat masks the favorable shape of the lip of the laugh line. This problem arose as a result of root resection and a larger bone defect. Despite the patient's satisfaction, the author is not satisfied, the treatment should have started with augmentation, formation of the alveolar ridge, and then continued with implantation after waiting at least 12 months. The mistake was made due to the fulfillment of the patient's request to get fixed work as soon as possible. However, the most important thing is that the patient is satisfied.

In the case shown in Figures 18.23-18.26, after eight months, the implants show good stability. However, experience suggests that the waiting period should be extended to 12 months by loading the implants with provisional acrylate crowns in mild subocclusion.

Can a similar unforeseen complication be expected in the lower jaw at the location of the central incisors?

Yes, always. For example, pictures 18.27-18.30. a patient case is presented in which the two central milk incisors remained until the age of 34. During this time, the crestal bone lost its function, which resulted in three-dimensional quantitative bone loss. The horizontal loss of the crestal bone was particularly pronounced, which after implantation is reflected in the quality of soft tissue formation. The formation of soft peri-implant tissues and the achievement of aesthetic results depends on the support of the crestal bone. In similar cases, in the frontal part of the lower jaw, the best results are obtained by installing one-piece implants, choosing the diameter according to the width of the bone (3 mm and 3.2 mm). In the presented case, even though narrow diameter implants (3 mm) were selected, fenestration occurred, because the width of the alveolar bone in that place was less than 2 mm. It was necessary to change direction towards lingual, although there are limitations. Augmentation was performed with xenogeneic bone substitutes mixed with autologous bone shavings taken from the retromolar space of the mandible.

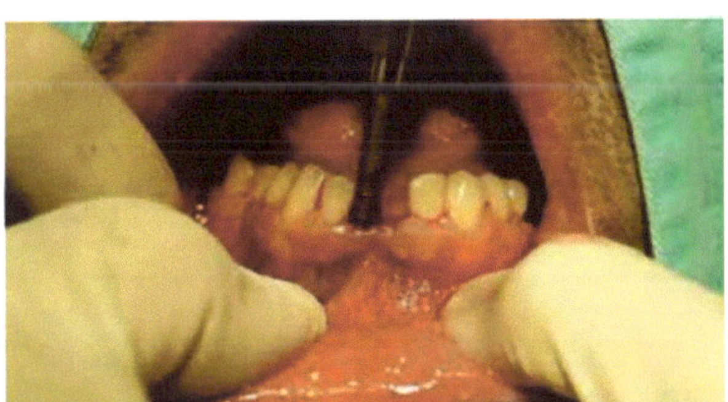

Figure 18.27. With a concave alveolar ridge in the frontal region of the lower jaw, there is usually a risk of fenestration in the labial part. The patient's milk teeth were removed at the age of 34.

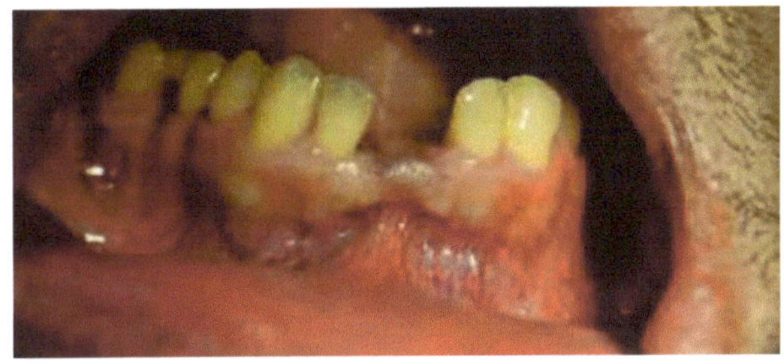

Figure 18.28. After the delayed extraction of milk teeth, an extremely concave remnant of the alveolar ridge was formed, which is a great risk for implant placement. The danger of lamellar bone fenestration always exists.

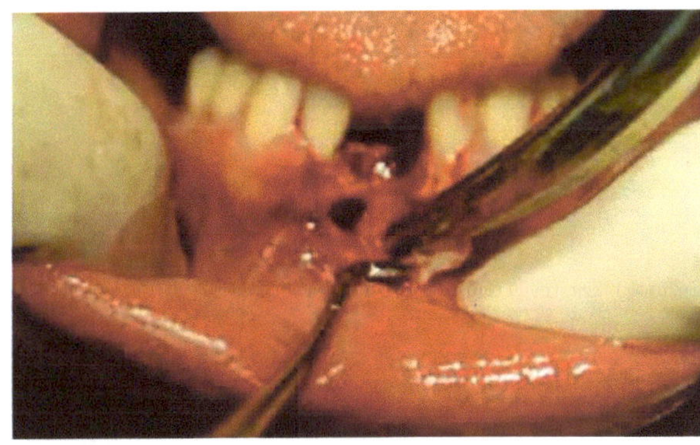

Figure 18.29. Fenestration in the frontal region of the lower jaw is a consequence of the concavity of the alveolar ridge.

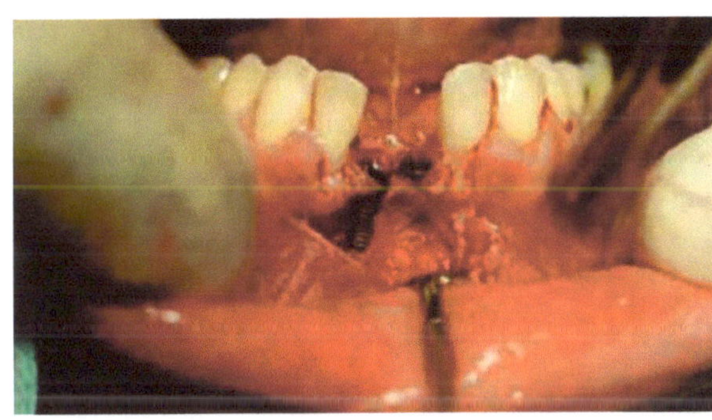

Figure 18.30. Preparation for augmentation with bone substitutes covered with a resorbable collagen membrane.

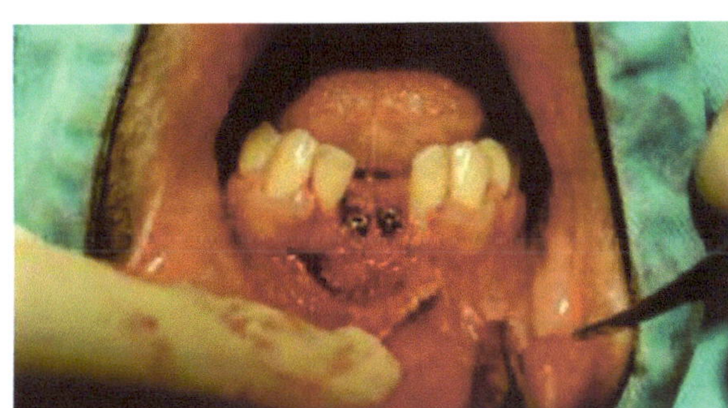

Figure 18.31. Appearance of the fenestrated portion of the alveolar bone covered by a bone substitute.

A similar problem can also occur if teeth are extracted due to periodontitis, and it is solved in the same way in principle.

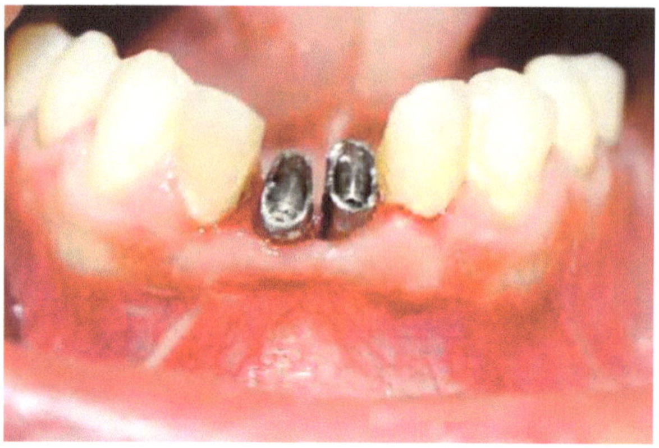

Figure 18.32. Treated brackets, after 8 months of augmentation.

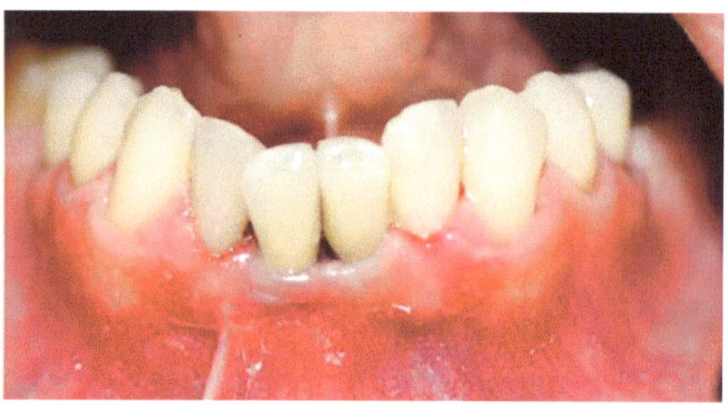

Figure 18.32a. Condition after 6 years. Endangered papilla due to poor oral hygiene and plaque deposition. Regenerated bone of the defect and achieved osseointegration.

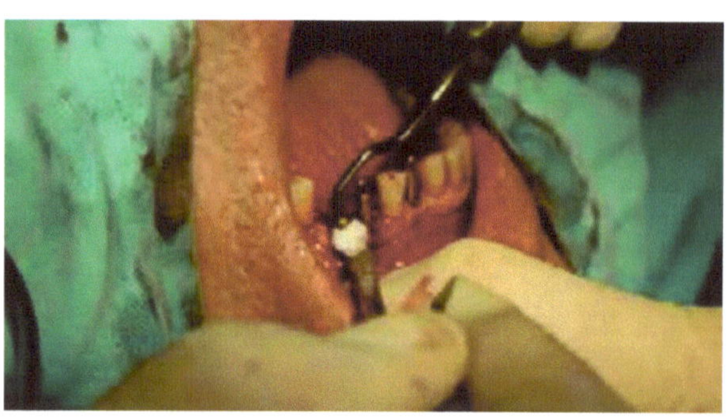

Figure 18.33. .A case that required shortening the treatment time. Immediate installation of implants at the site of loosened periodontopathic teeth.

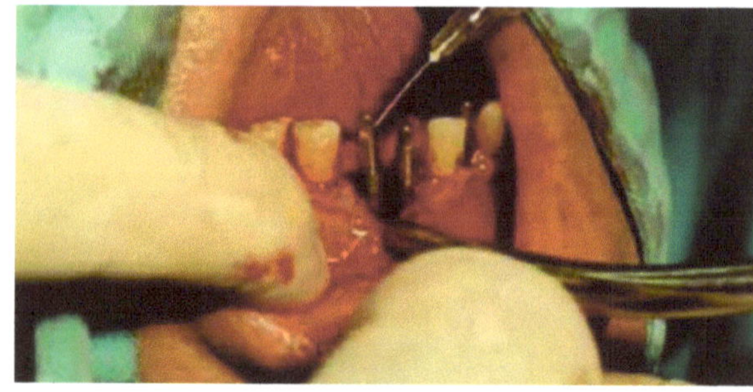

Figure 18.34. Implantation of a reduced-diameter implant in the preserved alveolus at the site of bone and soft tissue defects.

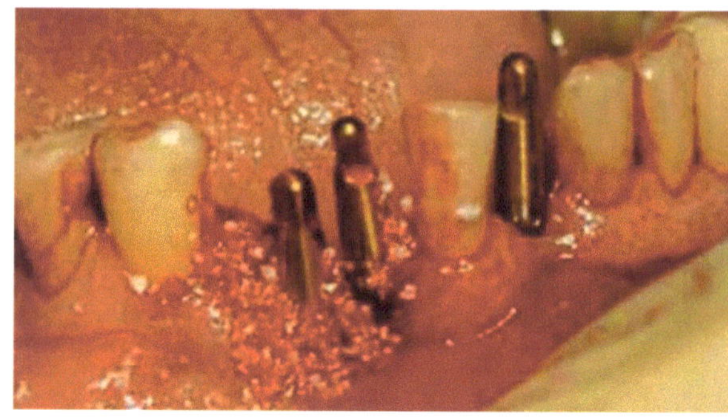

Figure 18.35. The success of the treatment depends on the "management" of the alveolar wound (preservation of the alveolus) by augmentation of the bone substitute. Destruction of soft tissues requires microsurgical interventions with subepithelial connective tissue grafts.

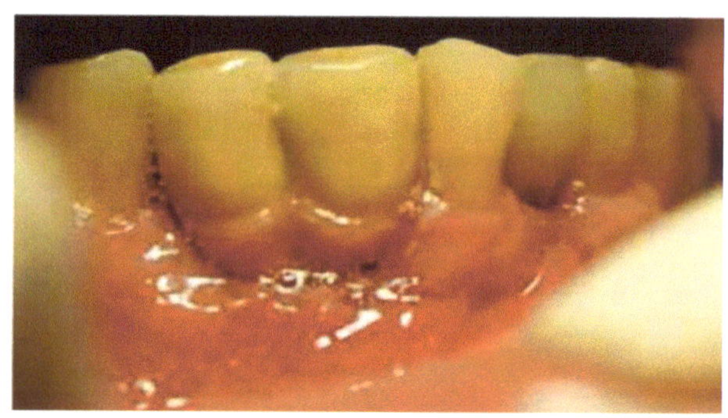

Figure 18.36. Aesthetic lack of soft tissues compensated by prosthetic work. The patient's available time did not allow periodontal microsurgical soft tissue reconstruction (he lives in Australia).

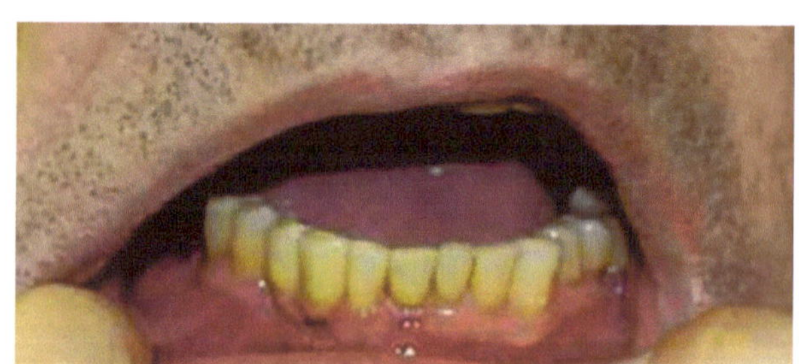

Figure 18.37. The patient presented after 9 years of implant-prosthetic treatment. Appearance of prosthetic work and soft tissues from immediate implantation and immediate loading of prosthetic work in metal ceramics.

What procedure should be applied in such cases?

One-piece implants should be installed, using the maximum length (16 mm) and immediately loading them with precise provisional crowns. The soft tissues are allowed to heal unhindered. A small number of clinicians will likely opt for a similar procedure. However, the author's experiences show good results.

Does this mean immediate loading is preferred?

Absolutely. I have been advocating that position for a long time, and it has been confirmed by successful results. However, some authorities take a different position, based more on theoretical considerations. Waiting for months for the patient to get fixed teeth (at first provisional) is a waste of both time and comfort for the patient. Also, it is not justified for several reasons: soft tissue healing and the osseointegration process. Figures 18.38 and 18.39 show a complicated case solved by immediate implantation, augmentation, and immediate loading. The gingiva is well-formed around the definitive brackets.

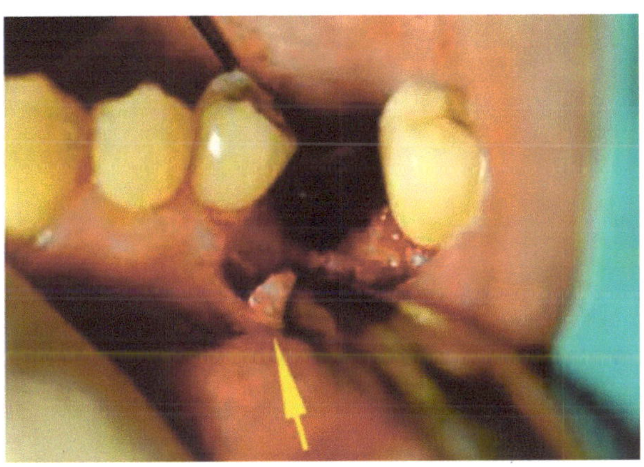

Figure 18.38. Installation of wide-diameter implants. Treatment of epithelial connective tissue and papilla formation with a special instrument.

With a different procedure, the treatment time would be significantly longer, more complicated and difficult for the patient, but not of better quality: by placing the healing caps after implantation and raising the flap again after a few months, the healing time would be prolonged, and the tissue formation around the support would not be better. There is no specific rule here, everything depends on the judgment and experience of the clinician. Optimal solutions are the result of good judgment.

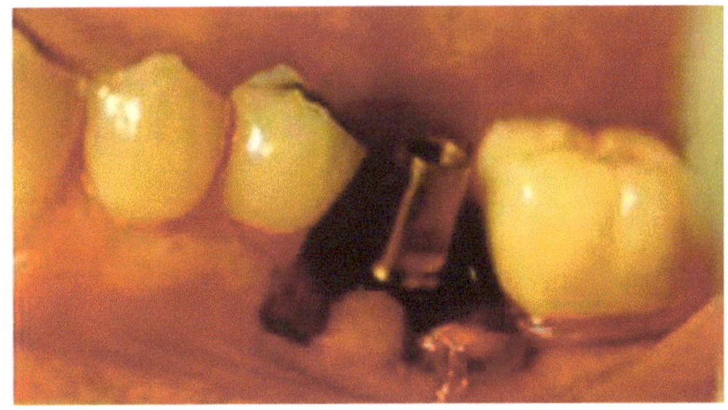

Figure 18.39. Placing a definitive bracket immediately after implantation, instead of healing caps, has multiple advantages. Shaping the papilla with a special instrument. (picture 18.79.)

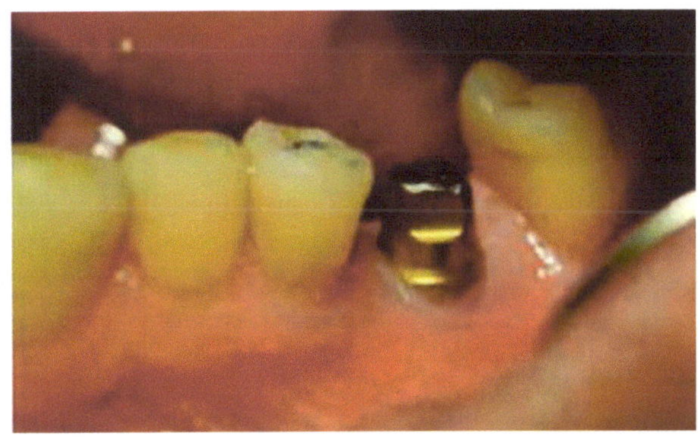

Figure 18.40. Appearance of formed soft tissues and papilla restoration after 8 weeks.

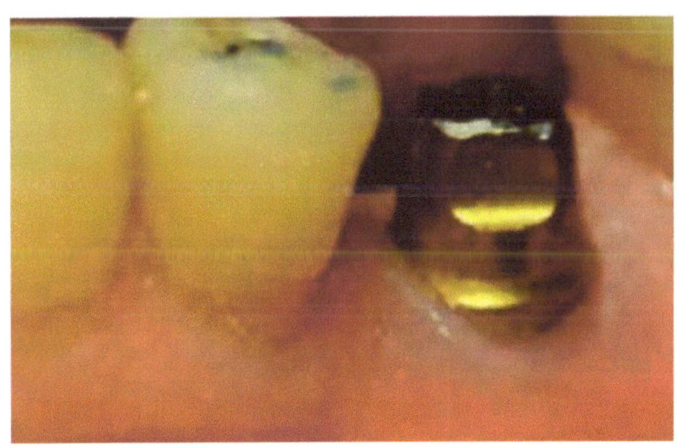

Figure 18.41. Appearance of formed soft tissues after 3 months. The author's opinion is that it is better to leave a definitive support for the formation of the surrounding tissues instead of using a gingiva-former, which requires unnecessary re-surgery.

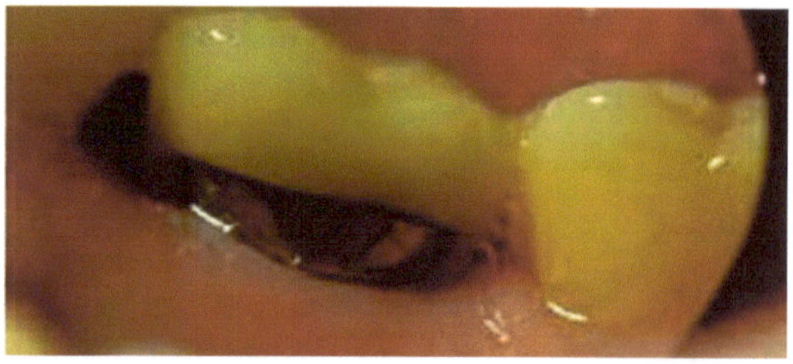

Figure 18.42. The condition of the gingiva and the appearance of the crown from the lingual side after 4 years. Leaving a high collar lingually maintains healthy gingiva because it prevents plaque deposition.

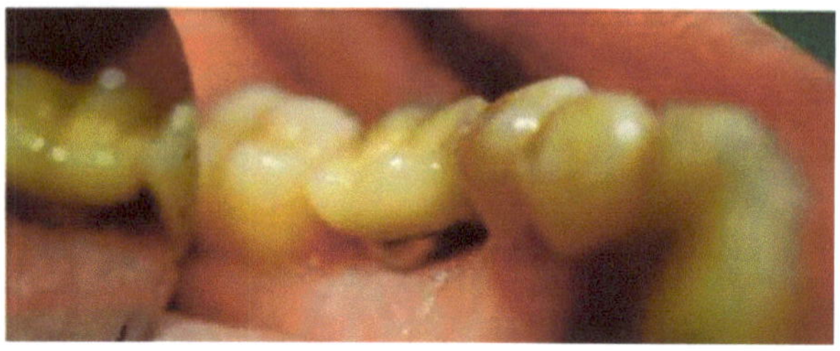

Figure 18.43. The appearance of definitive prosthetic work with the emphasis that a high metal collar should be left lingually for better maintenance of oral hygiene. Appearance of healthy gingiva from the lingual side after 6 years.

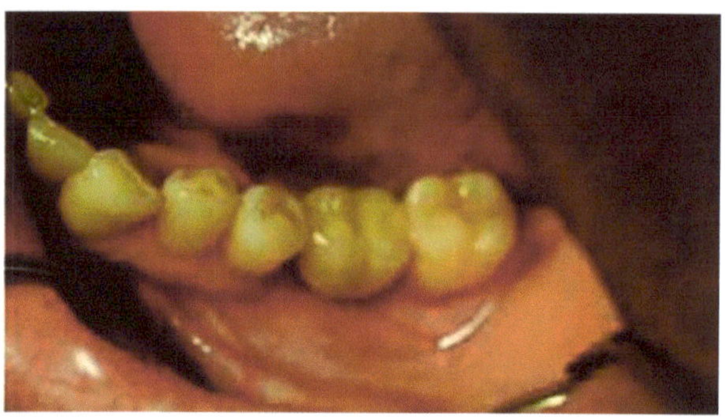

Figure 18.44. Occlusal appearance of the compensated molar. The cusps of the occlusal surface must be shaped according to gnathological principles, i.e. that during lateral movements of the lower jaws they do not make premature contacts.

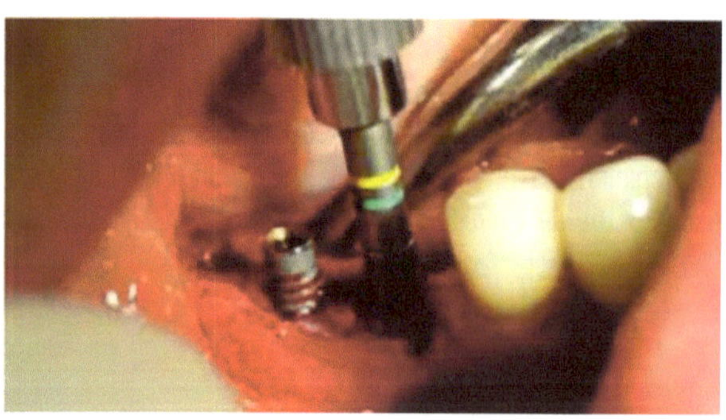

Figure 18.45. Achieving paralysis begins with the preparation of the bed for implant placement. The parity of the implant and the primary stabilization of the implant at the beginning of the procedure determine the outcome of the treatment.

The next picture (18.46.) further confirms the advantages of immediate loading of the installed implants.

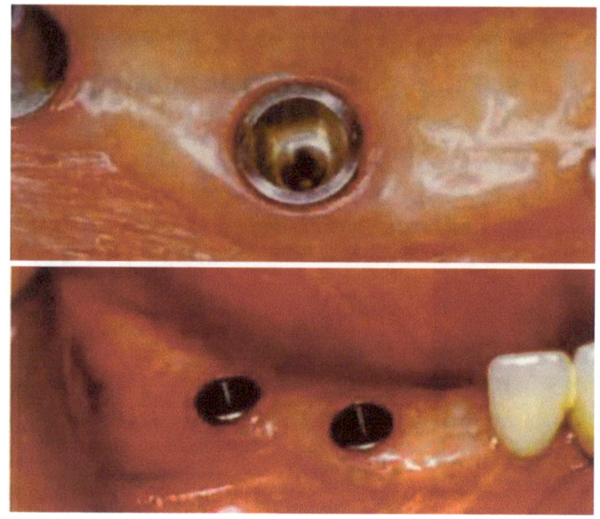

Figure 18.46. Appearance of soft tissue healing after 3 months of immediate implant placement. Good bone support results by the state of the soft tissues shown in the picture.

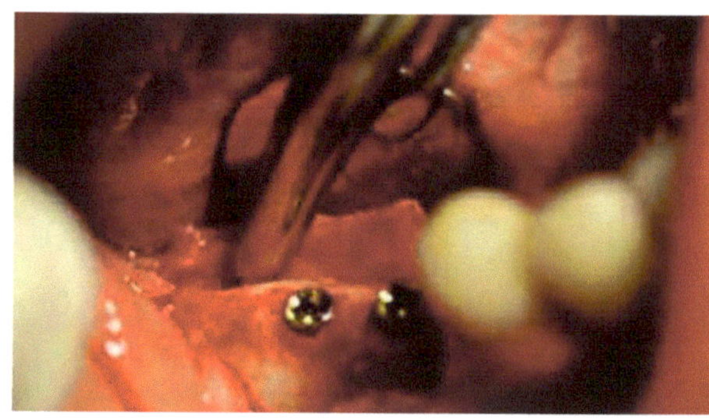

Figure 18.47. The decision to raise the flap and immediate implantation of the implant, as well as immediate loading, is made on the basis of tomographic analyzes (3D). When it comes to soft tissue healing and osseointegration processes, the results are the same after one year regardless of the loading method (immediate-delayed). The advantage of immediate installation of implants and immediate loading is in reducing the patient's discomfort and faster establishment of comfort in the mouth.

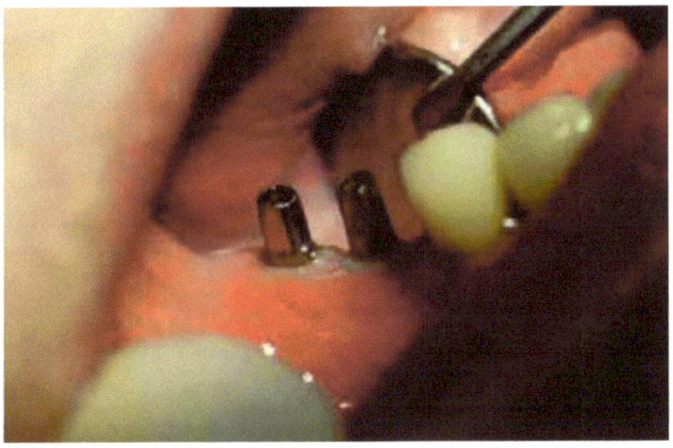

Figure 18.48. By positioning the definitive brackets instead of the gingivaformer, the gingival sulcus is formed better. Frequent unscrewing and screwing of the carrier traumatizes the surrounding soft tissues and increases the possibility of introducing bacterial content into the microcrack between the carrier and the body of the implant.

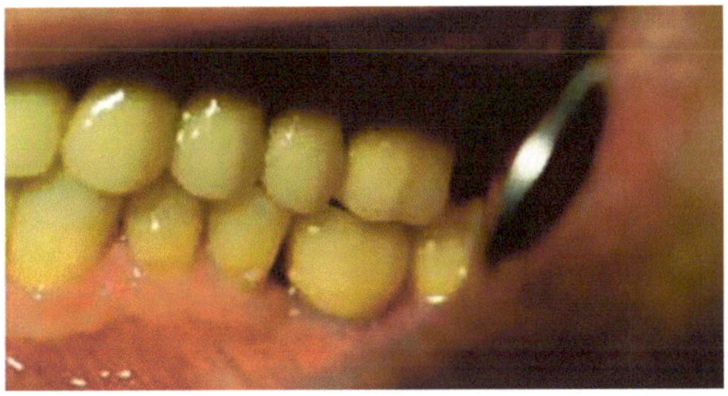

Figure 18.49. Replacement of molars on implants. The pressure of chewing forces requires the formation of the occlusal surface in accordance with gnathological principles: the height, slope and oblique plane of the cusp in accordance with biomechanical requirements.

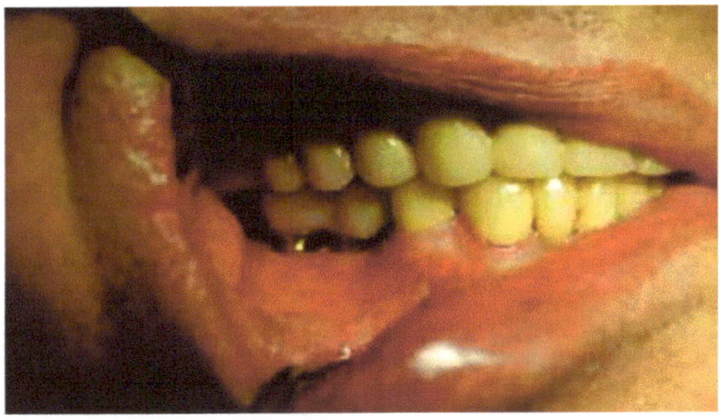

Figure 18.50. Provisional immediate restorations made of softer materials create favorable conditions for bone tissue healing and integration processes.

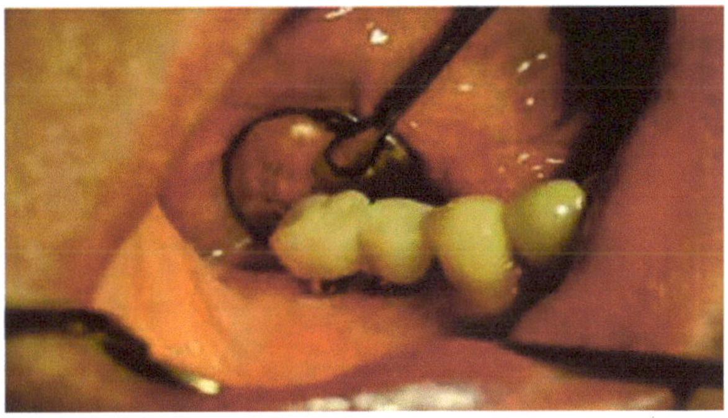

Figure 18.51. For provisional restorations in the lateral regions, it is primary that the biomechanical requirements are met and that the soft tissues are not traumatized during the healing period.

Do we have uniform answers to such and similar questions today?

Today's oral implantology has answered many questions with scientific confirmation and this is part of the great relief. Technical and technological possibilities are incomparably better than before. Also, the possibilities and methods of modern updating of knowledge and education are much better and faster. But practice and experience give the best answers to many questions. Of course, the way of thinking also depends on general knowledge.

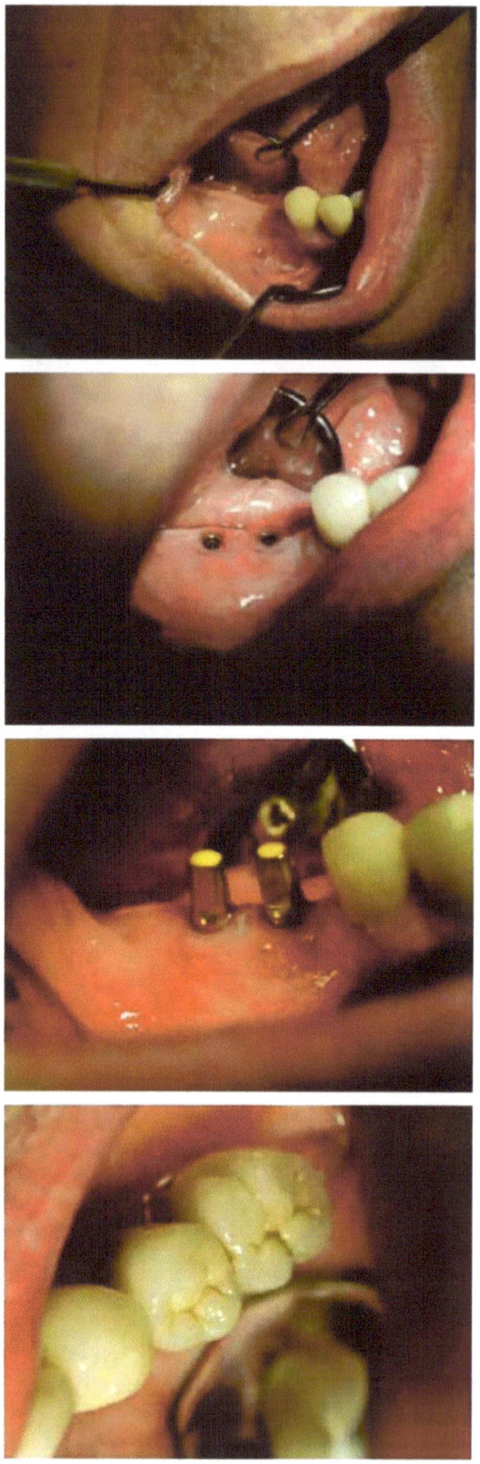

Figure 18.52. Embedded implants without raising the flap. The gingiva formed around the brackets placed immediately after the installation of the implant, with good paralysis. Condition of the gingiva after 6 months. The appearance of the formed gingiva around the support and the occlusal surface of the metal-ceramic crown. The inclination of the cusps is modeled according to gnathological principles so that the reception of chewing forces is axial. Fissure pigmentation is an imitation of the occlusal surface of a natural tooth.

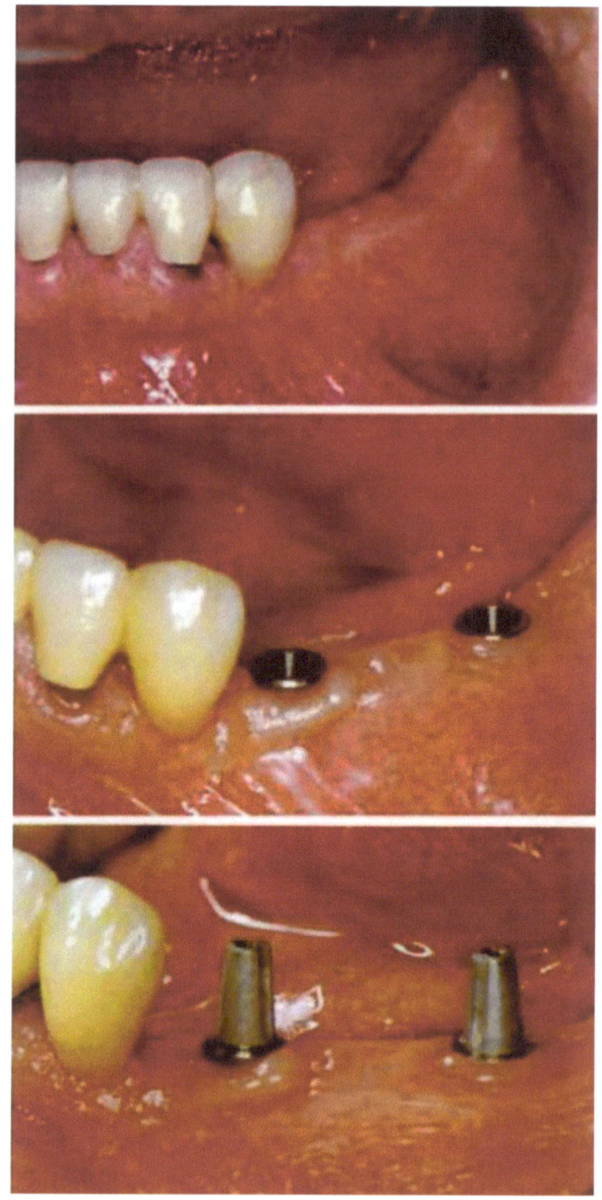

Figure 18.53. To achieve primary stabilization, the design of the implant must allow for subcrestal placement that leads to bone overgrowth and provide a safe, stable platform for prosthetic work. The greater slope at the shoulder allows the bone to grow the implant over its top. In the region of the molars, larger diameter implants should be placed if there is a wide alveolar ridge. Display of soft tissue appearance.

What is the essence of knowledge in cases where opinions differ, and are these differences justified from the aspect and principles of modern implantology?

The essence of good knowledge begins with the practitioner's theoretical thoroughness, perfect knowledge of anatomical structures and recognition of possible variations, and knowledge of physiological processes, in order to fully understand the process of bone integration, the process of healing soft tissues, and the like. Experience based on this will result in good planning and a successful solution.

Even though oral implantology has advanced significantly, a doctrinal position on many issues has not yet been developed. Therefore, each case requires a multi-faceted approach, and thinking about how to approach it depends on the clinician's attitude. The attitude stems from general medical and dental knowledge. There were similar differences in attitudes in the past. For example, once the oral surgeons for endosseous implantation, when it comes to surgical technique, the basic parameter was the sufficient amount of available bone! That point of view was especially important during the installation of Linkov-leaf implants. And often, from the prosthodontist's point of view, the implant should not have been installed in that place. For this reason, these two disciplines seek unity when it comes to indications and evaluation of the outcome of decisions made. A gap in thinking is still possible today, despite all the advantages offered by modern implantology, and mistakes are not excluded even today if the implantologist does not think multidisciplinary, and this is a condition for good planning, which is the basis of success.

How much does success depend on planning?

Experience confirms that good planning and preoperative diagnostics are the basic foundations of predicting success. The planning of the entire operation deserves exceptional attention, especially in terms of predicting possible failures that can, later, compromise the entire effort. The biggest damage from wrong planning is the patient because of the suffering, lost time, and invested money.

Can cases of a different approach, or attitude, be shown practically, when, perhaps, another clinician would act differently?

The following examples show the views of the authors of the book (Figures 18.54-18.65). The patient tried to wear full dentures for seven years. He could not tolerate them and they were more in his pockets than in his mouth.

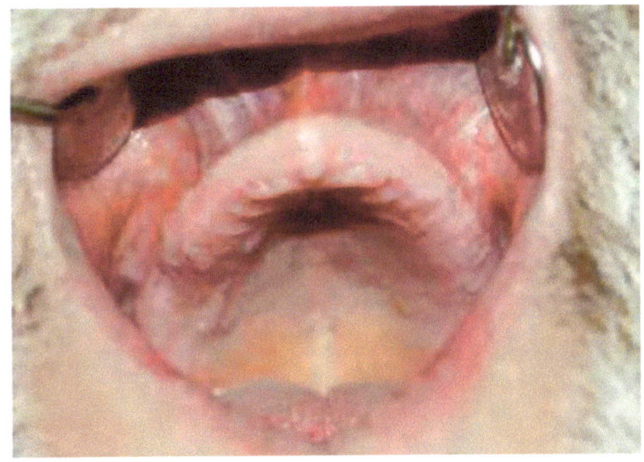

Figure 18.54. A patient who could not get used to total mobile prostheses. He states that he has been trying for 7 years. The full dentures were more in his pockets than in his mouth. The appearance of the destroyed tubers and dry palate were also factors in the instability of the upper total denture.

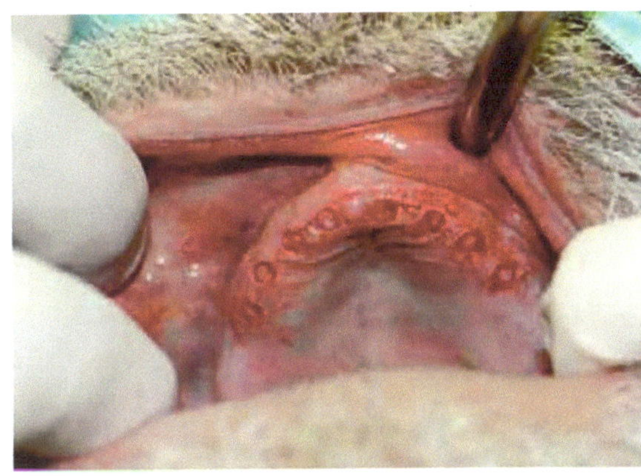

Figure 18.55. The patient's requests to receive fixed compensations as soon as possible and available time (he lived abroad) determined the plan and method of rehabilitation. It was decided not to lift the flap to save time. A special instrument for the processing of soft tissues was used to determine the position for implant placement, and the appropriate length and diameter of the implant was planned using 3D analyses.

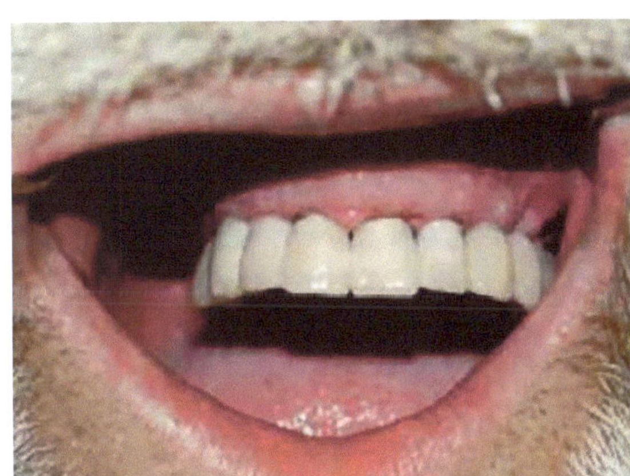

Figure 18.56. Provisional restorations immediately after the installation of implants in the upper jaw. Functional and aesthetic requirements of the patient are fully met.

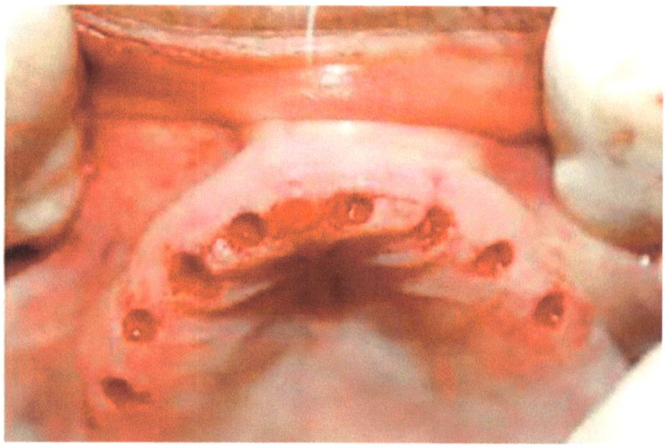

Figure 18.57. Using the WaxUp method in the laboratory, the implants are positioned in accordance with the tomographic measurement indicators. With a stent made in the laboratory (determined position of the implant, position and shape of the teeth), the place of installation of the implant is shaped with a special instrument. WaxUp is a method when fixed prosthetic work on a plaster model is indicated by modeling in wax the appearance of future prosthetic work is determined. With the WaxUp method, the shape and size of the future teeth are determined and seen in advance, and thus the place where the implants should be placed.

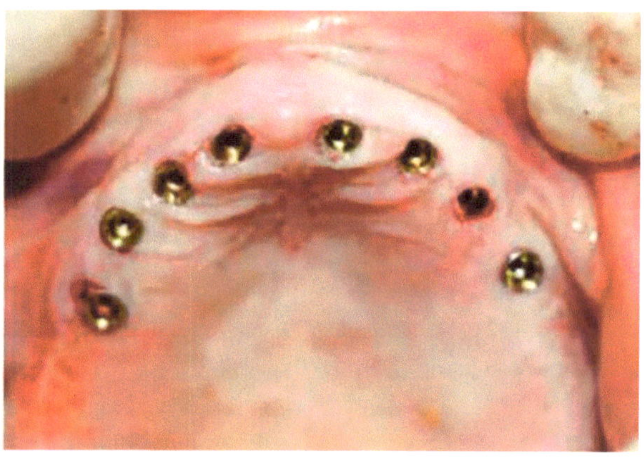

Figure 18.58. Appearance immediately after implant placement.

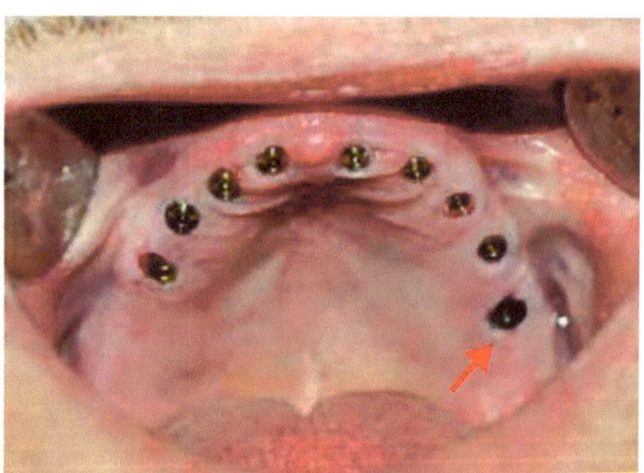

Figure 18.59. Appearance after a week. 8 standard-diameter implants were installed, and a wide-diameter implant was installed in place of tooth 25 (arrow).

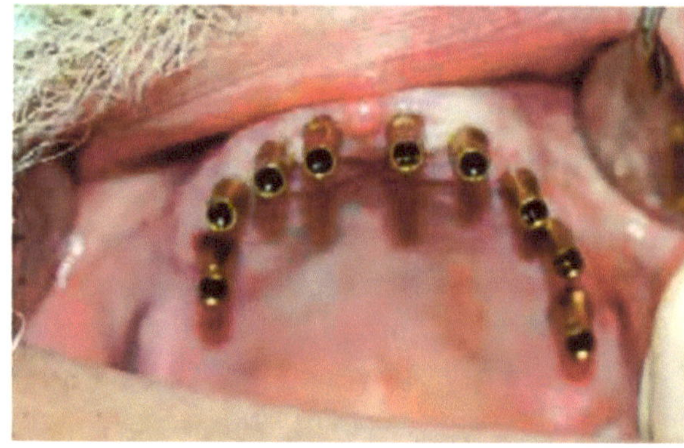

Figure 18.60. Placed supports on the same day after implant placement.

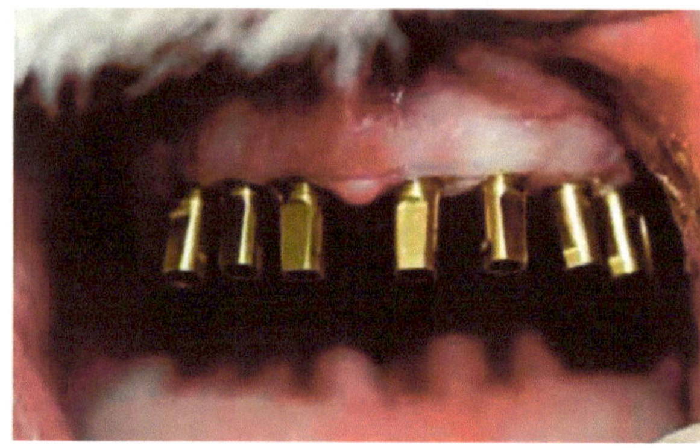

Figure 18.61. Control of carrier paralysis immediately after implant placement.

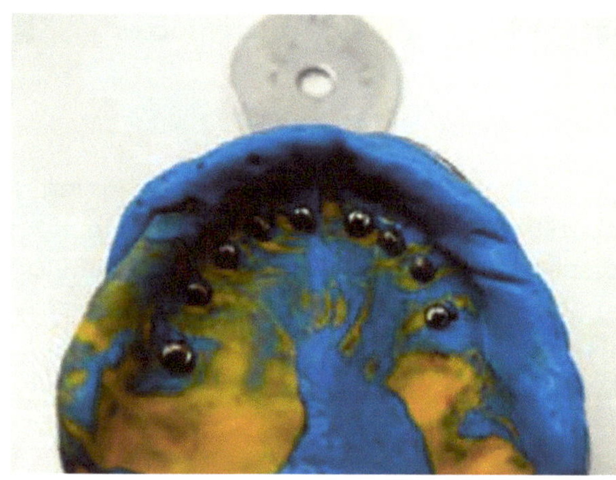

Figure 18.62. The position and parallelism of the implant can also be seen with a one-phase precise impression. Installed analogues on laptops.

The presented case shows that the positioning and installation of the implant by omitting the surgical incision and raising the flap has a special advantage in shortening the healing time of the soft tissues around the support. The implants are immediately loaded with a precise temporary acrylate bridge on a metal base.

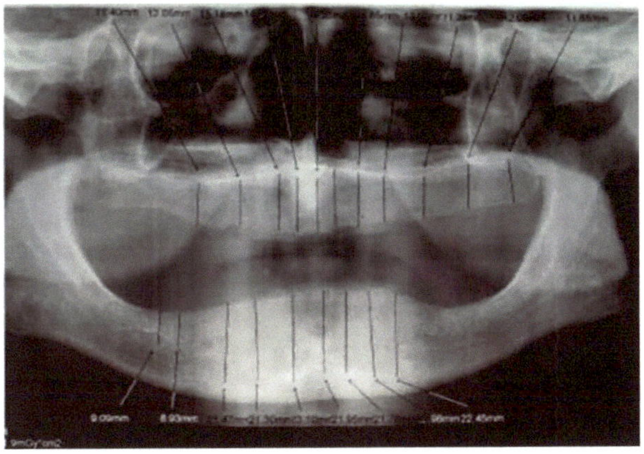

Figure 18.63. Detailed anamnesis and analysis of the tomographic image of 3D anatomical structures and details important for implantation are the basis for making a plan and its implementation.

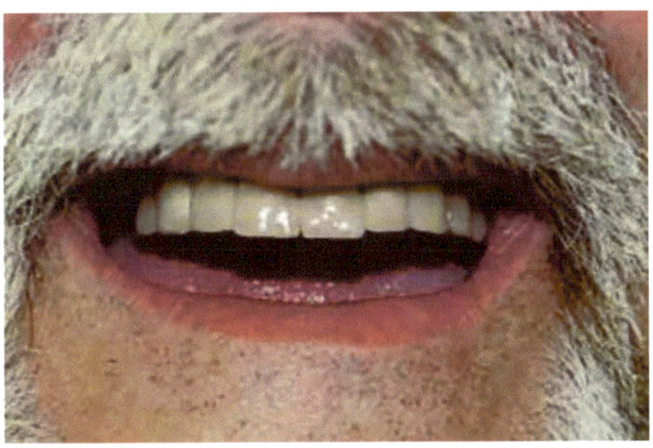

Figure 18.64. After 7 years of trying to wear several made-up total prostheses (he lives in the USA), he is satisfied with the temporary prosthetic work (to this day, 5 years later, he has not come for the definitive prosthetic work).

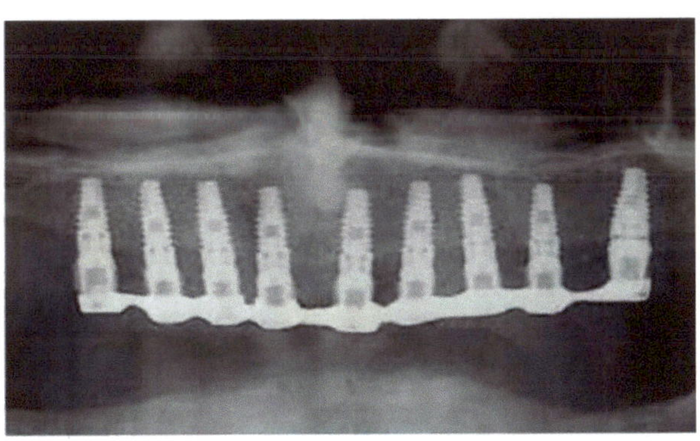

Figure 18.65. X-ray view of the position of implants treated with Laser-Lock technology, immediately installed without raising the flap.

In the same patient, the situation in the lower jaw required a different approach in the planning of the procedure, due to the condition of the alveolar bone and anatomical disadvantages: the razor-sharp shape of the crestal bone, strong cortical bone of sufficient height and insufficient width in all segments between the mental foramen, atrophy of the alveolar ridge in the lateral regions and position of sensitive anatomical structures (mandibular canal and mental nerve). The method of planning the procedure in the lower jaw depends on the condition of the alveolar ridge: the quantity and quality of the bone, anatomical structures (mandibular canal), width and height of the alveolar bone. For example, in the patient shown, the ridge width on individual segments was 5 mm (sufficient bone width to accommodate the selected implant diameter). In this patient, the lack of alveolar bone width was compensated by an implant length of 16 mm, and in some segments even 18 mm (diameter of 3.3 mm).

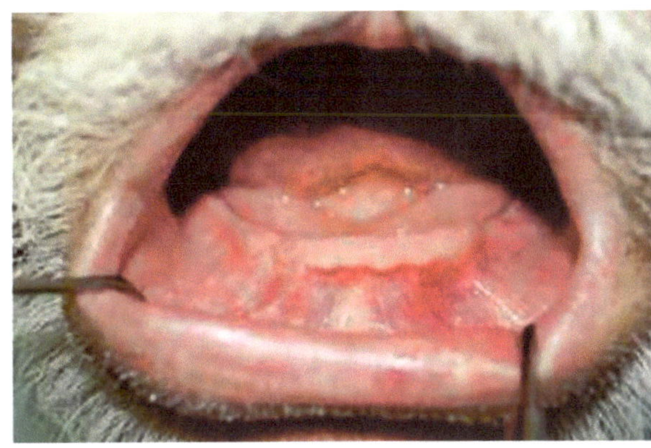

Figure 18.66. The situation in the lower jaw was significantly different from the situation in the upper jaw. Extreme atrophy of the alveolar ridge with pronounced concavity. In the lateral zone, the narrow dimensions of the crestal bone required a different implantological approach. Initial state.

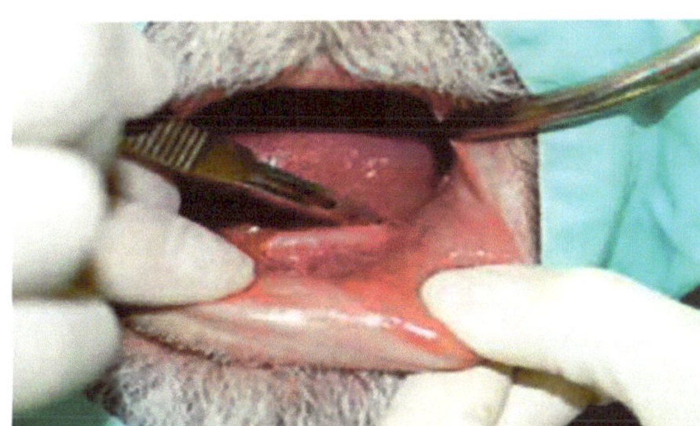

Figure 18.67. The sharp edges of the crestal bone and unfavorable horizontal dimensions required raising the flap for visibility and leveling of the crestal bone.

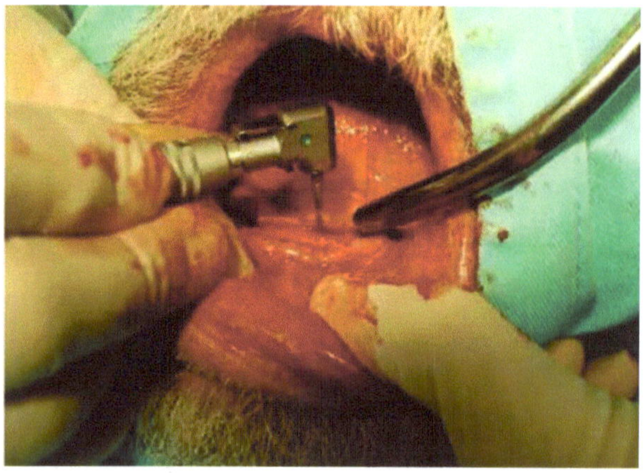

Figure 18.68. In the laboratory, a plan of the entire treatment was created using the WaxUp method. Marking the position of the implant with a pilot drill based on the WaxUp method, thus predetermining the appearance of the future fixed prosthetic work.

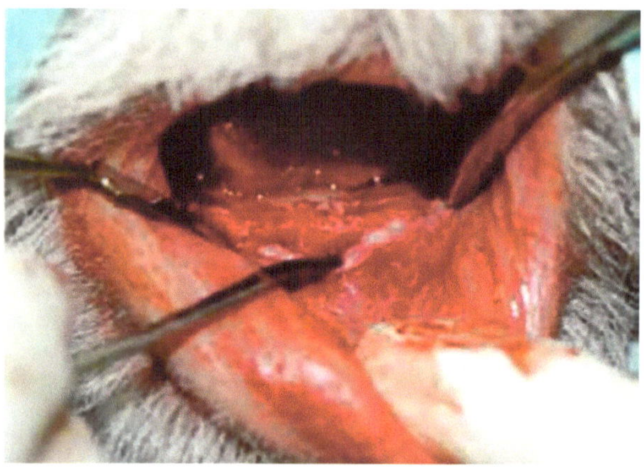

Figure 18.69. After raising the flap, the examination of the crestal bone is less favorable than it was found on the X-ray.

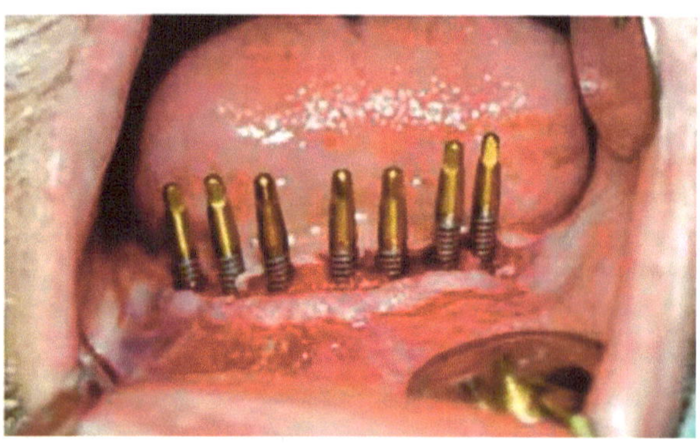

Figure 18.70. The dimensions of the alveolar bone determine the type and number of implants. By increasing the number of implants, micromovements of immediately loaded implants are reduced, which accelerates the integration process. Planning the position and number of implants is in accordance with the planning of future definitive prosthetic work.

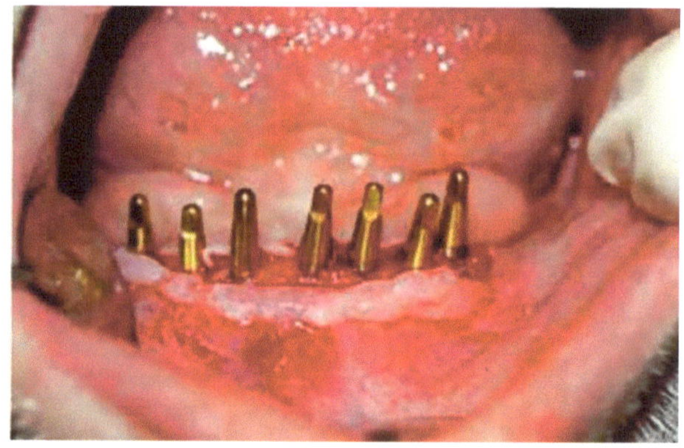

Figure 18.71. Built-in implants of reduced diameter. The supports are made of soft material, which enables adjustment and achieving parallelism without transferring thermal stimuli to the bone.

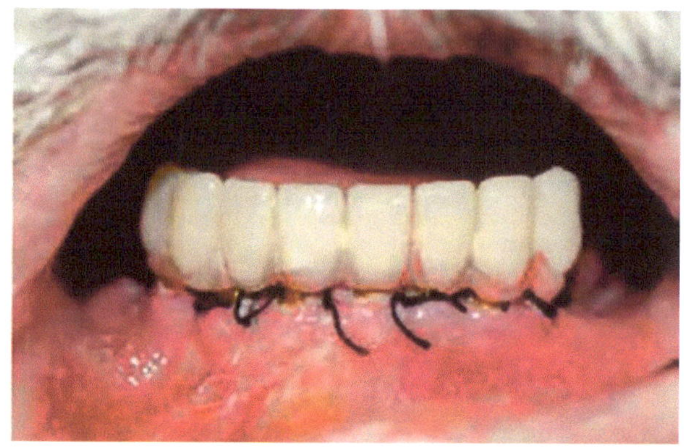

Figure 18.72. A provisional restoration was placed on the same day after the installation of the implant.

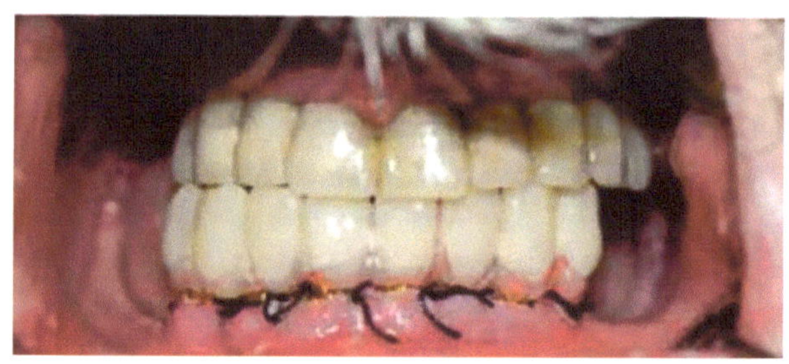

Figure 18.73. Provisional restorations in both jaws made immediately after implant placement.

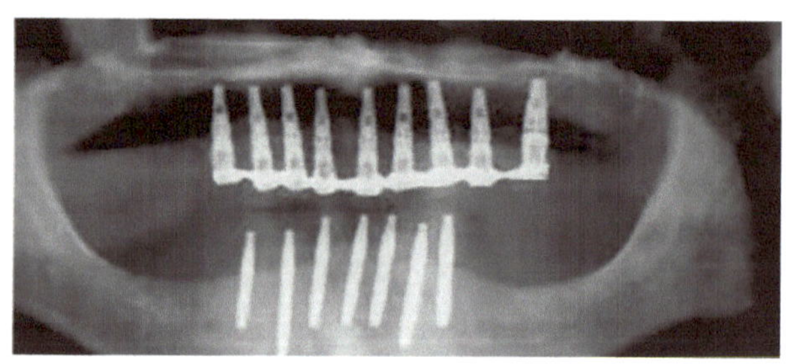

Figure 18.74. The number and position of the implants allow the addition of hanging members in the lateral regions. A wide diameter implant was used in position #26.

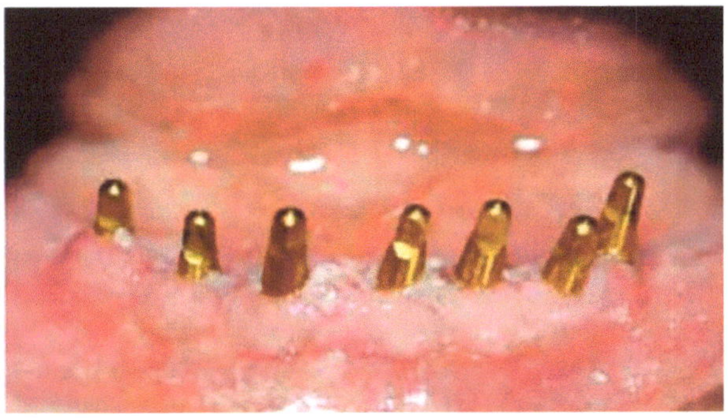

Figure 18.75. Condition ten days after removal of stitches.

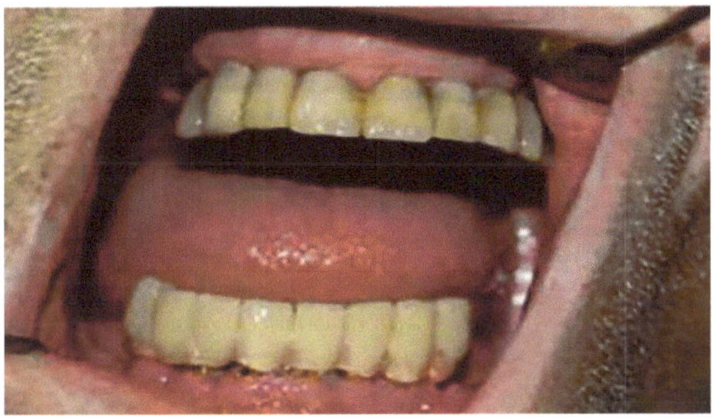

Figure 18.76. View of provisional restorations in both jaws ten days after implant placement. After 4 weeks, new, more precise temporary bridges were made in acrylate, with a metal base.

Can you show a complicated case where the approach and procedure of many implantologists would be the opposite of the one you applied?

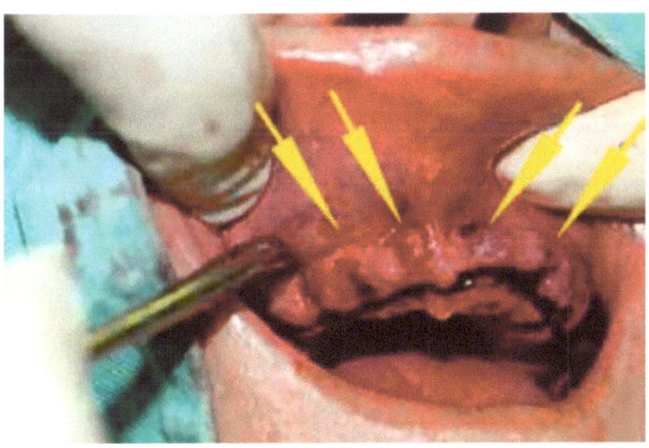

Figure 18.77. Presentation of a case where the patient's requirements and the condition of the mouth are extremely complicated. Destroyed lamellar walls and insufficient soft tissues are a major risk factor for fulfilling the patient's wishes. The experience of a dentist is crucial for solving such complex cases. The position of the extracted pathologically migrated teeth in the vestibule marked by arrows. The patient's request to receive teeth immediately due to professional obligations, with the express refusal of a total temporary prosthesis. Condition after removal of bridges and extraction of teeth. Arrows indicate the position of pathologically migrated teeth in the fornix.

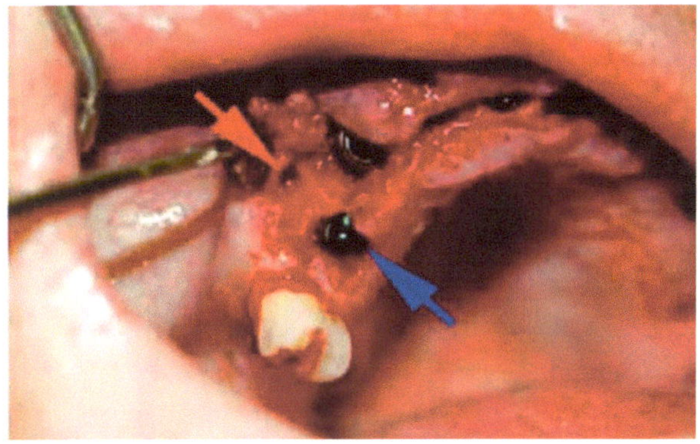

Figure 18.78. The position of the pathological migration of the buccal root of the first premolar is visible (red arrow), and the implant is placed in the solid palatal part of the bone (blue arrow).

For example, in the patient shown in Figures 18.77 and 18.78, solutions could be sought in the following procedures: after extraction of periodontal teeth positioned outside the ridges, leveling the ridge and augmenting the defects, suturing the wounds, and after removing the sutures, possibly making temporary total prostheses.

Another procedure would be the installation of implants of selected appropriate diameters and lengths based on tomographic images, augmentation of bone defects with bone substitutes, placement of caps on implants covered with a flap. It should be emphasized that it would be necessary to remove the frenulum that extended to the middle of the alveolar ridge. After the sutures were removed, the patient would receive a temporary total acrylic prosthesis. The soft tissue healing time and waiting for the implants to integrate would be six months.

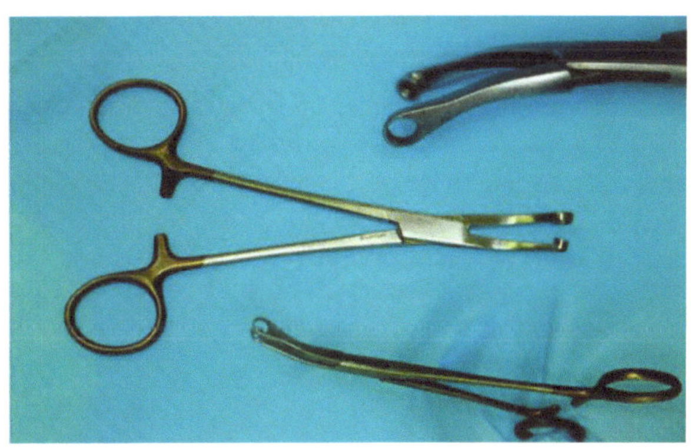

Figure 18.79. An instrument used to shape the interdental papillae.

However, the presented case was solved with the following procedures: extraction of the tooth, installation of the implant, placement of the bracket, formation of the gingival margin around the bracket, formation of the papilla with a special instrument (Fig. 18.79), treatment of the frenulum, suturing of the wound, taking an impression for immediate loading with a precise temporary bridge.

What parameters determined the planning of the solution?

The significantly changed position of the teeth outside the arch of the alveolar ridge of the upper jaw required their removal. The patient wanted to have teeth as soon as possible due to professional obligations, refusing a mobile total prosthesis at all costs, because the long-term torture with a total prosthesis in the lower jaw caused her not to fit another total prosthesis in her mouth, despite the explanation that it is a temporary solution.

Before tooth extraction, it was necessary to make a detailed treatment plan. The existing situation in the mouth was transferred to the laboratory. Interjaw relationships were analyzed, teeth were removed on a plaster model, on which the position of the implant was determined and the aesthetics of future prosthetic work was planned. Placing teeth in the laboratory on the formed toothless alveolar ridge, at a previously determined position of the implant, is of essential importance for the final aesthetic result.

In order to avoid raising the sinus floor, the second premolar on the right side was retained, which was very solid, because at position 16 the bony part of the floor of the maxillary sinus was about 3 mm. This would require a complete change of the planned plan and time of the restoration.

One day after tooth extraction, the implementation of the adopted plan based on tomographic calculations was started. By raising the flap, an insight into the true state of the alveolar bone was obtained. Verification of established tomographic calculations determines the method of implantation, the position of the implant and the type of load. Positioning the implant in place of the central incisors would be the first step.

By raising the flap in the lateral region at the position of region 27, a sufficient width of the ridge was seen, and an unfavorable height to the floor of the maxillary sinus. The quality and quantity of the bone determined the choice of the implant with the widest diameter. The primary stability of the "spare" implant was achieved, which was supported by the addition of a bone substitute, due to which loading was delayed for several months.

At the position of the first premolar (region 14), the implant was placed more palatally using the cortical part of the bone, which achieved good primary stability.

In case of loss of frontal teeth caused by trauma, can an implant be inserted and loaded immediately?

It depends on the judgment of an experienced clinician and the extent of the injury. Authors who deal with theoretical education will probably say that it is not possible and that it should not be done. From the point of view of the surgical protocol, such a claim has justification. However, there are situations where the decision is made following the experience of the clinician, and a possible risk can turn into a success. Theoretical propositions are important, but experience and practice dictate that in certain cases they should be supplemented or even changed, especially when it comes to integration processes in bone, where there is still a lot of uncertainty, at least when it comes to oral implantology.

The discovery of the integration of implants and bone, in the 1960s, led to a forced reconsideration of traditional concepts and attitudes about bone wound healing. Before that, it was thought that the body would, over time, reject any foreign body placed through the surface of the epithelium. Rejection would occur because the epithelium lining the foreign body would move apically and completely surround it, so the foreign body would be rejected.

This was also the thinking when it came to dental implants. The epithelium tends to swell, proliferate and to surround and reject the foreign body, because any disruption of the surface of the epithelium causes epithelial growth and its movement around the foreign body. The epithelium continues to expand and proliferate until it comes into contact with epithelial cells on the other side of the foreign body, when its further proliferation is prevented. The discovery of integration processes confirmed that the inert biocompatible material of the implant, when placed through the epithelial wall, does not cause an epithelial reaction as other foreign bodies do. The reason the epithelium does not continue to move apically when it comes into contact with the surface of such a "foreign body" (titanium) remains unclear. Consequently, in the case of traumatic injuries, when it comes to compensation with implants, assessments of the behavior of the epithelium can be variable, depending on the specificity of the case and the probable immunobiological potential of the organism.

Have you ever been in a situation to install an implant and primarily load it, and the attitudes were that you should wait four to six months?

Yes. This question reminds me of the period four decades ago when I had my first implants. There are rules and laws in medicine, and how they will be applied and respected depends on situations, often specific, as well as several other circumstances. In cases where the specific situation is required, an assessment derived from experience is essential, so that risk is replaced by successful predictability. Primary loading was considered a considerable risk. Only Linkov felt that his leaf implants should be loaded after four weeks. I immediately accepted Linkov's advice and all cases would end successfully. There was not much thought about the soft tissues around the implant carrier, and the design of the Link leaf implant part did not allow for the design of the endosseous part, especially in the lateral regions.

However, it happened that I applied immediate loading in an extremely complicated case where implant placement was not advisable, especially primary loading in a highly aesthetic region. Specific circumstances were the determinants for both implantation and primary loading. From the point of view of surgical principles and protocols, such a method was highly risky. However, experience prevailed in assessing the positive outcome of the procedure.

For example?

A 25-year-old female patient lost her central incisor in a traffic accident (Figure 18.80). The patient reported several days after the injury. The patient is an educator who needs daily communication, and the complexity of the treatment was increased by the purchased plane ticket for a trip abroad for ten days.

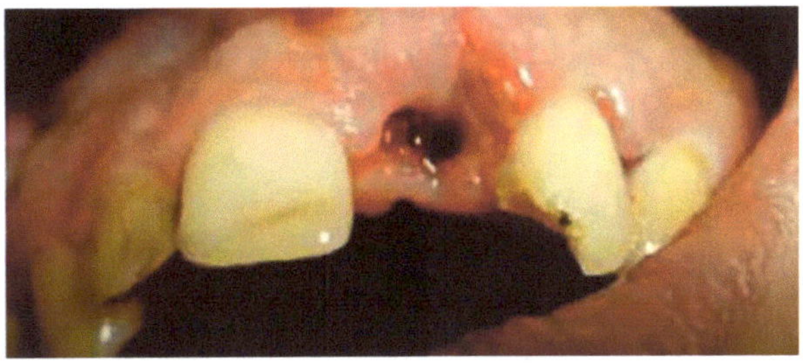

Figure 18.80. Upper left central incisor lost due to traffic trauma, with dislocated fragments.

A typical case where the clinician is faced with numerous dilemmas: how to shorten the treatment time and in what way to do it; how and what kind of provisional restoration to perform and for how long it should be in the mouth, primarily for aesthetic reasons; which final solution is optimal in terms of functional and aesthetic outcome?

Dilemmas:

The conventional procedure of grinding two teeth to compensate for one, has been overcome today by a prosthetic solution. At the same time, the lateral incisor is slightly dislocated due to trauma.

Making an immediate prosthesis ("frogs") in this case, is an impossible solution due to the dislocated fragments. An immediate prosthesis is contraindicated for several reasons: healing of soft tissues would be difficult and worsened, and bone resorption at the site of the lost tooth would be accelerated. It is essential to avoid such a solution, because the contours of the soft tissue surrounding the lost tooth would be completely damaged, especially since they have already suffered partial damage due to trauma.

Before considering which decision should be made, the criteria to be used must be established:

- the absence of fracture of the alveolar process, infection, and pathological inflammatory processes;
- radiographic assessment;
- to determine by preoperative sounding how well the alveolus is preserved, what is the condition of the cortical, labial, and palatal, alveolar bone;

- What are the possibilities for achieving the primary stability of the implant;
- Is the bone fragment mobile and dislocated (if so, how far is it dislocated)?

After consideration of the above criteria, in this particular case, the solution in the form of immediate implantation of the implant (pictures 18.83 18.85.) is justified for the following reasons:

- Healing of soft tissues and bone fragments requires a longer waiting time;
- While waiting for complete healing, implantation also solves a temporary aesthetic problem;
- Since the patient has a protrusion of the upper front with an open bite, there was no occlusal problem;
- immediate implantation activates the physiological function of the bone around the immediately loaded implant, which results in a better density of the newly created bone;
- The healing process will be assisted by guided regeneration of the bone substitutes used on this occasion.

On the radiograph, the bone fragment above the central incisor was not shadowed, and after raising the flap, the fragment was mobile. If this fragment is lost, a large bony defect would be created, which would compromise the aesthetic outcome.

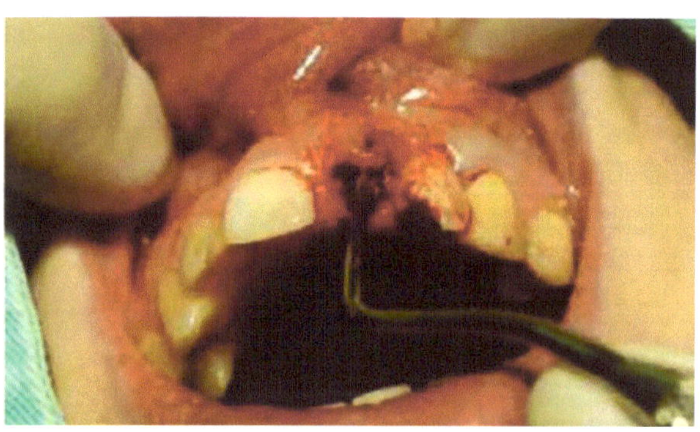

Figure 18.81. Initial situation after trauma and lost tooth, 3 days after the accident.

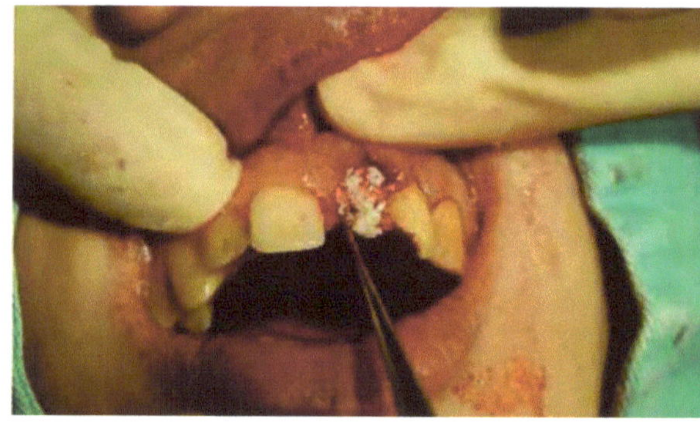

Figure 18.82. The patient's demands to immediately compensate for the lost tooth led to overlooking the objective state of the injury. After preservation of the alveolus, during the attempt to place the bone substitute, the mobility of a larger broken bone fragment was found (which was not clearly visible on the orthopan image), which required more extensive treatment, repositioning of the fragment, fixation with titanium screws and covering with bone substitutes.

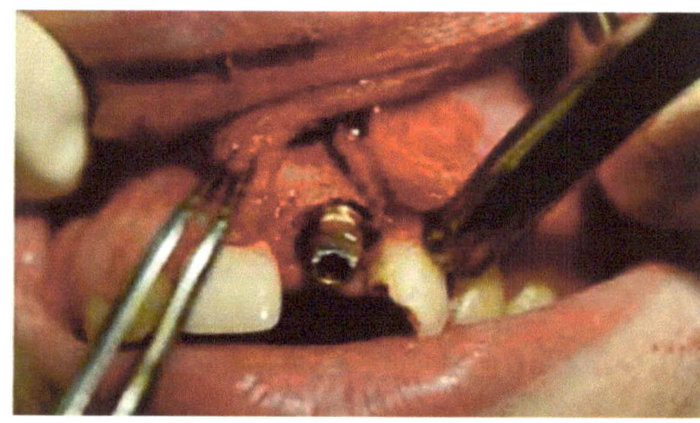

Figure 18.83. The condition immediately after the trauma, the implant was immediately installed.

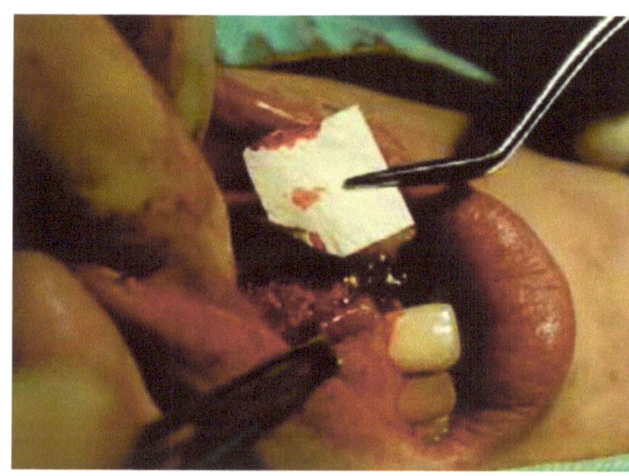

Figure 18.84. Covering the fixed fragment with titanium screws and a mixture of xenogeneic bone substitutes and autologous bone, covered with a collagen resorbable membrane.

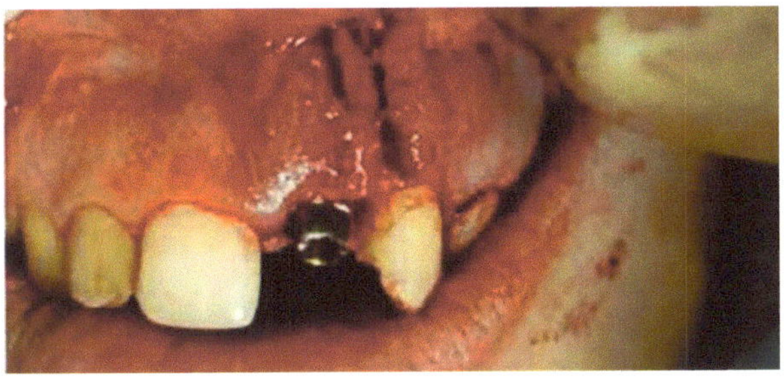

Figure 18.85. Clear dislocation of the bone fragment. Fixation of the fragment with titanium screws, placement of a mixture of xenogeneic bone substitutes with autologous bone chips covered with a resorbable membrane.

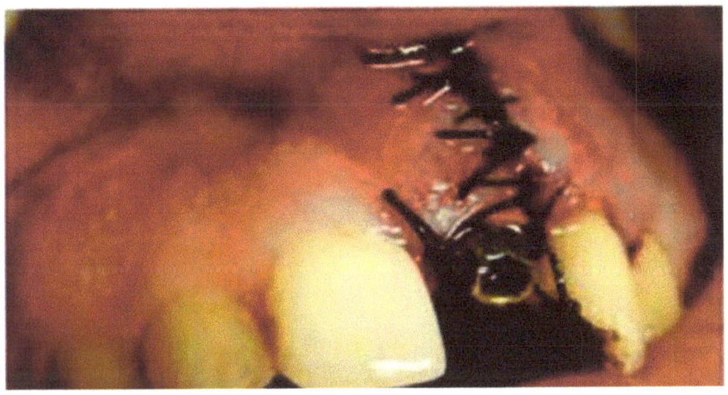

Figure 18.86. Stitched wound after immediate implant placement.

Conclusion:

Aesthetics in the frontal region of the upper jaw play an important role in making a decision. Of course, implant placement in a well-healed wound would be more precise and simpler. But, it turns out to be a big problem: to compensate for tooth loss with provisional work for a longer period of time needed for bony healing and soft tissue healing, without jeopardizing these processes? The protrusion of the frontal teeth was in favor of the selected and timely prosthetic rehabilitation procedure (Fig. 18.83).

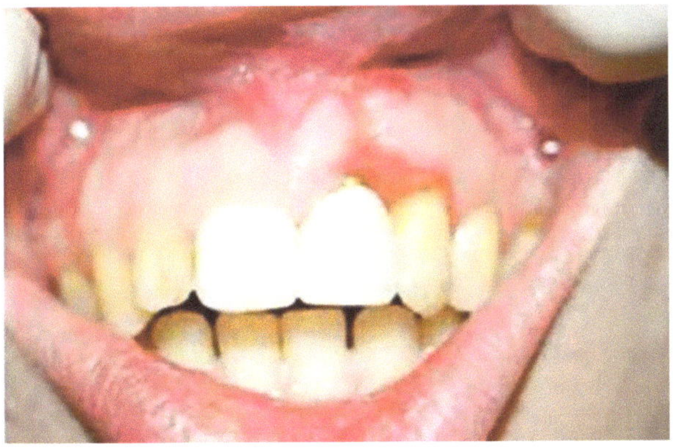

Figure 18.87. Condition after six weeks with a temporary crown.

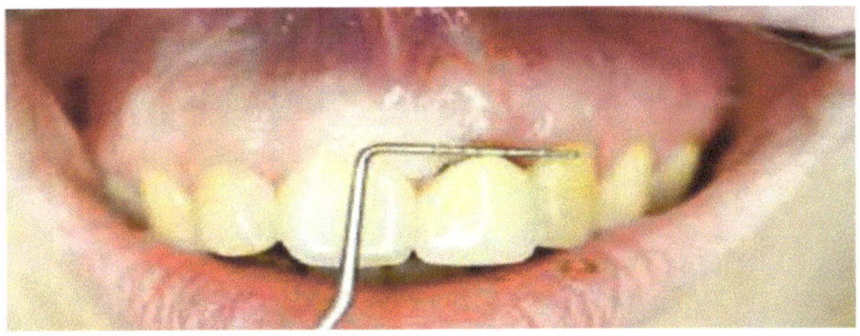

Figure 18.88. Condition after 6 weeks. Satisfactory stability of the immediately loaded implant. Soft tissue reconstruction with a subepithelial connective tissue graft is required.

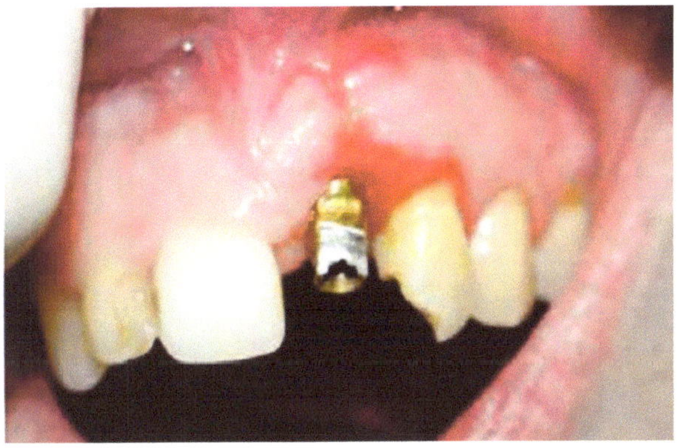

Figure 18.89. By adapting the edge of the provisional crown, it is necessary to shape the gingival edge.

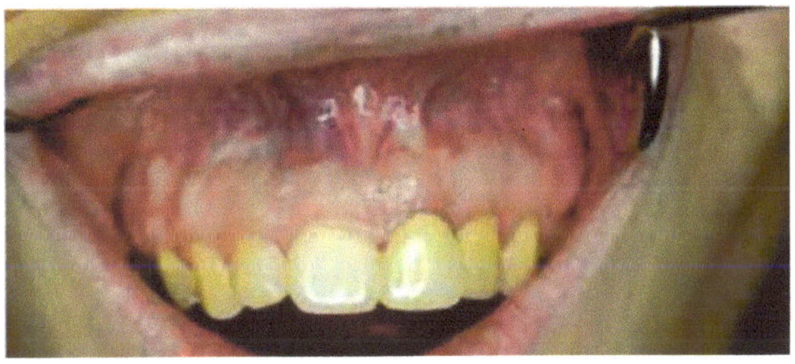

Figure 18.90. Appearance 12 months after injury and immediate implant placement. Mucogingival surgery with a subepithelial connective tissue graft significantly improved the appearance of the soft tissue.

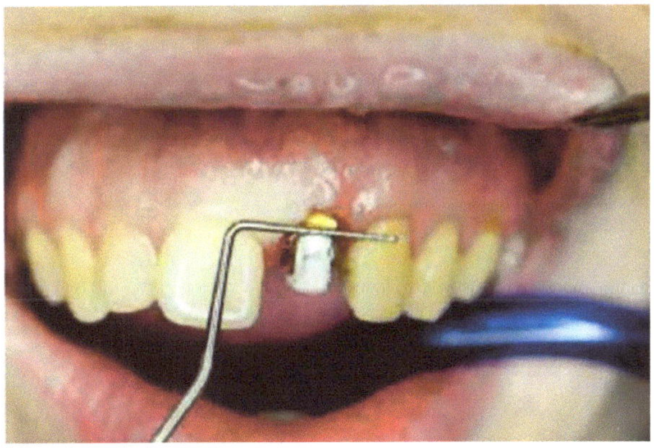

Figure 18.91. Condition after 12 months of reconstructed papilla. Gingival correction needed.

What should be paid attention to when planning the entire treatment in similar cases?

Good planning is considered an important phase of implant-prosthetic treatment. As seen from the previous case, the clinician finds himself in a dilemma as to which procedure to apply for the outcome to be successful. In practice, planning is most often done using routine, classic diagnostic methods. Any superficiality in this, the most important, phase is paid too dearly by compromising the results and mistreating the patient.

In the presented case, there were special aggravating circumstances after a traffic accident, where a tooth was lost. The patient had bought a plane ticket for an urgent trip abroad. Application of a movable acrylate immediate prosthesis (so-called "frogs") would cause compression trauma to the soft tissues, and thus to the complete augmentation procedure: to the bone fragment, filled with a mixture of collagen substitutes for bone and autologous bone sawdust, covered with a collagen resorptive membrane. A special circumstance is that the patient did not want to travel abroad without teeth at any cost. Taking into account the time that has passed since the injury (she reported on the fifth day) and the real state of the trauma, with the additional persistent demands of the patient, in addition to a well-thought-out treatment plan, it was necessary to have the courage to accept such a risky case. The reason for acceptance was to help the patient. The final result after 24 months confirmed that both the plan and the achieved implant-prosthetic treatment were correct.

In similar cases, you should not regret the time spent analyzing each case separately and very thoroughly. In the presented case, computed tomography of the cross-section of the traumatized segment and the density of the palatal compact cortical bone significantly facilitated the adoption of a therapy plan and treatment decision. During the treatment of the presented case, each stage of the procedure was controlled with a retroalveolar digital sensor (Figure 18.93).

Today, there are great opportunities for good diagnostics, which makes it possible to plan the best solution. The application of a digital intraoral sensor (RVG recordings), as a first step, is a very reliable aid. Also, three-dimensional (3D) radiographic analyses provide great relief in planning. It can happen that even with 3D analysis, during an oral surgical procedure, one unexpectedly encounters disadvantages that are not fully understood and predicted in the radiographic analysis.

It happens during the tomographic analysis of the alveolar ridge that the results of the section size do not correspond to the condition in the mouth. The unreliability of the obtained results is most often a consequence of outdated equipment, poor positioning of the patient, and the like. Because of such mistakes, the therapist unexpectedly finds himself in front of minor or major pitfalls.

In the future, we should expect a significant improvement in these technologies, which are still at a very high-level today. When planning, maximum caution is required in every case! It may happen that even after a detailed analysis and diagnosis, only by lifting the flap, it is concluded that it is not advisable to enter into a risky adventure in this specific case, even though all analyzed parameters pointed to a safe installation of the implant.

However, recently, the possibility of 3D imaging, with an additional image of the existing condition in the oral cavity, greatly facilitates the planning of the entire procedure.

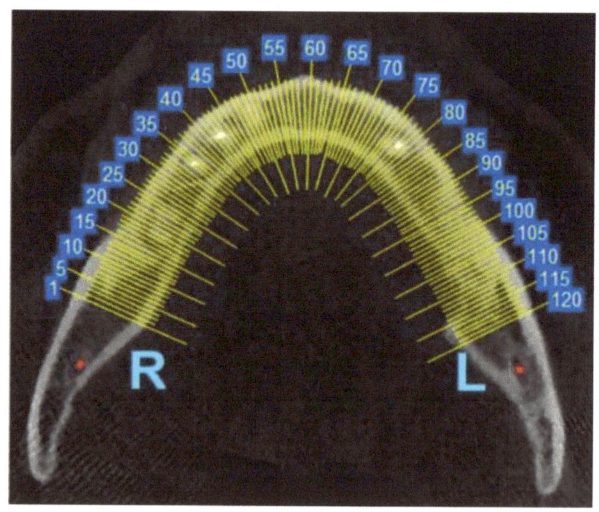

Figure 18.92. Tomographic sections of the segments make it much easier to plan the installation of implants.

Does it really happen that after 3D orthopan tomographic findings, by raising the flap, a deviation from the actual condition in the mouth is noted?

Yes. And there are several reasons for this: the quality and age of the equipment, the patient's positioning, the angle of the mandible and maxilla, the skills and experience of the X-ray technician, and more. Today, intraoral digital sensors (RVG technology, etc. 18.93.) provide considerable relief and check the course of implant installation.

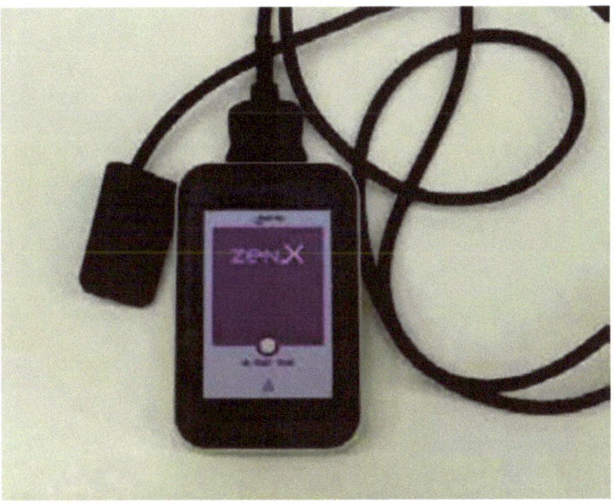

Figure 18.93. RVG technology significantly ensures the safety of implant placement during surgery.

An X-ray can be obtained by chemically developing and fixing the film or directly on the screen. The new generation of portable x-ray devices (ADX 400 Portable X-ray) enables viewing of the image immediately on the display, and more detailed answers to this question can be found in the chapter "The future of diagnostics in oral implantology".

How were implants installed in the past when there were no modern aids?

In the past, there was no predicting the outcome, and the results depended on the experience and skill of the practicing dentist. We acted exactly as they did in the world, we did not change the existing protocols of the then range of oral implantology. At the beginning of the installation of the first implants, there were only a few techniques, which is incomparable compared to today's scope and condition. The safe installation of the implant required good knowledge and mastery of the available technique prescribed by its creator. The doctor had to unconditionally comply with all the procedures and specifics of that technique. Even today, the application of each technique has details that must be strictly observed during implant placement. Each surgical technique has details that distinguish it from another. Those details are very important to ensure the conditions for good primary stability of the implant and bony integration, as well as the formation and healing of soft tissues around the neck of the implant, in the surgical phase of the work. In that phase of the work, there is a basic principle and law: during the preparation of the implant bed, the surgical procedure must be performed with minimal trauma to the surrounding bone, as well as to the soft tissues!

When you look at the past several decades, what and how was it done and what was installed? What does it look like from this time distance?

Very often I like to look at many of my works (on the next 15 or so pictures), I often wonder where the pioneers of oral implantology got so much courage to embark on many adventures by installing various implant systems, which are unproven in practice? A particularly aggravating circumstance was the imperfection of radiology and the ambiguity of the orthopan panoramic image.

What was the most perfect implant system that was applied at the time?

Of course, at that time subperiosteal implants were in the first place, but also the application of the so-called Combi implants, which was an attempt to combine subperiosteal and endosseous implants (Figures 18.94 and 18.95). With that implant, everything was missed, from the material (tantalum) to the execution, the part that lies in the bone and the part that rests on the periosteum. It must be said that tantalum was not a failure from the material aspect, but from the mouth manipulation aspect, due to excessive stiffness, it was.

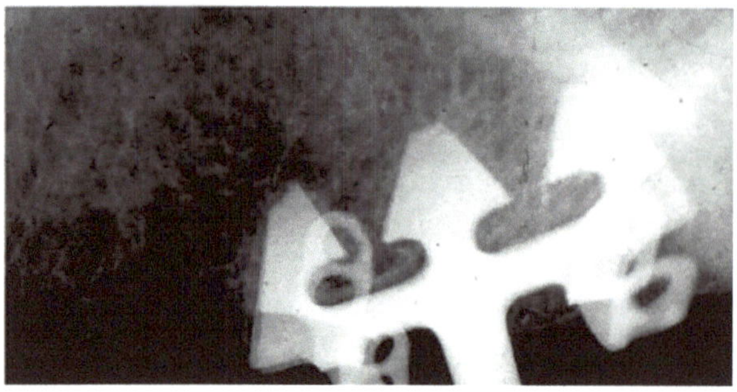

Figure 18.94. The development of oral implantology was full of many failures, and one of them was the use of Combi implants with subperiosteal wings.

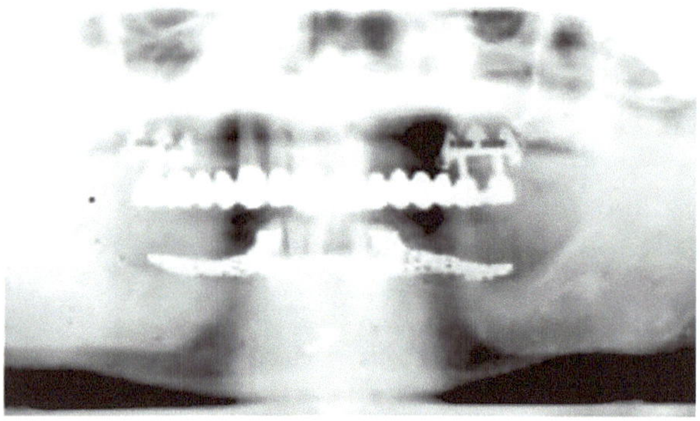

Figure 18.95. Heinrich's Combi implant with removed subperiosteal flaps, according to the author's idea. Regardless of this "improvement," the design of this implant was destructive to the bone.

Do all implants installed several decades ago deserve a negative rating?

Some implants, such as Tramonte's implant, should not be evaluated strictly even today. Such implants were kept in the mouth for years, and some of them last even today (Fig. 18.96).

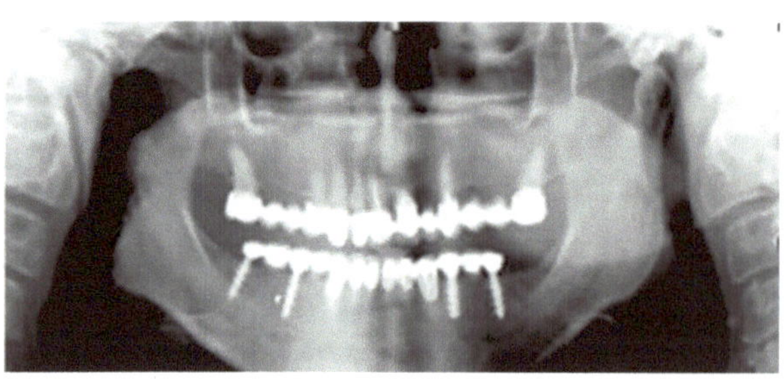

Figure 18.96. Tramonte's implants are still in the mouths of many patients after 18 years. The detail of this abandoned and outdated implant served as a guide to the design of the most modern forms of implants to achieve primary stability. The latest designs of many implant systems are based on Tramonti's idea.

When was the first time you saw an implant being installed by others and what impression did you get?

For the first time in Switzerland, Dr. Otto Buhler invited me to assist him in the installation of needle implants in order to stabilize the lower total prosthesis. It was the first attempt to stabilize a lower total prosthesis outside of standard methods in Switzerland. I tried to solve only a few cases of total prosthesis stabilization in this way, shown in pictures 18.97, 18.98, 18.99. and 18,100.

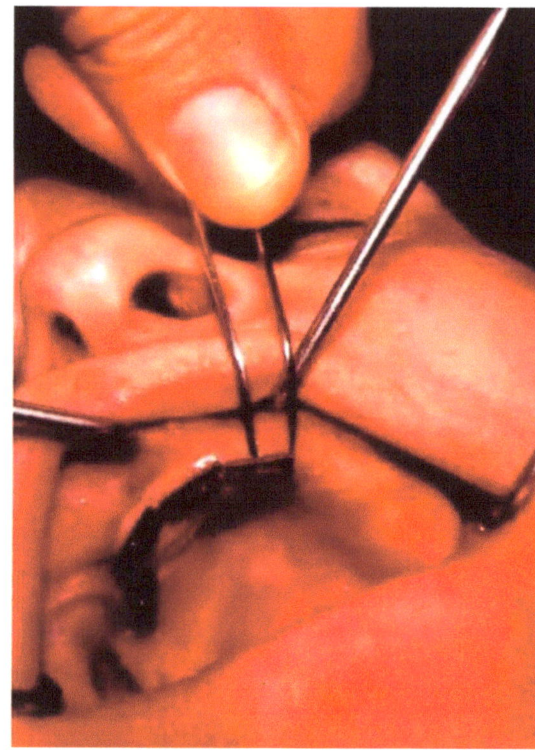

Figure 18.97. At the end of the sixties of the last century, by inserting needle-like tantalum implants connected by a metal arch with riders and grippers in the acrylate part of the prosthesis, the acrylate part of the prosthesis covering the palate could be shortened.

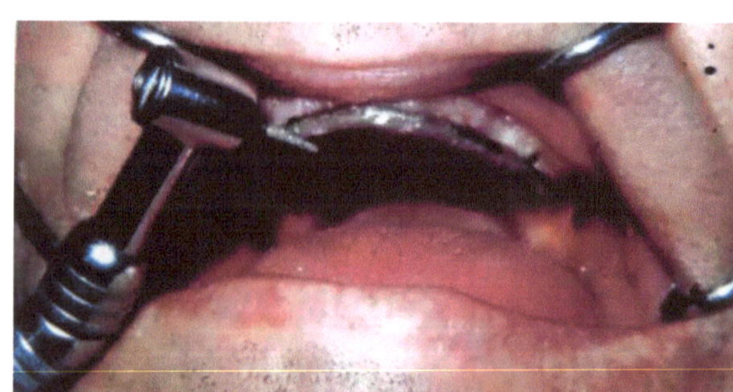

Figure 18.98. Insertion of needle implants was transmucosal. The implants are joined with a special apparatus for cold soldering in the mouth.

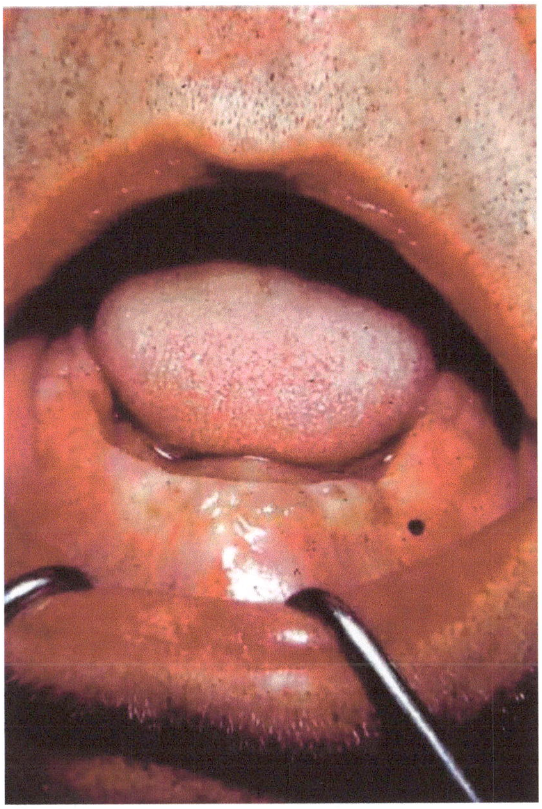

Figure 18.99. Despite the wide ridges, the prostheses were unstable. These are the initial "acrobations" of the author in the early seventies, when similar cases were dominated by subperiosteal implants. An attempt to fix the lower total prosthesis with endosseous needle implants.

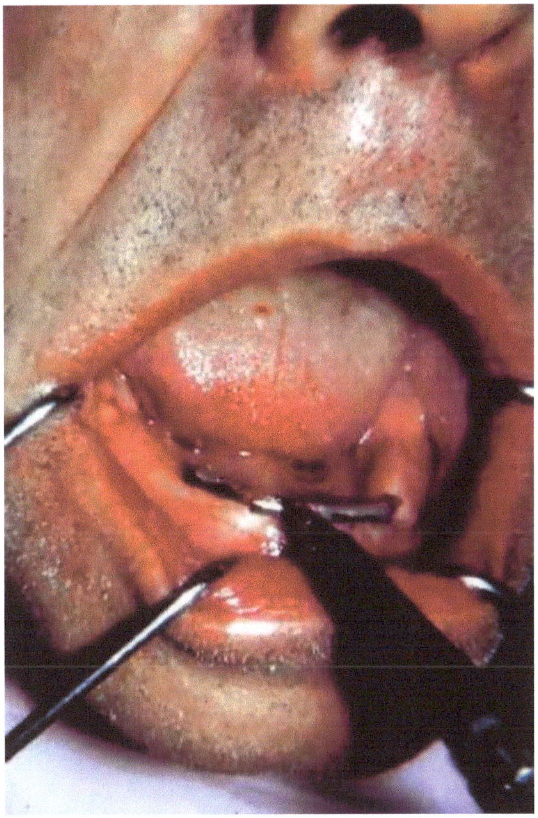

Figure 18.100. An attempt to remove the acrylate part of the total denture covering the palate and to stabilize the lower total denture with the patient's consent, the attempt satisfied the patient. Presenting the case at a local gathering in the canton of Ticino (Switzerland), colleagues laughed at this fabrication by fellow Swiss Otto Biller and the author of the book. At that time, few people thought of inserting a foreign body into a healthy bone. Pruin's needle-like tantalum implants were used, which were connected to an adaptable soft gold structure with riders. Laboratory-made gold riders are attached to the acrylic base of the lower total denture, shown in the picture. Such and similar interventions were the first steps in practical oral implantology, according to the idea; if we decide on a path, be it one long or a million steps, the most important is the first step, so that the journey begins.

Who are the youngest and oldest patients you have implanted?

The youngest patient was an eighteen-year-old girl from Dubrovnik who lost her right central incisor in the upper jaw due to trauma (Figure 18.101). A one-piece leaf implant was inserted (Figures 18.102 and 18.103). And the oldest patient who sat on my chair with implants was an almost hundred-year-old "well-behaved" and able-bodied Austrian woman.

It was fitted with Linkov-foliate tuber-implants on which Ackerman crossbars with riders were placed on which the prosthesis was retained (Fig. 18.105).

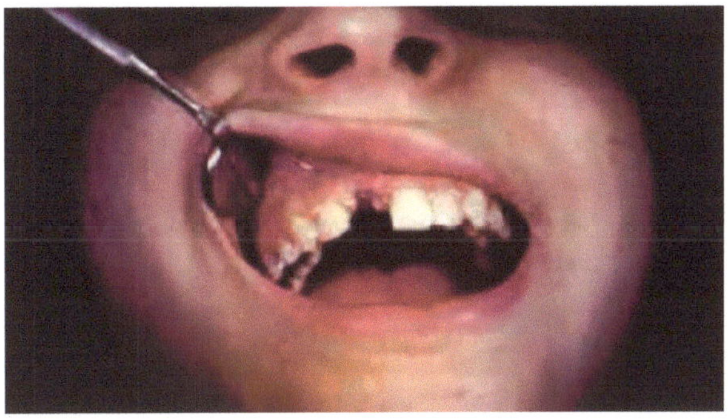

Figure 18.101. The right upper central incisor of an eighteen-year-old girl was lost due to trauma in the late seventies of the last century.

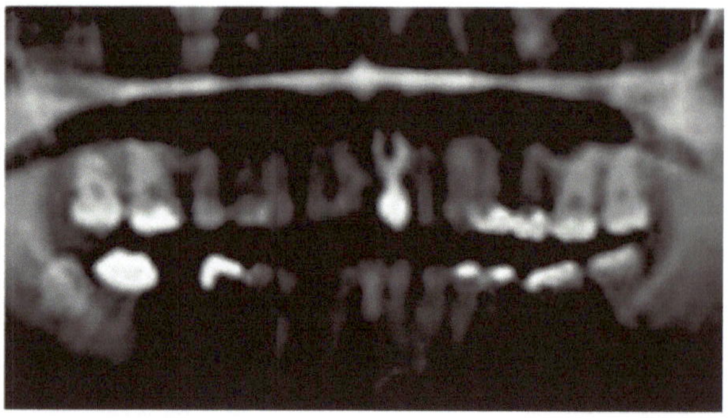

Figure 18.102. Leaf implant in the area of the central incisor. At that time, the author owned only a leaf implant designed for indications in the frontal part of the upper and lower jaw.

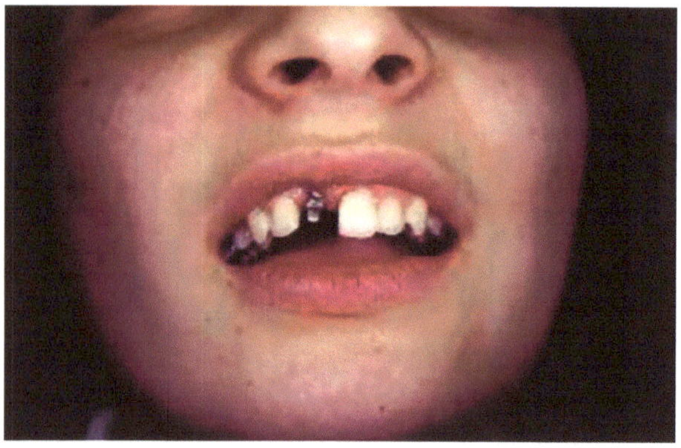

Figure 18.103. The appearance of the support of the one-piece leaf Linkov implant, which was not adapted to the shape of the soft tissues. This presentation confirms the lightning-fast development of oral implantology, in which way the oral surgical procedure of installing an implant with a design close to the root of a natural tooth is performed today.

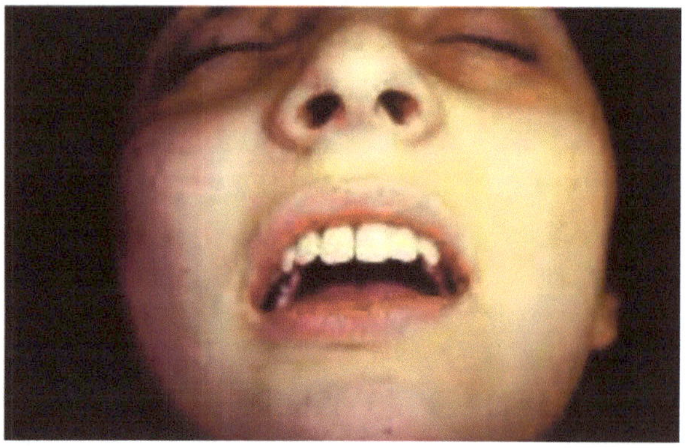

Figure 18.104. Definitive appearance of a crown on a one-piece embedded Linkov-leaf implant (Cavtat, 1977).

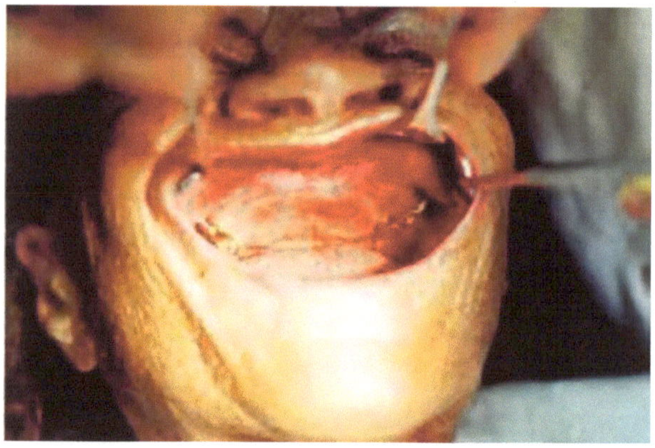

Figure 18.105. The biggest implantology "acrobatics" in the author's career, implanted leaf implants with two supports, between which an Ackerman retention bar was placed, in an almost hundred-year-old (96-year-old) patient from Vienna. The frontal part of the alveolar ridge does not exist. At the follow-up examination after two years, the patient was delighted because the prosthesis did not fly out of her mouth when speaking.

How do you look at all that today?

It may be funny; nevertheless, it remains memorable. From this time distance, I think about youthful enthusiasm and enthusiasm on the one hand, but also courage and craziness on the other. But it is somewhat justified by the saying that God helps the brave. Nevertheless, such "craziness" from the past, in a way, is a contribution to the development of oral implantology, forcing others to gather courage and start using implants. During that time, there were a lot of bright moments.

For example, in the case of an 18-year-old girl (picture 18.104), who lost her upper right central incisor due to trauma, avoiding the grinding of two healthy teeth or wearing a partial denture, installing an implant is the optimal solution even from today's point of view. As far as I am informed, even today, at the time of writing this book, that implant is in the mouth of that "girl", even though it was implanted almost thirty years ago.

How do you look at Tramonte's implant today and how do you explain the long-term "stay" of that implant in the bone?

The longevity of the Tramont implant in the bone aroused the interest of modern manufacturers to analyze the properties of this implant. It is considered that the greatest merits for longevity are the threads (which is copied in modern implants, of course processed with the latest technologies). Even today, special importance is attached to threads from the aspect of self-threading, biomechanical events and bone-integration processes (Figures 18.106 and 18.107).

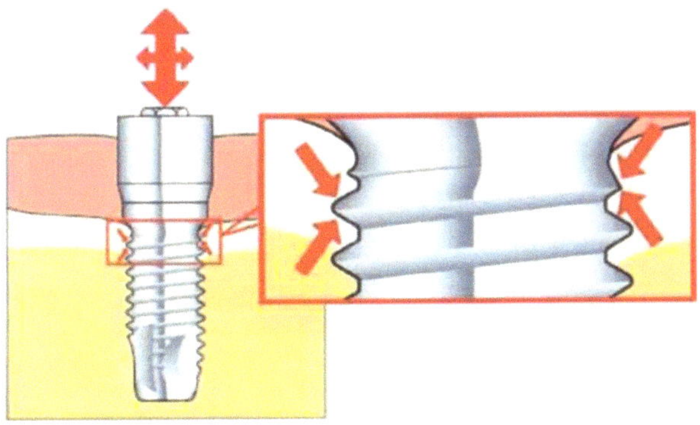

Figure 18.106. Axial forces are evenly received by the implant via the thread. The forces are evenly distributed. The highest stress of occlusal forces is received by the first thread.

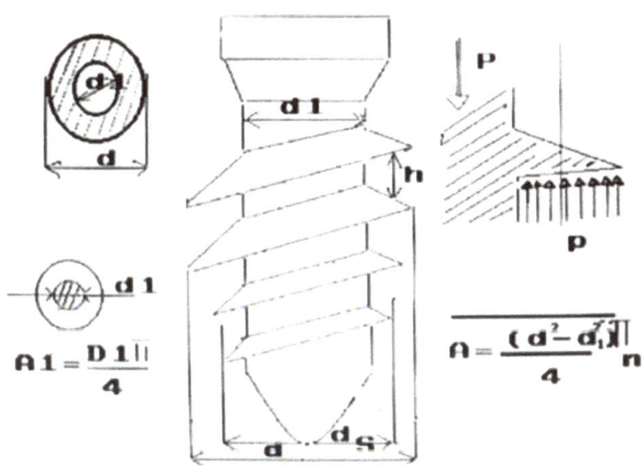

Figure 18.107. The reception and distribution of forces depends on several factors: the diameter and design of the neck, the position and angle of inclination of the threads, the length of the implant, the quality of the material and the treatment of the surface of the implant (from a lecture by the author of the book, Bologna, Italy 1984).

What set Tramonte's implant apart from others at that time was the minimal thermal aggression to the bone during carving. The threads of Tramonte's implants had their own course of easy cutting into the bone, and this is the most important characteristic of the most modern implants. Statistical data show that the failure of these implants was minimal compared to others that were applied during that period. My experience and the experience of other implantologists confirms this fact.

Which implants were installed almost from the eighties to the nineties of the last century?

The answer to this question is best explained in Figure 18.110. until 18,115.

More modern implant systems, compared to the ones shown, have been significantly improved: firstly, in design by imitation of natural roots, quality of materials, technological processing, and implantation procedure, with X-ray computerized diagnostics, which shows that progress is imminent. This progress enabled easier and more precise planning and installation of implants with significantly reduced trauma to the bone and surrounding tissues. Of course, thanks to these benefits, the percentage of success has also increased.

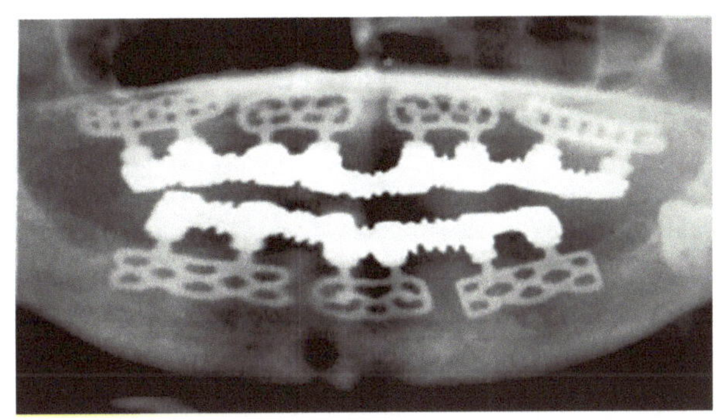

Figure 18.108. Restoration of total edentulism with leaf implants. The work of the author in 1980.

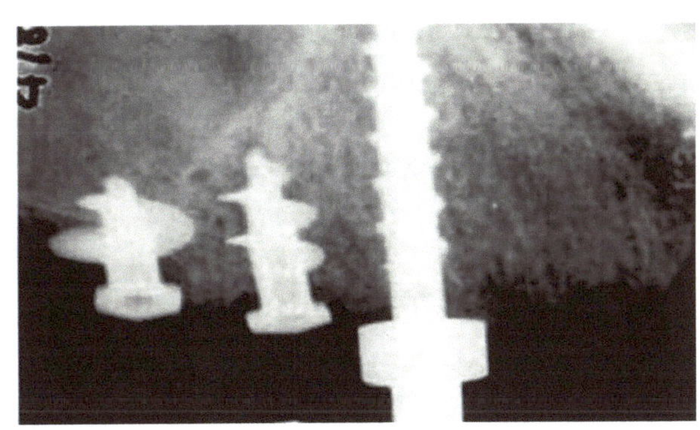

Figure 18.109. A combination of Muratori and Pasqualini implant screws.

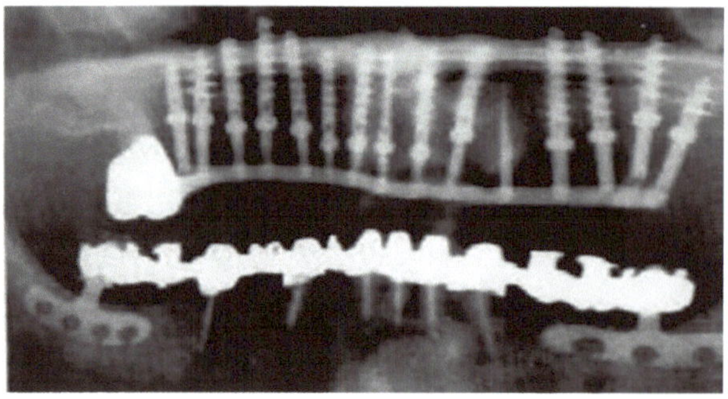

Figure 18.110. Combination of the first generation of open Link implants and cortical screw implants. All these implants had an aggressive thread, due to which they easily self-etched into the bone. A typical example of wandering and changing attitudes in oral implantology.

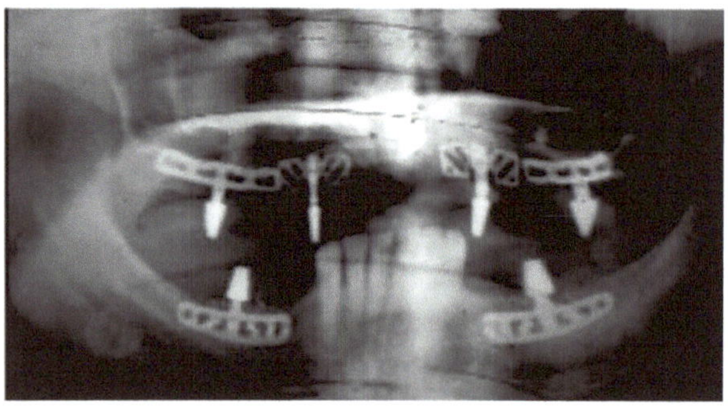

Figure 18.111. X-ray view of the position and shape of the closed leaf implants "V generation" whose surface is coated with "titanium plasma. Used bone substitute (Interpore). The work of the author in 1978.

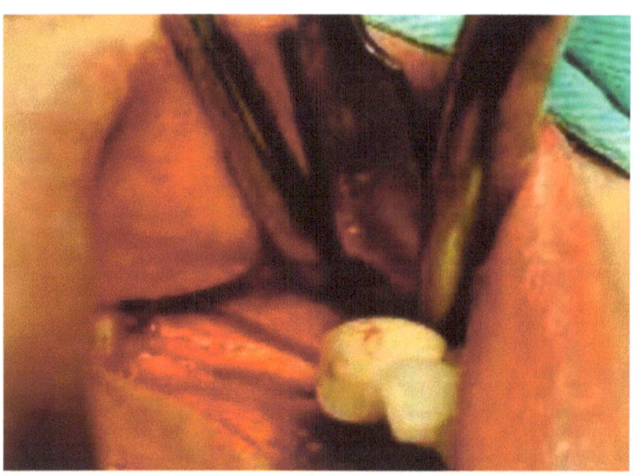

Figure 18.112. The preparation of the bed for the leaf implant was an extremely aggressive and risky phase of implant placement. Using inadequate instruments, there was a risk of injury to the surrounding tissues.

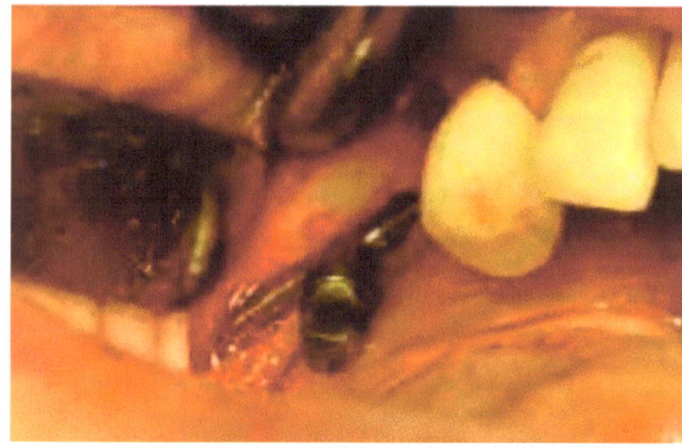

Figure 18.113. Insertion of the leaf implant into the implant bed was performed with aggressive rotary cutters and tapping.

What are the most common reasons for failure today?

Frequent failures can be caused already in the first stage of implantation by mechanical and thermal aggression on the bone. If the traumatic aggression on the bone is less, the bone damage is less, which improves all the conditions for bone regeneration and bone integration with the implant to be fast and complete. One of the most common reasons for premature implant loss is surgical trauma, that is, overheating of the bone due to an inappropriate number of revolutions of the drill and insufficient cooling with saline solution. Thermal trauma to the bone is also supported by the use of low-quality and dull drills. Damaged soft tissues are much easier and faster to regenerate than damaged bone. It should be emphasized that, for commercial reasons, to sell as many implants as possible, the representatives of certain companies borrow a surgical set (which circulates from office to office), which increases the wear and tear of the driller. Dull drills are the most common cause of bone overheating. Often, due to the short time for sterilization, such sets are not even sterile. A prerequisite for the successful application of a certain surgical technique is a well-coordinated team that knows all the details of a certain surgical technique, with strict adherence to the protocol of the entire treatment.

Failure can most often be caused by the choice of low-quality implants, which are not made of titanium type 4. Then, biomechanical reasons, poorly performed prosthetic work on implants, and occlusal and gnathological problems are frequent causes of implant loss. Of course, failure can be contributed to the patient himself, with poor oral hygiene and excessive smoking.

What makes implantation easier, less complicated, more precise today; how much does it depend on the implant technique and how to choose it?

You should choose only reputable manufacturers. The simpler the implant technique, the easier it is to apply. A little more than a decade ago, the first book was published in which the characteristics of all implant techniques available at the time were described (Orale Implatologie: A. Schroeder, F. Sutter, G. Krekeler. 1988). The author applied most of those techniques in his practice, not so much out of necessity, but out of curiosity, to learn the advantages of one technique over another. In truth, the offer of implant systems compared to today's was incomparably more modest.

Today, the situation has completely changed. Due to the great pressure of the implant manufacturing industry, it would not make sense to write such a book because it would have to be printed as a new edition, as it were, every month.

This fact is confirmed by the following example: the largest trade fair (IDS) in the world, which is held every other year in Cologne (Germany), is a place where you can get to know the latest and most modern achievements in the development of all dental techniques and technologies, starting with new materials and equipment, to the latest achievements in diagnostic aids in endodontics, jaw orthopedics, oral surgery, prosthetics and other branches of dentistry.

Three decades ago, there was not a single stand dedicated to implantology at that fair; in the following years, only a few stands were dedicated to implantology. At the last fair in Cologne (held in March 2017), it can be safely said that the subject of implantology was convincingly in the first place: about 70% of the stands were dedicated to implantology. Many implant manufacturers on the market were not represented at the fair. It should be emphasized that in Germany alone there are ten regular monthly magazines dedicated to oral implantology, and the number of millions of installed implants is reliably mentioned.

For example, Italy is one of the countries with the most implant factories. At the fair in Cologne, it was not represented in the scope of the implant systems it offers to the market. South Korea is among the world's most important manufacturers of implants. Several of its factories are exclusively engaged in the production of plagiarism. Such plagiarisms, on the market, are more competitive only in price, but not in quality. A little more than ten years ago, the Chinese launched their implant, calling it the "Bam-implant". This implant was heralded as a hit in implantology because the surface was coated with hydroxyapatite. After some time, however, the separation of hydroxyapatite from the titanium surface occurred, manifesting itself in the appearance of peri-implantitis with abundant granulations. After removing the granulations and filling the defect with bone substitutes, with the use of resorptive membranes, the bone-titanium connection was restored. This problem is given special consideration in the chapter on osseous integration (see Chapter 7).

The momentum of the development of oral implantology is shown by the following example: not so long ago, the use of implants in jaw orthopedics was unimaginable. Meanwhile, in Cologne, at the manifestation of the most modern achievements in dentistry in 2017, a large part of the exhibition space was dedicated to the application of implants in jaw orthopedics, which clearly shows that implantology is also becoming a part of modern orthodontics.

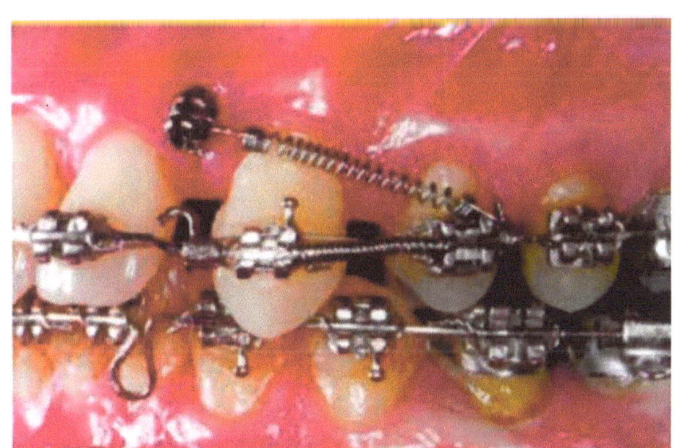

Figure 18.114. Application of one-piece implants as an abutment in orthodontic therapy.

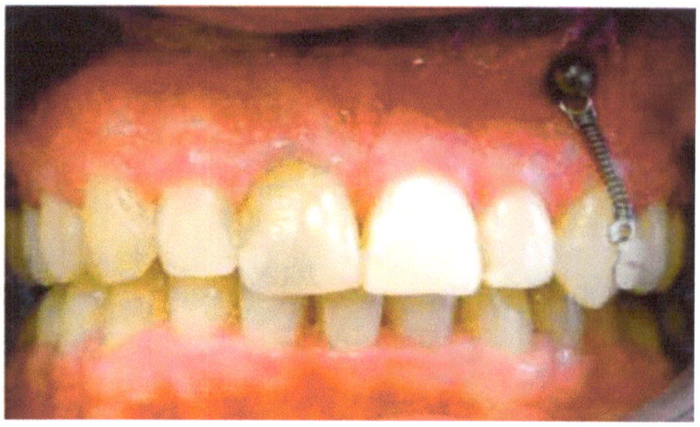

Figure 18.115. Presentation of the application of implants as an abutment in orthodontics.

Has the application of implants in jaw orthopedics moved the limit of implant application, when it comes to age, and above all, the application of implants at the age before 18 years of age?

Until recently, the answers to questions from and up to what age of life that implants can be inserted were that before the age of 18, the use of implants is contraindicated. A separate chapter in this book is devoted to the latest understanding of changing restrictions at younger ages. (Application of implants in children and developing persons).

When it comes to the application of implants in orthodontics, how much is the effect of chewing forces on the implant itself?

When the implant is used as an abutment in orthodontics, the forces of action are of a different direction than the forces that act on the implant during chewing.

In addition to the aforementioned recommendations for the success of the entire implant application procedure, a very important requirement is a good knowledge of biomechanical events in the oral cavity. The forces acting on the implant are very important for the long-term survival of the implant in the bone. For oral implantology, biomechanics in the oral cavity encompasses much more than the concepts of implant loosening and the comfort of wearing an implant-anchored restoration. An implant in jaw orthopedics serves as a support for moving not only one tooth, but a whole row. In orthodontic treatment, these forces, especially traction with shear stresses, are not small. When applying implants in orthodontics, a constant dilemma has been resolved: whether the implant should be loaded immediately or wait. However, there is still not enough bibliographic data when it comes to the application of implants in jaw orthopedics.

How much does the application of implants in orthodontics contribute to the attitude of justification of immediate load?

The experience of many implantologists and the author says that in many cases where the implants were loaded, the immediate outcome was successful. Experience confirms that immediate loading shows better and faster integration processes than is the case with implants that are not immediately loaded.

Of course, the experience of the implantologist is crucial in the assessment: first, in achieving maximum primary stability, with a previous assessment of bone condition, quality and quantity. In the book, attention is paid to the author's position on the justification of immediate burden in several places.

The benefits of implants in orthodontics can only exist if the planned implant is well integrated and only as such can correspond to the orthodontic treatment goals.

Practice has confirmed that the action of forces within physiological limits is manifested by stimulation of osteoblasts, and rapid remodeling of trabeculae, and deposition of new bone. The effect of these forces is attributed to the thickening of the new compact bone tissue around the implant, and over time the bond between the bone and the surface of the implant becomes more and more intimate, and the implant is more and more solid. This process, when the implant is completely integrated with the surrounding bone, is determined as achieved bone integration.

Will science have to provide additional explanations and answers to the mechanism of stimulation of the creation of novelty around the dental implant? Is the mechanism of stimulation of new bone formation around the implant with immediate loading completely clarified?

Recently, increasing importance has been attached to the processing of osseoinductive surfaces of implants, the so-called. nanoosteoinductive implant surfaces. Implant surfaces are processed by applying nano millimicron deposits of crystalline calcium phosphate particles. It has been shown that the bone should be put into physiological activity as soon as possible, which accelerates physiological processes, and activates osteoblasts and vitreous, with better blood circulation in the milieu around the implant. This is achieved by loading the bone within physiological limits. In modern orthopedic surgery, patients are mobilized much earlier after surgery and implant placement (knee or hip replacement), to stimulate metabolism in the injured area. Research has shown that after a fracture, callus formation is faster and of better quality if the part affected by the trauma is activated. These studies and experiences are in favor of early postoperative loading of implants

How much space in the literature is devoted to early postoperative stress?

Several books have even been written about it. A group of authors (Matteo Chiapasco, Claudio Gatti, Jan Gottlow, Anna Karin Lundgern, Paulo Malo, Neil Meredith, Giovanni Polizzi, and Lars Sennerby), based on long-term studies on the benefits of early post-operative loading, wrote the book "Bone integration and immediate loading biological basis and clinical applications" (Oseointegratione e carico immediato. Fundamento biologici e applicazione cliniche. Carl Misch calls early loading progressive (Contemporary Implant Dentistry, Mosby, 1993.) The scientific basis for these studies also gave Claudio Gatti. Enriched with knowledge and scientific evidence, my personal experience has shown that the immediate load is justified It is necessary to use implants with wide diameters if there is enough bone in the horizontal direction, since good primary stability is often not achieved. Such implants should not be used as immediate support for provisional prosthetic work. Most often, in such cases, the lateral bony walls should be increased by augmentation, and then delayed loading is justified.

How much and when is the clinical application of thin implants and their early loading justified?

A narrow alveolar ridge, its shape, horizontal and vertical dimensions, and the quality and arrangement of the spongiosa and the compact, are conditions that indicate the choice of an implant. In patients where the width of the alveolar ridge in the platform (favorable bone width) is in the range of 3 to 4 mm and case of greater bone loss, the width in the crestal part usually ranges from 1.5 mm to 2 mm. Then, for a possible solution, there are two choices:

The first is to create favorable conditions for the installation of implants of standard diameters by augmentation, which significantly extends the treatment time and increases the price. The quality of augmentation and the healing time depend on how it will be performed: whether with autogenous grafts, or bone substitutes, or a combination of both (Figures 18.117 and 18.118).

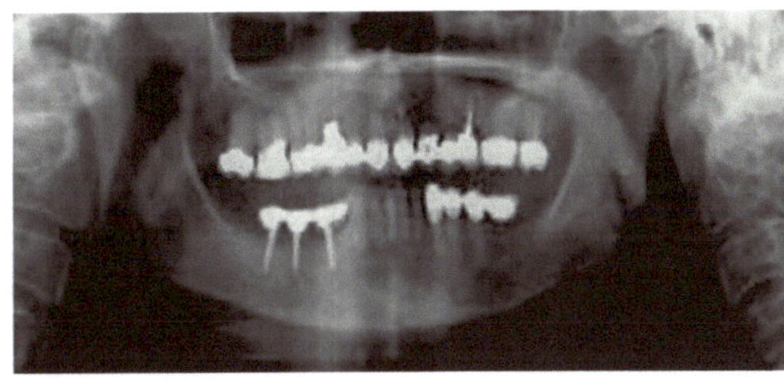

Figure 18.116. Narrow-diameter implants (diameter 3mm) embedded in an extremely narrow alveolar ridge. Condition after 10 years.

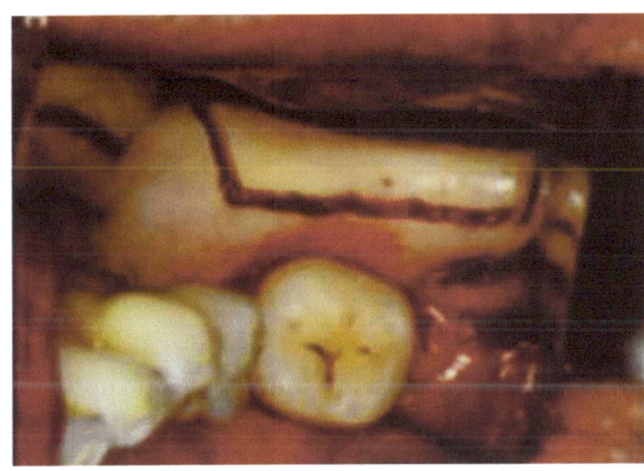

Figure 18.117. Preparation for taking an autogenous bone block graft for augmentation.

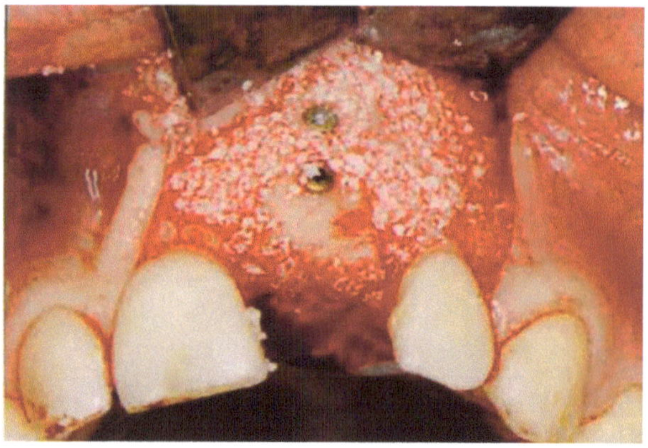

Figure 18.118. Autogenous bone graft attached with titanium screws to bone, with added xenogeneic bone substitute. A case of presented traumatic tooth loss.

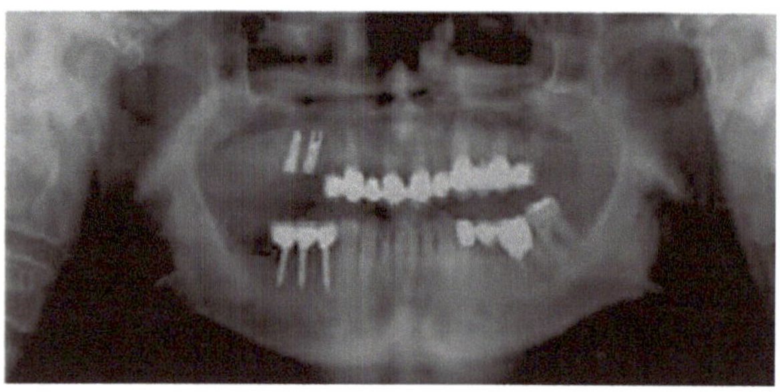

Figure 18.119. The application of thin implants for fixed restorations is conditioned by two factors: alveolar bone insufficiency and the patient's finances (if extensive augmentation is to be performed). Implants of standard diameters are installed in the upper jaw by raising the sinus floor.

Another choice is the installation of thin implants with a width of 2.4 mm to 3 mm. In cases where there is a sharp, narrow, and high alveolar ridge of insufficient width, the installation of a thin implant with a diameter of 2.5 mm has proven to be justified in practice, especially if the maximum height of the ridge, i.e. the maximum length of the implant, can be used. The length of one-piece implants is very important. For this reason, there are no one-piece narrow implants shorter than 10 mm. Application of narrow implants is possible for quick solutions, with immediate loading (Figures 18.120 and 18.121).

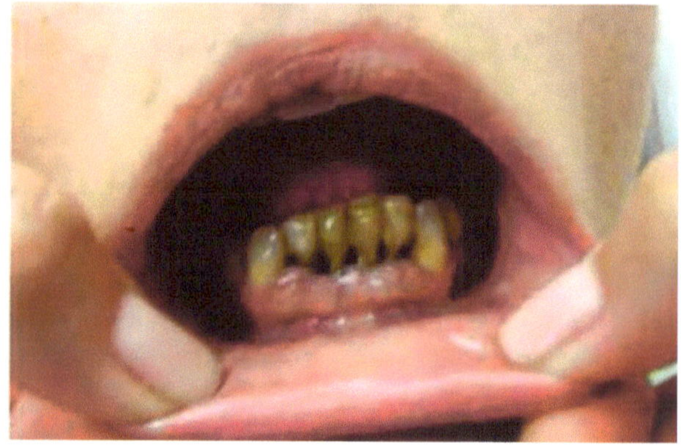

Figure 18.120. Clinical appearance of the gingiva in the frontal region of the lower jaw, active periodontal pockets with a predominance of inflammation of the productive-exudative type.

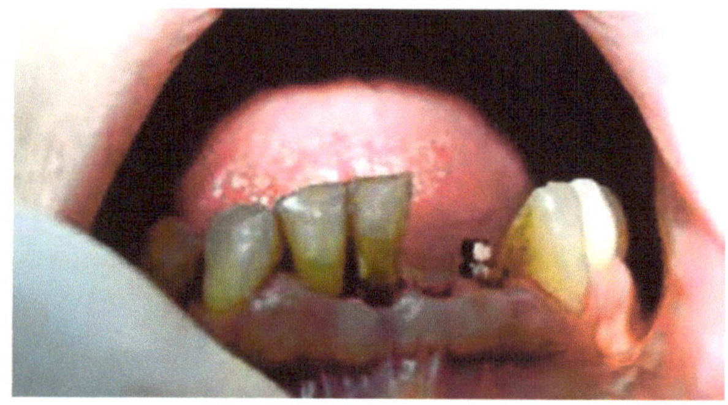

Figure 18.121. Simultaneous extraction of teeth and installation of narrow-diameter implants.

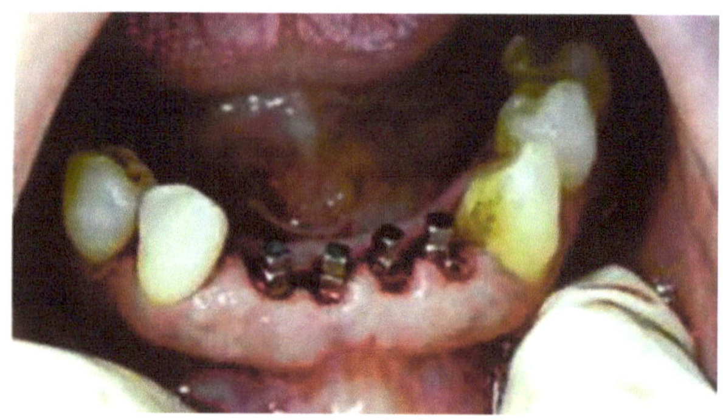

Figure 18.122. Embedded NDI (Narrow Diameter Implants) implants.

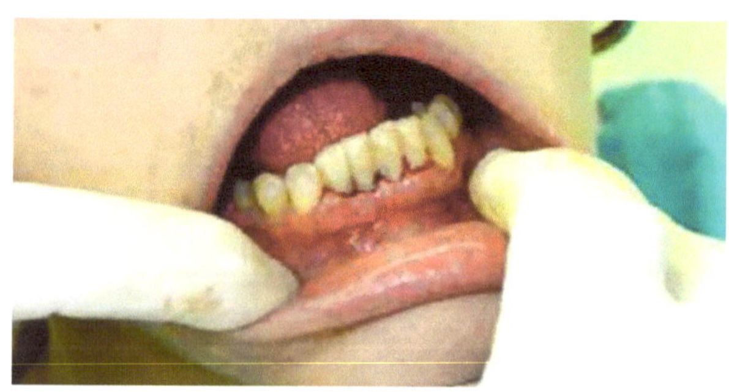

Figure 18.123. Temporary bridge (a copy of the extracted teeth immediately after implantation).

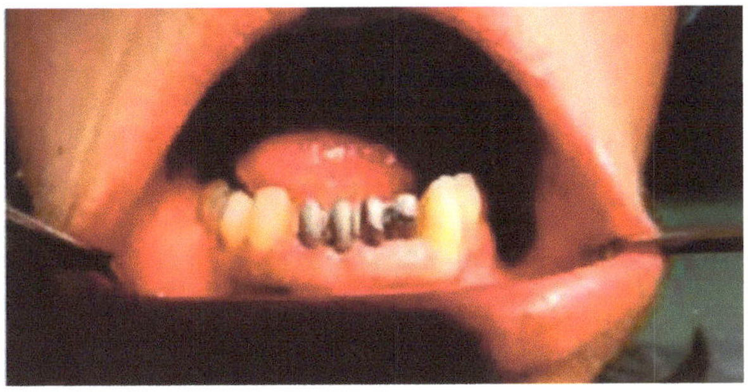

Figure 18.124. Test of metal construction. The metal structure in the gingival area must rest on the implant.

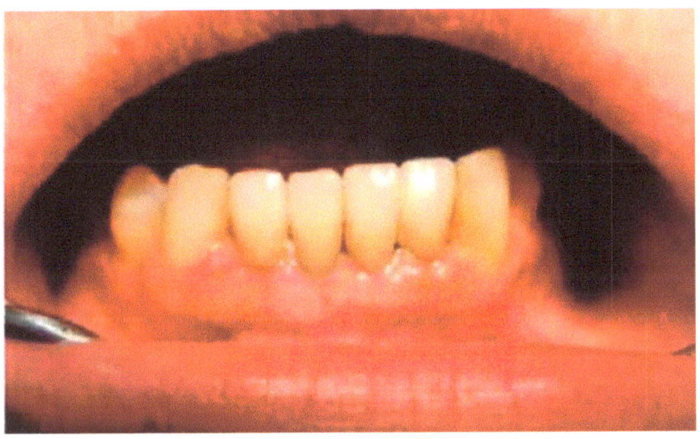

Figure 18.125. Definitive prosthetic work. Achieved function and aesthetics. With this method of implant-prosthetic treatment, complete comfort was achieved in the mouth during the treatment (the patient received temporary teeth immediately after the extraction) and definitive prosthetic work in metal ceramics.

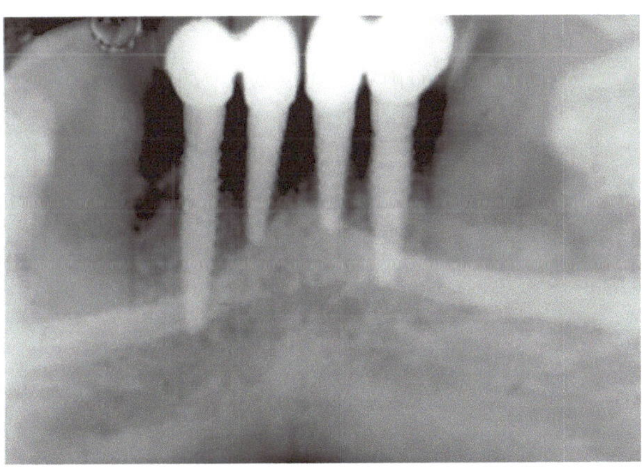

Figure 18.126. Control shot after 12 years. Prosthetic work is stable.

By using the maximum available length of the alveolar ridge, favorable preconditions for prosthetic rehabilitation are created, by creating a favorable ratio between the length of the crown and the part of the implant that lies in the bone. The longer the implant, the more resistant it is to receiving chewing forces, reducing the risk of loss.

For example, in the case of an alveolar ridge with a width of 3.5 mm to 4.2 mm and a length of 10- 15 mm, it is not recommended to install implants with a standard diameter of 3.5 or 3.75 mm due to the insufficient amount of available bone. If the implant is not surrounded by a sufficient amount of bone due to insufficient blood supply to the surrounding bone, bone integration processes cannot occur. There is a high probability that fenestration of the implant thread from the vestibulo-oral side will occur during implantation.

When are the thinnest diameter implants most often used?

Using one-piece, thin implants, with different diameters (1.8 mm, 2.4 mm, or 2.8 mm), the bone quality of the narrow and high alveolar ridge is used, because the amount of cancellous bone is much smaller, which allows for better primary stability. With a wide alveolar ridge, the amount of cancellous bone is greater, which makes it less possible to achieve primary stability. Misch and Judy stated in their research that narrow alveolar ridges are more compact; they most often belong to bone type D2, which is the most favorable for implant placement.

Application of thin one-piece implants in regions where this is only possible and connection with implants of standard diameter has proven to be successful in practice.

What to do if the patient in such cases is persistent and requires the installation of implants at his own risk because he cannot tolerate the lower total prosthesis?

If the patient is persistent, the doctor should evaluate whether to follow the patient's persistence. Pictures 18.127, and 18.128 show such a case. and 18,129. In a 34-year-old patient, the alveolar bone from the top of the ridge to the plateau at 5 mm was 1 mm. The possibility of augmentation with bone grafts or granules was one of the possibilities, but such a procedure would require a longer period of treatment, which the patient could not support in terms of time and money. The patient's request for fixed work at any cost was met. A fixed bridge was made on narrow-diameter implants, which after 7 years meets the patient's aesthetic and functional requirements. The solution is justified because the patient would keep the total prosthesis in his pocket.

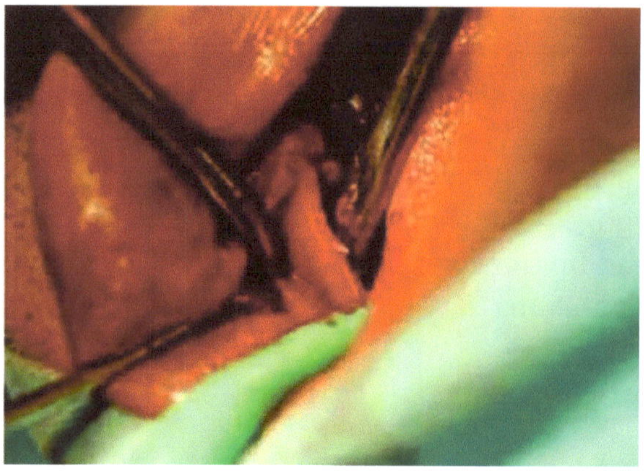

Figure 18.127. Extremely narrow alveolar bone is observed after raising the flap. In such cases, care should be taken if the patient's wishes are respected.

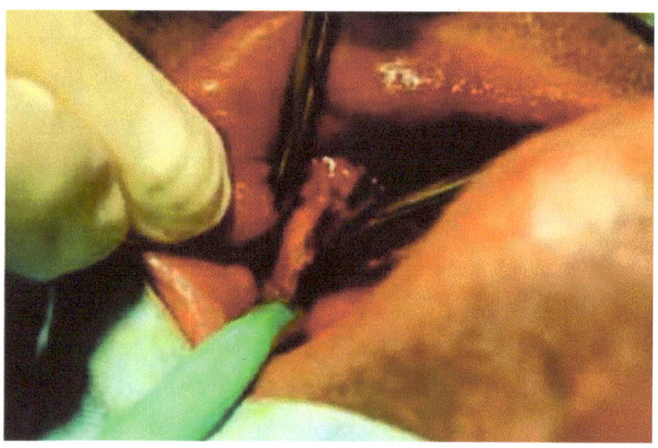

Figure 18.128. In the case of unfavorable anatomical structures - razor-shaped crestal bone in the same patient from the lingual side - one should not risk implantation or use the PRF method to shape the alveolar ridge, which is a serious procedure that this type of patient will not accept.

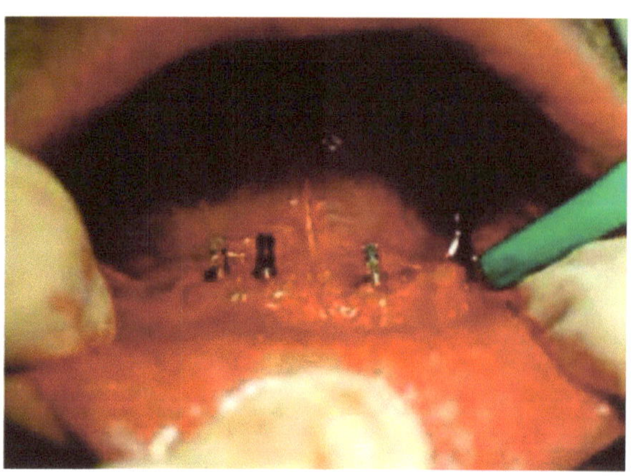

Figure 18.129. A patient with an extremely narrow alveolar ridge in which only reduced-diameter implants can be inserted, and the patient's financial situation was in favor of this.

Implants with a diameter of 3 mm are increasingly used in conditions of insufficient horizontal bone diameter and in patients who want a faster solution.

The use of thin one-piece implants with a diameter of 1.8 or 2.4 mm, in the case of total toothlessness in the lower jaw, gives extremely good results in stabilizing the total prosthesis. Most often, with a severely atrophied alveolar ridge in the lower jaw, stabilization of the total prosthesis with thin one-piece implants, with spherical retention attachments, is one of the solutions, and in many cases the only one. If there are conditions, the use of implants with a wider diameter (3.0 mm) is a more favorable solution.

Is the application of thin one-piece implants in the upper jaw contraindicated?

It depends on the case, the position of the anatomical structures, the quality and quantity of the bone and the condition of the antagonist. If the quantity and quality of the bone and the position of the anatomical structures allow the application of a 3.0 mm diameter implant, success can be predicted. Combination with implants of standard diameters is possible. In the upper jaw, most often, the vertical dimension of the alveolar bone is more problematic than the horizontal dimension. If the height of the alveolar bone is insufficient, near the floor of the sinus, the application of thin implants is absolutely contraindicated.

It depends on the case, the position of the anatomical structures, the quality and quantity of the bone and the condition of the antagonist. If the quantity and quality of the bone and the position of the anatomical structures allow the application of a 3.0 mm diameter implant, success can be predicted. Combination with implants of standard diameters is possible. In the upper jaw, most often, the vertical dimension of the alveolar bone is more problematic than the horizontal dimension. If the height of the alveolar bone is insufficient, near the floor of the sinus, the application of thin implants is absolutely contraindicated.

In which cases is it justified to apply narrow diameter implants in the upper jaw and can they be loaded immediately?

A New York dentist's challenge to apply a thin implant was this: He had titanium posts available to insert into the roots of devitalized teeth, when a Broadway actress needed a temporary bridge quickly installed so that the premiere performance would not be canceled. This was also the inspiration for some American implant manufacturers to create implants with narrow diameters.

Most often, the decision is made to use narrow-diameter implants in the frontal regions of the upper and lower jaw for two reasons: the patient's request to get teeth as soon as possible and the financial factor. The financial possibilities of patients whose width and height of the alveolar ridges allow the installation of implants of standard diameters may indicate the implantation of thin one-piece implants, because they are significantly cheaper. Augmentation, especially the application of the PRF method, would significantly extend the treatment time and increase the price.

Are there cases where small diameter implants can be successfully applied and immediately loaded with fixed prosthetic works?

If there are certain reasons for the insufficient amount of bone and the faster realization of the patient's wishes, the use of one-piece implants with narrow diameters may be indicated. In that case, it is advisable to install a larger number of longer implants, using the cortical bone and the benefits it provides in primary stability.

How important is the surface of the implant, i.e. its processing, for the reception and distribution of chewing forces on the jawbone, and what are the recent technological improvements?

The balanced load of the peri-implant bone is highly dependent on the degree of bony integration achieved. When it comes to new knowledge about the processing of the implant surface, which is in intimate contact with bone and soft tissues, there are different interpretations by manufacturers. Renowned implant manufacturers provide scientific explanations of the treatment of the implant surface with the new Laser-lock technology (Fig. 18.130).

What is the essence of that technology?

Laser-lock technology (Fig. 18.130 and 18.131.) is characterized by magical grooves (canals) in which bone cells are deposited, creating a solid connection between the bone and the implant.

Laser-lock technology consists of micron gutters - grooves (Fig. 18.131), which are laser-engraved with great precision on the surface of the implant. This newly patented surface (engraved with Laser-lock technology) is a surface on which a thin layer of Laser-lock gutters (laser-applied tubes) is located and is unique in the industry, making it the only surface treatment that can achieve periodontal connective tissue attachment. It is claimed that this technology can preserve and integrate both hard bone tissue and soft tissue.

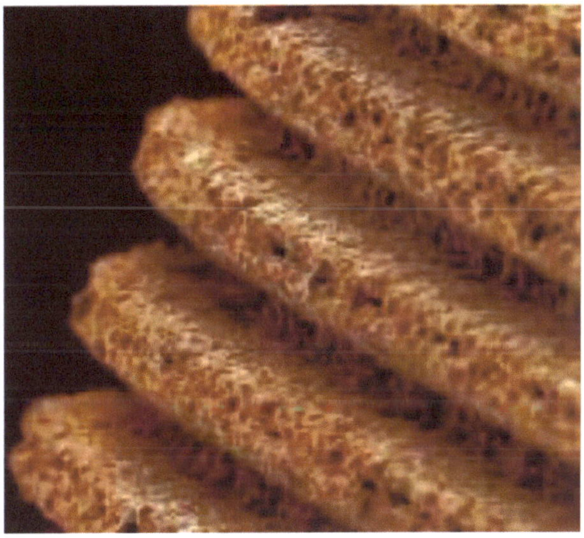

Figure 18.130. Laser-lock microscopic gutters of grooves on the implant surface treated with Laser Lock technology.

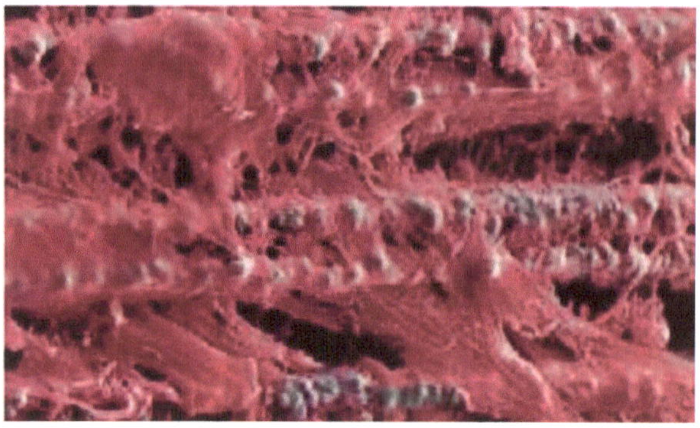

Figure 18.131. The appearance of the microscopically enlarged laser-treated surface of the implant - Laser lock technology

Laser-lock micro-gutters (Fig. 18.131.) are the result of fifteen years of research and documented studies at leading universities. As part of that research, numerous animal, human, and laboratory studies were performed to understand how bone and soft tissue respond to different surface geometries and to evaluate how micron surface geometries affect crestal bone and the biologic surface around the implant over time. reception of chewing forces.

Evaluations of the advantages of implants treated with Laser lock technology are the result of numerous experiments on humans and a series of scientific studies in the group (around Tarnau, Salama et al.) for scientific research. It has been proven that after 37 months of implant placement, the loss of crestal bone was only 0.59 mm for implants treated with Laserlock technology, while for other implants this loss amounted to 1.94 mm. The advantage of implants processed with Laserlock technology is the formed stable, solid dam of periodontal soft tissue above the crestal bone that surrounds the implant processed with this technology.

Research was also performed on fifteen patients who had two BioHorizonts implants and two Nobel Replace Select implants implanted in the frontal part of the mandible. One of each type of implant was loaded with masticatory forces, while the other two were not loaded. After one year, pocket depth and crestal bone loss were significantly lower in implants whose bone contact surface was treated with Laserlock technology, regardless of whether the implant was loaded or not. So, Laserlock microchannels improve the attachment of bone and soft tissue along the entire length of the implant neck, and they form a much more stable attachment of soft tissue above the crestal bone, compared to other implants.

The German manufacturing implantology industry has recently launched the "ICX-Templant" implant (Figures 18.132 and 18.133).

However, such claims by the manufacturer should be taken with a grain of salt as they may be part of normal marketing.

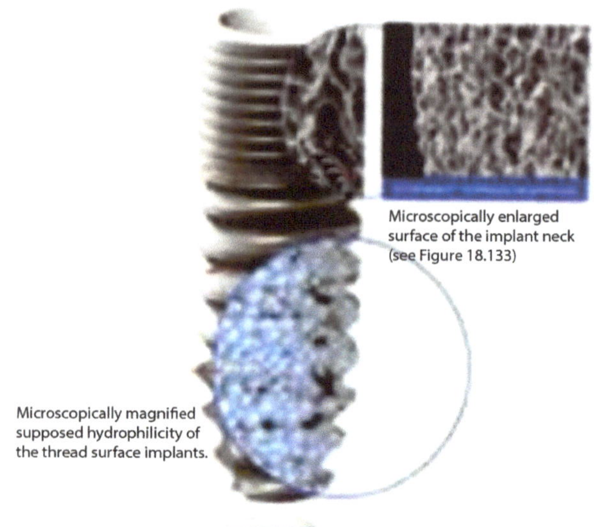

Figure 18.132. Schematic and microscopic view of the "ICX templant" implant.

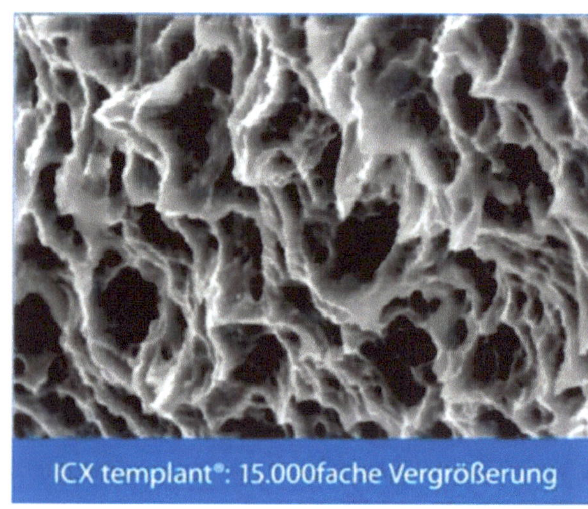

Figure 18.133. The surface of the ICX template magnified 15,000 times.

According to the manufacturer's claims, the surface of this implant is also treated with a special technology, called hydrophilic. It is stated that it has been clinically proven that the hydrophilic surface structure significantly affects the tissues surrounding the implant, which heal much faster and more reliably compared to contact with implants whose surfaces are treated with another technology. With a hydrophilic implant, an additional possibility is that it absolutely can and must be loaded as soon as possible. In contrast, hydrophobic implants only achieve maximum bone integration with the bone after a year, which a hydrophilic implant achieves in a few weeks.

The specific micro-roughness of the implant surface, in addition, provides a good milieu in which new bone mass develops and is deposited on the implant. The special surface refinement technology of the ICX template achieves good hydrophilic properties, which is important for promoting faster healing in the first weeks. The characteristics presented by the manufacturer for this implant (pictures 18.132 - 18.134) about the hydrophilicity of this implant should be taken with a grain of salt, because they are part of the manufacturer's marketing. For this reason, the author gave up on applying this implant system.

For the production of "ICX templant" (which also has the additional name "VOLKS implant", which means people's implant), the manufacturer states that only high-quality pure American titanium (grade 4 quality) is used. The processing of the titanium surface is subject to a special technological procedure: irradiation and etching of the material. After that, the creation of a special protective layer is continued and the surface of the implant acquires the characteristics of hydrophilicity. The implant retains these properties, remaining constantly hydrophilic, which is manifested by a fast and high degree of bone integration and faster healing of the surrounding tissues. A similar characteristic of the implant surface is offered by the Strauman hydrophilic Roxalid implant, a combination of titanium and zirconium.

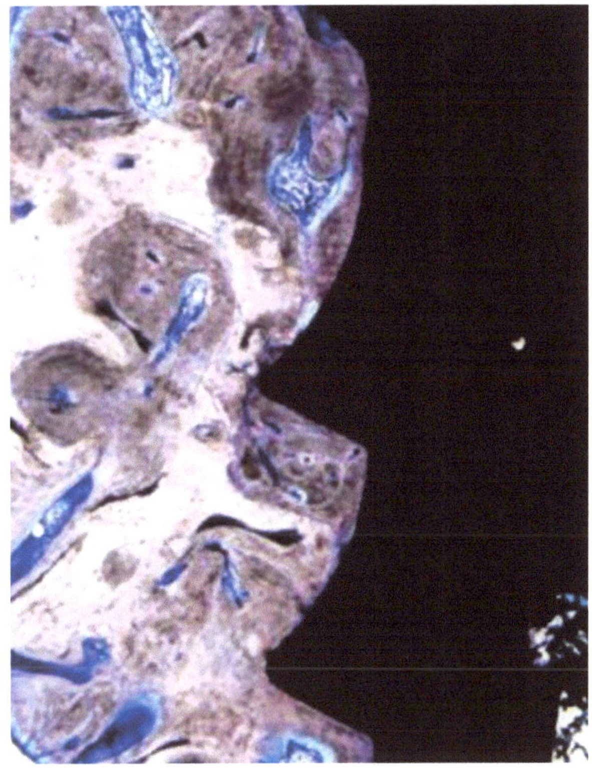

Figure 18.134. Histological presentation of the relationship between the implant surface and the bone in "ICX templant". Manufacturer's marketing presentation.

However, the above is stated in the manufacturer's recommendation when it comes to processing the surface of the implant ("ICX templant") which is in contact with the bone.

The author, applying this implant system (pictures 18.135 to 18.143), noticed that, due to the design at the junction of the prosthetic work support and the first thread, plaque accumulates in that place, which can be the reason for failure (pictures 18.146 and 18.147).

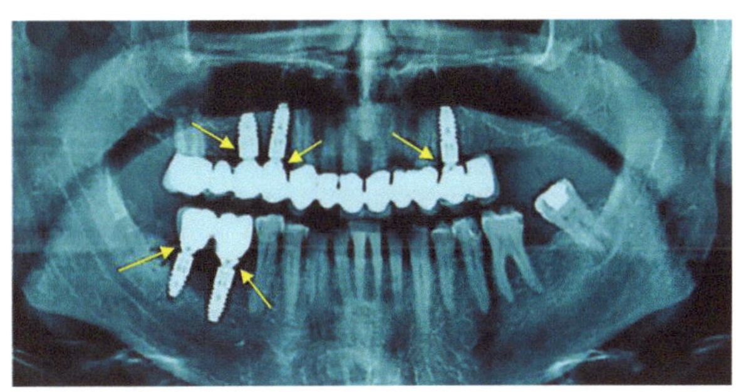

Figure 18.135. "ICX templant"-implants installed by immediate installation without raising the flap, immediately loaded.

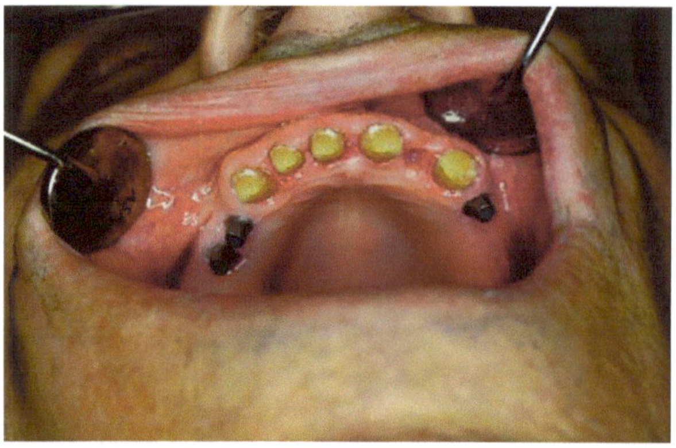

Figure 18.136. Formed tissues around the definitive supports, without the application of a cap for the formation of the gingival sulcus. ("ICX Implant").

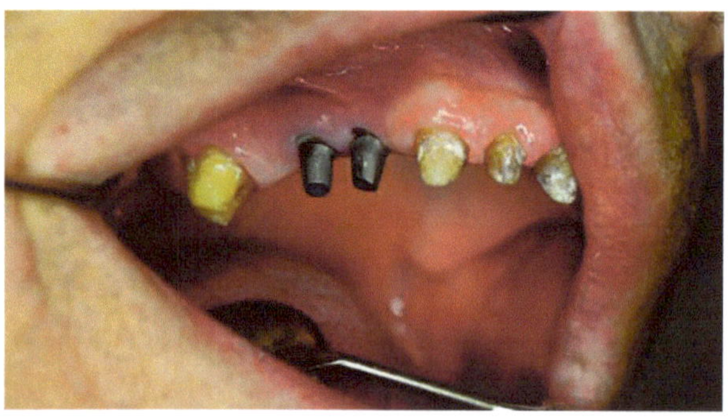

Figure 18.137. Soft tissue appearance around definitive supports in region #14 and #15.

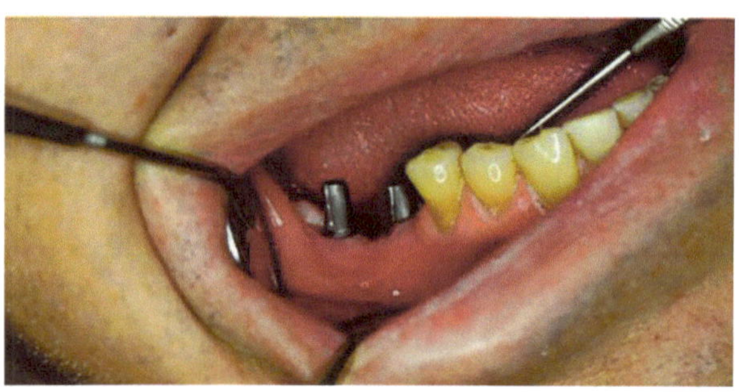

Figure 18.138. Built-in "ICX implants" in the lower jaw.

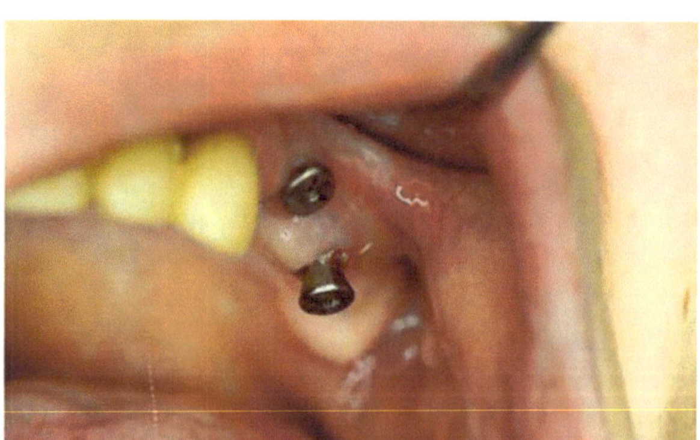

Figure 18.139. Built-in "ICX templant" in the upper jaw.

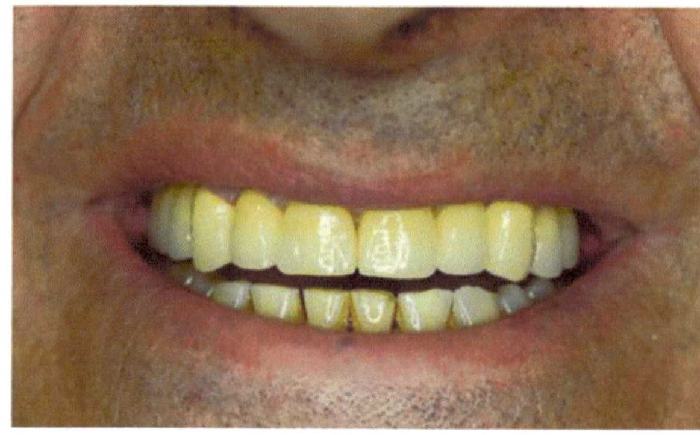

Figure 18.140. Definitive prosthetic works in the distal regions anchored to "ICH" implants. A good occlusion has been achieved, the morphology of the cusps enables occlusal contacts that are in accordance with gnathological principles during lateral movements of the lower jaw.

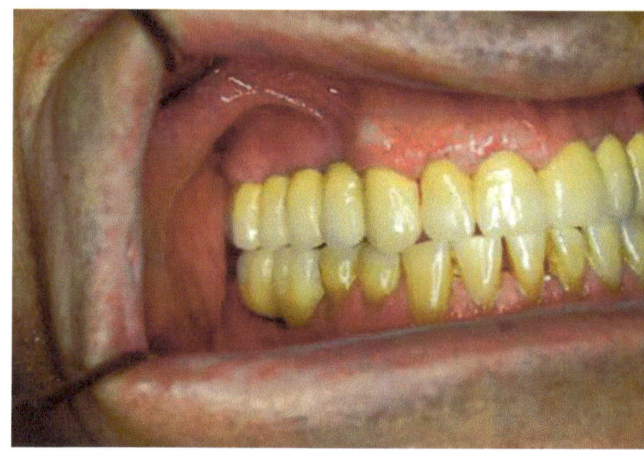

Figure 18.141. Definitive prosthetic works in the upper jaw. With the immediate installation of the implant, immediately loaded, the time of the entire implant-prosthetic treatment was significantly shortened. Good function and aesthetics were achieved.

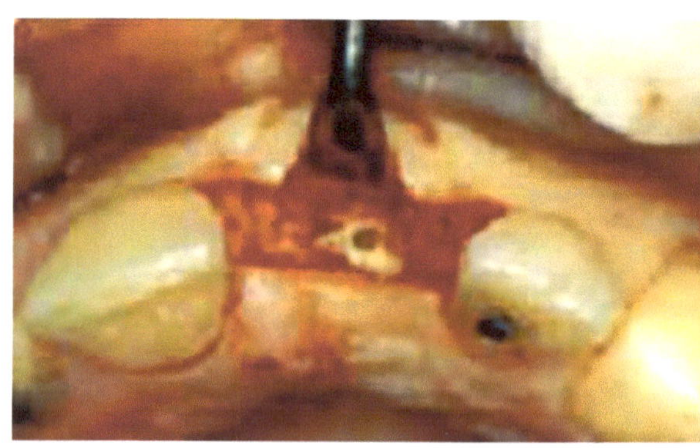

Figure 18.142. Exposing the "ICX" implant with a mucoperiosteal flap from the palatal side with the tip of the ridge with a labial movement of the mucoperiosteal flap.

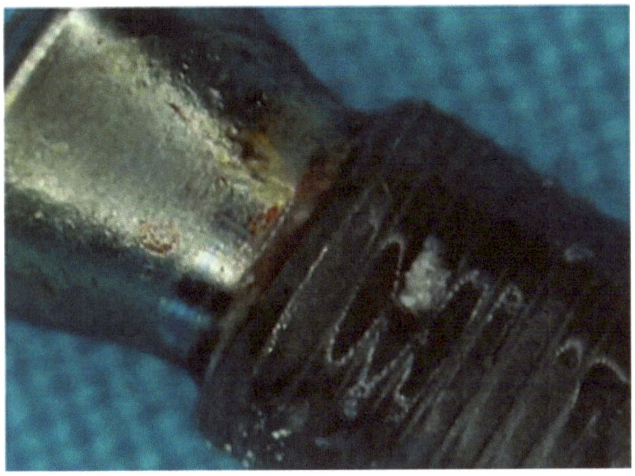

Figure 18.143. The design of the "ICX templanta" neck and the processing of the threads do not correspond to the biomechanical requirements, especially the first thread where the stress of occlusal forces is the strongest. To achieve primary stability, this implant lacks aggressive apical threads that are easier to cut into the softer spongiosa, which achieves good primary stability.

The following example, with the "Astra-Tech" implant, shows how far marketing advertising goes. In an oversupply, marketing advertisements should be received with a grain of salt, and confirmation should be sought in practice and the exchange of experiences with colleagues, primarily considering long-term clinical results and evidence.

The manufacturer of this implant states that a successful implant system cannot be determined by only one characteristic, but that there must be several internal independent characteristics that are combined into one whole. The following are the key features of the "Astra-Tech" implant: Manufactured by Ti Oblast tm, Osseo Speed Is the first and only implant with a chemically modified titanium surface that also stimulates early bone healing; the micro-roughness of the titanium surface coated with fluorides affects bone formation and strengthening of the connection between the implant and the bone; the neck of the "AstraTech" implant is designed with small threads (Micro Thread), which provide optimal reception of forces and their distribution, converting these loads into lower pressure values. This detail of the implant neck design also has the "El Esthetic" implant system.

The manufacturer of this implant claims in its documentation that the "Astra-Tech" implant is the only one that, with its design and conical shape of the neck, protects the marginal bone from adverse effects of forces, where the force stresses are the highest.

Which implant system has the most reliable evidence, scientifically confirmed over a long period of time of testing and obtained by clinical results?

All manufacturers while presenting their implant system as an advantage over other implant systems, use the same term "unique surface treatment with special technology". Of course, all advantages are directed towards the same goal: faster and better integration process of implant and bone, fulfilling the requirements of function and firmer formation of soft tissues around the neck of the implant, satisfying the requirements of aesthetics. So, everyone strives for faster healing so that the implant can be useful as soon as possible.

A particular problem is that the market offers many failed copies of almost all high-quality implant systems. The weak side of the copy is in the low-quality material from which the implant is made, the quality of titanium (type IV) and the surface treatment determine the quality of the implant.

Strauman's implant is the most copied implant system from many manufacturers, which can also be said for Nobel Biocare implants. Today, in the implant manufacturing industry, some factories deal exclusively with copies of all implant systems. It is difficult to say how faithful those copies are to the quality of the technological processing of the originals. All copies deviate from the original by 15 to 20 percent. If the copy were faithful to the quality of the original, the production cost of the copy would be much higher than the cost of the copied implant, that is the reasoning given by the copy manufacturers. That data clearly speaks of the dubious quality of plagiarism. Due to the difference in quality, only implants from reputable manufacturers should be installed for a successful outcome.

For example, Nobel Biocare and Strauman added additional terms to their new editions. Biocare Nobel added the term "Active" and Straumann the term Bone Level, which for both systems means an improvement over the previous versions.

What are these improvements?

Many years of experience and knowledge of the details of many implant systems, now obsolete, can provide the following explanation to this question: for example, both systems (Nobel and Straumann) copied some details of the endosseus part of the once-tried Tramonte implant.

Some researchers have come to the conclusion that the long-term presence of implants in the bone determines some details that should be studied and copied. They did that by modifying the thread from Tramonte's implant. See Figure 18.96 showing four Tramonte implants after 18 years with almost negligible marginal bone resorption. The first copy of this implant was made by Muratori, calling it his name.

The multi-decade longevity of Tramonte's bone implant was one of the valid reasons that something could be copied on new designs. It can be said that the researchers and creators of new forms of Strauman and Nobel Biocare implants Tramonte paved the way and stimulated thoughts towards the improvement of new forms of their implants. It should be emphasized that the surfaces of Tramonte's implant, which are in contact with the bone, were exclusively machined.

What is the essential difference of that improvement?

With the Nobel Biocare TiUnite implant, we are talking about the unique treatment of the implant surface with titanium oxides. Branemark's MkIII TiUnite surface has been tested for over 30 years. All clinically proven principles and obtained results speak of the success of this system. The overall goal of Branemark's implant surface treatment research was to create such surface features to accelerate the bone healing process, which also accelerates the process of osseous integration.

Faster bone healing is achieved by a controlled increase in the thickness of the titanium oxide layer on the surface of the implant itself. Thus, Ti Unite maximizes risk-reducing features by accelerating the bone integration process. The speed of healing is the most important factor for the stability of the implant, and by gradually increasing the titanium oxide surface enriched with phosphates, the body responds by creating a new bone layer. Ti Unite (enriched titanium oxide with a high concentration of phosphate crystals) is characterized by a micro-structural surface with open pores and this affects the acceleration of bone healing, unlike implants whose surface is machined.

The regenerative process was just as well achieved with implants with machine processing, but after a certain time, which also depends on the quality of the titanium itself. The TiUnite surface is chemically the same type of titanium dioxide as the surface of the Branemark implants. The difference is that the machined surface has a layer that is 2 mm thick, while the TiUnite surface is only 10 μm thick. The TiUnite surface is not added to the implant but is an integral part of it, and it is created by causing oxidation of the surface through an electrochemical process. From this comes the conclusion, which also applies to other implant systems, that the advantages of the TiUnite surface are: an increase in the titanium-oxide layer, as well as a porous and increased implant surface.

Bearing in mind everything that has been said before, one gets the impression that the processing of the implant surface has not yet reached the final stage, and excessive marketing advertising can only cause suspicion in an experienced implantologist.

The claims of many manufacturers, especially those whose products are plagiarized, are often not supported by scientific evidence. Also, it is very important which scientific team and which names are behind a certain project.

Manufacturers realize their marketing interest, very often and very skillfully, at many scientific symposia and congresses, using some authorities from dental faculties. They give lectures colored by marketing, which the manufacturer imposed on them, and with the absence of personal experience, verified in practice.

From the above, what is the general conclusion?

From all this, one gets the impression that even today, the greatest attention and scientific discussions are devoted to the improvement and acceleration of bone integration.

And how much importance is attached to the attachment of soft tissues at the neck of the implant?

In the past, no implant system paid even minimal attention to soft tissues. That was a big pain and a permanent problem of all previous implant systems. It should be noted that, a few decades since Tramonte launched his implant, renowned manufacturers manage to improve the endosseous parts of their implants by improving self-cutting into the bone, but the problem of soft tissue attachment still remains.

With those implants, how much care was taken of the soft tissues, that is, of the gingiva that surrounds the neck of the implant?

Copying certain details of Tramonte's implant (thread pitch, length and inclination of the thread in contact with the bone) proved to be successful, as the cutting of the implant into the bone was significantly improved, and the stress on the surrounding bone was reduced. Tramonte's implant drew attention for its long duration in bone, with emphasis on the fact that the threads in the endosseous part received and distributed masticatory forces within physiological limits, which is one of the explanations for the long duration in bone. However, there was not a single detail that could be copied when it came to the relationship of the gingiva to the implant crown support.

What are the current knowledge and attitudes when it comes to soft tissues, i.e. soft tissue to implant neck relationship?

Today, modern oral implantology deals, to a large extent, with soft tissues. More and more attention is paid to the technological processing of the part of the implant that surrounds the soft tissues. Laser treatment, created with micro-threads, significantly improved the ratio of implant surfaces to soft tissues. Figure 18.144 shows the processing of the surface of the implant that is in contact with soft tissues.

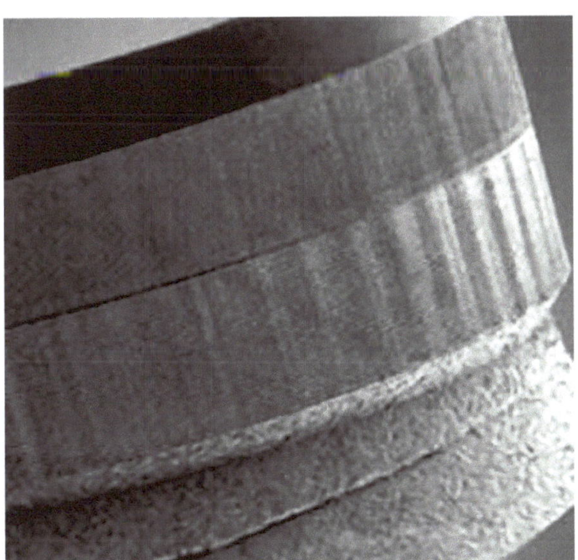

Figure 18.144. Microscopic view of the laser-treated part of the implant that is in contact with soft tissues.

Today, opinions have completely changed. The PINK ESTHETIC SCORE (PES) is increasingly in the center of attention, i.e. attention is increasingly focused on the behavior and restoration of soft tissues, i.e. the morphological type of gingiva (thin and thick). Already during planning, in order to achieve optimal success, the mentioned requirements and factors must be given great importance. That is the imperative of aesthetic implantology.

How did earlier understandings change when it comes to implant contacts with soft tissues?

Today, we can confidently claim that our implants, especially in the mandible, remain incorporated for 15, 20, and even more years. The function of the implant is still an important criterion for determining success, which was the first and basic condition for the development of oral implantology. But today, that criterion is not the most important, especially about frontal restorations, where aesthetic requirements must be fulfilled to the maximum.

Aesthetics, especially with a wide smile, requires attention to every millimeter of soft tissue, regardless of all circumstances.

For this reason, implantology has made a big breakthrough here. Bony integration is no longer the only dominant factor. Oral implantology has risen several levels higher, with the conclusions that, in addition to the contact of the implant with the bone, the contact of the implant with the soft tissues is just as important.

For that topic, Dr. K.A. Schlegel (2007), a practitioner, says: "the subject of soft tissue and implant relationships represents an old wine in a new blend." The truth of these words will be confirmed by many implantologists, and the author's personal experience supports this.

Does this mean that, when it comes to the neck of the implant, which is in contact with the soft tissues, there is still no final solution?

And from an aesthetic, periodontological, and even functional point of view, for implantology, in the future, it will be the most important task.

Is this also one of the risks in oral implantology?

Despite the enormous progress of oral implantology, the answer to this question requires an exhaustive explanation. Peri-implant mucositis, as an inflammatory process, is always a risk that can lead to complications. We can classify any progressive soft tissue inflammation as a risk factor. Chapter 13 - Risks in oral implantology is dedicated to that topic.

What are the criteria by which we can evaluate the success of installed implants?

Those criteria have changed over time. At the time when I was installing the first implants, those criteria were different from today's. With the development of modern implantology, however, the criteria also changed.

Today, implants can be said to have met the criteria of success if they meet the following conditions:

a) provided chewing and speaking functions;
b) psychological satisfaction of the patient;
c) absence of pain;
d) aesthetic suitability;
e) achieved stable bone integration;
f) absence of inflammation of the surrounding soft tissues;
g) fulfillment of all gnathological principles of prosthetic work;
h) fulfillment of biomechanical requirements.

If any of the mentioned criteria are not met, the implant treatment can be considered unsuccessful.

Have these criteria been changed or supplemented in accordance with innovations in implantology?

Yes. In the past, the only criterion for success, according to the Harvard Convention, was that the implant should stay in the bone for five years. It's funny today. Today, Albrexton sees those criteria in the following parameters:

a) that there is no clinical mobility of individual implants that are not connected in a block;
b) that the mandatory control radiological findings, in the first two years after implantation, do not show peri-implant radiographic lightening;
c) that the vertical bone loss after one year of loading is below 0.2 mm;
d) that there are no permanent pains, paresthesias, and similar neuropathic problems;
e) that there is no perforation of the upper wall of the mandibular canal and no pressure on the lower alveolar nerve.

Some authors draw the following conclusion based on the mentioned criteria: a few years ago, success was considered satisfactory if all these criteria were met and the percentage of success was 85% after five years, and around 80% after 10 years. Based on the thoughts I gave through the answers to the questions in which direction the development of implantology will go, I am convinced that the above percentages will increase even more. I emphasized this in all my lectures at a time when oral implantology was fiercely contested

Does the success rate depend on the region where the implants are placed?

The success rate depends on many factors and is variable; it depends on the position of the implant in the dental arch, the quality of the bone, as well as the number, arrangement, and condition of the remaining teeth, if any. Of course, the most important thing is which region it is.

In the frontal region of the lower jaw, in edentulous patients, the space between the two mental openings belongs to the most suitable region for implant placement. For fixed benefits in that region, the success rate after five years is more than 90%. There is not enough valid data for mobile restorations in that region, or combined with partial edentulism.

In the frontal region of the upper jaw, between the mesial borders of the maxillary sinuses, the percentage of success with fixed prosthetic works after five years is at least 85%. The experiences of many dentists say that implants installed in that region, burdened with fixed compensations, show an even higher percentage of success for 10 years or longer.

For fixed-mobile restorations in partial toothlessness, we also do not have enough reliable clinical research and valid data on success.

The percentage of success in the lateral regions in the lower jaw, distal to the mental foramen, ranges as high as 98%. Of course, if there is enough bone and when larger diameter implants are used. In this case, too, there are no long-term clinical results, but the results in daily practice are very promising.

When it comes to the lateral regions in the upper jaw, especially when they are in the region of the tubercle and under the maxillary sinuses, we do not have long-term valid results when it comes to the percentage of success. Calculating the percentage of success is made much more difficult by the patients themselves, who do not attend regular check-ups.

There is also the question of how to classify those implants where the bone breakdown is above 1.5 mm, and the clinical condition is completely stable.

When can it be considered that the cause of implant failure is an inadequate prosthetic solution?

For the exact gradation and sequence of failure, when it comes to prosthetics, a reliable answer could not be given, because it is about different solutions in different conditions. It would be logical to consider prosthetic procedures unsuccessful in the case of:

a) changes in the adopted prosthetic solution due to poorly placed implants;
b) failure to achieve the planned prosthetic solution;
c) frequent corrections of prosthetic work due to biomechanical problems;
d) loosening of screws or breakage of parts of the bridge;
e) dissatisfaction of the patient due to unrealized aesthetics;
f) existence of speech impediments;
g) created problems for maintaining oral hygiene due to the inaccessibility of cleaning around implants, remaining food residues, and difficult removal of dental plaque.

How to explain this to the patient?

First, judge well where mistakes were made; in the doctor's office or laboratory. If there is an error in the laboratory, do not hesitate to ask the dental technician to redo the work. The possibilities of prosthetics in his case must be explained to the patient, with a lot of patience, because the patient's wishes are often at odds with his objective condition, the position of the teeth or alveolar ridges.

How to perform it and what is the success rate of prosthetic works on implants?

Some authors suggest that such prosthetic works should be constructed that could be removed once a year in order to examine the mobility of the implants. Practically speaking, this proposal is in many cases difficult, even impossible. Experience and obtained results confirm that prosthetic work fixed with adhesives on implants is a better solution than screwing. On the other hand, screwing also has an advantage, because there is no possibility of cement residues causing pre-implantitis and implant loss.

Why?

Many long-term analyzes confirm this view because the production is much more complicated and expensive, and the number of dental technicians who can perform such precise work is small. The condition for prosthetic work to be performed correctly is that the clinician emphasizes all the important details to the dental technician. The percentage of success of prosthetic works on implants can only be hypothetical, because patients who are satisfied for years do not come for regular check-ups. No research on this topic has been completed.

What period do you consider the beginning of modern implantology?

I think it's the second half of the 80s from 1985. Many implantologists call the period the era of the Swede Branemark. This researcher from Gothenburg, who is not a dentist but an anatomist, flawlessly laid the scientific foundations of modern implantology. Since then, understandings about implantology have changed, new terminology has been introduced, new books have been published, many periodontological-implantological journals have been launched, the technology industry has changed, and the design of implant manufacturing has improved. Implantology is increasingly being accepted by universities that have long been skeptical of this branch of dentistry.

What is modern implantology today?

Today's implantology can respond much more easily to the increasing demands of patients, and the installation of implants is much easier than in the past.

Installing an implant is no longer an aggressive oral surgical procedure, but a simple and painless method. By installing implants, aesthetic and functional requirements are met.

The implant approximately imitates the root of a natural tooth. It completely takes over its role, i.e. all its functions from reception and transmission of chewing forces to the bone, to the fulfillment of aesthetic requirements. The "root" is made of titanium, a material biocompatible with bone, with which it integrates after a certain time. Metal-ceramic or zirconium crowns are placed on such an implant, be it one or more, which should completely replace natural teeth aesthetically and functionally. The position of the author of the book is that zirconium prosthetic work on implants should not be used in the lateral regions for biomechanical reasons. The function also depends on the design of the implant, and the conical form best meets those requirements.

What replaces the ground tooth on which the crown is placed?

The ground tooth replaces the continuation of the implant, which is placed above the level of the bone and is called an abutment. If there is a disparity of supports during the installation of several implants, such a situation can be adjusted by choosing supports of different angles. However, the angle of inclination of the support must not exceed 25 degrees.

Are the crown supports the same for the frontal and lateral regions?

They are essentially the same. In the frontal region, especially in the upper jaw, special attention must be paid to aesthetic requirements. But this must be foreseen when installing the implant.

Which and what kind of prosthetic work is preferred when it comes to the front regions, especially in the upper jaw and how are the aesthetic requirements met?

If prosthetic rehabilitation is performed with metal-ceramic crowns, a titanium support is indicated. If the crowns are made of zirconium in the front, the titanium supports are screened, so this can compromise the aesthetics in the neck area, which is especially visible if the laugh line is high. To avoid this, it is necessary to use zirconium supports, the price of which is high (Figures 18.145 and 18.146).

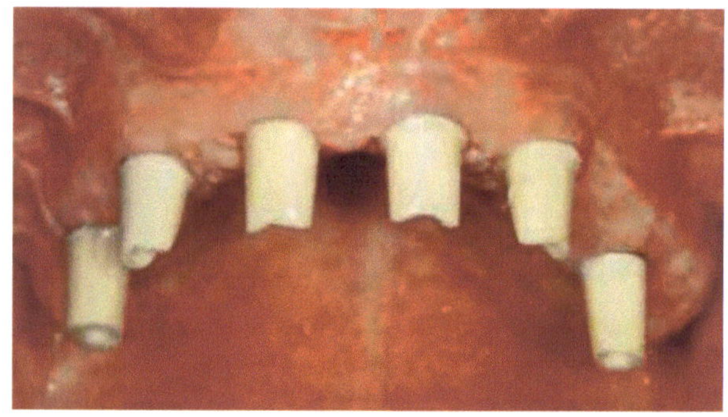

Figure 18.145. Supports (abutments) made of zirconium in the front of the upper jaw have an advantage if prosthetic work is performed with metal-free crowns.

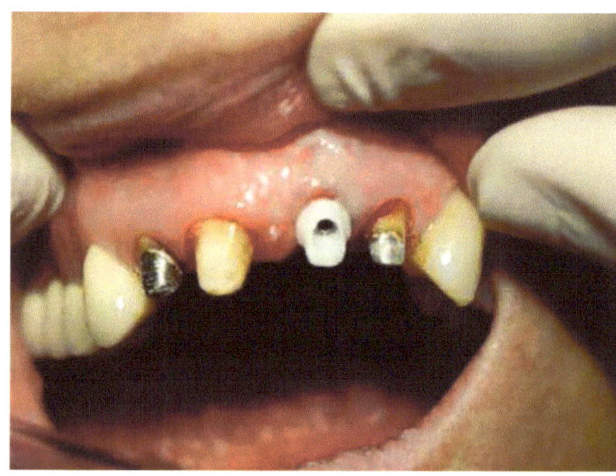

Figure 18.146. Existing metal abutments on the lateral incisors and provisional support on the implant. Metal extensions can compromise aesthetics if the prosthetic work is performed in zirconium. In similar cases, metal-ceramic restorations are a more justified and successful solution.

Can implants harm the body and can they be discarded?

Such questions are primarily asked by lay people, patients. But it is not uncommon for dentists who do not deal with implant placement to ask a similar, layman's question. It has been scientifically proven that quality implants are biologically neutral and cannot cause harmful effects on the body. Unlike transplants (from organ donors), there is no immune rejection with implants, and the failures of individual implants are caused by surgical error or low-quality implants, of which there are over 500 forms on the market. Choosing the highest quality implant, a renowned manufacturer, with a scientific certificate, as well as the experience of the implantologist, are a guarantee of success, which then ranges up to 98%!

Is the surgical implantation procedure painful and how long does it take to install one implant? What is the waiting period to replace lost teeth?

The answer to this question is more for the patient. Implant placement is performed painlessly under local anesthesia. The extraction of impacted wisdom teeth is a much more complicated procedure than the installation of implants. The average time of installation of one implant is about 20-30 minutes, or even less, depending on the experience of the dentist. The time it takes for a patient to get teeth on implants depends on the assessment of the implantologist. The author's knowledge and experience confirm that the treatment plan is mainly focused on the immediate burden.

Shortened treatment time is a great advantage for the patient for several reasons, especially because of better comfort. Of course, which procedure will be implemented depends on the case by case, where the experience of the doctor is crucial. Sometimes a waiting time of three to four months is needed, sometimes more, in patients where there is a larger bone defect and where it is necessary to perform bone augmentation with bone substitutes, in order to then install an implant. The author's experience confirms that it is more justified to perform the entire intervention procedure at the same time. Which procedure to apply depends on a good assessment of the bone condition (quantity and quality), which is different in many patients. Also, the waiting time depends on anatomical convenience. Experiences confirm that good results are achieved with simultaneous implantation and augmentation.

Which implant system is suitable and where one does not have to wait several months for the patient to replace one or more teeth?

Wolff's rule in orthopedics, pronounced almost a hundred years ago, is more relevant today than in the time when it was created: that the bone should be put into function as soon as possible. The same principle is absolutely applicable today in oral implantology.

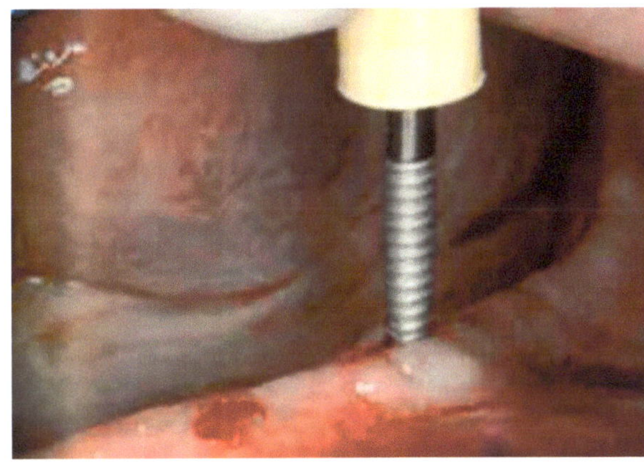

Figure 18.147. Installation of one-piece implants in the lower jaw without raising the flap is a simple surgical procedure.

Are there any restrictions on implant placement?

Like all other surgical branches, implantology is not immune to risks. Thanks to the enormous progress of implantological science, the number of general contraindications has been significantly reduced, but there are patients for whom the installation of implants is not suitable. In the case of a risk group of patients, all parameters should be carefully evaluated, without being guided by the patient's ability to pay, if he wants to fulfill his wishes at all costs, and for which there is no realistic basis. Some diseases of the body exclude the possibility of installing implants, which is assessed by an implantologist. This topic is described in more detail in the chapter "Indications And Contraindications For Implant Placement".

Can implants be installed in pregnant women?

It can. But the position of modern science is that implantation should be avoided during that period

Is the durability of oral implants a common question asked by patients?

It is. If everything is carried out according to the protocol, from the selection of a quality implant, a suitable patient, an experienced implantologist, precisely performed prosthetic work, and all this is followed by extremely good maintenance of oral hygiene and regular controls, such work can last 15-20 years, or even more.

It should be emphasized that every organism is exposed to degenerative changes and aging for years, so it must be reckoned with a certain degree of bone loss (resorption) around the implant, mostly in the marginal part, which also happens with natural teeth. Likewise, with implants there is a certain physiological bone resorption, which amounts to about 0.1 or 0.2 mm per year. Any major loss on an annual basis is an alarm to look for and eliminate the cause of accelerated bone loss at regular check-ups.

How to answer the patient if he asks if the implant can "get sick" like a natural tooth can get sick?

It can. But this disease is both similar and different. The most common "implant" disease is caused by two factors: the first reason is inadequate load, due to poorly executed prosthetics, and the second reason is the accumulation of bacterial plaque around the implant due to inadequate oral hygiene. Bacterial plaque penetrates along the implant and the bone, causing inflammatory changes in the surrounding tissues, peri-implantitis, and smoking is an additional risk factor that accelerates those unfavorable processes that threaten the stability of the implant.

It is still debatable which of the causes of decay and loss of bone around the implant has priority: biomechanical pathological stress, inadequate pathological load on the bone, or accumulated bacterial content around the implant. Although today there are divided opinions about that.

What is the basis of success in implantology?

Modern implantology has the ability to predict success. That success can be 97-98%, but only with respect to certain principles described in this chapter.

Explain the causes of failure?

You will find partial answers to this question in the answers to the previous questions. But it is useful to repeat some. Modern implantology has significantly reduced the number of lost implants. However, something happens that we didn't want to happen, and it did! That is the definition of risk!

The most common causes of risk are determined by anatomical factors, the lack of sufficient amount of available bone, where the primary stability of the implant has not been achieved.

Primary stability can also be compromised if the bone is of poor quality. The causes of failure can be found in: surgical error, poorly and unprofessionally performed prosthetic work, or poor oral hygiene, the negative effect of which is enhanced by smoking. This should be emphasized and often repeated to patients.

Failure to comply with the agreement by the patient can be one of the causes of failure. If the principles are respected, in the international literature, a failure rate of 2-4% is recorded!

The biggest guarantee of success is when the implantologist analyzes the case in detail, and good planning is the basic starting point for a successful outcome. It is also important that the implantologist knows without hesitation what not to do in a specific case. Any venture into an adventure with unpredictable success is a big risk.

Maxillary cavities in the upper jaw, low sinuses, are these insurmountable obstacles for the installation of implants today, as in the past?

Such obstacles are no longer insurmountable. This is where the big advances offered by modern oral implantology have taken place. Elevating the floor of the sinus cavity and inserting a bone substitute has become a routine operation. However, it must be emphasized that this procedure always requires caution and is one of the more complicated procedures. A longer waiting period is also required for loading the implant. If there are favorable conditions in the frontal region for implant placement (sufficient amount of available bone), where implant placement can be performed safely and good primary stability of the implant can be achieved, with adequate planning of the prosthetic work, the patient's requirements for fixed work can be met. Planning prosthetic work also depends on the state of inter jaw relationships. Patients often put aesthetic requirements first, which can be achieved with distal hanging members. By adding one or two hanging members to the fixed part carried by the implants, which also depends on the length and diameter of the installed implants, the desired goal can be achieved.

And what is done when there is too much bone loss in the lower jaw with all the anatomical disadvantages?

Augmentation of the alveolar ridge is attempted, which means raising the ridge in height and width in order to compensate for the lost part of the bone to the extent necessary to accommodate the implant. After the development of regenerative and reconstructive techniques, it is possible to perform directed bone regeneration (GBR) and tissue regeneration (GTR). Directed bone regeneration is often combined with local bone grafts taken from the chin or ramus of the mandible.

With the discovery and development of molecular biology and histochemistry, bioactive preparations are used that activate osteocytes, and due to the presence of bioactive polypeptides, growth factors are also promoted, which induce the formation of new bone.

Questions About Surgical Procedures

Why is it that surgical techniques for installing different implant systems are not described in the book, as it was done in some textbooks and earlier books?

First of all, the first books written about implantology were mainly concerned with describing various techniques of several implant systems. Today, when numerous surgical techniques are described, it is a matter of permanent education, which is mandatory in modern implantology.

For example, modification of the H-shaped incision to move the proximal part of the soft tissue above the implant is important for shaping the soft tissues, primarily the papilla.

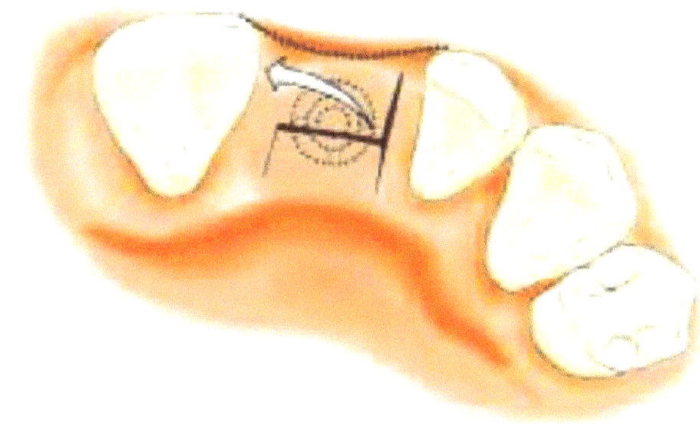

Figure 18.148. A modification of the H-shaped incision to move the soft tissue laterally above the implant, useful for shaping the papilla.

In picture 18.148. the occlusal appearance of the H-shaped incision is shown, which can be used for the installation of implants with planned immediate loading and at the same time preserve the papilla. The second picture (b) shows the position of the flap after placing the abutment on the implant. The soft tissue that covers the implant is pushed labially and forms the labial contour of the gingiva.

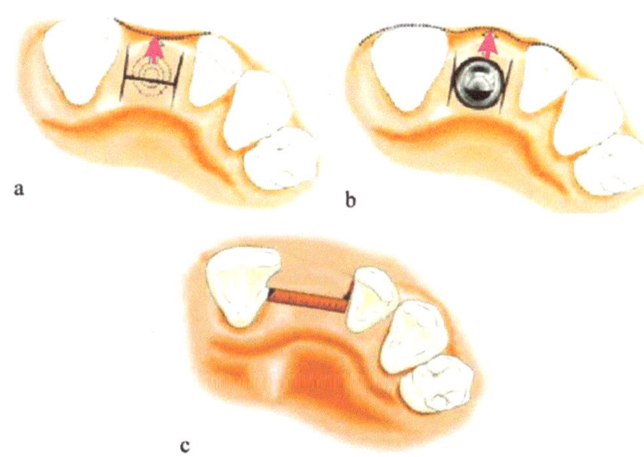

Figure 18.149. Schematic representation of the H-shaped incision for an implant with delayed loading, a) this incision shape can also be used when installing an implant with immediate loading; b) incision after placement of the support on the implant. The soft tissue that was above the covering cap for healing is pushed labially (arrow) with which the labial contours of the gingiva are formed; c) shaping the incision for immediate implantation and immediate loading. An incision with the crestal part towards the palatal side is considered ideal for better contouring of the labial part of the gingiva. This incision can be converted into an H-shape if a more transparent approach is necessary for implant placement.

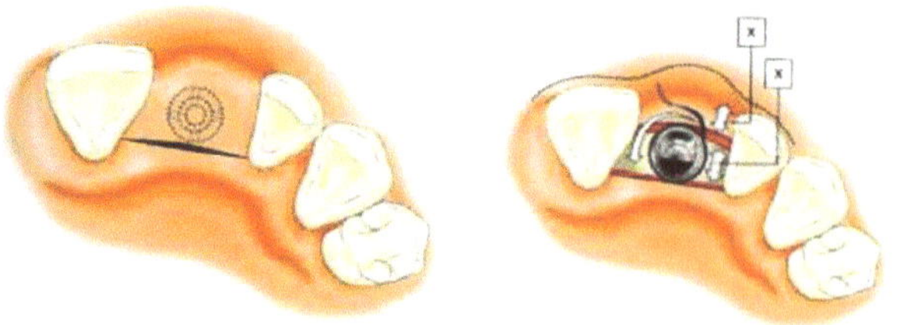

Figure 18.150. Schematic representation of a palatal incision for delayed loading. The incision is made in two parts: an incision on both sides of the edentulous part perpendicular to the alveolar ridge about 10 mm.

Figure 18.151. shows the occlusal appearance of the S-shaped incision performed when processing individual implants. The second picture is a view with the bracket installed. The soft tissue flap is displaced labially. An alveolar ridge was revealed mesial and distal to the support. The mark X indicates the direction of soft tissue movement. The solid line indicates the part of the S-shaped incision that completely cuts through the periosteum. The dotted line represents the part of the S-shaped incision that is performed subepithelial. The S-shaped incision forms a small petioled flap that covers part of the exposed ridge.

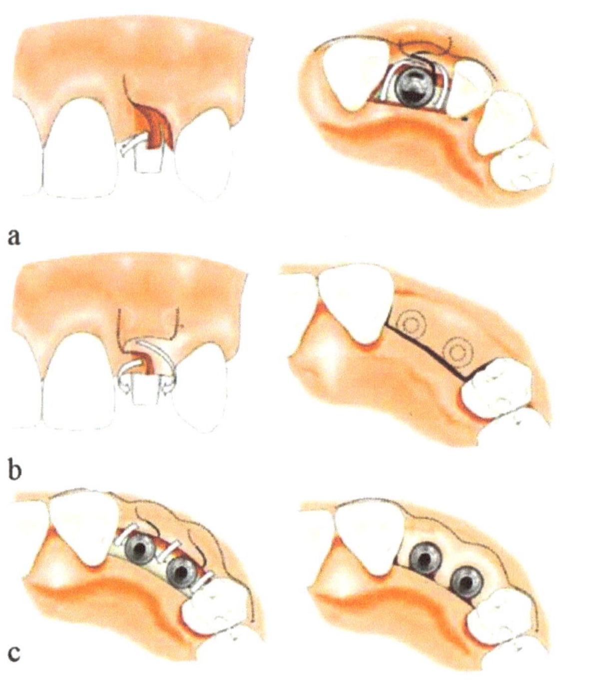

Figure 18.151. Labial and occlusal views of the double S lobe. The direction of movement of the two separate petioled lobes is shown by the arrow. Diagram of an S-shaped incision when revealing a large number of implants. Demonstration of abutment placement, the incision is made so that the pedicle flap can be moved mesially to allow papilla formation. Displaced flap pedicles that allow reconstruction of the papilla. A pedunculated papilla-forming flap displaced mesial from each implant.

Figure 18.151. shows a double S-shaped incision view with a schematic view of the mucoperiosteal and subepithelial components. Image b shows an S-shaped incision when multiple implants are exposed. The picture shows the occlusal view of the left lateral incisor and canine with brackets in place. The incision (mucoperiosteal and subepithelial) is performed so that the pedicle flaps can be moved mesially and closure is possible in the direction of the arrows. The image shows a displaced pedicle flap that allows closure of the exposed ridge and reconstruction of the papilla. The pedunculated lobes that form the papilla are displaced mesial from each implant. The fifth picture explains covering the wound by breaking the open part of the ridge around the implant.

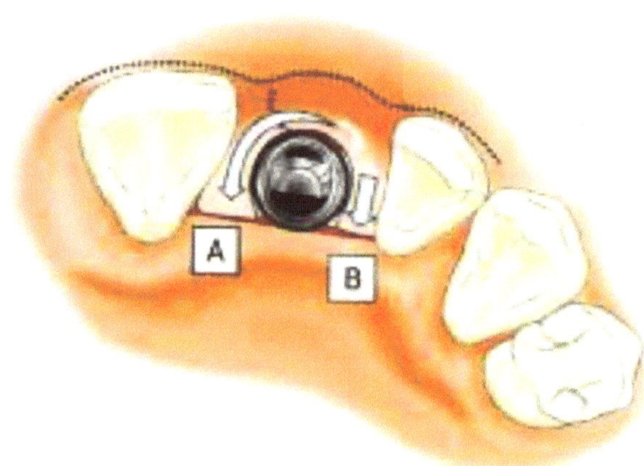

Figure 18.152. Wound closure by returning the flap to the ridge. By moving the pedicle flap mesially (A), the entire distal flap can be returned to its initial position.

Figure 18.152. shows that by moving the small pedicle flap mesially (A), the distal part of the flap (B) can be moved to its original position. It is important to know that performing an S-shaped incision is indicated when the papilla needs to be reconstructed, which is extremely important to achieve a favorable aesthetic result. The incision is made in such a way as to create a narrow petioled flap that is placed in the interdental space, which is explained in the attached pictures.

When installing a large number of unilaterally placed implants (Fig. 18.153), the pedicle lobes are shaped in such a way that they are repositioned mesially. The height of the alveolar ridge, the size of the interdental space, and the thickness of the tissue affect the width of the flap. The S-shaped incision is started in the distal area of the support after its placement. An experienced clinician should be able to visualize the final position of the flap mesial to the carrier. The first part of the cut separates the mucoperiosteal flap, and the second part of the cut is performed subepithelially in the area of the periosteum, without separating the epithelial part. In this way, the petiole lobe acquires the necessary mobility without creating a split in the area of the marginal epithelium. The position of the first incision is in the interdental space to determine the starting point for the incision in the area of the second bracket. After completion of the second incision and positioning of the miniature flap, the mucoperiosteal flap distal to the second carrier will lead to spontaneous gingival healing. The S-shaped incision can be performed bilaterally when there is only one support, if there is enough soft tissue.

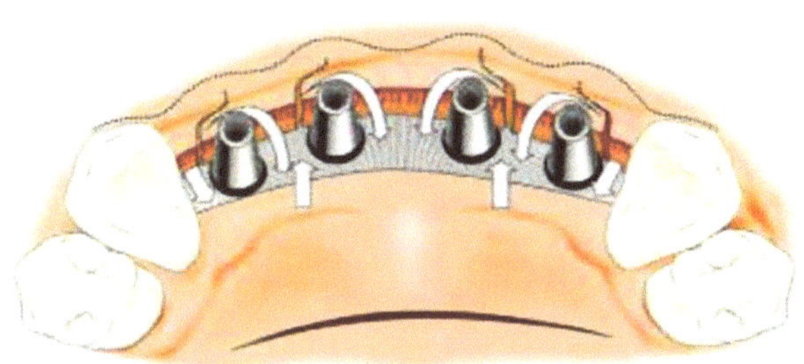

Figure 18.153. Schematic representation of a mucoperiosteal incision to reveal four implants in the frontal region of the upper jaw. The incision is made in an S shape in the midline so that the flaps can be moved mesially. Two pedunculated flaps are pushed into a larger inter-implant space, and in patients who underwent augmentation, the amount of keratinized attachment mucosa was reduced. Full flap shaping is done palatally. This creates the possibility to obtain more keratinized tissue for the reconstruction of the papilla, while at the same time ensuring better coverage of the exposed bone.

In order to promote the new formation of the papilla between the natural tooth and the implant, what should be paid attention to?

Care should be taken not to place the implant too close to the natural tooth, because it will prevent the new formation of the papilla and, as a result, an unfavorable aesthetic result will be obtained in that interdental space (Fig. 18.154).

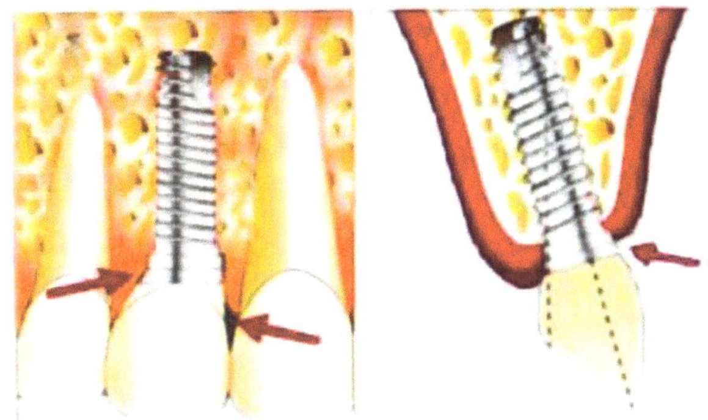

Figure 18.154. It is preferable to place the implant so that its axis is in the center of the alveolar ridge. If the implant is inclined too labially, the axis of the implant will cause an unaesthetic exit point.

When it comes to surgical procedures in oral implantology, what should you pay attention to?

The essence is knowing the surgical techniques that can be used to install implants with as little trauma as possible to all tissues in the shortest possible time. The team must be coordinated so that the duration of the procedure is as short as possible and constant attention must be paid to avoid trauma to the bone due to overheating during bone preparation, especially if the procedure is performed with blunt drills. Preparation of the implant bed should be carried out intermittently with abundant wetting with saline solution. Use only quality sharp drill bits. Surgical techniques must be performed with minimal trauma to all tissues and all surgical protocol procedures must be followed. This would be a short answer to the question asked, a more extensive answer requires more space.

What is the first surgical step in oral implantology?

The first step is to prepare patients for surgery. The patient should be prepared by meeting all the requirements of the surgical protocol. This preparation should be done in the following order:

- Premedication of the patient, antibiotic, antiphlogistic, and if necessary prescribe some of the anxiolytics;
- Wipe the face with an antiseptic solution such as merfen (this procedure used to be done with iodine tinctures, and despite its reliability, it is

used less and less in oral implantology because of the unpleasant smell and possible allergy);

- Rinse the mouth well with a solution of chlorhexidine or a similar antiseptic before administering anesthesia;
- This is followed by the preparation of the implant installation region with an antiseptic solution;
- A sterile disposable cap is placed on the patient, and the patient's face is covered with a sterile compress.

The surgical instruments must be sterile, and the sets must be well distributed in order for the entire surgical intervention to be rational and the duration of the operation as short as possible.

What kind of incision does the operation start with?

The direction of the cut changed with the development of implatology. Since 1985, the Branemark school has changed the positions of the cut direction in the lower jaw between the mental foramina, and in the upper jaw medial to the first molars.

Today, it is recommended to guide the incision along the alveolar ridge, more orally, in the attached gingiva with vestibular or oral relaxing incisions (Fig. 18.155) without injuring the marginal free gingiva of the adjacent teeth. After that, the mucoperiosteal flap is raised with a raspatory to obtain complete visibility of the bone of the alveolar ridge. The raised oral flap is attached with surgical thread to the necks of the teeth or the opposite alveolar ridge so that it does not interfere with further work. The surface of the bone must be well prepared and smooth before the drills start working in the bone.

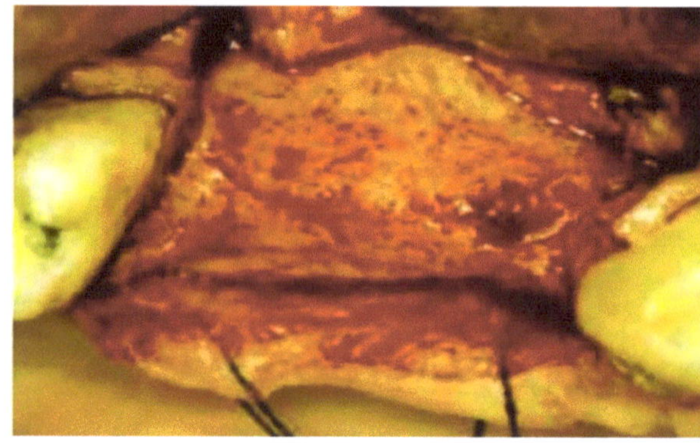

Figure 18.155. An orally relaxing cut without damaging the edge of the marginal gingiva of the adjacent teeth. Tightening the flap with a surgical thread enables unhindered bone preparation, thus creating the conditions for papilla reconstruction.

What is the next step in the surgical procedure?

It is a preparation for inserting the drills into the bone. Drill bits must be sharp and sterile. At the beginning, it must be emphasized that during work with bone drills, all the time, the bone must be intensively cooled with physiological solution in order to avoid overheating of the bone.

What is the sequence of further procedures?

The sequence of procedures is shown in pictures 18.156 - 18.158. This order means:

- raising the flap of the cortical part of the bone and marking the position of the implant with a pilot drill;
- deepening of the opening of the implant bed;
- expanding the edge to 3 mm;
- definitive check of the prepared implant bed;
- entering the canal with an incision of the appropriate diameter if the bone is very hard;
- in the case of weaker resistance to the drill, that is, if the bone is softer, make incisions with the implant itself.

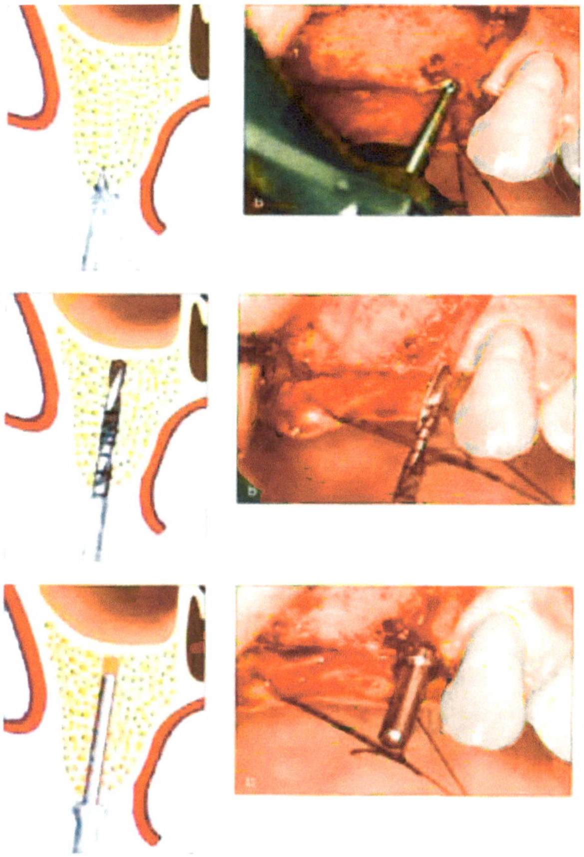

Figure 18.156. Schematic representation of the implantation sequence: marking the implant position with a pilot drill (a), working with a dimensioned drill (b), implant parallelism indicator (c).

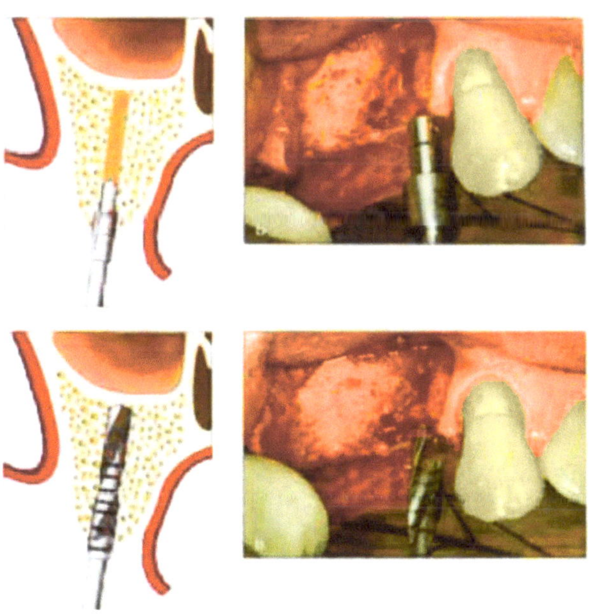

Figure 18.157. Schematic representation of the selection of drill bits of the appropriate diameter and length.

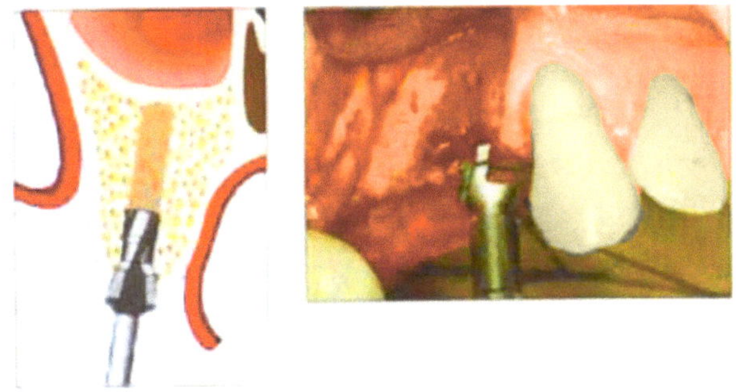

Figure 18.158. Final processing of the bone of the implant bed.

Marking Of The Implant Position And Sequence Of Surgical Procedures

How is the implant position marked?

The implant site must be precisely determined and marked before starting the bone dissection with a pilot drill. How this phase will be carried out depends on whether the implant installation will be carried out with the raising of the mucoperiosteal flap or not. If it is done without raising the mucoperiosteal flap, the mucoperiosteal part of the soft tissue is removed with the instrument for that purpose until it reaches the bone (pictures 18.158, 18.160, and 18.161). Adjust the speed of the pilot drill to open the hard marginal bone layer (lamina corticalis) without thermal trauma at the very beginning of the procedure.

To avoid overheating the bone, the bone filings from the bone packing drill should be immediately removed with saline and collected in a bowl as valuable augmentation material instead of suctioning them. If the temperature during work in the bone rises above 47°C, bone necrosis may occur after one minute.

During the first procedure with a pilot drill, if it is a single implant between the remaining teeth, care must be taken that the center of the osteotomy is far enough from the anatomical structures of the adjacent teeth to avoid their damage when working in the bone when preparing the implant bed. If it is noticed that the border zone of the neighboring tooth is threatened by the osteotomy, which is best controlled visually, it is necessary to make corrections to the bone preparation immediately so that the implant of the selected diameter of the socket is placed in the appropriate position. If the implant is placed incorrectly it can only be noticed in the prosthetic phase of work. If the implant is placed too vestibular, the consequence may be dehiscence in the region of the carrier and the implant, which will affect the aesthetics. If the implant is placed too palatally, unwanted occlusal problems may occur during prosthetic work. An occlusal problem can result in both implant loss and lamellar bone resorption. To avoid unwanted consequences, the implant must be placed in the middle of the alveolar bone. Therefore, it is required to maintain a minimum distance of 4 mm from adjacent teeth and 7 mm from adjacent implants.

For example, if the implants are 3.5 mm in diameter, the distance from the adjacent teeth must be at least 2 mm and more than 3 mm from the adjacent implant. After marking with a pilot drill, the implantation procedure continues with a 2 mm spiral drill. The bed in the bone is deepened to a predetermined depth with spiral drills of slightly larger diameters of 2.5 mm and 2.8 mm. Then the gradual preparation of the bed continues with the change of drills of larger diameters by the diameter of the implant with occasional interruptions. More often, the direction of the drill bit and the implant should be controlled three-dimensionally: using a surgical stent and a direction indicator, and the depth should be examined with a precise millimeter gauge, and maybe with a marked periodontal probe.

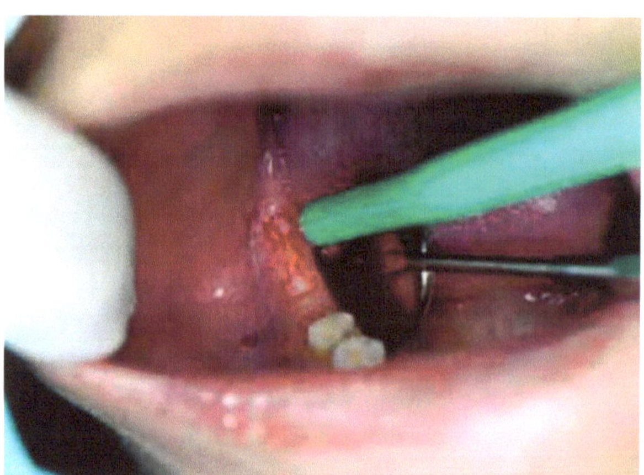

Figure 18.159. Marked places of the implant position without raising the flap. According to previously determined parameters, sufficient horizontal and vertical available bones.

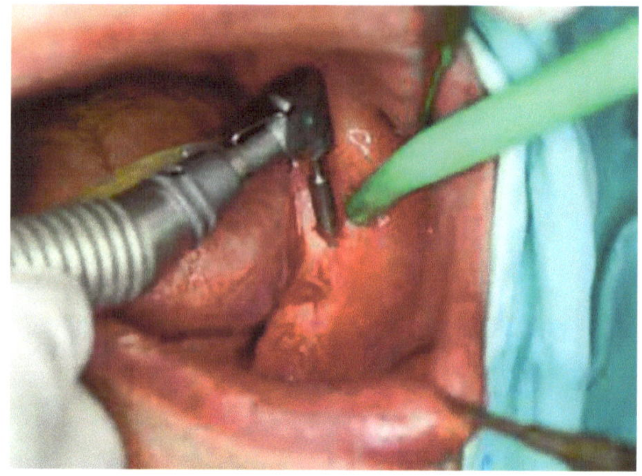

Figure 18.160. An instrument used to form access to the bone by removing soft tissues. First by hand, then by machine.

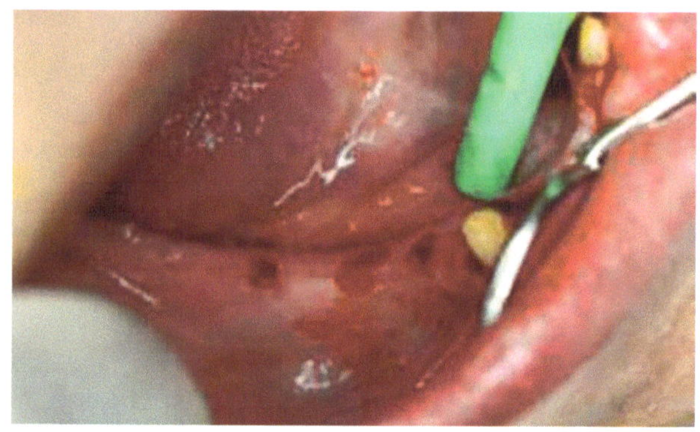

Figure 18.161. Prepared implant positions. Strive for the implants to be placed in a tripod position due to the fulfillment of biomechanical requirements.

The spiral drill should be 1 mm longer than the length of the implant itself. During bone preparation, if the procedure is performed in the lower jaw in the lateral region, care should be taken not to compromise the safe distance of 2 mm above the mandibular canal. If the procedure is performed in the upper jaw near the maxillary sinuses, this safe margin of 2 mm depends on the assessment of the use of the cortical bone of the sinuses. Therefore, the surgical intervention in that region can be performed in two ways: if there is sufficient bone height, the best solution is found by resting the tip of the implant on the strong cortical bone, or the other more complicated and risky way, raising the sinus floor.

What's next?

After expanding the bed with 2 mm, 2.5, or 2.8 mm drills, expand the bed to 3 mm with the next drill. Recently, a Korean company has launched a drill that processes the hard marginal bone layer, so that the expanding peripheral part of the bone bed collects bone chips that, mixed with allogeneic bone substitutes, can be usefully used later. With the previous way of preparing the bone for the implant bed, that precious material was lost by removing it and washing it with a saline solution. The number of revolutions must be reduced so much that the bone files do not overheat. Always pay attention to the direction of the drill bit. Before that, it is important to gradually use three drill bits with narrow diameters to expand the bed the implant was introduced gradually, with as little trauma to the bone as possiblse, and the entire course of the procedure must be constantly followed by copious cooling with physiological solution.

Definite Bearing Expansion

When is the deposit definitely expanded and how is it finally processed?

In a definitively expanded bed, a 3 mm drill bit is used to the bottom if it is an implant with a wider diameter of 3 mm. Recheck the drilling depth with a gauge. If very hard bone is encountered, a slightly wider diameter 3.15 mm or 3.25 mm spiral drill can be used. It is necessary, if required by the work phase, to use a drill that collects bone shavings that, mixed with allogeneic bone substitutes, can use to strengthen the bone walls where the implant lies. Each implant set has typed drills for its implant. But the principles are similar in all of them. When installing standard implants in bone types III or IV, the diameter of the drill must be at least 3 mm.

With a special drill bit, prepare the implant neck in the hard marginal margin. The implant should be inserted by self-cutting, gently, with pauses, so that the stress on the surrounding bone is gradual. The intensity of cutting into the bone depends on the inclination and length of the thread, and of course the primary stability of the embedded implant also depends on it.

Definitive Processing Of The Prepared Implant Bed

What should be paid attention to when finishing the prepared canal in the bone?

The final processing of the shape of the bone canal is achieved with appropriate drills whose diameters correspond to the diameter of the selected implant. In all sets, there are also taps for the corresponding diameters. Use the cutting tool only at the beginning of the prepared bed, and continue the installation of the implant by self-cutting into the bone. For this reason, the characteristics of the implant threads (inclination and angle) are important, on which the achievement of good primary stability depends.

In case of poor bone quality, preparation of the bed must be done carefully, and the depth of the bed should not be identical to the length of the implant, which would prevent good primary stability. For example, if a 3.8 mm diameter implant canal is being cut, drills and taps of the same diameter should not be used. The manufacturer's instructions do not emphasize the quality of the bone. That is why, with poor bone quality, it is necessary to use drills with a narrower diameter than the diameter of the implant for bed preparation. Do notching with the implant itself, of course if it is a self-tapping type of implant.

Implant Placement

Are there any specifics for implant placement?

Most of the newer generations of implants are self-tapping. As previously emphasized, incisions should be avoided, except in cases of high bone density. In such cases, the drilling speed should be adjusted to 15-20 revolutions per minute. When working with dense bone, the burr should enter the bone canal without applying pressure to prevent overheating at the beginning of the procedure. This step must be carried out carefully to avoid changing the preparation direction and damaging the threaded part, as this could compromise the implant threads.

When using an incisor for multiple prepared bone beds, it is essential to constantly clean it of bone filings. Additionally, the site should be rinsed well.

It is important to avoid undercuts whenever possible. The implant itself, through its threads, performs this function, and the design of the threads is crucial for ensuring primary stability and supporting the forces acting on the implant.

The next procedure is the installation of the implant. The implant is placed in the socket to follow the prepared direction of the bone socket. The initial screwing, without excessive force, should be done by hand and again carefully see if the implant is in the correct direction. The screwing is continued manually or mechanically. If it is done by machine (knee), directed machine twisting should be done slowly (15-20 revolutions per minute).

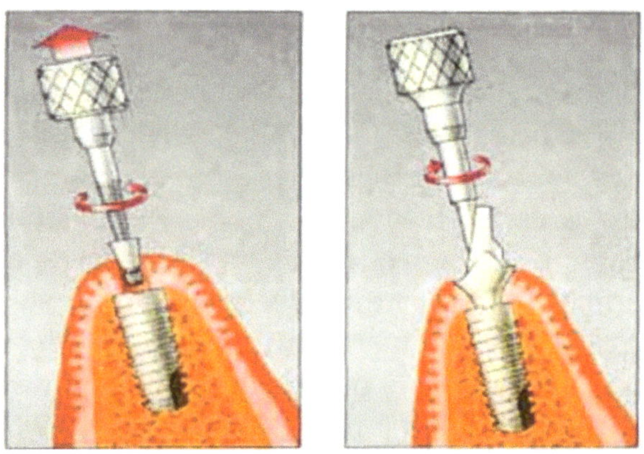

Figure 18.162. After the installed implant, the further sequence of procedures depends on the set treatment plan: placing a cap for healing (gingiva former) and waiting for a certain time or setting a temporary or definitive support (abutment) and making a temporary prosthetic work.

Is it necessary to follow this sequence of procedures?

After screwing the first apical third, you should stop to let the bone "rest", and in order to reduce the trauma of the pressure on the bone walls, screw two should be unscrewed. After a short break, continue twisting to the coronary edge. The screwing of the implant is finally completed with a screw wrench. Wrenching requires some application of vertical force. The most suitable are wrenches that can measure that vertical force in newtons, which should not exceed 35 N cm.

When placing implants, what must be paid attention to?

The implant must not be tightened too much, as this can cause microcracks in the bone.

The conclusion is that during the definitive placement of the implant in the socket, the bone should be "rested" so that the bone can reduce that tension with its elasticity. Fast twisting with a wrench and tightening too hard without resting, makes the bone suffer a lot of pressure, which is not recommended.

When the placement of the implant in the bone is completed, if the implant is not primarily loaded, a covering cap is placed on it. It is good to put some of the antibiotic ointment in the implant (in the bed for the covering cap), not only to prevent local infection, but also to make the cap easier to unscrew after healing.

Reso-pac collagen-based packing remains elastic all the time, thus protecting the wound from compression, and food deposition after surgery, which accelerates and slows healing.

After placing the caps on the implants, the operative site should be thoroughly washed with saline solution, and cleaned of all bone and soft tissue remains. At the end, the mucoperiosteal flap should be returned, and tightly pressed against the bone and the wound should be closed well with several sutures. At the same time, give the patient a roll of sterile gauze to bite over the wound.

Discovery Of Implants – A Small Surgical Operation

What to do next if waiting time is required?

The following procedure can be said to be the second surgical procedure. After three to six months (healing time depends on the assessment of the implantologist and the manufacturer's recommendation), the second surgical procedure is the removal of the implant. When opening the soft parts around the implant covering cap, it is necessary to remove the deposited parts of bone and soft tissue formed above the covering cap. The covering cap is replaced by unscrewing with a cap for the formation of gingiva that corresponds to the output profile of the implant (Fig. 18.162).

The correct choice of cap for healing is determined by the thickness of the gingiva, which can be measured with a gauge or a periodontal probe. The healing cap should be left 2 mm above the mucosa.

When screwing the cap, you should pay attention to the direction in order not to damage the thread on the implant. After placing the cap, the surrounding tissue should be precisely shaped around the cap, and if necessary, secured with one or two stitches.

The gingival formation cap should be left in place for four to eight weeks. This duration can be shortened if a definitive support is immediately placed instead of using healing caps. The author's experience suggests that this method is more effective, as it allows for any additional small surgical procedures aimed at improving aesthetic and functional outcomes to be performed on a definitive profile.

After this period, prior to prosthetic rehabilitation, it is essential to assess bone integration. Even minor mobility of the implant indicates that osseous integration has failed. Peri-implant pain, despite local anesthesia, suggests that soft granulation tissue has built up around the implant. A control X-ray is mandatory to check for any peri-implant lightening. If lightening is detected, consideration should be given to removing the implant with thorough curettage, and, if conditions permit, to replacing it with an implant of a wider diameter.

The author of the book has noted that many previously described procedures have been simplified or abandoned in favor of immediate installation of implants, the use of supports (abutments) instead of healing caps, and immediate loading of the installed implants.

What mucogingival procedures can be performed to improve the quality and thickness of the peri-implant mucosa in order to improve aesthetics?

It depends on a case by case basis. Various mucogingival procedures can be undertaken to meet aesthetic requirements.

These interventions include the following actions:

a) apical positioning of the buccal lobe;
b) application of a lateral or displaced flap;
c) free gingival graft;
d) free connective tissue grafts; e) gingivoplasty.

Are there new approaches, that is, new methods, which can influence the shaping of soft tissues around implants for aesthetic reasons?

Yes, there are. The latest methods are as follows:

- Controlled wound healing;
- Regeneration of the papilla;
- Guided soft tissue regeneration; and
- Positioning of interdental contact points.

All this belongs to the domain of modern periodontology. However, knowing some details from the field of periodontology is also important for an implantologist. For example, crowns on natural abutment teeth protrude 0.5 mm to 1 mm into the sulcus. Crowns on implants, often for aesthetic reasons, go into the sulcus, which is a big mistake. Keratinized tissue is essential for the aesthetic and functional result of rehabilitation.

Several techniques are available for controlled tissue healing, and this concept is to improve aesthetic results. Of course, this process must be accompanied by proper oral hygiene. In controlled soft tissue healing, the so-called EPS concept (eruption profile system). This concept consists of the fact that the cap for healing and transfer caps must match the diameter of the implant, as well as the width of the intended crown. In this way, the prosthetic result of the derived crown aesthetically approaches the natural crown.

What method is used to achieve this?

In this procedure, a healing cap, which matches the exit profile of the planned crown and has a diameter of either 5.6 mm or 7 mm, is securely attached to the implant. After the healing period, a transfer cap that corresponds to the healing cap is placed on the implant. This transfer cap allows for the accurate replication of the peri-implant tissue through an impression, which is then transferred to the working model.

This process is extremely important because it provides the dental technician in the laboratory with a precise representation of the situation, enabling them to shape the intended crown aesthetically and optimally. When the dental technician sculpts the eruptive profile of the soft tissue on the working model, they no longer need to rely solely on experience or improvisation. Instead, they have access to very precise details, which enhances the quality of the gingival attachment.

Ultimately, when the definitive crown is placed, there is no need for additional treatment around the gingiva. This is because the risk of crown oversizing is minimized, and the transfer caps provide an accurate representation of the external part. It is important to ensure that the healing caps are not overly wide, as this could put pressure on the soft tissues.

Depending on the subgingival depth of the embedded implant, the exit profile of the placed healing cap must be adjusted to the bone level. For this, there are special trepanning drills that are adapted to individual output profiles. Recently, there are also specially made anatomical caps for healing, which can individually form peri-implant soft tissue.

Imprint Taking

How important is imprint taking?

Taking an impression is a very important stage of the work to fully achieve the functional and aesthetic requirements. Modern implantology seeks to improve the aesthetic appearance of the patient as much as possible.

Taking impressions on implants must be similar to taking impressions for classic prosthetic fixed works. With conventional prosthetics, after the teeth are ground, an impression is taken and the situation of the mouth must be accurately transferred to a working model in the laboratory. The same principle applies to prosthetic work on implants (pictures 18.163 to 18.168).

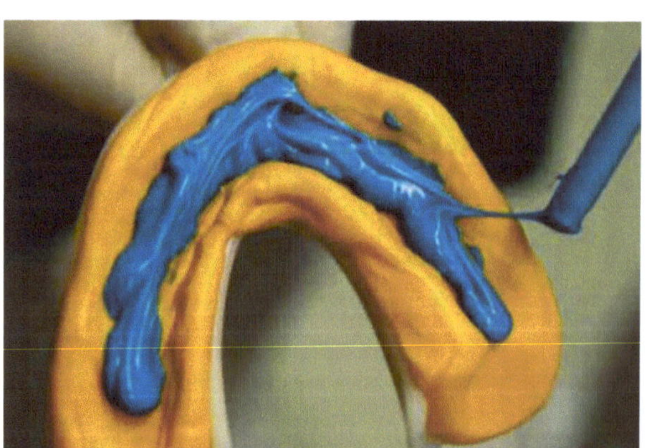

Figure 18.163. Single-phase impression taking.

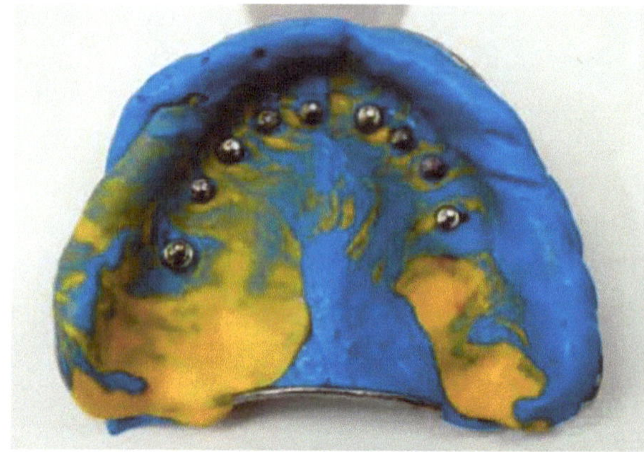

Figure 18.164. The analog bed in the impression must be thoroughly checked before sending it to the laboratory.

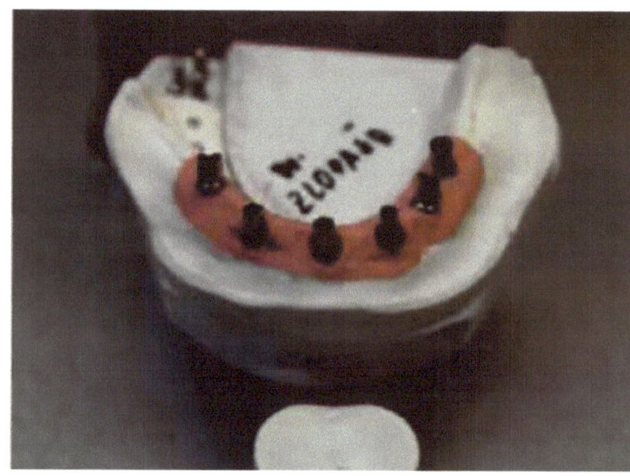

Figure 18.165. Branemark system supports mounted on a plaster model. The achieved parallelism enables more precise fabrication of prosthetic work.

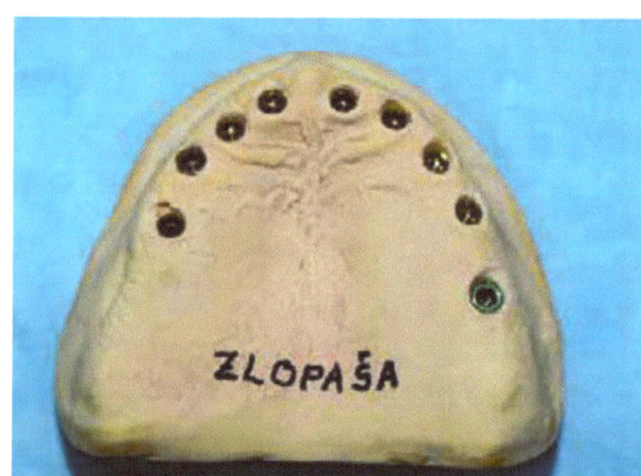

Figure 18.166. Molded analogues in a plaster model; correct position and arrangement of the installed implants.

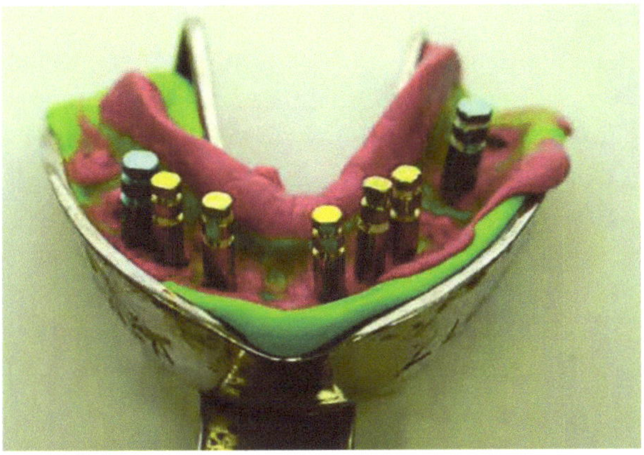

Figure 18.167. Placed analogs of the implants in the impression show the parallelism of the positioned implants.

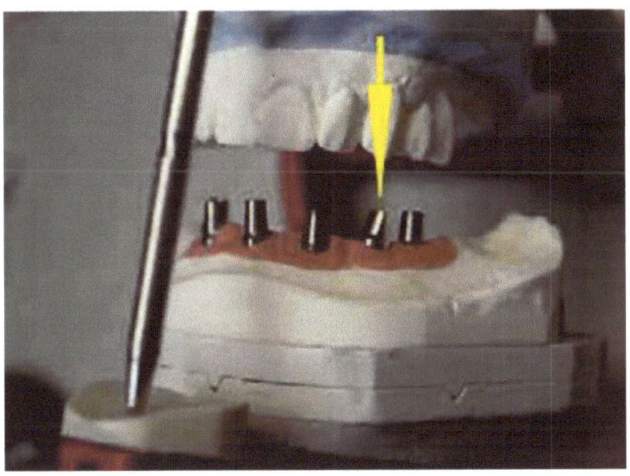

Figure 18.168. On the cast impression the disparity of the supports corrected by using an angled support. For primary loading, avoid using implant supports whose angle is greater than 15 degrees.

When transferring an oral situation to the laboratory, even the most accurate impressions can lead to a series of errors, which may have serious consequences. Variations in dimensions can occur, either in the impression materials or during laboratory processes, due to several factors: the method of pouring the model, the type of material used for the working model, the waxing technique, the use of inappropriate varnish to coat the stump, the maintenance of the interspace between the metal and the tooth surface, the choice of cuvette mass, errors during metal casting, or contractions during porcelain firing.

All these errors can impact the quality of the prosthetic construction and lead to imprecise placement on implants. If metal constructions are poorly fitted onto the implants, this can jeopardize not only the supports of the prosthetic superstructure, risking broken screws, but also the integration of the bone. It is crucial to remember that metal structures are not elastic; thus, achieving precise positioning on the implants is essential for the overall success of the treatment.

The testing of the construction in the mouth should be painless and should not cause any tension on the supports. It is important to document any errors that occur, from the transfer of the situation from the mouth to the working model to any mistakes made in the laboratory, as these represent common issues. Additionally, a separate section emphasizes the significance of accurately transferring the in-mouth situation to the articulator.

When should I take an imprint?

The impression can be taken immediately after the installation of the implant, or after several months. It depends on whether the desire is to load the implant immediately or postpone it for later. Postponing impression-taking depends on assessing whether primary stability suitable for immediate loading has been achieved. This procedure should be approached with good judgment and a lot of caution to avoid complications. The decision whether to perform immediate loading depends on clinical judgment as well as the experience of the dentist.

The immediate loading of an individual tooth with a larger number of implants requires a different approach. In the first case, the position of the antagonist and occlusal forces that may endanger the entire procedure should be evaluated. The ideal situation for immediate loading exists when the bony alveolus is completely filled with the implant. For immediate loading to be successful, it must be ensured that lateral movements of the mandible avoid displacement of the implant in the bone during healing.

The decision to immediately load the implant depends on whether the primary stability of the implant has been achieved, which depends on several factors: bone quality and quantity, design, diameter and length implants, and occlusal load of temporary prosthetic work. All these factors add to the importance of the performed surgical intervention by the clinician and his experience.

Immediate implantation of implants has recently been given more and more importance for several reasons: shortening the duration of treatment and simplifying treatment compared to delayed implantation are obvious advantages for the patient. A further documented advantage of immediate loading is the maintenance of bone volume and the stimulating action of forces within physiological limits on the formation of new bone. After all, replacing a tooth that cannot be preserved with an implant and putting it into function immediately without disturbing the aesthetic appearance, as a basic thought, is very tempting. The clinical results of implants that are installed immediately after tooth extraction, and also in case of long-term toothlessness, confirm the view that it is a technique that results in a high success rate.

Connecting a larger number of implants with provisional prosthetic work has the advantage that the implant is put into operation, and an additional quality is that the physiological stress on the implant stimulates the healing process, accelerating bone integration.

To achieve this, the temporary work is placed outside the occlusion avoiding interference during lateral movements of the mandible. If the implants have cortical anchoring, the situation is even more suitable for immediate loading.

When it comes to the immediate installation of implants, it can be said that it is a reliable procedure, but that decision should be preceded by a thorough analysis and assessment, which essentially depends on the knowledge and experience of the clinician.

When evaluating the benefits of immediate loading, the clinician must also have in mind the risk assessment related to the procedure that should be applied if complications occur.

What is important to do before the definitive handover of prosthetic work?

The healing period (depending on which procedure is chosen) lasts approximately two to three months. Many clinicians suggest waiting six weeks for definitive loading. Experience shows that the healing period and bone integration process should be longer; especially, if the temporary restoration is made very precisely, there is no need to hurry with the definitive prosthetic work, because in this way the condition that the condition of the soft tissues is stable will be fulfilled. This is concluded by assessing the condition of the gingival margin and papillae, with the provisional work being used as a reference. Definitive construction should not be started until the soft tissues have achieved complete stability. With immediate implantation with implants of reduced diameter (3 mm, 3.3 mm), the healing of soft tissues is much faster and of better quality.

Soft tissues, primarily the papillae, must not be endangered by the definitive fabrication of the prosthetic work, because all of this endangers the aesthetic appearance.

Can the papilla be reconstructed?

One of the significant achievements in modern implantology and periodontology is the regeneration of the interdental papilla. Successfully regenerating the lost papilla contributes greatly to the aesthetic outcome of dental treatments. In 1992, M. Palacci first described a method for papilla reconstruction during a secondary surgical procedure. Later, researchers such as Spikerman and Saša Jovanović made important contributions to this technique.

To reconstruct the papilla, vertical incisions are made at least 3 mm mesial and distal to the implant. These vertical incisions are then connected by buccal or lingual horizontal incisions, which extend only to the periosteum. After these incisions are made, the mucoperiosteal flap is lifted to expose the covering caps of the implant (see Fig. 18.154). Once the covering caps are revealed, they are removed and replaced with healing caps, which should be positioned at least 2 mm above the soft tissue.

It is essential that any excess buccal flap tissue measures between 3 to 5 mm. Following this, a circular incision is made around the implant, extending to adjacent caps and the marginal gingiva, allowing for proper alignment with the healing cap. The flap is then rotated 90 degrees, filling the 3 mm space between the implants and creating the new papilla. This papilla is then sutured to the periosteum.

Special attention must be given to the suturing of the flap stem, ensuring that it is fixed with stitches that are not under tension. Careful suturing of the petioles is critical, as excessive tightening can lead to necrosis of the papilla, significantly compromising the aesthetic results of the treatment. For this technique to be successful, it is crucial to have sufficient keratinized tissue available.

How successful are guided soft tissue regenerations today?

It depends on a case by case basis, and it all depends on many factors. Nevertheless, a general conclusion can be drawn that they are successful in a large percentage.

Does this mean that the bone ridge has a decisive role for the function of the interdental papilla?

Yes. The bony ridge has a decisive role for the function of the interdental papillae. Its visible regeneration depends a lot on how far the interdental contact point of the prosthetic crown is from the bone, i.e. the edges of the crown in the neck area should not touch the bone (Fig. 18.162).

In one study (D.Tarnow et al.) the following data were given: in 288 teeth, the papilla was completely regenerated in cases where the distance from the point of contact to the bone was below 5 mm. When the gap was 6 mm, the percentage of papilla regeneration was reduced to 56%, and with a gap of 7 mm it was only 27%. Today, guided soft tissue regeneration is becoming increasingly important. The concept of guiding soft tissue regeneration has been developing since the end of the last century. The concept consists in an augmentative method that enables the creation of a new interdental papilla, and thus the achievement of outstanding aesthetic results, especially in the frontal regions. The method is contraindi cated in the following cases:

a) when there is a large bone resorption;
b) when the mucous membrane is very thin;
c) when there is too little keratinized tissue.

What kind of cut should be used with this method?

The incision is made palatally in the shape of the letter II (see Fig. 18.148) with a fine raspatoria, partially separated flap at 3-4 mm, which then turns into a complete flap. In this way, we also stimulate primary healing, that is, better healing.

After raising the flap, the covering caps of the implants are reached, in the place of which caps are placed for healing, and the length of the caps should correspond to the height of the lost tissue. After the first suturing, a small space remains in the narrow operative site between the bone and the healing cap, which must first be filled blood coagulum, and after that it turns into additional soft tissue. It is mandatory to wait 8 to 12 weeks for the soft tissue to heal completely and only then can the secondary support part be placed.

It should be noted that for this method it is sometimes necessary to perform several reoperations, so delaying the placement of the secondary part (carrier) for several weeks is inevitable. The problem is the relatively difficult sewing of the flap. In addition, based on clinical results so far, it cannot be concluded how long one should wait for new soft tissues to form. Also, subsequent soft tissue recession due to the absence of a bony substrate cannot be ruled out.

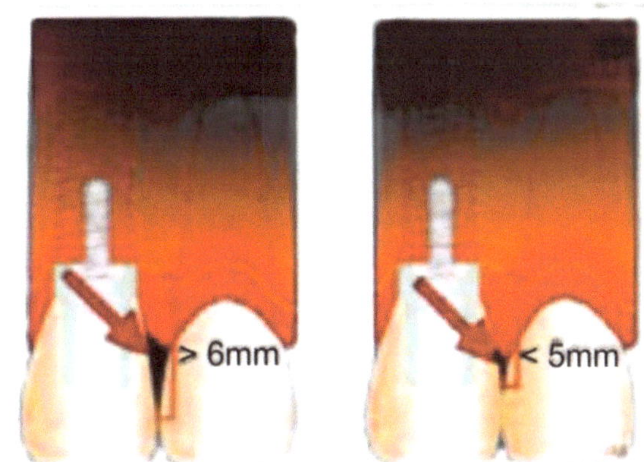

Figure 18.169. The possibility of regeneration of the papilla depends on the state of the crestal bone.

In addition, the quality and precision of temporary crowns plays a big role. Temporary crowns must exert pressure on the soft tissues from the sides after placing the supports.

The aforementioned study, however, dealt with research on natural teeth and their periodontium. If we start from the assumption that this rule also applies to implants, it seems that we should look at it with some reserve. With well-placed interdental contact points, with a distance of less than 5 mm from the bone ridge, the papillae are completely regenerated.

For this reason, the importance of placing temporary prosthetic work is decisive, which could help in evaluating the success of the treatment. All such studies have the same drawback: the time of consideration of peri-implant soft tissue structures is still too short. For this reason, the obtained results are insufficient to draw a definitive conclusion.

Questions About Implant Diameter And Length

What dilemma does the practitioner most often face when it comes to choosing the diameter and length of the implant?

The implantologist often finds himself in a dilemma as to which diameter and length of the implant to use in a certain situation without endangering any anatomical structure. For example, for an implant with a diameter of 3.75 mm and a length of 10 mm, the volume of the bone, that is, the width of the alveolar ridge, must be at least 2 mm larger than the diameter of the implant, that is, it should be at least 1 mm larger on each side.

And as for the height in the lower jaw, it should be at least 12 mm. So, this height enables a safe distance of 2 mm from the mandibular canal to be preserved (Figure 18.170). If this minimum required height is smaller, the shorter length of the implant can be compensated by a wider diameter if the volume of the bone allows it.

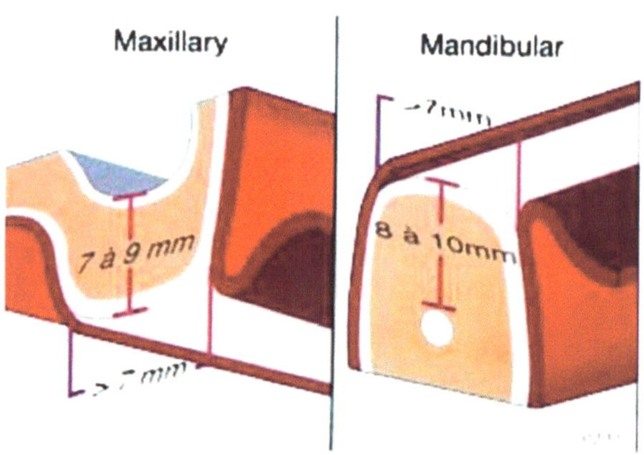

Figure 18.170. In the lower jaw, there must be a safe distance of 2 mm above the mandibular canal, so short implants with an aggressive thread, with a larger diameter, are indicated. If the bone in the upper jaw is of insufficient height, larger diameter implants are indicated.

What about cases in the upper jaw?

The height of the alveolar ridge should be at least 10 mm, and if it is less than that height, implants with a larger diameter (5 mm) are indicated. In the case of lower quality bone, a larger diameter implant is more stable (Fig. 18.171). However, the width of the ridge must be taken into account in order to prevent perforation of the lingual cortical wall due to the width of the implant.

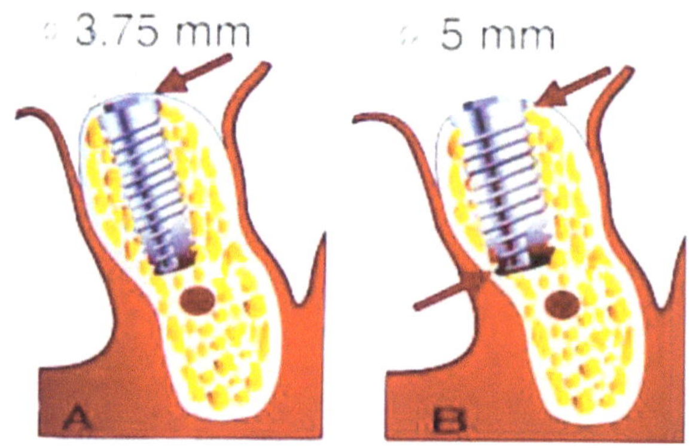

Figure 18.171. If the bone is of poor quality (type IV), when spongiosis is dominant, larger diameter implants should be used

What should be done in the upper jaw to avoid the "adventure" of raising the sinus floor?

Unlike the mandatory safety distance of 2 mm above the mandibular canal, a safety distance of 2 mm is not required in the upper jaw near the maxillary sinus. The best solution is to insert the implant up to the cortical part of the sinus floor. If the volume of the alveolar crest allows the installation of a larger diameter implant, it is a far simpler and more successful option than raising the sinus floor to install a longer implant.

What should be the mesiodistal distance between two implants?

In the case of the edentulous part of the alveolar ridge, the number and size of the implants is chosen according to the available bone and the planned prosthetic reconstruction. For individual implants, the mesiodistal width of the bone between the two teeth must be at least 7 mm. Between two implants, a gap of 3 mm should be provided for prosthetic work, and between the implant and the natural tooth, the gap should be 2 mm to preserve the bone and gingiva.

The diameter of the implant (Fig. 18.172.) affects the functional and aesthetic result. Wide diameter implant (A) 5 or 6 mm, with adequate thickness in the neck. Implant with a standard diameter (B) of 3.75 or 4 mm and a neck thickness of 4.1 mm. Implant with a reduced diameter (C) of 3.25 mm and a reduced neck thickness of 4.1 mm. The implant has a narrow diameter (D) of 3.25 mm and a reduced thickness around the neck of 3.4 mm.

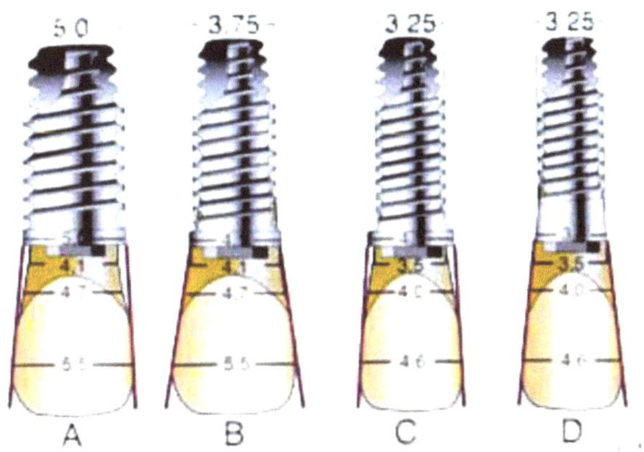

Figure 18.172. The functional and aesthetic result depends on the choice of implant diameter. The shaping of the gingiva and the reconstruction of the papilla depend on the width of the implant in the neck area, especially in the upper frontal region ("aesthetic zone").

What period is considered the beginning of thinking about the importance of implant diameter?

Until the end of the 1980s, implantology did not reach the point where the importance of implant diameter became the focus of interest. Much attention was paid to bony integration, and this problem was sidelined. In the last ten years, more and more attention has been paid to aesthetic requirements. In that period, new surgical techniques and new prosthetic achievements advanced significantly. Thanks to the variety of implant diameters, aesthetic results are increasingly successful. The ideal diameter of the implant depends on the quality and quantity of available bone, the type of prosthetic work (partial or en bloc), as well as aesthetic and biomechanical requirements.

When should smaller diameter implants be used?

There are limitations when implants of standard diameters cannot be inserted. Implants with a smaller diameter than 3 mm should be avoided if fixed prosthetic works are planned. In anatomically limited situations, it is sometimes possible to apply only this type of implant, but there is always a risk, because it is very easy to get into complications that have an inevitable outcome, the failure of the entire treatment.

This type of implant can be applied in places where there is a thin bone ridge, razor-shaped at the top of the alveolar ridge, or if the mesiodistal available space is less than 7 mm. Then implants with a reduced diameter of 3 mm or 3.4 mm are indicated. The advantage of using these implants is avoiding a major and complicated surgical intervention: increasing the width of the alveolar ridge with bone grafts, or avoiding expensive and long-term orthodontic treatment to create a favorable mesiodistal space. However, when deciding whether to apply a narrower implant, all biomechanical requirements must be thoroughly examined to avoid risks.

What conclusion can be drawn?

Narrow implants, i.e. implants of reduced diameter are indicated in cases of:

1. narrow bone ridge; and
2. reduced cervical diameter of the crown.

If the first case is considered, in the frontal region of the mandible, if the intra-radicular distance is less than 7 mm, 3.75 mm implants are contraindicated due to possible damage to the adjacent root. If this mesiodistal space is reduced to 5-7 mm, several possibilities are available: to increase this space by orthodontic displacement, to use an implant with a narrower diameter (2.4 mm and 2.8 mm), but a longer length, or finally, to treat the specific case with a classic prosthetic solution.

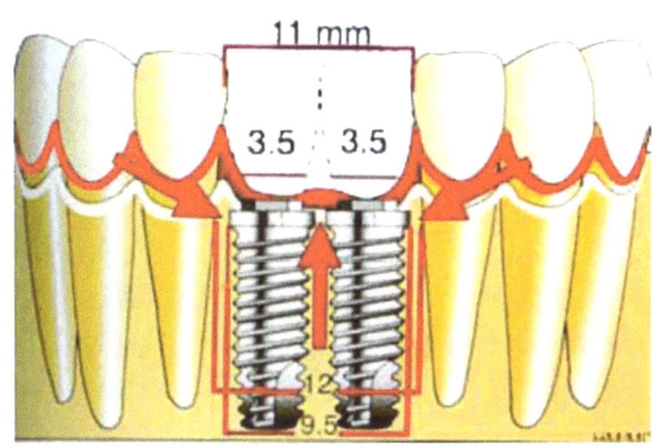

Figure 18.173. Implants of standard diameter in the place of central incisors in the lower jaw are not indicated because they can create an aesthetic problem. Good aesthetic results are achieved with a reduced diameter.

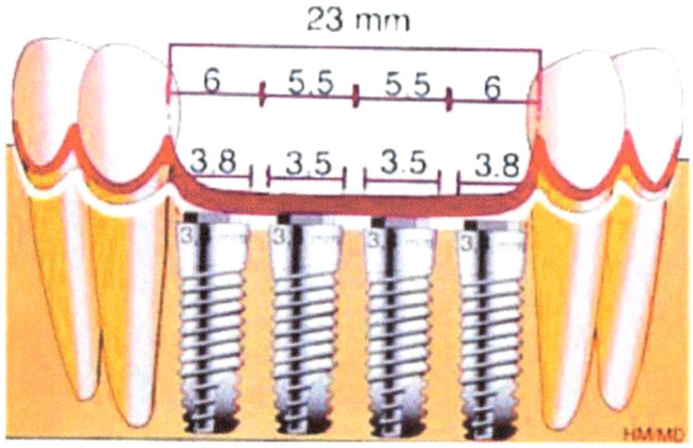

Figure 18.174. Smaller diameter implants in the frontal region of the lower jaw achieve a good aesthetic result.

It all depends on several factors: the place of edentulism, the width of the alveolar ridge, the time required for orthodontic movement and the distribution of occlusal forces.

Which implant diameter should be chosen if two middle incisors are missing in the lower jaw?

There is always enough bone in that place in terms of length. Aesthetics must be taken into account when choosing the diameter of the implant for the restoration of the central incisors. Standard diameter implants are not suitable (Fig. 18.160). If four incisors are missing in the lower jaw, implants of a smaller diameter (reduced neck thickness) should be inserted, which will enable a good aesthetic appearance (Fig. 18.161).

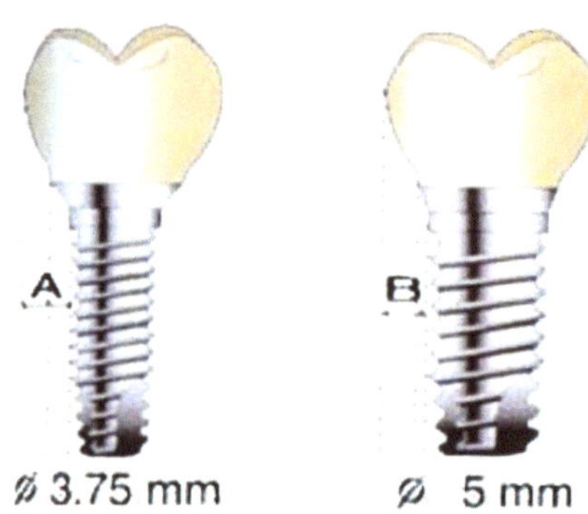

Figure 18.175. Implants with a larger diameter should be used with poor bone quality. Implants with an increased diameter enable shaping of a more natural exit profile of the crowns in the lateral regions.

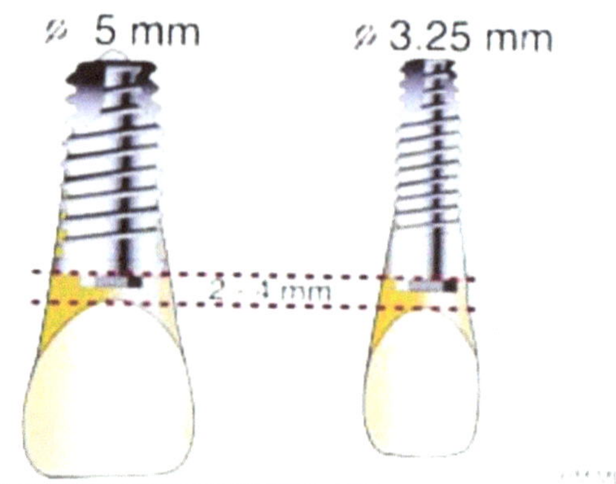

Figure 18.176. The replacement of central and lateral incisors requires the selection of implants of different diameters.

If there is a narrow bone ridge, what kind of implant should be chosen?

If the width of the alveolar ridge is less than 6 mm, implants with a reduced diameter can be considered. It must be known that the exit profile of the dental crown significantly affects the aesthetic appearance. Buccal concavity or strong central bone resorption can cause the direction of the implant to lie too lingually, i.e. for its exit point to be in that direction. This can jeopardize the entire intended treatment.

For example, in the upper jaw in the frontal region, such decomposed bone must first be treated with a reconstructive method, then think about the installation of the implant and its diameter. Otherwise, it may lead to bone fenestration during implant placement and treatment failure.

With a reduced mesiodistal space, which implant should be chosen in order to obtain a good aesthetic result?

It depends on the cervical and coronary diameter of the crown of the future prosthetic work and the output profile of the implant. In the region of the lower incisors, often also with the lateral upper incisors, the mesiodistal space is less than 4.5 mm, so a standard implant cannot be placed in those places, because the cervical diameter is around 4.1 often even a little smaller, so there then it cannot achieve a good aesthetic appearance (Fig. 18.161).

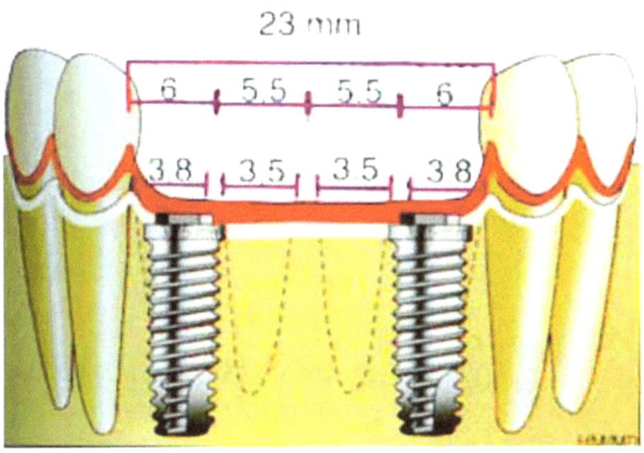

Figure 18.177. In the frontal region of the lower jaw, for compensation of central and lateral incisors, never apply implants of standard and wide diameters. It is impossible to achieve the desired aesthetic result. Installing two standard implants for the purpose of compensating 4 incisors can damage the aesthetic appearance.

In order to achieve a good aesthetic result, what should be paid attention to?

From an aesthetic point of view, the cervical mesiodistal diameter of the implant must be slightly less than the diameter of the intended crown. In its apico-coronal dimension, the implant should lie 2-4 mm below the enamel-cementum border of the adjacent teeth. The diameter of the natural root lies at this height below the enamel-cement border.

For individual implants, in places where the mesiodistal distance is a maximum of 4 mm, only implants with a narrower neck diameter are indicated. This allows the output natural diameter to achieve a full aesthetic effect.

What determines the choice of implant diameter and how to choose the appropriate diameter?

The choice of implant diameter depends on the type of crown. Of course, it will not be the same for the central incisor as for the lateral one (Fig. 18.178). When replacing central incisors in the lower jaw, smaller diameter implants should always be chosen.

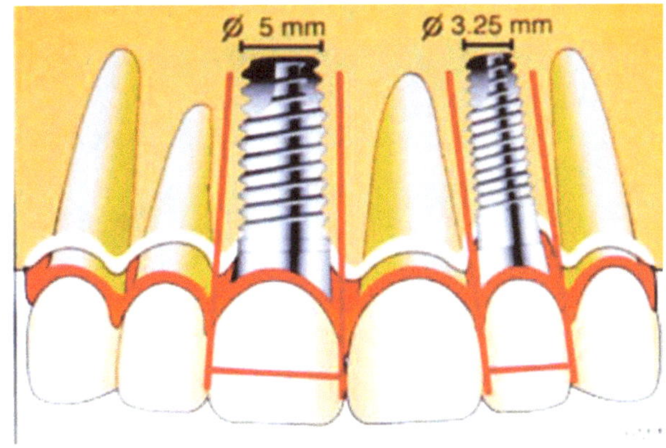

Figure 18.178. The choice of implant diameter depends on the width of the crown.

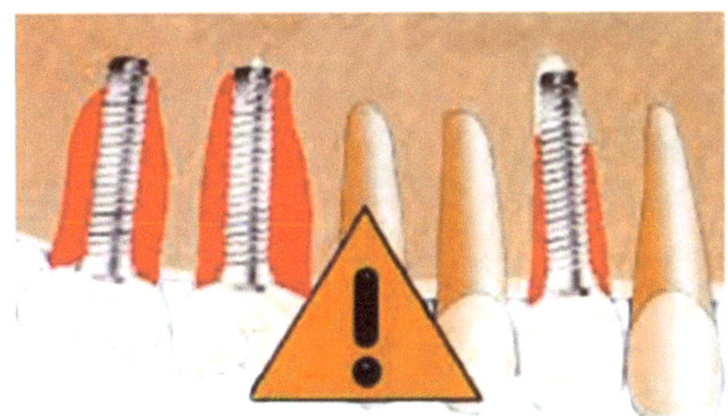

Figure 18.179. In the lateral region of the upper premolars, the use of implants with a smaller diameter is not indicated.

In which cases are narrower diameter implants contraindicated?

It is not recommended to place implants with a narrower diameter in regions where masticatory forces are strongest. These are the regions of premolars and molars (Fig. 18.179).

How much does tooth morphology affect aesthetics, especially in cases where the morphology cannot be completely restored?

The choice of the diameter of the implant significantly affects the aesthetic result of the implantation. But there are cases where the volume of the bone is reduced because there was not even a germ of a permanent tooth in that place. Such a case is most common with upper lateral incisors, when there is convergence of adjacent teeth, crowns and roots (Fig. 18.180). In such cases, it is usually necessary to decide on orthodontic displacement in order to obtain a suitable mesiodistal space. A narrower diameter implant is most often indicated in that area.

In the frontal region, the morphology must be adapted to the morphology of the opposite tooth, in order not to compromise the aesthetic result. In the frontal region at the place of incisors and even premolars, cervical and coronary dimensions require the installation of implants of a smaller diameter.

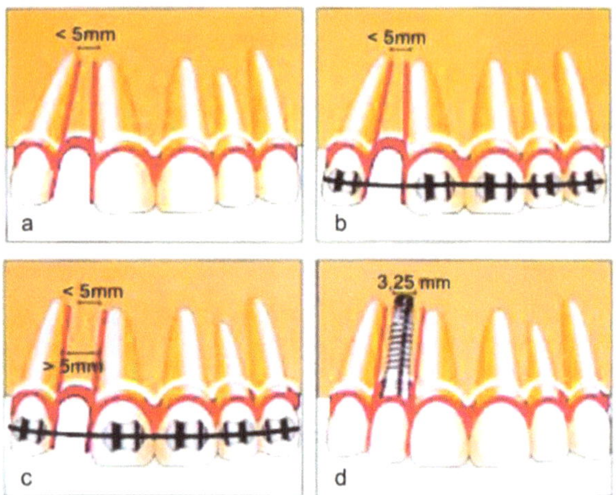

Figure 18.180. With a reduced interdental space, orthodontic displacement can create a space of 5 mm for the installation of implants with a diameter of 3 mm to 3.25 mm.

From a biomechanical point of view, when it comes to implant diameters, what should be paid special attention to?

The reception and distribution of occlusal forces depend on the diameter of the implant. Before deciding on implant diameter, it is necessary to analyze in detail what occlusal forces the implant will be exposed to. Occlusal forces are strongest in the region of the molars, and implants are indicated in these regions with larger diameters. These implants better receive and distribute occlusal forces provided they are surrounded by a sufficient amount of bone. With implants of smaller diameter, the distribution of forces is less favorable, and the load on the bone is greater. Moreover, small-diameter implants may fracture under unfavorable forces, which is a higher risk. One study gave the following results: implants of different lengths (7.8 and 15 mm) and diameters (3.0, 3.3, and 4.0 mm) were examined. It turns out that the twisting force increases proportionally to the length of the implant, while the traction forces, independent of the diameter of the implant, remain constant.

For example, Nobel Biocare withdrew its 3 mm diameter implant from the market and replaced it with a 3.3 mm diameter implant to meet biomechanical requirements. The obtained results showed that the fracture resistance of this implant was significantly lower compared to the earlier form.

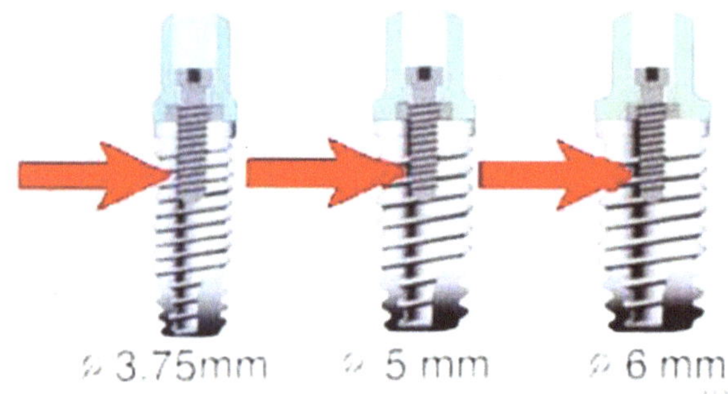

Figure 18.181. With wide-diameter implants, the risk of screw breakage and separation of the support (abutment) is significantly reduced.

Is there any knowledge of how the diameter of the implant affects the surrounding tissues?

Setnax (in 1992) investigated the relationship between surrounding tissues and implants with a diameter of 3.25 mm and 4.0 mm in 50 implants. He found that the soft tissue around the implant with a reduced diameter reacted more favorably over a period of three years. He advocates the thesis that there can be a critical diameter with accompanying bone breakdown followed by inflammatory processes. What is the critical diameter, the author does not know for now.

In the early 1990s, several scientists investigated how and how much implants of different diameters load the bone. They came to the conclusion that the reception and distribution of forces depends on the size of the diameter. For example, in the case of a cylindrical implant with a diameter of 3.75 mm loaded with vertical and lateral forces of 100 N/cm in the horizontal and vertical directions, the highest load was on the cortical part of the bone around the neck of the implant. Therefore, if the diameter of the implant is larger and the bone is wider, the reception of the forces is more favorable.

All these views for now are still more at the level of theoretical considerations when it comes to the biomechanical basis in relation to different diameters and cortical bone loss around the implant neck. For this reason, with some implant systems there is also a different design of this part of the implant.

How reliably smaller diameter implants guarantee the stability of bone and bone changes and what is the impact on soft tissues, reliable results can be given by long-term tests. However, it should be concluded that implants with a narrower diameter compared to standard implants have a reduced anchoring surface and bone-implant contact surface, and thus reduced fracture resistance. Uncontrolled occlusal forces should be eliminated.

In place of canines and molars, implants of reduced diameter are absolutely contraindicated.

Does this mean that wide diameter implants have an advantage?

If the width of the alveolar ridge enables a larger anchoring surface, which also achieves better primary stability, all conditions are created for faster and better bone integration. Such claims also led to the development of wide implants of 5 mm and even 6 mm for certain cases where the quality and quantity of bone is reduced.

What is the scientific evidence on this topic?

There are few published research results on this topic. The first research results can be found in the NobelBiocare multicenter studies in which 35 clinics from 13 countries participated. 977 implants with a diameter of 5 mm were installed in 614 patients. 605 implants were installed in the upper jaw, and 372 in the lower jaw. The percentage of success was 97.7%. The causes of 22 failures were not commented on.

Research with Branemark implants with a diameter of 5 mm was performed in 30 patients who had partial edentulism. After the healing phase, 48 implants were loaded for more than 12 months, and 43 for more than 18 months. Success after 12 and 18 months was the same, about 96%. During detection, bone degradation of two threads was observed in five implants, and in one implant of three threads, which remained clinically and radiographically stable in all cases after 6, 12 and 18 months.

A study of 51 patients, in whom 84 Branemark implants of increased diameter were inserted, showed six failures in the first year, the cause of which was bone quality. The success rate after one year was 88.2%.

133 wide Branemark implants (Bahat) implanted in the lateral regions, which were partially connected to standard implants, were examined. Results obtained: four failures in the lower jaw. The overall success rate was 97%. No data were recorded on prosthetic complications or peri-implant bone breakdown.

From these examples, we can draw the conclusion that a general position cannot yet be drawn.

Why?

At the beginning of the procedure, we cannot reliably determine the quality of the bone. The width of the implant depends on the quality of the bone. The worse the quality of the bone, the larger the diameter of the implant should be. In case of insufficient height of the crest to the anatomical structure of the mandibular canal, implants with a wide diameter are indicated, but the width of the available bone ensures good blood supply.

What are the indications for using the largest diameter implant?

The application of the largest diameter implant should be coordinated with the quality of the bone. If the bone is of poorer quality, better primary stability is achieved with a larger diameter implant, which is a prerequisite for successful bone integration. The width of the alveolar ridge must not be less than 8 mm (Fig. 18.163). For example, with type IV bone quality, good primary stability cannot be achieved with implants with a diameter of 3.75 or 4 mm. One must think about a 5 mm implant, and even a wider diameter.

In the lateral region where there is a width of the alveolar ridge of 8 mm and more, but the height is missing. A solution in that case can be sought in two ways:

- First, apply shorter implants with a larger diameter, because this achieves a larger anchoring surface, i.e. a larger surface of contact between the implant and the bone, thus compensating the shorter length of the implant with a larger width;

- Another method of bone height compensation is augmentation with autologous bone blocks or autologous bone granules mixed with xenogeneic bone substitutes.

Applying the first method will avoid complicated surgical procedures for augmentation with grafts, raising the sinus floor, etc., as well as reducing the cost of the procedure.

Practical experience points to the conclusion that it is simpler and safer to install an implant with a larger diameter, if the volume of the bone allows, and a smaller length and rest it on the cortical part of the bone, than to opt for a sinus lift, which is a more complicated procedure and requires larger financial investments

What is the danger in placing the largest diameter implant in the lower jaw where there is not enough bone height to ensure the necessary safe distance (2 mm) from the mandibular canal?

There is a danger in the possibility of perforation of the lingual cortical wall when installing implants of the largest diameter (Fig. 18.182).

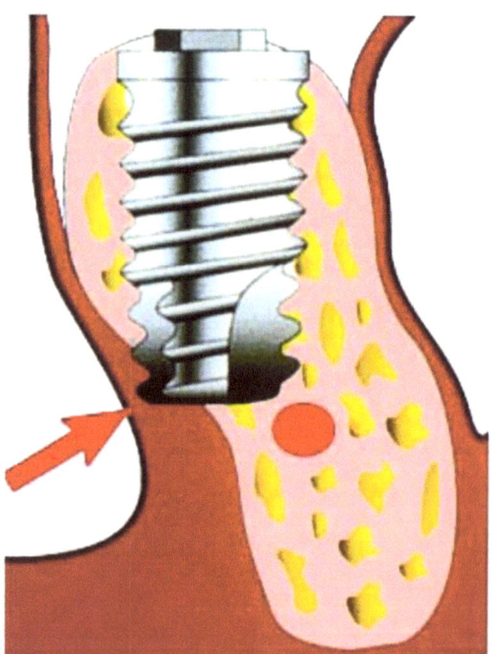

Figure 18.182. In the case of insufficiently available bone in terms of height and width, the lingual cortical lamella of the mandible can be perforated by installing a larger diameter implant.

What are the results of installing implants immediately after tooth extraction?

By exchanging opinions with my colleagues, I gained the impression that by installing implants immediately after tooth extraction, extremely satisfactory results can be obtained.

Success depends on a good assessment of the extraction wound. First, it should be assessed whether the required primary stability can be obtained. Many extraction wounds are larger than standard diameters implants, so in such cases achieving primary stability is not certain.

With implants of a larger diameter, which can be used to close the extraction wound with the addition of osteoinductive grafts, a good result can be achieved, but with patient waiting. It is recommended that fresh extraction wounds be closed with implants with a larger diameter of 5 to 6 mm.

In the case of implants with a larger crown base, the diameter of the implant significantly affects the reduction of occlusal forces (Fig. 18.183).

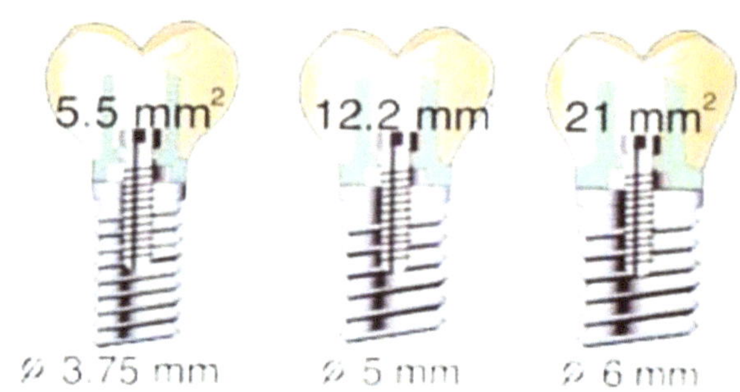

Figure 18.183. The greater the support of the crown, the more evenly distributed will be the reception of occlusal forces during chewing.

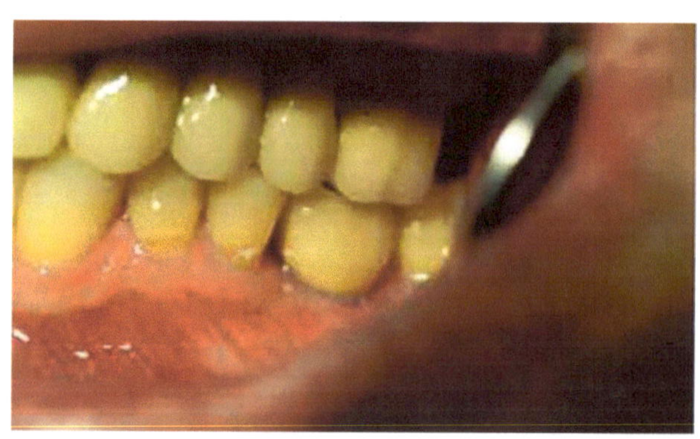

Figure 18.184. The wide diameter of molar restorative implants ensures a more even reception of occlusal forces over time chewing excellent aesthetic result.

The width of the implant neck in molar replacement can enable a similar exit profile that the natural tooth had, which results in an outstanding aesthetic appearance (Fig. 18.184).

Thanks to the width of the implant, the natural morphology of the teeth can be modeled in laboratories. Biomechanical complications in the reconstruction of individual molars can be avoided with larger diameter implants, but on the other hand there is a risk of fenestration on the lingual side (which was emphasized in the answer to the previous question).

What is the concept of applying large diameter implants?

The application of implants with a larger diameter is becoming more and more important, especially in cases where there is insufficient height of the alveolar bone, which avoids endangering the adjacent anatomical structures. These are, first of all, cases where there is limited bone volume and reduced interocclusal space and cases where there is insufficient bone volume and there is sufficient interocclusal space. A similar situation exists if the interocclusal space is reduced and there is not enough bone (Fig. 18.185).

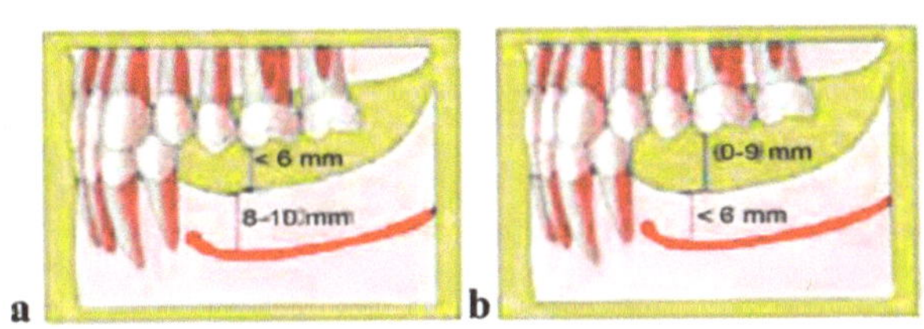

Figure 18.185. Limitations for implant placement due to reduced position compared to antagonists (a). Insufficient amount of bone in height, but sufficient interocclusal distance (b).

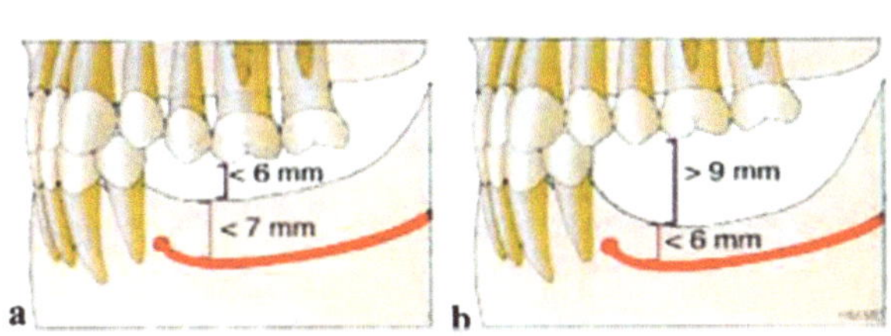

Figure 18.186. Insufficient available bone 7mm (a) risk for implant placement with reduced unfavorable intermaxillary relationship. The second image (b) shows the disadvantage for implant placement, the distance from the top of the ridge is 6 mm, and there is a favorable interjaw relationship.

Figure 18.186. explains that there are cases where there is not enough bone volume, and the interocclusal interjaw space is reduced, or there is insufficient bone volume, and the interocclusal interjaw space is increased.

What are the advantages of large diameter implants from a biomechanical point of view?

Large-diameter implants, when it comes to meeting biomechanical requirements, have the following advantages:

- better distribution of reception of occlusal forces;
- better primary stability;
- optimum exit profile of the crown and aesthetic effect;
- better stability of prosthetic work;
- lower risk of loosening and breakage of the support screws; and
- there is no risk of implant breakage.

What are the selection criteria for the replacement of individual molars?

To successfully replace a lost molar, 3 conditions are required:

- Sufficient area of the anchoring place;
- Sufficient mesiodistal space;
- Sufficient width of the alveolar ridge.

Molars usually have a larger mesiodistal dimension than the diameter of standard implants. An accurate assessment of that space is very important, because the choice of implant width also depends on it, which entails the analysis of chewing forces, which are very intense in the lateral regions. The decision to install standard implants in the place of molars should be carefully evaluated to see if there are factors that could affect the primary stability, and overloading can cause significant complications (looseness of the support screws or breakage, and due to the uneven distribution of chewing force can cause bone destruction).

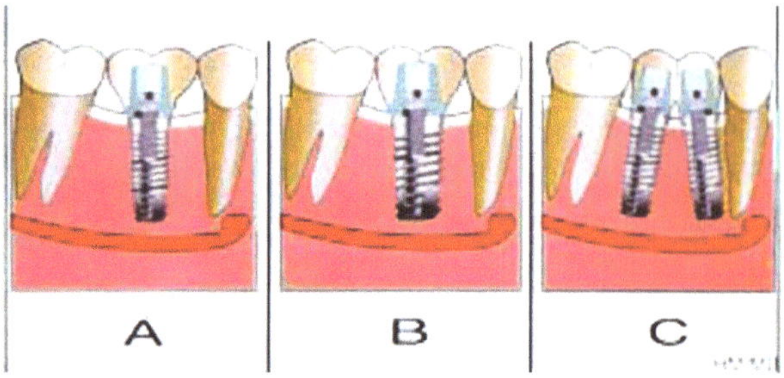

Figure 18.187. For the replacement of molars, a different choice of implants is possible: implant of standard diameter (A), implant of larger diameter (B), installation of two implants of standard diameter (C).

There are two basic choices for molar replacement:

1. implant of increased diameter; or
2. two standard diameter implants.

If the mesiodistal space is about 12 mm, two standard-diameter implants should be inserted (pictures 18.187 to 18.190).

A three-year trial of the installation of Banemark implants (Balsch et al.) as a replacement for molars gave the following results: in 22 cases, the molar was replaced with one implant of a larger diameter, and in 25 cases, two implants of standard diameter were installed to replace the molars.

The success rate in both cases was 98.6%, but with the difference that significantly more prosthetic complications were recorded in the group with one implant than in the group with two implants (48% vs. 8%).

From a biomechanical point of view, two implants for the reconstruction of one molar reduce occlusal overloads and prosthetic complications. The anchorage is significantly stronger, and the occlusal biomechanical forces are better distributed. But, on the other hand, the bone between two standard-diameter implants can show a higher degree of resorption, because the bone in that part loses its function, and this does not happen with implants that are in function. The disadvantage of installing two implants in the place of one molar is also reflected in the fact that the morphology of a natural tooth in the neck area cannot be adequately copied.

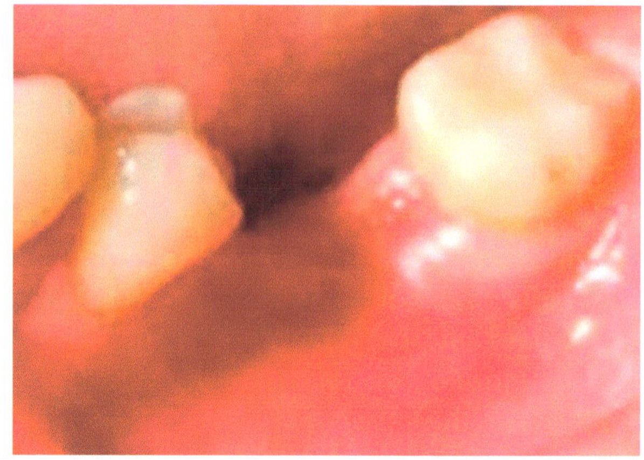

Figure 18.188. The mesiodistal space, width and height of the alveolar bone determines the type of implant.

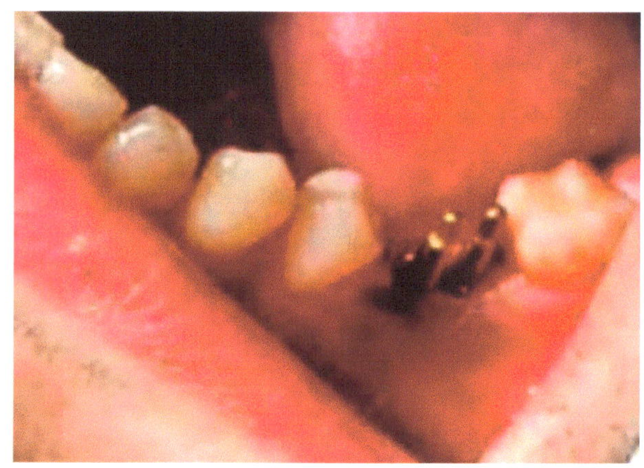

Figure 18.189. The mesiodistal space required the installation of two standard diameter implants.

Are the diameters of the implants aligned with the diameters of the natural teeth in the mesiodistal and buccolingual direction?

There is a match with some teeth. The size of the premolars in the upper jaw in the mesiodistal direction is about 5 mm, and the diameter in the buccolingual direction is 8 mm.

In both molars, the mesiodistal diameter is about 8 mm, the buccolingual dimension in the first molar is slightly larger and amounts to 10 mm, and in the second molar it is 9.0 mm.

In the lower premolars, the mesiodistal space is 5 mm, and the buccolingual dimension in the first lower premolar is 7 mm, and in the second 8 mm.

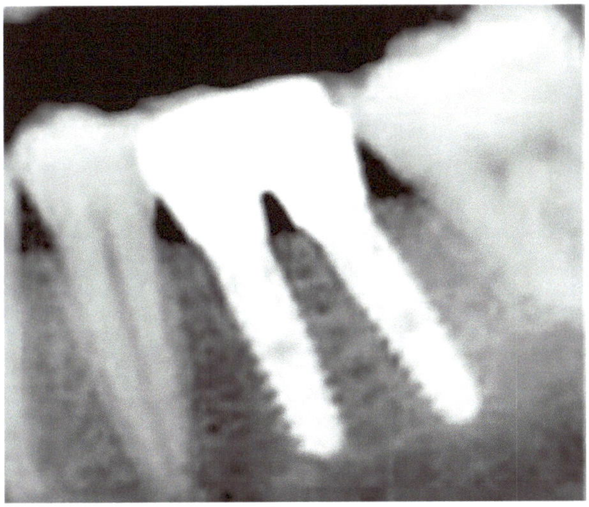

Figure 18.190. Replacement of molars where there is a larger mesiodistal gap with two implants of standard diameters. Control image after 4 years, marginal bone preserved.

In the case of the lower first molar, the mesiodistal space is 8.5 mm, and the buccolingual space is 9.0 mm. In the case of the second molar, the mesiodistal space is 8 mm, and the buccolingual space is identical to the first molar.

What are the parameters that the practitioner should know in order to choose the most optimal implant diameter?

The diameter of the implant should be chosen depending on the status of the existing teeth, the quality of the bone, the available space in both directions (mesiodistal and buccolingual), as well as the type of output profile (to achieve a good aesthetic result). The choice is influenced by the type of occlusion and the position of the antagonist.

It can be said that the era of consideration of the importance of implant diameters began in the mid-1980s. For a long time after that, there were no credible studies when it comes to the application of implants of different diameters. Even today, all results on this topic are based on short-and medium-term research, but from which satisfactory conclusions can still be drawn.

Most manufacturers offer a wide range of implants of different diameters and lengths. All these differences have one goal, which is to adjust the thickness of the implant to the bone circumference.

In order to choose the optimal implant diameter for a successful outcome, all clinical parameters must be taken into account:

- Quality and quantity of available bone, position of edentulous space;
- available space for prosthetic work (crown);
- type of occlusion;
- The position of the antagonist.

The diameter must satisfy all operative-prosthetic requirements.

From a surgical point of view, the available bone volume should be used to achieve the primary stability of the implant. From a prosthetic point of view, a satisfactory range and exit profile of the implant should be provided that will match the intended crown and meet aesthetic requirements.

Is it possible to conclude, from the previous answers, about the indications for the use of implants of a smaller or larger diameter?

To summarize the answer to this question: smaller diameter implants have indications in the following cases:

a) reduced interradicular bone width;
b) narrow alveolar ridge;
c) limited cervical diameter of the crown.

Larger diameter implants have been used in the following cases:

d) poor bone quality;
e) insufficient height of the alveolar ridge;
f) single-phase implant replacement where bone integration failed;
g) one-phase replacement of fractured implants;
h) immediate installation after tooth extraction, lack of single molar.

When it comes to the amount of bone for standard implants, the mesiodistal and buccolingual width should not be less than 7 mm. Standard implants should always be avoided in situations where there are biomechanical and anatomical limitations.

Complications most often occur due to poor assessment, which compromises the entire treatment.

When the alveolar ridge is narrow, it is far better to use an implant with a smaller diameter, of course with a satisfactory length. If even then the doctor is not sure that he has made a good assessment, then considerations should be directed towards increasing the width of the alveolar bone (with bone grafts or guided regeneration). Unfavorable occlusal forces and biomechanical loads should always be excluded.

In the lateral regions, the width of the bone is often around 8 mm, and sometimes more. But there is not enough bone height due to anatomical limitations (maxillary sinus and mandibular canal). What decision to make in such cases?

The only orientation in such a case is the choice of short implants. From the experience and review of the literature and presented clinical results, it has been shown that implants with a standard diameter and a length of less than 10 mm have a higher percentage of failure. In that case, it is better to install an implant with a larger diameter, because a larger area of contact between the implant and the bone is immediately provided, so that the shorter length of the implant is compensated by a larger width. Such an implant can avoid an invasive procedure in the case of the upper jaw: raising the sinus floor or bone transplantation, and in the lower jaw - lateralization of the lower dental nerve.

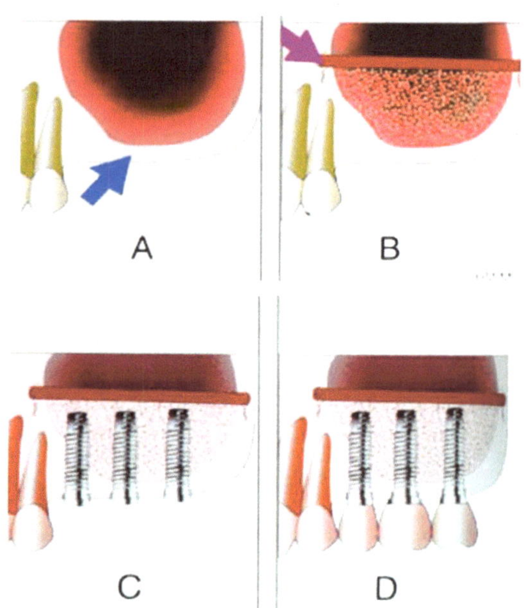

Figure 18.191. Schematic representation of sinus floor elevation and implant placement: (A) insufficient alveolar crest height, (B) elevation of the sinus floor with bone substitutes, (C) embedded implants in the upgraded bone, and (D) prosthetic work on the implants.

In the picture 18.190. a schematic representation of raising the sinus floor is given, which enables the installation of a larger number of implants of standard length. Picture (A) shows an insufficient amount of bone, and picture (B) shows the elevation of the sinus floor with a cortico-spongy block, i.e. installation of the implant (C) in the healed bone, prosthetic work on the implants (D). The raising of the sinus floor (sinus lifting) is discussed in more detail in the chapter on augmentation (Chapter 10).

With low bone density, can good primary stability be achieved with implants of a standard diameter of 3.75 mm?

Most often not. But not only with that standard diameter, but also with a slightly wider diameter of 4 mm. In low-quality, low-density bone, that diameter is closer to an unsuccessful outcome than to a successful outcome. It happens that the X-ray shows that there is enough bone to install a shorter, wider diameter implant. By raising the flap, however, low-quality cancellous bone is encountered and in such situations it is not worth trying implantation.

What is the failure rate of standard implants versus larger diameter implants?

In the literature 10 years ago, a high percentage (35%) of the failure of standard implants (3.75 mm) in low-quality bone of low density in bone structure type IV was recorded. That percentage of failure is significantly lower today. With larger diameter implants, better bicortical stabilization is achieved. If the clinical condition and bone volume or prosthetics require the use of a smaller diameter implant, in that case the smaller diameter must be compensated by a longer length and high-quality surface treatment of the implant. Of course, if the anatomical conditions allow it. To a great extent, a lot depends on the skill of the dentist

In order to ensure a satisfactory anchoring surface of the implant, and on the other hand to reconstruct the morphology of the tooth, what does the choice of implant diameter depend on?

In order to meet the indicated requirements, the width of the implant should correspond to the surface of the lost root. However, that width is individually different. The problem of the anchoring surface has been investigated by many implantologists and their conclusion is that the middle width of the implant should be applied. Today, the implant market offers a large number of implants that could meet these requirements. The surface of the anchorage depends on the shape and anatomy of the incision, as well as on the surface properties of the implant.

In order to ensure a demanding anchoring surface, it is necessary to adhere to the following concept:

- standard implants for: incisors, canines and premolars;
- Smaller diameter implants for upper lateral incisors and lower incisors, which is different from patient to patient;
- incisors in the lower jaw can rarely be compensated with the same number of implants of standard diameters;
- Larger diameter implants for molars. This would be a general estimate, but deviations are possible, depending on the case by case.

What are the criteria to achieve this?

In order to best achieve this, when it comes to replacing molars, three criteria must be met:

1. anchoring surface;
2. mesiodistal space;
3. quality and quantity of bone crest

When it comes to the installation of implants in place of molars, what should you pay special attention to?

First, you should know that during lateral movements of the lower jaw, the chewing forces in that area are the most intense and further aggravate the condition. Molar crowns are larger than standard implants. If we replace molars with a standard implant, poorly located, or if we expose it to overload at the very beginning, several complications can follow: screw breakage, and in the worst case, weakening of the bone-integration connection.

To avoid unwanted consequences, two options are available:

- use two standard implants;
- provided that the mesiodistal space allows the use of only one implant with a larger diameter.

In case of partial toothlessness, it is necessary to use as many implants as there are missing roots. That would be a logical conclusion. However, realistically, the number of implants replacing the number of roots will be limited due to the altered mesiodistal space and anatomical limitations. In that case, the volume of the bone and the planning of the construction of the prosthetic work determine the type and number of implants.

In the case of partial tooth loss, if there is enough available bone, the number of implants may correspond to the number of lost teeth, not the number of lost roots, as this is dictated by the dimension of the mesiodistal space.

And what happens when it comes to the region where the four lower incisors need to be compensated?

The application of standard implants in the frontal region at the place of the lower incisors makes it difficult to make correct aesthetic prosthetic work. An implant with a standard diameter would violate the ratio of the diameter of the neck of the natural tooth, that is, the output profile of the implant would not correspond to the cervical diameter of the natural tooth and would impair the aesthetic appearance. In the lower jaw, an additional problem is the middle of the face. By moving that line through the wide neck of the implant, the aesthetic requirements could not be met. The necks of implants are often much wider than the necks of natural teeth, so it is impossible to install one implant on one missing tooth. It is not just an aesthetic reason. Due to the insufficient mesiodistal distance, the standard diameter of the implant would jeopardize the osseous integration due to the reduced blood supply and the insufficient volume of the labial and lingual bone around the implant.

Two options are available: installation of two standard implants near the canines, or three to four implants of small diameter. Implants that approximately correspond to the diameter of the neck of the lost natural tooth enable the realization of complete aesthetics.

In order to achieve a good aesthetic result, the cervical mesiodistal diameter of the implant should lie slightly below the diameter of the intended crown. In the case of a natural tooth, the diameter at this height is slightly below enamel-cement boundaries.

In the upper frontal region of the lateral incisors, the optimal exit profile of the implant will be obtained if the anatomy of the lateral incisor on the opposite side is well analyzed.

In the lower and upper lateral incisors, the mesiodistal space is less than 4.5 mm, and in the standard implant the cervical diameter is 4.1 mm, which makes it impossible to obtain a good aesthetic result.

However, when it comes to the upper jaw, in the region of the incisors, the exit profile can be improved with a wider implant. This can be achieved by parallel installation of implants and modeling of the prosthetic work, so that the natural appearance of the crown is obtained. Aesthetic restoration of natural teeth with wide crowns of central incisors can also be achieved with larger-diameter implants

Theory is one thing, practice is another. Of course, for good success, it is necessary to realize theoretical assumptions through practical work. What would you suggest if practice confirmed it?

Experience verified through practice imposes more advice. For the lower incisors, apply implants of a smaller diameter, and for the lower premolars, implants of a normal diameter. Also, for upper incisor implants of standard diameter, with the fact that, due to the aesthetic effect, an implant of a slightly narrower diameter should be installed in place of the lateral incisors, as this enables the technician to successfully carry out the envisioned project.

The diameters of the implants that can be applied in the frontal upper region are also suitable for the upper premolars. But when it comes to aesthetics and biomechanics, the approaches are different. The aesthetic requirement of the premolars can be fulfilled by the diameter of the implants corresponding to the upper frontal region. But, from a biomechanical point of view, and to the detriment of aesthetics, it is far better to install a wider implant. Of course, depending on many factors: quality and quantity of bone, anatomical conditions, etc.

But there are details to which you should always pay maximum attention when choosing the diameter of the implant. These are biomechanical reasons, which depend on the position of the implant in the dental arch, the type of occlusion and possibly existing parafunctions.

Always when deciding to install a smaller diameter implant, occlusal forces should be carefully analyzed and evaluated, especially in the lateral regions where they are most intense.

Therefore, a narrow-diameter implant for the replacement of canines and molars is always contraindicated. For example, by reducing the diameter of the implant, i.e. reducing its diameter by 20% (from 3.75 mm to 3.0 mm), the resistance to chewing forces is reduced by 50%.

When replacing one molar, from a biomechanical point of view, all complications can be easily avoided by installing a larger diameter implant. But there is also evidence that with two Branemark implants of a small diameter, in the same situation, better results are achieved than with one implant of a wider diameter. The conclusion is that two implants in place of one molar reduce the occlusal loads on the implant itself and the prosthetic construction. In order to obtain a stable replacement of molars, one should have an increased crown base, which can be achieved by choosing a larger diameter implant that increases the neck of the implant.

For example, with implants 5 to 6 mm wide, complications are reduced three to ten times, which cannot be achieved with standard diameter implants. The area of the crown base increases by 122%, i.e. up to 281%, which enables a better distribution of occlusal forces. It is reported that the occlusal load is reduced by 20% for implants with a diameter of 5 mm, and that the load for implants with a width of 6 mm is reduced by 33%.

What conclusion should be drawn from all this?

Implants of standard diameters still remain the standard needed in everyday practice. The existence of implants with a reduced or larger diameter enriches the variety of the offer, and thus their choice for certain clinical cases. And this is where the experience of the implantologist is crucial, and his good judgment and surgical dexterity, along with a good knowledge of biomechanical requirements and prosthetic knowledge, are the keys to success.

For some new implants of various diameters, final evaluations cannot be given, because long-term studies are lacking, but some short-term ones have satisfactory results.

However, when the topic is implant diameter, there are still many questions that need answers:

- Why can narrow implants break and what is the percentage and long-term average of staying in the bone?
- How and to what extent does the smaller or larger diameter of the implant affect the peri-implant soft tissues?
- How does the wide diameter affect the peri-implant bone and how can the occlusal forces be optimally distributed during lateral movements?

There are no valid statistical data on all these questions (a separate chapter is devoted to this issue).

What diameters are most adequate for bone structures of types I to IV?

There are enough theories about all these questions, but for now we have no long-term valid scientific evidence. I emphasize, long-term!

It gives the impression that you give priority to the primary (immediate) load. What factors influence the decision to load the implant primarily, or should we wait for healing for several months before putting the implant into operation?

The most important assessment is whether a good primary stability of the implant can be achieved, and therefore several conditions must be met:

1. if there is a sufficient amount of bone, apply longer implants;
2. if there is not enough length, use the width of the bone by using shorter implants and larger diameters. One of the methods to increase the primary stability is to insert the graft into the implant bed, which is condensed by tamping and then the implant is installed;
3. the prepared implant bed must have a smaller diameter than the implant, which means the last drill must have a smaller diameter than the diameter of the implant;
4. if good primary stability is not achieved, fill the bed with a bone substitute graft and leave it for several months for the graft to calcify, and then insert the implant.

In cases involving larger operations in both jaws at the same time, the basis for predicting success starts from the first step of the imagined plan of the entire implantological treatment.

Patients who have been toothless for a long time and wear full dentures permanently, or occasionally, are different from cases where there are teeth. With the former, there is the possibility of implantation without making an incision and raising the flap, which avoids postoperative pain, hematomas and possible infections. So, traumatization of soft tissues is avoided, which is very important for the healing and formation of soft tissues, both from the functional and even more from the aesthetic aspect. This is especially important when it comes to the front region of the upper jaw.

It happens that implant therapy is extremely complex, as is the case shown in the following images (images 18.192-18.200). The case was complex for the following reasons:

- 15 decayed teeth in the terminal phase had to be extracted;
- the patient did not want to be without teeth due to business obligations;
- she did not want to wear immediate prostheses as a temporary solution due to strong urges to vomit (even when choosing a spoon for the impression, she felt nausea with the urge to vomit, and taking the impression was extremely difficult).

It should be taken into account the fact that in cases where the teeth are strongly protruded and are held in the bone almost only by the tip of the root, after extraction there is a significant part of the bone above the apex, which is very favorable for implantation and achieving primary stability.

If the patient cannot tolerate and use total prostheses, the associate is all the more favorable. Advantages of anatomical structures and available bone in edentulous jaws also determine the procedure plan. At the same time, in the case where there are teeth and disturbed interjaw relationships, the complexity of the entire treatment increases. In these cases, in addition to pain in the joint, there may also be a deviation of the position of the lower jaw by moving the middle line, with a unilateral increase in the volume of the musculature.

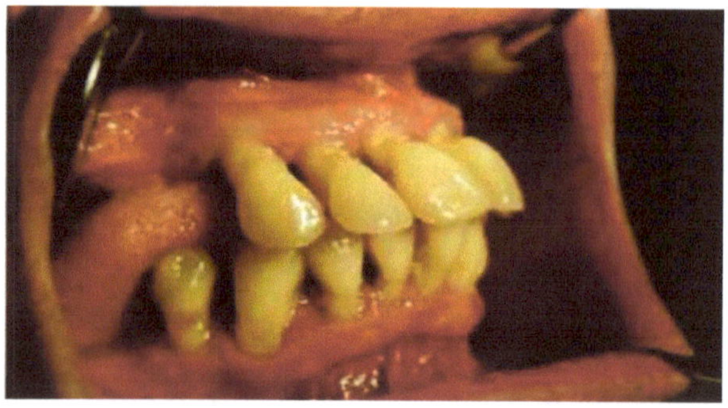

Figure 18.192. Initial condition, with extreme pathological migration and loosened teeth. Clinical appearance of gingiva with active periodontal pockets and productive exudative type of inflammation.

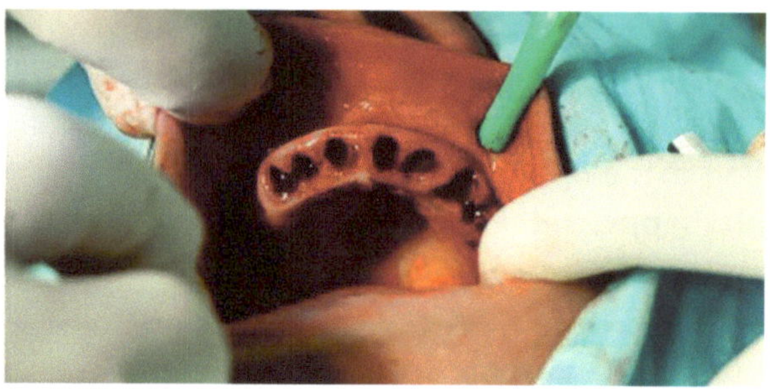

Figure 18.193. Extraction of pathologically migrated teeth. Planned installation of the implant in a fresh alveolus.

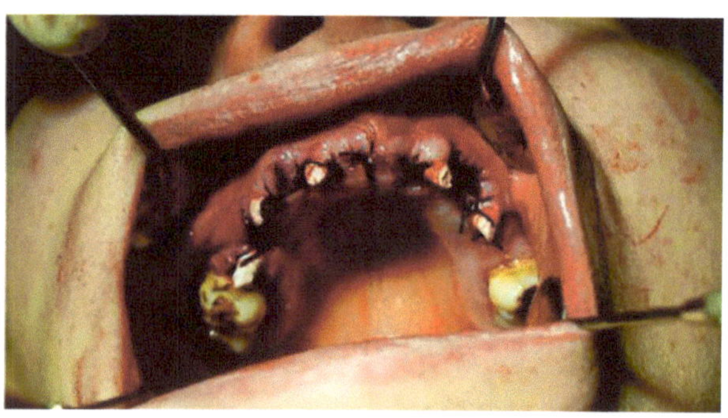

Figure 18.194. Immediately installed implants of standard and wide diameters with temporary PEEK supports for the production of fixed immediate prosthetic work. Immediate implantation of the implant is supported by the augmentation procedure.

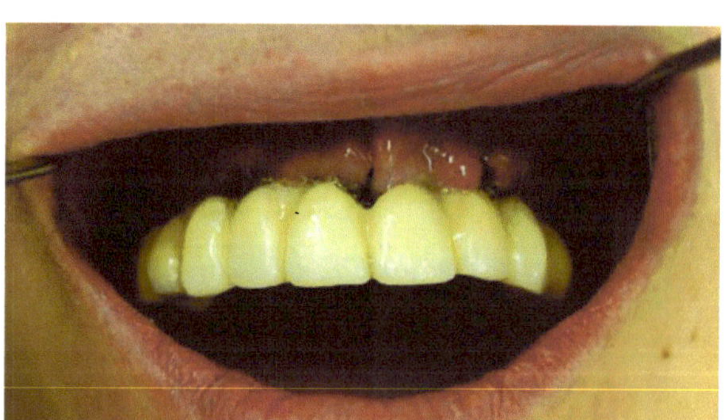

Figure 18.195. Temporary prosthetic work immediately after immediate implantation.

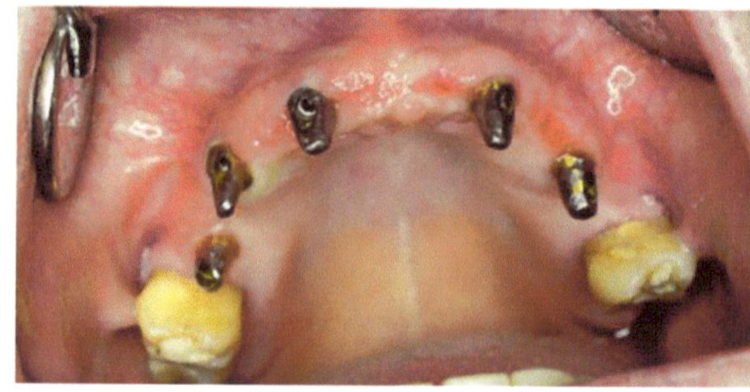

Figure 18.196. Appearance of soft tissue healing after 6 months.

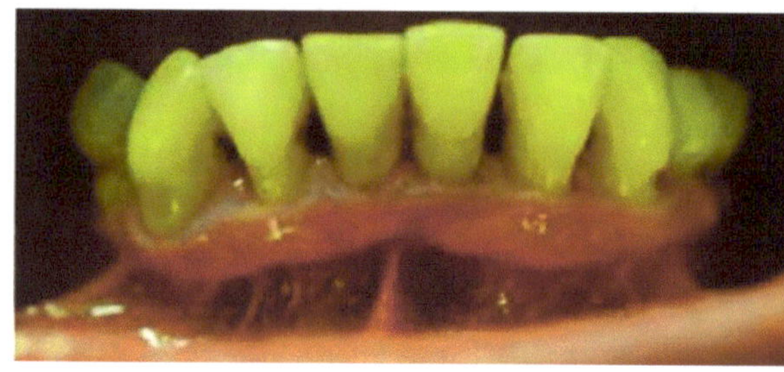

Figure 18.197. Clinical appearance of the gingiva in the frontal and lateral region of the lower jaw with active periodontal pockets, dominant inflammation of the productive type and pronounced exudative inflammation in the region of all teeth. The treatment procedure in the lower jaw was identical to that in the upper jaw.

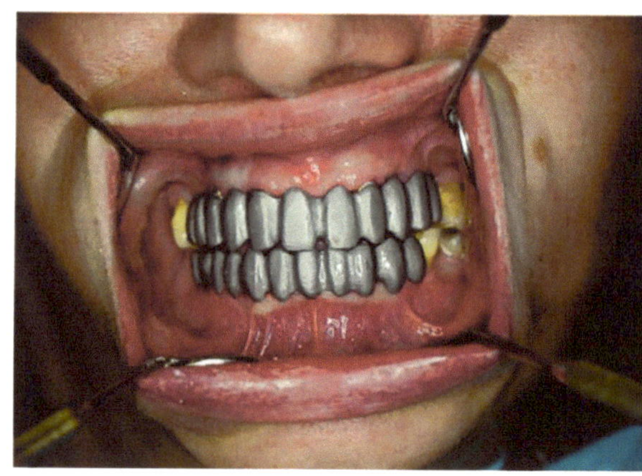

Figure 18.198. One of the stages of definitive restoration. Compare with the initial state.

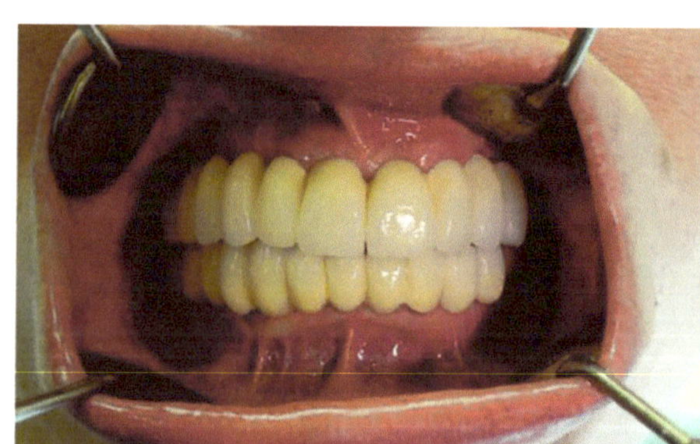

Figure 18.199. Fulfilled functional, aesthetic and biomechanical requirements. Compare with the initial state.

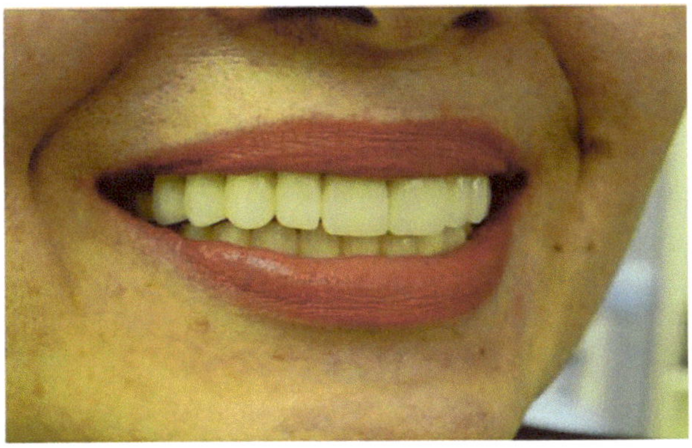

Figure 18.200. Achieved patient satisfaction with treatment procedures; from the beginning to the end of the treatment, the fixed prosthetic work was in the mouth.

What serious problems can be caused by poor occlusion if it is a compensation on implants?

Bad occlusion on prosthetic work, regardless of whether it is placed on implants or natural teeth, can cause unilateral mastication, so that when chewing, the patient uses only one side. In most cases, unilateral mastication leads to an imbalance in the temporomandibular joint.

The success, that is, the survival or loss of the implant, will depend on how the mechanical tensions are transferred to the bone surrounding the implant. How the occlusal forces will be transmitted and affect the bone surrounding the implant depends on many factors: the type and strength of the force (functional, parafunctional), the position, length and diameter of the implant, the technological treatment of the implant surface, the shape of the neck, the surface treatment of the implant neck, the quality of the bone around the implant, geometry of the suprastructure (form, dimensions of occlusal surfaces, occlusal relationships).

All these parameters are known and can be influenced. But parafunctional forces are often unpredictable, unlike functional forces, whose action is known and can be influenced by correcting the direction of the forces (Figure 18.201).

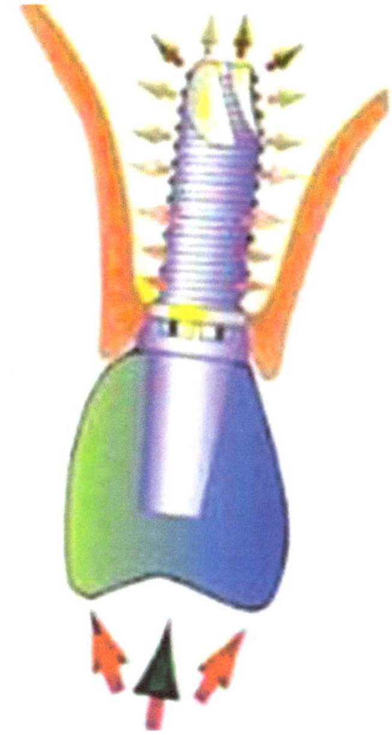

Figure 18.201. Directed axial forces that are received through the central fissure of the crown are evenly transmitted and neutralized, and the morphology of the cusps of the artificial crown depends on how the impulses of the given forces will be received and decomposed during contact with the antagonists, reducing or increasing the load.

Can the question be asked, what is the specificity of implants in such a biological milieu?

The specificity of dental implants lies in their role as substitutes for the root of a natural tooth. However, unlike natural tooth roots, implants lack the periodontal ligament, which significantly alters the relationship with the surrounding bone and is crucial for functionality. The materials used (primarily metal), along with the different shapes, volumes, dimensions, and designs of the implant body and neck, contribute to varying biomechanical properties. Consequently, implants cannot be entirely compared to the characteristics of natural tooth roots.

The absence of the periodontal connection limits the implant's ability to adapt in relation to the central nervous system. Without the receptors and impulses that a natural tooth root receives through the periodontal ligament, there is an increased risk of microtrauma. This lack of nerve receptors means that patients cannot sense excessive forces, particularly during lateral movements of the lower jaw, which may lead to potential complications.

Furthermore, the phenomenon of microtrauma transmitted to the bone via the implant is exacerbated by the absence of the periodontium. The periodontal ligament allows the root of a natural tooth to absorb axial forces up to 28 micrometers (µm), while the elasticity of occlusal contacts in implants is about 5 µm. The amortization mobility of natural tooth roots was calculated by Parfitt in 1960, while Glicerman calculated that of implants in 1994 (Fig. 18.202).

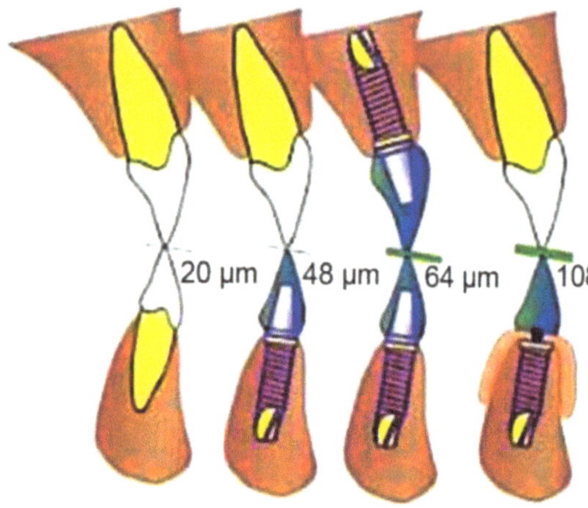

Figure 18.202. The absence of a periodontal connection significantly reduces the cushioning capacity during occlusal contacts. For this reason, the dentist must know the principles of gnathology.

Clinical tooth mobility varies from 56 to 108 micrometers (Parfitt, 1960); relative to the implant, it can vary from 10 to 50 micrometers (Sekinc, 1986), and the mean value of tooth mobility is about 25 micrometers (Sullivan, 1991).

What is the difference in the elastic connection of the periodontal ligament in the tooth compared to the implant?

The new conclusions are:

- The connection of the periodontal ligament enables cushioning of occlusal and parafunctional forces;
- The periodontal ligament increases the mobility of the tooth and in case of overload, it allows the tooth to regain its initial position after the end of the force;
- With implants, it is completely the opposite.

The mobility of the implant (during the absorption of forces), caused by the excessive load on the occlusal surfaces transferred via the implant to the surrounding bone, is an irreversible process.

The difference in force transfer significantly impacts how stress affects the occlusal surfaces, the implant body, and the surrounding bone tissue. Natural tooth roots transmit transverse forces more effectively during lateral movements due to their conical shape and position. The presence of the periodontal ligament allows for physiological mobility, enabling rotation from the center towards the apex and preventing forces from concentrating near the crestal bone area.

In contrast, dental implants have limited mobility, causing forces to be transferred from the center of rotation directly to the neck of the implant. If an implant is improperly positioned or if the occlusal scheme is not correctly executed, the resulting occlusal forces may concentrate on the marginal area of the crestal bone near the implant's neck. This information is crucial for practice; during follow-up examinations where significant marginal bone loss is observed, it is essential to identify the underlying causes of this loss.

Transverse forces acting especially during lateral movements of the lower jaw, due to the above reasons, increase the risk of excessive transverse forces, and lead not only to the loss of marginal bone, but also fracture of the implant itself (fracture of the support screw). For this reason, the diameter of the implant is extremely important. If the implant has a narrow diameter, there is a greater risk of transverse excessive forces. The conical shape of certain implants can partially neutralize this risk by distributing lateral forces similar to what happens on the root of a natural tooth.

What does the practitioner need to know in overcoming this difference between natural root and implant? How to amortize excessive forces, that is, reduce them to physiological tolerance, which is made possible by the elastic periodontal connection to the natural root?

First, most dental technicians have little or no knowledge of this issue. Due to the work system (distance from the laboratory), the dentist does not have the opportunity to control and give instructions when making the model and shaping the size of the crown, as well as the cusps of the biting surface. It would be desirable if the dentist knew how to direct the dental technician how to shape the morphological details that are extremely important for biomechanical events during chewing.

It starts in the doctor's office. The shape of the alveolar ridge during the installation of the implant requires that the body of the implant be placed in the region of the lingual cusps, as is advantageously solved with natural teeth. The lingual contour of the cusp can remain the same, and whether and how much it will be reduced depends on the lateral movement.

However, the buccal cusp must be reduced in height and adjustable slope, and the occlusal surface must be reduced from the buccal side for the implant to have an axial load. In the case of a natural tooth, this condition is fulfilled by the buccal cusps of the lower teeth lying in the central fissure of the premolars and molars in the upper jaw, in intercuspation, directing the load axially. For this reason, care must be taken when forming an artificial crown on an implant. If the contact were on the palatal cusp of the upper teeth, then the action of forces would also be directed outside the axial direction. In a natural tooth, these forces are accepted by the palatal root.

Why is there so much emphasis on the importance of tubercle height?

This is where the biggest problem is when it comes to biomechanical events dependent on prosthetic work anchored on implants (the same applies to natural teeth when they are the carriers of prosthetic work). It happens that the dentist evaluates the work by the beauty of the appearance of the occlusal surfaces in the lateral regions, convincing the patient (layman) that his new teeth look natural, especially with accentuated cusps which, however, in the contacts of the dental arches can cause a whole confusion and be unpleasant for the patient from from the very beginning. More experienced clinicians know very well that patients often do not provide accurate sensation information at the beginning, when adjusting the occlusion. It is only after a few days that very dangerous, premature contacts are detected in certain places.

The occlusal height of the cusp directly aids and influences the load moment resultant (see Chapters 8 and 11). The height of the cusps directs the components of forces coming from the facio-lingual angle and the components of forces that are directed from the mesio-distal angle. At the same time, the components of the lingual forces can produce a torque, acting around the neck of the implant if the height of the cantilever receives forces along the entire length of the implant.

It should be emphasized that the load moment always tends to induce rotation of the implant in three planes: clockwise rotational forces, counterclockwise forces and mesio-distal forces. In these three planes, the forces result in six moments: lingual transverse, partial transverse, occlusal, apical, facial and lingual. These forces are always three-dimensional, with components directly related to one or more clinical angular coordinates. It is important to know these events because experience shows that the occlusal height can affect the resultant load moments

Why is that important?

When there is sufficient available bone, the forces involved create a smaller moment of load on the crestal part of the bone. This is in contrast to ridges with limited bone height, which must be considered when determining the height of the crown. The crown should be designed in proportion to the action of these moment forces. This understanding is crucial for dentists during follow-up examinations, especially if they observe marginal bone loss around an implant, as biomechanical factors may contribute to this loss.

The fixed height and slope of the cusp, along with the hardness of the material, can adversely affect the implant and the surrounding bone. At the World Implantology Meeting in Bologna in 1986, I discussed this issue by graphically comparing it to a "lying policeman," which is used to limit speed and enhance safety (see Figure 18.203). This analogy highlights the role of the inclined plane and the hardness of the material (concrete) that has historically led to damage in the vehicle's suspension systems. Traditionally, these "recumbent policemen" were constructed from solid concrete with two high, slanted surfaces and a sharp edge running along their length. When vehicles pass over this obstacle, they experience force pulses, the intensity of which depends on the height, slope of the plane, and the material of the "lying policeman."

Hypothetically, instead of using soft and abrasive tires, a vehicle is equipped with solid metal wheels. This configuration results in a very high and destructive amplitude of forces when the vehicle moves and encounters obstacles. The stresses on the car are evident throughout all its components, leading to complete glass breakage.

If we were to replace the metal wheels with porcelain ones, the impact amplitude would be somewhat reduced, as the porcelain would break upon impact. This breakage would absorb some of the force, resulting in significantly less damage to the vehicle. However, the damping parts of the car, referred to here as the "periodontium," would still struggle to absorb the forces, leading to major damage.

Ultimately, it was concluded that the severe damage caused by these hypothetical rigid obstacles, akin to "lying policemen," should be addressed with a more effective solution aimed at reducing speed and increasing safety, in line with the principles of mechanics.

The solution involved rounding the height of the obstacle and, crucially, changing the material used. Solid concrete was replaced with elastic rubber. This change eliminated the amplitude of destructive impacts (noted in green in the accompanying illustration). In contrast, when the obstacle was made of solid material with an inclined plane, the impact amplitude (indicated in red in the figure) remained high and destructive.

The reception of impact forces on the car when encountering various disadvantages on the road (potholes, unevenness, etc.) depends on the quality of the damping system and on the driver's ability to spot the obstacle in time. The first factor of shock absorption (unpredictable "parafunctional forces") is the tires on the wheels. The comfort and safety of driving depend on the quality of the rubber, its softness, and its abrasiveness. What conclusion can be drawn from this hypothetical pictorial representation if compared to the events in the oral cavity during prosthetic rehabilitation?

Depending on the knowledge (contractor and designer) and experience in modern prosthetics, the hair plane ("lying policeman") is successfully influenced by the creation of prosthetic work, whether it is worn with natural teeth or implants. However, as far as other factors are concerned, the strength of the material from which the artificial crown is made and the modeling of the biting surface have not gone far in approaching nature. Porcelain is two and a half times harder than enamel, and especially zirconium restorations.

For example, the author's experience confirms that with immediate loads, softer materials (acrylate) achieve faster and better bone integration and predictability. The softness and abrasiveness of the material favored the integration process during the period of adaptation of the biotolerant material in living and very dynamic bone. The softness of the material of the biting surfaces reduces all chewing forces to functional physiological values. When it comes to loading implants with prosthetic works, the author's position is that zirconium in the lateral regions it is not the material of choice. The above suggests, from the point of view of theory, that composite materials have an advantage over ceramics. Prosthetic works on zirconia implants are justified only in the front of the upper jaw for aesthetic reasons. Also, the support (abutment) must be made of the same zirconium material so that the metal of the titanium support does not show through.

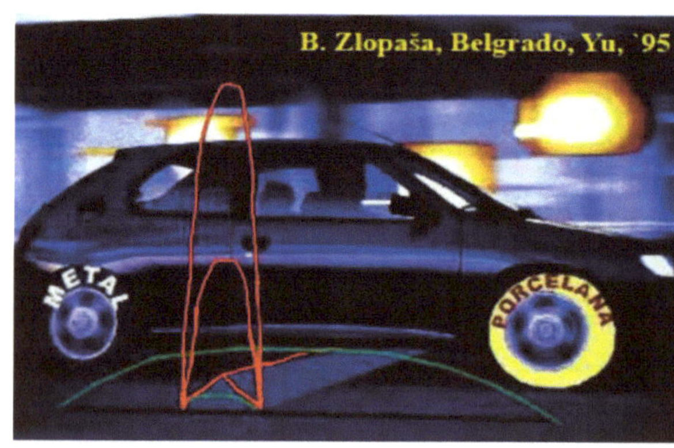

Figure 18.203. Demonstration of occlusal problems depending on the formation of oblique planes of the cusps and the hardness of the material on the occlusal surfaces.

How to explain the latest knowledge about the preservation of the crestal bone, the formation and preservation of soft tissues around implants?

Preservation of crestal bone and soft tissues depends on the design and processing of the implant neck. Processing with Laser-lock technology is a significant improvement in the conservation of the crestal bone and the formation of peri-implant soft tissues. A specially designed laser creates micro-channels on the neck of the implant that are 8 and 12 microns in size, which corresponds to the size of the osteoblasts and fibroblasts that vertically attach to the laser-treated surface and make a connection that is most similar to an epithelial connection, i.e. imitates the attachment of a natural tooth. Long-term studies (by M. Nevis) published in 2010 show on a human model that crestal bone loss is less with implants technologically processed with the Laserlock method, and comparisons were made on several implant systems.

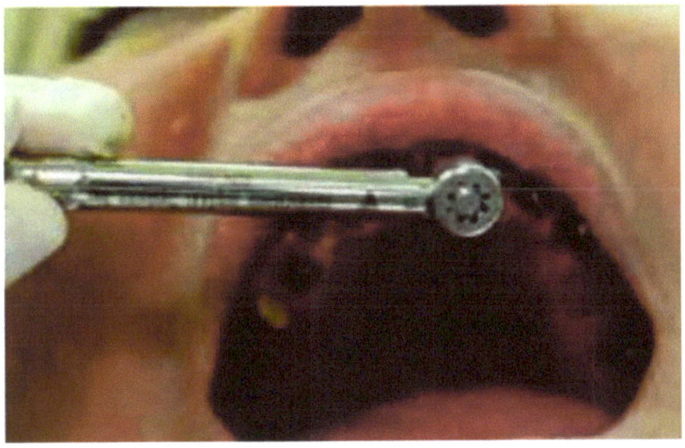

Figure 18.204. Torque wrench (Dynatorq Torque Wrench) for definitive tightening of the bracket. Tensile strength values range from 20 to 50 Ncm. A tensile strength of 35 Ncm is considered sufficient, especially when achieving primary stability. In the same way, the degree of integration of the implant is checked at the follow-up examination after 6 months.

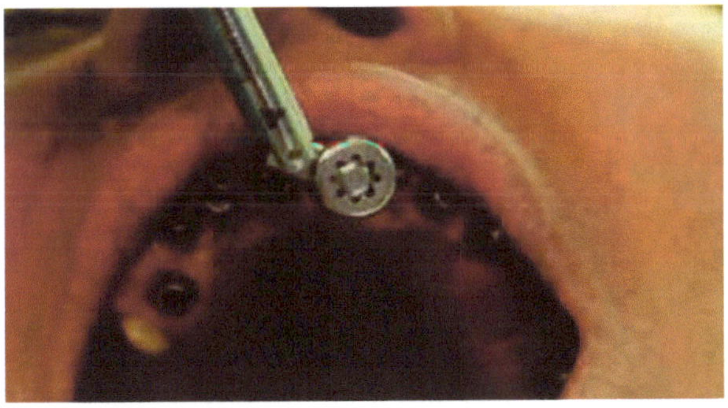

Figure 18.205. Checking the degree of implant integration after six months. A tensile strength of 35 Ncm is sufficient.

However, methods to improve the formation of the soft tissue and biological collar around the neck of the implant are constantly being sought. For this reason, more and more importance is attached to the micro-gap between the implant and the support. A crack between the implant and the support of the artificial crown is a suitable place for the deposition of microorganisms (over 500 types of potentially pathogenic microorganisms in the oral cavity). That space between the carrier and the implant can also be a place for the growth of connective tissue around the neck of the implant, which can spread to other peri-implant tissues. For this reason, it is mandatory to use a torque wrench for tightening the bracket screws with an adjustable tightening force (Figures 18.204 and 18.205).

What happens if the implant, during installation, is too inclined or "rests" on the root of the natural tooth?

Too inclined position of the implant can lead to biomechanical and especially aesthetic problems during prosthetic restoration. If the implant is placed too close to a vital tooth, blood supply to both is compromised. Due to the ischemia of the surrounding bone, the osseointegration processes are endangered, and by resting the implant on the root of the natural tooth, necrosis of the pulp may occur due to the ischemia of the surrounding bone. Overheating the bone during preparation with blunt drills near the natural root can also cause necrosis of the pulp. If this is overlooked, and the symptoms are usually not manifested at the beginning, more serious complications can follow with the consequences of losing both teeth and implants. Such a tooth should be endodontically treated or extracted. If a periapical lesion occurs due to the devitalization of the tooth near the implant, the spread of the periapical lesion can cause the loss of the implant and compromise the entire implantological rehabilitation.

But the loss of implants can also be due to the following reasons:

a) by placing the implant too close to the root of the natural tooth, or if it rests on the root of the tooth. Due to the compression on the surrounding bone and the periodontium, both the tooth and the implant are at risk;
b) contamination by microorganisms during implantation;
c) overheating of the bone;
d) intrusion of a foreign body file into the stuffed bone;
e) contact of the implant bed with gloves or instruments before implant placement

What should be done to avoid periapical changes on the teeth with the installation of implants?

X-rays are used to determine the exact position of the roots of adjacent teeth and their angulation. Ideally, the distance between the surface of the implant and the root of the tooth should be 1.5 to 2 mm.

When the depth of the bone is 5 mm, it is necessary to check the parallelism with an instrument for checking the parallelism in cases where a ridge has been formed and the bone is healthy. If the implant is to be inserted into the alveolus immediately after tooth extraction, never insert the implant into an infected wound. It is necessary to preserve the alveolus and postpone the installation of the implant. Also, augmentation should not be performed in an infected wound. You need to be patient and wait for complete healing

What is the rate of wound healing?

Epithelium forms 0.5-1 mm per day, connective tissue 0.5 mm per day, and bone 1.5 mm per month. Fibrin collagen is formed up to 24 hours, and after one week the coagulum turns into granulation tissue.

In the second week, the flap is attached to the periosteum with collagen connective fibers. If one of the bone substitutes (artificial bone) is added to the alveolus, it is necessary to wait 4-6 months for the graft to calcify in order to insert the implant.

What happens if the membrane of the sinus floor is perforated and the implant enters the sinus or nasal cavity by a few millimeters?

Most often it passes without complications. The implant should be left, and infection should be prevented with antibiotics, amoxicillin 500 mg one capsule every 8 hours or augmentin 1000 mg. one tablet every 12 hours. Just in case, it is good to accompany all this with the use of nasal drops. If the patient has an allergy to penicillin, then prescribe another appropriate antibiotic from the tetracycline group (doxycycline), or erythromycin.

What is a routine complication of a sinus floor lift?

Membrane perforation occurs in 25 to 40% of cases. Pay attention to bleeding. Complications can be prevented with antibiotics, but already in the anamnesis it is necessary to find out from the patient whether he is allergic to antibiotics.

What should be paid attention to if the patient takes certain medications, uses anticoagulant therapy, etc.?

Patients taking aspirin should stop taking the drug 7 days before the intervention. Nonsteroidal anti-inflammatory drugs can sometimes increase bleeding. Then alternative herbal remedies, ginkgo biloba, ginger, fish oil, garlic and vitamin E can prolong the bleeding time.

A few hours before the intervention, the patient should have a blood analysis, namely: blood count, bleeding time, coagulation time, prothrombin time (INR) and glycemia.

What is the basic principle of flap lifting?

Flap lift should be performed with as little trauma as possible and as shallowly as possible.

If the flap elevation is too deep towards the fornix, the following complications can occur: hematoma, greater edema with signs of hematoma, bleeding, greater possibility of infection, dehiscence and necrosis.

Can the question be asked: "What are the golden rules that a dentist must follow when it comes to raising a flap?"

There are ten basic rules:

1. flap design planning before the procedure itself;
2. make a minimally invasive incision in the aesthetic zone. In the lateral regions, a wider field of view and a longer incision that heals at the same speed as a short incision are needed;
3. the flap should be as simple as possible;
4. the base of the flap should be wider than the coronary part to maintain maximum vascularization;

5. the shorter the treatment time, the less edema, or none at all;
6. the flap should be sutured without tension, because necrosis may occur due to strong tension, and also the sutures should not be tightly placed;
7. the flap should be constantly moist, moistened with physiological solution;
8. when processing soft tissues, perform the procedure as gently as possible;
9. take care of vital anatomical structures (blood vessels and nerves);
10. if a vertical relaxation incision is made, the submucosa containing blood vessels should be included to ensure good blood supply to the flap.

What is more primary today in modern oral implantology: bone integration or healing and formation of soft tissues?

Considering the problem of bone integration, since the appearance of Branemark in the early sixties of the last century until today, science has paid great attention to it. Even today, there is no scientific research in this field. In the last few decades, the application of osseointegrative implants, whether it is about total or partial toothlessness, has proven to be a proven and successful method of oral rehabilitation. Thanks to knowledge about bone integration, the indications for implantation have expanded considerably.

However, according to seda, that is the end of the story. Of course, if all prerequisites are met. Gone are the days when failure in front of the patient was justified with a lack of bone. The doctor is the one to evaluate and decide whether the implant should be placed, after a thorough evaluation of the place where the implant should be installed. If the treatment requires augmentation, then you should wait until the conditions are created for the installation of the implant and the achievement of good primary stability, and thus the conditions for the continuation and completion of the integration process. So the question of a solid connection between the implant and the bone is no longer a problem from the aspect of function, which must not be threatened by anything, but science is paying more and more attention to the integration of soft tissues and implants

On the basis of the presented views on bone integration, can an explanation be given for the behavior of bone implants after installation?

In the first two weeks, the primary stability decreases, and after that it begins to stabilize and increase over time. The author's thoughts and recommendations are based on experience. In order for the bone to function as well as possible as a future support for the implant, it should be restored to the role that nature determined for it, the bone should be restored as soon as possible to the function it lost due to tooth loss. So, in order for the implant to take over its role as a substitute for the lost root and tooth, it is considered that one should not wait several months. Thanks to new implantation techniques and many innovations in the development of modern prosthetics, the immediate installation of implants has significantly expanded the indications. But there are cases where such a treatment concept should not be applied, because the healing of bone and soft tissues requires waiting time

Contemporary implantology places aesthetics, especially in the frontal region of the upper jaw, as a priority. How much time is needed in the highly sensitive aesthetic zone for the formation of peri-implant tissues around the neck of the implant?

The issue of aesthetics in oral implantology is a priority challenge today. For this reason, more and more attention is paid to the treatment of soft tissues. It takes at least 6 weeks to assess how well the plan is being implemented and the expected outcome.

In some cases, tissue treatment requires a longer time to achieve a successful aesthetic result.

If augmentation with a graft was performed before that, does the graft slow down the healing of the wound?

Yes. With a graft, wounds heal much more slowly. If the graft is placed in the extraction wound, the healing time is much slower. Cortical bone heals in about 6 months.

How long does it take for bone to heal depending on the type of bone quality?

TYPE I bone heals in 8 weeks, and TYPE IV bone much slower, in 24 weeks, hence the risk for implantation in this type of bone. An experienced implantologist already recognizes this bone quality during the preparation of the bone for the implant bed.

What should be paid attention to during implantation in order to reduce postoperative pain?

The operation should be performed with as little trauma as possible to soft tissues and bones. Drills should be sharp, because blunt drills increase the pressure on the bone, which causes it to overheat. If the temperature exceeds 47°C, in 1 minute the bone will be overheated and the bone chips will be brown and dark in color. The change in the color of the bone can sometimes not be noticed immediately if it has occurred in deeper parts, but it will be accompanied by stronger postoperative pain. Bone trauma will affect the health of the soft tissues and their formation around the implant neck itself.

When it comes to the aesthetic success of the implant procedure, what is given priority today to fulfill high aesthetic requirements?

Achieving aesthetics in modern implantology is a significant challenge, even for the most experienced dentists. To achieve an aesthetically pleasing result, the entire implant procedure must be approached as a complex treatment that requires a solid understanding of the biological processes within the body.

Historically, the primary goal of implantology was to fulfill functional requirements. However, there is now a growing emphasis on aesthetic considerations, particularly in the visible areas— especially the frontal region of the upper jaw. These visible areas are aesthetically sensitive, making the pursuit of a harmonious appearance in the soft tissues quite complex.

Successful aesthetic outcomes depend on key factors such as the formation of the gingival margin and the preservation of intact papillae, alongside maintaining the convex contour of the alveolar ridge. The peri-implant tissues must harmonize in volume, color, and contour with the healthy soft tissues of adjacent teeth.

The process should begin with a bracket that closely resembles the characteristics of a polished natural tooth in terms of color, shape, composition, and size, in order to meet aesthetic standards. Any violations of aesthetics may result in issues such as compromised papilla condition, discoloration of the peri-implant soft tissue, mismatch in the color of the abutment, and gingival recession.

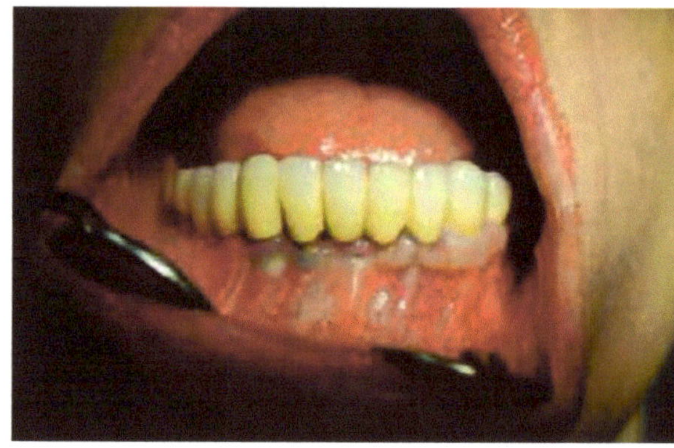

Figure 18.206. Screening of the color of the implant neck support in thin gingival biotype. Figure 18.206. Screening of the color of the implant neck support in thin gingival biotype.

What is important for fulfilling the aesthetic appearance of peri-implant soft tissue?

The fundamental factor is bone, as the basis on which soft tissues are located. Computed tomography (CT) or digital volume tomography (DVT) can be used to analyze a three-dimensional representation of the bone base and, based on that, plan the realization of aesthetic requirements. When there is enough available bone in the horizontal and vertical dimensions, the aesthetic result of soft tissue formation and papilla reconstruction can be predicted. Achieving a satisfactory aesthetic result depends on whether one or more teeth are missing in the front region of the upper jaw. If it is a single tooth replacement, the formation of peri-implant tissue and preservation of the papilla will depend on the distance of the bone to the gingival edge of the crown. When several teeth are missing, the formation of inter-implant papillae in most cases is not adequate for the papillae when one tooth is missing or for the papillae that are prestylized in natural teeth.

What does aesthetic success in the front region of the upper jaw depend on and what are the basic starting points for aesthetic requirements to be met?

The existence of a buccal bone lamella is the first condition for aesthetic success in a sensitive region such as the front of the upper jaw. After tooth extraction, the buccal alveolar wall in most cases is thin and that part of the alveolus is resorbed very quickly because the blood vessels of the periodontal ligament are cut off by tooth extraction. In patients who were treated for orthodontic anomalies of protruding frontal teeth with a fixed method, after the treatment, the buccal lamella was significantly weakened. By retruding the crown in the palatal direction, the root moves labially, exerting compression on the lamellar bone, causing its resorption.

Very often, such treatment of orthodontic anomalies is performed at a late age (even in the third and fourth decade of life), when the bone is definitely formed. In such patients, before implantation, augmentation of the alveolar ridge in both horizontal and vertical dimensions is mandatory.

By exchanging opinions with orthodontists about the aforementioned observations, a frequent answer is obtained "that it should not" occur that the lamellar wall weakens or completely disappears with fixed orthodontic therapy of tooth movement. However, the author's claims are based on the findings of a patient who underwent orthodontic treatment. In a patient at a younger age, completely different physiological processes occur in the bone compared to patients at a late age. In people at a late age, the bone loses its reparable properties and does not have time to compensate for the bone loss that inevitably occurs due to permanent compression of the periodontal tissues as root support.

In explaining such treatments, two terms are often used: socket-preservation and socketsealing. Explain their meaning?

"Socket-preservation" is a therapeutic method when a fresh alveolus is filled with bone substitute material after tooth extraction in order to stop the physiological processes of resorption and maintain the convex contour of the alveolar bone. Placed bone substitutes inserted into a fresh alveolar wound can act osteoinductively and result in preservation of alveolar ridge dimensions.

"Socket-sealing" is a method when the filled alveolus is covered with a mucous graft taken from the tuber in order (for the planned implantation) to create the conditions for a sufficient volume of soft tissue and to optimize the formation of the peri-implant mucous gingival sulcus. There is research evidence for the "socket-preservation" concept, but no such evidence for the "socket-sealing" concept.

When it comes to implant rehabilitation and the time needed to replace lost teeth, what are the most common requests from patients?

One of the characteristics of modern man is the speed of life and impatience. After the loss of teeth, loss of function and deterioration of aesthetic appearance, the priority request of patients is to shorten the treatment time. Most patients do not want a mobile acrylic prosthesis even as a temporary restoration. The patient's desire to regain the lost comfort in the mouth as soon as possible is one of the big challenges for the doctor as well. Patients' demands for shortening the therapy time led to the concept of immediate implant placement and immediate loading. Immediate placement of a definitive crown support, instead of a cap or gingiva-former (healing abutment), has proven to be a proven and successful procedure. The formation of gingiva around the neck of the implant and the support is far better. During the entire treatment, the bracket should be unscrewed and screwed as little as possible, thus avoiding microtrauma to the already-formed gingival margin. On this occasion, the position of the carrier changes or is insufficiently tightened and a larger micro-crack remains between the implant and the carrier, in which bacterial plaque can be deposited.

What is the success rate of immediate implant placement in the aesthetic zone compared to delayed implant placement?

The percentage of success of immediate installation of implants with immediate loading, compared to the percentage of success of delayed implantation, as well as the conditions of soft tissues in both procedures, are approximately the same.

Implantology therapy in a highly aesthetic area such as the front of the upper jaw aims not only to achieve good tissue integration, but also to obtain an aesthetic contour of the soft tissue, i.e. to establish both function and aesthetics. It often happens that this cannot be achieved due to unfavorable conditions of the alveolar ridge. Disadvantages are caused by periodontal diseases, pathological migration of frontal teeth, loss of teeth due to trauma and destruction of the alveolar wall by extraction.

All this means that insufficient available bone, in both dimensions, makes implant placement impossible in the aesthetic zone. Then, to create favorable conditions, augmentation of the alveolar ridge is required.

In order to satisfy the esthetic requirements in the frontal region of the upper jaw when replacing one tooth, what is the ideal position of the implant?

Replacement of one tooth in the frontal region of the upper jaw is one of the most complicated, demanding, and fascinating implant prosthetic procedures. Evaluation of the success of the procedure has two points of view: the patient's point of view and the dentist's point of view. From the patient's point of view, success is based on only one parameter, aesthetics. That criterion is the appearance of the peri-implant tissue, and the shape and color of the prosthetic work of the crown.

However, the assessment of success by dentists has many more parameters based on which the criterion of treatment success is determined. There are several starting points. For example, Meier et al. (2004) proposed the so-called "white esthetic score" white esthetic score (WES) for evaluating the aesthetic success of the crown and soft tissue appearance documented with nine parameters. However, Furhauser et al. (2005) took only one index for assessment only, the appearance of the peri-implant tissue, the so-called. "pink aesthetic score" (PES). Belser et al based the assessment of success on the equal importance of both PES and WES scores. From practical experience, the evaluation of the aesthetic result also depends on the patient's smile line. A low smile line in patients where 75% of the frontal teeth in the upper jaw are visible is advantageous. At the middle laugh line, in the front of the upper jaw, the teeth are exposed from 75% to 100% and a part of the papilla, and at the high laugh line, the teeth and facial soft tissues are completely exposed. Visibility of the facial soft tissues of patients is found in about 10% of cases, where the female population is more numerous, about 20% of patients have a low laugh line, and about 70% have a medium one.

The result of the implant treatment for the replacement of an individual tooth in the frontal region of the upper jaw depends on several factors. The first factor is the reason for the loss of a natural tooth (trauma or periodontal disease).

What is the bone defect and condition of the laminar bone wall?

The situation is less favorable if the three-dimensional bony defect is larger vertically, and is accompanied by a soft tissue loss. In that case, it is necessary to replace the lost bone with an autologous bone graft and bone substitutes, with the use of a resorbable membrane. Bone support is extremely important for vertical shaping and soft tissue condition. From practical experience, after augmentation, you should wait at least 6 months before installing the implant. It should always be kept in mind that buccal recession of the soft tissues is possible, resulting in major aesthetic problems. For this reason, caution and waiting time are necessary. In such cases, a two-phase method of implant placement is indicated.

Immediate installation of the implant can only be performed if the buccal lamella is intact, with a minimum thickness of 2 mm, and when the peri-implant tissues are thicker periodontal types of gingiva. The author's experience recommends that the buccal area should be augmented in such cases as well.

When replacing one tooth with an implant, care should be taken to position the implant in relation to the edges of the gingiva of the adjacent tooth. The appearance of the peri-implant tissues around the implant also depends on the condition of the gingiva and papillae of the adjacent teeth. For aesthetic success, the thickness of the marginal periodontal tissue is extremely important, which in most patients, according to some statistics, about 75% of cases is below 1 mm, while only 25% shows a thickness over 1 mm. Clinical and practical experience shows that the thin type of soft tissue of the gingiva reacts to surgical trauma sooner with scars and recessions than the thick type of gingiva. The shape and appearance of the papilla also depends on the thickness of the tissue in the proximal area of the papilla. In the thick biotype of the gingiva, the papilla is better shaped and larger, which significantly increases the aesthetic effect. In the case of immediate implant placement in a region with a thin periodontal biotype, recession is more pronounced than in patients with a thick gingival biotype.

The implant should be positioned directly under the incisal edge of the crown of the adjacent tooth that extends in two planes, including the buccal bone loss that existed before the implant was placed. The greatest bone loss occurs when the implant is positioned 2-4 mm below the cementoenamel border. The implant should be placed in a position with an optimal inclination.

If the slope of the implant is not optimal, this can be corrected with an angled bracket, which creates a condition for the formation of peri-implant soft tissue and achieving good aesthetics. When replacing multiple teeth in the anterior region of the upper jaw, the formation of soft tissues is a very complex procedure.

In order to achieve good esthetics of the soft tissues, the following criteria must be met: the depth of the gingival sulcus, the appearance of the interdental papilla, a good attachment of the gingiva, the thickness of the soft tissue and the location of the gingival margin.

What are the parameters for assessing the state of soft tissues on which aesthetics depends?

The occurrence of facial soft tissue recession on the labial side, the quality of the peri-implant tissue, the condition of the surrounding tissues and possible inflammatory processes are important parameters for evaluating the success of the aesthetic result. All these changes usually occur in the first year after implantation.

What are the advantages, disadvantages and possible complications of immediate implant placement and immediate loading?

A similar question has already been discussed in the book. The advantages of immediate loading are more numerous than the disadvantages:

- significantly shorter treatment time;
- preservation of the proximal bone;
- higher quality and faster integration processes;
- better and faster formation of the gingiva around the support;
- reduced number of implants;
- reduction of the number of surgical interventions.

If it can be said that it is a disadvantage, then it is the fact that it requires more experience and routine of the therapist. Determining the direction and position of the implant, i.e. achieving parallelism is an extremely important planning phase. The concept of implant-prosthetic treatment requires careful selection of patients, recognition of suitable cases. The planning of implant-prosthetic treatment must include predicting the outcome. When it comes to the disadvantages of immediate installation of implants with immediate loading, I would rather say that it has multiple advantages that I have previously emphasized: first of all, shortening the treatment time for the patient is a great relief, faster return of comfort in the mouth and improved quality of life. And when it comes to the physiological processes of the bone-implant relationship, the immediate installation of implants with immediate loading is in accordance with Wolf's rule in orthopedics, which today in modern orthopedics has been transformed into Wolf's Law: that the bone should recover as soon as possible lost function. With the loss of teeth, the jawbone also lost its basic physiological function of supporting something with physiological stress and renewing itself due to reactivation. With implantation, the basic physiological processes manifested by bone integration of bone cells around the implant are achieved. The concept of immediate implant placement and immediate prosthetic restoration requires the experience of a therapist.

Give one example from practice where the dentist is in a dilemma as to which implant installation concept to apply?

For example, a patient living abroad. The doctors explained to the patient, shown in Figure 18.207, pictures from a) to n), that his problem can only be solved by installing an implant. Extraction of one molar in the upper jaw on the left bearing the distal part of the bridge was proposed. It was proposed to install only one implant in the place of the first premolar and, after healing for 3 months, connect it to the canine with the addition of a hanging member. It was explained to the patient that later metal-ceramic crowns will be made on all the teeth in the upper jaw. The patient explained that he only had five days at his disposal and that he did not want to return to work without teeth. Another requirement was that it does not fit a removable prosthesis even as a temporary solution. After a detailed analysis and planning of the implantology-prosthetic treatment, the first step of the treatment procedure was the removal of the bridge and the extraction of the decayed molar, and the entire further procedure is shown in Figure 18.207. marked with letters from "a)" to "n)".

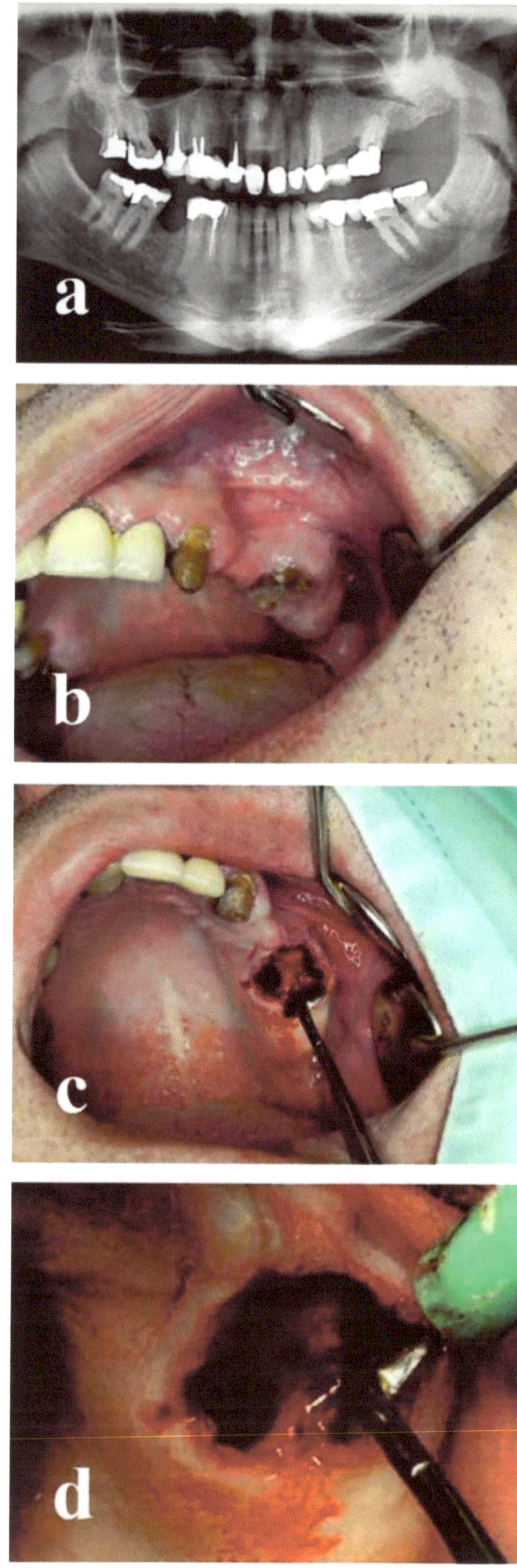

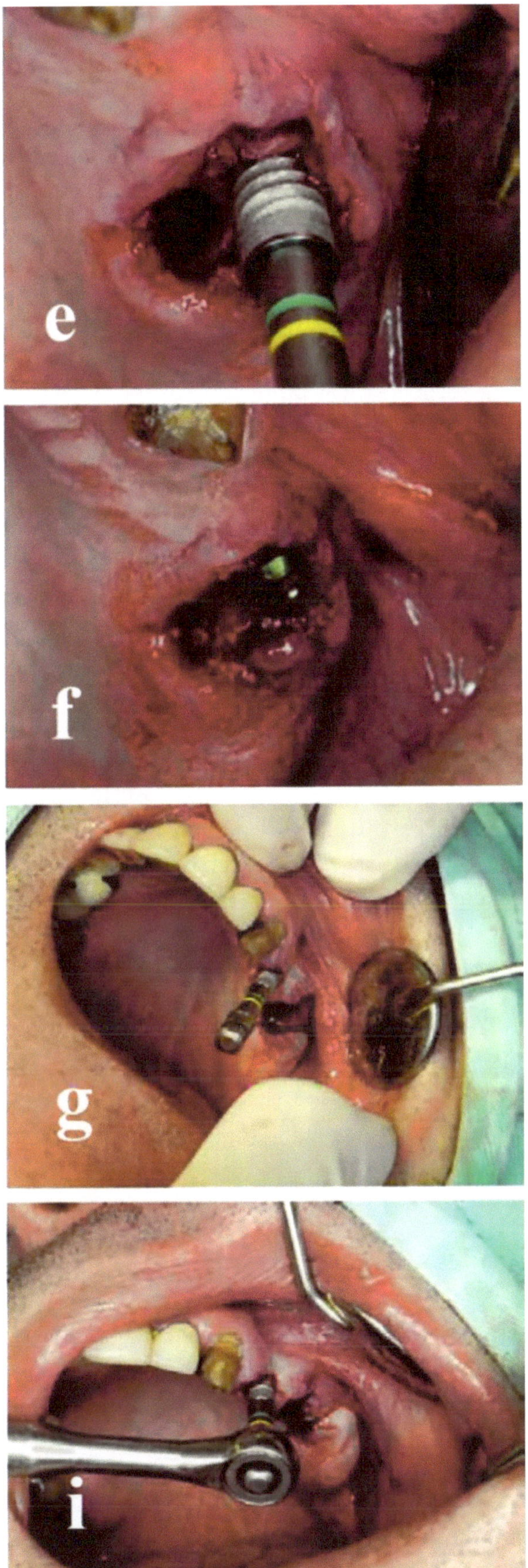

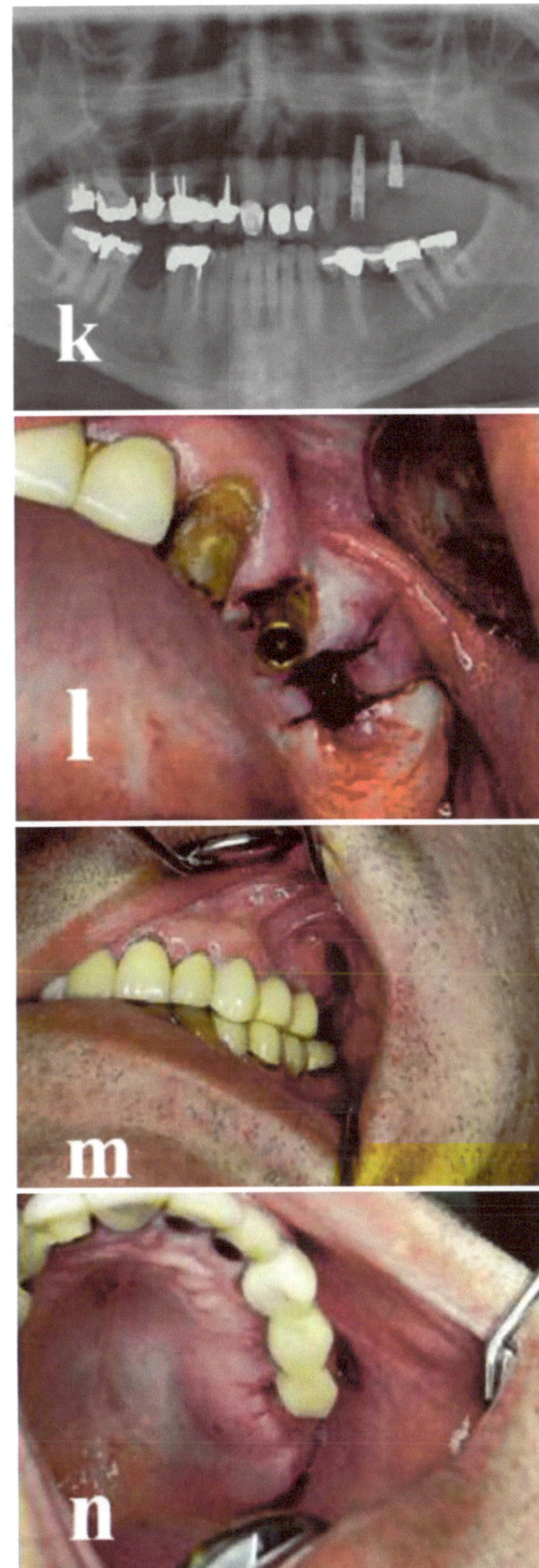

Figure 18.207. a) Initial condition; b) Molar extraction is indicated; c) Extracted molar; d) Appearance of the extraction wound and bony septum; e) Installation of implants in the septum; f) Built-in implant with healing cap; g) Installation of the implant at the site of the second pre-

molar without raising the flap; i) Achieved tensile strength of 35 Ncm; k) Presentation of installed implants; l) Definitive support placed and bone substitute covered with a resorptive collagen membrane placed; m) Temporary bridge placed on the same day after implant installation; n) Temporary bridge view from the palatal side.

Does delayed implantation create more favorable conditions for a better aesthetic result than immediate implantation?

It all depends on the size of the bone defect. Many patients have labial bone defects. It is very important to establish how big that defect is and how and in what way it will be compensated. After 6 to 8 weeks of healing, a sufficient volume of soft tissues is obtained and the procedure of buccal contour formation by augmentation continues. Whether the guided regeneration of the bone defect will be performed with autologous bone or xenogeneic (bovine) bone substitutes depends on the size of the defect and the therapist's assessment. In any case, covering the augment with a collagen resorptive membrane is a mandatory procedure. Shaping the labial contour of the alveolar bone with augments compensates for physiological resorption and forms a sufficient bone base for soft tissues and a successful aesthetic result.

There is no valid long-term research and evidence on the advantages of delayed implantation over immediate implantation. There is a short-term study by Buser and associates that talks about the stable relations of bone and facial soft tissues in delayed implantation of implants after 3 years in function. However, delayed installation of implants is a more complicated procedure, requires a longer time and a higher price. Guided bone regeneration with autologous bone blocks is one of the more complicated oral surgical procedures. After that, soft tissue augmentation is needed. All this is accompanied by pain and swelling, and often a hematoma, with an uncertain outcome.

Assuming that guided bone regeneration was successful, followed by successful soft tissue transplantation, what should we focus our attention on next?

The optimal position of the implant ensures a high-quality aesthetic result. If the implant is placed too labially, there are two risks: the difficulty of making the labial part of the artificial crown and the increased risk of soft tissue recession and sieving of the mucous membrane around the neck of the implant. If the implant is placed too palatally, prosthetic restorative problems arise. The position of the implant in the mesiodistal direction must ensure a sufficient distance from the adjacent teeth to create favorable conditions for the preservation of the interdental papilla or its repair. The mesiodistal position of the implant is also important for preservation of the proximal part of the bone, which preserves the height of the papilla. An implant placed too apically can increase vertical bone resorption, because that part of the bone then loses function and is susceptible to resorption. In order to place the implant in the optimal position, modern implantology offers various aids (CT and DVD, special software programs) in order to plan the optimal position and angulation of the implant, the depth of implantation, and accordingly also the planning of prosthetic work. It is complicated work that increases costs for the patient.

However, in practice, the therapist's experience is crucial. With a minimally invasive procedure without raising the flap, the postoperative risk is also reduced. With the immediate installation of the implant, extraordinary aesthetic results are achieved even in cases where a flap lift is not required. The immediate installation of implants, first of all, significantly shortens the time of the procedure and reduces pain due to the avoidance of surgical intervention.

The placement of precise temporary prosthetic work enables the gradual formation of peri-implant tissue, which is accompanied by the comfort and satisfaction of the patient that during all that time he has a lost tooth, or several teeth, compensated for.

How much does the aesthetic result depend on the type of gingiva, which has a decisive role in the behavior of the soft tissue around the implant?

The type of mucosa plays a crucial role in the formation and behavior of soft tissues. The greater the thickness of the fibrous soft tissue and the wider the keratinized gingiva, the more resistant the peri-implant tissue is to pulling and better covers the dark color of the carrier. On the support (abutment) made of titanium, the artificial crown can be adapted and its relationship with the soft tissues adjusted depending on the type, width and thickness of the mucous membrane. Aesthetics also depends on the type of support, that is, on the material from which it is made. It has been shown that the titanium bracket already shows a dark screening on the labial side at a soft tissue thickness of 3mm. In contrast to the titanium support, the zirconium dioxide support does not cause any changes in the color of the soft tissues, even in soft tissues with a thickness of 2 mm.

Practical experience shows that ceramic supports made of zirconium dioxide achieve better aesthetic results. This is especially important in patients with a thin layer of soft tissue. Clinical research at Harvard University in Boston says that front teeth in the upper jaw with titanium supports on implants, compared to adjacent natural teeth, show clearly visible discolored soft tissue.

What is the average soft tissue recession with implants?

The average recession of the peri-implant tissue is 0.5 to 1 mm. Some studies have shown that soft tissue recession is greater than 1 mm in 17% to 40% of cases. The morphological difference between periodontal and peri-implant tissue is caused by the absence of an enamel-cement border on the implant, which is why the long-term stability of the soft tissues surrounding the implant is not guaranteed. For this reason, mucogingival surgical interventions are often required for a good aesthetic result. In modern oral implantology, more and more attention is paid to this issue, both in practical and in scientific research work.

What are the results of augmentation of soft tissues compared to bone?

Correction or compensation of soft tissues in order to achieve aesthetic requirements, by whatever method it is performed, is a far more complex procedure than augmentation of bone defects. Augmentation of soft tissues is all the more complex in cases where periodontal microsurgical interventions are required. The collection and adaptation of subepithelial connective tissue grafts, or free mucosal grafts, whether taken from the tuber or the palate, are very delicate microsurgical procedures so that a successful end result can always be predicted. Despite solid knowledge and experience, many dentists stumble over this problem. The author's experience speaks in favor of a satisfactory aesthetic result using a coronary displaced flap.

In order to fulfill aesthetic requirements, the path is often complicated and uncertain. The main goal of soft tissue augmentation is to improve the volume of the mucous membrane. A submucosal connective tissue graft taken from the palate or tuber can be combined with coronary flap displacement. By redoing the edge of the marginal gingiva and the asymmetric relations of the mucous membrane, new peri-implant soft tissue contours would be created.

Preservation of the papilla is one of the important conditions for achieving aesthetics in the front region of the upper jaw. What does papilla regeneration depend on?

When replacing single teeth with an implant, the papilla is dependent on the approximate bone height of the adjacent teeth. The widest part of the implant is flush with the bone, but it is also below the crestal part of the proximal bone of the tooth, which affects the resorption of the surrounding bone. This difference in bone height determines the height of the papilla between the natural tooth and the implant. In addition, it should be taken into account that the existence of the papilla, its quality, color, volume, and attachment depend on the age of the patient, the shape of the teeth, the contact point, the type of con tact (surface or point), as well as the thickness of the interdental gingiva.

Reconstruction of the destroyed papilla is still a big challenge not only for implant dentists but also for periodontists.

According to my knowledge, modern implantology has not yet given an answer as to whether successful papilla reconstruction is possible with long-term stability and predicting the duration of success. Also, in the case of peri-implant tissue recession, with transplantation and covering with soft tissues, the predictability of success is uncertain. These considerations may be related to the lack of bone to support the papilla.

Preservation of the papilla in its shape, color, volume, and especially the reconstruction of the destroyed, therefore non-existent papilla, its compatibility with the tissue around the healthy tooth is a great challenge for the implantologist and periodontologist, but the predictability of the final outcome is very limited.

What does the healthy, harmonious appearance of the peri-implant tissue with the surrounding tissues depend on, and what is the condition for a good aesthetic result?

It must be borne in mind that the healthy appearance of the peri-implant tissue also depends on the condition of the keratinized mucosa. If the mucosa is keratinized around the implant, the quality of the gingiva is much better, there is less plaque deposition, less bleeding after probing and less recession of the peri-implant environment. For easier maintenance of oral hygiene and stability of the gingival peri-implant sulcus, a certain width of keratinized mucosa and minimal loss of marginal bone is required. Regarding the expansion of keratinized mucosa by vestibuloplasty and free mucosal autologous graft taken from the tuber, these methods have been shown to be more successful than the application of allogeneic materials. The mucosal graft taken from the tuber is significantly different in color from the mucosal graft taken from the palate, although these differences diminish over time. However, due to the healing period and pain, repeated surgical procedures on the palate should be avoided. A great relief for the patient is the application of allogeneic materials whenever possible.

The author's conclusion is that, for now, there are still dilemmas when it comes to the reconstruction of the non-existent papilla to meet the aesthetic requirements of implanted implants. Although there are possibilities to apply various microsurgical techniques (coronary flap displacement, combined with subepithelial connective tissue grafts, then attempts with free mucosal grafts to encourage the formation of keratinized mucosa), this is a topic of the future, which has yet to be confirmed by successful evidence in practice

Can prosthetic work influence the formation of peri-implant tissue in order to establish a harmonious appearance and achieve high aesthetic requirements in an aesthetically sensitive region?

As much as surgical techniques enable the rehabilitation of soft tissues, prosthetics have the ability to shape soft tissues in the visible area and significantly contribute to their harmonious appearance. Application of temporary restorations on implants is of great importance for optimizing soft tissue. Provisional compensation enables the gradual adaptation of soft tissues to prosthetic work and gives the possibility for the peri-implant mucosa to form ("tissue-shaping" tissue shaping; "tissue guiding" tissue guidance). Occasional corrections on the temporary crown in the contact area with soft tissues can influence the shaping of the gingival margin and the formation of peri-implant tissue.

The application of ceramic supports (abutments) represents a great advance in the creation of aesthetics. Ceramic supports are particularly advantageous in cases with thin, transparent mucous membranes. Placement of a zirconium oxide bracket has a great aesthetic advantage over a titanium metal bracket due to the screening of the metal color. Zirconium oxide, in addition to good technical properties, also has good biological properties. Due to its good biological properties, with the application of zirconium oxide, there is much less discoloration of the peri-implant mucosa compared to metal ceramics.

Color intensity, i.e. The transparency of the gingiva depends on the thickness of the gingiva. If the gingiva is about 3 mm thick, the aesthetic result is better. Next, zirconium oxide fits better into the periodontal environment of the natural tooth, especially when dealing with individual restorations in the anterior region of the upper jaw.

How many implants does a person need to chew well and look good?

This has become somewhat of a philosophical question. The multitude of indications, the desire to achieve success in various situations and the possibility of choosing an implant, exceeds all previous expectations. Despite this fact, for example, in the edentulous mandible with extreme atrophy of the alveolar bone and unfavorable anatomical structures in the lateral regions, the front region between the mental foramina remains the only possibility for implant placement. If there is a sufficient amount of available bone in the horizontal and vertical dimensions to be able to install implants of sufficient length and diameter, the question remains with how many implants will achieve an optimal functional solution. In addition, the question arises as to which method of prosthetic rehabilitation on implants should be chosen.

Should the stabilization of the total prosthesis be done with retention ball elements on the implants or should it be decided to connect the implants with crossbars (according to Dolder or Ackerman)? If the decision is to perform the procedure with Dolder's retention bars with riders, the question of the number of implants also arises.

In general, I think that the previous claim that a larger number of implants is a better solution is not correct. True, thanks to these attitudes, the author of the book also made mistakes. Those were established positions. For example, it is better to insert four implants than two. That was, apparently, the axiom for the stabilization of the lower total prosthesis. I remember that a similar rule was valid for a long time in prosthetics, when anchors had to be installed for anchoring partial dentures in order to avoid unsightly hooks: the recommendation was that two teeth must be ground down and the crowns must be connected as supports for the anchors.

However, after a long period of validity of that rule, that attitude has been completely changed. Why? Due to the action of forces during chewing, the lever twisting forces acted on the attachment. Regardless of the quality of the attachment in receiving and amortizing those forces, the involved tooth that did not carry the attachment suffered because the tooth carrying the attachment assumed the role of a lever, transferring twisting forces to the adjacent tooth.

The position that it is more justified to stabilize the lower total prosthesis with four instead of two retention elements has been changed. At an educational meeting in the USA (New York, 2012), the opinion was expressed that support with four supports on implants with spherical heads and attachments is much more rigid than with two implants.

Regarding these claims, the author's experience confirms: the number of implants in such solutions does not play a decisive role, but the quantity and quality of the available bone, as well as the length and diameter of the implant. The author's experience confirms that long-term stability can be achieved with two as well as with four. Even, a good result is recorded with one implant of maximum length and wide diameter. In any case, the therapist's surgical experience and knowledge of prosthetics play a crucial role, because implatological treatment requires a multidisciplinary approach, concludes the author of the book.

That explanation refers, conditionally, to fixed-mobile prosthetic work. But when it comes to fixed prosthetic works, bridges, for example in the case of total toothlessness in the lower jaw, what is the layout of the implants and how many implants are needed?

The number and arrangement of implants depends on several factors: the quantity and quality of available bone and the position of anatomical structures. In the lower jaw, optimal solutions can be achieved with 8 implants. If in the lower jaw the width and height of the alveolar bone allow the installation of implants with standard diameters, and in the lateral regions with wider diameters, but not less than 12 mm in height, the number of implants can be reduced to 6. In the frontal region of the lower jaw, if there are conditions to install implants with a length of 15 and 16 mm, the installation of standard diameter implants in place of central and even lateral incisors should be avoided. The implants should be positioned in place of the lower canines. If the distance between the implants is greater, it is sufficient to install one implant in the middle.

In the upper jaw, the number and placement of implants, in the case of total toothlessness, also depends on the shape of the alveolar ridge, the available bone and the size of the sinus cavities. Due to cancellous bone, avoid using implants with narrow diameters. The number of implants in the upper jaw can be variable, from case to case. Due to the quality of the bone and the weaker cortical bone, if possible, larger diameter implants should be used in the lateral region, provided that good blood supply to the surrounding bone is ensured in order to achieve faster and better integration processes.

Fixation of prosthetic works on both natural teeth and implants is extremely important. What is the best way to fix prosthetic work on implants?

There are two concepts for fixing prosthetic works on implants: screwing and cementing. Both procedures have advantages and disadvantages. At one time, preference was given exclusively to screwing, which was used for a long time. According to some data, 90% of cases were fastened with screws, and only 10% were cemented. Over time, based on the observed results, the procedure for fixing crowns and bridges has changed, and today the relationship is almost reversed in favor of cementation.

The emergence of new adhesive materials, with strong metal-to-metal adhesion, has contributed to giving advantages to cementation. Today, there are very few dentists who fasten prosthetic works on implants with screws.

The advantages of cementing prosthetic works on implants are as follows:

- the creation of the work is simpler;
- the aesthetic result is better;
- fewer components are required;
- putting on and taking off work with temporary cements is simplified;
- it is possible to adjust the occlusal surfaces;
- the crowns fit more easily and precisely on the supports;
- it is easier to correct inaccuracies, and as much as possible
- lowers production costs;
- good stability and retention;
- ceramic breakages are smaller;
- the load on the implant is more favorable;
- the number of visits and the cost of work are reduced.

Disadvantages of cementing prosthetic works on implants are:

- the impossibility of removing and controlling the state of the soft tissues under the prosthetic work and around the support (subgingival embossing);
- impossibility of checking the stability of the implant;
- the duration of the temporary cement is unpredictable;
- there is a danger of cement lagging.

The advantage of screwing is the easy removal of the prosthetic work during periodic control of the condition of the implant. First of all, it should be pointed out that the concept of screws was forced at a time when there was talk about the survival rate of implants and the uncertainty of predicting the final result.

It should be emphasized that the design and technological processing of the implants did not ensure the predictability of the outcome. Therefore, screwing enables not only easy removal of the prosthetic work in order to check the condition of the implant, but also possible reconstruction due to loosening of the support, whether the loosening was caused by unscrewing the screw or peri-implant changes. Many experienced dentists emphasize the advantage of screwing over cementation because of the strong adhesiveness of the fixation material, which makes it very difficult to remove the remains of stuck cement, which can cause peri-implantitis.

Disadvantages of the bolting concept are:

- laboratory production is very complicated, which significantly increases the cost of work due to the greater number of components, the larger size of compensation;
- production in the laboratory must be precise, because if there is even the slightest error in precision, it is very difficult or impossible to make corrections;
- the abutment of the metal is not intimate with the support of the prosthetic work. With the concept of cementation, greater tolerance is allowed regarding the position and axis of the implant and easier correction of inaccuracies;
- when screwing, it is not possible to adjust the occlusal surfaces due to possible damage to the screw;
- in the crack at the place of the screw there is a space for the deposition of bacterial content, which can cause unpleasant breath from the mouth.

Using screwing, the aesthetic result is worse. Leaving space for the screw will cause the ceramic to crack and the veneers to fall out. The materials covering the screw abrade and fall out. Due to the action of rotation forces, the screw is unscrewed. In addition to all the listed disadvantages, screwing works are significantly more expensive. However, the advantages of screwing have been replaced by new materials for fixation, such as "implantlink" (semi, forte and transparent), which has the properties of good retention and easy removal (Figures 18.208 and 18.209).

The great "danger" (risk) of burying should be emphasized. Whether this is done with conventional zinc phosphate, carboxylate or composite cements, there is always a risk of cement retention. It happens that due to the difference between the diameter of the implant and the size of the crown to be replaced, the edge of the crown lies too subgingivally or medially where, due to inaccessibility, the probing is impenetrable and therefore the removal of cement remains is difficult. Due to this discrepancy between the diameter of the implant and the prosthetic work, the edge of the crown lies too sublingually and rests on the soft tissues. Experience suggests that after cementation it is necessary to take an OPT-image to check for cement residues (Figure 18.209).

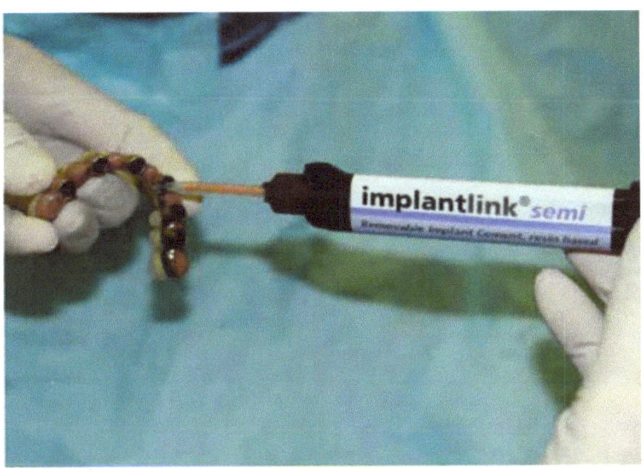

Figure 18.208. Temporary fixation of the bridge with implantlink.

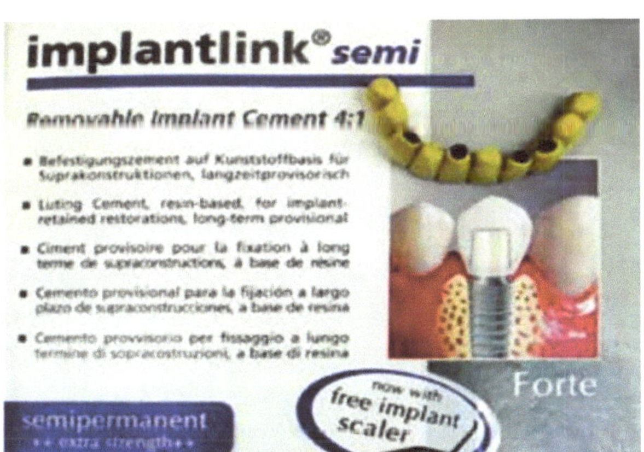

Figure 18.209. Implantlink-semi is for temporary cementation, and Implantlink-forte is for permanent cementation, and Implantlink-transparent is for zirconium restorations. The characteristics of these adhesives: good fixation, and easy removal if necessary.

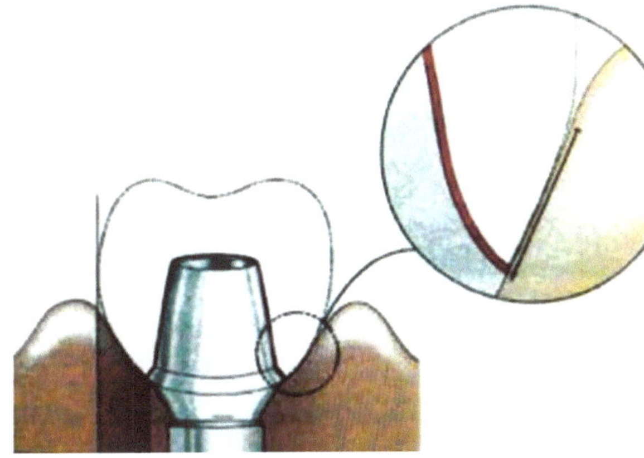

Figure 18.210. Retention place where it is possible to retain the remains of cementing material due to inaccessibility.

What should be done to avoid cement retention around the implant?

When cementing the crowns on the implant, care must be taken that the edge of the crown lies only slightly sublingual, so that it is easily accessible when removing cement residues. Before cementing, the crown should be tried and carefully checked to ensure that it does not exert pressure on the soft tissues (pictures 18.210 18.211, 18.214-18.215).

For this reason, it is necessary for the sublingual metal collar of the artificial crown to be as thin as possible, so that it does not rest on the soft tissues and exert pressure on them with the thick edge of the collar (four layers: metal, opaque, dentin, and glaze). The author's experience confirms that a small number of doctors in our country do not follow this rule. By justifying that patients don't like it.

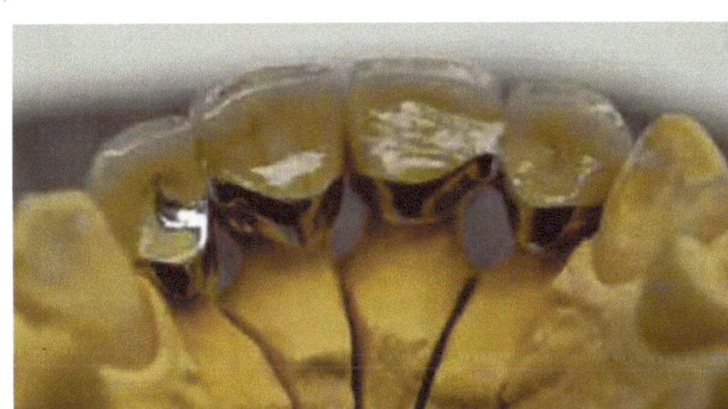

Figure 18.211. Correct construction of restorations on implants. Space left for papillae.

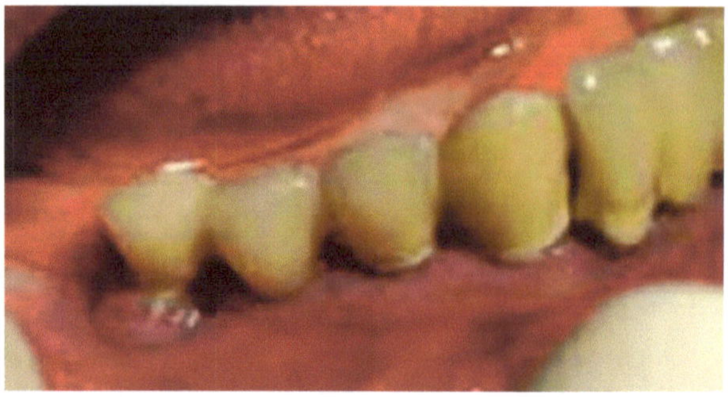

Figure 18.212. Peri-implantitis caused by retention of glass ionomer residues during bridge cementation.

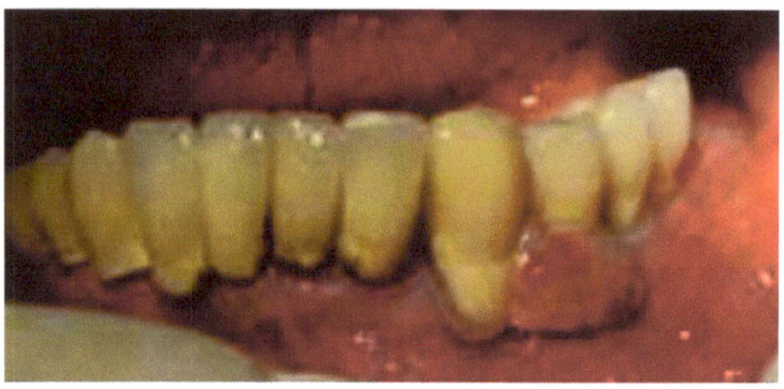

Figure 18.213. Ignition due to unremoved cement residues.

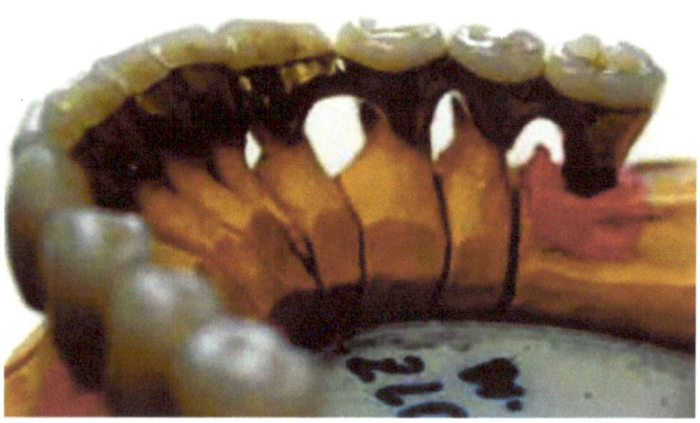

Figure 18.214. Prosthetic work supported by implants must be adapted to maintaining oral hygiene.

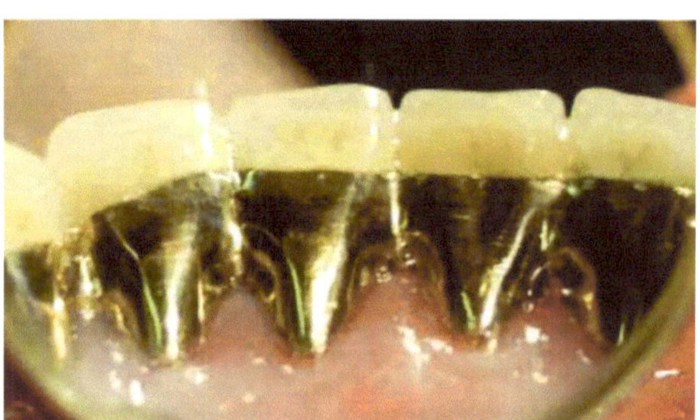

Figure 18.215. Prosthetic work on implants must be performed from the lingual side so that the space between the edge of the crown and the implant is not a place for plaque to settle.

What should be concluded when it comes to cement residues around the neck of the implant?

Great care should be taken when removing cement residues. Their presence can cause inflammatory reactions of the most severe form (18.212 and 18.213). The inflammatory process can spread and cause peri-implant bone destruction. One study shows that peri-implantitis was caused by submucosal cement residues in as many as 81% of cases. The risk of developing peri-implant inflammation is particularly noticeable when cementing with fast-setting, highly adhesive metal-to-metal cement. If the excess cement is not removed during bonding, the residues stick so strongly to the metal part of the support that removing the cement residues with a probe is extremely difficult, so the removal must be done with a turbine. For this reason, this type of cementing material should be avoided. The most common retention of cement residues is in the area of premolars and molars, and this can be complicated by peri-implantitis. If the unremoved cement residue is deep in the gingival sulcus, the complication is more severe. Since the fixation of prosthetic works on implants today is mostly done by cementing, there is always a risk of iatrogenic error and consequent inflammation of the peri-implant tissues. For this reason, for now, the material of choice is implantlink (semi, forte and transparent), which has the characteristics of zinc-oxide pastes for provisional cementation, and implantlink semi has this characteristic. Implantlink forte is used to fix definitive prosthetic works for a longer period, and Implantlink transparent is used to fix prosthetic works in zirconia. The characteristic of this material is that it has greater elasticity for good fixation of prosthetic works in function. It is especially important that the excess material is easily removed during cementation, because it is elastic. Fixation of prosthetic works in this way, whether provisional or definitive, has an advantage over screwing.

How are individual crowns fixed on implants?

Only by cementing. A single replacement of a lost tooth is in most cases in the front of the upper jaw. Installing a screw into a single crown would increase its volume, which would compromise aesthetics.

Restoring individual teeth in the anterior region of the upper jaw is a great challenge for the practitioner. Today, it is unthinkable to replace one tooth by grinding two healthy teeth, or to do it with the famous movable "frog". An increasing number of patients are informed that the installation of an implant is the best solution when replacing a single tooth. Patient awareness increases aesthetic requirements.

Which parameters in that highly aesthetically demanding area can influence the good or negative outcome of implantological treatment?

This outcome is primarily influenced by the condition of the alveolar bone, the biotype and condition of the gingiva, the height of the papilla, the width of the attached gingiva, the condition of the periodontium, the structure and condition of the adjacent teeth. The laugh line is a very important parameter. Attention should also be paid to the interocclusal space - is the flap horizontal or vertical?

An important parameter is the dimension of the mesiodistal edentulous space when one or more teeth are missing. The endodontic and periodontal status of adjacent teeth and the quality of adjacent crowns are very important for the final aesthetic result.

The radiological status determines the vertical and horizontal height of the alveolar bone, the position of the anatomical structures, the position of the root of the adjacent tooth, the illumination of the alveolar ridge, possibly the rest of a foreign body (the rest of amalgam fillings, broken burrs, lentules, etc.).

Neglecting just one of the listed factors can lead to more or less failure, despite the success rate ranging from 96% to 98% percent.

The replacement of one or more teeth with implants represents a set of procedures: from the achievement of good bone integration, to the achievement of aesthetic requirements, ideal attachment of soft tissues and ideal occlusion

As a precaution, what should you know and what should you pay attention to?

At the beginning, tooth loss patterns should be analyzed; whether the loss was caused by trauma or was caused by an acute or chronic infection (periodontitis, periapical lesions, granulomas, etc.). The lack of one tooth can also be congenital anodontia, and in that case it is most often the lateral incisor in the upper jaw.

The tooth extraction itself represents a traumatic intervention, after which, as a consequence, a defect in hard and soft tissues occurs. The vestibular lamellar bone wall is particularly susceptible to strong resorption. Resorption is manifested already two weeks after tooth extraction, and after eight weeks the loss of bone height amounts to about 2 mm. After one year, the alveolar bone loses about 50% in width, which is an average of 5 to 7 mm per year. It should be emphasized that most of the bone resorption process occurs in the first three months after tooth loss.

The condition of the vestibular lamella is of crucial importance for the final result of the entire procedure. According to numerous studies and data from the literature, the thickness of the cortical alveolar wall is from 0.1 to 1.9 mm, with an average of 0.6 for upper incisors and canines.

Explain the physiological processes after tooth loss and its replacement with an implant?

The state of lamellar bone depends on vascularization. Bone is nourished through spongiosa, periosteum and desmodont. The thin and compact buccal lamella is mainly fed by desmodonts and periosteum. The extraction of teeth damages the desmodont and then the nutritional deficiency of the lamellar bone occurs. If this is added to a full-thickness flap lift, nutrition is not only impaired but interrupted, which inevitably leads to bone resorption. This physiological process has attracted, in the last few years, a lot of attention from scientists and clinicians. In order to slow down that process, numerous new techniques and materials have been developed, and in the first place immediate implant installation, socket preservation, implant installation techniques without raising the flap ("flapless surgery"), methods of moving the platform ("platform switching"), and new augmentation materials are also used.

However, numerous possibilities can cause confusion among practitioners, because today many attitudes often arise from marketing dictates. Therefore, the choice of conception, implants and materials for therapy is not at all simple, but the experience of the clinician is important, which is especially highlighted in situations where work is done in an aesthetically highly demanding region, when each case requires caution and detailed analysis.

For example, is immediate implant placement indicated in a patient who has had a tooth extracted due to an acute or chronic periapical lesion?

In such cases, immediate implantation or augmentation with bone substitutes is not indicated. It is a principled position that such a wound should be covered with soft tissue augments, a free mucosal graft, in order to prepare for future implantation and augmentation with bone substitutes. It is important that after tooth extraction, the alveolus is carefully excised, and the gingival edge is refreshed slightly with a diamond drill, or cut with a scalpel obliquely undercut in the direction towards the alveolar cavity. Before closing the wound with a mucosal graft and before suturing, the extraction wound must be filled with fresh blood. The soft tissue graft should be carefully sutured with a thin suture for freshened edges. After the entire procedure, there is a delicate question about what kind of temporary restoration the patient should wear, because at the beginning no pressure must be applied to the graft and the wound. Healing takes at least eight weeks, when the procedure can be continued.

What should be done in cases where a tooth has to be extracted and there is no alveolar infection and buccal bony wall defect, but the gingiva is of a very thin biotype?

In cases with a thin biotype of the gingiva, where there is no infection of the alveoli and there is no pronounced defect of the lamellar wall, one should be careful about the aesthetic result. In such cases, bone resorption is more pronounced due to poor blood supply, and gingival recession can often be expected. After extraction, detailed curettage of the alveolus and refreshing of the gingival margin, the alveolus is filled with a mixture of autologous bone with some of the bone substitutes ("socket preservation"). Taking the autologous bone from the retromolar region is done with a special instrument for scraping the bone. (Fig. 18.216 and 18.219), and it is usually mixed with xenogeneic bone substitutes (Fig. 18.220 - 18.222).

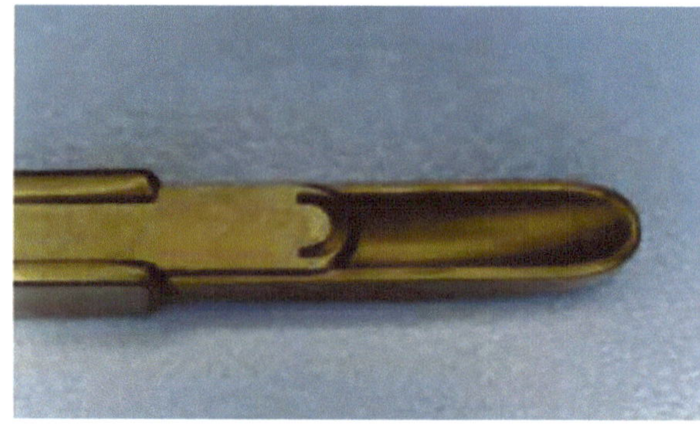

Figure 18.216. Instrument for taking autologous bone chips.

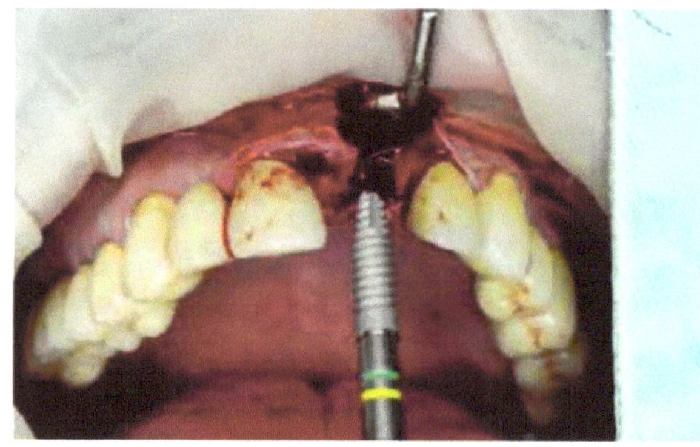

Figure 18.217. Installation of implants immediately after tooth extraction. Caution, do not insert the implant if the wound is infected and if the granulation tissue has been radically removed. Preservation of the alveolus is the foundation of successful treatment.

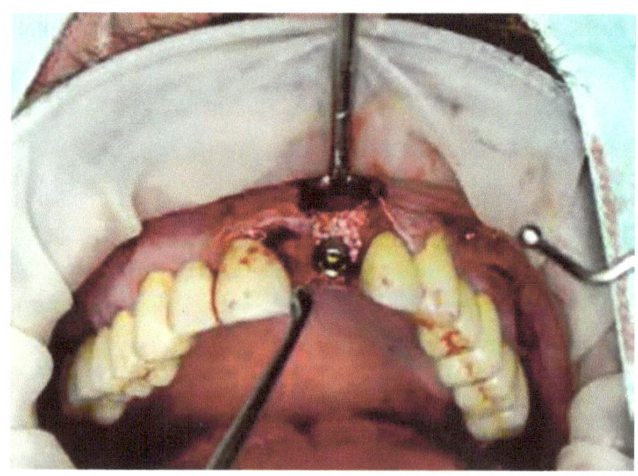

Figure 18.218. Replacement of the lamellar wall with a mixture of xenogeneic bone substitute with autologous bone chips.

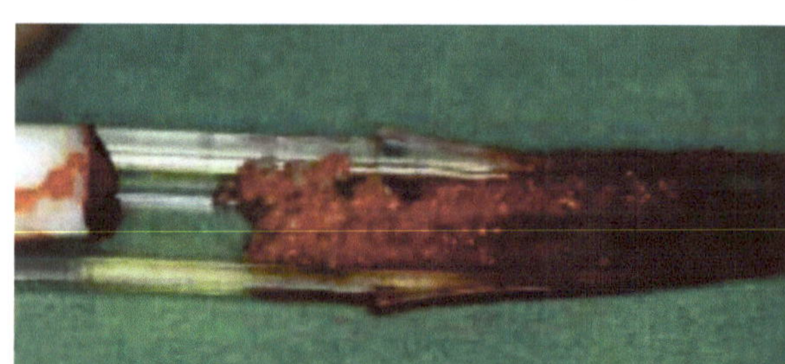

Figure 18.219. Autologous bone scratches.

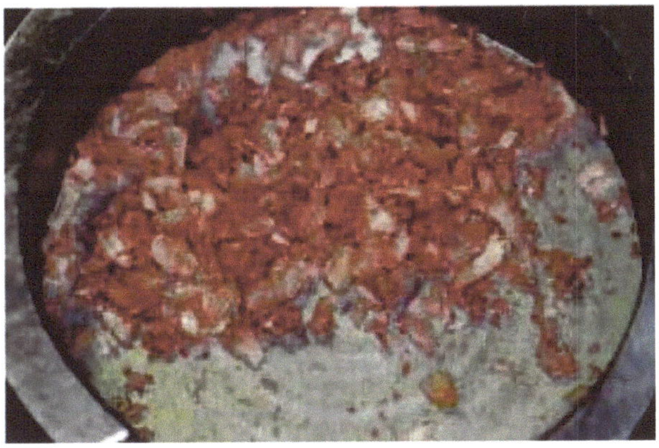

Figure 18.220. Analogous bone mixed with xenogeneic bone substitutes. The material (white) of the xenogeneic (bovine) bone substitute can be seen.

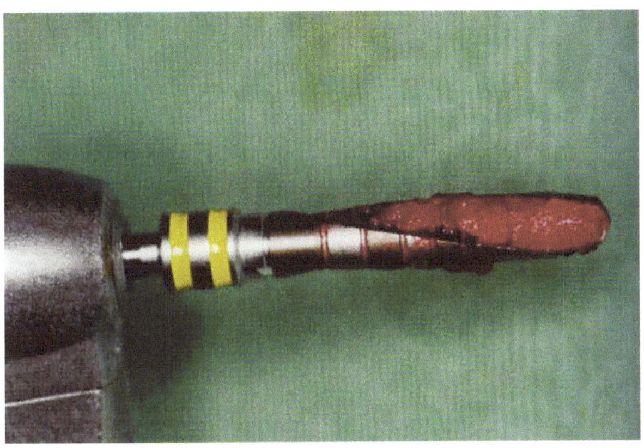

Figure 18.221. Taking autologous bone with a special drill with minimal slow motion. The drill is dimensioned to the depth to which the bone can be drilled for taking autologous files. With this procedure, the bone can be taken from several places.

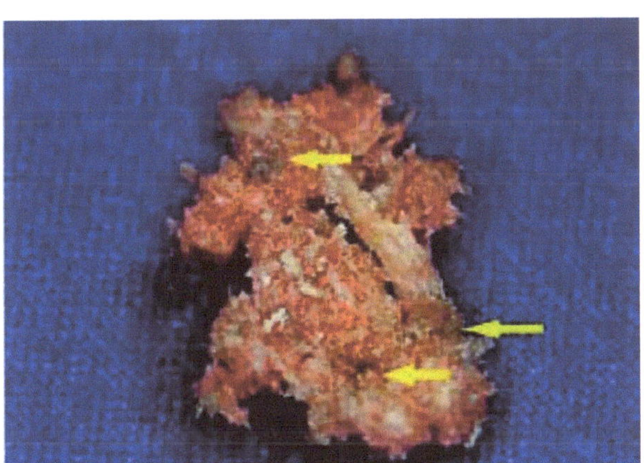

Figure 18.222. Autologous bone filings marked with an arrow.

For coronary closure of the alveolus, there are several techniques in the literature, but none have proven reliable. Finally, it is recommended to take a mucosal graft from the palate. The author also applied this procedure to several patients, but without much success. It is best not to enter into an uncertain adventure with soft tissue transplants, but perform augmentation ("socket preservation") and wait 6 to 8 months for the augment to be stable for implant placement, provided there is enough keratinized gingiva. How to perform the augmentation, whether with a mixture of autologous bone granules and bone substitute, depends on the size of the bone defect.

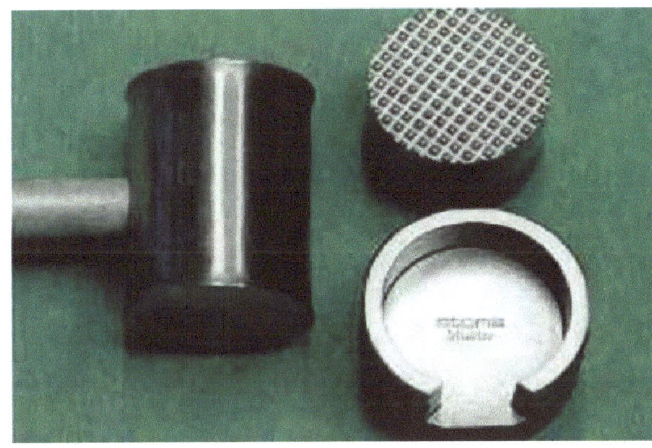

Figure 18.223. Container for shredding autologous bone sawdust.

If the defect is larger, when the entire bone lamella has been lost, it must be compensated with a bone block taken from the retromolar area and covered with a mixture of augments and closed again with soft tissue. Then the healing is faster. The augment mixture is made by crushing one part of the bone block in a special container and mixing it with some xenogeneic bone substitute (Fig. 18.221). Then, the alveolar ridge is shaped for the needs of the implant procedure. Finally, when looking at the entire procedure, it can be concluded that the treatment of cases with a thin gingival biotype is very complicated to achieve a good aesthetic effect.

In a case where there is a well-healed alveolar ridge, but with a visible bone defect, and with a thin gingival biotype, what should be done to achieve a good aesthetic result and is it possible to fully achieve good aesthetic requirements?

It is possible. But the treatment is complicated. First of all, healing takes time. Augmentation must be done first. Different methods are used, depending on the judgment and experience of the clinician. Augmentation with autologous bone block, or bone-guided regeneration, have proven to be the most successful techniques. After bone block augmentation, implant placement can be done after 4 months, and if guided bone regeneration was performed, then after 6-8 months. As protection against late resorption, i.e. recession of the gingiva of a thin biotype, it is necessary to create a thicker biotype of the gingiva by augmentation of the connective tissue. This can be done immediately after installing the implant, or when opening the cap that covered the implant.

What is the procedure if it is a thin gingival biotype?

In that case, the thin gingival biotype should be converted to a thicker one, which can be achieved with a connective tissue transplant. A healthy gingiva with a wide keratinized zone is important for aesthetics, but it is even more important functionally. Keratinized gingiva more easily resists biomechanical stimuli, reducing the possibility of peri-implantitis.

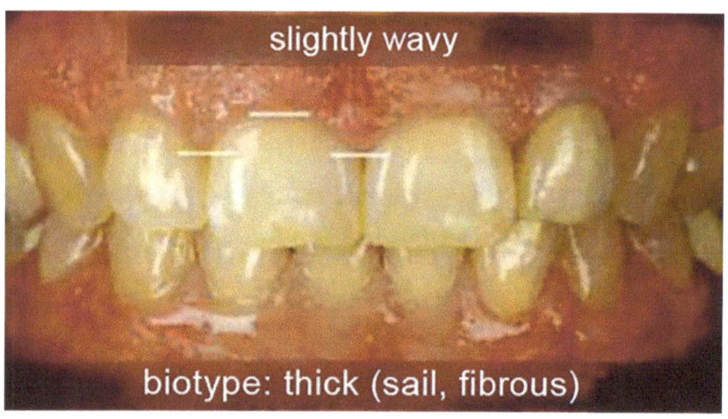

Figure 18.224. Appearance of gingival types.

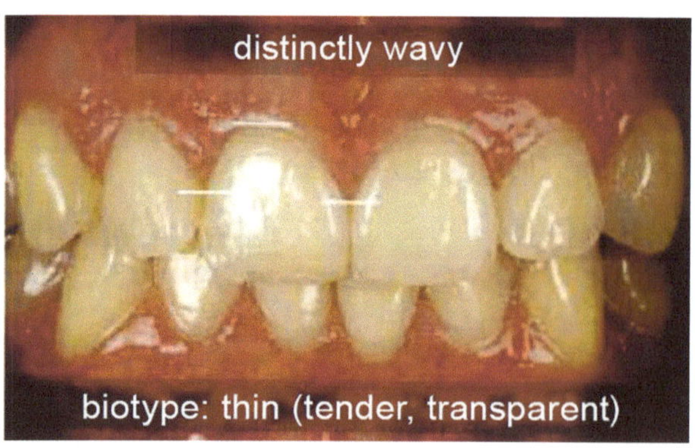

Figure 18.225. Appearance of gingival types

If a tooth has to be extracted, and there is no alveolar infection, but a larger buccal bony defect is present, with a thick gingival biotype, what procedure is recommended?

If there is a larger buccal defect, augmentation must be done using the "socket preservation" method, filling with bone substitutes and applying a collagen resorbable membrane. The protocol indicates the position that one should wait 6 months for healing and then insert the implant. However, the second position, which the author most often applies, is to insert an implant using the "flapless surgery" technique without raising the flap. This is especially indicated if a minor buccal bone defect is present after tooth extraction, and there is a thicker gingival biotype of soft tissues. Such a favorable situation allows the simultaneous installation of implants and augmentation of the buccal wall with protection by a collagen resorbable membrane. After that, according to the protocol, it is necessary to cover the implant with a cap for healing. However, the author of the book sets a definite abutment. The author's experience indicates that a more optimal solution in such cases is to place a definitive support instead of a healing cap. Whether the implant will be loaded immediately is decided individually, and the author's position is that the implant should be loaded, which puts the bone into function and promotes healing.

In cases where the alveolar ridge is shaped and the analysis of the 3D tomographic image shows that there are favorable parameters for inserting the implant, which surgical procedure has the advantage: raising the flap or without?

First, it depends on the experience of the implantologist. Both implantological surgical procedures have advantages. The lifting of the flap has an advantage for the following reasons: during the installation of the implant in the prepared bed, there is a clear view of the bone, which allows visibility to which bone level the implant should be placed. This detail is significant, because the implants of the latest implant systems are designed in the neck of the implant to enable the growth of cortical bone, which is the basis for soft tissues for good and faster healing and shaping in the first row and interdental papillae.

The installation of implants without raising the flap in order to meet all the parameters that are necessary for a successful outcome of the implant-prosthetic treatment, as in the case of raising the flap, requires the experience of an implantologist. The implant installation procedure without increasing the flap is a great relief for the patient: less morbidity and faster achievement of comfort in the mouth due to avoided trauma by surgical intervention on soft tissues, as well as a faster course of soft tissue healing.

The initial stage of the intervention procedure: determination of the location of the implant with wax up templates, preparation of soft tissues with a special instrument in the form of a "plug" for the preparation of the implant bed (Fig. 18.226). Implants of selected diameters and lengths are positioned in the prepared beds (18.227.)

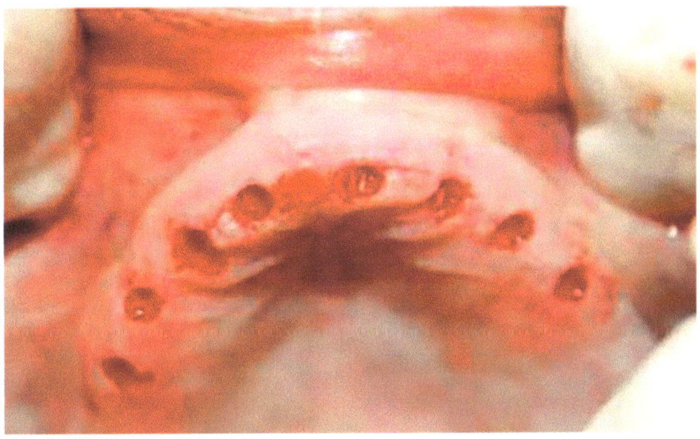

Figure 18.226. Soft tissues prepared with a special instrument for the preparation of the bed in the bone.

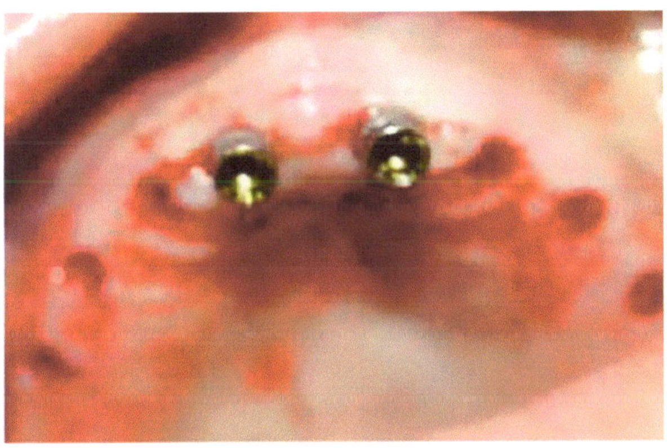

Figure 18.227. Wax-up template determines the start of positioning of the implant without raising the flap.

If the tooth has to be extracted, and there is no infection of the alveolus, the buccal lamella is preserved by careful extraction, but with a thin gingival biotype, what should be done then?

The distinction is made when there is a thin gingival biotype with a buccal bone defect, or a thin gingival biotype with a favorable bone situation. In the first case, it is necessary to perform augmentation with the installation of implants. In the case of excessive bone defects, augmentation should be performed in two stages, which depends on the evaluation and experience of the therapist. Soft tissue augmentation is not required.

In cases where there is a favorable bone condition after extraction, immediate implantation can be performed. This procedure poses significant challenges and requires extensive experience. It is essential to assess the size of the gap between the implant surface and the alveolar bone. If this space is no wider than 2 mm and is filled with fresh coagulum, it will heal spontaneously. However, if the gap is wider, augmentation is necessary to prevent resorption.

To prepare for augmentation in front of the buccal lamella, a mucoperiosteal pocket should be created without raising the gingiva. This pocket, along with the space between the implant surface and the buccal lamella, should be filled with augmentation material. Filling the area with autologous bone chips from the retromolar space or using bone substitutes is recommended.

The decision to proceed with immediate implantation depends on the experience of the doctor, as an experienced practitioner can accurately assess the thickness of the labial lamella. Overall, it is preferable to use a minimally invasive approach, such as the flapless technique, which avoids raising a flap. Achieving aesthetic results involves successfully thickening the mucous membrane on the vestibular side.

The best prognosis and the greatest success are achieved in cases where after tooth extraction there is enough lamellar bone with the absence of infection and a thick gingival biotype. With the immediate installation of implants without opening the gingiva, and when good primary stability is achieved, it is preferable to apply immediate loading, but in subocclusion.

In cases of optimal conditions of sufficient lamellar bone thickness and a thick gingival biotype, the author's experience confirms that the best result is achieved if the implant is placed without raising the mucoperiosteal flap. Regardless of the doctor's experience and mastery of the flapless technique, before starting the procedure, it is necessary to plan the procedure with a good orthopantomographic image and computerized tomography (3D). If these prerequisites are not met, there are great risks of vestibular perforation and incorrect implant location. However, for practitioners with less experience, it is easier to apply a flap lift, if possible as minimally invasive as possible.

What should the practitioner know when it comes to patients who need implants in a highly demanding aesthetic region?

When it comes to implant-protest rehabilitation in a highly demanding aesthetic region, in the front of the upper jaw, the practitioner should let the result depend on how he starts the implantation, that is, on the created plan.

Mistakes made at the beginning of implant installation are difficult or impossible to correct later. Due to the extended therapeutic possibilities of implantation and its indications, the most important thing is to make a detailed treatment plan and stick to it. Not even the smallest cut can be started until the final work plan is established. How to start the procedure depends on the practitioner's experience and knowledge of the chosen method. Whether immediate or delayed implant placement will be used in a particular case must be known before the surgical procedure begins.

When dealing with cases in a highly demanding aesthetic region, which method is preferable, immediate or delayed implant placement?

The success of dental implants largely depends on the condition of the alveolus. If the labial lamellar bone wall is sufficiently thick (around 2 mm) and a good primary fixation can be achieved with an appropriately sized implant, evidence suggests that immediate implant placement is beneficial for several reasons.

Firstly, it creates more favorable conditions for preserving interdental papillae. Recent research emphasizes the importance of soft tissues, which can only be reliably maintained with adequate bony support. Experienced practitioners ensure that during implant placement, the implant is positioned to keep the labial lamella as thick as possible while preserving a 2 mm gap between the implant surface and the bone. Attention must also be given to maintaining the integrity of the labial bony lamella, since the health of the surrounding soft tissues depends on the quality of the underlying bone structure.

Successful periodontal surgical techniques rely on having a stable bone foundation. Recent studies have demonstrated that thickening the gingiva positively affects the preservation of the bone, particularly the vestibular bone lamella. The active regeneration of periodontal tissues through tissue engineering marks the beginning of a new era in periodontal tissue restoration. This approach is based on biological principles aimed at creating and reconstructing the form and function of damaged tissues. The core concept of tissue engineering involves utilizing a tissue matrix, progenitor cells, and growth factors to promote healing and regeneration.

Who are the carriers of the latest concept of periodontal tissue regeneration using tissue engineering?

The bearers of the concept of active regeneration of periodontal tissues are:

- Platelet-rich plasma (PRP);
- Bone morphogenetic protein-rh BMP;
- Platelet growth factors-rhPDGF;
- Osteogenetic protein;
- Tissue culture and transplantation of autogenous stem cells;
- Gene therapy.

In the active regeneration of periodontal tissues using tissue engineering, the most important role is played by growth factors. So far, it has been possible to isolate several types of growth factors from the tissue that participate in the regeneration of periodontal tissues:

- Platelet growth factor;
- Transformational growth factor;
- Insulin-like growth factor;
- Fibroblast growth factor;
- Osteogenic protein;
- Bone morphogenetic protein; and
- Angiogenetic growth factors.

Most of these growth factors are released at the site of injury or in the surgical wound and play an extremely important role in wound healing. Growth factors are cell-specific, each factor acts on a specific type of cell. It should be emphasized that with implant restorations today, emphasis is placed on the soft tissues surrounding the implant. The regeneration of the periodontium is a very complex process, even in the case of the application of growth factors, because the regeneration of both non-mineralized and mineralized tissues must be affected at the same time. The regenerative potential increases with the combination of individual growth factors.

Pathological processes of the periodontium in natural teeth in the course of periodontopathy destroy all periodontal tissues, and the pathological process continues with the destruction of the alveolar bone. For this reason, to fulfill aesthetic requirements during implantation, the support of bone tissue is important, which we create in bone defects by augmentation, whether achieved with autologous bone or bone substitutes.

What advice should be given to the practitioner when it comes to surgical periodontal interventions on soft tissues as part of implant-prosthetic rehabilitation?

Surgical periodontal interventions on soft tissues are extremely complicated and often do not give satisfactory results. Such interventions can be undertaken by a practitioner with extensive experience in implantology-prosthetic treatment.

Especially demanding are cases with thin gingival biotype and with a high smile line. For this reason, patients with a low smile line should be selected at the beginning, and cases with a thin gingival biotype should be left to a more experienced periodontologist. Several important details must be emphasized here, on which a successful result depends. The surgical intervention with which everything begins is the most important. But the importance of choosing an implant should not be overlooked. When it comes to soft tissues, it is a big mistake to apply implants with a polished neck. The shaping of soft tissues also depends on the superstructure on the implants. Ultimately, all of these procedures can be significantly compromised if the input of the dental technician is poor. The final work of every implantological-prosthetic therapy is imitating nature. So, compensation on implants, an artificial crown, can only be recognized by an expert eye. Hard and soft tissues should be aligned, ie. in harmony with the surrounding tissues, in terms of color and shape. An inflammatory process of the marginal gingiva must not occur around the implant. It can be said that an ideal result has been achieved if the marginal gingiva is partially keratinized, which achieves the full aesthetic effect and function. When making a plan before starting the procedure, the practitioner must know what to do if complications arise. Very often this happens in the dental laboratory. The author experimented so that the same patient case is solved by two dental technicians separately, without referring to the material costs. The differences were striking!

In which cases can immediate installation of implants not be applied?

For a practitioner with extensive experience, there are few cases where immediate implant placement cannot be applied. This is also confirmed by the research of Scharf and Tarnau. It depends on how much risk you want to take on the procedure. The greater the experience, the lower the proximity to the risk. An experienced practitioner knows what not to do. Good judgment and planning move away from risk. Shortening the treatment time by immediate installation of the implant increases the comfort of the patient. But there are cases with large defects of the buccal bone lamella and thin gingival biotype, when delayed implantation should be applied.

Are longitudinal tooth root fractures in the frontal region of the upper jaw a common reason for tooth extraction?

Yes. Probably the most common causes of longitudinal root fractures are: endodontic root canal treatment, extensive cavity preparations, root canal treatment with abutment expanders and driving cast abutments into the resected root. A tooth with a longitudinal root fracture is lost and should be extracted as soon as possible. The longitudinal fissure of the root is an ideal space for the settlement of bacteria, which leads to the resorption of alveolar bone. If a tooth with a longitudinal fracture is not extracted in time, the vestibular cortical lamella can be completely lost. Bone breakdown continues towards the apical part and onto the surrounding bone. The presence of granulations is abundant. Such a situation is considered a typical contraindication for implant placement, and especially for immediate and immediate loading with prosthetic work.

What position, based on experience, does the author advocate when a tooth with a longitudinal root crack should be replaced with an implant?

The author's opinion is that in the case of longitudinal root cracks, there is no need to hurry with implant placement. After thorough treatment of the wound, it is necessary to carry out augmentation using the "socket preservation" method, and if there is a pronounced bone defect, it is necessary to carry out subsequent augmentation and only after a wait of at least 6 months to proceed to implant installation.

This is the concept that the author followed in the long-term treatment of cases with a pronounced defect of the buccal lamellar bone. The position that neither augmentation nor implantation should ever be performed in an infected alveolus was respected. As such cases are a big challenge for an experienced dentist, I tried to apply some new views advocated by individual authors in my practice.

The patient (58) was resected by the practicing dentist at the apex of the canine root with an existing metal abutment. The patient was rehabilitated with a metal-ceramic circular bridge. However, she persistently complained to the dentist that she felt pain in the canine area. He delayed the solution with the use of antibiotics. On the tomographic image, the longitudinal crack of the root was not visible. The intraoral image was repeated and, again, the longitudinal fissure was not visible. As soon as we made the incision and started lifting the mucoperist, a clear crack appeared, and the labial lamellar bone was destroyed. Removing the entire bridge for the patient would be a great expense, abuse, and trauma to the remaining teeth and surrounding tissues. Healing of the alveolus required augmentation with bone substitutes and the application of a collagen-resorbable membrane. All this required time, which the patient did not have due to an already scheduled trip and an absence of at least a year.

The following procedure was applied: the tooth was cut from the bridge and carefully extracted. The root was split along its entire length, the longitudinal crack was filled with granulations, and the vestibular lamella was completely destroyed. The patient's available time and longer absence also determined the procedure. The patient did not want to be without teeth for a year, so immediate implant placement remained the only option, although this was not recommended in the current situation for the following reason: a radical curettage was performed, and the amount of available healthy periapical bone was sufficient to achieve a good primary stability. Simultaneously with the installation of the implant, augmentation with a mixture of autologous bone and xenogeneic bone substitute was performed without raising the flap (as soon as a longitudinal crack of the root became visible, the previously started incision was stopped). An incision was made from the middle of the ridge towards the palatal side, while preserving the marginal edge of the gingiva that had already been interrupted by the initial incision (about 0.5 mm), and a flap was cut from the palatal side in order to obtain an overview of the palatal cortical bone. The bone preparation for the implant bed was performed palatally, and the apical part of the bone was also used. By installing a standard-diameter implant, the direction of the implant's axis followed the axis of the root it replaces. The implant is inserted 0.5 mm below the surface of the palatal bone. After that, for the reconstruction of the buccal bone lamella, the mucoperiosteum was carefully raised with a narrow raspatorium and augmentation was performed with autologous bone mixed with a xenogeneic bone substitute. As the bony buccal lamella was completely missing, during the last screwing of the implant 0.5 mm below the surface of the palatal cortical bone, primary stability up to 35 Ncm was achieved. A temporary crown was made on the definitively placed support, and the patient was able to leave without removing the circular metal-ceramic bridge.

What should be done after tooth extraction to preserve the alveolus and the alveolar ridge in order to create optimal conditions for the implant bed?

If the bone lamella is preserved, the installation of the implant in the alveolus, with the simultaneous compensation of a smaller bone defect, is the best solution, because the soft tissues are repaired at the same time.

Satisfactory horizontal and vertical dimensions of the alveolar ridge are the basic prerequisites for implant placement to be successful. Preservation of alveolar bone after tooth extraction depends on how the extraction was performed, whether the vestibular cortical lamella was traumatized to a large extent or not. Extracting a tooth inevitably endangers the part of the bone that is connected to the periodontium. By tearing and separating the periodontium from the buccal bony lamella of the alveolus, bone resorption occurs, which leads to the loss of the horizontal and vertical dimensions of the alveolar ridge. The loss of the alveolar bone, especially its vestibular wall, is most pronounced in the frontal part of the upper jaw. Since the atrophy is greatest in the first 4, that is, in the first 12 weeks, the question arises, what is more effective: to carry out implantation, or augmentation, or simultaneously combining both. The more complex the procedure, the greater the loss of tissue volume.

In practice, the loss of bone and soft tissue volume can be compensated by filling the fresh alveolar wound with bone substitutes. By filling the alveolus with bone substitutes with osteoinductive action, bone support for soft tissues and their preservation is also ensured. It is best to use a mixture of autologous bone with xenogeneic bone substitutes. This preserves tissue volume in all three dimensions. The bone substitute mixture acts osteoinductively so that new bone formation maintains the volume of hard and soft tissues completely. This procedure, when the bony walls are intact, is called socket preservation, and when there is greater loss, or the absence of bone walls of the alveolus, it is called ridge preservation.

What is achieved by preserving the alveolus and the alveolar ridge after tooth extraction, and does immediate implant placement stop tissue loss?

When there is a loss of the buccal bone wall of the alveolus, the soft tissues no longer have a support and they "collapse" into the alveolus. Preservation of the alveolus prevents such behavior, i.e. the sagging of soft tissues and preserves their volume. If the success of preserving the alveolus by augmentation with bone substitutes is evaluated, the evaluation of success is also manifested by the quality of preservation of soft tissues and their volume. It is logical that tooth extraction leads to tissue loss through resorption, and whether this process can be stopped by immediate implant placement, we do not yet have research and statistical data to draw a conclusion.

However, if the immediate installation of the implant shortens the treatment time, increasing the comfort of the patient, the subjective opinion of the author of the book is that the physiological processes in the bone and its remodeling are supported by the immediate installation of the implant. This procedure promotes better and faster bone integration with the surface of the implant. If the patient chews well and there are no disturbances, it means that the implant is stable in the bone and that its presence brings the surrounding milieu back into function. Physiological function is the basis of establishing homeostasis of the milieu around the implant, and bone resorption is a pathophysiological phenomenon, so it is logical that they exclude each other. The author's considerations are based on experience, because almost 90% of implantological-prosthetic cases are solved by immediate installation of the implant and immediate loading.

The goal of the adopted plan of every intervention in oral implantology is to facilitate the surgical procedure, i.e. the installation of implants. The relief starts with shortening the treatment time if the walls of the alveolus are preserved, there is no reason to delay the installation of the implant; or, if a part of the buccal bone lamella is preserved, and there is 2-3 mm of good apical bone, with the immediate installation of the implant and the simultaneous augmentation of the buccal wall with a mixture of xenogeneic bone substitute and autologous bone sawdust, with the application of a collagen resorbable membrane, all the conditions for a good bone integration. Extensive augmentation procedures require complex surgical techniques, prolonging therapy time, and when implant placement is delayed, the risk of complications increases.

One gets the impression that you favor immediate implant placement and immediate loading. Why?

With the development of oral implantology, the spectrum of indications has been significantly increased, and contraindications have been reduced. If after installing the implant in the bone, a primary stability of 35Ncm is achieved, it is reason enough to safely complete the adopted treatment plan. More than thirty years ago, I visited Philip Ledermann, one of the pioneers of implantology, and then he presented to me the concept of immediate loading of implants connected by a bar for stabilizing the lower total prosthesis. Then I showed him the cases I solved in Cavtat with immediate loading of one-piece Linkov implants. He completely agreed with my views. At that time, not much was known about bone integration. Later, with the advent of Brennemak's discoveries, Linkov and Grafelman make a two-part leaf implant, coated with the so-called titanium plasma, calling them the "Fifth generation of Linkov leaf implants" and representing the position of delayed loading of the implants for 6 months, which was not the case for the previous generation of one-piece leaf imiplants, which were loaded after three weeks.

At the meeting of implantologists in Munich (1980), in my lecture, I presented the opposite view that one-piece implants should be loaded immediately after installation. I based my attitude on personal failures. Despite the well-achieved primary stability of the sheet one-piece implants, after two weeks the implants loosened and fell out. The loss of the implant was caused by strong lingual forces and their moments on the post of the implant carrier of the prosthetic work. Comparing the results with both one and the other form, good primary stability was achieved, but the final results with two-phase implantation were no better, confirmed by radiographic analyzes and the condition in the mouth. From the above, it can be concluded how long the wandering lasted when it comes to loading and putting the implants into operation. If lessons are learned from the past, it can be said that today's implants achieve outstanding primary stability thanks to the micro-structure of the implant surface treated with new technologies, the conical shape, the design of the double thread, the processing of the neck part with Laser lock technology... All this fully justifies the concept immediate installation of implants.

What can lead to risks and complications, negating the previous claims?

Most often it is bad prosthetics. This justifies the author's opinion that a dentist who deals with implantation must be equally competent in dealing with both oral surgical procedures and prosthetic works. The prosthetic plan is set before the implant installation. Non-compliance with gnathological principles can be a special factor of risk and failure of the entire imagined project. But there are a lot of details that the clinician needs to know and show the dental technician how to do prosthetic work on implants.

Which procedure to apply in cases where the alveolar ridge is extremely narrow, the crestal part is about 1 mm, the width of the platform is from 3.5 to 4 mm, and the patient's wishes and possibilities are not in accordance with the complicated and expensive augmentation procedure. Can such cases be solved by installing thin (so-called mini) implants and how reliable and long-lasting is this solution?

Experience will answer this question. Often, theory answers "no" or "maybe" to some questions, and practice says "yes". It depends on the characteristics of the alveolar bone (shape, ridge size, length and height), as well as on the arrangement of cancellous and cortical bone. This also determines the choice of implant. It happens that the thickness of the crestal bone is barely 1 mm, and the height is more than 20 mm, then the clinical application of mini-implants is justified. If the alveolar ridge is minimally thick (from 3 to 4 mm), it is impossible to insert implants of standard diameters, because fenestration will appear. Further treatment depends on the degree of fenestration, and it is possible to successfully continue it with augmentation, or bone block grafts, or bone substitutes with a resorbable membrane. Experience confirms that thin implants with a diameter of 2.5 and 3 mm can be equally loaded as implants with larger diameters, especially if they are 15, 16 or 18 mm long.

The length of the crown on the implants is determined as the vertical distance from the occlusal plane to the top of the residual ridge bone. The greater the vertical bone resorption, the longer the length of the crown will be, and since the length of the implant is the same, the ratio of the length of the crown and the implant changes. The most ideal ratio is 1:2 in favor of the implant, and the minimum is 1:1. If this ratio is greater in favor of the clinical crown, then the action of unfavorable forces and their moments, twisting and rotation of the implant itself, as well as the action of the lever comes to the fore.

By using the height of the alveolar ridge for the installation of implants of maximum length and smaller diameter, favorable relations between the length of the crown and the body of the implant are created in favor of the body of the implant. This fully satisfies the biomechanical requirements.

With narrow and high alveolar ridges, the alveolar bone is much more compact, and thus more favorable for the installation of implants with narrow diameters. The thin alveolar bone contains little spongiosa and a lot of compact, which is why the primary stability is outstanding. Misch and Judy (1990) stated that with narrow alveolar ridges according to the classification bone type D2 is the most favorable for implantation. The wider alveolar ridge has more cancellous bone, and the buccal and palato-lingual cortical bone provide good primary stability, which is of utmost importance for successful treatment.

What are the advantages in cases where it is only possible to use implants with smaller diameters?

The advantages are:

- ease of installation of implants;
- good primary stability;
- the possibility of immediate encumbrance;
- there is no lifting of the flap and no trauma to the soft tissues;
- no additional surgical procedures;
- there is a possibility of self-incision, which avoids traumatizing the bone;
- good bone integration; and
- Lower cost of treatment.

What is the success rate of small diameter implants?

There are cases where the application of narrow implants is only possible.

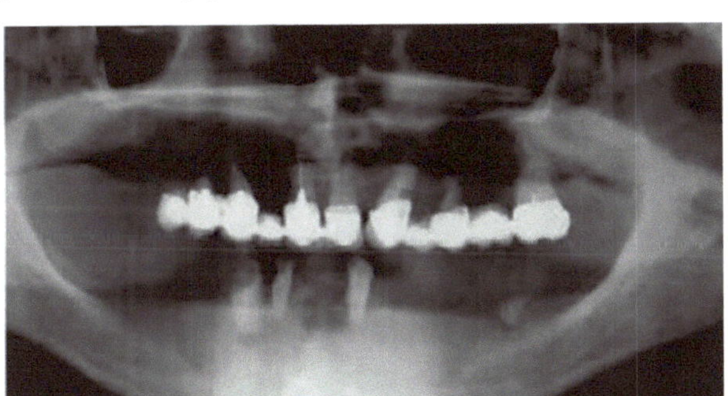

Figure 18.228. Orthopan-tomographic image of the found condition. The picture shows: bad prosthetic work, inflammation of soft tissues, bad oral hygiene, avid smoker. Limited financial possibilities determine the rehabilitation plan.

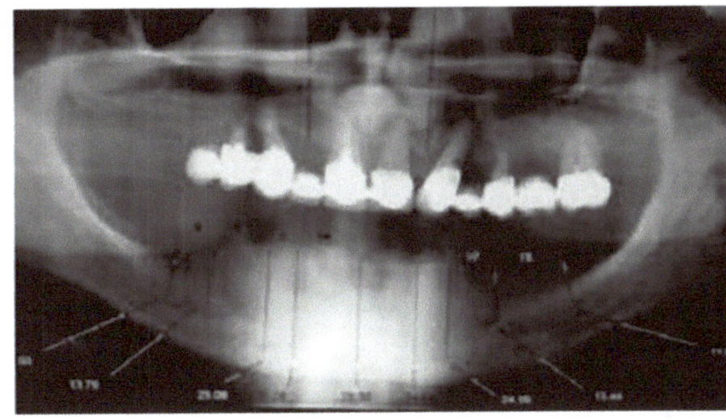

Figure 18.229. Tomogaph findings show the complexity of the case; critical width and sufficient height.

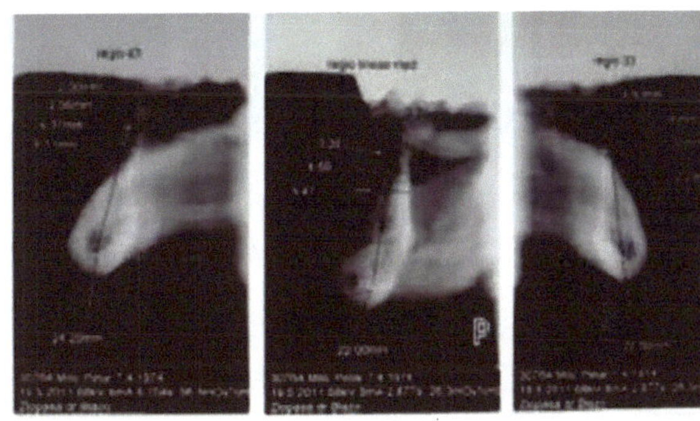

Figure 18.230. Computed tomography shows an extremely unfavorable width of the alveolar bone (1 mm from the top of the ridge, and the distance of 4 mm from the top of the ridge to the platform is 3.36 mm. The height is favorable from 19, 20 and 24 mm).

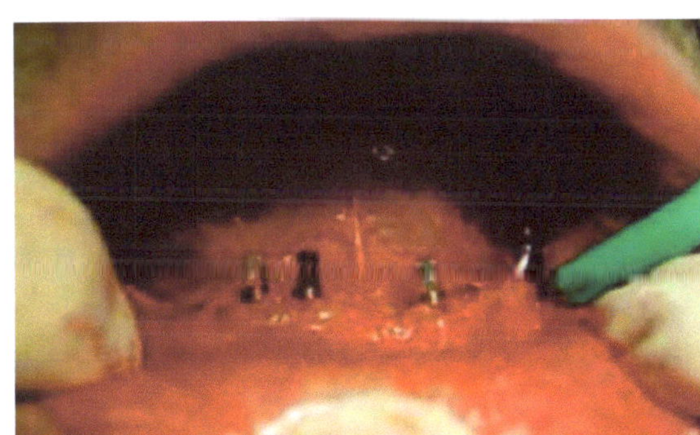

Figure 18.231. The only possible solution is the installation of NDI implants of the smallest diameter and longest length (18 mm). The parallelism of the installed implants is important.

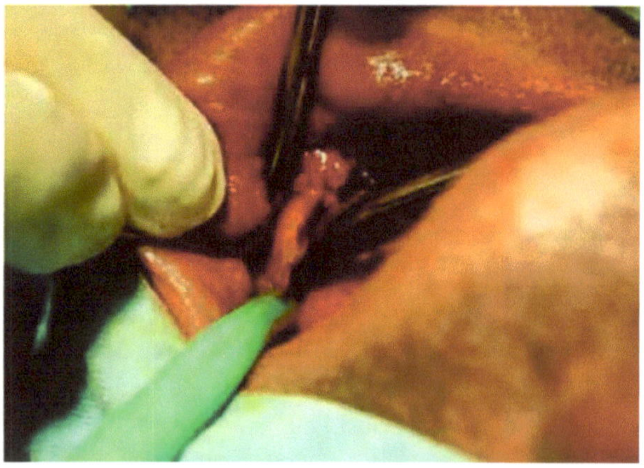

Figure 18.232. Raising the flap in the posterior region shows the appearance of the alveolar bone from the labial and lingual side. The patient was presented with the initial condition based on the analysis of radiographic images. Even, with such extremely unfavorable findings, an attempt to insert an implant by going back in time; the installation of thin leaf implants would end in trial and error.

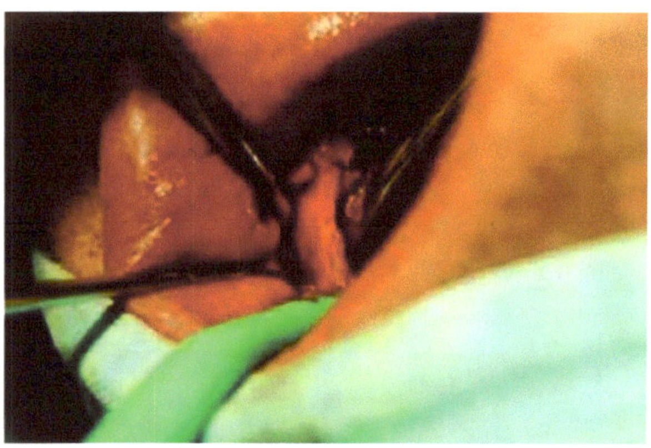

Figure 18.233. Extremely narrow alveolar ridge in the retromolar region lower jaw.

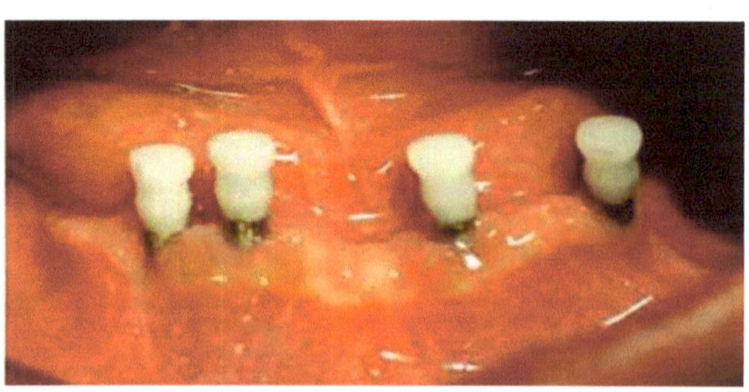

Figure 18.234. An extremely narrow alveolar ridge is also risky for the installation of implants for the narrowest diameter.

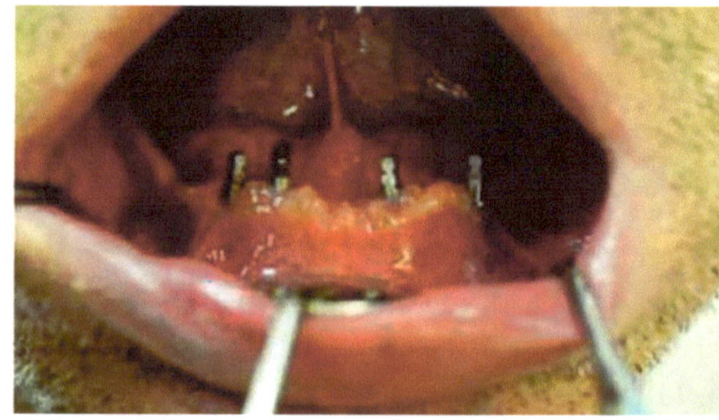

Figure 18.235. Appearance after implantation.

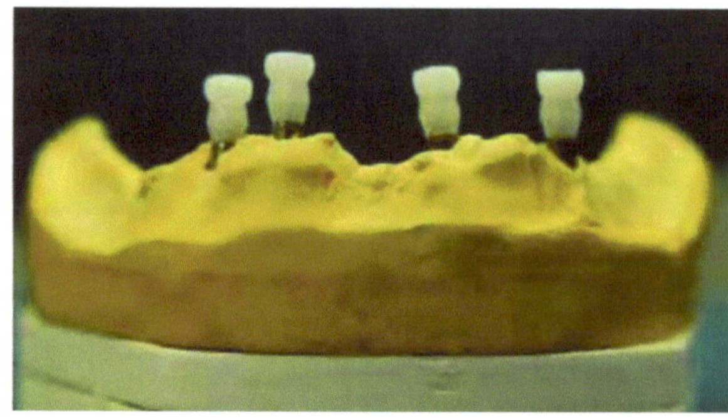

Figure 18.236. And on the plaster model, the relief of the alveolar ridge, which is unfavorable for implant placement, can be clearly seen. The persistence of the patient's request was respected.

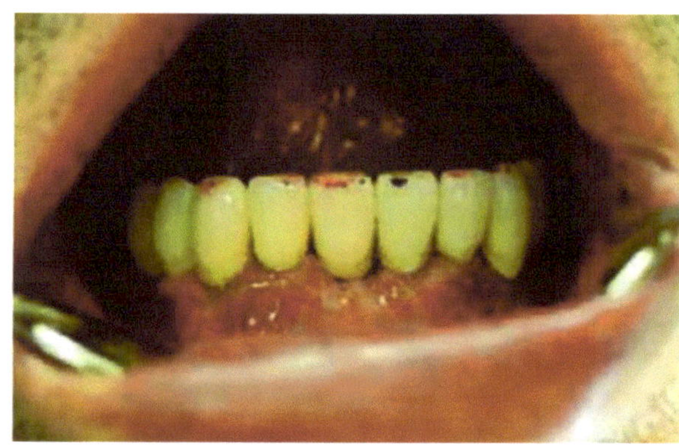

Figure 18.237. Condition after 3 years of prosthetic work on narrow-diameter implants maximally stable despite smoking and poor oral hygiene.

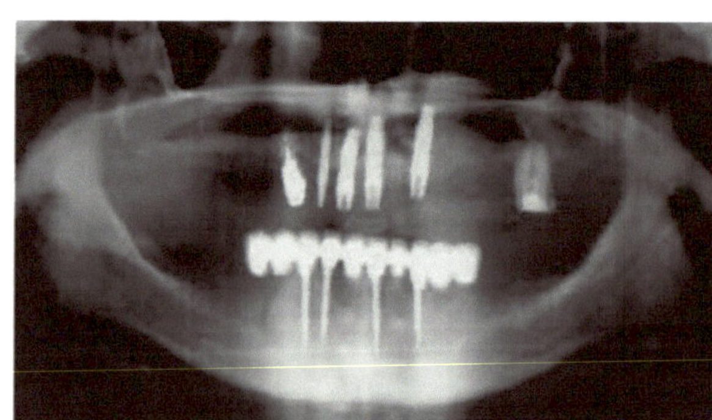

Figure 18.238. The control image shows the state of the lower jaw after 3 years and the installed implants in the upper jaw. Implants positioned according to available bone. The patient was advised to replace the right

upper canine with an extension with an implant, to install an implant in the position of the left molar, if possible also in the position of the left upper molar. Experience confirms the benefits of using implants of small diameters, the success of which approaches absolute, if implants of longer lengths (from 14 mm to 18 mm) are used.

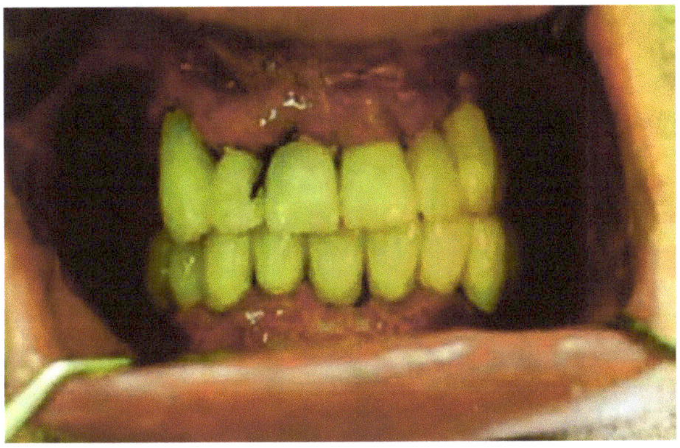

Figure 18.239. Immediate loading in the upper jaw with an acrylate provisional bridge. The patient was satisfied with what had been achieved, and after three years he did not come forward for definitive prosthetic work (a common occurrence among patients in these areas), which is proof that implant-prosthetic procedures should be avoided in such patients. The fact that the patient is a heavy smoker and poor oral hygiene are major risk factors.

Did you ever change the plan during the surgical procedure?

Despite the detailed analysis and adopted plan, it happened that objective findings necessitated the change of the planned procedure. For example, in the following patient, shown in Figures 18.240-18.248, who requested retention of canines which was complied with.

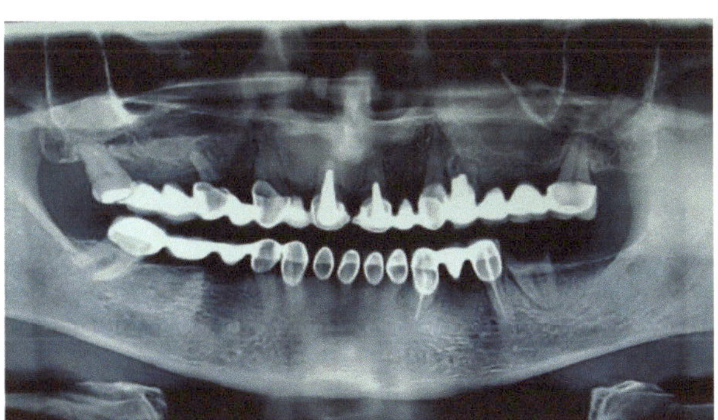

Figure 18.240. The condition found, on the basis of which an agreement was made with the patient, which procedure and how many implants will be needed for the entire treatment.

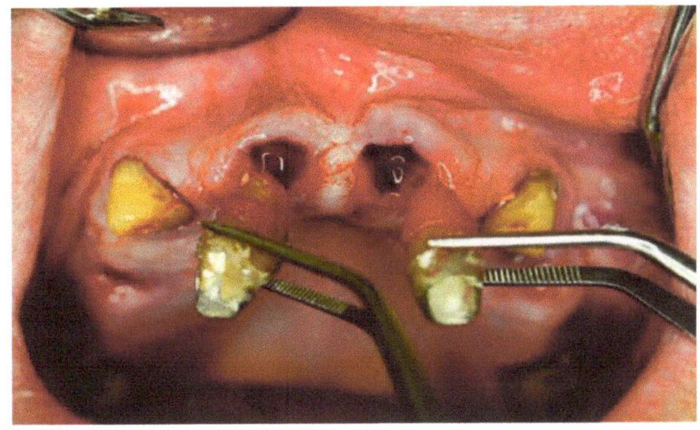

Figure 18.241. When extracting the central incisors, maximum care should be taken to preserve the vestibular lamellae, using primarily rotating movements.

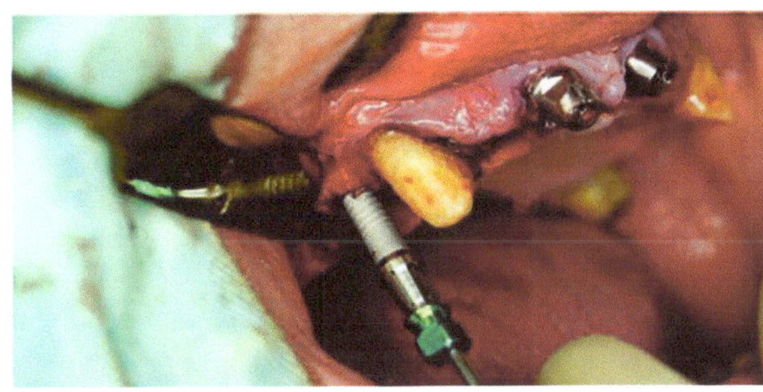

Figure 18.242. Installation of the implant in the place of the first premolar (Direct Implant system) - definitive support (abutment) with transfer.

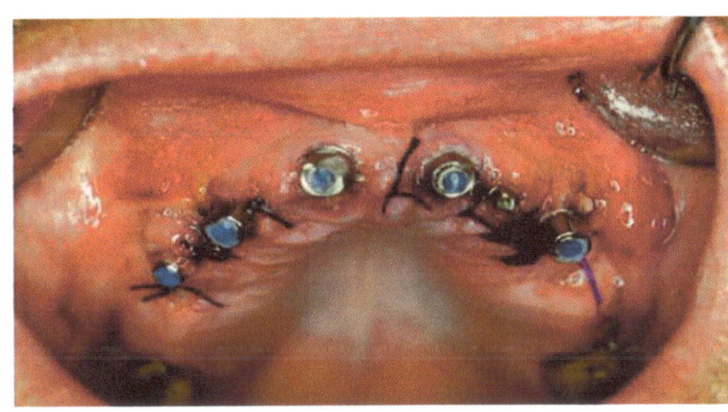

Figure 18.243. Position of implants with fixed transfers, which were transferred by impression to the working model for the creation of temporary prosthetic work.

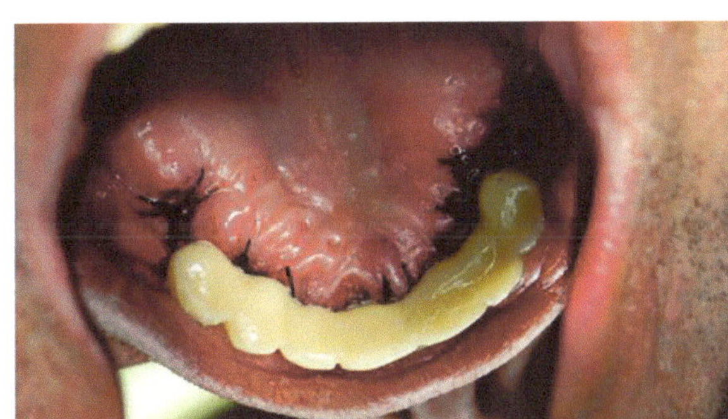

Figure 18.244. Augmentation of bone defects using collagen resorbable membranes. Appearance of the immediate prosthetic work from the palatal side.

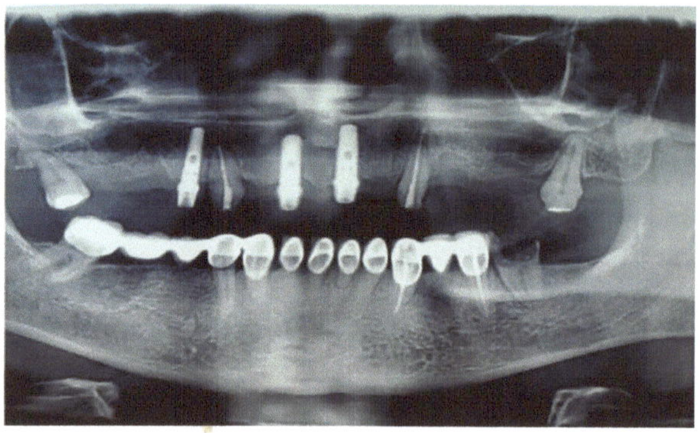

Figure 18.245. However, the canines showed mobility. It was explained to the patient that devitalization can lead to some strengthening of the teeth, but that there is a high risk after a certain time.

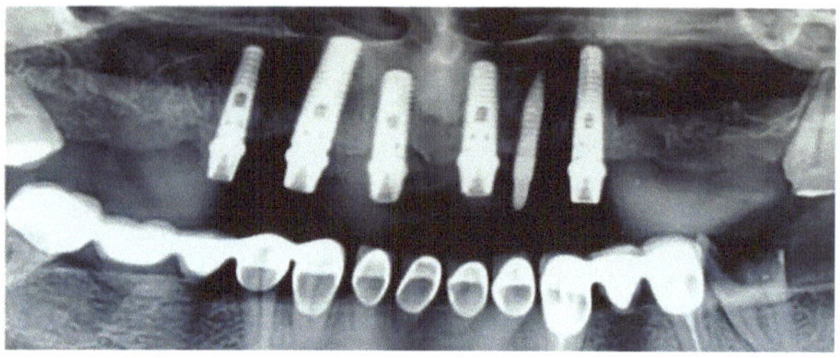

Figure 18.246. Immediately after the extraction of the canine, larger diameter implants were inserted, a region 13 vocabulary implant 5.2 mm and 16 mm long, and a 4.7 mm diameter and 16 mm long implant was inserted in place of the left canine.

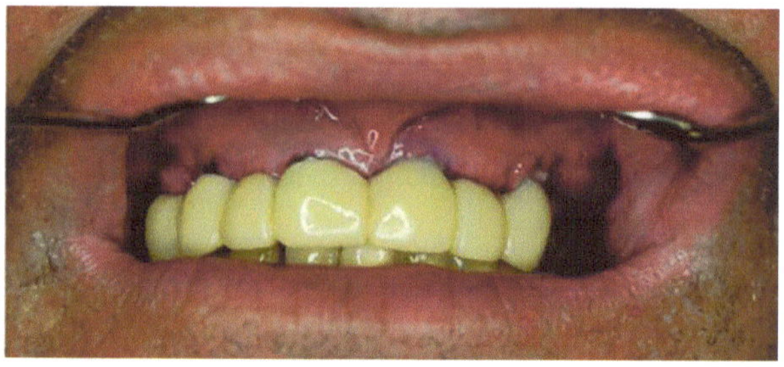

Figure 18.247. Immediately after the installation of the implant and placement of the temporary acrylate prosthetic work, the patient regains security in communication and function. The predictability of success with this treatment is based on decades of experience of the author.

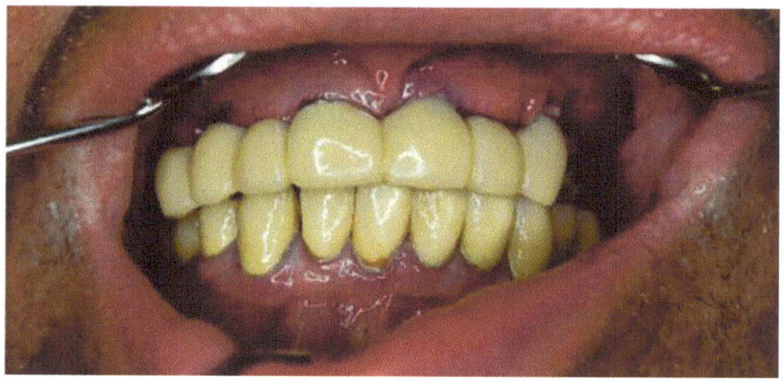

Figure 18.248. By achieving good primary stability of the immediately installed implants, immediate temporary prosthetic work was set, the patient was comfortable in communication and chewing food.

After such implant-prosthetic procedures, the patient is always given a form with instructions to be followed after the treatment (Figure 18.248).

- UPUTSTVA POSLE OPERACIJE -

Kod Vas je upravo završen hirurški zahvat. Nakon operacije normalno je krvarenje u prvih nekoliko dana. Ako je krvarenje prekomerno, držite **hladnu** oblogu na mestu gde je izvršen hirurški zahvat. Takođe, česta je i normalna pojava otoka koji se može povećati, naročito trećeg dana nakon operacije.

Kod nekih osoba može se pojaviti bledilo lica i malaksalost. **NE BRINITE!** To je takođe normalno.

Prvi dan:

- Za donju vilicu, obloge (led) stavljati ispod vilice sa obe strane.
- Za gornju vilicu, obloge stavljati preko usana, nosa i obraza.

Obloge držati 15min., prekinuti 10 minuta i ponavljati postupak do odlaska na spavanje.

Najbolje je spavati na dva jastuka u toku noći.

Drugi dan:

Prestanite sa stavljanjem obloga.

Rastvoriti 1/2 kafene kašike soli u jednu šolju vode. Ispirajte usta sa mlakom slanom vodom svaka dva sata. Vrlo je važno da ne mućkate, kako ne bi došlo do odvajanja šavova rane od zarastajućeg tkiva što bi moglo izazvati ponovno krvarenje.

Treći dan:

Nastavite ispiranje sa mlakom slanom vodom. Ispiranje usta možete kombinovati sa mlakim čajem od žalfije i kamilice i rastvorom koji Vam Doktor propiše. Nastavite sa ispiranjem . Mućkajte tečnost u ustima jačim pokretima svakih nekoliko sati.

Stavljajte **tople** obloge na oteklinu i nastavite ispiranje četiri puta dnevno do kraja nedelje. Istovremeno počnite da održavate higijenu usta, četkicom koju će Vam asistentkinja pokazati i objasniti postupak. Moguća je pojava postoperativnog bola.

Za smirenje bola uzimajte *Brufen, Nimulid ili Movalis* od 7,5 mg. jednu tabletu na svakih 6 sati.

Nabavite u apoteci "*CURASEPT*" pastu i tečnost ADS-220 koja je namenjena upotrebi posle hirurških zahvata. Ispirajte po uputstvu. Počnite da održavate oralnu higijenu specijalnom mekanom četkicom za zube "*CURAPROX SURGICAL MEGASOFT*", upotrebljavajući prvu nedelju dana pastu za zube "*CURASEPT ADS 712*", potom nastaviti pranje zuba sa pastom "*LACALUT ACTIV*" i istoimenom tečnošću.

NE ZABORAVITE DA UZIMATE PROPISANE LEKOVE!

Uzimajte lekove za smirenje bola samo kada je to neophodno. Molimo da uzimate propisani antibiotik DOK NE ZAVRŠITE DOZU!

Jedite sve što želite od kuvane hrane (mekih namirnica).

Ne uzimajte čvrstu hranu, naročito onu sa tvrdom korom. Izbegavajte prve dve nedelje: keks, kifle, kosti, tvrdo meso i lepljivu hranu.

PUŠENJE MOŽE DA ISKOMPROMITUJE ČITAV ZAHVAT!

PUŠENJE NE DOZVOLJAVA PRIMARNO ZARASTANJE RANE I ZNATNO USPORAVA ČITAV PROCES LEČENJA.

MOLIMO, NAGLAŠAVAMO I UPOZORAVAMO: NE SMETE PUŠITI BAREM PRVE DVE NEDELJE NAKON HIRURŠKOG ZAHVATA!!!

NAPOMENA ZA VAŠU SIGURNOST:

Posle povratka iz Švajcarske, naša ordinacija je prva privatna ordinacija na prostoru bivše Jugoslavije (1975god.), a poznata po tome što su u njoj usađeni prvi implantati.

Mi Vam stavljamo na raspolaganje veliko iskustvo, a Vi nama poklonite Vaše poverenje. Samo obostrana saradnja rezultira uspehom.

STOMATOLOŠKA ORDINACIJA ZA ESTETSKU STOMATOLOGIJU
IMPLANTOLOGIJU - PARADENTOLOGIJU, ORTOPEDIJU VILICA

"Dr Zlopaša"

Tamara B. Zlopaša-Jovanović

doktor stomatologije

Bulevar dr.L. Đinđića 211 (Bul. AVNOJ-a), tel: 011/2691 932, 011/2601 969

Figure 18.249. Instructions after surgery, which must be given to the patient after surgery.

Is it unusual for a book with the topic of oral implantology to emphasize so much the events in the temporomandibular joint, i.e. to talk about temporomandibular dysfunctions?

Perhaps at the beginning of the answer it could be said that they overemphasize. Our practice, i.e. implant-prosthetic rehabilitation of disabilities in the oral cavity, can directly influence the events in the TMJ. Disturbances in the TMJ are most often caused by poor occlusion, which is noticed by the patient after a certain time. Implant placement is only one phase of complex implantological treatment, which has become a routine procedure today. Everything after that is a more complicated process. Prosthetic solutions can affect the improvement, or deterioration, of both the state of the implant in the bone and its duration, as well as the health of the TMJ. Temporomandibular disorders include a number of clinical problems and symptoms in the head and neck area. Masticatory muscles and jaw joints are primarily affected. In Figure 18.250. it is shown where attention should be directed and where problems can start. (Gnatology, Prof. Dr. G. Graber, Basel, 1981). Among the most common symptoms are tension and pain in the masticatory, facial and neck muscles, accompanied by sounds in the temporomandibular joint, with limited movements of the lower jaw.

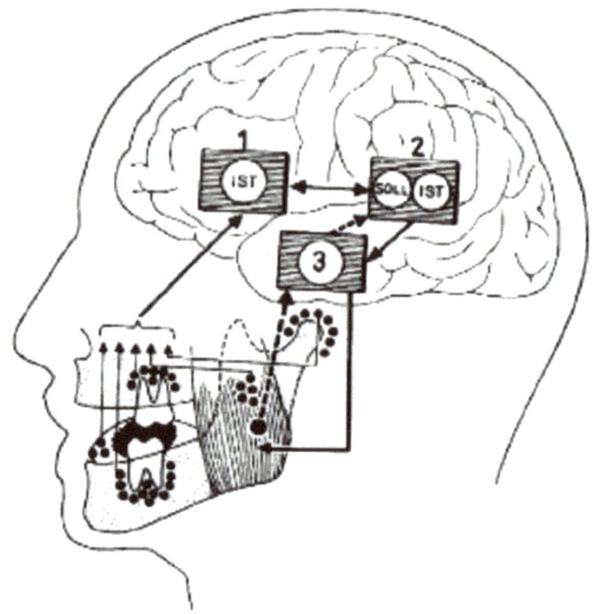

Figure 18.250. Spreading pain caused by poor occlusion.

Temporomandibular disorders (TMD) can manifest as headaches, migraines and tinnitus (ringing in the ears). The clinical symptoms of TMD are based on myopathy and arthropathy. Myofacial pains in painful regions ("trigger points") are reflected in muscles, tendons and muscle sheaths and are symptoms of myopathy. Arthropathies are manifested by dislocation of the articular disc, luxation of the condyle, and inflammatory changes in the jaw joints.

The distribution of complaints caused by TMD is illustrated in Figure 18.251. (Gnathology, G. Graber, Basel). The areas where pain caused by TMD can spread are shown in Figure 18.252.

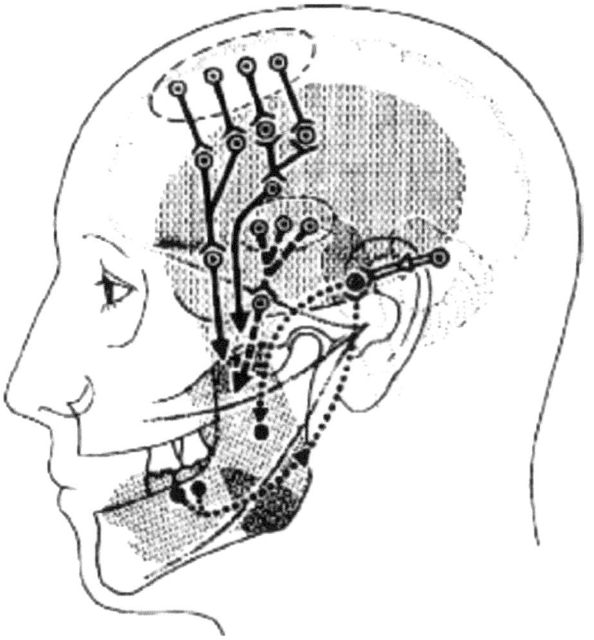

Figure 18.251. Zones of pain transmission caused by changes in the temporomandibular joint.

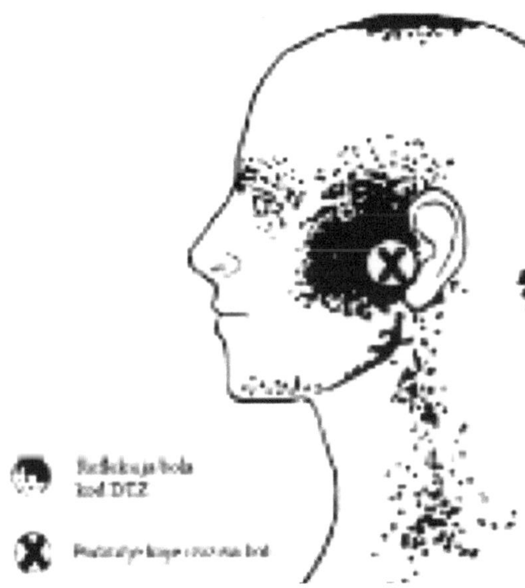

Figure 18.252. Representation of the spread of muscle pain due to disorders in the TMJ indicated in black (Prof. Dr. G. Garber).

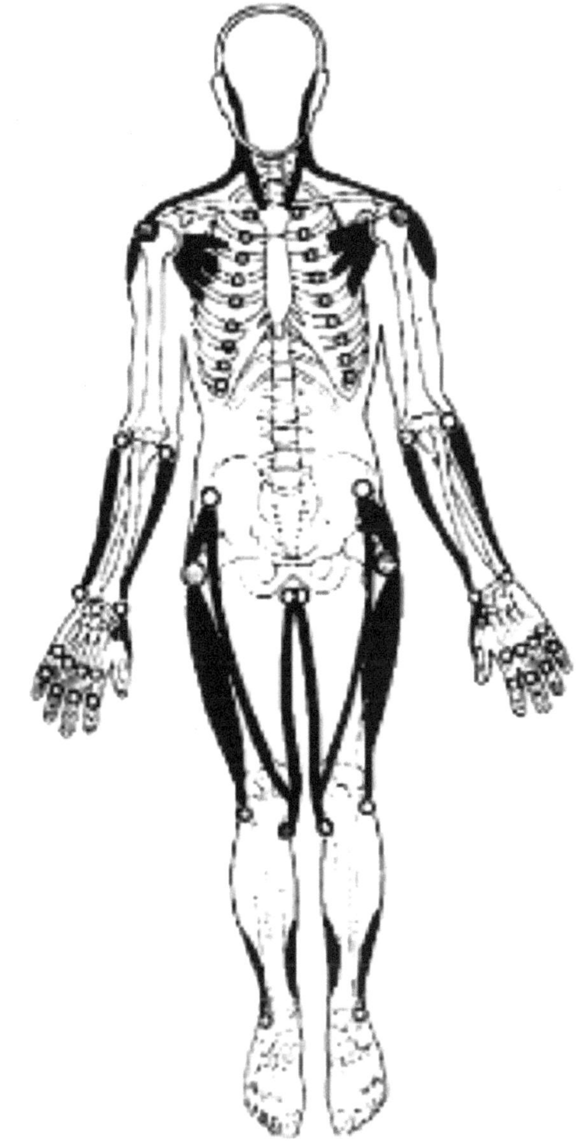

Figure 18.253. Spread of pain caused by changes in the TMJ: in the occipital, occipital, frontal, neck and facial area and lower jaw.

Generalized tendomyalgia (according to Muller) due to interjaw dysfunctions and disorders in the TMJ itself can be manifested by painful points, muscle tightness and a feeling of pressure on those painful points. It is very difficult to single out the factors that are primary for the occurrence of myofascial pain and the involvement of musculoskeletal structures. Targeted therapy cannot be determined without a well-established diagnosis. Factors that are considered to be influential in the occurrence of functional disorders of the craniomandibular system can be different: predisposing, initiating, or supporting. Predisposing factors of disorders in the craniomandibular joint increase the risk of TMD.

Initiating factors of TMD have a direct and sudden impact on the masticatory system, such as trauma to the head and neck, or a sudden involuntary movement when eating, yawning or holding the mouth open for a long time in the dental chair.

Additional factors that cause TMD in the first place are parafunctional movements. For example, if bruxism is a chronic phenomenon, the stress caused by bruxism leads to increased muscle tone and hyperactivity, causing myopathy, or arthropathy.

When researching the causes of TMD in the last few years, genetic factors are also being sought as possible causes of TMJ dysfunction. Even 15 different genes have been identified that can affect the individual pain modulation. However, all this is still at the level of assumptions. However, most research into the causes of TMD has been attributed to mechanical changes in condylar position due to tooth loss, or intermaxillary occlusal events.

Does this mean that occlusion is attributed as the primary factor in the development of TMD?

There are many factors that can cause problems with TMD, and which of them should be singled out as the primary cause in each case depends on the degree and scope of the dysfunction, which requires a detailed analysis. Malocclusion and unbalanced occlusal interjaw relationships may be the most common factors for the development of TMD and, combined with other factors, worsen the symptoms of TMD.

In the implementation of the prosthetic plan, whether the prosthetic work is supported by natural teeth or implants, occlusion is the most important factor for good function. It should be known that occlusion is not only a static intercuspid relationship of the intermaxillary arches, but a very dynamic relationship between all the tissues of the masticatory apparatus. Occlusion is much more than simple physical contact of occlusal surfaces, because it represents coordinated functional interaction of different tissues of the masticatory system, i.e. tissues of different histological composition, which differentiate, model, remodel, decay and regenerate.

Dysfunctions in the TMJ caused by occlusal factors can influence changes in the way the mandible moves. The TMJ tries to accommodate occlusal interference, but this is possible to a certain extent. For example, the lateral movements of the lower jaw depend on the height of the cusps and the inclination of their oblique planes. The height of the cusps and the depth of the fissure depend on the vertical movement of the rotating condyle during translational movement of the lower jaw.

Occlusal morphology also depends on the form of lateral movement of horizontal lateral movement. So, if it is about prosthetic restorations on implants, the prevention of iatrogenically causing TMD starts in the laboratory only on good and individually adjustable articulators.

Chewing is the initial stage of digestion and must be pleasant, including the sense of taste, touch and smell. Along with the masticatory muscles, the morphology of the biting surfaces is also extremely important in the chewing process it must not be formed arbitrarily, according to the "taste" of the dental technician.

Chewing is an automatic action and is usually not subject to voluntary control, although sometimes it can be a voluntary action. Chewing consists of well-coordinated rhythmic movements when opening and closing the mouth and occlusal contacts. This activity is under the control of the CNS (18.149) which is responsible for and from which the coordination for all other muscles originates.

Temporomandibular dysfunction (TMD) is a common name for a number of pathological conditions that manifest themselves with similar symptoms and lead to disturbances in the function of the stomatognathic system. Most of these pathological conditions in the TMJ can be of multifactorial etiology, which makes it difficult to make an accurate diagnosis.

Patients most often complain to us about subjective complaints, such as pain when chewing in the joint itself. Sometimes the patient cannot accurately determine the pain, so he complains of pain in the oral cavity, ear, shoulder or head, as well as the limitation of certain functional movements, for example, pain when opening and closing the mouth, pain when chewing, etc.

In contrast to the symptoms, there are certain signs that indicate that there are pathological changes in the joint itself: pain on palpation, limited individual movements of the lower jaw, sounds in the joint, abrasions on the teeth, insufficient periodontal tissues that promote tooth mobility, even pathological migration, which is inevitably reflected in the events in the joint itself. Such joint disorders can be accompanied by frequent headaches and severe migraine pains. The spread of pain can also be outside the masticatory system

Are there cases of TMD without the patient experiencing any subjective symptoms?

There are also cases of TMD without significant subjective symptoms, when the stomatognathic complex is compensated within the limits of physiological tolerance despite the existence of the disorder.

How long can such a condition last where the patient does not feel any discomfort?

Such a condition can last for a long time, and in some cases even for life. But it also depends on the type of person and the tolerance towards TMD. Research has shown that in 40-60% of patients there is at least one sign of TMD, and that only 5-10% of cases have pronounced symptoms and complaints, which is why they come for examinations. In principle, TMDs are quite a complex pathology even for a well-trained dentist

What therapy should be used for TMD?

The masticatory system is so complex that you need to know it well in order to preserve its health, that is, its good function.

Certainly, the state of health of the entire masticatory system is closely related to occlusion.

If the disorders are caused solely by occlusal factors caused by the loss of teeth, or if it is necessary to perform prosthetic work for functional, aesthetic, or other reasons, then all gnathological requirements must be met.

If the disorders are complex, a multidisciplinary approach is often required. There are complicated disorders that do not belong to the domain of dental therapeutic procedures.

What are the principles that should be followed when it comes to prosthetic work on implants?

In order to avoid disruptions in the TMJ, or if there are already TMDs, the following principles apply during the fabrication of prosthetic works:

- prosthetic works must be performed in good individually adjustable articulators, so that the transmitted situation of interjaw relations is as close as possible to the situation in the mouth;
- modeling of cusps on occlusal surfaces must be coordinated with maximum intercuspation during all movements;
- the shape and inclination of the cuspid surfaces should be carried out in such a way that premature wounds, the so-called, are removed by control in the mouth. traumatic contacts;
- if there are symptoms of TMD, definitive prosthetic work must not be done in the present condition. It is necessary to carry out additional diagnostics, in order to achieve the best function and aesthetics with prosthetic work.

The previous questions and answers related exclusively to fixed compensation. When it comes to total mobile prostheses versus TMJ, is there a difference?

The differences in treatment procedures are great. The goal is to bring the condyles to the central position. It is very important to accurately determine and convey the interjaw relationships, when the condyles are brought to the maximum distal position. When it comes to total mobile restorations, the procedure depends on several factors: from the alignment of the teeth to the stability of the prostheses. Stability during chewing is significantly affected by reocclusion, which also depends on the position of the condyle. If there is a possibility of stabilization, especially of the lower prosthesis, with retention "clips", then the chewing function is better, which is also reflected in the function of the TMJ.

How many implants are enough to stabilize the lower total prosthesis with retention "clips"?

The application of two implants with spherical heads is considered the minimum standard therapy for the stabilization of the lower total prosthesis (Fig. 18.254).

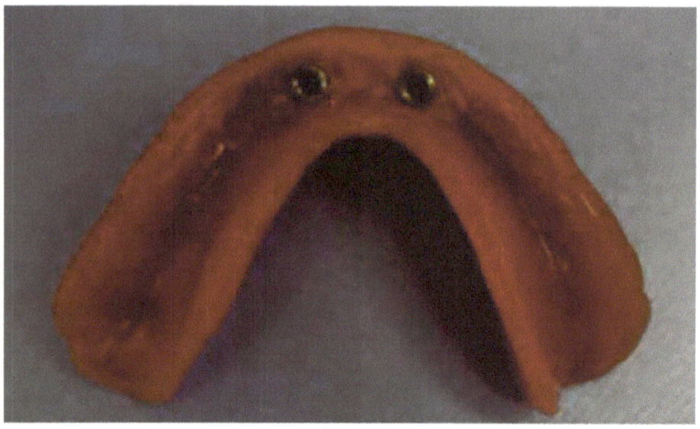

Figure 18.254. Custom acrylic prosthesis with modified soft base and built-in mini-implant caps.

If it is not possible to use two implants, can only one be used?

There are two reasons to attempt stabilization with a single implant: anatomical conditions and the patient's ability to pay. There are cases where the patient cannot afford the installation of two implants, especially if prior augmentation with bone substitutes is required. In order to obtain a quantitative increase of the alveolar ridge in the horizontal and vertical direction, time and patience are required, accompanied by the morbidity of the patient (Fig. 18.255).

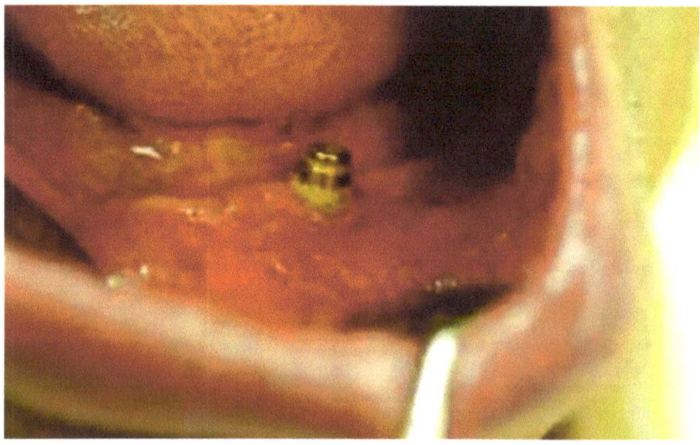

Figure 18.255. A wide-diameter implant after 3 years in extreme atrophy of the alveolar bone of the lower jaw is the only possible position of the implant

How long can such an implant last given the overload?

Based on experience, using implants with the best technological treatments (Laser-lock technology) of standard and larger diameters (extremely rare indication), as well as smaller diameters, the survival rate is from 5 to 10 years, and often longer. Nevertheless, rehabilitation in this way, even after the eventual loss of the implant, helped the patient to get used to the total prosthesis more easily, adjusting the movements of the masticatory musculature.

Does the length of time also affect whether the implant is immediately loaded or the load is delayed?

I used both methods. It has no effect whether the implant is primarily loaded or not. The duration in bone is the same. However, in elderly people, with a large atrophy of the alveolar ridge, the implant should be applied as a retaining factor at least for a certain period of time. How long it will last depends on the type of bone. If the bone type is D4, the implant will not last long in such an environment, whether it is processed with the best surface technology or not, immediately loaded, or with delayed loading.

Does it happen that, despite well-integrated implants, implant-prosthetic treatment fails, and what are the reasons for the failure?

It happens that the entire implant-prosthetic procedure is compromised, in which the implantologist and the patient did not participate. The error was created in the dental laboratory. Often, those errors that are created in the laboratory can be in aesthetics (Fig. 18.156) and even more serious, caused by occlusal problems. Aesthetic problems are much simpler and easier to eliminate. Occlusal problems created in the laboratory can cause serious consequences, even with the loss of the implant. Both complications are manifested by patient morbidity. In the presented case, an aesthetic problem, the patient is exposed to the trauma of removing the prosthetic work by cutting (Fig. 18.157) and the repetition of procedures that are not pleasant.

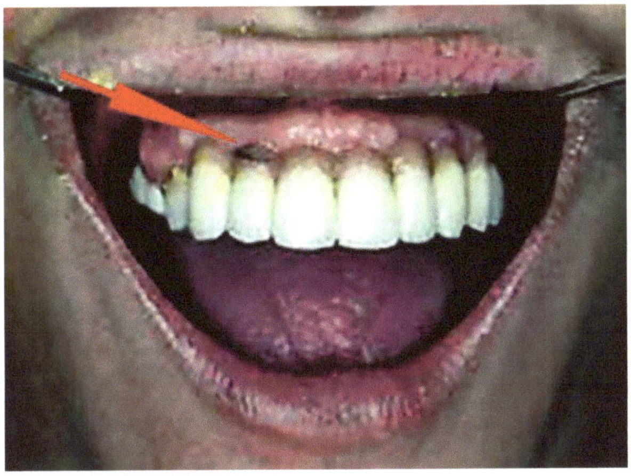

Figure 18.256. Laboratory errors are a big risk. The patient suffers from the mistakes of the dental technician.

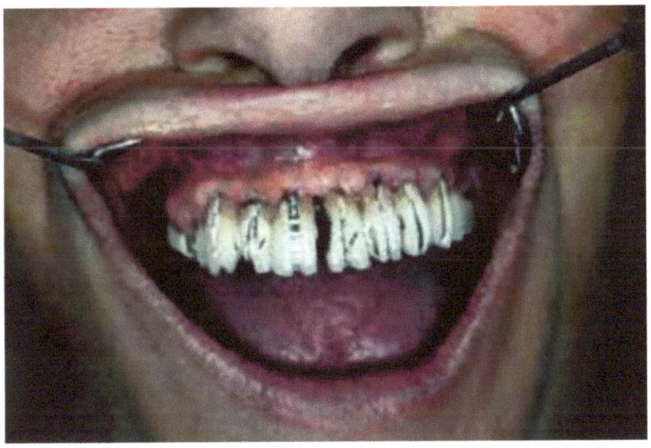

Figure 18.257. Removal of prosthetic work due to laboratory errors, in addition to torturing the patient, is at the same time a trauma to the already integrated implants. Removal of the cemented work should be performed carefully, with as little trauma as possible to the implants and the surrounding soft tissues. Error cementing with glass ionomer instead of "implantlink forte"

What do practice and experience say, and what does theory say, regarding the installation of an implant in the alveolus immediately after tooth extraction, with immediate loading?

Theory cannot be far from practice, because it essentially relies on practice and experience. The theory is there to explain what is important in some practical solution, and ignore the unimportant details.

For example, in physics, the equation of free fall is taught, which explains the mechanism of fall. Air resistance to a falling object exists, but is negligible. Practical knowledge and experience are important and useful, but they do not give great knowledge without theoretical design, and this knowledge is most often a truncated one. But, also, practice is vital, and despite knowing a lot of theoretical details, much of what is achieved through practice often cannot be explained. The practice is endless, very diverse. Often, successful achievements in practice are the result of experience, and the reasons for success or failure can, in the end, be recognized by theory. And it also happens that theory is sometimes unable to explain what practice has achieved. Albert Einstein humorously explains it with these words: "Practice is when everything works." A theory is when nothing works and you can't explain why." The conclusion of the author of the book is that a good and successful practice creates a good theory, so that such a theory would create a new good practice, where this one was not like that.

The above may be the answer to the question about implant placement immediately after tooth extraction. Insertion of implants into healed bone in edentulous or partially edentulous patients is an established implantological procedure in dental practice and the positions are clear. However, when it comes to installing an implant immediately after tooth extraction, in a fresh alveolus, opinions are divided. In the pursuit of shortening the time of implantological treatment, which significantly increases the patient's comfort, the moment of implantation and prosthetic rehabilitation is being discussed more and more.

The experience of the author of the book suggests that the installation of implants immediately after tooth extraction is justified for several reasons:

- practice and experience have shown that the installation of an implant in a fresh alveolus, immediately after tooth extraction, slows down the resorption of the alveolar bone, especially its buccal walls. At the same time, it is extremely important to perform tooth extraction with as little trauma as possible in order to preserve the anatomy of the alveolus and the dimensions of the bone structure;
- by simultaneously filling the alveolus with a bone substitute, the horizontal dimension of the alveolar bone is formed better and faster;
- immediate load, function is restored to the bone tissue and bone remodeling and bone integration of the implant and bone are enhanced;
- with immediate implantation, the formation of soft tissues is coordinated with the physiological processes of wound healing, because

the most important time for the formation of soft tissues after immediate implantation occurs in the first three months. Complete stabilization of soft tissues is achieved after six months. Some studies have shown that the formation of soft tissues continues even after six months, and the papilla takes its final shape only after a year.

However, some studies claim the opposite: that implant placement immediately after tooth extraction in a fresh alveolus does not prevent resorption, especially of the buccal wall.

The author's objection to these claims, when talking about the fact that bone resorption cannot be prevented by immediate implantation, is a wrong determination. Aging, and especially tooth loss, the accompanying resorption is a physiological process. Therefore, in this case, a more appropriate term is that resorption can be significantly slowed down by implantation.

What should be taken into account during the immediate installation of the implant in a fresh alveolus?

Achieving primary stability is most important. For immediate implantation and immediate loading, it is extremely important to limit micro-movements within the tolerance limits of the implant and the bone. Achieving good primary stability creates the conditions for the implants to adapt faster and better to the biomechanical loads of chewing forces, and the primary stability of the implant is one of the basic factors for successful osseointegration. In the case of immediate loading, the tolerance threshold must not exceed 100 micrometers, and this depends on the treatment of the implant surface. If the mechanical load is not reduced to the limits of physiological tolerance, the formation of fibrous encapsulation of the implant may occur. At the same time, one should take care of the stability and formation of soft tissues, especially when it comes to the aesthetic region. With immediate implantation in the aesthetic region, care should be taken not to cause gingival recession. It depends on several factors: the biotype of the gingiva, the bucco-lingual or bucco-palatal position of the implant, the state of the bone around the adjacent teeth, the dimensions of the alveolar ridge in the region of implantation. Thickening of the buccal marginal soft tissue, especially in the aesthetic region, is achieved with a subepithelial soft tissue graft, which reduces the possibility of gingival recession and stabilizes the soft tissue formation. The more lingual or palatal the position of the implant, the better the stability of the soft tissues.

Why is more and more attention being paid to implant placement in a fresh alveolus immediately after tooth extraction and primary loading of the implant?

To many answers, during the writing of the book I tried to use English expressions as little as possible in the explanations. But the answer to this question requires me to use them, because they are used in the literature in the Serbian language: "socket preservation" and "alveolar ridge preservation". What does that mean? The preventive principle is that after tooth loss, the width and height of the alveolar ridge should be preserved and the alveolar ridge whose arch has been destroyed by larger bone defects should be reconstructed. Filling the alveolus immediately after tooth extraction with xenogeneic bone substitutes and reconstructing the ridge with autologous bone blocks is an established procedure in everyday practice. It should be emphasized that reconstruction of the alveolar ridge ("alveolar ridge preservation") represents morbidity for the patient. After tooth removal, resorption is an inevitable biological process that occurs as soon as the periodontium from the inner side of the vestibular bone lamella is broken, and thus its blood supply. As soon as the vascularization of the vestibular and lingual bony lamellae of the alveolus is interrupted, resorption necessarily occurs, but its speed depends on several factors. Chewing forces have a significant impact.

The measured thickness of the labial bony lamella, especially in the upper jaw, usually ranges only from 0.5 to 1 mm. Also, there is evidence that after 6 months after tooth extraction, the average loss of horizontal bone is about 4 mm, and vertical bone loss is slightly above 1 mm. After 6 months, resorption processes are significantly reduced.

From the understanding of the above, the explained advantages of installing an implant in a fresh alveolus arise:

- strive for the extraction to be performed with as little tarum as possible (do not use levers);
- as the periodontium was interrupted by the extraction, and thus the blood supply of the inner side of the lamellar bone, the blood vessels of its front side are not torn when the implant is inserted into the fresh alveolus;
- root extraction leaves the position and direction that the implant will inherit using the apical bone to achieve primary stemness;
- the arch of the alveolar ridge is preserved, without the need to apply "socket preservation" and "alveolar ridge preservation";
- extensive augmentation is avoided, and patient costs are reduced;
- the patient receives fixed provisional prosthetic work immediately after tooth extraction and implant installation;
- healing of bones and soft tissues is performed in function and significantly shortens the time of the entire treatment.

Is there scientific evidence or statistical data for the success of this method of implant rehabilitation?

They do not exist in the literature, not even valid statistical data. What has been said above stems from the author's experience of successfully solving cases of this kind of implantological-prosthetic approach. The fact that there are no scientific confirmations and sufficient statistical data is not important. Many years of practical application and successful results confirm this.

After all, aspirin was synthesized in 1899, when it was officially presented by the Bayer company. But, despite such long-term use, the mechanism of aspirin's therapeutic effect was discovered only in 1971., and John Vane received the Nobel Prize and a knighthood for that discovery. Similarly, in oral implantology, many successful solutions have not yet been scientifically explained.

When you mentioned aspirin, explain the mechanism of its action, which explanation was waited for several decades?

A dentist, and especially an oral surgeon, before every surgical procedure, must find out in the anamnesis whether the patient is taking anticoagulant and antiplatelet drugs (which includes aspirin).

Aspirin inhibits cyclooxygenase, an enzyme involved in the synthesis of prostaglandins (which are produced during inflammation, causing pain) and thromboxane. In addition to analgesic, antipyretic and anti-inflammatory effects, aspirin also inhibits platelet aggregation. Recent studies have proven that there are two groups of cyclooxygenase and that aspirin inhibits the synthesis of pro-aggregation prostaglandins and thromboxane, but not prostaglandins in the blood vessel wall, which act as vasodilators and anti-aggregators. Since thrombi in the arteries are mainly made of platelets, aspirin in low doses inhibits their aggregation and maintains patency of the arteries. For antiplatelet purposes, in the first line of heart attack prevention, in the last few years, an optimal dose of 81 mgv (Low dose safety coated Aspirin), cardiopirin 75 mgv has been established.

When it comes to immediate implantation, can you show any such case?

The displays in the following pictures show the sequence of procedures and the success of the entire intervention.

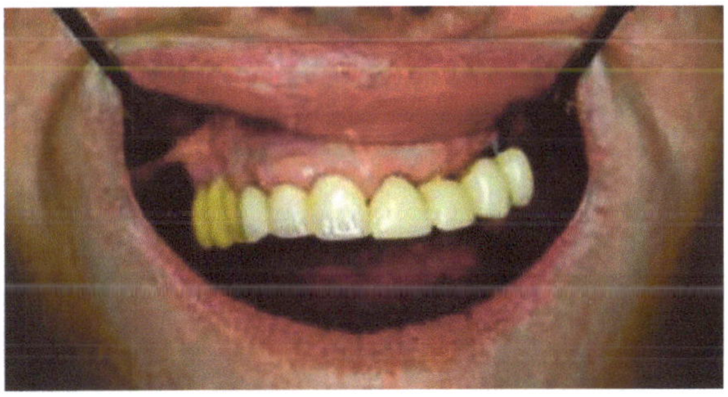

Figure 18.258. Initial state.

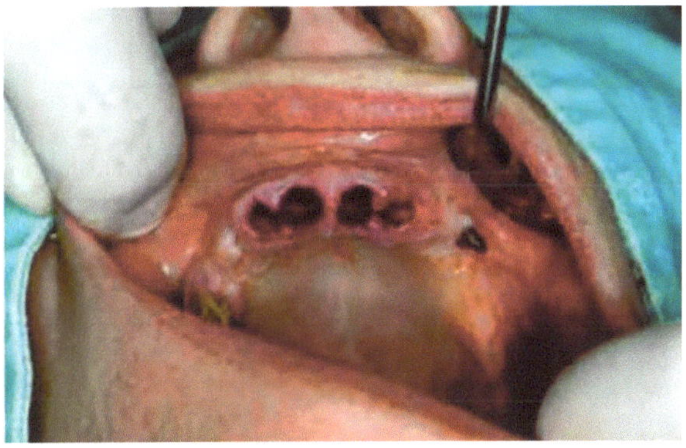

Figure 18.259. Extracted teeth, alveoli prepared for immediate implantation and primary loading.

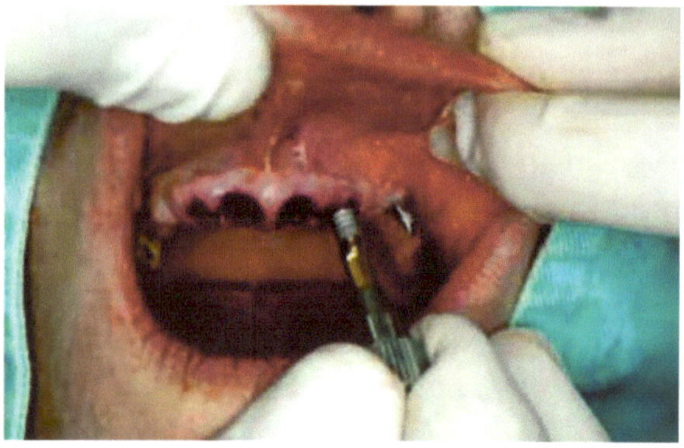

Figure 18.260. Immediate installation of the implant in a fresh alveolus. The first thing the implant is allowed to touch is blood.

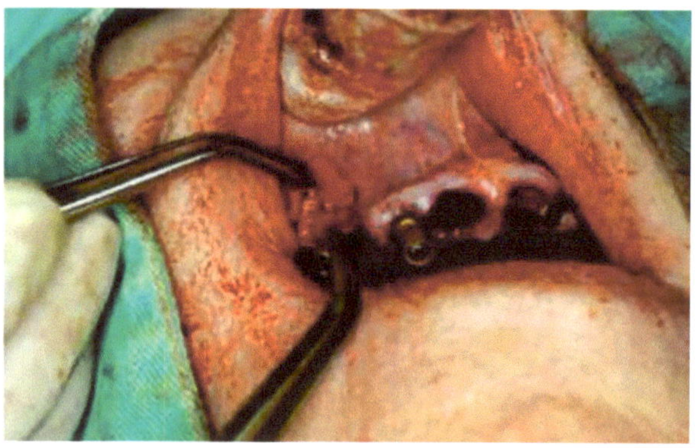

Figure 18.261. Performed sinus lifting with immediate installation of implants.

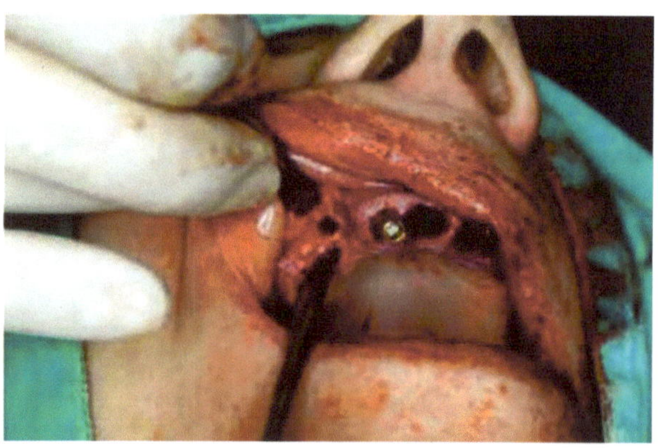

Figure 18.262. Augmentation in area 15 for sinus lifting. Installing the implant in that place requires a healing period of 6 to 8 months.

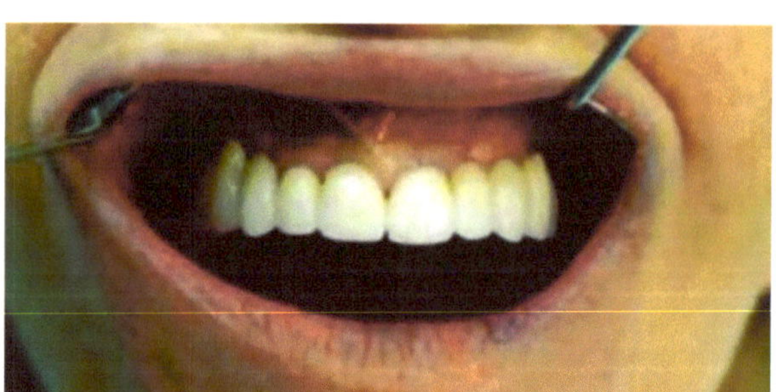

Figure 18.263. Aesthetic appearance of prosthetic work and formed soft tissues.

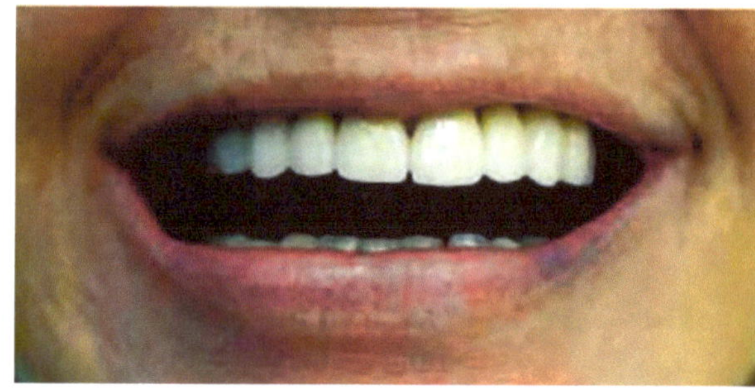

Figure 18.264. Definitive prosthetic work with a favorable upper lip line.

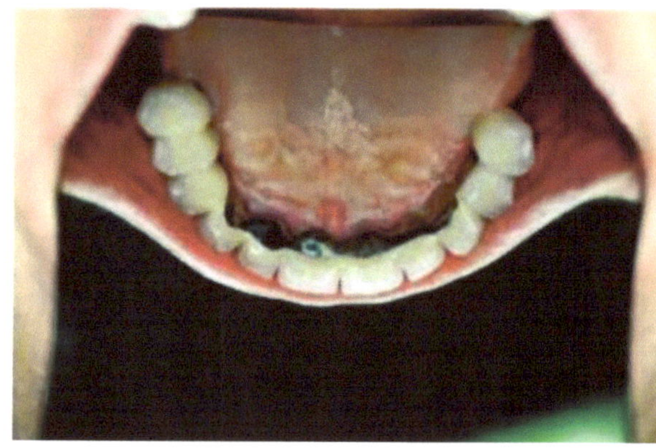

Figure 18.265. Appearance from the palatal side after 2 years. Absence of soft tissue inflammation.

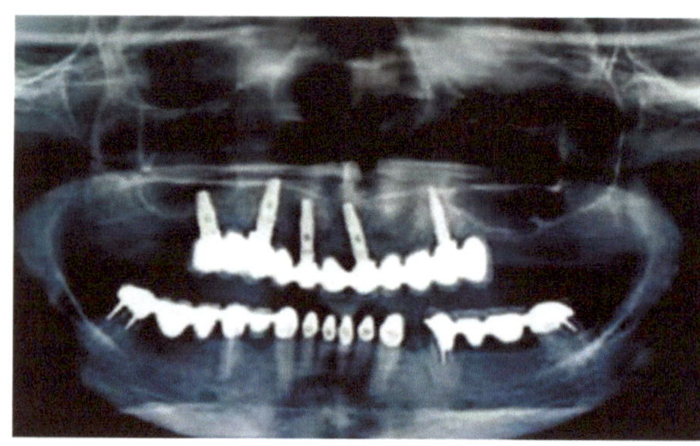

Figure 18.266. Control X-ray after 3 years. In place of tooth #24, the only possibility was the installation of a reduced-diameter implant. Cortical bone was used to achieve primary fixation.

A case of solving immediate implantation and immediate loading in a patient with limited time for complete rehabilitation

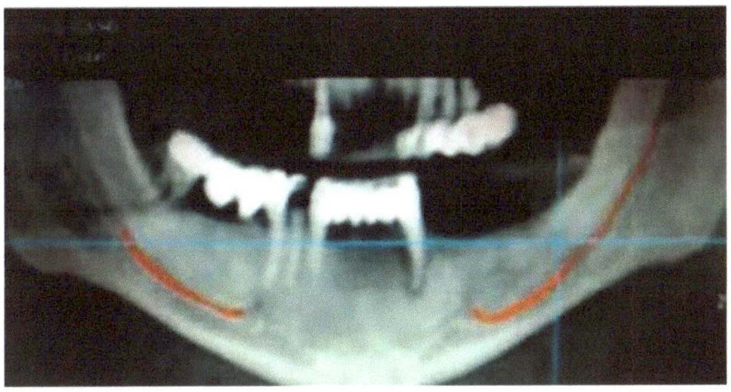

Figure 18.267. Tomographic representation of the position of the lower dental nerve.

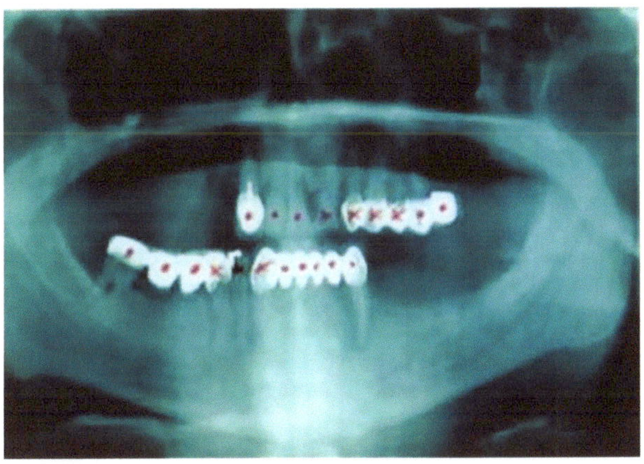

Figure 18.268. Assessment and intervention plan done on the second place. However, due to the high price, the patient opted for treatment at Dr. Zlopaš's office, but with limited time.

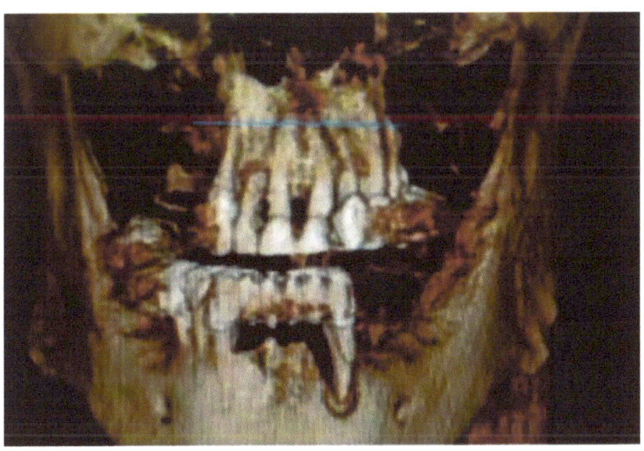

Figure 18.269. Tomographic visibility of the existing condition.

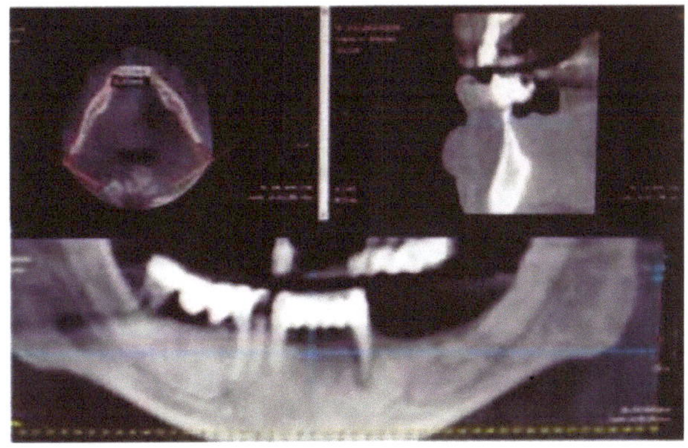

Figure 18.270. Radiographic visibility of affected teeth.

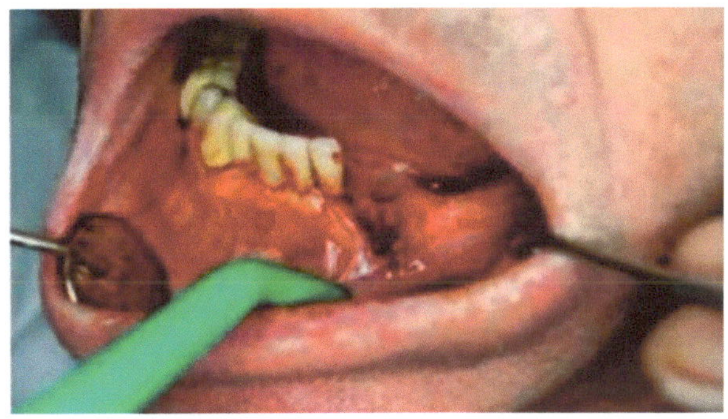

Figure 18.271. After extraction of the canine, a larger bone defect is visible.

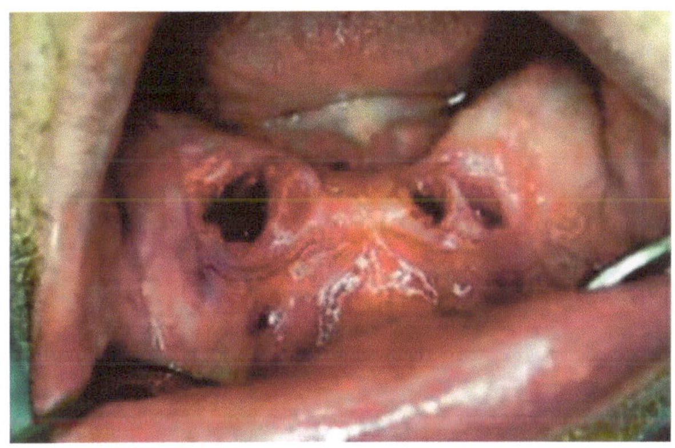

Figure 18.272. The appearance of the extraction wounds after extraction requires the preservation of the alveolus.

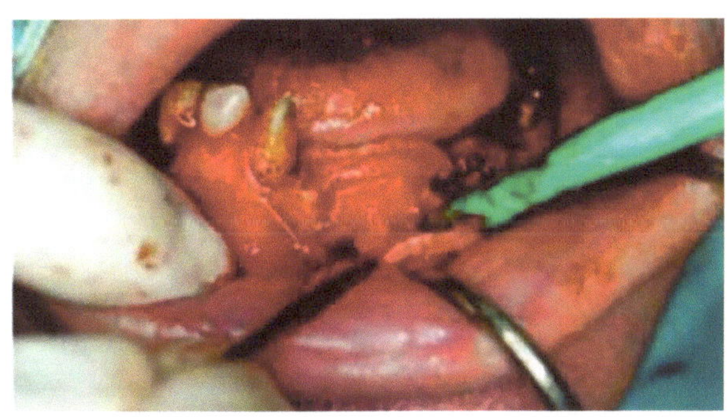

Figure 18.273. The doctor's assessment is extremely important for choosing the diameter of the implant, which is in line with the size of the bone defect.

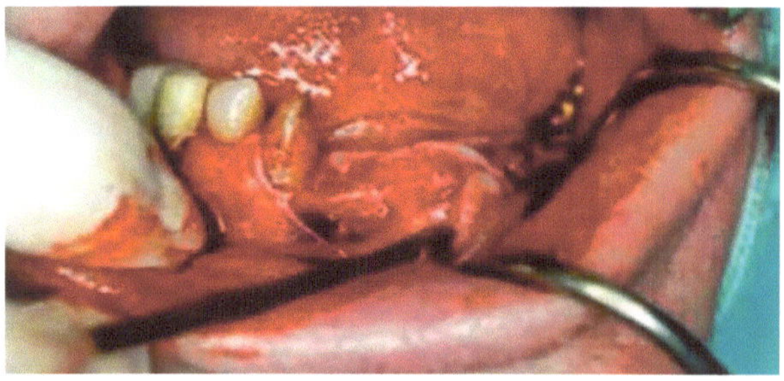

Figure 18.274. By raising the flap, it is observed that the condition of the available amount of bone enables the installation of an implant of smaller diameter and longer length (15mm).

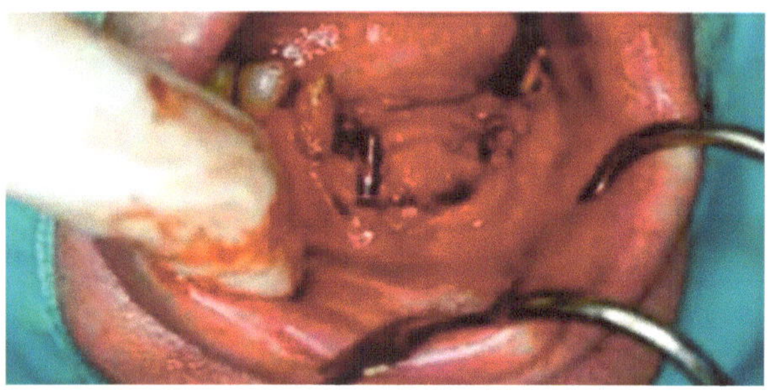

Figure 18.275. Achieved primary stability with augmentation of bone defects with a xenogeneic bone substitute mixed with autologous bone and covered with a collagen resorbable membrane.

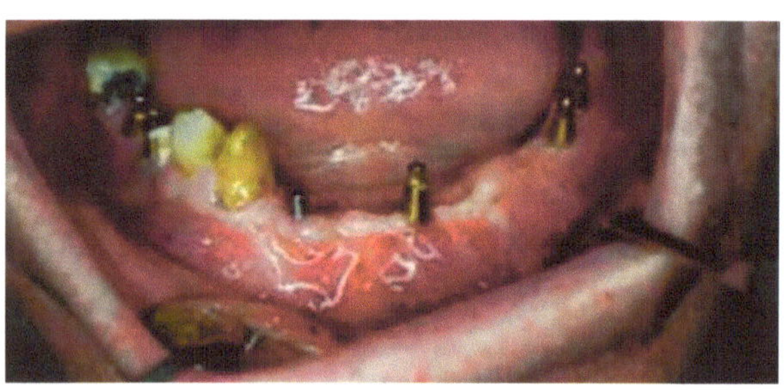

Figure 18.276. Appearance after 6 months. Good bone integration achieved and soft tissues formed.

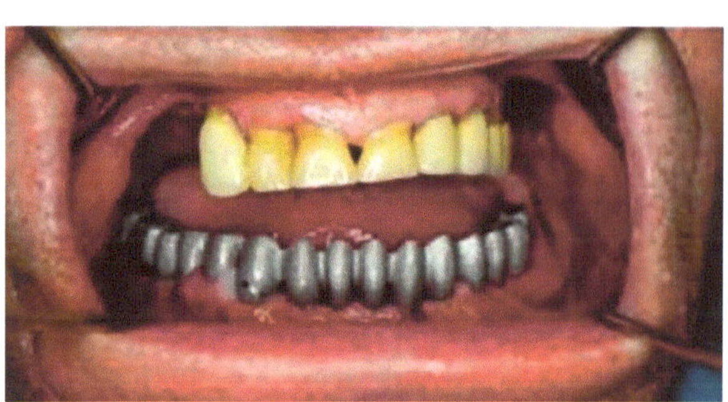

Figure 18.277. Test of metal construction.

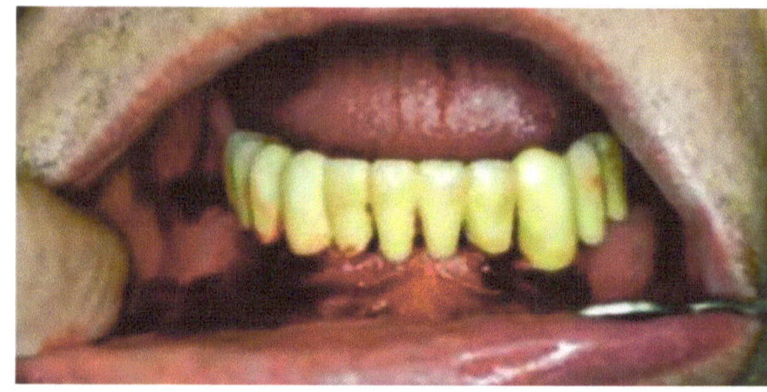

Figure 18.278. Placed implants in places 23, 26, 27, 43, 46 and 47. Temporary prosthetic work made in acrylate on a precise metal structure immediately after implantation. Adjusted to the patient's available time due to return to the US. The temporary orthotic work must be stable for the bone and soft tissue healing period for a period of 6 months.

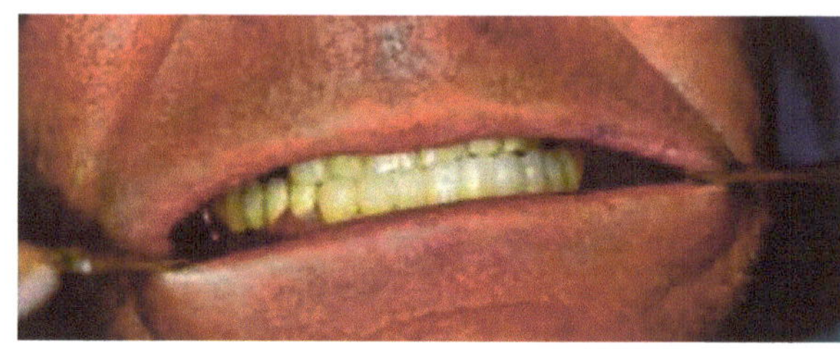

Figure 18.279. Definitive prosthetic performance in metal ceramics.

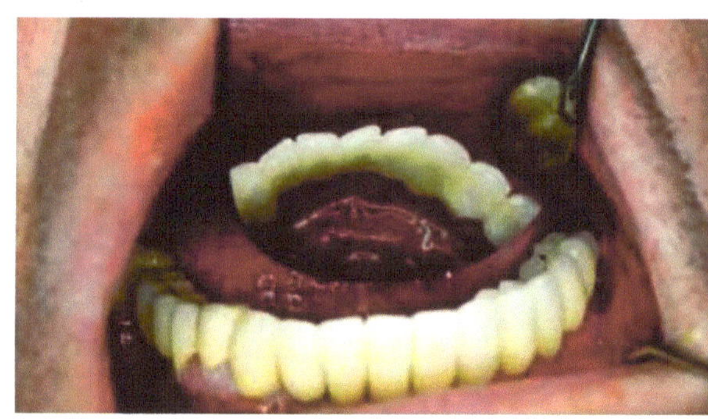

Figure 18.280. Appearance of definitive prosthetic work from the lingual side.

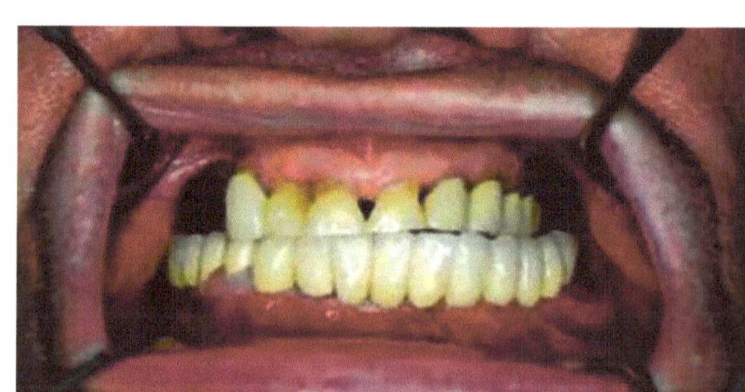

Figure 18.281. Achieved functional and aesthetic satisfaction of the patient.

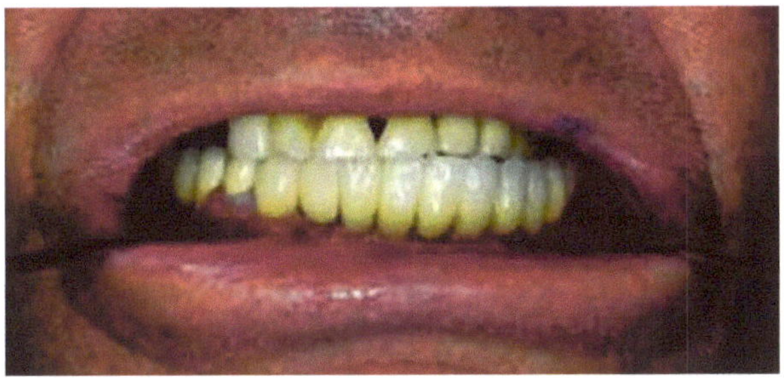

Figure 18.282. Restoration of the upper jaw was also proposed to the patient.

The case of a patient with a request to get fixed prosthetic work as soon as possible

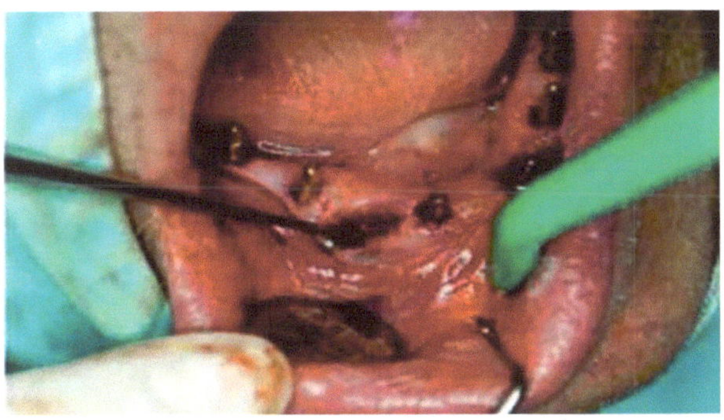

Figure 18.283. Immediately placed implants with good primary fixation.

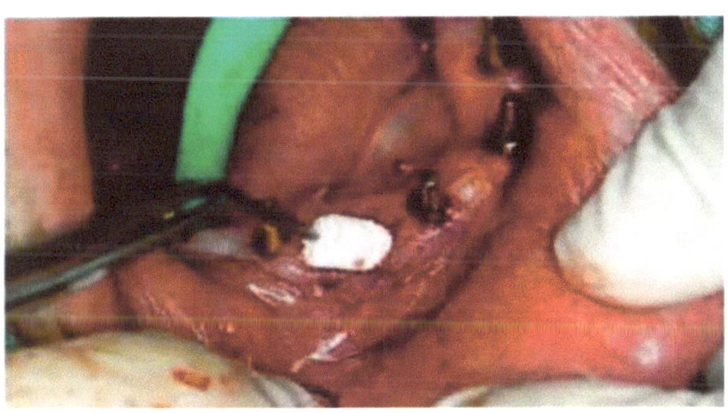

Figure 18.284. Treatment of a larger bone defect at site 43.

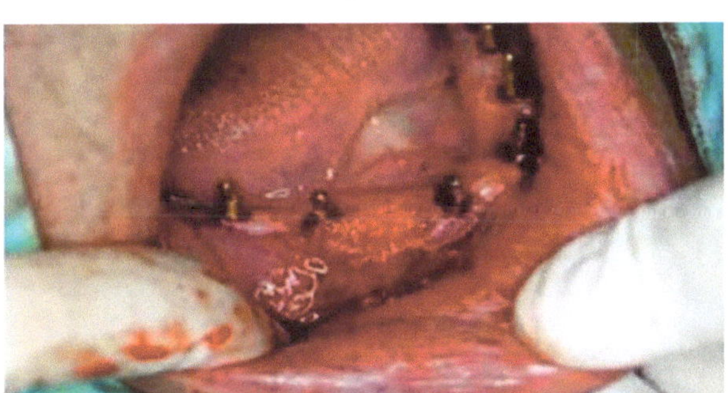

Figure 18.285. Augmentation of a bone defect with a bone substitute covered with a collagen resorbable membrane.

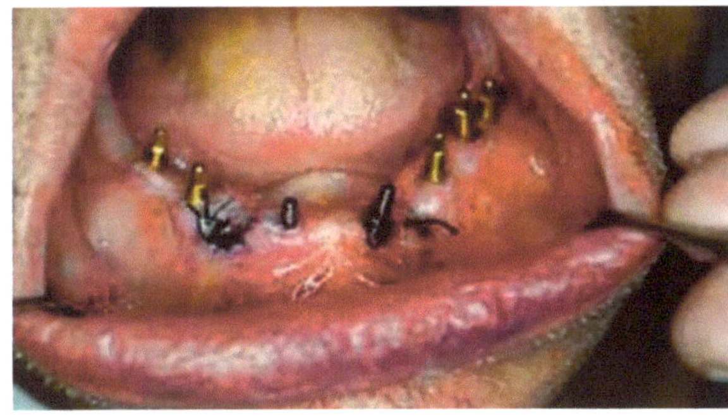

Figure 18.286. The situation after 10 days.

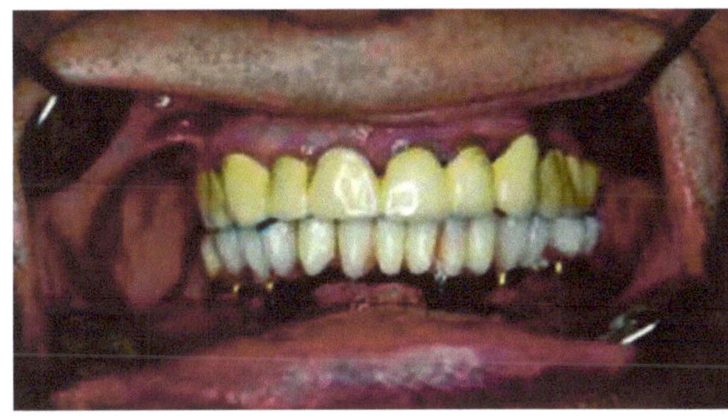

Figure 18.287. Temporary prosthetic work in which the implants are immediately loaded.

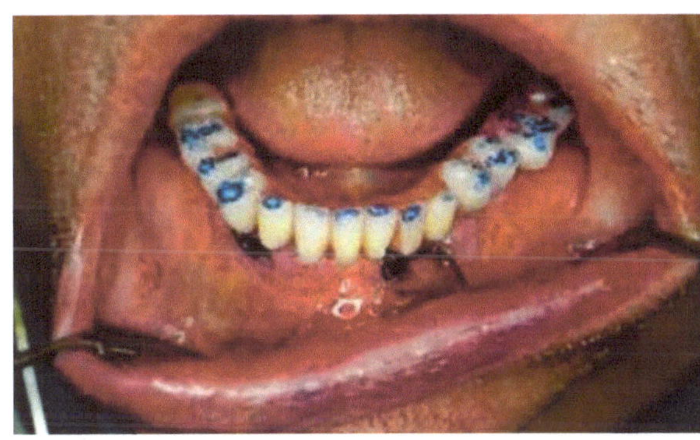

Figure 18.288. Micro-movements of tolerance must not exceed the threshold of 100 micrometers. The dosed load is achieved by good occlusion, elimination of premature contacts and the softness of the material of the temporary work, which accelerates the integration processes.

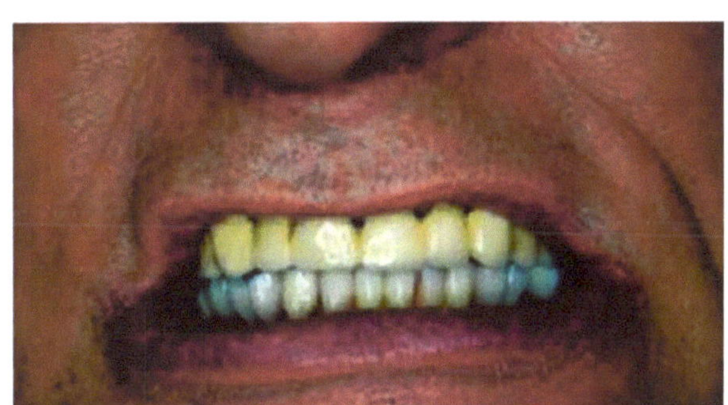

Figure 18.289. Good chewing function was established with immediate prosthetic work

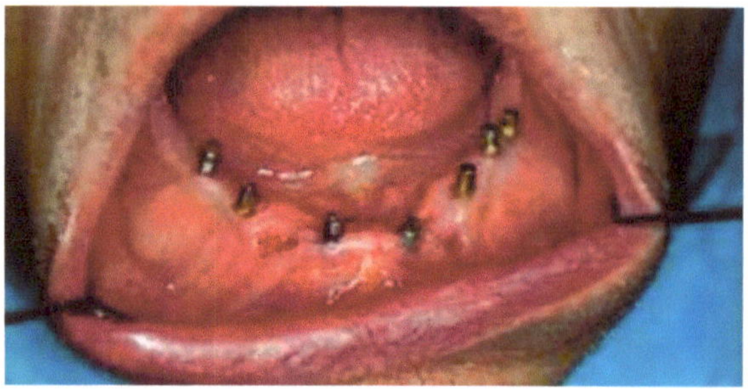

Figure 18.290. Rehabilitated tissues, integrated implants and shaped soft tissues are a condition for a successful result.

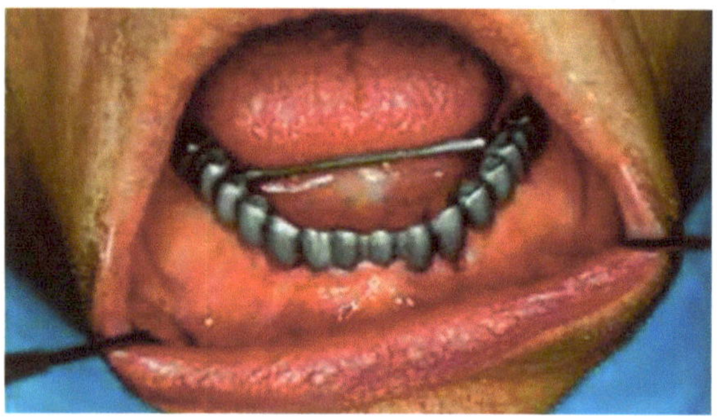

Figure 18.291. During the test, the metal structure must not exert pressure on the supports.

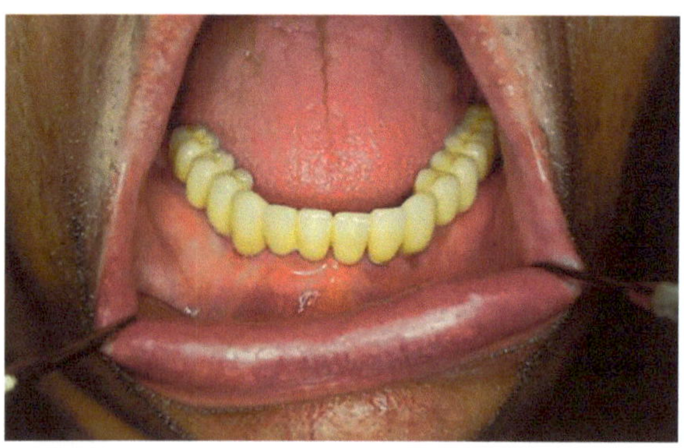

Figure 18.292. Definitive prosthetic work in metal-ceramics. Compare with the initial state. The time of implant-prosthetic treatment is significantly shortened, as is the patient's morbidity.

Presentation of a complex case typical for the fulfillment of the patient's wishes; due to professional obligations and daily communication, immediately after the extraction of all diseased teeth, he immediately receives fixed prosthetic work.

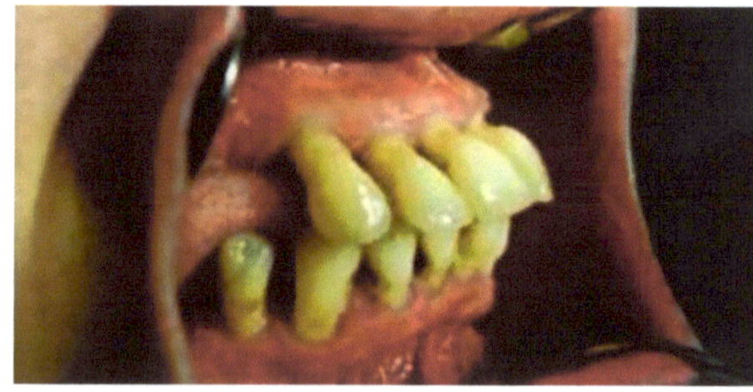

Figure 18.293. Extreme pathological migration in both jaws, with soft tissue inflammation present.

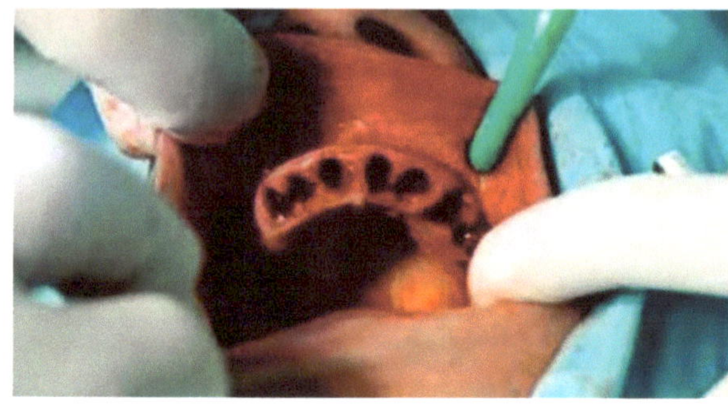

Figure 18.294. Extracted pathologically migrated teeth.

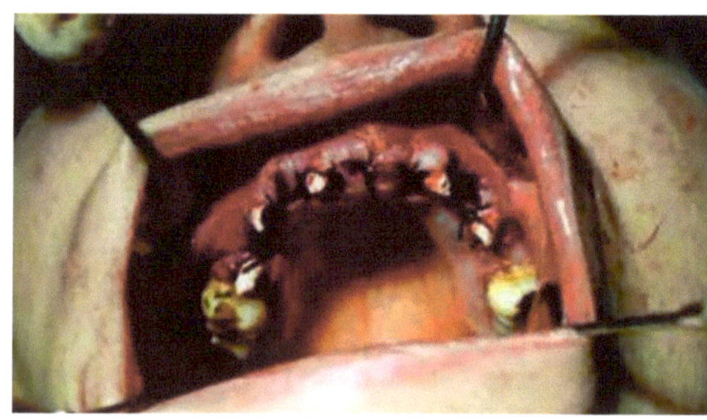

Figure 18.295. Immediate implant placement with immediate temporary PEEK plastic supports.

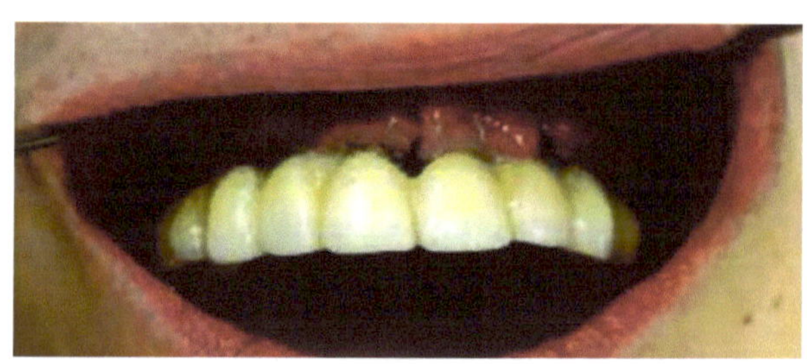

Figure 18.296. Immediate temporary restoration with sutures still present.

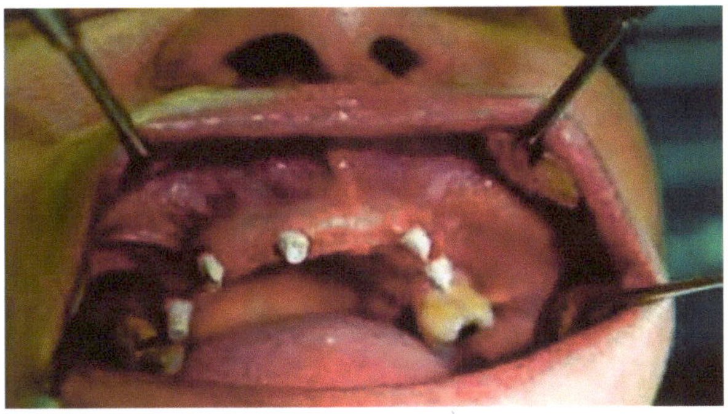

Figure 18.297. Appearance of temporary PEEK brackets after 3 months.

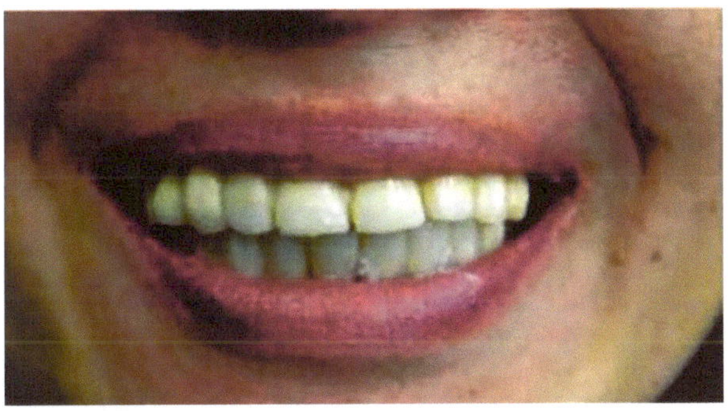

Figure 18.298. Fulfilled the requirement from the functional aspect.

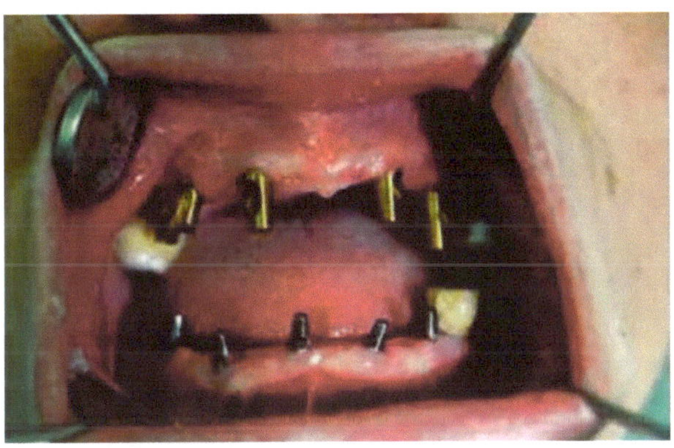

Figure 18.299. The stability of implants and soft tissues is extremely good.

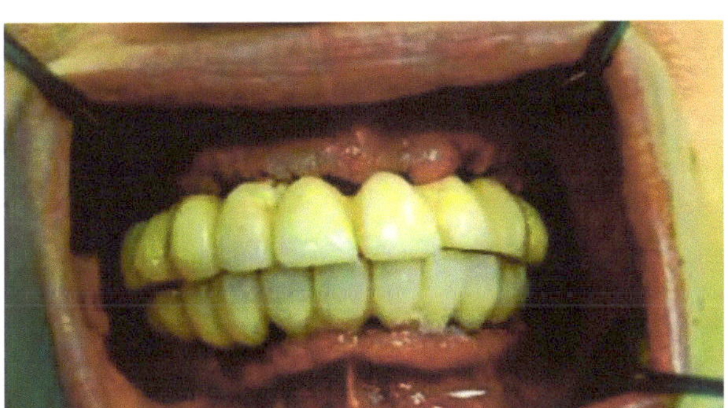

Figure 18.300. The same procedure was performed in the lower jaw.

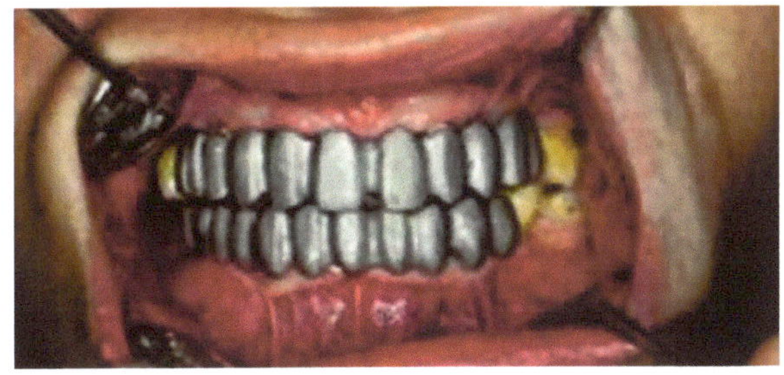

Figure 18.301. Properly established interjaw relationships are the foundation of the entire treatment.

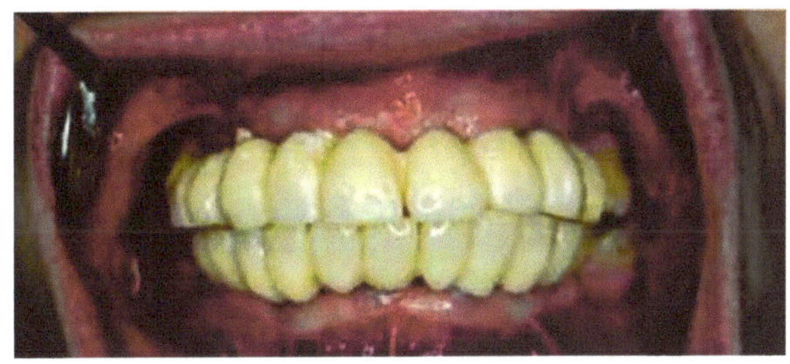

Figure 18.302. It is extremely important not to traumatize the implants and surrounding tissues during the removal and placement of temporary restorations.

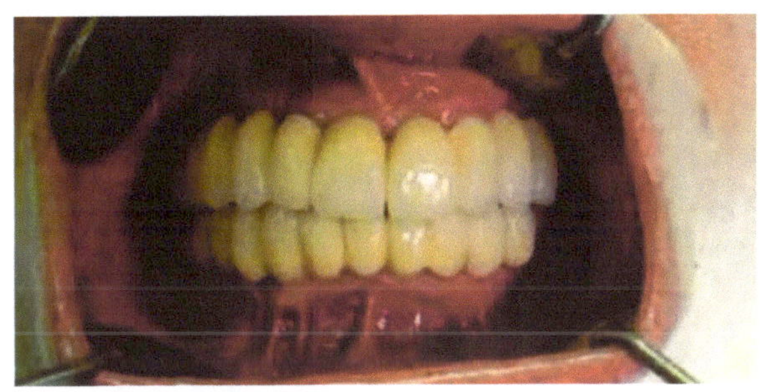

Figure 18.303. Established good occlusion with definitive prosthetic works promotes integration processes.

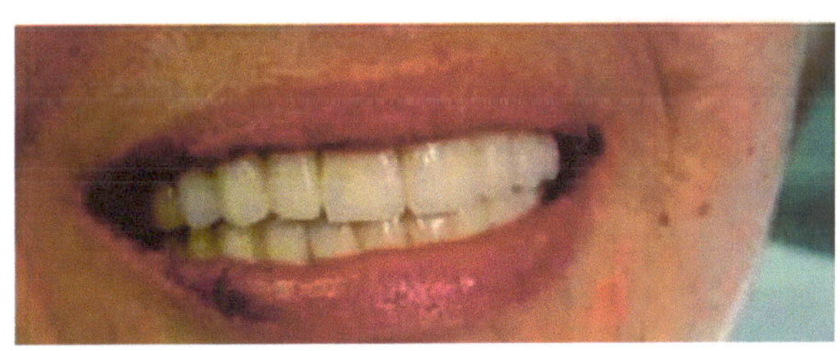

Figure 18.304. With definitive prosthetic work, the patient's satisfaction with aesthetics and function was maximum.

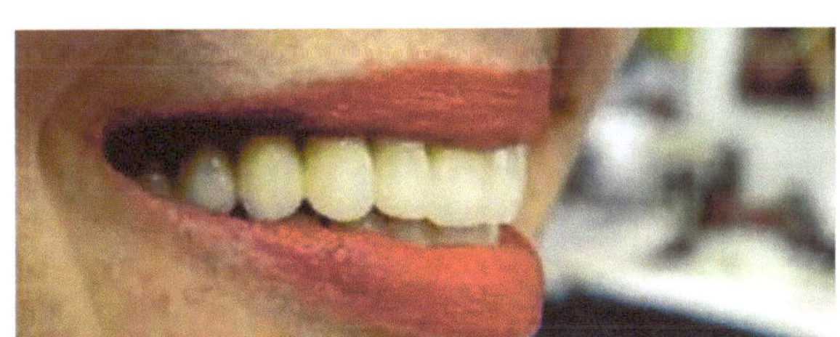

Figure 18.305. Profile view. Compare with the picture of the initial state (picture 18.293).

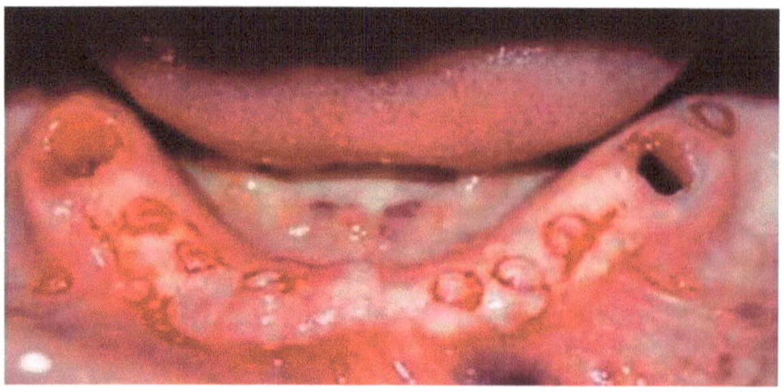

Figure 18.306. Using the wax-up method, the position of the implant was determined and it was planned to install the implant without raising the flap.

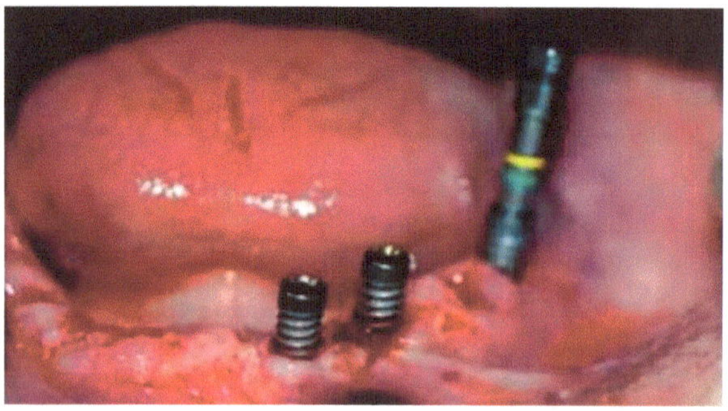

Figure 18.307. Beginning of the procedure without raising the flap.

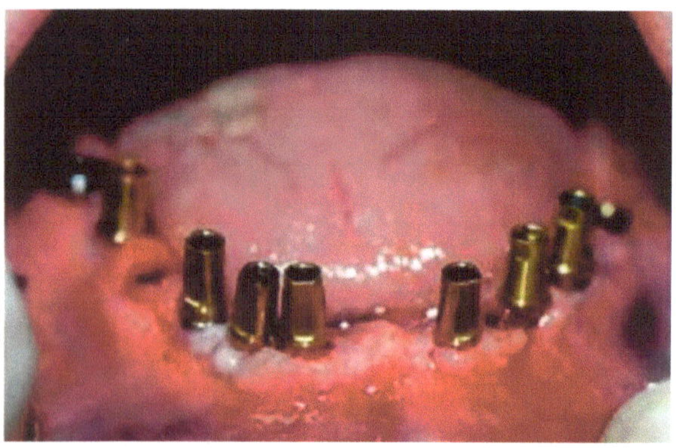

Figure 18.308. Installed definitive supports. Avoided placement of locking caps and gingiva-formers. Experience confirms that the sulcus of the gingiva is formed better in this way, than when the soft tissues are traumatized by constant twisting and turning of the gingiva-former or carrier.

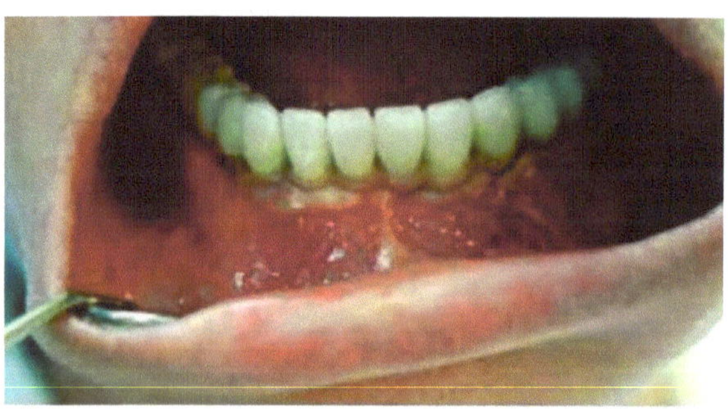

Figure 18.309. Appearance of definitive prosthetic work in metal-ceramics. Solving a complex case - inconsistency of the condition in the mouth and the patient's requirements.

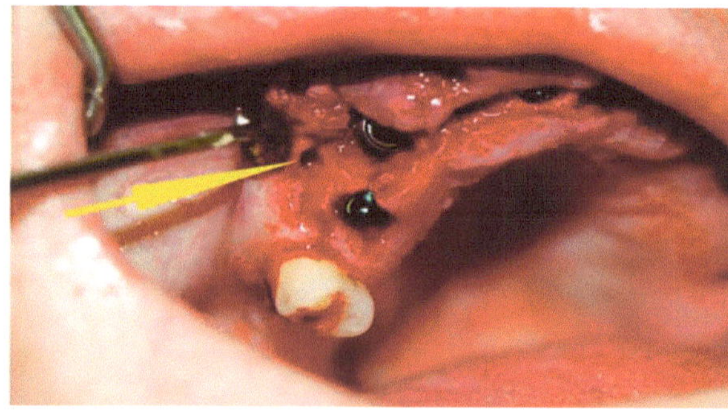

Figure 18.310. The available bone also determines the positioning of the implant.

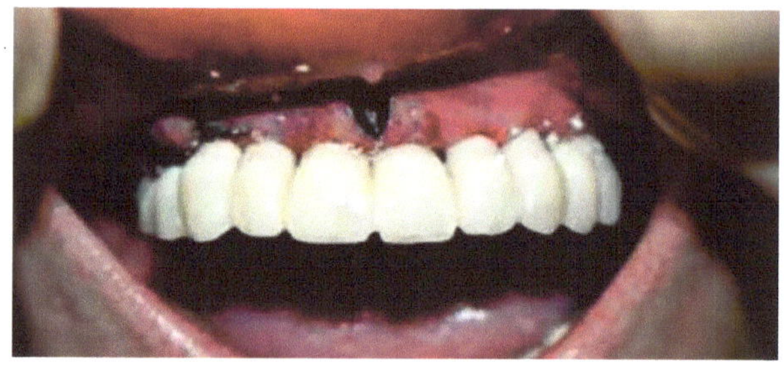

Figure 18.312. Temporary prosthetic work must enable the formation of soft tissues, on which the aesthetic result depends.

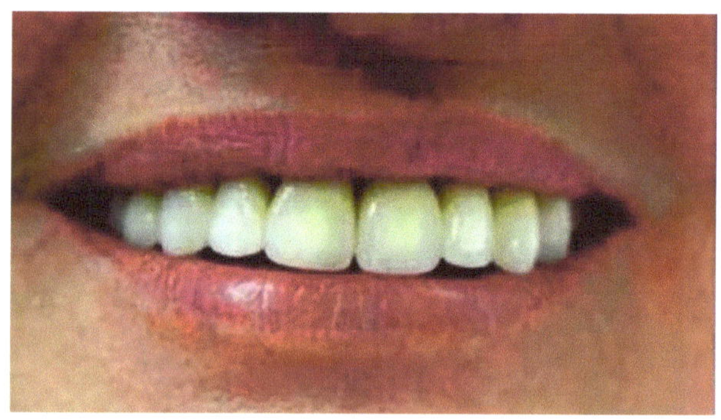

Figure 18.314. The shape of the lips and a favorable smile line contribute to the success of the aesthetic appearance.

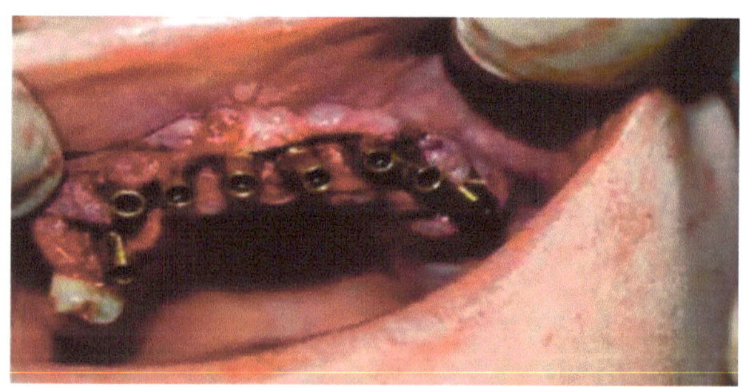

Figure 18.311. The planned treatment must shorten the time to restore the masticatory function.

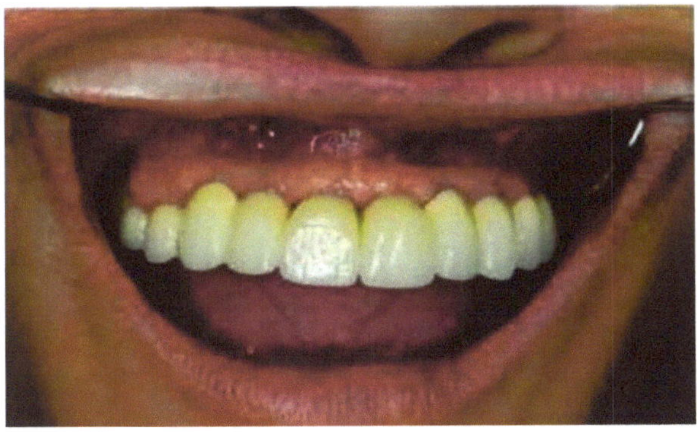

Figure 18.313. Appearance after one year. Compare with the initial state of extreme pathological migration in the frontal region of the upper jaw (Chapter 7, Figure 7.29).

How to slow down bone resorption after tooth extraction?

Since the subsequent processes of alveolar bone resorption occur after tooth extraction, it is always desirable to take measures that will alleviate this process.

The installation of implants in edentulous jaws is an established and routine therapeutic procedure with a success rate of 95% after 5 years, and 89% after 10 years, depending on whether the implantation is performed in the lower or upper jaw.

At the time when oral implantology was disputed, it is clear that these disputes (and their method) were not only unargued but also layman; claims about the inadmissibility of inserting a "foreign body into living bone". However, today it is known that the installation of implants slows down the resorption of the bone that has lost its function with the loss of the tooth. With the installation of the implant, it is possible to continue the action of masticatory forces on the bone, which restores the lost function.

From this logical thinking comes the answer to the question, and the position on the advantage of immediate implant installation in a fresh alveolus immediately after tooth extraction. By installing the implant immediately after extraction, it is possible to preserve the anatomy of the alveolus and the dimensions of the bone structure of the ridge. Preservation of bone structure and bone dimensions is supported by the addition of bone substitutes, and integration processes are enhanced thanks to the formation of coagulums mixed with osteoinductive bone substitutes. The immediate installation of the implant has an exceptional advantage in terms of resorption flow and bone remodeling processes.

In oral implantology, there is more and more debate about the appropriate moment of implant placement; not only because of the bone-implant relationship, but also because of the stability of the soft tissues. The stability of soft tissues becomes extremely important for the entire implant-prosthetic rehabilitation, especially if it concerns the aesthetic region. The author's experience shows that the risk of immediate implant placement and an unfavorable aesthetic result can occur due to buccal soft tissue recession. How pronounced this soft tissue recession can be depends on: gingival biotype, implant position, bone dimensions in the implant region, bone level around adjacent teeth, and soft tissue level.

It should be emphasized that if the implant is placed as lingually/palatally as possible, a good basis is created for the thickening of the buccal marginal soft tissue with a soft subepithelial connective tissue graft, thus creating the conditions for a good aesthetic result.

In this regard, care must also be taken to fill the gap between the implant surface and the alveolar bone wall with a bone substitute or PRF procedure. The justification for the immediate installation of the implant in the alveolus immediately after a tooth extraction is confirmed by some studies on the percentage of success (98.4%) and failure (0.82%), and after four years the percentage of success was 97.5%.

To evaluate the success of the immediate installation of implants and immediately loaded implants, I compared those results with the results of installed implants in the edentulous region with a long wait after implant installation by performing an immediate implantation with immediate loading in the same patient at the same time on one side of the jaw. On the long side, in the edentulous region, implants are installed with a long wait to load. The results after 12 months were the same, which was confirmed in many similar cases.

In what period of time do the most intense changes occur in the soft tissues?

The main changes in the soft tissues occur in the first three months after implant placement, and six months after implant placement, the soft tissues stabilize. However, by monitoring the patient with follow-up examinations, it can be stated that the remodeling of soft tissues continues even after six months; while the papilla with a good bone base tends to gain height over time, which certainly improves the aesthetic result. Marginal recession also occurs, and to prevent a recession, thickening of the buccal marginal soft tissue with a subepithelial connective tissue graft can be attempted, thereby reducing the possibility of recession.

Which attitudes are correct when it comes to prosthetic work in the front of the upper and lower jaw. Should prosthetic work be done in metal-ceramic or zirconium?

When it comes to the immediate installation of implants, especially if it is done immediately after tooth extraction in the frontal regions, a fixed provisional prosthetic restoration should be made of soft material, in acrylic. In both jaws, the aesthetic risk due to soft tissues should be taken into account. For this reason, it is not indicated to set temporary mobile allowances. Definitive prosthetic works can be done in metal ceramics or zirconium. Zirconium has a certain aesthetic advantage in the aesthetic region of the upper jaw. However, the possibility of its application also depends on the position of the antagonist, because zirconium, due to its high hardness, can affect the osseointegration processes. In the lateral regions, where the occlusal forces are the strongest, prosthetic work on implants made of zirconium is not desirable. The dimension of the available horizontal alveolar bone in that region is often insufficient to receive and distribute the forces of mastication. Thus, a bad prosthetic solution can compromise the entire effort.

In cases where there is root malformation with a fistula where it is not possible to perform endodontic treatment, and a bent root is not an indication for an apicotomy. What procedure to apply?

When it comes to the case shown in the following pictures, the only possible procedure that can be applied is the extraction of the central right incisor and the immediate installation of the implant with the immediate loading of the provisional crown. When it comes to root resections, personal attitude root resection is an outdated method of treatment considering the high range of oral implantology. In decades of practice, I have never seen lamellar bone restored after root resection. By resecting the root, many bundles of tubular infected canals are opened, which disturbs the biological homeostatic balance in that part and compact bone is never formed in that place, and the periapical space is filled with fibrous tissue due to biological imbalance, i.e. disturbed homeostasis. Oral surgeons probably have a different opinion, and the opinion of the author of the book stems from several decades of experience. Tooth extraction, preservation of the alveolus, augmentation with bone substitutes (the PRF method is the ideal solution for the restoration of the lamellar bone wall), immediate installation of implants with immediate loading is the only correct course of treatment. The treatment shown in the following pictures (18.315 to 18.329.) justifies what has been said before.

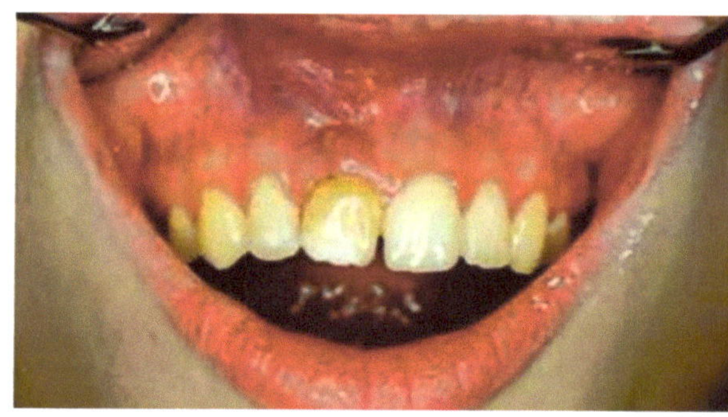

Figure 18.315. Due to the malformation of the root of the right central incisor, there was a loss of laminar bone in the lower third of the root with entrapped processes of the buccal soft tissues.

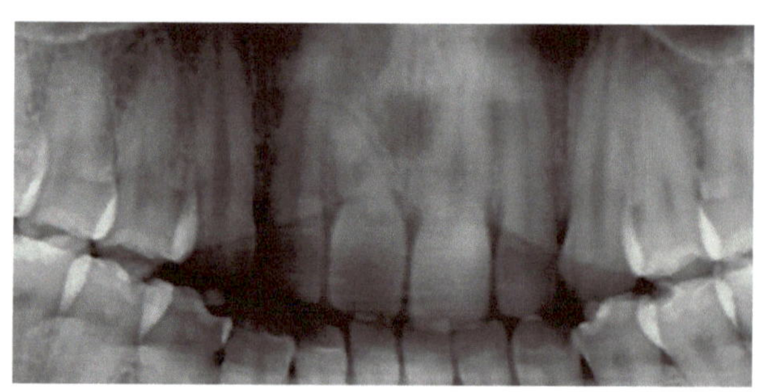

Figure 18.316. The root is curved distally, and there is a considerable amount of compact apical bone above the root of the central incisor.

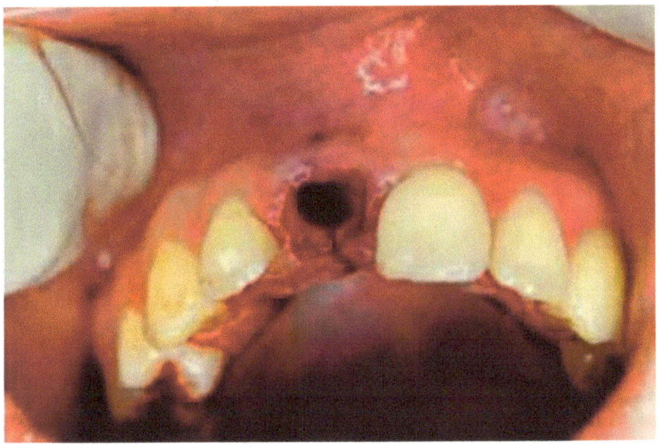

Figure 18.317. Extraction of the central incisor (11).

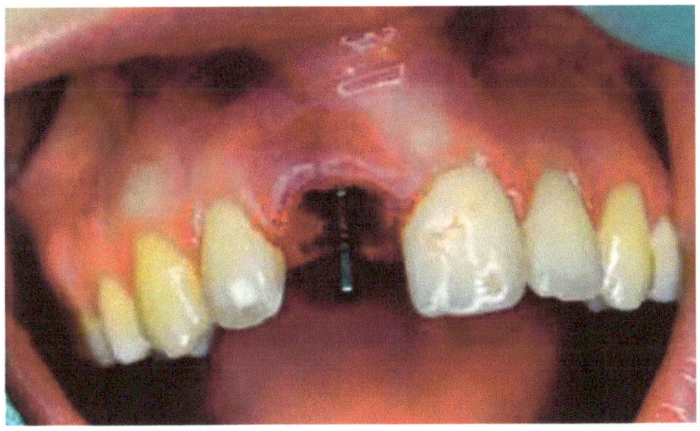

Figure 18.318. Checking the depth of the implant bed and the position towards the palatal.

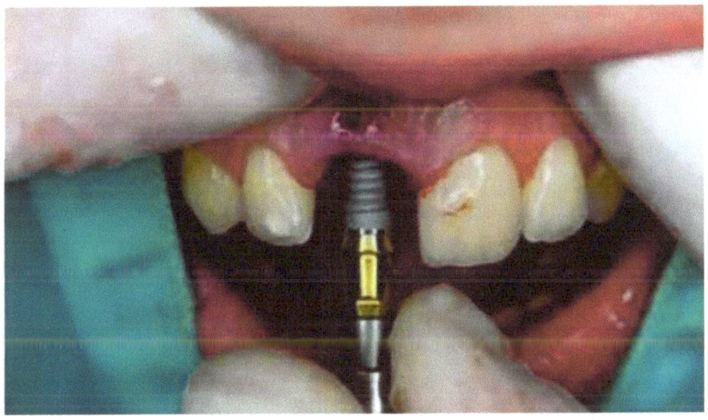

Figure 18.319. Installation of implants immediately after tooth extraction.

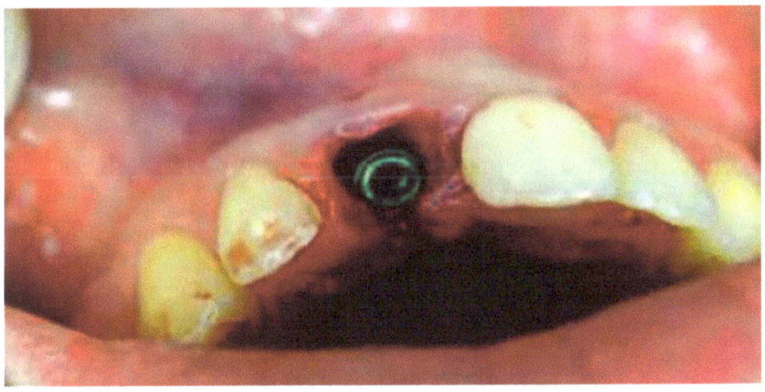

Figure 18.320. Immediately after the extraction, an implant with a diameter of 4 mm and a length of 15 mm was inserted. Implant positioned more palatally.

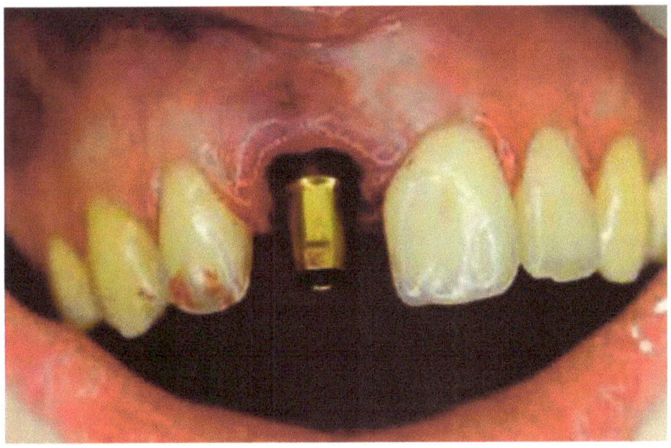

Figure 18.321. Positioned bracket more palatally.

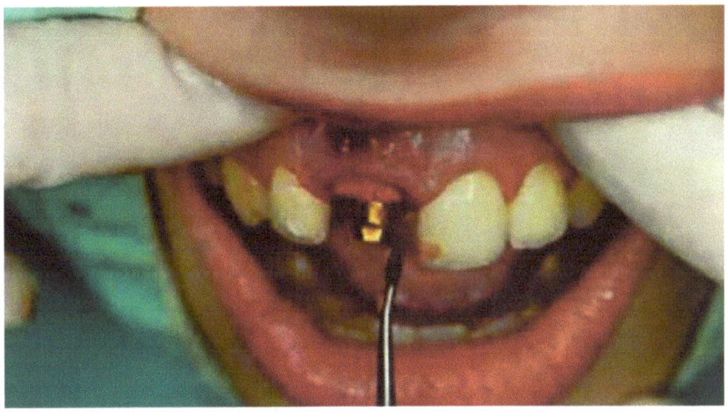

Figure 18.322. Without lifting the flap, soft tissue treatment is performed, the collagen resorptive membrane is drawn at the beginning of the destroyed lamella, and the space of the destroyed lamella is filled with a bone substitute.

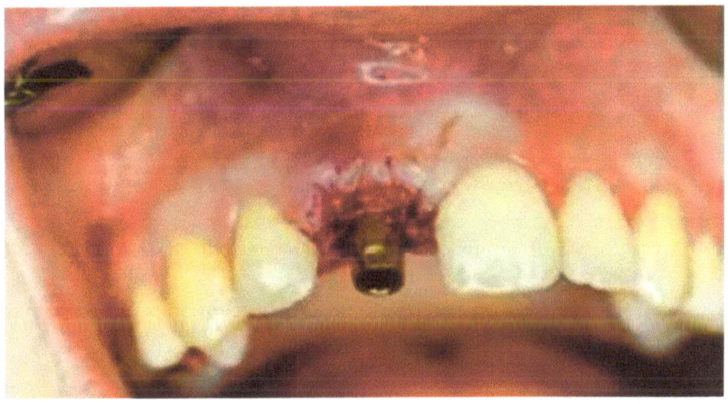

Figure 18.323. Processing of soft tissues in preparation for shaping the marginal edge with a provisional crown.

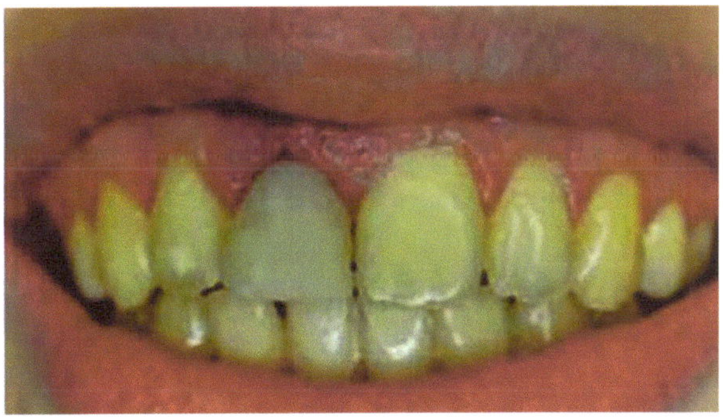

Figure 18.324. Temporary crown immediately after tooth extraction and implant placement.

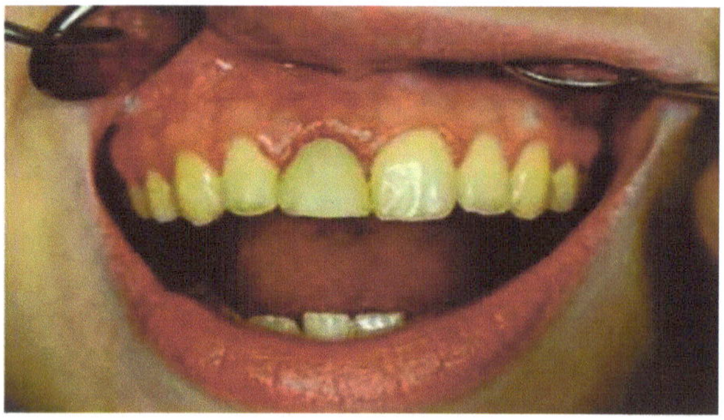

Figure 18.325. Condition after two weeks of immediate implantation with immediate loading. A shortened procedure with one surgical intervention is a great relief for the patient. Avoided temporary mobile compensation and traumatization of soft tissues.

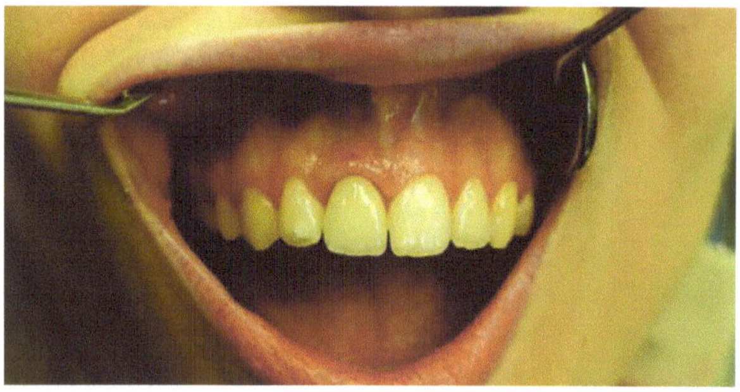

Figure 18.326. Preserved interdental papilla. Control after 12 months.

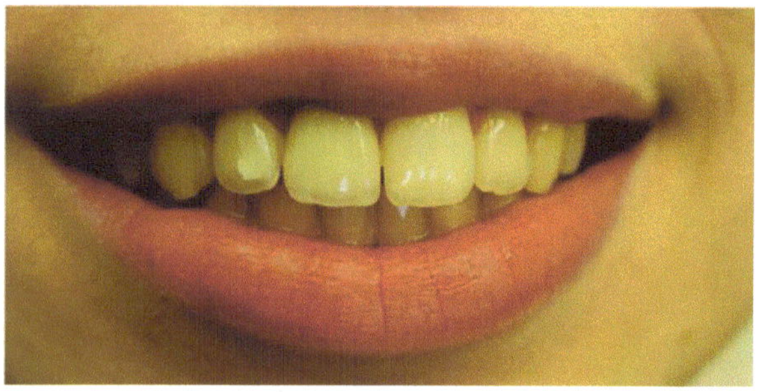

Figure 18.327. Coordinated harmony with definitive prosthetic work, and the aesthetic effect is supported by a favorable laugh line.

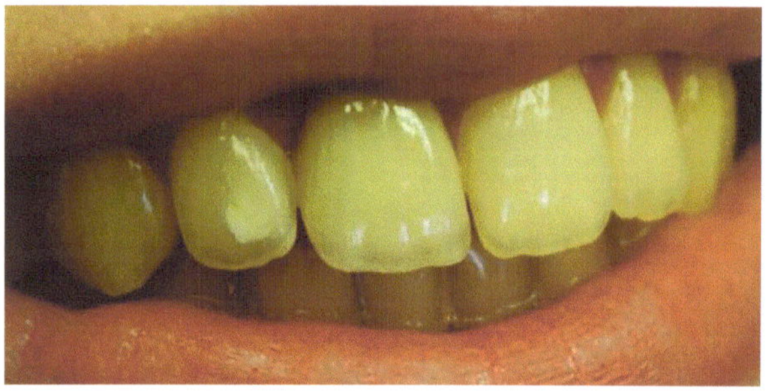

Figure 18.328. The result of implant prosthetic treatment: functional and aesthetic satisfaction of the patient with immediate implantation and loading immediately after tooth extraction.

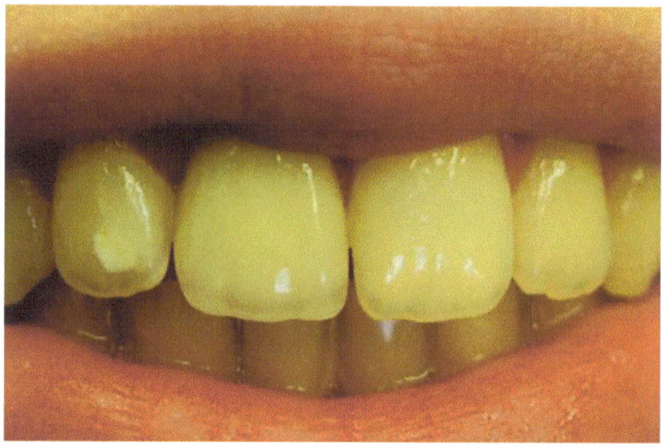

Figure 18.329. Esthetic result Appearance of definitive zirconium central incisor crown (11) on implant and zirconia crown support. Copied all the details adjacent to the tooth: shape, color and pigmentation effects.

When it comes to implant treatment, more and more attention is paid to aesthetics, especially in the frontal region. Despite a good prosthetic reconstruction, it happens that the aesthetics are compromised by the recession of the soft tissues around the neck and the implant support. What microsurgical procedures can be undertaken to meet the aesthetic requirements of patients?

When the position was advocated that oral implantology had the only role in the return of chewing function, the role and formation of soft tissues around the support of prosthetic works were not considered. However, after gingival recessions in natural teeth began to be solved in periodontology with soft connective tissue grafts through a microsurgical procedure taken from the palate, the indications for gingival recession therapy after implant placement were expanded, especially in the aesthetic region. Plastic reconstructions of soft tissues when covering recessions around implants also fulfill aesthetic requirements.

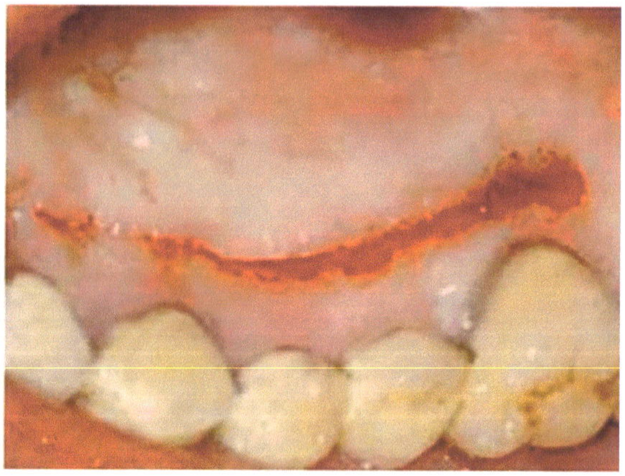

Figure 18.330. The incision from where the subepithelial graft of the palate is to be taken.

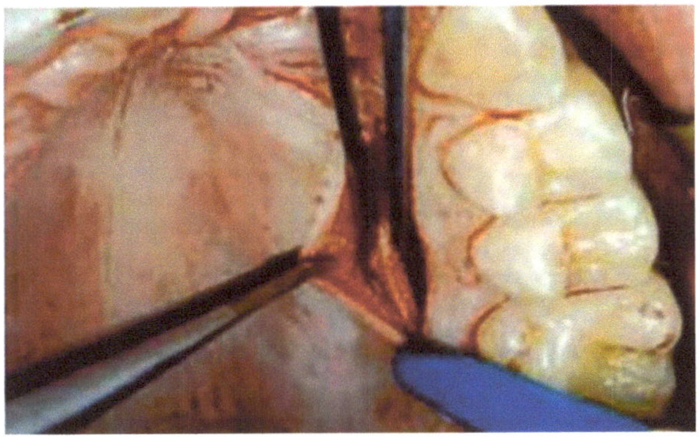

Figure 18.331. Connective tissue grafting procedure.

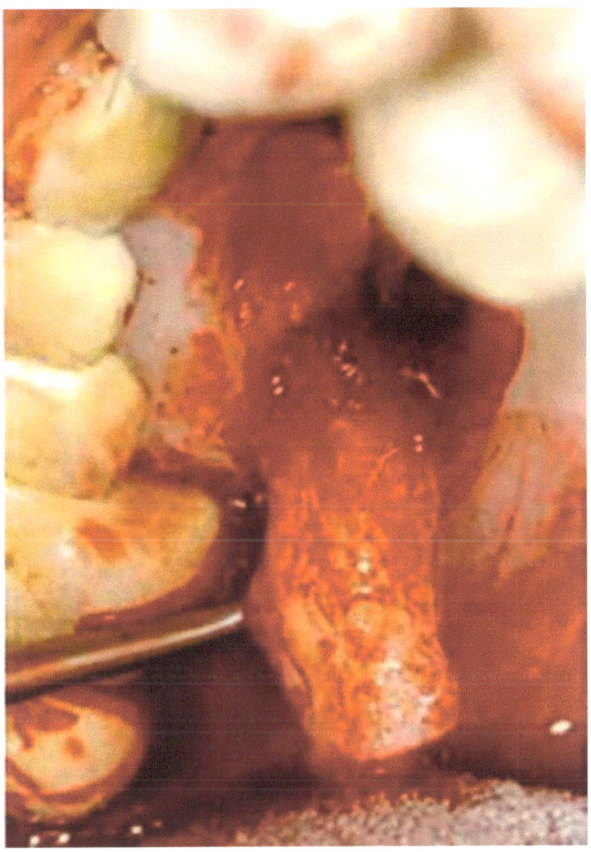

Figure 18.332. A prepared connective tissue graft taken from the palate.

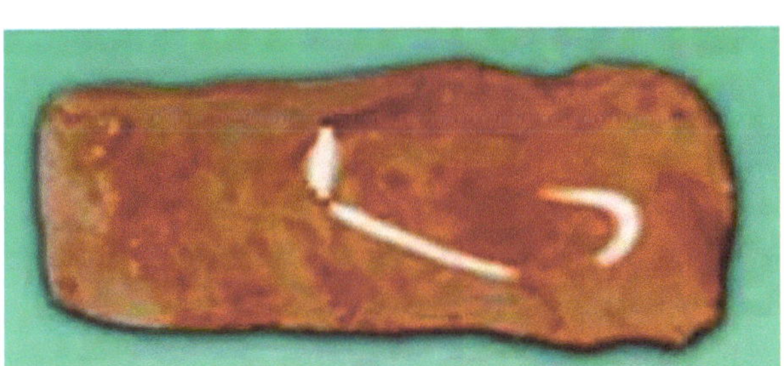

Figure 18.333. Prepared subepithelial connective tissue graft from the palate.

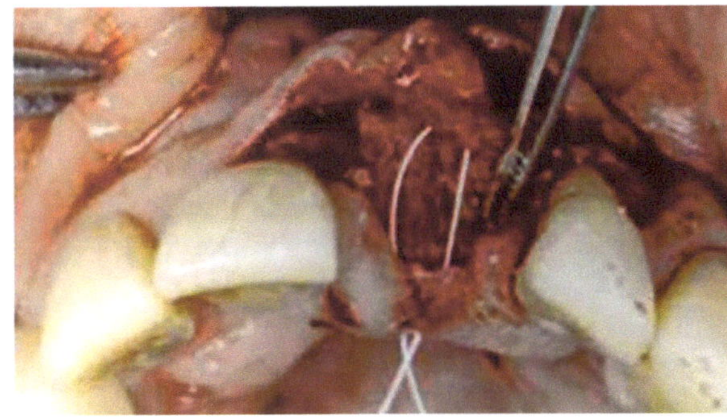

Figure 18.334. Preparation of the undermined soft palatal tissue, and the flap is tied with a return suture.

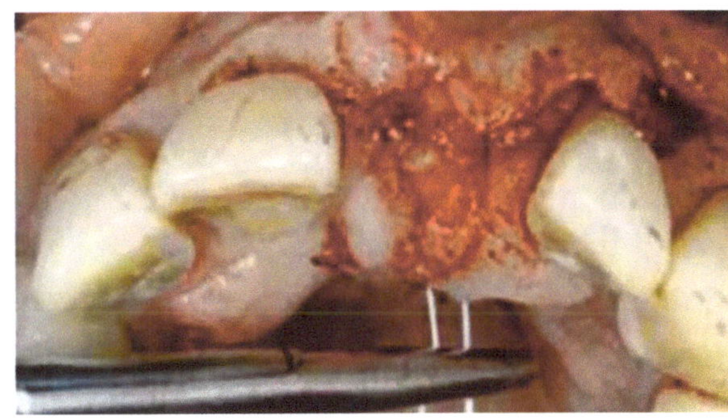

Figure 18.335. The petiole-shaped buccal flap should be pulled towards the palatal side with a return suture, i.e. into the palatal pocket, in order to cover the augmented field with bone marrow and collagen resorbable membrane.

The application of connective tissue grafts and microsurgical techniques has changed attitudes not only in periodontology but also in implantology. Connective tissue grafts, whether free or stalked (Figures 18.330-18.334), can be used in various cases in oral implant therapy. For example, after tooth extraction and implant installation (if delayed implant installation is planned), during implantation in a fresh alveolus immediately after extraction, and during soft tissue correction, prosthetic reconstruction, whether it is carried by a natural tooth or an implant, create space for papilla reconstruction.

Burgund and Linde's research showed that the thickness of the soft tissue shaping beyond the biological width significantly affects the crestal bone For this reason, many authors recommend the use of connective tissue grafts, which helps the reconstruction of alveolar ridge defects in augmentations with bone substitutes, which is also manifested by thickening of the soft tissue. It has been proven that the risk factor of tissue recession around the implant depends on the thickness of the soft tissue; at the same time, with a thin biotype of the gingiva, the dark parts of the implant material show through, which worsens the aesthetics.

Recessions of soft tissues on implants, when they appear after placement of prosthetic works, manifest as visible aesthetic defects, especially in the aesthetic region, which cannot be predictably corrected with connective tissue transplants. Experience shows that the key risk factor for the occurrence of soft tissue recession and sieving of the color of the implant material (door and support) is the thin biotype of the gingiva, and the positioning of the implant (Figures 18.336- 18.340).

If the implant is positioned too vestibular, then the recession of the soft tissues can no longer be affected by microsurgery. That is why the most important thing is the exact three-dimensional positioning of the implant so that there is no forward-emphasized risk.

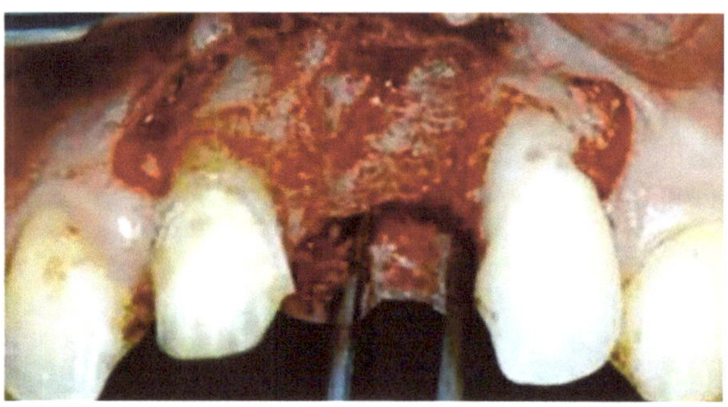

Figure 18.336. By raising the flap, visibility of the bone defect is obtained, and a mucoperiosteal flap is shaped by a microsurgical intervention.

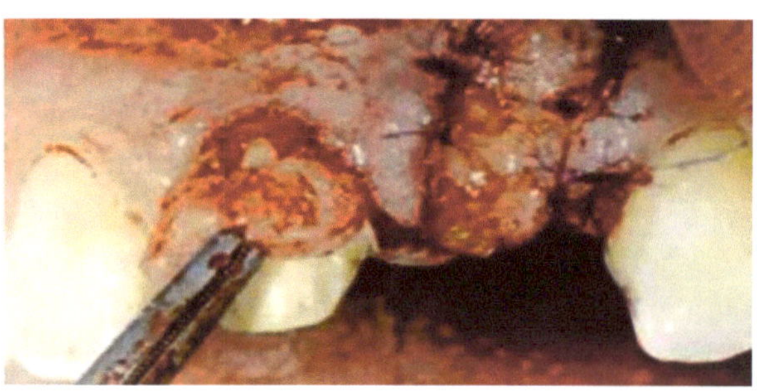

Figure 18.337. Immediately after the extraction and closure of the wound with a connective tissue graft, the soft tissue defect of the left central incisor (#21) is reconstructed, and on the right incisor (#22) it is necessary to prepare the vestibular pocket in order to place the graft in it with a return suture.

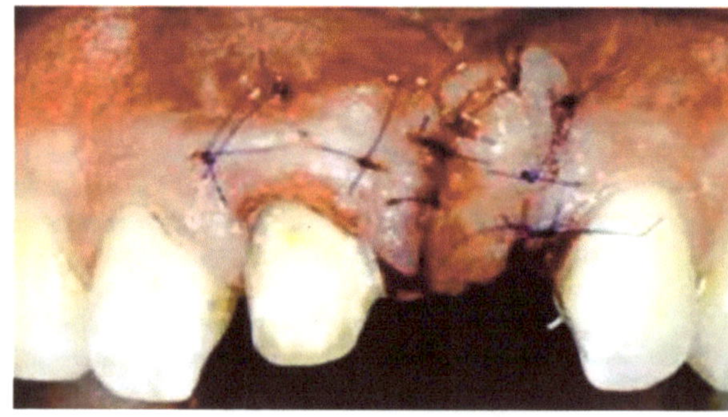

Figure 18.338. Microsurgically reconstructed soft tissue.

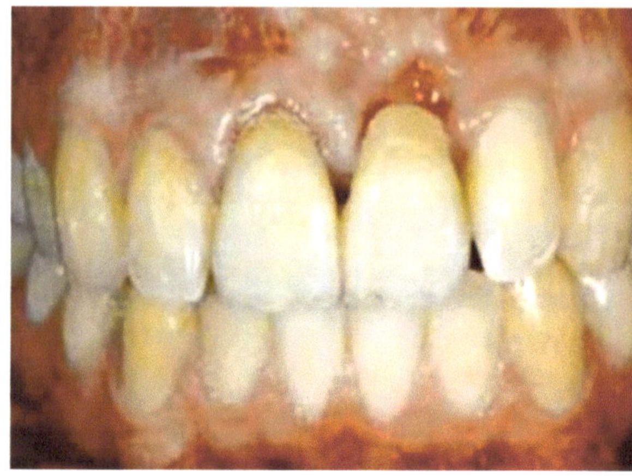

Figure 18.339. Appearance of reconstructed soft tissues with connective tissue graft after 6 weeks.

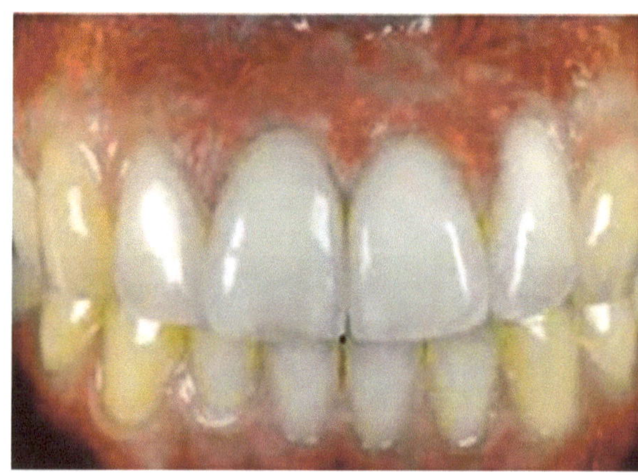

Figure 18.340. Appearance two years after placement of definitive compensation.

From the previously presented cases, it can be concluded that pre-implant management of the extraction wound is very important in order to determine which procedure should be applied; whether to use free mucosal grafts at the same time as bone reconstruction with autologous bone or a xenogeneic bone substitute covered with a collagen resorbable membrane in order to create conditions for later delayed implantation of the implant, or to perform the entire procedure with immediate procedures. It is a matter of judgment and experience of the therapist.

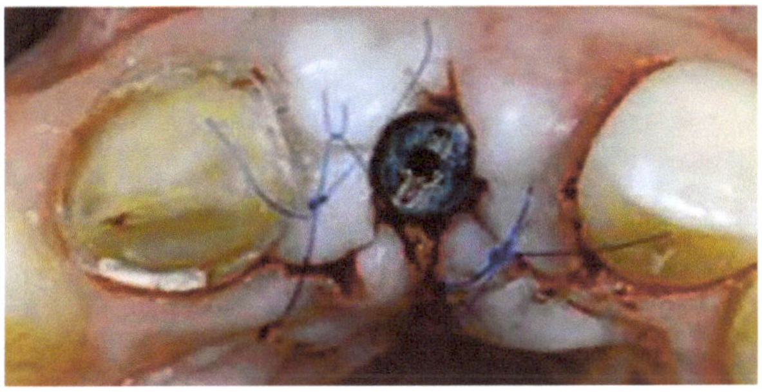

Figure 18.341. Positioned implant in the augmented region with soft tissue reconstruction with a connective tissue graft.

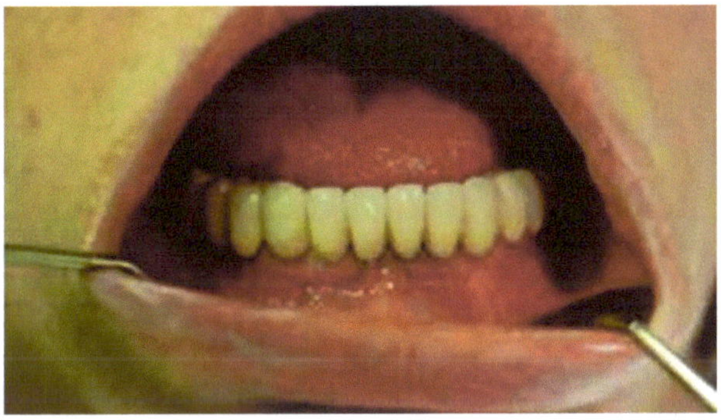

Figure 18.342. Screening of implant material when the gingival biotype is thin.

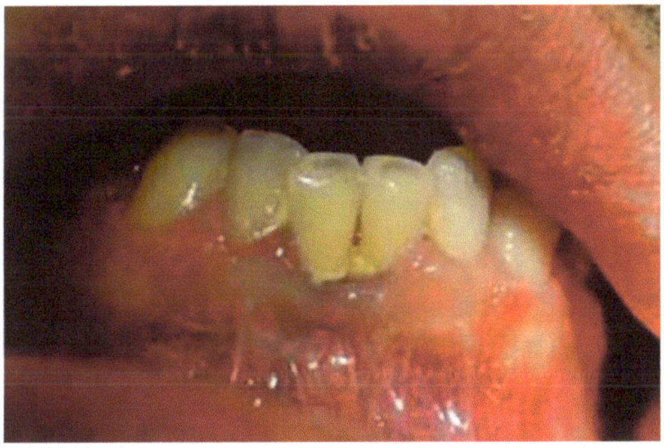

Figure 18.343. Thin gingival biotype and poor oral hygiene can cause recession. A case of a patient with delayed primary teeth, alveolar ridge perforation and augmentation. Condition after 8 years.

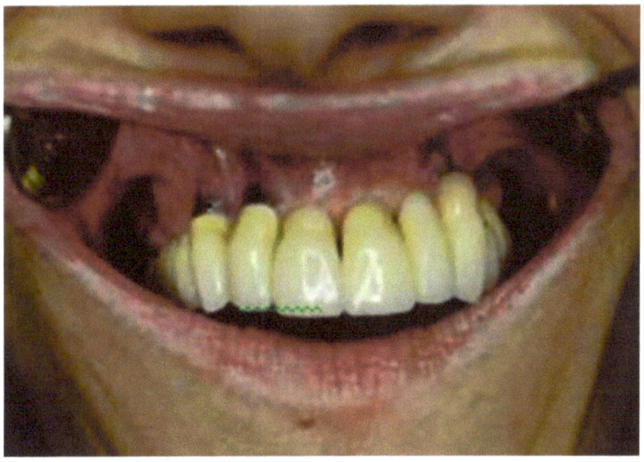

Figure 18.344. Soft tissue recessions caused by implant positioning too vestibular, poor prosthetic performance and insufficient oral hygiene. It is not possible to perform soft tissue correction with connective tissue transplants.

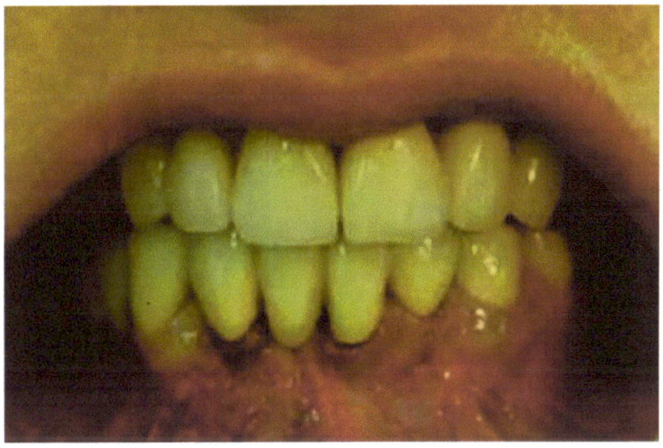

Figure 18.345. Too labially positioned implants and thin gingival biotype are aesthetic risk factors SIfting dark materials and substrates for soft tissue recession.

It can be concluded that in several places in the book attention is paid to precautions, risk and complications. Why?

Indications for the installation of endosseous implants are expanding more and more, and thus the number of implant installations, is increasing so much that even the biggest supporters of oral implantology could not have predicted it. Installing implants has become a part of daily routine practice. Oral rehabilitation in modern dentistry is unthinkable without reliable implant-prosthetic solutions, with predictable long-term successful results. Of course, such a Himalayan jump in the application of implants is not always accompanied by a successful outcome.

The number of complications will also increase. For this reason, the author devoted four chapters to this problem: "Knowledge of anatomical structures important for oral implantology", "Risks in oral implantology", "Contract with the Patient" and virtual "Conversation with the Patient".

With the daily routine application of implants, there is a danger that also follows the pharmaceutical industry: only the manufacturer benefits from a large percentage of the drugs produced. The way of marketing is so developed that many swallow pharmaceutical products in large quantities, without thinking whether their liver can handle it without consequences. This phenomenon also appears in oral implantology; sites are published with bad taste, low prices, and false promises. Of course, behind this is the installation of untested, cheap implant systems without certificates, scientific analyses, and confirmations. This is mostly done by young, inexperienced dentists, which is against the moral code of the medical profession.

For this reason, the author of the book draws attention to the complications that can occur when it comes to oral implantology. Nerve injuries may present with transient symptoms such as paraesthesia, but permanent nerve disruption can result in a lawsuit with unpleasant consequences. In highly developed industrial countries, where the number of implanted implants increased to hundreds of thousands, the number of lawsuits also increased.

What does practice say, what are the most common complications of oral surgery and in what order could they be ranked?

The spectrum of oral surgical complications as a result of the installation of endosseous implants can be from minimal ones, such as pain and swelling, to more serious ones, such as iatrogenic nerve injuries (lower dental nerve, chin nerve), injury to the lingual artery, injury to the sinus mucosa with severe bleeding from the sinus cavity and the resulting hematoma, infection and a very serious complication by inserting the entire implant into the sinus cavity (Fig. 18.346).

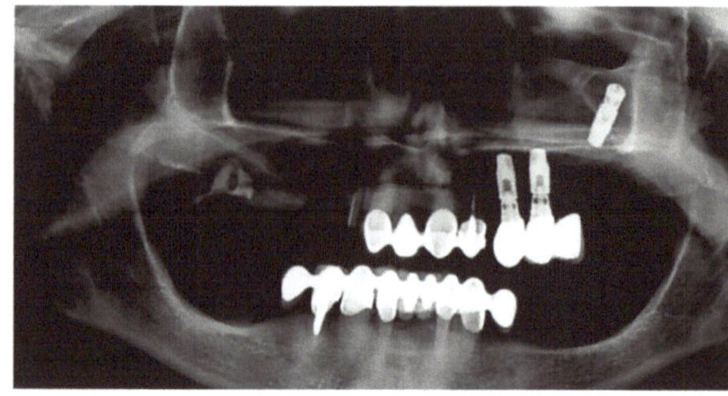

Figure 18.346. Complicated incident of inserting an implant into the sinus, which is a consequence of the dentist's inexperience. In addition to professional and ethical failure - the patient was not informed about the incident.

Inserting the implant into the sinus is a consequence of surgical inexperience. Repairing this complication is extremely complex. Implant removal can be performed in several ways: transnasal, transanal or intraoral surgical approach.

Major complications during the installation of implants in the lower jaw include profuse bleeding during the procedure, along with the formation of an extensive hematoma of the floor of the oral cavity, which can also lead to airway obstruction. For this reason, the installation of implants in the lower jaw must be approached with great caution and bearing in mind the proximity of the sublingual artery in the lingual periosteum. Even minimal perforations can cause profuse bleeding due to injury to the sublingual artery or its branches.

Also, injuries to the submental and mylohyoid arteries can cause profuse bleeding that can only be stopped by ligation of the injured arteries. However, more often minor complications occur that pass quickly: hematoma caused by rough manipulation and soft tissue trauma, nerve compression, which is manifested by transient paraesthesia, swelling that passes quickly with the use of dexamethasone, and minor infections.

The most important thing for a practicing dentist is to be aware of all possible complications and to recognize them early. The doctor remembers mistakes, and the patient suffers!

In which complications would the author classify damage to the root of the adjacent tooth?

The contact between the implant surface and the root of an adjacent tooth is a rare but serious complication. This issue typically arises from inexperience or a poorly planned surgical procedure. Such complications can be avoided by conducting a detailed radiological analysis and studying model analyses prior to the operation. Additionally, selecting the appropriate diameter for the implant is crucial.

This complication may stem from unfavorable anatomical structures, as well as a lack of knowledge about them. Therefore, I have paid special attention to the anatomical structures that are essential for the safe placement of implants.

Based on my many years of experience, I believe that a realistic assessment of mistakes made during surgery is vital for preventing more serious complications. Throughout the book, the reader will notice a recurring emphasis on caution and my acknowledgment of past mistakes to ensure they are not repeated.

I must admit that with insufficient bone quantity—especially if it is accompanied by poor quality type IV bone—the effectiveness of augmentation procedures is not always reliable. Consequently, some augmentations, whether in the upper or lower jaw, may end in failure despite advancements in bone substitutes.

However, practice and experience say that it is possible to achieve the desired results in another way. Thanks to the technological development and improvement of implant systems, by choosing an adequate implant design, augmentation can be avoided. The question is how and in what way to realize the predictability of a successful solution; whether by choosing a reduced-diameter implant (one-piece of 3 mm, so-called "mini-implants") or two-piece, with a diameter of 3 mm, 3.2 mm, 3.3 to 3.5 mm. The use of reduced-diameter implants requires sufficient ridge height.

Another procedure to avoid extensive augmentation is the use of shorter implants with a larger diameter, if there is adequate width of available bone. The author's experience shows that the use of narrow diameter implants (Narrow diameter implants NDI) has multiple advantages. Their biggest advantage is that they expand the indications for implantation in extremely narrow alveolar ridges, i.e. in patients in whom implant therapy would be impossible. The use of these implants, in addition to significantly reducing the patient's morbidity, shortening the time of implantological treatment, also significantly reduces the costs of the entire treatment. Also, the installation of NDI implants can be applied in cases where the interdental space is less than 6 mm, especially in the frontal region.

Implants with a reduced diameter, in addition to the indicated advantages, also have a major disadvantage in terms of increased biomechanical risk. The cortical load with NDI implants is significantly higher than with implants of standard diameters. At the junction of the bone and the surface of the implant, there are far greater stress loads, which can lead to the fracture of the implant. For example, it has been proven that the stress loaded at the junction of the bone and the surface of a reduced diameter implant is greater when the diameter of a 4.1 mm implant is reduced to a diameter of 3.3 mm than when a 4.8 mm implant is reduced to a diameter of 4, 1 mm.

What are the author's experiences with the use of reduced-diameter implants?

Despite the satisfactory results with this type of implant and the fact that it is also a "social solution", the author's opinion is that implants of standard diameters, due to biomechanical risk factors, have an advantage.

When there are unfavorable dimensions of the available bone, implant placement can be risky. In order to avoid augmentation, what are the more recent attitudes to the installation of implants in those places?

Many attitudes in oral implantology are constantly changing. They are changed by practice, that is, the search for reducing the time of implantological-prosthetic treatment, the patient's morbidity, and also for reducing the costs of the entire procedure.

More and more attention is being paid to the question of how to avoid the risk of injury to anatomical structures in cases where it is desired to install implants with an insufficient amount of available bone in those places. Even though we have several surgical techniques available to increase bone height, there are still dilemmas which one to choose. Attempts are made to simplify the procedure by avoiding augmentation, either with bone graft blocks or guided bone regeneration (GBR). Of course, one could list some other surgical techniques that are more in the domain of theory, but not in practice, I don't see the practical application of taking bone blocks from the thigh and similar procedures. It is not applicable in wider dental practice.

To shorten the treatment time and reduce the material costs of the patient, solutions in the application of short implants are increasingly sought.

The principles established by Carl Misch, as presented in his various books, regarding the minimum bone height of 10 mm have been definitively abandoned. He emphasized that 10 mm implants are not recommended, and at that time, short implants were not discussed. While I somewhat agree with Misch's views, my perspective also depends on the quality of the bone. For instance, if the bone type is classified as quality I or II, the use of newer designs of shorter implants, specifically those less than 10 mm in length, is justified.

Even today, there are varying definitions of what constitutes a short implant and differing opinions on the matter. Some authors categorize implants under 11 mm as short implants, while others restrict this classification to those under 8 mm.

In my experience, implants shorter than 8 mm, which are usually classified as short implants, can yield predictable outcomes, although they always carry a certain level of risk.

Furthermore, there is no consensus on what defines standard implants. One perspective states that implants with a diameter above 3.5 mm are considered standard, while another viewpoint considers short implants with a diameter above 5 mm and lengths of 6 mm, 7 mm, and 8 mm to be standard.

However, паст short implant designs cannot be compared to the more recent creations. Newer technologies have significantly improved the treatment of the implant surface, and thus better integration relationships in the lateral regions, where the bone is of poorer quality (type III or type IV). The length of the implant, the surface of which has been treated with laser technology, is one of the decisive factors for achieving good integration between the implant and the bone.

The latest research comparing implanted short wider implants without augmentation and implants implanted with augmentation in order to increase the vertical amount of bone showed that the percentage of survival after 5 years is the same. There was no difference in marginal bone loss. For the above reasons, and mainly due to the shortening of the rehabilitation procedure, the views on the advantages of installing short implants and avoiding augmentation are increasingly advocated.

What is the reason for using short implants explained from a biomechanical point of view?

For the long-term predictability of the success of short implants, two prerequisites must be met: the horizontal width of the alveolar bone must not be less than 9 mm, and the diameter of the implant must be greater than 5 mm.

In the book, readers will encounter previous views that the length of the implant and the height of the crown should at least maintain a 1:1 ratio. However, recent insights suggest that this postulate has changed; the diameter of the implant can compensate for its shorter length.

From a biomechanical perspective, occlusal forces during chewing are strongest at the shoulder of the implant and on the first thread. A larger diameter implant results in lower forces acting on the bone. Therefore, the width of short implants compensates for the height of the crown. A control radiological examination performed after one year can reveal whether the occlusal load from lateral forces is physiological or indicative of overload.

The first thread of the implant helps absorb the tension from occlusal forces and directs these forces towards functional actions, leading to less bone breakdown around the shoulder of the implant. It has been observed that in the first year of functional load, the average loss of marginal bone is about 0.50 mm. However, after five and ten years, the height of the crestal bone remains stable.

If the views that the ratio of the length of the implant and the crown must be 1:1 are abandoned, how should the crown replacement be performed?

In response to this question, the author would recommend that one should always try to achieve that relationship. Why? Biomechanical considerations in oral implantology follow the laws of physics, which are based on the principle of lever action. The shorter the arm of the lever (crown) on the implant, about the length of the implant, the more favorable the biomechanical effects of occlusal forces on the implant. It follows from this that the unfavorable effect of the lever due to the height of the crown and its relationship to the length of the implant should be neutralized to prevent the breakdown of the marginal bone, due to the unfavorable effect of occlusal forces on the shoulder of the implant. It is convenient to connect short implants in a block because in this way favorable conditions are created for an even reception and distribution of chewing forces.

What is the author's conclusion, advice and recommendation to colleagues when implant placement should be applied in limited conditions?

In the time of initial enthusiasm and prestige, I solved cases with insufficiently available bone in various ways. Most leaf implants were available and I can emphasize that the percentage of survival was satisfactory. Disappointing results with the so-called "disk" implants made me stop using these implants at the beginning of the eighties of the last century. For this reason, I am not a supporter of Ihde's so-called "basal implant" which has recently been advertised, first of all, because of its extremely aggressive implantation. Perhaps this opinion is subjective, but the opposite view has not yet been proven by any valid statistical data.

In the case of insufficient ridge height and proximity to anatomical structures in the lateral regions, primarily in the lower jaw, a newer design of short implants with an aggressive thread should be tried. A crucial condition is the satisfactory width of the alveolar ridge for the placement of larger-diameter implants. In the lateral regions, the occlusal forces are the strongest, and by installing implants with a larger diameter, the necessary biomechanical requirements are met.

It is known that many periapical changes can be successfully resolved by endodontic treatment instead of surgery. Is it significant for possible implantation in a later period? How does all this relate to oral implantology?

A healthy and compact bone is required for the successful installation of an implant in the jawbone. By shortening the roots when periapical lesions are treated surgically, primarily from the biomechanical aspect, a lever action is obtained that affects the remodeling of the bone tissue traumatized by the surgical procedure. Countless open channels remain on the cut root, in which pathogenic content can be retained. Homeostasis is definitely disturbed in that place. Compact bone is usually not formed in the periapical space of the cut root. If such a shortened root were used for prosthetic work, it would never be a reliable support. Of course, the resorption processes of the rest of the roots should not be neglected. In cases where the resected tooth must later be extracted (most often due to recurrence of infection and existing inflammation), and the installation of an implant is planned in that place, augmentation is mandatory due to the lack of compact bone, with a longer waiting period for the healing of the bone and surrounding tissues. Immediate installation of implants in such a milieu would lead to unwanted consequences.

How to explain the success of this method, verified in practice?

If periapical lesions are treated endodontically, a better biological balance is achieved between the forces that attack the tissues in the organism and the organism as a whole and the immune defense forces to establish homeostatic harmony. This is how homeostasis of the tissues of the periapical space is maintained, supported by the immune (defense) forces of the organism (Fig. 18.298). I believe that these thoughts on the concept of biological balance are the forerunners of the PRF method, which consists of a high concentration of growth factors extracted from the blood of the person to whom it is applied. The concept of a biological boundary between the local apical defense and infectious agents in the root canal leads to an understanding of the special pathology of the periapical space, and it is especially important to understand why the damaged apical region returns to normal restored bone structure as soon as the infection is removed from the canal. SECANTE CAUSSA, SECANTE EFFECTUS! (Remove the causes, the consequences will disappear by themselves).

In chronic apical periodontitis, there is a fine line between the destabilization of the apical region and the number of bacteria in the root canal. This equation can be represented as follows: canal infection = (f) defense of the organism, because local resistance is expressed only to the extent necessary to stop the virulence of bacteria from the canal to the periapical region. Local defenses do not have the power to reach infectious agents and their toxins within the ducts.

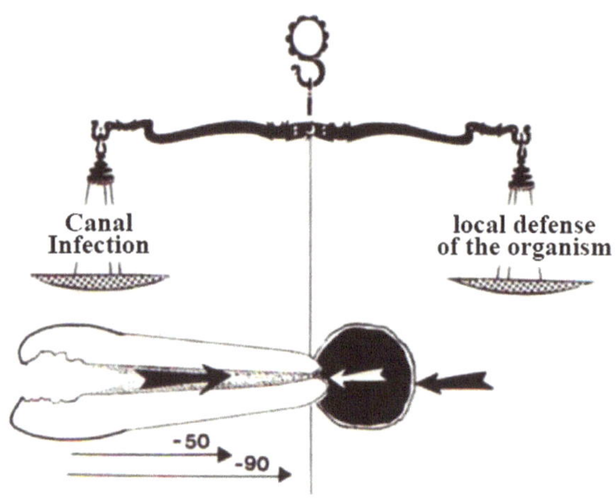

Figure 18.347. Establishing the biological balance of canal infection and local defense of the organism. This relationship of biological balance is disturbed by the resection of the roots, the possibility of retaining pathogenic residues in the tubular canals.

This concept of the biological equation shows how the local defense in the periapical region is economically organized, its activity always corresponding to the number of bacteria in the root canal and their virulence. As soon as, with appropriate endodontic treatment, the number of bacteria in the root canal is reduced, the apical defense is in a more favorable situation. By removing only 50% of the bacteria from the canal, the recovery of the bone structure in the periapical region is manifested. If 80% or even 95% of the bacterial content is removed from the canal, the recovery process of the periapical region will be even faster. The body's defenses can at a certain point overcome the canal infection and lead to complete healing and the formation of compact bone in the periapical space. In this way, the disturbed homeostasis is restored in that space (Fig. 18.347).

Why was this problem found in a book on oral implantology?

I was thinking about whether it is appropriate for such a topic to be found and take up space in a book on oral implantology. Since this book is written by a practitioner, experience was the guideline for writing, both about successes and failures in practice. The dentist often finds himself in a dilemma, whether the tooth should be extracted or saved. Given that oral implantology is increasingly applied in everyday practice, patients must be viewed from several aspects: professional, ethical, and not exclusively from a profitable aspect. For example, a patient recently came to whom a younger colleague, with a prominent advertising site, recommended extracting 11 teeth and replacing them with implants. The "treatment" plan was enacted based on profitable greed, not professional conscience. Of course, there was also the high cost of treatment. However, a detailed examination revealed that the case can be solved in another way, with prosthetic care without tooth extraction. The first reason is not only a significant reduction in the material costs of the patient, but also the unnecessary morbidity of the patient with the creation of disability in the mouth. I am sure that the attending physician would not apply that procedure to himself. The case was successfully resolved with prosthetic work without tooth extraction. The proposed "treatment" is a typical example of abuse of oral implantology for profit motives contrary to medical ethics. For this reason, this topic was included in the book on oral implantology

At the end of this conversation, when you have already decided to write this book and collect your experiences, what would you conclude using the treasury of memories: where is oral implantology today?

The answer to this question would be a summary of what was written in the book. In many places, as many answers as possible, and more with representations of solving complicated cases, the conclusion I emphasized can be drawn: oral implantology is in constant development, and its development is based on scientific knowledge and practical confirmations. From an unrecognized, long-contested branch of dentistry, oral implantology has become one of the most important disciplines without which the rehabilitation of disabilities in the oral cavity is unthinkable today. Toothlessness is a great handicap for a person, teeth mean multiple things for his overall health, both from the physical and psychological aspects.

In addition to the two fundamental goals of establishing function and restoration of aesthetics, the third goal is to restore the power of a smile to a person. About the first two goals, the third one will be considered by some as negligible and not so important. What this means for a person can be seen in the chapter "Returning your smile, security, and self-confidence with implants". I thought for a long time whether this chapter also belongs in this book. Eventually, I saw that it belonged. The same question could be asked about some other chapters in this book. Since the book is intended not only for practitioners, I am convinced those chapters are also very important (prosthetics, occlusion, lateral movements, events in the temporomandibular joint, etc.).

In the time of the pioneers of oral implantology, much information was unavailable to dentists, and not much could be learned from the very scarce literature. The only way to find out and learn something new was to visit many places where implantology took its first steps.

How informed was the patient?

Today, patients can find information about the possibilities of oral implantology via the Internet. This is their great advantage, while advertising sites are dangerous traps for the patient. Oral implantology, thanks to the development of science, has expanded its indications, and the demands of patients and their impatience to get prosthetic work as soon as possible have increased significantly.

It seems that the priority request of the patient is to shorten the treatment time to the smallest possible extent. Despite the increasing importance given to immediate loading in the last ten years, I started thinking about this problem in the late 1970s when Linkov's sheet endosseous one-piece implants dominated. At expert meetings, there was no opinion on how long to wait for the implant to be loaded, 3 to 4 weeks or three or six months.

Linkov himself changed his views. At first, he advocated the position that his one-piece implant can be loaded after 3-4 weeks, since with sheet implants, by tapping into the prepared bed, extraordinary primary stability was achieved.

However, in the practice of the author of the book, it happened that, despite the achieved good primary fixation, the implants, unloaded, after a few weeks of installation, were completely disintegrated and eventually removed.

Thinking about the reason for this failure, I came to the conclusion that in certain patients the lingual forces and their torques had a very unfavorable effect on the implant carrier and that this was the reason for the loss of the implant.

After several failures, I loaded the leaf implants on the same day after installation with acrylic temporary bridges, which the patients used for 6 weeks. After that, there was never a single loss of the implant, standing the test of time for several decades. I wrote to Mr. Link with my observations and he agreed with my views. At the scientific meeting in Liège (Belgium, 1980) I gave a lecture about the failures I had with the application of leaf implants, explaining the reasons for their occurrence.

Based on the experience gained at that time, I started solving the most complicated cases with immediate implantation and primary loading. The leading predictor of success was experience gained. Several cases are presented in the book. Based on the experience gained, it can also be said of proven courage, the primary load in most operations has priority. Implants that can be loaded with prosthetic work on the same day are a great benefit for the patient as well.

In most cases there is no need for delayed loading, because all research proves that the waiting time, in fact the resting time of the implant, is lost time for the patient, after a few years the results are the same.

What does immediate load success depend on?

The success of immediate loading depends on several factors: achieved osseointegration, which depends on the quality of the implant, i.e. from the type and shape of the implant, the laser technological treatment of the implant surface, the available bone and its quality; it is crucial that the surgical procedure is performed with as little bone trauma as possible during the preparation of the implant bed.

The author emphasized in many places in the book why he is forcing the primary burden. According to Wolff's rule that the bone should be put into function as soon as possible, we can determine the immediate load as functional, because this stimulates the regeneration of bone tissue, that is, faster and better osseointegration.

In orthopedics, it has been proven that in case of bone fractures, the callus is of better quality if the bone is put into function as soon as possible.

Based on the above, the conclusion would be that the immediate load has two goals:

- biological
- logistic.

Biological target:

- achieving faster and better osseointegration;
- action of forces during healing, by primary loading through precise temporary prosthetic work made of softer material (acrylate);
- reducing the action of those forces to physiological limits, which has a stimulating effect on the processes of osseointegration;
- shaping of the surrounding soft tissues with a definitive abutment.

By unscrewing the gingiva-former and screwing the carrier when taking impressions and samples in the mouth, as well as by repeating these procedures several times, the soft tissues are traumatized. The author explained this position in more detail in the book.

Logistics objective:

That is, the prosthetic and surgical phases are performed simultaneously. The difference between the protocol of immediate installation of the implant with immediate loading and the conventional solution with waiting for several months to load the implant, apart from the biological advantage of stimulating faster osseointegration, also aims to shorten the interval between the surgical and prosthetic phase.

For both phases, the experience of the practitioner and the coordination of the entire team, including the dental nurses and the dental technician, are important.

When it comes to the immediate installation of implants, the book shows very complicated cases in which the implants were installed without raising the flap, and in some cases the flap was raised. What is the decision on the method of intervention based on?

There is certainly less trauma to the soft tissues and a much more comfortable procedure for the patient if the flap is not raised. However, there are principles that must be respected, as well as principles when installing an implant in a fresh alveolus.

When installing implants without raising the flap, the dominant experience is gained. But regardless of great experience, one must always be careful. Before the procedure, a 3D image must be taken and the width of the ridge must be carefully assessed. Only with wide ridges is this procedure safe. Even when the ridge, at first glance, has width for implantation without raising the flap, a hasty decision can lead to bone perforation due to the concavity of the ridge. Rapid deterioration of the burr is a warning sign of poor quality bone. In the frontal region of the lower jaw, the flap should always be raised cautiously, for several reasons, primarily due to the proximity of blood vessels such as the sublingual artery. Likewise, when it comes to the immediate installation of the implant in a fresh alveolus, caution is needed in order for the result of the intervention to be successful. Here we are mainly talking about situations where periodontal teeth should be removed. Experience shows that the best results are when "delayed" implantation of implants is applied. What does that mean? After the extraction of the tooth, the alveolus should be treated radically so that it bleeds well and is closed by the primary coagulum. After that, it should be closed with a surgical suture and wait 3-4 weeks (the time when reparable processes are strongest) and then insert the implant. A condition for a successful outcome is good primary stability of the implant. The conclusion would be: be careful, and coordinate the ways of solving procedures with gaining experience.

You have explained the advantages of an endodontic approach to the treatment of periapical lesions. Still, why is it discussed in a book on oral implantology?

There are two basic reasons to talk about it in a book like this: practical and ethical. A long time ago, at a congress held in the former Yugoslavia, I asked: why such a strict separation of disciplines in dentistry, when in practical work it is not good, neither for the doctor nor for the patient. Acquiring knowledge can be in several ways. Paper as an administrative document (diploma) does not have to be a confirmation of fundamental knowledge. I also presented the following example: a dentist who only treats teeth pays attention to the treatment of a gangrenous tooth for a long time. After therefore, if the treatment fails, the dentist refers the patient to an oral surgeon for root resection. After the resection, the prosthetist concluded that that tooth should be extracted, because it is an unreliable support for prosthetic work. The result: wasted time and "mistreatment" of the patient.

Another reason is ethical. As oral implantology has reached a high level in dentistry, it is being misused for commercial reasons. I have always considered the profession, to which I have dedicated most of my life, to be humane, in the interest of people who need our help. The spirit of the new age, in many activities, puts profit first, which in medicine is opposed to the Hippocratic Oath.

Can you give an example that indicates the abuse of oral implantology for profit?

We are witnessing the fact that doctors are being punished for accepting bribes. The punishment is justified, because a doctor must not use someone's illness for financial gain. It is not only inhumane, but also a criminal act.

Recently, a patient in his sixth decade of life came to check the condition of his oral cavity and the treatment proposal he received in another office. In the aforementioned office, it was suggested to him to remove all ten teeth in the upper jaw and install nine implants (picture 18.348).

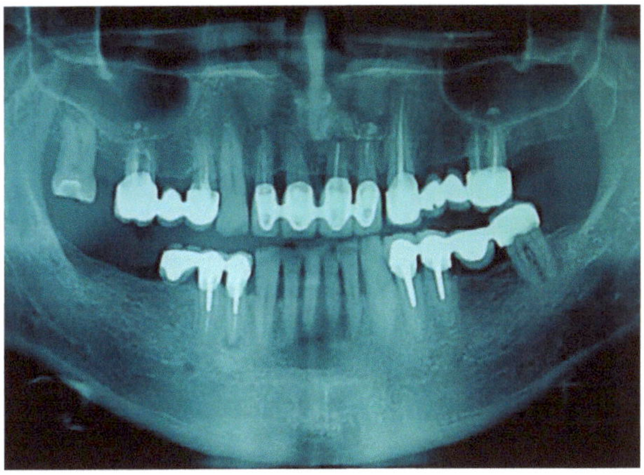

Figure 18.348. The orthopan-tomographic scan of the patient shows the condition in which it was proposed to extract 11 teeth in the upper jaw and install 10 implants. This professional and ethical failure is the answer to the review of endodontic treatment in this book of oral implantology.

After a detailed analysis of the video and the situation in the mouth, I realized that the answer should be based on three positions: philosophical, ethical and professional.

Philosophical thinking concerns the age of a person and it is not the same approach to the problem when the patient is in the second or third decade of life as when he is in the sixth. "The river does not flow, but the water"; "Time does not pass, but we pass in time," Ivo Andrić would say. Instead of helping a man to maintain his existing comfort in his mouth, or to make him a disability out of greed at an advanced age, it is more than a professional failure. Why make someone 80% disabled in the oral cavity in the sixth decade, when a simpler solution can maintain comfort for the next decade or more? Not only that, treatment costs, long recovery and the risk that the outcome will not be successful are significantly reduced. Doubt about the success of the outcome stems from the fact that money was put in the foreground.

The case was resolved in the following way: after an endodontic revision, the patient had cast extensions made on all devitalized tubes. Periodontal treatment was performed. The procedure and the result of the treatment are shown in pictures 18.349-18.356.

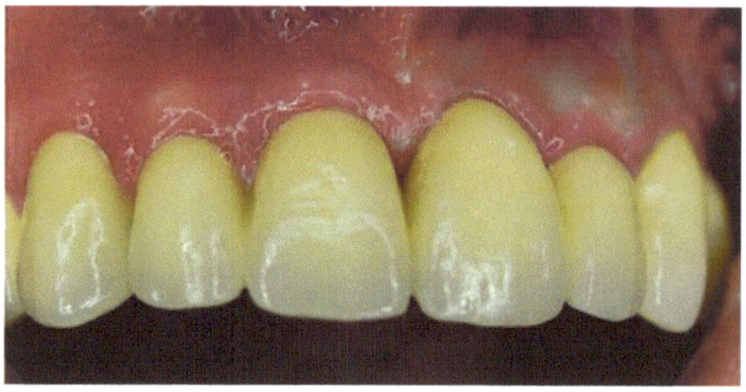

Figure 18.349. After the endodontic revision of the endodontically treated roots, cast extensions and periodontal microsurgery were performed. Temporary prosthetic work 4 weeks after healing of the soft tissues, definitive prosthetic work was done.

Presentation of mistakes by dentists: from filling, endodontic treatment, root resection, extraction to prosthetic replacement

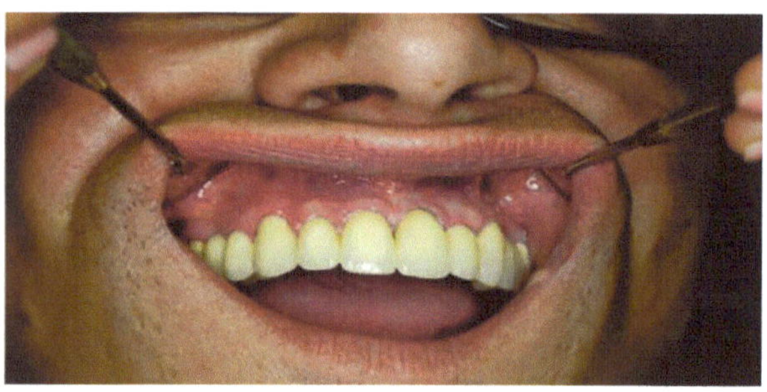

Figure 18.350. Appearance of healed soft gums and preserved interdental papilla, which would be more difficult to achieve with implant therapy.

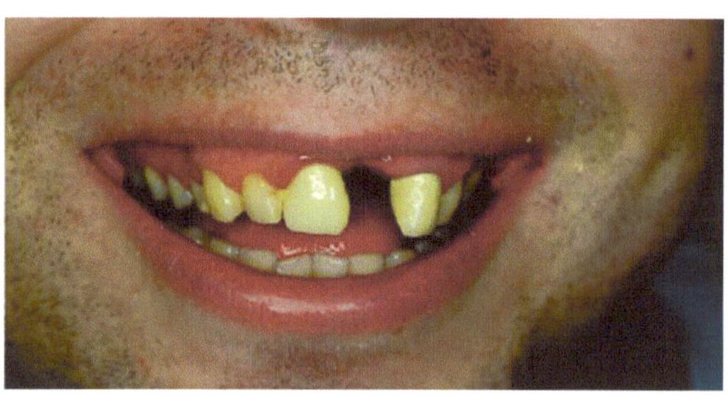

Figure 18.351. Anamnestic data indicate that a root resection was performed on the extracted tooth.

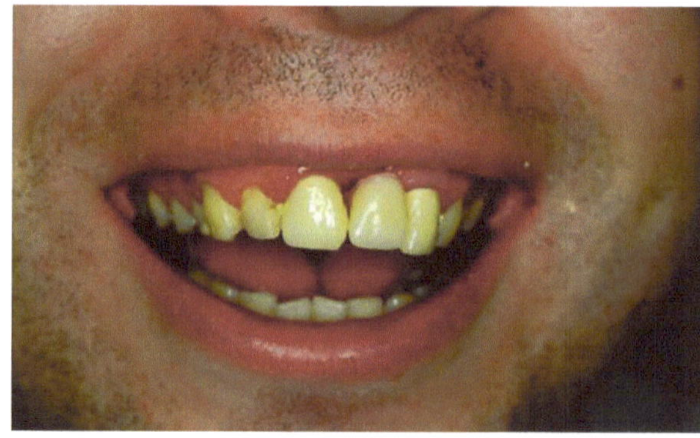

Figure 18.352. Destroyed lamellar bone by resection, and enhanced alveolar bone resorption by compression with a temporary acrylate prosthesis (the so-called "frog"). Implant restoration would be extremely uncertain from both a functional and aesthetic point of view. The augmentation procedure would require a longer period of treatment and increased material costs.

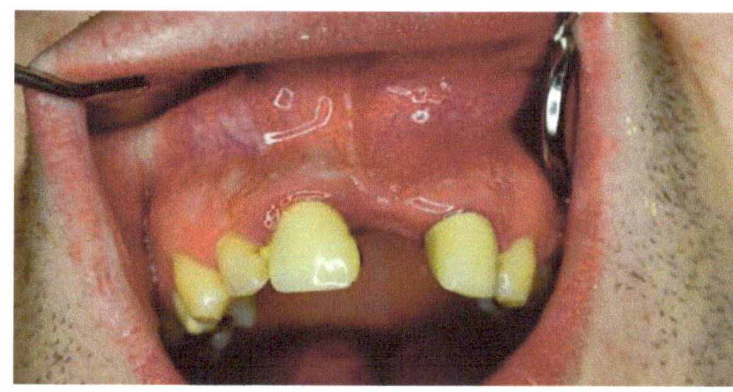

Figure 18.353. Extreme loss of alveolar bone at the site of lost left central incisor and narrowed interdental space implant placement contraindicated.

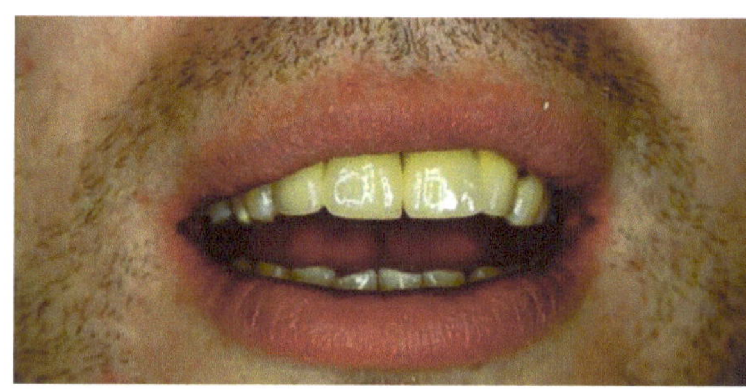

Figure 18.354. Complete satisfaction of the patient from both functional and aesthetic aspects with a classic metal-ceramic prosthesis.

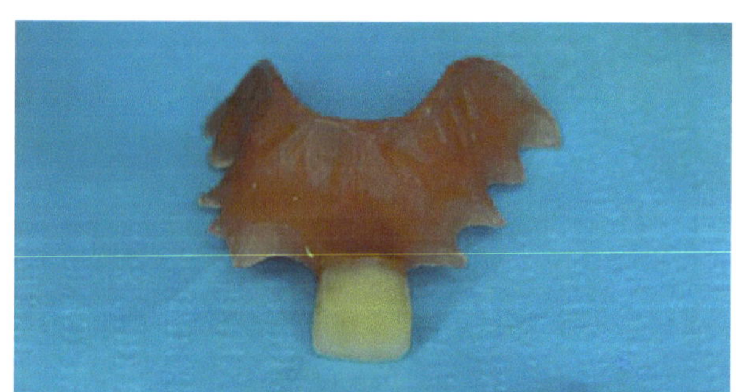

Figure 18.355. Catastrophic interim compensation, the "frog".

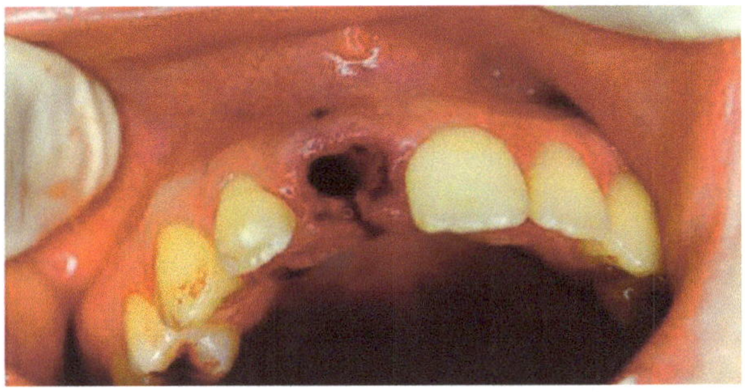

Figure 18.356. It is more justified to install an implant in a fresh alveolus than to resect a root with greater periapical pathological changes!

Finally, a question about titanium, the material from which the endosseous implant is made and its properties in relation to bone integration and the whole organism. The literature is increasingly discussing the possibility of zirconium oxide replacing titanium as a building material for implants?

Through decades of practice, practice has verified and confirmed that titanium is the material of choice for making implants. Thoughts and dilemmas as to whether titanium, as a building material of implants, should be replaced by some other material, can be raised for two reasons: scientific and marketing. Every scientific research has full justification in order to progress oral implantology. For now, when it comes to the material from which the endosseous implant is made, the dilemma does not exist due to the biocompatible and biomechanical properties of titanium. There is some thought that titanium can cause adverse reactions, such as allergy, and that it can lead to an increase in metal titanium ions near the implant, as well as in the lymph nodes. Such hints are only at the level of theories, without proof of the harmfulness of titanium in the body. Such assumptions are already denied by the application of titanium implants in orthopedic surgery (knee or hip replacement), because the weight of a dental implant is about 5 g, and the weight of an orthopedic implant is about 1000 g.

As for the disadvantages of titanium, we can only talk about an aesthetic disadvantage due to the screening of the carrier through the thin biotype of the gingiva in the region of the implant neck. But when it comes to the contact of titanium with the cells, tissues and tissue fluids of the human organism, titanium has shown all the properties of biocompatibility. Biocompatibility in the body is characterized by a strong affinity of cells to the surface of the implant. There are a large number of materials, which, from a purely theoretical aspect of materials engineering, are ideal for making implants. Non-toxicity is an important characteristic of titanium, because so far no release of metal ions or any other products that could affect the occurrence of cancer, allergies or inflammatory processes has been observed.

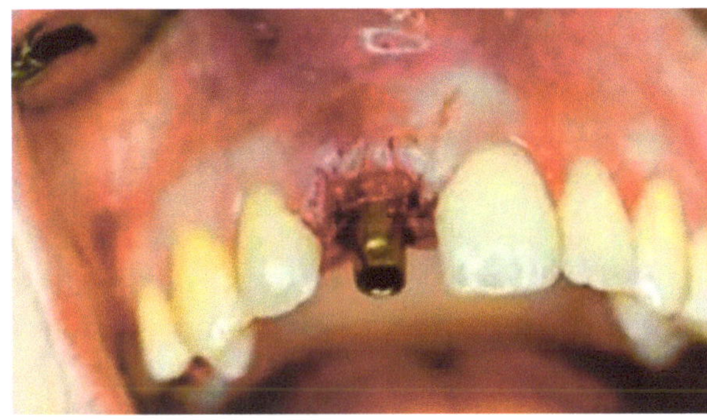

Figure 18.357. The indisputable advantage of immediate implantation with immediate loading.

For now, the quality of titanium for use in oral implantology is indisputable: resistance to corrosion, mechanical resistance, i.e. endurance when performing the function without any damage to the surrounding tissues.

Titanium is an extremely reactive element, which is found in the earth's crust in the form of a stable oxide, which is the reason for the very difficult separation of titanium and oxygen.

Its exceptional properties are: relatively high specific gravity, biocompatibility and extremely low level of toxicity. Thanks to the rapid reaction of titanium with oxygen at room temperature, a very stable passivating oxide layer is formed on the surface of the implant, as a protective oxide film.

Commercially pure titanium and alloys Ti6 Al-4V are used today. Due to minor, but strictly controlled differences in composition, titanium is produced in four basic compositions, which are numbered from 1 to 4. As the number increases, the value of strength and purity that characterizes the composition increases.

Citing the characteristics of titanium, as the material from which the implant is built, the question arises as to what properties zirconium should possess in order to surpass and replace it as the material of choice.

It would be ideal if a non-metallic implant could replace a metallic one, while possessing all the properties that titanium possesses.

Zirconium dioxide (ZrO2), chemically and biologically, is inert towards all tissues and fluids in the body. It has extremely high stiffness and this property is one of the disadvantages of zirconium dioxide. Due to the high rigidity of zircon, if the stress exceeds a certain limit, it will break. The endosseous part of the implant must be connected to the support similar to the components of the implant made of titanium. However, the components that bind the endosseous part (body) of the implant must be extremely precise and easily adjustable due to the extremely high coefficient of tension in that part of the implant system.

If a two-part implant were to be made from zirconium oxide, due to its extreme rigidity and brittleness, the superstructure, the support (abutment) would have to be made of metal. This would revert to the disadvantage that titanium has: metal screening in thin gingival biotype.

Therefore, implants made of zirconium dioxide would have to be designed exclusively as one-piece. The problem would arise with disparallelity of the implants and correction of the angles of the supports.

As zirconium dioxide is increasingly used in prosthetics due to its exceptional strength and high inelasticity, prosthetic works made of zirconium dioxide, supported by implants, are not justified in the lateral regions, unlike in the frontal regions, when aesthetic reasons are decisive.

It can be concluded that, for now, there are no valid statistical results on the application of zirconium dioxide implants in practice and on the percentage of success. Everything, for the most part, boils down to theoretical assumptions and in the experimental phase there are no pre-clinical, and especially clinical, results.

Could a certain implant system be chosen as the best after several decades of experience?

In the chapters at the beginning of the book, a lot has been said about the historical development path of oral implantology. For a long time, there was a lot of confusion in the design of implants. The beginning of the author of the book is marked by needle implants, and for a time subperiosteal. A longer period of application of endosseous implants was marked by the installation of leaf-shaped, Linkov implants.

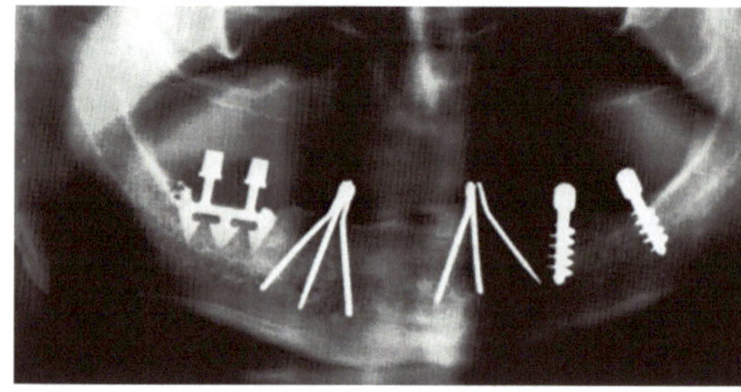

Figure 18.358. A typical example from the time of wandering in the development of oral implantology: Kombi, needle and screw-shaped implants.

The period of installation of the "first generation" of open one-piece endosseous Link implants was marked by both successes and many failures in general, including the failures of the author of the book, due to the breakage of the support. It happened that when solving total toothlessness in the lower jaw, all brackets broke and the patient brought a fixed bridge in his hand, and the endosteal part of the implant would remain in the bone. Extraction of the rest of the implant was extremely aggressive and resulted in bone defects. Bone substitutes were not in use then.

However, there are cases of application of leaf implants, so-called. "fifth generation" of closed Linkov-sheet implants that survive in the bone for more than three decades. This type of implant is the first endosseous implant in general, in which the endosseous part is plasma coated with titanium particles, and they are designed as two parts.

An unsuccessful period is considered the application of the so-called "Implant Van". At that time, with a lot of success, I applied implants designed in the form of a "screw", which were launched by Tramonte, Muratori, Pasqualini, Garbaggio and others. With Tramonte's implants, I recorded a very successful period after 15 or more years, the changes in the marginal part were minimal.

The period of cylindrical implants (insertion of implants performed by tapping) is the period with the most failures. The most frequent failures were related to the application of cylindrical implants coated with hydroxyapatite (due to the failed technological processing of the joint of the implant surface with hydroxyapatite). The author of the book records an extremely successful period with the use of Branemark implants.

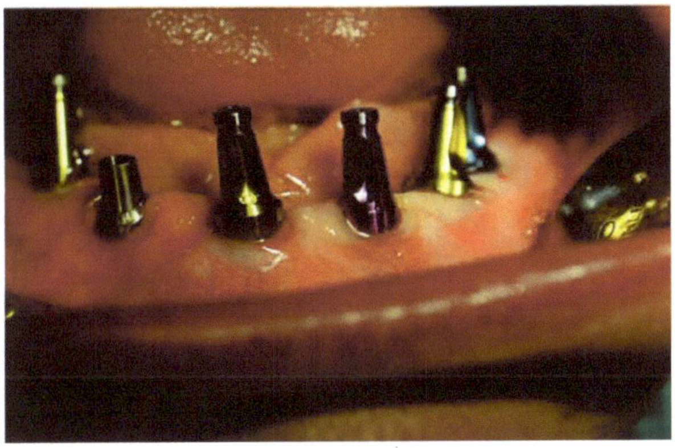

Figure 18.359. Brackets placed on immediately placed Brenemark implants placed immediately with immediate placement instead of gingiva former. Presentation of healed pre-implant soft tissues.

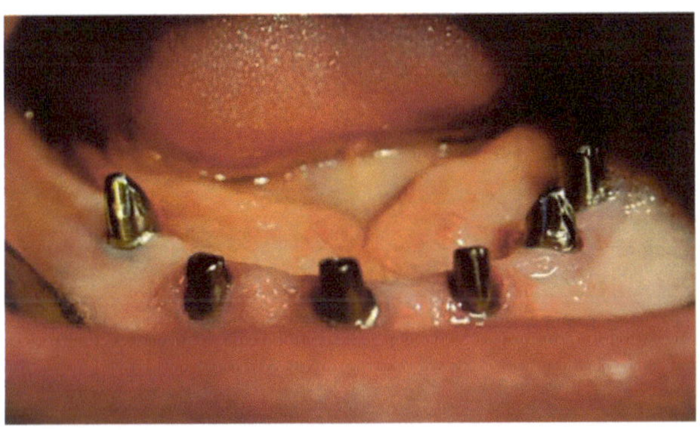

Figure 18.360. Brackets placed on immediately placed Brenemark implants placed immediately with immediate placement instead of gingiva former. Presentation of healed pre-implant soft tissues.

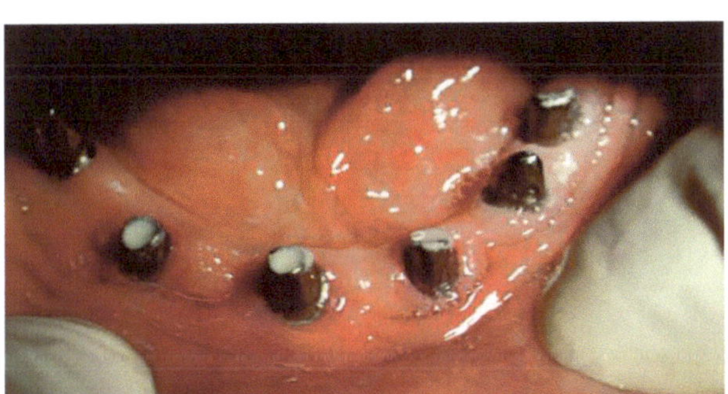

Figure 18.361. Definitive processing of supports (abutments) before taking impressions. Display of healing around the support of prosthetic work.

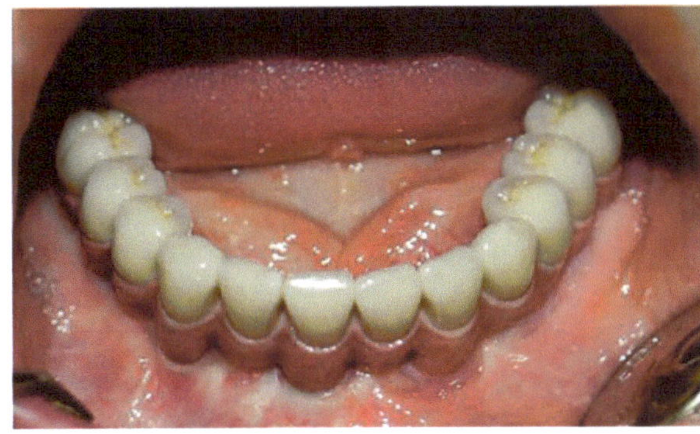

Figure 18.362. Definitive prosthetic work in the lower jaw. The morphology of the cusps and teeth is determined by the mixed teeth, when the condyles are in the maximum distal position - that is, the teeth are in central occlusion. Position of the condyles Interjaw relations when the condyles are placed in the maximum distal position, i.e. teeth in central occlusion.

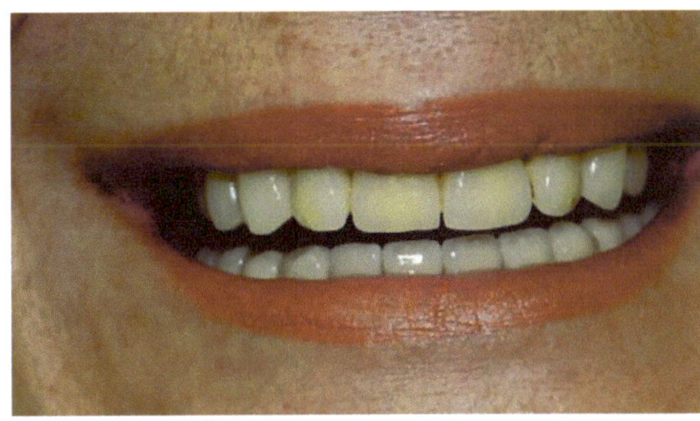

Figure 18.363. Definitive prosthetic work in both jaws, achieved good function and aesthetics.

In the mid eighties of the last century, an extraordinary success was marked by the installation of Pit-Easy implants (picture 18.364), with which the author of the book did not have a single loss! When one looks at such a long path of installation of various implant systems (successful and unsuccessful), then an authoritative answer can be drawn from the experience gained in the assessment of implant systems.

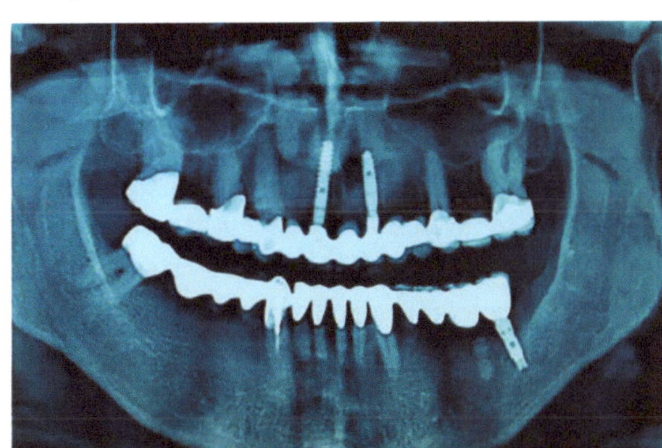

Figure 18.364. Control image of the Branemark implant after 20 years.

It is not possible to give a concrete answer to the question and to say that a particular implant system is the best, because there are numerous high-quality systems today. However, several implant systems can be singled out that I have applied the most and for the longest time, with extremely good results: Nobel Replace, Strauman, Biohorisonts, Esthetic. The application of the Astra implant was also successful. I have noticed that the occurrence of peri-implantitis is less frequent when one-piece implants are used in an edentulous mandible. This observation of the author of the book is confirmed by other authors. The probable reason is the absence of a micro-crack (gap between the support (abutment) and the body of the implant) in one-piece implants (Fig. 18.365).

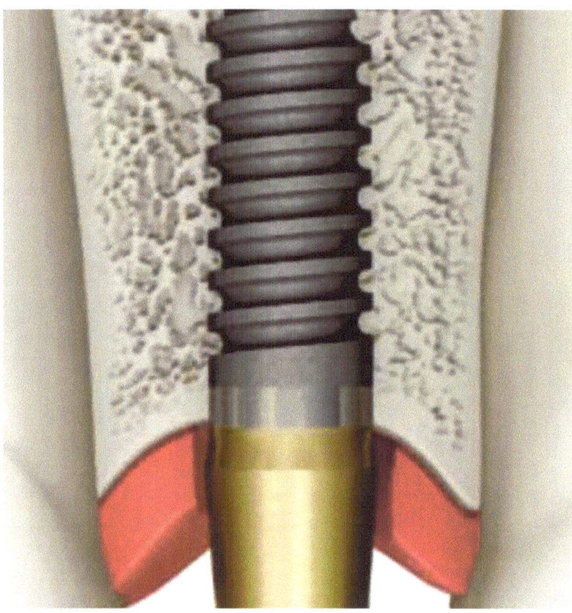

Figure 18.365. Appearance of the one-piece BioHorizonts implant. In the rehabilitation of total toothlessness, especially in the lower jaw, they proved to be very successful.

On the basis of these observations, the design of one-piece implants was improved, which refers to the diameter of the implant. One-piece implants were designed only as reduced (narrow), and the largest diameter was 3mm. However, today there are forms of one-piece implants with standard diameters (see chapter "Role and design of implants").

One-piece implants appeared at the end of the 70s in the form of screws, but they did not find wider application due to the limitations of the application, the supports could not be placed at different angles. That shortcoming is "solved" because the support (abutment) is made of a much softer material than the body of the titanium implant. In this way, it is possible to establish the parallelism of the support by grinding without transferring thermal stimuli to the body of the implant and the bone.

Advances in technology have changed the reality of using dental implants. The first serious education in the domain of oral implantology was organized by the American and German Academy of Oral Surgery and Implantology, and the author of the book was a regular participant, as the literature for deepening knowledge was extremely scarce.

The first implant system to receive much attention was the Branemark implant system. In the beginning, Branemark tied the application of its system to a license which it issued at a very high price. Acquaintance with Brennemak in Washington and education about his system, he offered me a "reasonable price with a discount" for his implant system, which at the time cost (surgical set and 40 implants) "only" 40,000 US $. I have had all 40 Branemark implants placed with nothing but success.

In the middle of the 80s of the last century, the Screw-Vent system was launched, and in 1999, with the support of this system, the Zimmer Implant system with good characteristics was launched. A major advance in design and technological processing in 2008 was the implant launch by the Nobel manufacturer Nobel Aktiv Implantat. This implant system is characterized by internal entry bevels with an internal hexagonal connection. The Nobel Aktiv Implant was announced as the "implant of the future". The installation of these implants, I can emphasize my own experience, I can count among the most successful installation of implants in decades of practice in oral implantology. The only "disadvantage" of this implant system is the high price.

The attachment of many dentists to a specific implant system persists even today. Transitioning to a different system requires not only education but also the acquisition of new instruments, which leads most dentists to develop a routine with one or two systems.

Advancements in oral implantology have significantly transformed this practice. Historically, the name most associated with oral implantology was Leonard Link, who was known for creating a variety of endosseous implant designs—64 in total. Today, that legacy has been continued by Gerald Niznick, the founder of

Implant Direct Sybron International. With thirty years of experience in developing dental implants and holding 35 patents that have modernized implant systems, Niznick advocates for simplicity in design. His philosophy is that the simpler a system is, the smarter and more practical it becomes.

As a prosthetist aware of the challenges posed by prosthetic superstructures placed on implants, Niznick established the Implant Direct system based on this principle. Following decades of experience, he emphasizes that the design of prosthetic platforms within the Implant Direct system has addressed and eliminated many issues present in various implant systems. Ultimately, poorly executed prosthetics can undermine even the best implant systems.

If a dentist stops using a well-known implant system, such as Nobel Biocare, Straumann, BioHorizons, Astra, or Zimmer, it is likely due to the high costs and the limited purchasing power of patients. While some manufacturers address this issue by offering implants at much lower prices, the quality of these implants can be questionable.

The implant industry has advanced significantly, and many implant products are now produced on a mass scale. This mass production results in costs that can be 30 times, or even more, lower than the retail prices of implants. Consequently, the largest profit margins are enjoyed by the manufacturers and marketing intermediaries, while dentists earn the least.

To maintain the quality of renowned implant systems while making them more affordable, Dr. Niznick has developed a solution that allows more patients to access dental implants.

The Implant Direct system has advanced implant surface technology significantly compared to many other systems. The roughness of the implant surface is achieved through a soluble hydroxyapatite medium. The question remains about the practice results this technology will yield.

One of the biggest challenges for dentists is rehabilitating the edentulous lower jaw. The author of the book highlights that when using one-piece implants to treat toothlessness in the lower jaw, the occurrence of peri-implantitis is extremely rare or even non-existent. This can be attributed to two main factors: the absence of microgaps between the body of the endosseous part of the implant and the supporting structure of the prosthetic work, as well as the laser processing of the occlusal part, which enhances the connection of soft tissues to that section of the one-piece implant.

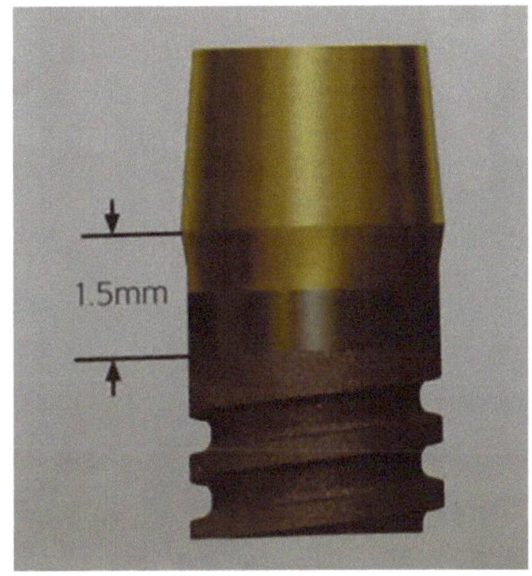

Figure 18.366. Treatment of the neck of one-piece implants with new technologies enables a better connection of soft tissues with the implant. The absence of a gap between the supports (abutment) is a prevention of the occurrence of peri-implantitis. The experience of the author of the book shows that with implantological treatment with one-piece implants, the frequency of peri-implantitis is significantly reduced.

The Implant Direct system, by launching a one-piece implant with standard and wider diameters, made the treatment simpler, with a lower cost for both the doctor and the patient, be it for fixed or mobile prosthetic works (Figures 18.364- 18.370).

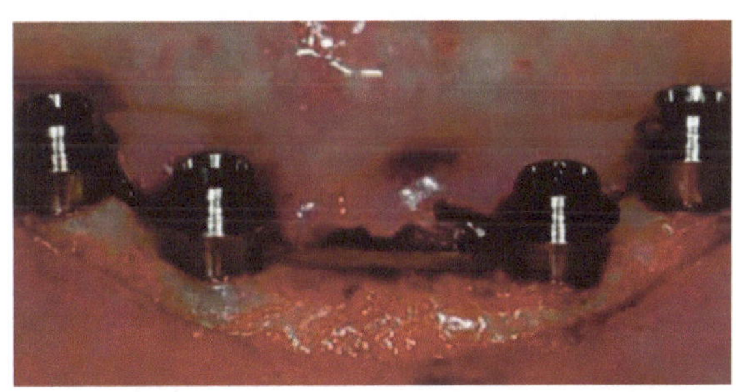

Figure 18.367. Built-in one-piece implants of standard diameters.

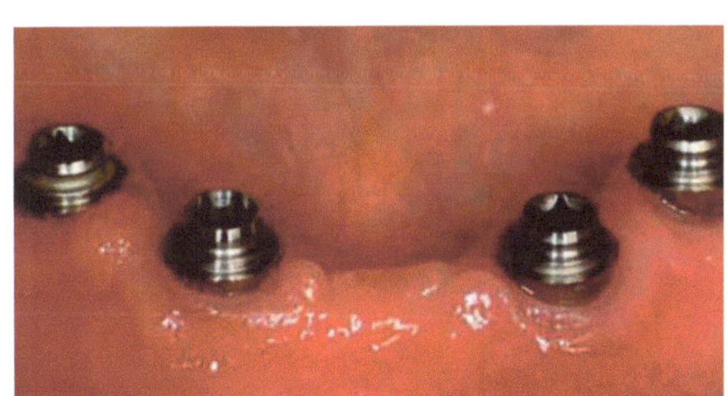

Figure 18.368. Appearance of healed tissues after 6 weeks.

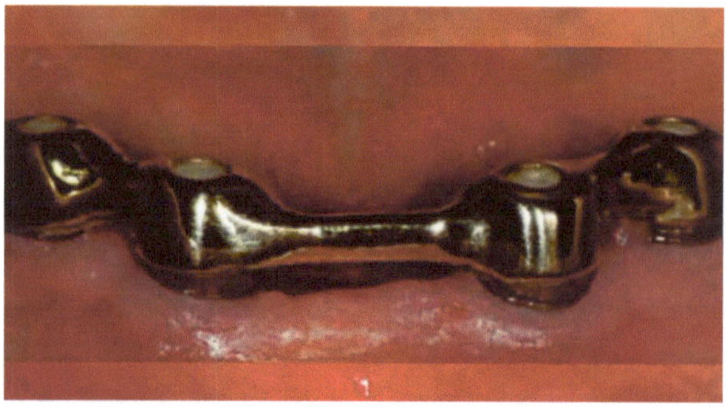

Figure 18.369. Dolder's retention bar on embedded implants.

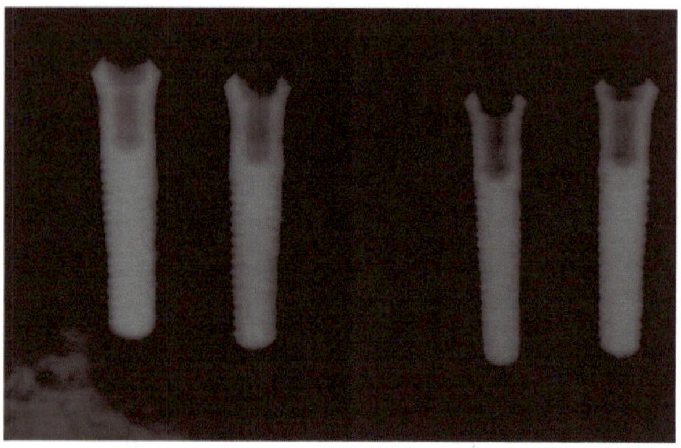

Figure 18.370. Control shot after implant installation.

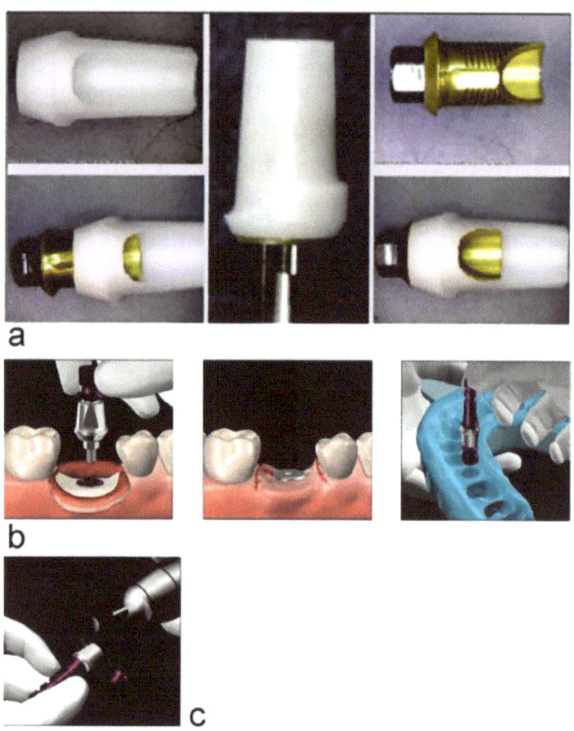

Figure 18.371. The advantage of the Direct implant system in all forms, in addition to the simplified surgical protocol, also increases the precision of transfer of the implant position in the laboratory (c). The support (abutment) of the prosthetic work is connected with the transfer, which is returned to the taken impression and is cut in the laboratory (d), with the possibility of processing the supports (abutments), i.e. if it is necessary to establish the parallelism of the carrier. The author's experience shows that instead of placing a cap for healing, after laboratory processing, a definitive support should be placed around which soft tissues are formed better and faster. This procedure avoids trauma to soft tissues. The procedure of immediate implantation should also be loaded immediately, which accelerates the integration processes.

The ultimate goal of oral implantology is the replacement of lost teeth, and the ultimate goal of treatment must be closer to nature. But it is equally important that the benefit offered by oral implantology is accessible to a larger number of patients. Until now, this has been denied due to the high cost of implants, not the cost of knowledge of stomatologists and dental technicians.

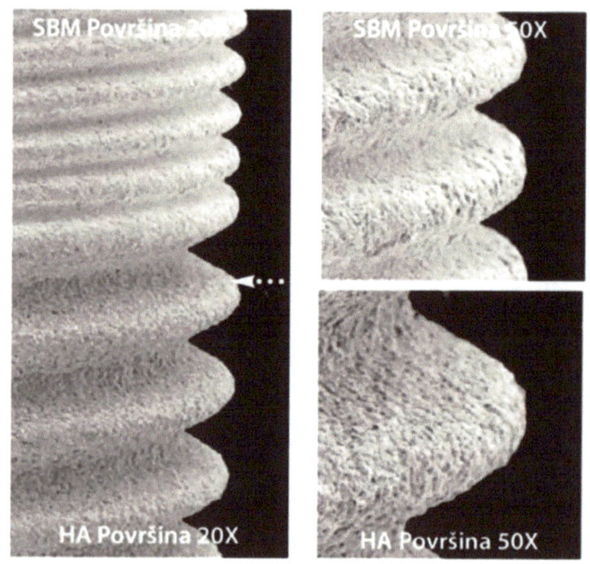

Figure 18.372. The microscopic appearance of the Implant Direct workable surfaces is similar to the laser surface treatment of the Biohorizons implant system, with the fact that the implant surface of the Implant Direct system was created using a soluble artificial medium of hydroxyapatite crystals to create a rough texture. Using a soluble artificial medium of hydroxyapatite crystals is a new technology that was worked on from 1982, when research began, to 2006.

With the development of the Implant Direct system, Branemark's protocol was changed, which required four to six implants to stabilize the lower or upper total denture in the front, which made the treatment too expensive and inaccessible. Especially parts of such systems increased the cost of treatment.

Treatment of total toothlessness in both jaws with fixed prosthetic works is a more natural and comfortable solution. The Implant Direct system offers supports at an angle of 40 to 20o.

Oral implantology has become a reality in the daily practice of dentists. For this reason, it is very important to know the implant system, which will enable the simplest implant installation and faster healing. The Implant Direct system made it possible to have "everything in one yen", which is a great relief for the patient and for the dentist, due to the simplicity of application and compatibility with several high-quality implant systems

Three decades ago, what were the attitudes when implants were placed in the aesthetic region, since the function was primary?

When it comes to implant-prosthetic treatment in the aesthetic region, especially in the upper jaw, treatment attitudes 20 years ago cannot be considered from any aspect. Moreover, in the last few years, new points of view have appeared when it comes to implant therapy in the aesthetic region. Decades ago, the most important determinant was the survival rate of implants. The technological development of implant manufacturing, the quality of the material from which the implants are made, and especially the technological treatment of the implant surface, have made implant placement a safe procedure in terms of implant and bone integration. When it comes to bone integration, failures are mostly the result of medical errors during implant placement.

Many implantation procedures in the aesthetic region are focused on the aesthetics of soft tissues, because the issue of successful integration is practically solved (Figures 18.373 to 18.379).

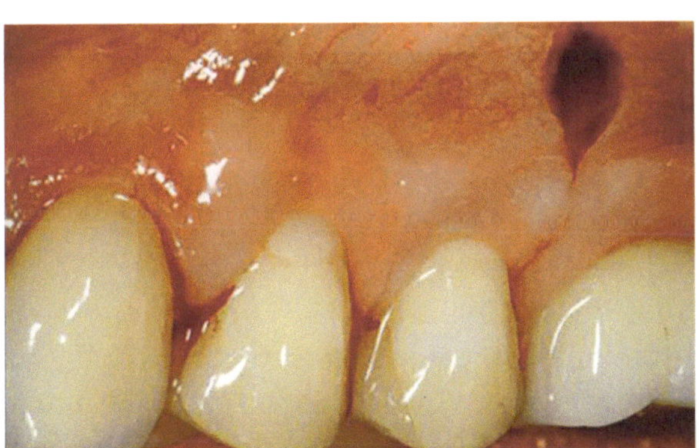

Figure 18.373. In order not to endanger the vascularization and the formation of a scar, a vertical incision is not made in the front area, but a C-shaped incision is made distal to the second premolar.

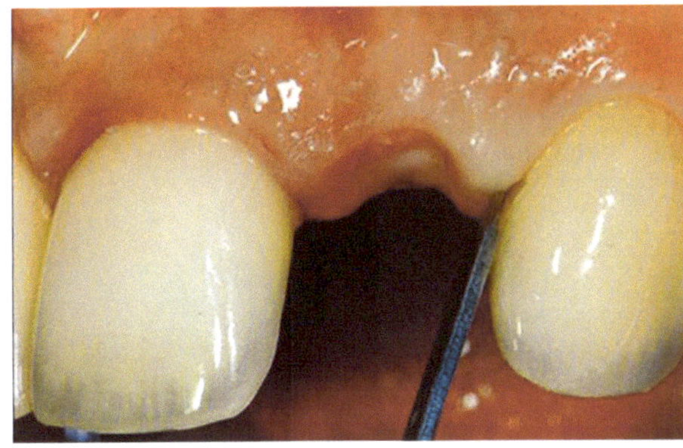

Figure 18.374. When raising the flap, start with making an interdental intrasulcus incision.

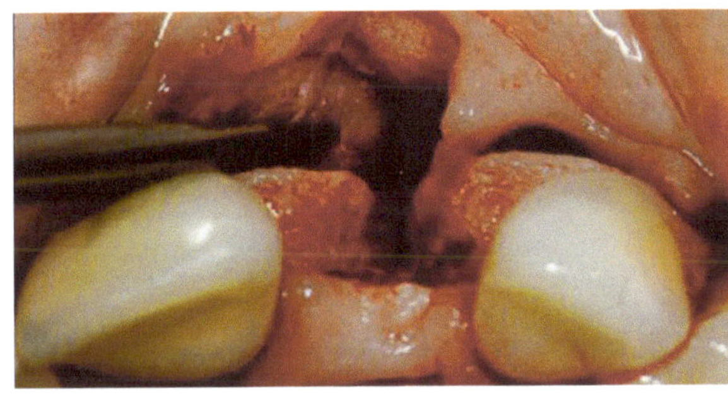

Figure 18.375. It is very important to create conditions so that the papilla is not damaged. In order to increase the mobility of the flap, the incision is made vertically and stuffed to the middle of the central incisor. Care should be taken to ensure that the papilla remains intact when pulling it out.

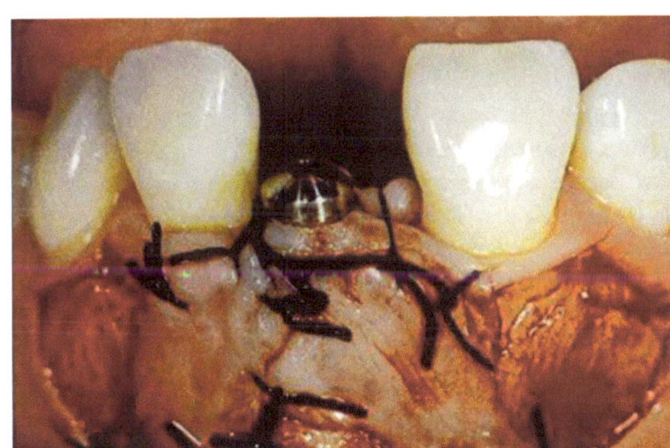

Figure 18.376. After placing the bone substitute, two laterally displaced flaps are sutured so as not to create a scar. With displaced flaps, reconstruction of the papilla is possible.

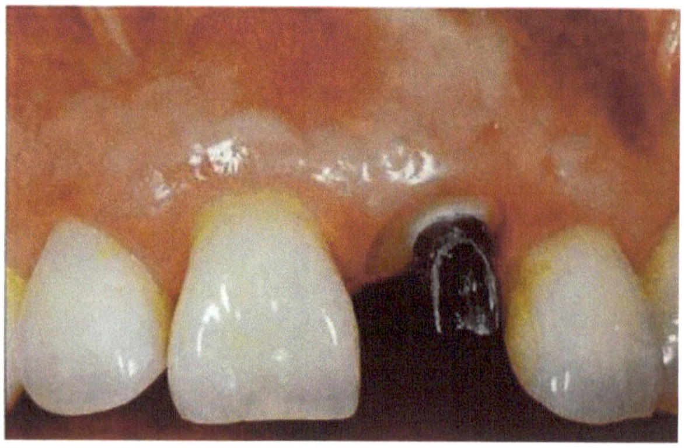

Figure 18.377. Appearance after healing of the placed implant in place of the central incisor (#21). The appearance of the healed tissues after 3 months, with the support (abutment) placed for the fabrication of the prosthetic work (crown).

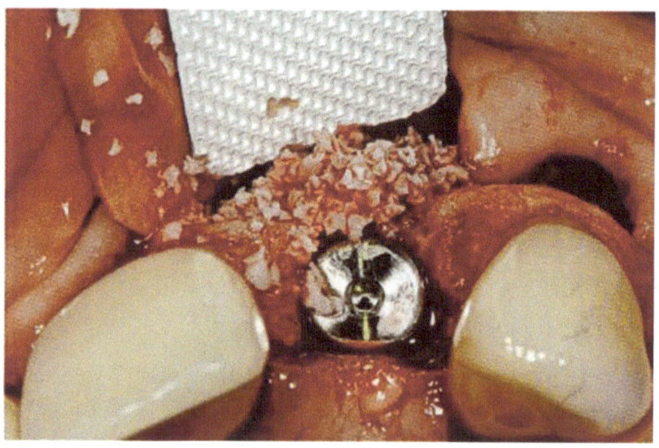

Figure 18.378. Appearance of deproteinized beef bone as a bone substitute.

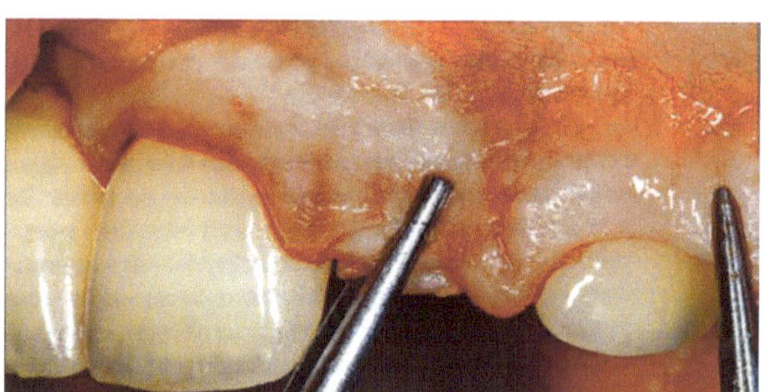

Figure 18.379. The prepared flap needs to be taut to allow good primary wound healing over the augment.

Progress has also been made when it comes to hard and soft tissue augmentation techniques (Figures 18.380-18.381). The development of new synthetic augments for the compensation of bone defects is increasingly successful and is increasingly used in everyday practice. Preservation of the ridge, bone regeneration by augmentation, shaping of soft tissues by micro-surgery, provides f new opportunities to prioritize aesthetics, especially in the frontal region.

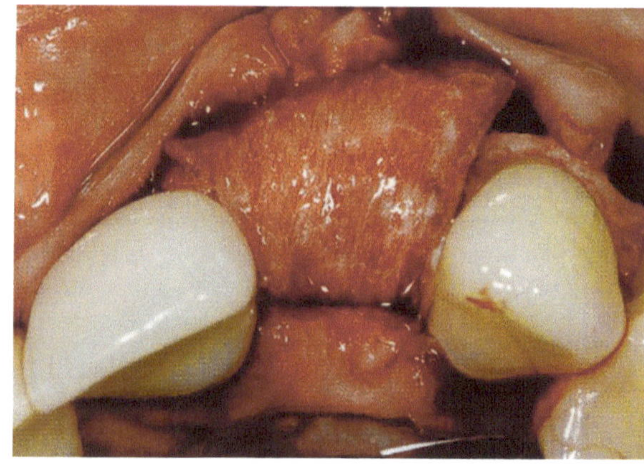

Figure 18.380. The placed augment (substitute for bone) should be completely covered with a resorptive membrane.

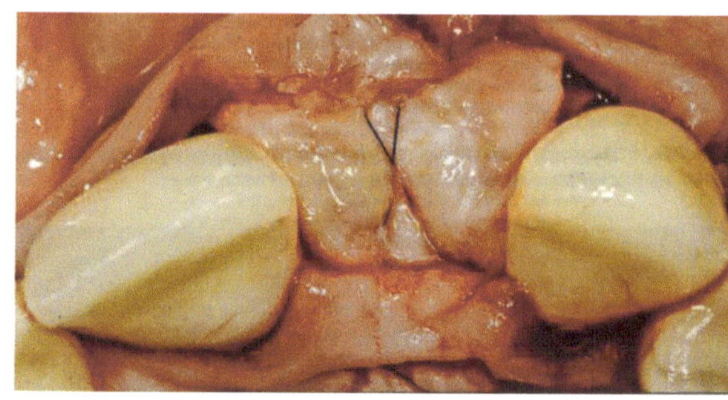

Figure 18.381. In order to increase the volume of the soft tissue and enable faster healing of the augment, the subepithelial flap should be fixed to the buccal part of the flap with a cross stitch.

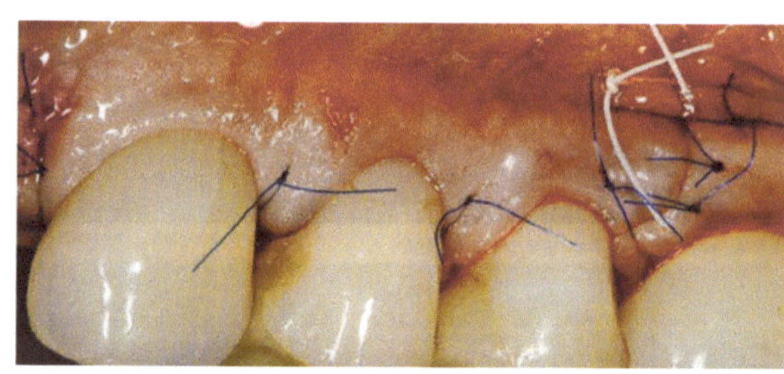

Figure 18.382. Sutures should be performed in the area of keratinized gingiva with the thinnest possible sutures.

Osseointegration implants have moved the implant survival rate to two decades, and it can be said more. The percentage of success when it comes to bony integration is up to 98%, but the percentage of success when it comes to soft tissues is still lower and with greater unpredictability of the outcome. But also in this regard, significant improvements have been achieved recently. Starting with the application of the CBCT radiography technique, which can obtain precise information about the available bone as a support for the soft tissues. To ensure good vascularization of the flaps, modified flap shapes are recommended. When installing an implant in the aesthetic region, the incision should start at the top of the ridge and intrasulcus on the adjacent teeth. This prevents the creation of a scar in an aesthetically visible area. In order to ensure a good visibility of the field where the implant is to be inserted, the mucoperiosteal and mucosal flap should be prepared so that it can be moved by two teeth towards the distal.

If augmentation coverage is required, a coronary mobile flap can be prepared. Twenty years ago, this procedure would have failed, because collagen membranes were not available. The materials of collagen membranes have been significantly improved, and the integration process, as well as the degree of complications, depends on the quality of the membranes. In case the membrane is exposed, the area can be covered with a subepithelial skin graft taken from the palate. The success of soft tissue healing depends on the perfect adaptation of the wound edges to achieve the best possible primary healing. This is achieved with delicate microsurgical instruments and very thin surgical sutures.

Resorbable threads should be avoided and used in exceptional situations, because they always break down with accompanying inflammatory processes, which also depends on maintaining oral hygiene during the healing period. Sewing with mattress seams has been abandoned. As for the sewing technique, a simple double loop stitch worked best.

All these improvements resulted in the long-term stability of transplanted soft tissues, which significantly improved the fulfillment of aesthetic requirements. The entire procedure was accompanied by a reduction in morbidity and significantly shortened time of implant therapy. The progress in the development of material technology for prosthetic works also contributed to the success of implant-prosthetic treatment. The improvement of osseointegrative implants and all the aforementioned techniques has improved the prevention of peri-implant diseases, as well as the treatment of peri-implantitis when it occurs.

What parameters are important for planning the entire implant-prosthetic treatment and the predictability of the outcome if the patient requests not to be without teeth and to have fixed prosthetic work on the same day after the extraction of the remaining teeth, and there are regions of the alveolar ridge with greater bone destruction?

Presentation of the following case will provide an answer to the question. First of all, it is a very complex case, where the patient requests to have fixed dental compensation on the same day due to professional obligations.

The risk must be presented to the patient when it comes to such a complicated case. The dentist must not take a risk if he has not informed the patient in detail.

To engage in such complicated operations, knowledge, experience, dexterity and a vision of the outcome are needed. The realization of the plan and the expected outcome of the treatment depends on the selection of a high-quality implant system whose quality (titanium type IV) has been confirmed by certificates and verified in practice. The El Estethic Line implant system was applied.

The design of the implant has a conical shape, and in the apical third, aggressive double threads that ensure maximum primary stability, especially in cases where there is soft bone (Fig. 18.322). The design of the micro-threads in the neck part enables the reduction of stress, i.e. trauma to the cortical bone during implant insertion. This design detail in the neck part of the implant, in the initial phase of implant insertion, reduces the stress on the cortical bone, because it directs and cushions the chewing forces, transforming the intensity of the forces into the limits of biological action. The characteristics of the implant are as follows: beveled shoulder in the neck of the implant, processed with the latest technology. This detail enables easier growth of new bone over the shoulder of the implant, which is important for its long-term stability, because it enables the biological distribution of forces on the cortical bone. The growth of new bone over the shoulder of the implant is a good support for the formation of soft tissues and the papilla.

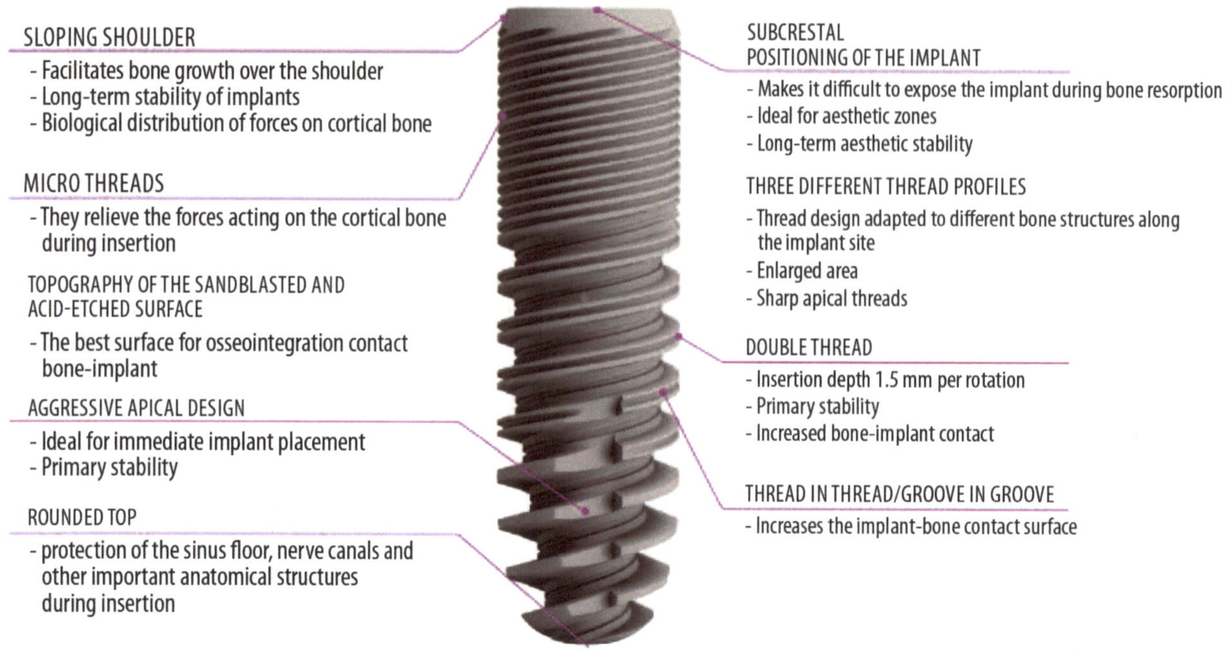

Figure 18.383. The characteristics of the EL Estethic Line implant system are: the design of this implant is the fifth generation of this system, with double aggressive threads, especially in the apical third. The surface designed in this way enables the achievement of good primary stability in many indications of oral surgical treatment.

In the presented case, the implants are positioned subcrestally, which prevents exposure of the implants if marginal bone resorption occurs. This must be considered in similar complicated cases. This also predicts a good aesthetic result after the immediate installation of the implants. The bracket is designed to show the maximum primary stability of the installed implant after placement and tightening to 25 Ncm, thus eliminating micro-movements and micro-space (microcrack) between the implant and the bracket.

For faster and better healing and shaping of soft tissues, the design of the support (abutment) is concave, which will allow platform-switching, i.e. the concavity of the abutment enables the desired shaping of soft tissues, and thus a successful aesthetic result.

"EL ESTETHIC LINE" implant system is an implant system that meets the stated needs (pictures 18.382 - 18.384). This implant also has an extremely important design detail: the apical part of the implant is rounded, which is extremely important for cases where sinus lifting is required.

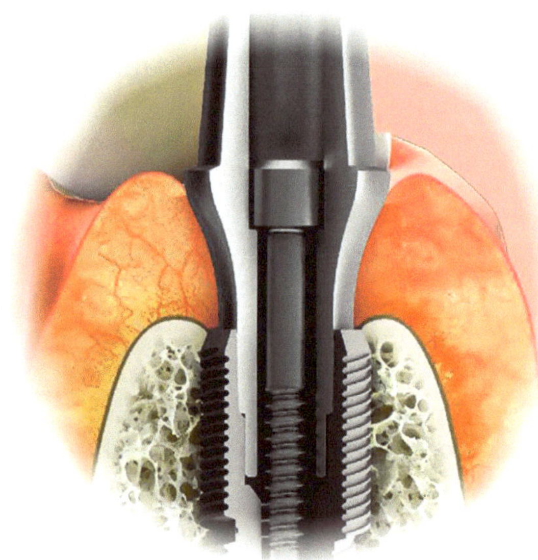

Figure 18.384. The design of the support (abutment) of the EL Esthetic implant has an advantage over many renowned implant systems, because its concavity enables the shaping of soft tissues and promotes the reconstruction of the papilla. PLATFORM SWITCHING enables prevention of bone mass loss, better biological width is achieved, and thus long-term stability of soft tissues. The conical design of the abutment eliminates micro-movements and unscrewing.

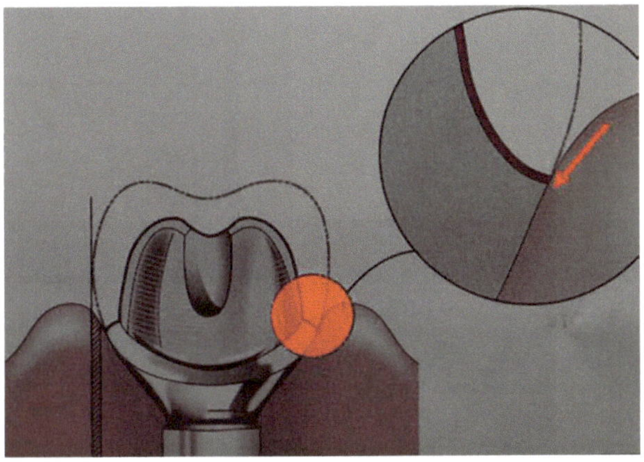

Figure 18.385. The design of the support (abutment) of many implant systems has a micro-crack (red arrow) a convenient location for the deposition of plaque and microorganisms, which can cause peri-implant changes. Residual cement in the space between the support and the crown can cause inflammation of the surrounding tissues (red circle).

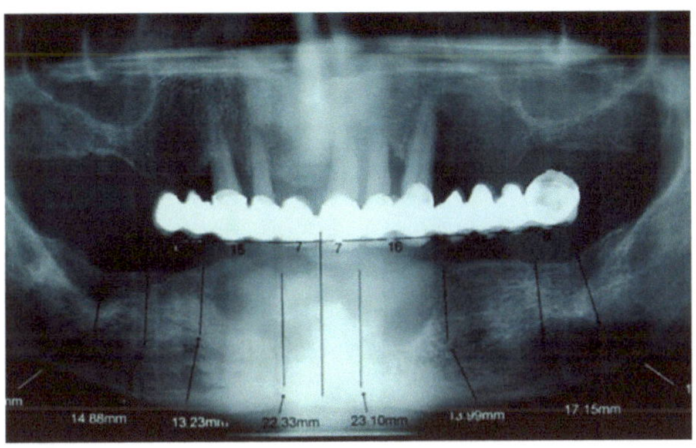

Figure 18.386. Tomographic analysis of the child's anatomical structure of the lower jaw, made 6 years ago in the same patient.

The answer to the question begins with the presentation of the case of the same patient who made similar requests 7 years ago for implant-prosthetic rehabilitation in the lower jaw (Figure 18.385).

The patient was then advised to treat both jaws at the same time, taking into account the situation in the upper jaw. In the upper jaw, the teeth on which the poorly planned prosthetic work was placed showed periodontal changes. Prosthetic work placed on five teeth, with six extensions (hanging members), from the aspect of biomechanical fasteners, was a bad prosthetic solution. At that time, the patient did not accept the advice to solve the problem in the upper jaw, but only in the lower one. When the patient came again, who wanted to solve the situation in the upper jaw, the condition in the oral cavity, thanks to the patient's negligence - poor oral hygiene, was not favorable (pictures 18.387 and 18.389).

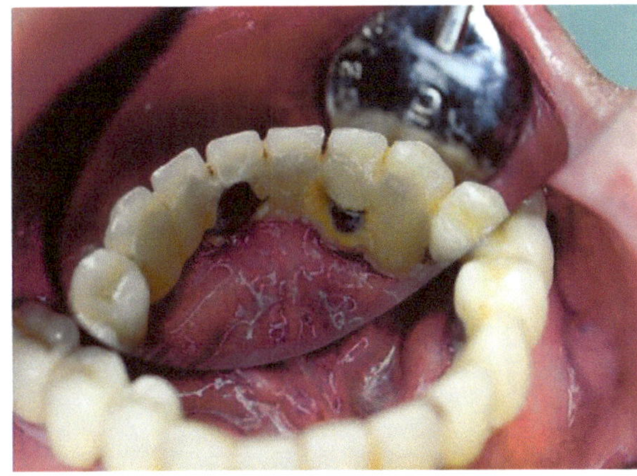

Figure 18.387. After 7 years of waiting, the patient came to solve the problem in the upper jaw. The prosthetic work was no longer in the mouth. Apparently satisfied with the implant-prosthetic treatment in the lower jaw, he did not attend the regular mandatory check-ups. However, poor oral hygiene resulted in an abundance of accumulated calculus and plaque.

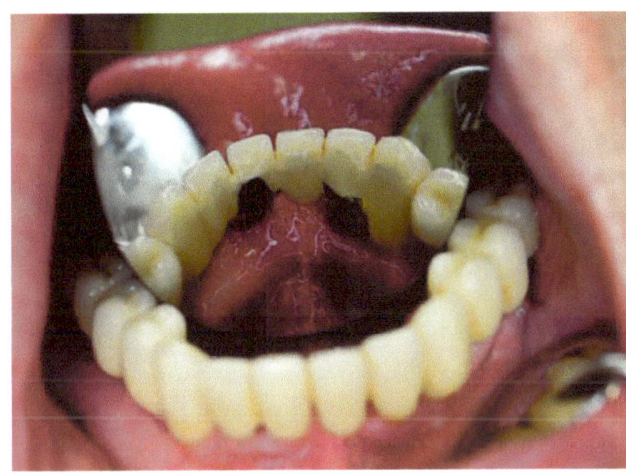

Figure 18.388. Appearance after ultrasonic removal of calculus and plaque deposits around all supports of prosthetic work.

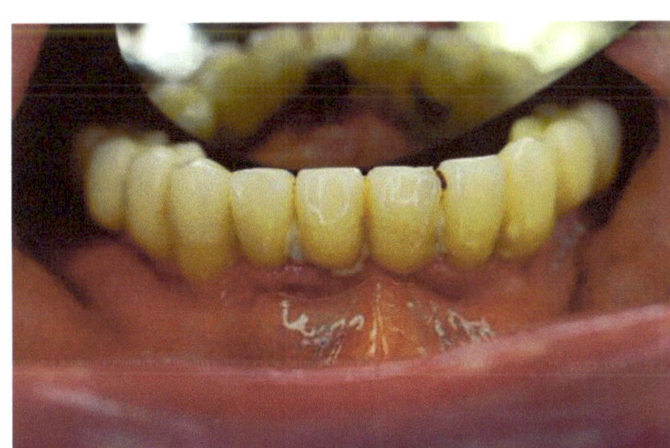

Figure 18.389. Considering the past carelessness and poor maintenance of oral hygiene, the patient was told to come for check-ups and plaque removal every three months. These tips are set as a condition for accepting treatment in the upper jaw, which is confirmed in writing (so the dentist is not responsible for any unwanted consequences).

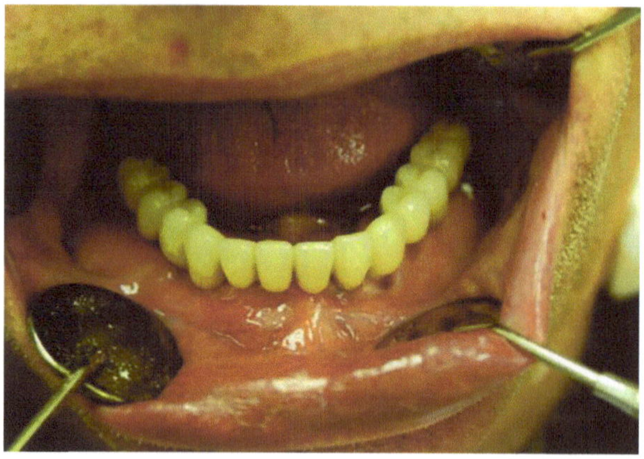

Figure 18.390. The result of mechanical cleaning of plaque and unsettled concrements is visible already after 10 days: stable soft tissues, without symptoms of inflammation.

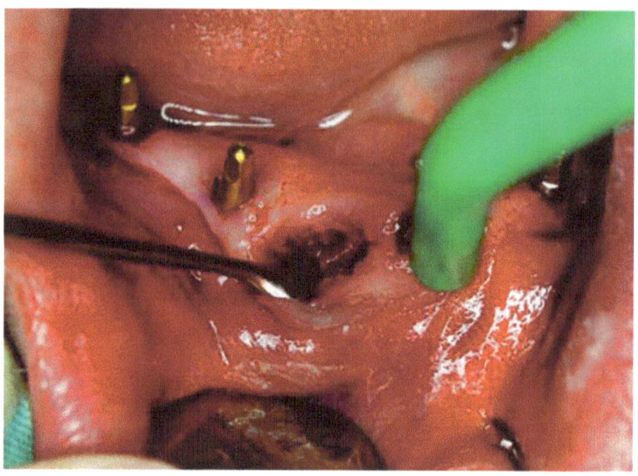

Figure 18.391. The beginning of treatment in the lower jaw 7 years ago in the same patient. Abundant granulation tissue with a larger bone defect.

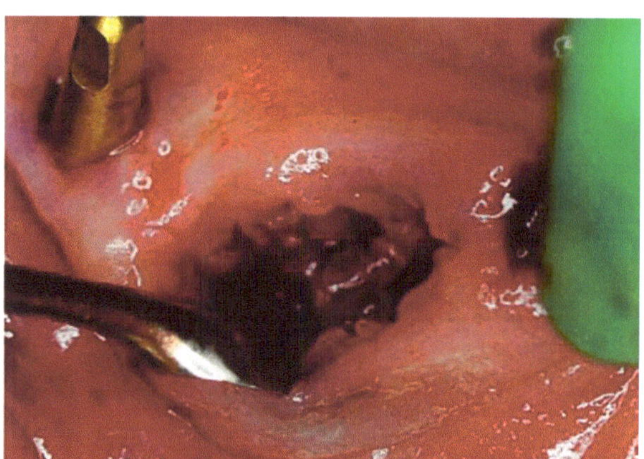

Figure 18.392. The presentation of the appearance of the objective state completely deviated from the theoretical implant surgical protocol of implantation and the fulfillment of the patient's request for immediate fixed prosthetic work.

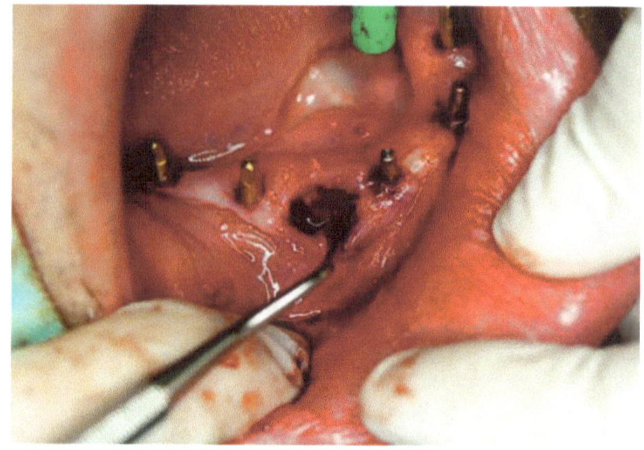

Figure 18.393. For embarking on similar implant surgical procedures, the decisive factors are the establishment of a good planning of the entire implant-prosthetic treatment; that the clinician possesses the knowledge of an oral surgeon and prosthetist. All of this is accompanied by experience, skill and judgment in predicting a successful treatment outcome.

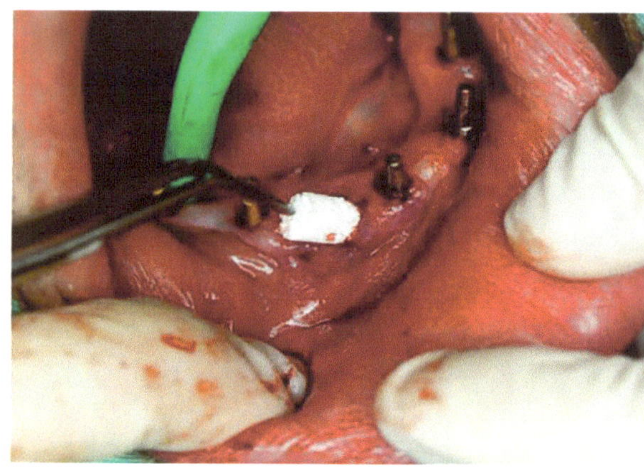

Figure 18.394. After preservation of the alveolus: abundant granulation tissue was removed, and larger bone defects were augmented with xenogeneic bone substitute blocks.

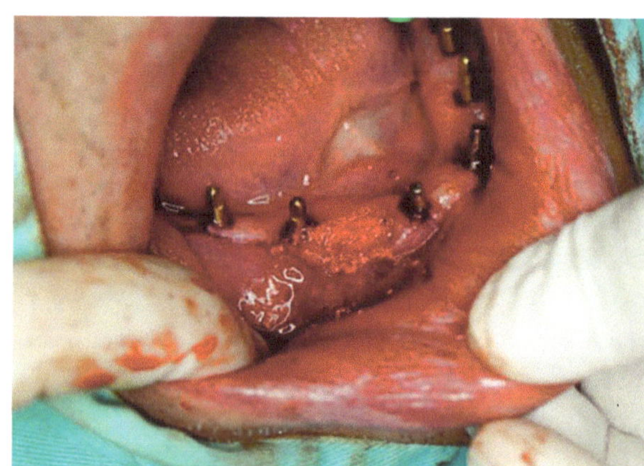

Figure 18.395. Xenogenic blocks covered with bone substitute granules, covering the augmented material with a collagen resorbable membrane. The implants were immediately implanted in the retromolar region next to the bone defect in the healthy bone without raising the flap, thus reducing the patient's morbidity and faster healing.

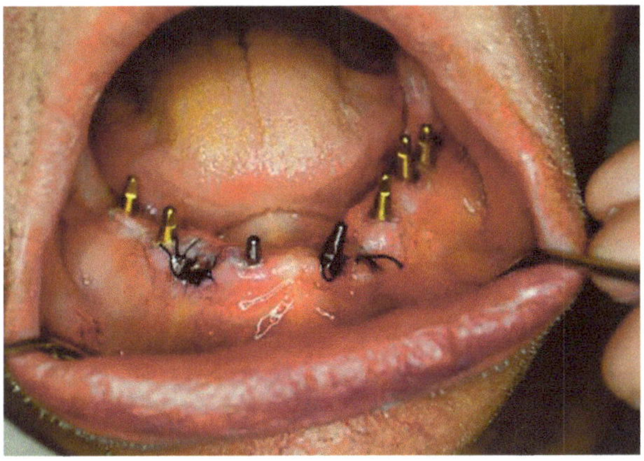

Figure 18.396. Condition after 7 days. Due to a larger bone defect, the implant in region 32 was placed in a healthy part of the bone.

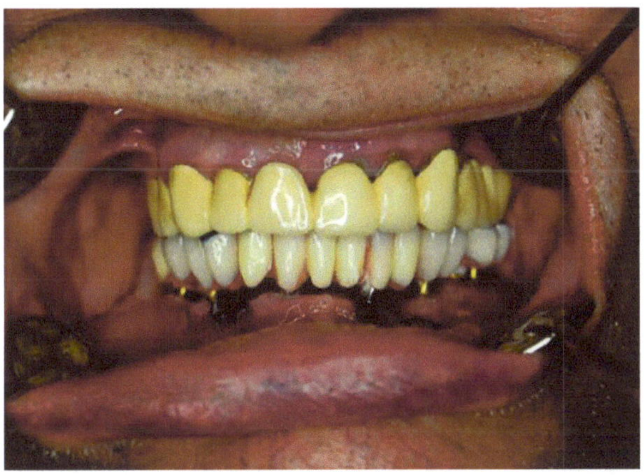

Figure 18.397. The patient's requests were fulfilled: on the immediately installed implants, a temporary acrylate fixed prosthetic work was placed. Appearance of found prosthetic work in the upper jaw with extensions in the premolar and molar regions.

At the moment when the patient came for implant-prosthetic rehabilitation in the upper jaw, the previously existing prosthetic work was no longer in the mouth. Due to the lack of antagonists, before treatment in the lower jaw, the existing prosthetic work in the upper jaw, on the periodontal teeth, remained in place. However, with the finalization of the implant-prosthetic treatment in the lower jaw and the established occlusion and articulation, the chewing forces and moments of those forces conditioned the action of the lever on both sides of the long extensions of the prosthetic work (suspending members), so that, after some time, the prosthetic work fell out of mouth.

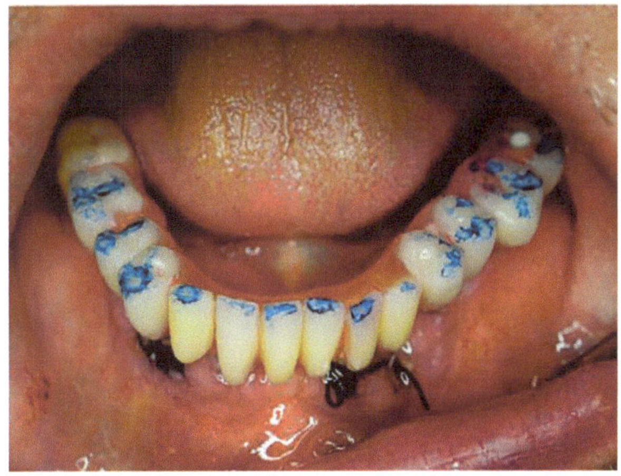

Figure 18.398. By establishing a good balanced occlusion, unfavorable chewing forces during lateral movements of the lower jaw are eliminated, it has a stimulating effect on the osseointegration processes of immediately installed and immediately loaded implants.

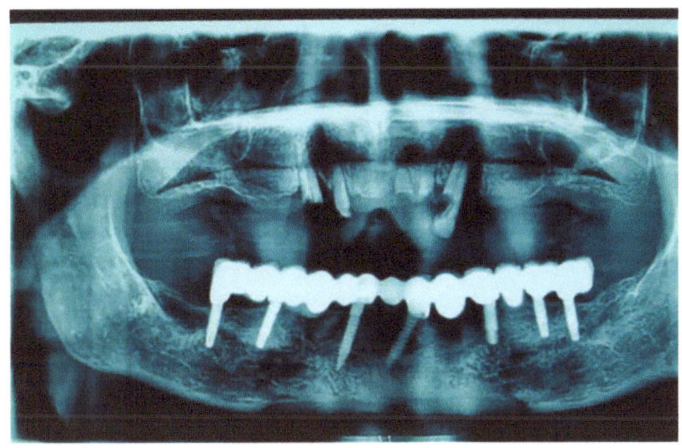

Figure 18.399. The condition found in the upper and lower jaw and the condition after 7 years. Despite poor oral hygiene, (Fig. 18.387 and 18.389) the condition of the lower jaw after 7 years: no bone resorption, while the soft tissues are stable. See image procedure steps 18.391 to 18.398. Procedure plan in the upper jaw: extraction of the remaining teeth is required. The condition after tooth extraction will determine further treatment procedures.

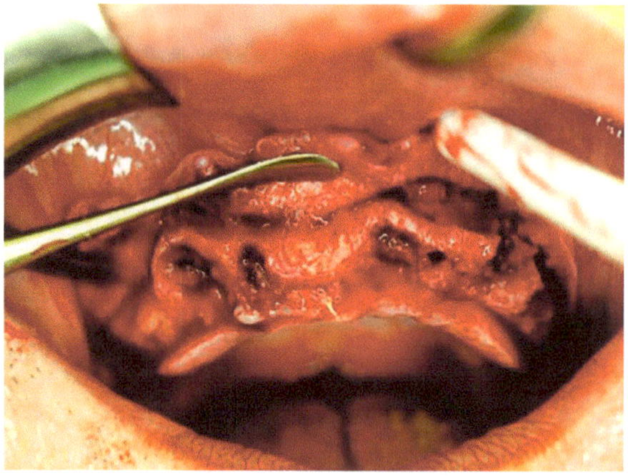

Figure 18.400. View after extraction of the remaining roots. Pronounced larger bone defects with abundant granulation tissue.

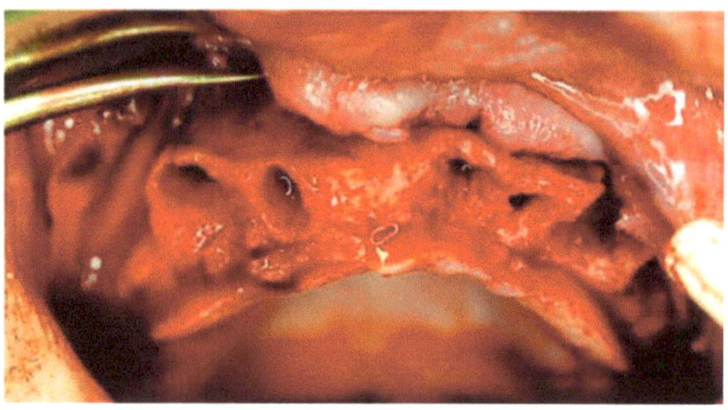

Figure 18.401. Appearance after preservation of alveoli removed abundant granulation tissue. Larger bone defects. The appearance of the condition seems worrying for the fulfillment of the patient's wishes; to have immediate fixed compensations. When solving such complicated cases, the most important light that represents the road to the desired result is the knowledge and experience of the dentist and the vision of the outcome of the implant-prosthetic treatment.

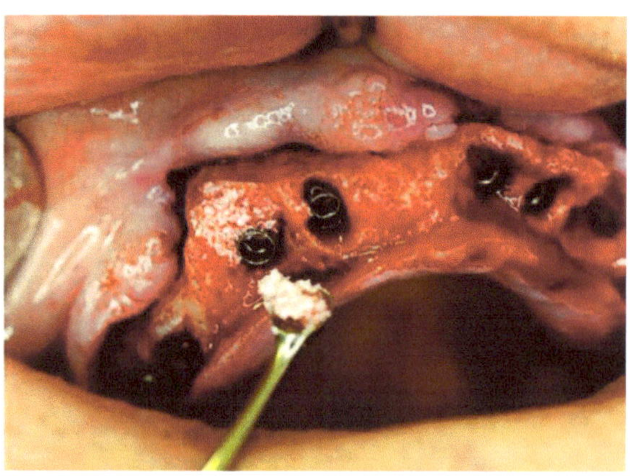

Figure 18.402. Augmentation of bone defects around immediately installed implants.

Further procedures of implant-prosthetic rehabilitation in the upper jaw are shown in pictures 18.403-18.413.).

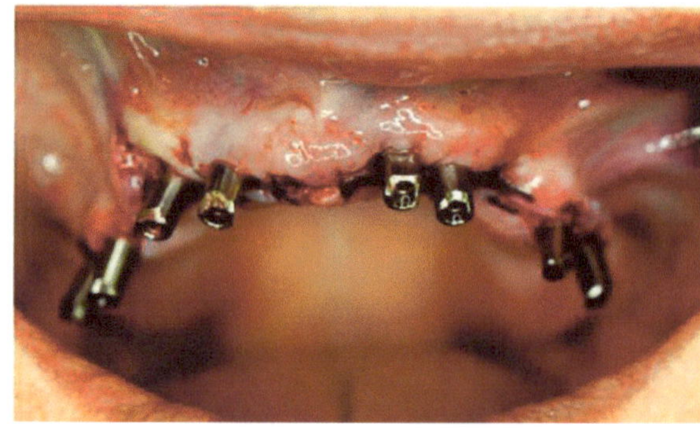

Figure 18.403. Immediately installed implants of standard diameters. The soft tissues around the implant were also treated with the Linkow papilla forming instrument. Adjusted parality of supports that are tightened with a dynamometer up to 35 Ncm. If the establishment of paralyticity of the brackets (abutments) cannot be achieved with brackets at an angle, the adjustment must not be performed in the mouth due to the transfer of thermal stimuli to the bone.

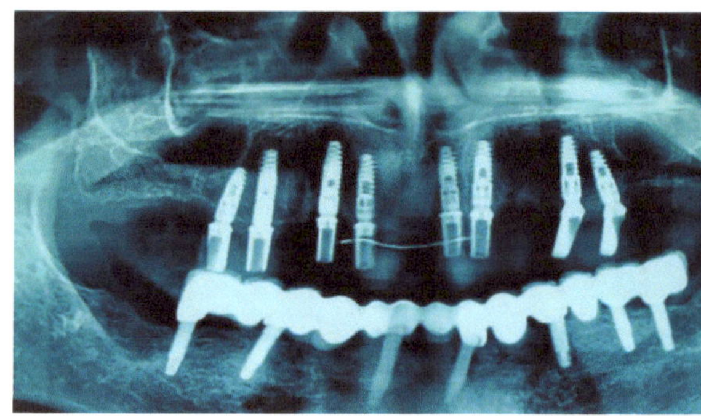

Figure 18.404. Radiological image after immediately installed and immediately loaded EL Estethik implants in the upper jaw, with augmentation of bone defects. Condition in the lower jaw after 7 years, stable bone condition around the implant (diameter 3.3 mm), with complete absence of marginal bone loss. This confirms the opinion of the author of the book that the micro-crack space between the support (abutment) and the body of the implant can be a place for the deposition of microorganisms that cause bone resorption and peri-implant changes.

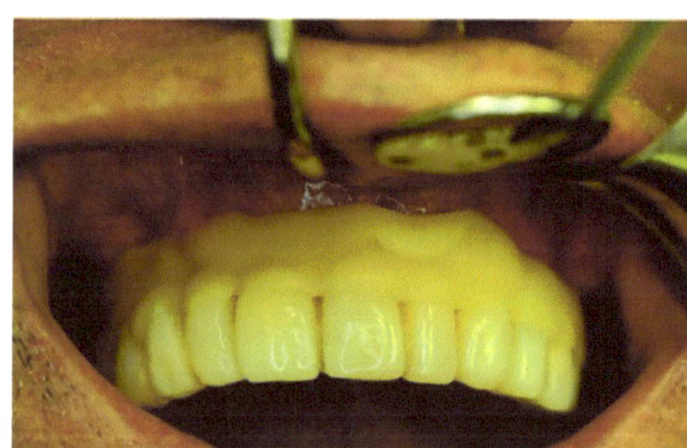

Figure 18.405. View after immediate installation of implants immediately loaded with a provisional bridge. Covering soft tissues with Reso-pac resorbable packing (Hager Werken, Germany) accelerates soft tissue healing).

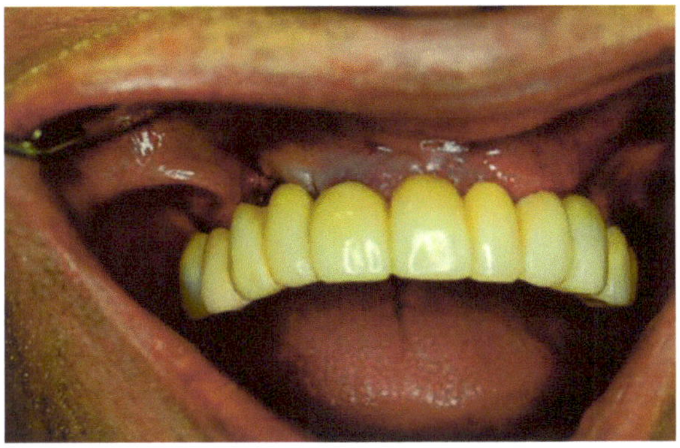

Figure 18.406. Provisional prosthetic work was placed on the same day after implant installation. Immediate loading stimulates osseointegration processes according to Wolff's rule (Wolf's Law): "The bone should be put into function as soon as possible!" With the loss of teeth, the jawbone loses its function, which is manifested by the quantitative loss of the alveolar ridge. At the same time, better and faster formation of keratinized gingiva is promoted around definitively placed supports (abutments). A favorable outcome also depends on the quality of the implant system.

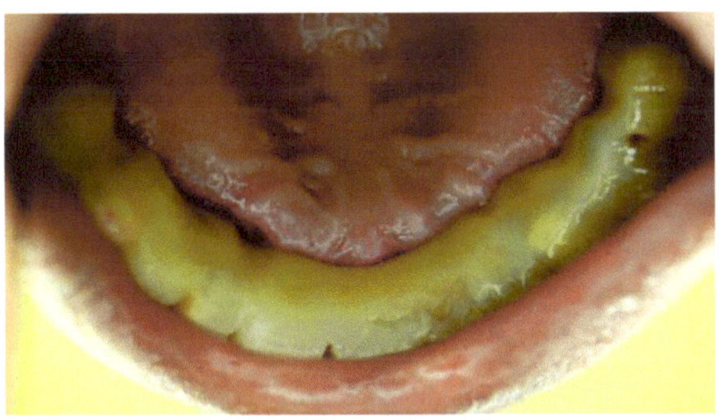

Figure 18.407. Appearance of the provisional bridge from the palatal side after 7 days. It is necessary to repeat the temporary prosthetic work with precise processing around the support to enable good soft tissue formation.

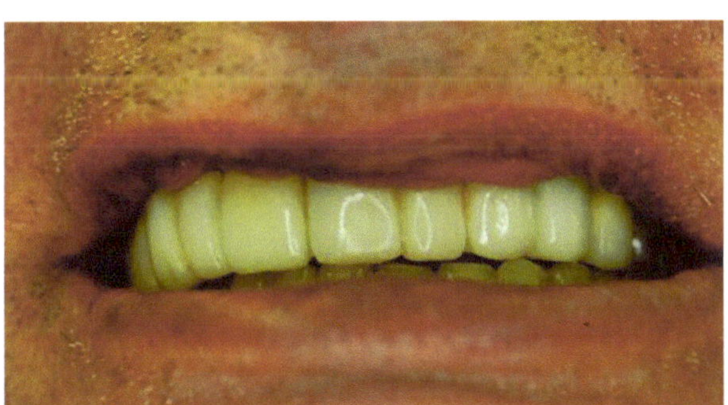

Figure 18.408. Immediately loaded implants with a provisional bridge, on the same day after a complicated oral surgical procedure, is a great feeling and the fulfillment of the patient's wishes. At the same time, morbidity was significantly reduced, good chewing of food and smooth business communication and cooperation were made possible.

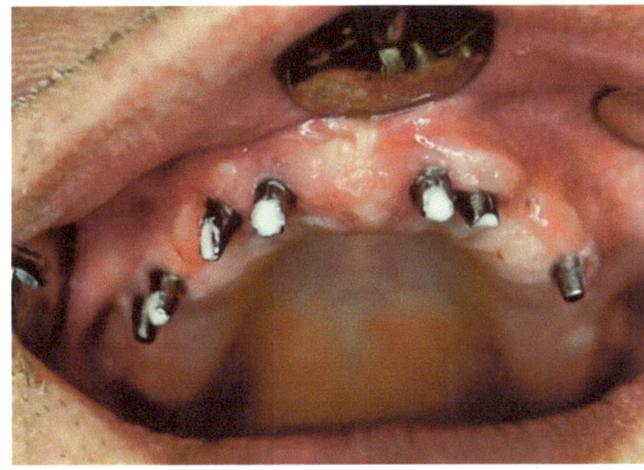

Figure 18.409. Appearance of the state after 6 months of immediate installation of the implant and immediate loading with fixed acrylate prosthetic work.

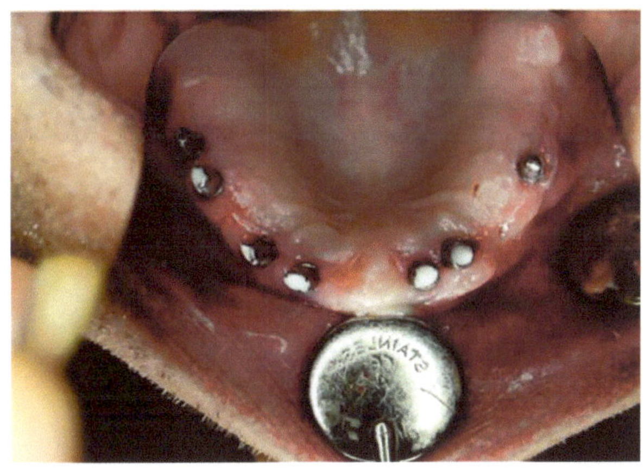

Figure 18.410. The arch of the alveolar ridge was also reconstructed by augmentation of larger bone destructions. Immediately placed implants are well integrated. Appearance of healed soft tissues. Compare with images 18.399, 18.400 and 18.401. Picture

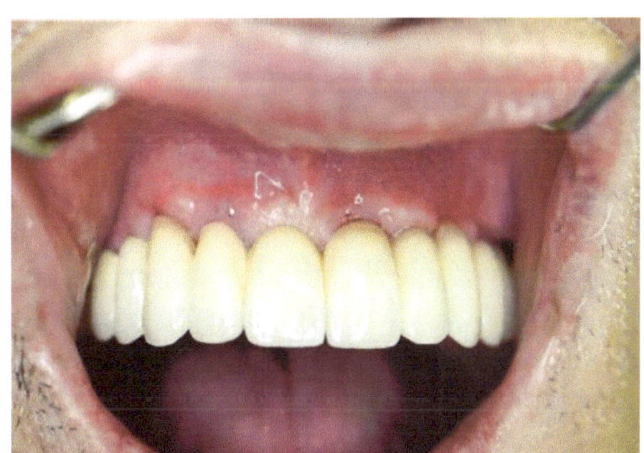

Figure 18.411. Definitive fixed prosthetic work in metal ceramics. Appearance of well-healed soft tissues vestibularly.

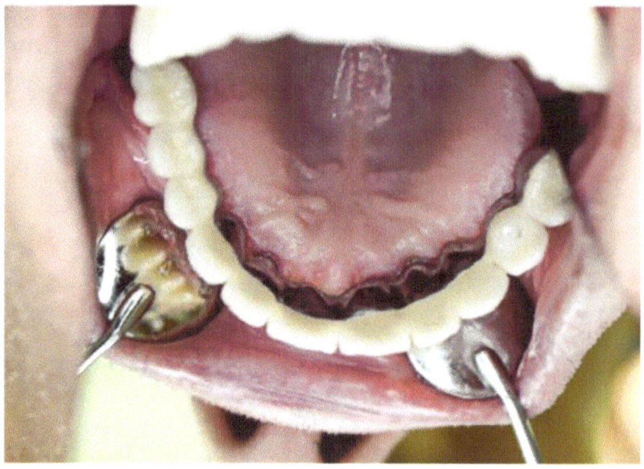

Figure 18.412. Appearance of healed tissues palatally.

Recently, on the market of implant systems, brand awareness has been given to implants built with a combination of two different materials, titanium and zirconium (Strauman's "New Roxolid implant system"). It is stated that the application of this new "hit" significantly accelerates the time of osseointegration processes from 8 to 4 weeks?

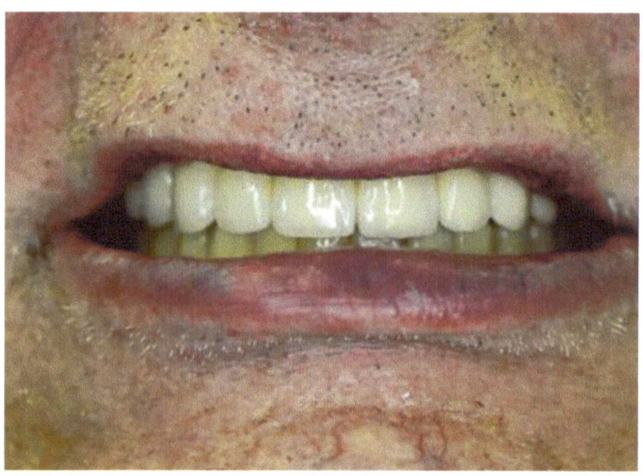

Figure 18.413. With the applied implant-prosthetic procedure, the patient's comfort was not compromised from the beginning to the end of the treatment.

It is indisputable that the technology of implant surface processing, when it comes to osseointegration processes, has reached a high level. New details on the implant and abutment are being designed, which have an impact on the osseointegration processes and on the soft shaping processes tissues. The industry of implant systems, so to speak, branched out like lightning, and thus the competition on the market increased significantly. All this process of development and offers is accompanied by the development of marketing. Marketing praise should be taken with a grain of salt until science confirms it, and practice verifies it. The author of the book, during his decades of practice in oral implantology, accepted and abandoned various implant systems that were given an advantage by marketing over all other implant systems at the time.

For example, in one period, the Markentian "hit" was cylindrical implants coated with hydroxyapatite. Even the author of the book presented cases solved with implants at a world congress where the titanium surface was coated with hydroxyapatite; of course, with the emphasis that this technological innovation promotes biological processes in the peri-implant milieu. According to data from the literature, there were no critical views, except praise. This is how the manufacturers explained the advantages of the combination of titanium and hydroxyapatite. However, after a few years, numerous cases of periimplatitis appeared.

When, later, I visited Professor Ferrai in Florida, who was installing similar implants coated with hydroxyapatite, the results of the implantation were the same as the author of the book, unsuccessful. It has even been documented that hydroxyapatite, separated from the titanium surface, was deposited in the kidney glomeruli. The conclusion is: technologically it was not possible to unite these two different materials.

It is indisputable that the technology of implant surface processing, when it comes to osseointegration processes, has reached a high level. New details on the implant and abutment are being designed, which have an impact on the osseointegration processes and on the soft shaping processes tissues. The industry of implant systems, so to speak, branched out like lightning, and thus the competition on the market increased significantly. All this process of development and offers is accompanied by the development of marketing. Marketing praise should be taken with a grain of salt until science confirms it, and practice verifies it. The author of the book, during his decades of practice in oral implantology, accepted and abandoned various implant systems that were given an advantage by marketing over all other implant systems at the time.

For example, in one period, the Markentian "hit" was cylindrical implants coated with hydroxyapatite.

Even the author of the book presented cases solved with implants at a world congress where the titanium surface was coated with hydroxyapatite; of course, with the emphasis that this technological innovation promotes biological processes in the peri-implant milieu. According to data from the literature, there were no critical views, except praise. This is how the manufacturers explained the advantages of the combination of titanium and hydroxyapatite. However, after a few years, numerous cases of periimplatitis appeared.

When, later, I visited Professor Ferrai in Florida, who was installing similar implants coated with hydroxyapatite, the results of the implantation were the same as the author of the book, unsuccessful. It has even been documented that hydroxyapatite, separated from the titanium surface, was deposited in the kidney glomeruli. The conclusion is: technologically it was not possible to unite these two different materials.

The answer to this question is: the way of marketing is adapting to the ever-increasing offer of implant systems on the market. It is stated that the combination of titanium and zirconium reduces the time to achieve the osseointegration process, from 8 to 4 weeks, thanks to the hydrophilic surface of the Roxlolid implant.

With the same Marchenti praise about the hydrophilicity of the titanium-implant surface, which enables faster and better integration of the implant and the bone, a few years ago, the "ICH templant Implantat", a Swiss-German creation, was launched. (picture 18.346). The difference in marketing approach for these two systems was the price offered:

"ICX-tempplant" even started with an extremely low price. Strauman, offered the "Roxolid Implants System" with an extremely high price, regardless of this time of weakened patient's ability to pay. Although it is a serious manufacturer, experience points to a cautious approach to innovation of all implant systems.

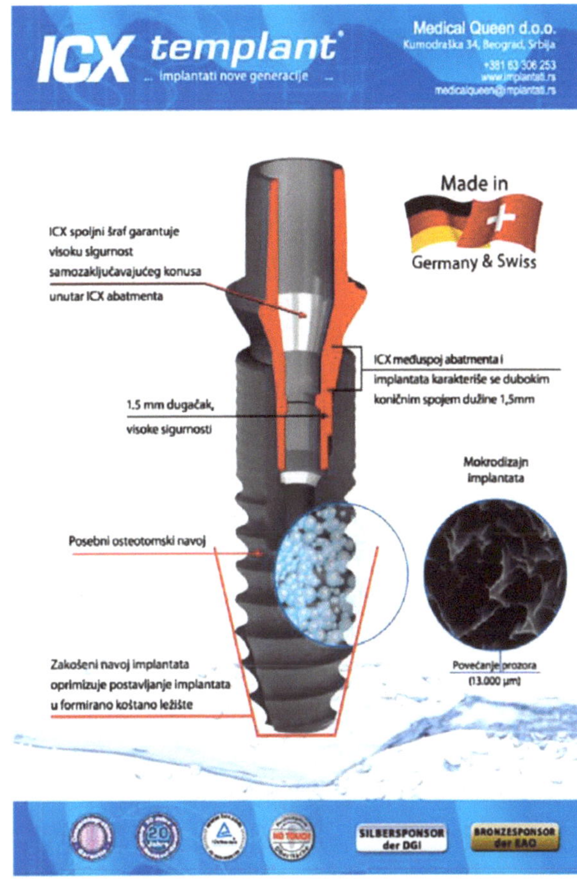

Figure 18.414. Schematic representation of the "ICX templant" implant showing the microstructure of the "hydrophilic" surface.

Everything that today's marketing emphasizes for the newest line of Straumann's implant system ("Roksolid implant system"), the hydrophilicity of the surface, is also emphasized for the "ICX template" implant, which has already been written about in the book. However, the results in practice were different from the manufacturer's promises (Fig. 18.415).

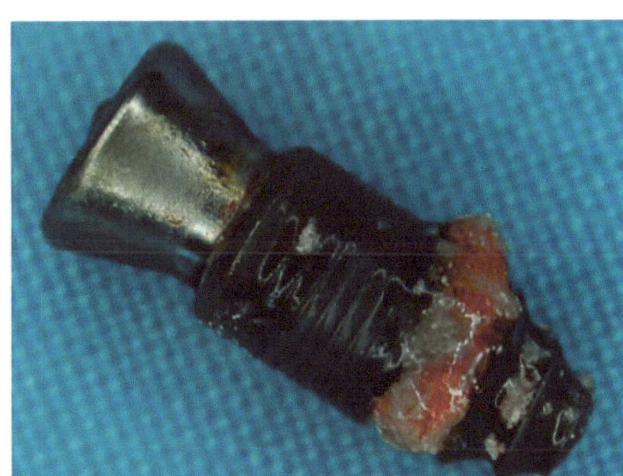

Figure 18.415. "ICX-template after 12 months." Implant loss caused by peri-implantitis.

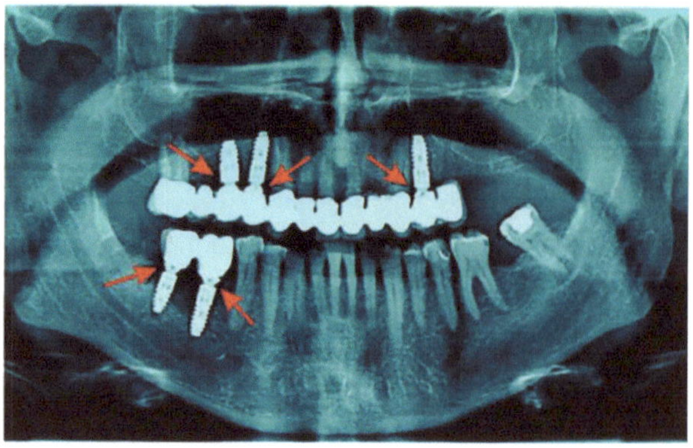

Figure 18.416. A major drawback of the "ICX system" is the junction (microcrack) of the support (marked by arrows) and the implant body, as well as the design of the abutment. "ICX-template after 12 months." Implant loss caused by peri-implantitis.

Since a lot of peri-implant problems are caused by poor prosthetic work and insufficient oral hygiene, to what extent can the performance of the prosthetic superstructure prevent such problems from occurring?

Prosthetic work that is anchored on implants can have both stimulating and destructive effects. Stimulating, if the construction of prosthetic work is carried out, first of all, in accordance with gnathological principles. Realized biomechanical requirements will stimulate osseointegration processes. Bad prosthetic work is the "tomb" of even the best implant systems. The long-term durability of bone implants ensures the stable formation of soft tissues, which depends on several factors, including the performance of the prosthetic work, explained in the book in several places, and will be documented in the following pictures (pictures 18.417-18.426).

Disease of peri-implant soft tissues (peri-implantitis mucosis) is an irreversible inflammatory process caused by poor oral hygiene. Prosthetic work must be performed in such a way that in the inter-implant spaces it provides access for easy cleaning and good maintenance of oral hygiene. The prevention of peri-implant changes also depends on this detail of prosthetic work.

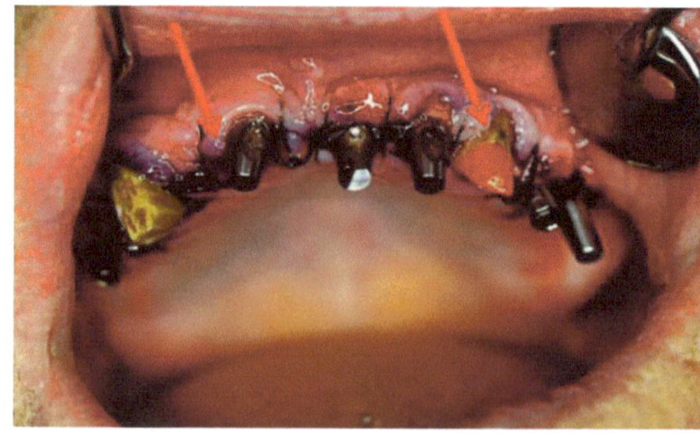

Figure 18.417. The fulfillment of the requirements for the realization of "legie-artis" prosthetic work depends on the planning and position of the installed implants. Implant positioning depends on the quality and quantity of the alveolar bone (width and height), which also determines the diameter of the implant. Display of immediately installed implants with definitive supports. The left canines (at the express request of the patient) are in good condition. Canine (#23), endodontically repaired, with acrylate modeled (red color) future cast replacement in metal.

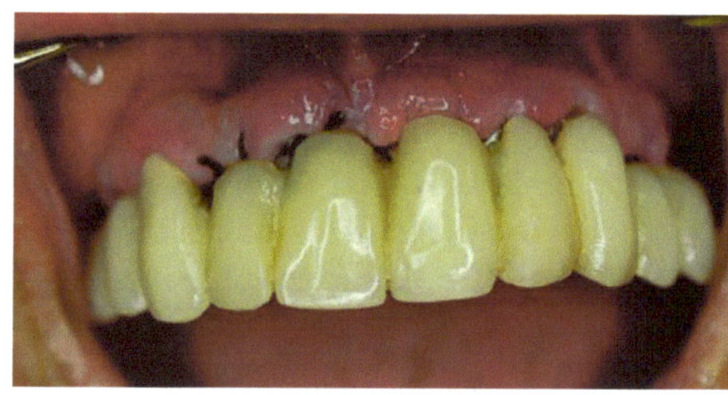

Figure 18.418. Immediately placed temporary acrylate bridge immediately after installation of the implant, with definitive supports (abutments). Papillae formed with the Linkow-instrument.

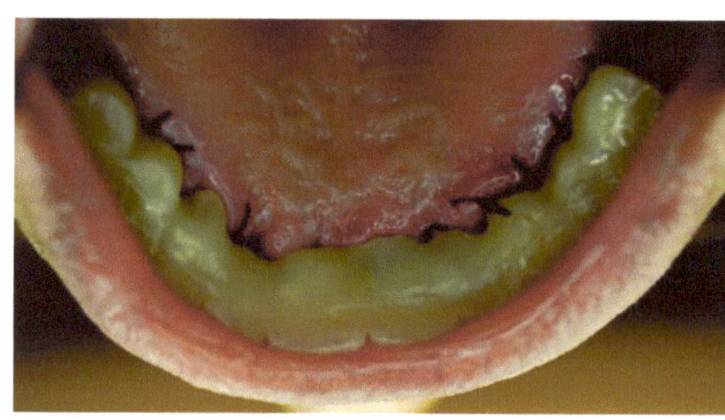

Figure 18.419. Appearance of the immediately placed temporary prosthetic work from the palatal side.

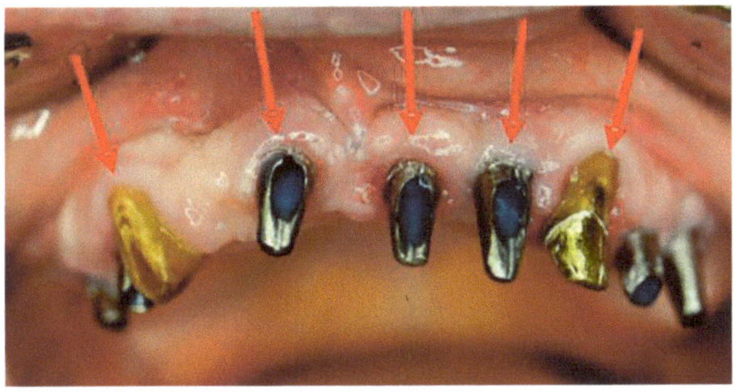

Figure 18.420. Appearance of the gingiva after 12 months. Extremely stable soft tissues (indicated by red arrows) formed around the definitive supports on which the temporary bridge is anchored.

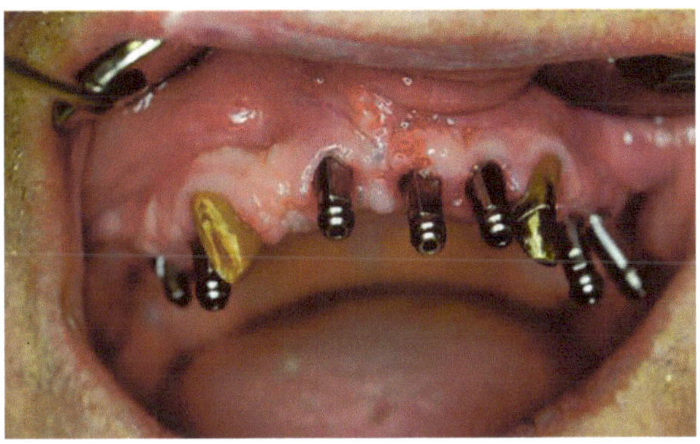

Figure 18.421. Transfers for transferring the position of the implant to the laboratory for parallelizing the supports (abutments), taken with a single-phase impression.

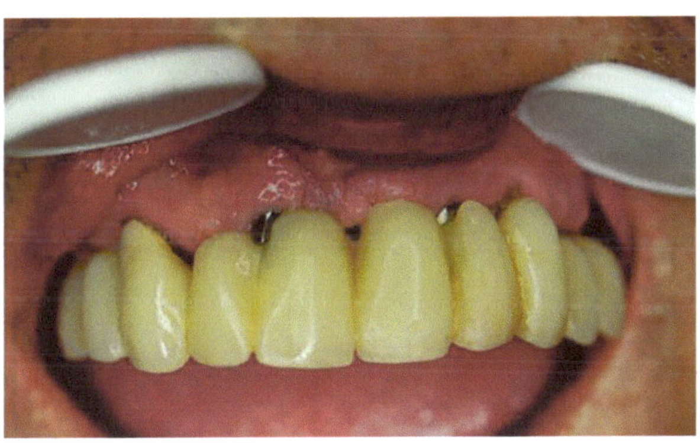

Figure 18.422. Condition after 12 months with temporary prosthetic work.

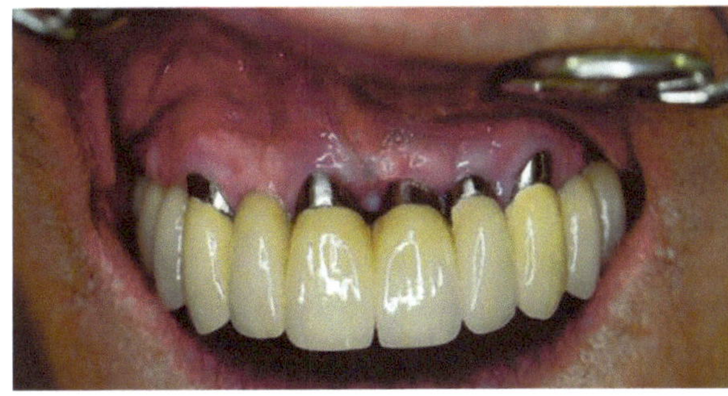

Figure 18.423. Control shot after 24 months. Stable soft tissues ideal maintenance of oral hygiene. Formed interimplant papillae.

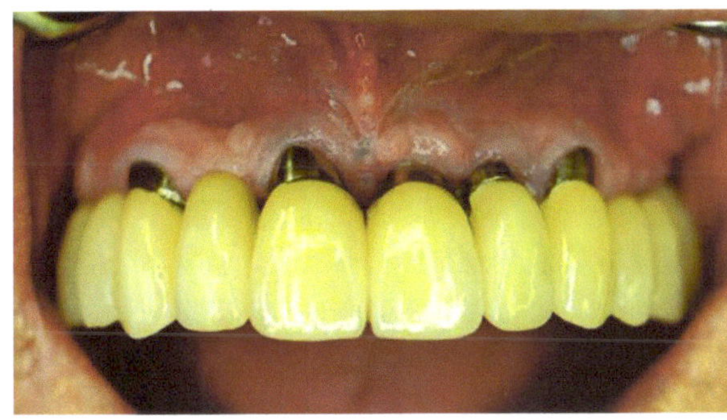

Figure 18.424. Ideal prosthetic work; enabled saliva circulation and access of the interdental brush between the implant spaces. Metallomics on gold for the prevention of peri-implant diseases. Good oral hygiene is facilitated by the circulation of saliva and the provision of brush access. A favorable smile line and lip position make this solution possible.

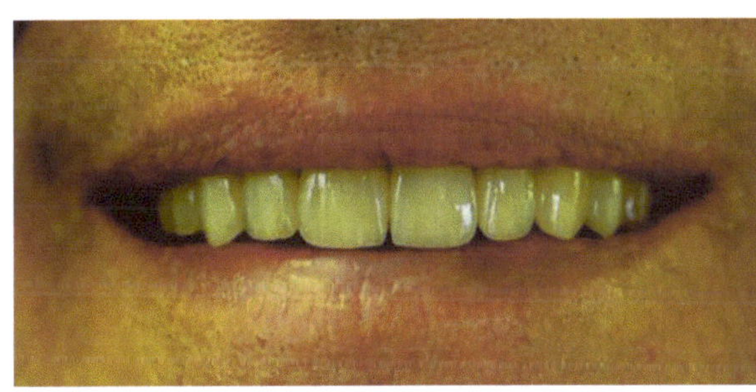

Figure 18.425. The aesthetic effect is determined by the shape of the lips and laugh line.

Conclusion:

Prevention of peri-implant diseases depends on prosthetic work.

In order to know how far you have come, you must know where you started from.

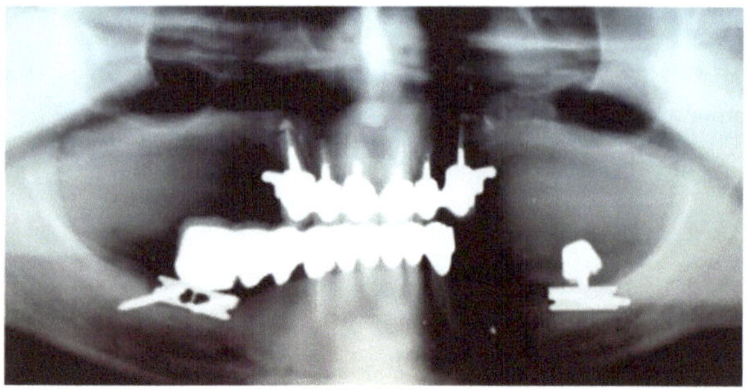

Figure 18.426. The author of the book does not know whose hand this was the work of, but it was the beginning of implantology!

To know that we know what we know and to know that we do not know what we do not know - that is true knowledge.

Nicolas Copernicus

Blessed is he who knows that he does not know, but wants to know!

Biblical wisdom

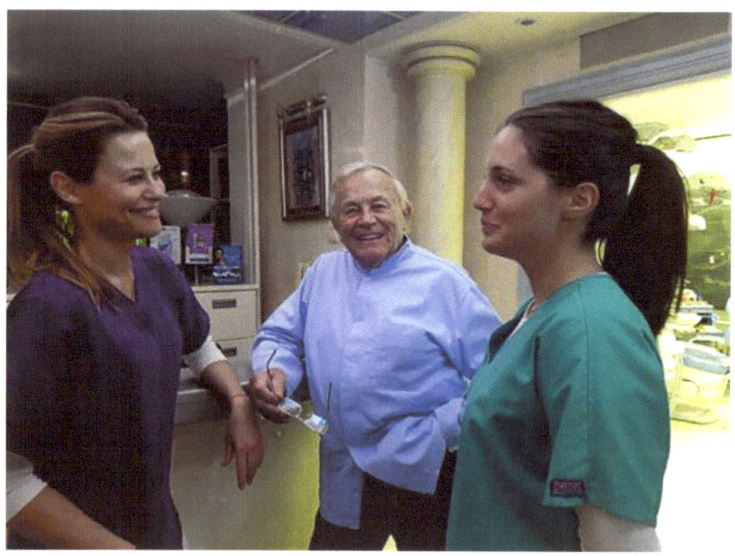

There are things we think we know, and that prevents us from learning what we should know.

19

Conversation With The Patient

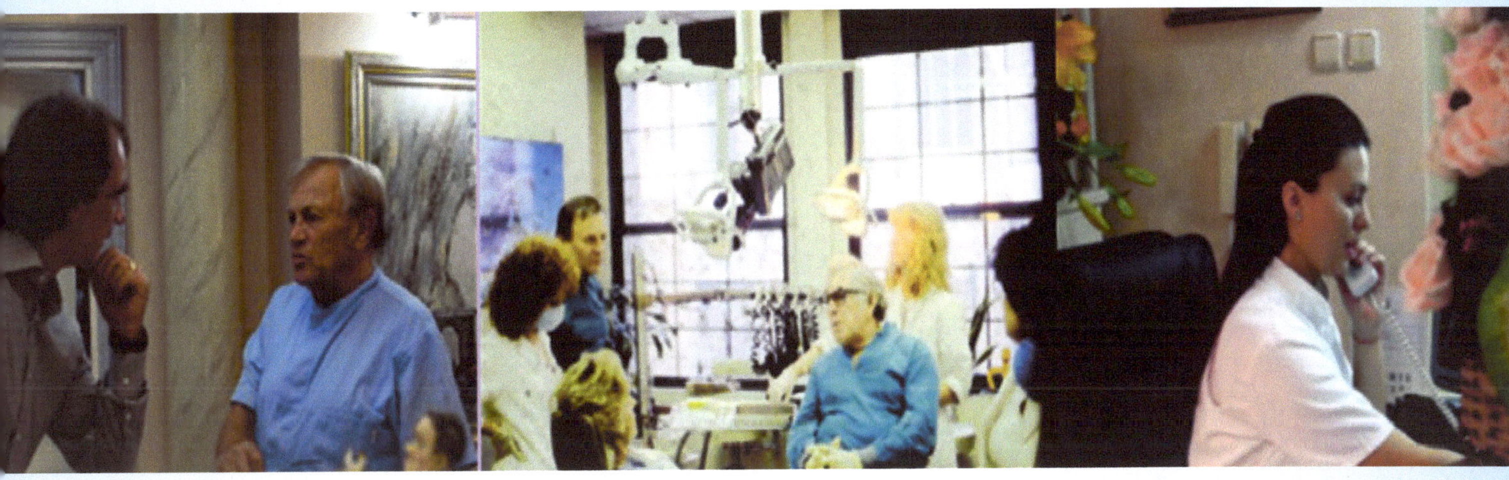

The aim of this chapter is to familiarize patients with the basic principles and real possibilities of oral implantology. Both students of dentistry and dentists, who did not have the opportunity to become familiar with the complex surgical-prosthetic procedures of this specialty through education and practice, will be able to learn about it relatively easily through this chapter, that is, to understand the basic principles, possibilities and indications of oral implantology.

Teachers, who teach oral implantology in any form and scope, can extract adequate questions from this chapter to test the knowledge of students and residents.

A special, and not so rare, problem for dentists is the so-called psychogenic pain, which is not described in dental and implantology textbooks and books, pain that, after a successful dental procedure, without a real cause and a real pathogenesis, is reported by mentally unstable persons who overcome it. empty pain" and justify their manifest or hidden failures, dissatisfaction and their frustrations. If the dentist does not understand what it is about in time, he will have big problems and, under the pressure of the patient, will make major or minor professional mistakes. Decades of experience and examples from practice led the author of the book to devote himself to this problem as well.

During the first examination of a patient interested in installing an implant, the dentist must not be superficial. The patient will ask many questions to which accurate and very clear answers must be given. It often happens that the patient visits several dentists, asking all of them for detailed information about the entire implant installation procedure. If he also brings extensive radiographic documentation, it is a sure confirmation that such a patient visits several surgeries. Patients without an appointment, or "passers-by", should not be admitted for an interview that requires a certain amount of time.

The patient's determination will depend not only on the clarity of the answer but also on the gain of trust. The dentist must have the patience to listen carefully to each question and think carefully about what answers the patient's questions require. The conversation must not be superficial, especially since it, at the same time, represents mutual testing. The dentist should conclude what kind of patient it is and whether it belongs to a suitable group for implantation, from several aspects. Without the patient's trust, as an important indicator that he will be a good collaborator, during and especially after the treatment, there is no desired success.

The patient's most common questions are related to the procedure itself—"What is tooth implantation, how is it performed, is it a painful operation, and how long will it last?" The patient should be explained in detail how the implant replaces the lost tooth. Some models show the patient how the implant lies in the bone (pictures 19.1 to 19.4).

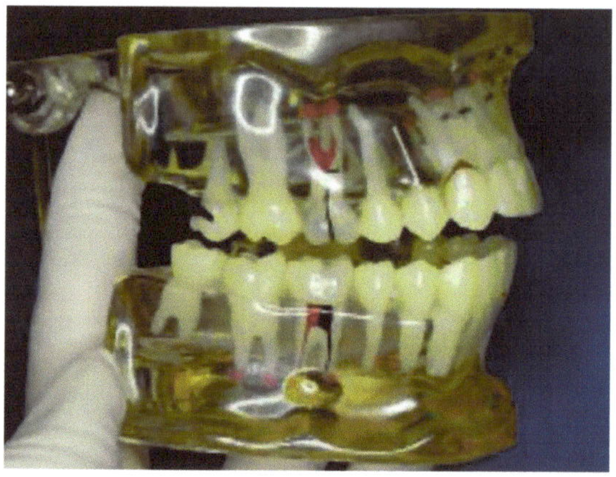

Figure 19.1. Model of jaws with "built-in" implant.

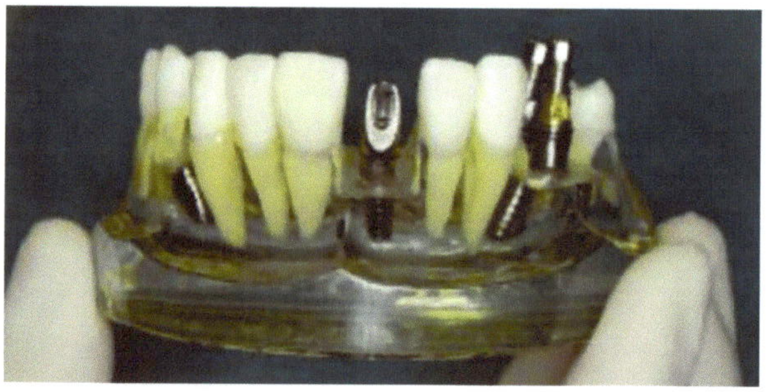

Figure 19.2. Jaw model with implant present - detail.

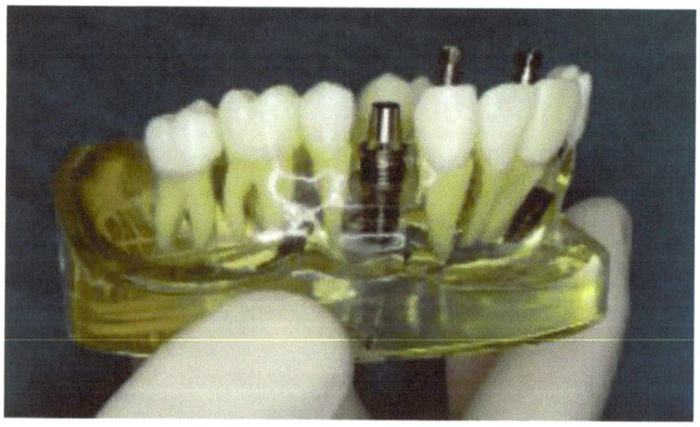

Figure 19.3. Jaw model with implant present - detail.

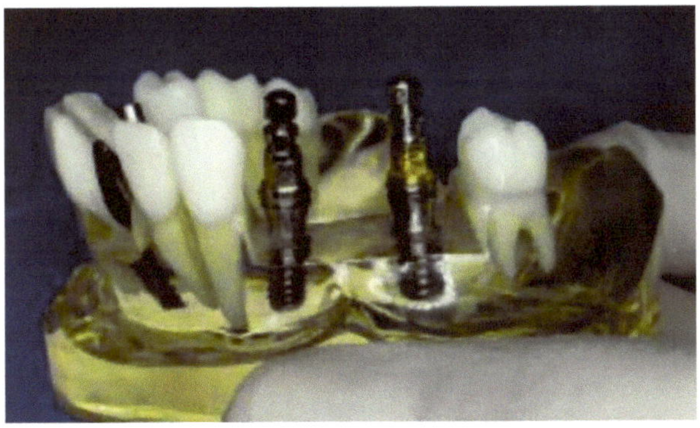

Figure 19.4. Jaw model with implant present - detail.

After the explanation, the patient, as a rule, asks the most important questions to him: how long it will take to get "new" teeth and how much the entire treatment will cost.

When he gets an answer about the cost of the implants and how many implants are needed for his case, the next question is: what will happen if the body rejects one or two implants?

The answer must be clear. If one of the implants fails, it must be emphasized that it is not a "rejection" reaction, because the organism cannot receive several implants and reject one. The loss of one or two implants is conditioned by other causes, namely anatomical obstacles, quantity and quality of bone, etc. It must be explained to the patient that there are ways to overcome the eventual loss of one or two implants.

In order to explain the entire procedure to the patient, dentists are greatly facilitated by atlases that explain the entire oral surgical procedure and prosthetic work in the most vivid and clear way.

With the help of such aids, the dentist must also expect additional questions, which he should answer accurately and precisely.

If the patient asks for the procedure itself to be explained in more detail, it should be done briefly, possibly with the help of photographs, which show the entire procedure in abbreviated form.

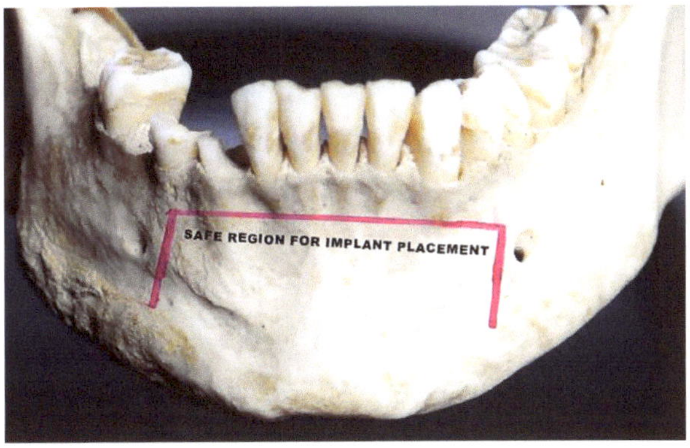

Figure 19.5. In the conversation with the patient, depending on the case; whether it is partial or total toothlessness, explain why certain regions are safe for implant placement, and others with risk factors and even the impossibility of implant placement.

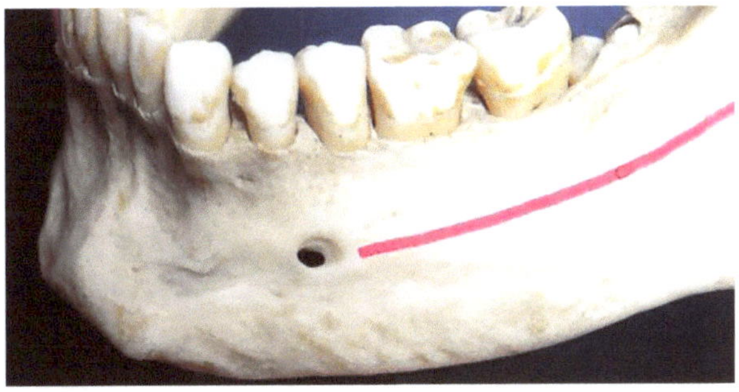

Figure 19.6. Unlike the frontal region in the lower jaw, in the posterior regions the possibility and application of implantation depends on several factors: the time of tooth loss, the shape of the alveolar bone and the condition of the available bone. In cases of extreme atrophy, the limiting factors are injury to the foramen mentalis and n. mandibularis inferior.

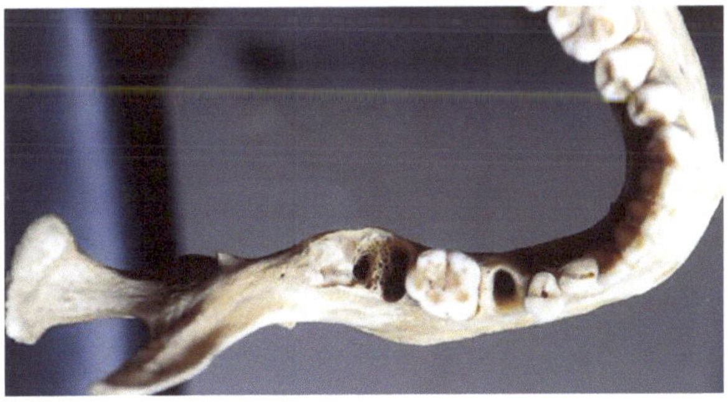

Figure 19.7. In the case of loss of individual teeth, it is possible to immediately install an implant at the same time as replacing the extracted tooth with a temporary crown.

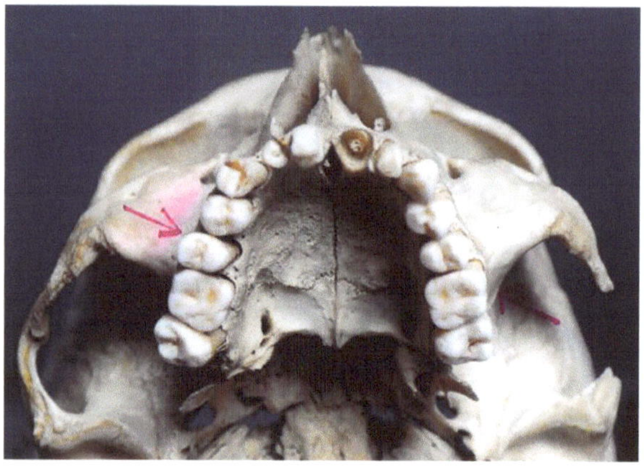

Figure 19.8. Explain to the patient why the indications for implantation in the upper jaw differ significantly: the quality of cancellous bone, anatomical structures - sinus and nasal floor, condition and quality of lamellar bone in the frontal region.

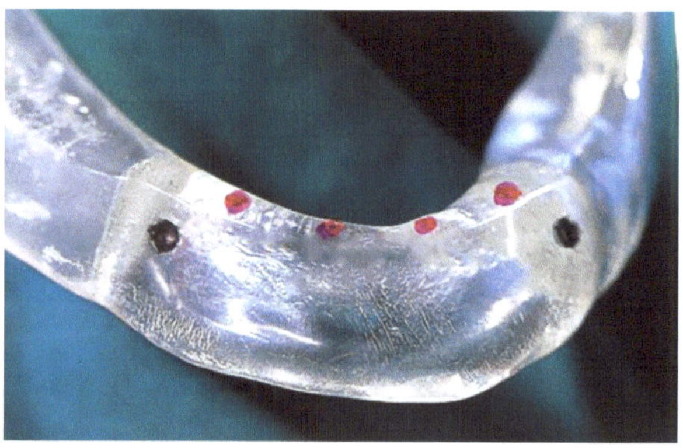

Figure 19.9. Implant-prosthetic rehabilitation in the oral cavity begins with a conversation with the patient and an explanation of what needs to be done with a presentation of the sequence of procedures. Explain the treatment plan for the entire procedure. The first step is to assess the quality and quantity of available bone. Then, determining the position of the implant, whether it is partial or total toothlessness. There are regions where implantation is indicated and the opposite - contraindicated. Explain this to the patient, especially if it is his case.

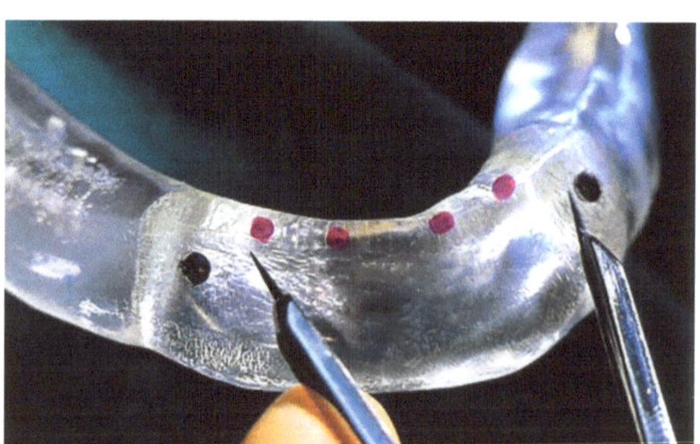

Figure 19.10. In the region between the chin (mental) openings, the implant system and implant selection procedure follows: diameter and length based on a 3D image. The diameter and length of the implant is determined by the horizontal and vertical available bone.

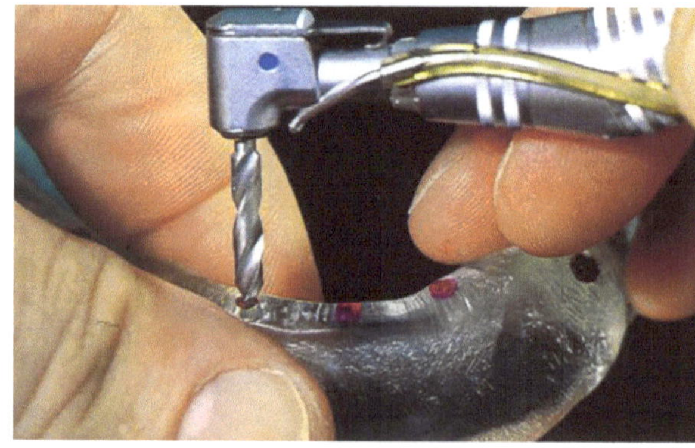

Figure 19.11. The preparation of the implant bed begins by marking the position of the implant with a "pilot drill", and after that, the direction of preparation of the implant bed is determined with a wider drill of 2 mm. With adequately sized drills, bone preparation is adjusted to the diameter and length of the implant.

The answer to the first question should be clear - tooth implantation means a replacement in the place where a tooth that was lost for any reason used to be. The surgical procedure is performed painlessly under local anesthesia, and the actual surgical procedure of installing the implant requires, on average, 20-30 minutes per implant, if no unexpected complications occur during the intervention.

In a conversation with the patient, by showing the following pictures, it can be explained to him what tooth "implantation" is and how it is performed. Likewise, this chapter can serve the dental student as well as the dentist who wants to know the first steps in oral implantology.

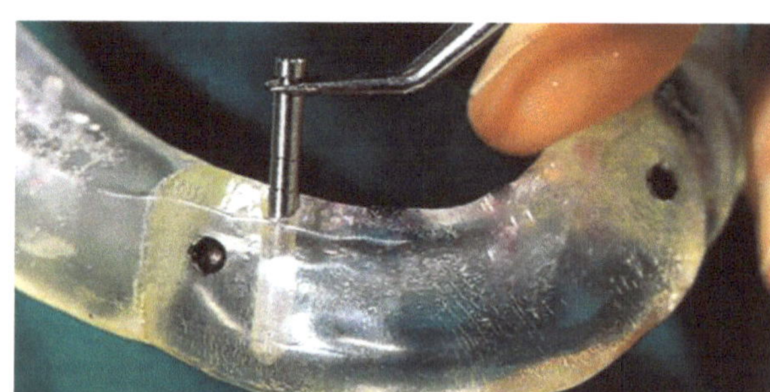

Figure 19.12. After the initial preparation of the implant bed, the direction of the prepared implant bed is checked.

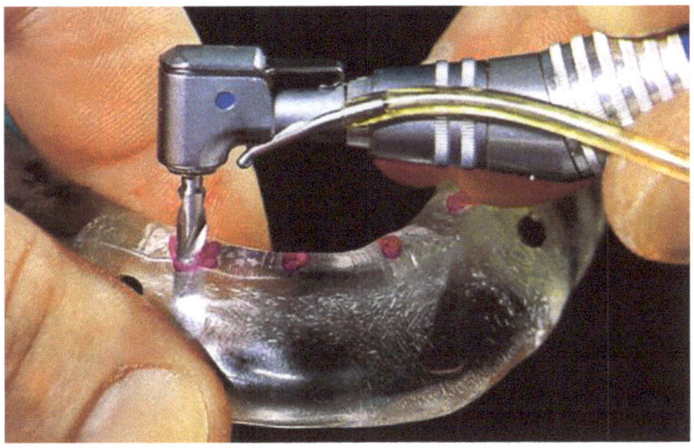

Figure 19.13. Definitive preparation of the implant bed with drills of a diameter that is identical to the diameter of the implant that is installed in the prepared bed. It is preferable for the drill bit to have a slightly narrower diameter in order to achieve primary fixation by self-tapping the implant.

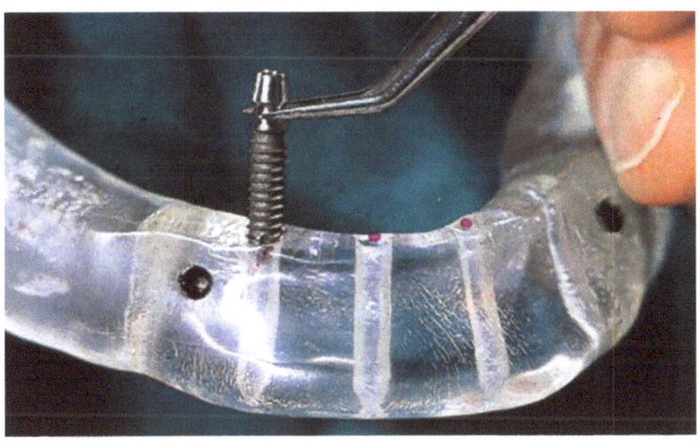

Figure 19.14. Placement of an implant of a certain diameter and length in a prepared bed.

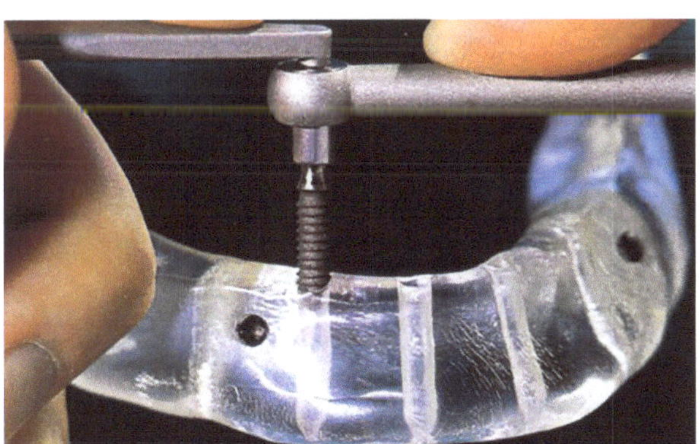

Figure 19.15. Placement of the implant in the prepared bed is done from the original packaging of the implant system by manual tightening (see picture 19.24.) and the first contact of the implant surface must be with blood, and the tension is tightened with a gidor - dynamometer up to 35Ncm. Tightening is done gently with short breaks to avoid tension on the surrounding bone.

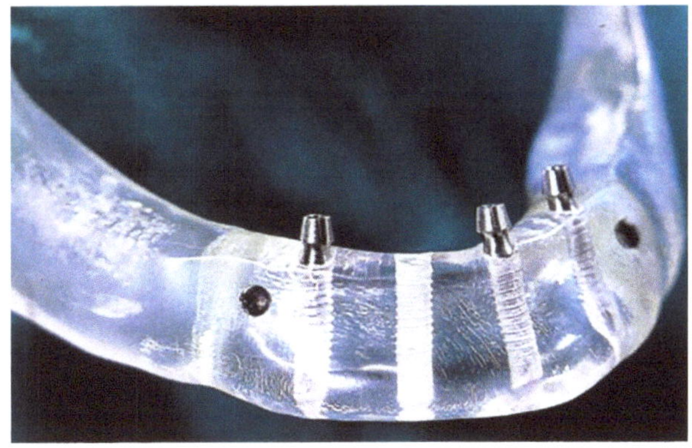

Figure 19.16. The parity of the installed implants is extremely important; whether they will be carriers of retention clips, Dolder and Ackerman retention bars or fixed prosthetic works. Display of the implant bed.

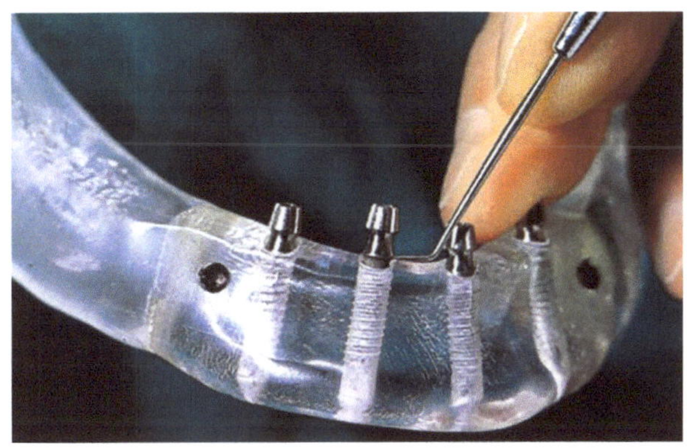

Figure 19.17. The endosseus part of the implant must be embedded 2 mm below the cortical bone level. The decision of which prosthetic retention method should be applied (retention brackets or crossbars) depends on the case, knowledge and experience of the dentist. In similar situations, it is possible to think about making a fixed prosthetic work with extensions, but with risk factors that depend on the quality and quantity of the jawbone, which should be explained to the patient.

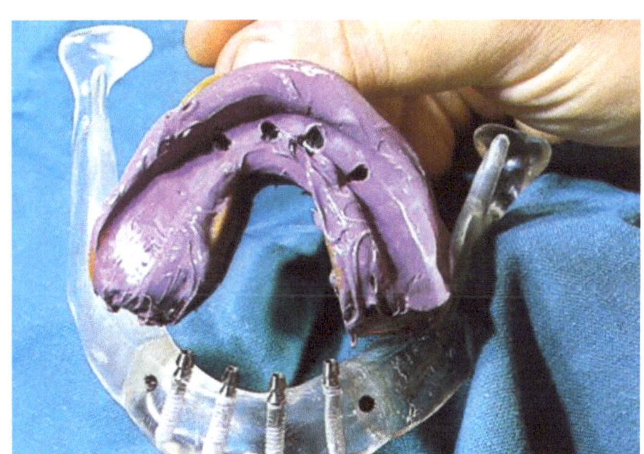

Figure 19.18. Take an impression of the placed supports (abutments).

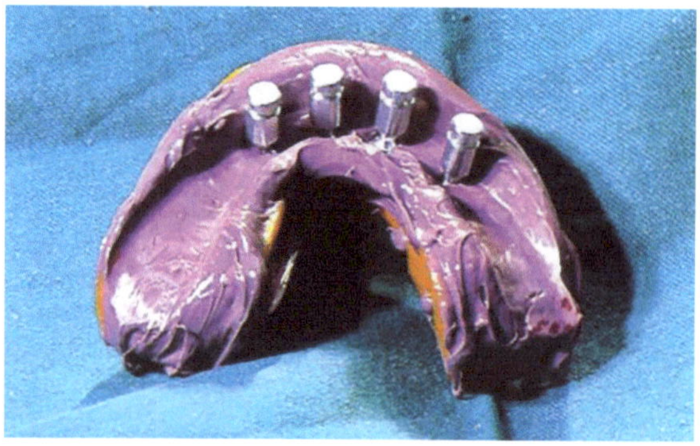

Figure 19.19. One-phase impression with transmitters (transfers) of the position of the implant, with which the situation in the oral cavity is precisely transferred to the laboratory on a plaster model.

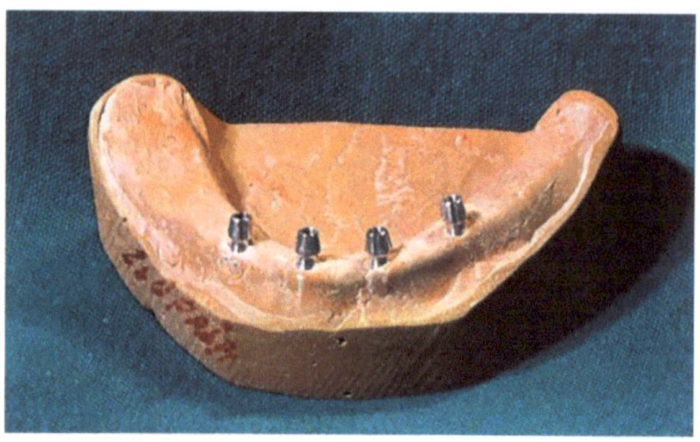

Figure 19.20. Appearance of the implant position on the plaster model on which the future retention Dolder bar is modeled in wax.

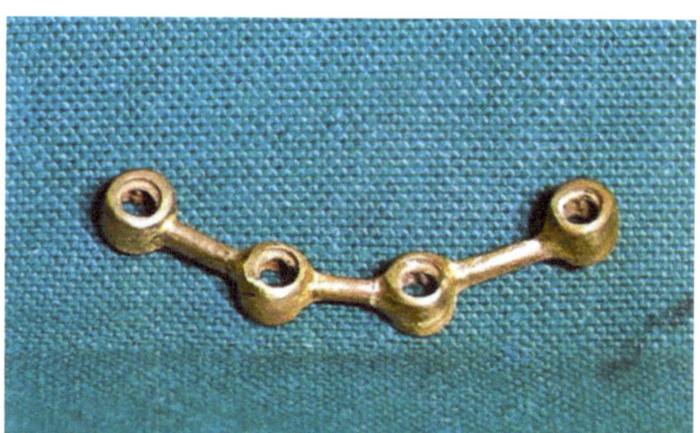

Figure 19.21. Appearance of Dolder crossbar after casting, rough machined which must be polished

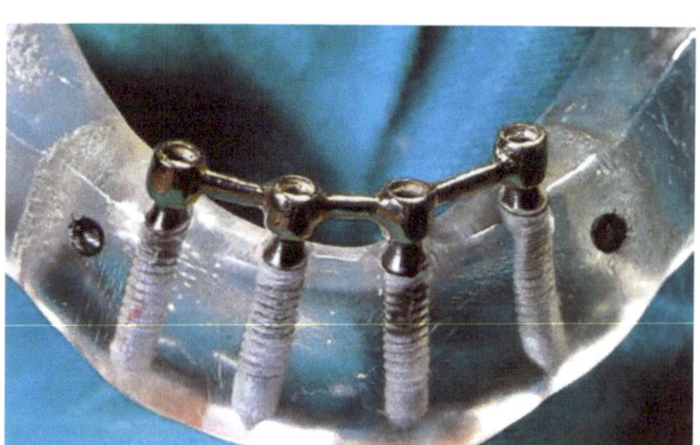

Figure 19.22. Placed Dolder bar on the supports (abutments).

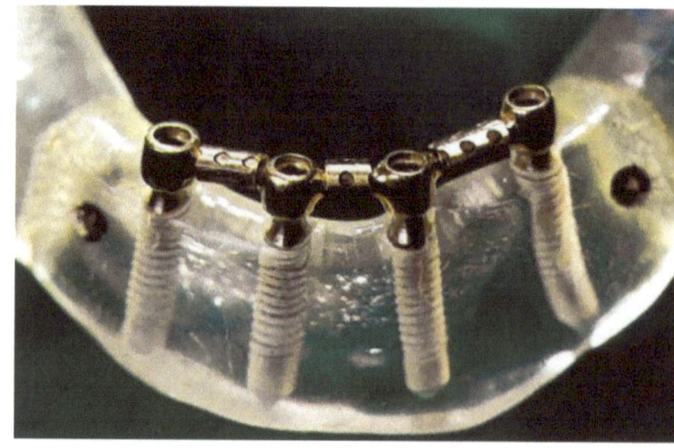

Figure 19.23. Appearance of Dolder's retention bar with mounted riders (handles), which are transferred to the acrylic part of the total prosthesis.

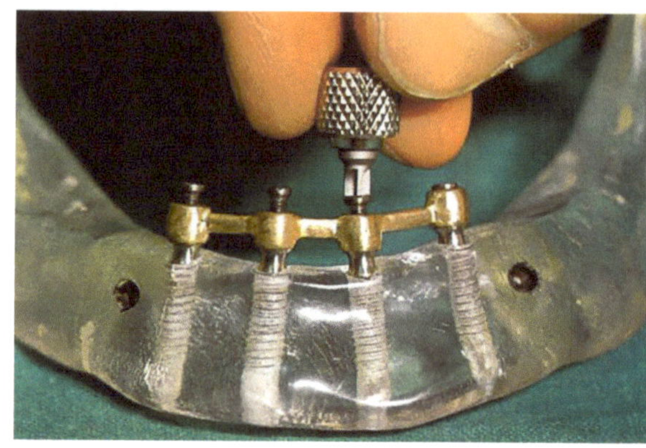

Figure 19.24. Initial manual screwing of the retention bar.

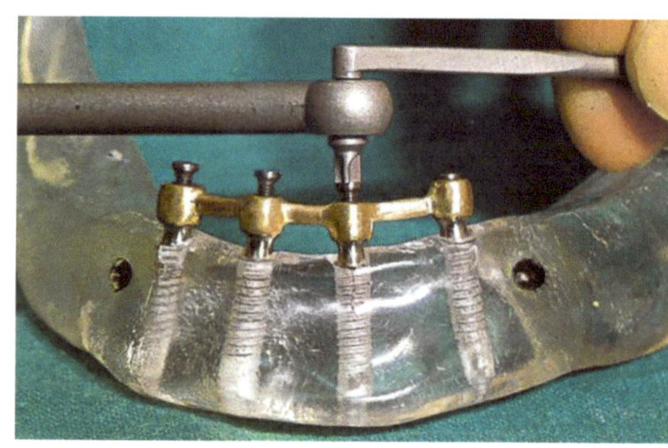

Figure 19.25. Definitive screwing with a dynamometer up to 35 Ncm, simultaneously checking the stability of the prosthetic design.

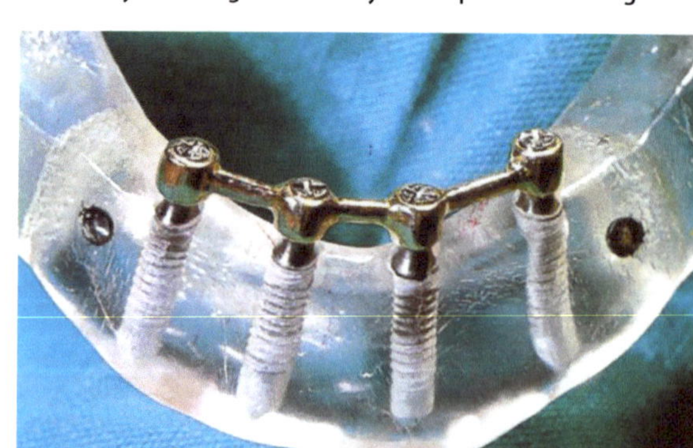

Figure 19.26. The appearance of a definitively screwed retention Dolder bar.

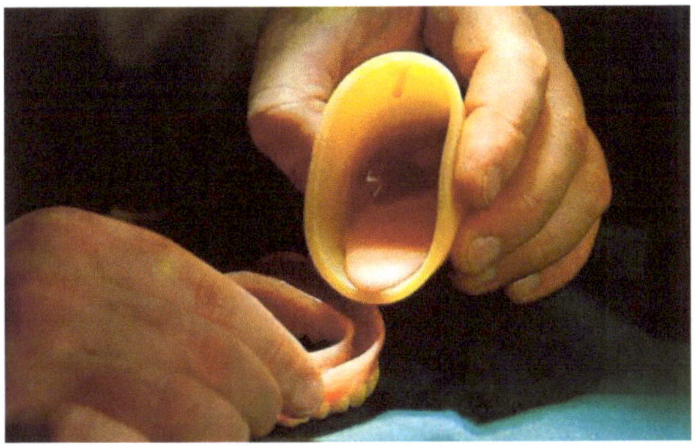

Figure 19.27. With self-polymerizing acrylate, the retention riders (handles) on the parts of the crossbar are fixed in the acrylate total prosthesis.

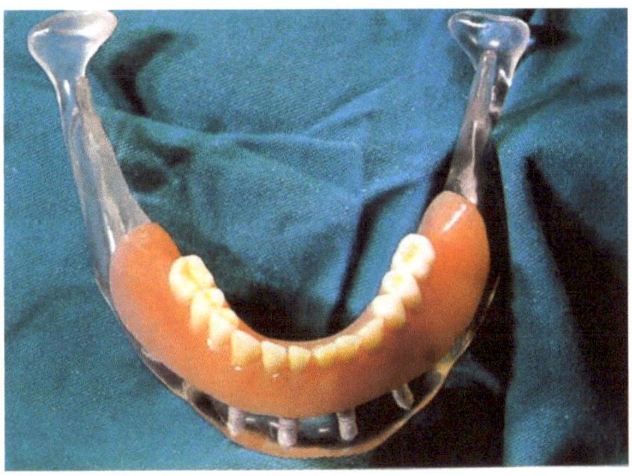

Figure 19.28. The lower total prosthesis anchored on Dolder's retention bar is one of the most optimal solutions for stabilizing the lower total prosthesis.

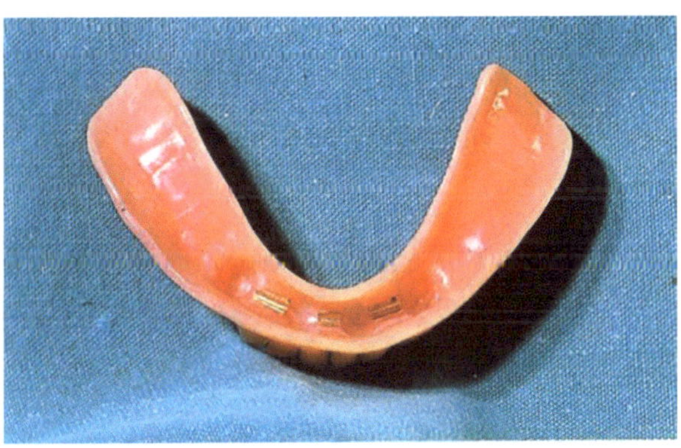

Figure 19.29. The appearance of the rider-grippers in the axillate prosthesis.

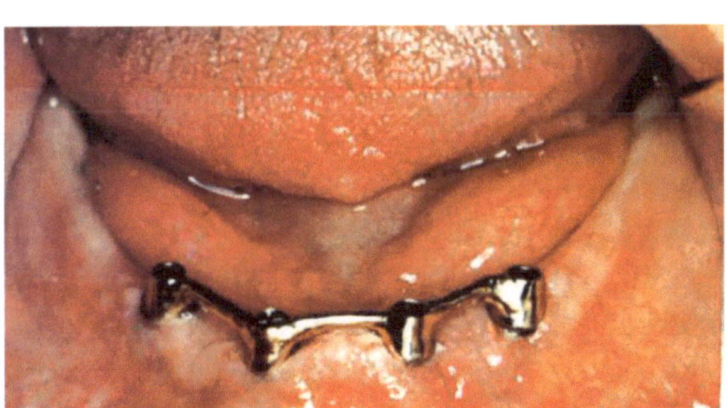

Figure 19.30. Appearance and condition in the mouth after 10 years.

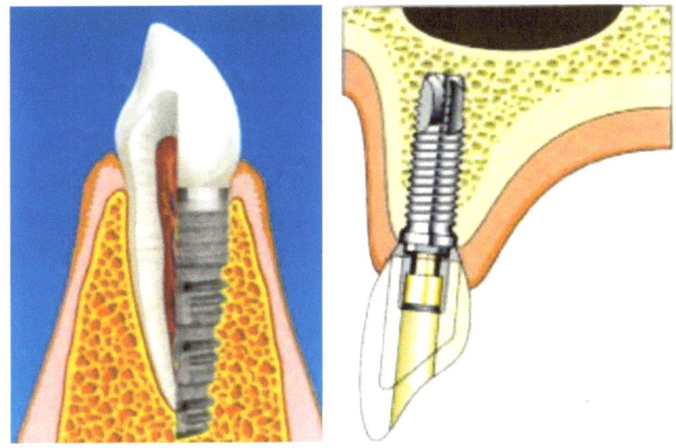

Figure 19.31. Explain to the patient how the implant replaces the role of the tooth and how it works, and with a schematic picture explain individual parts of the implant that are ordered separately.

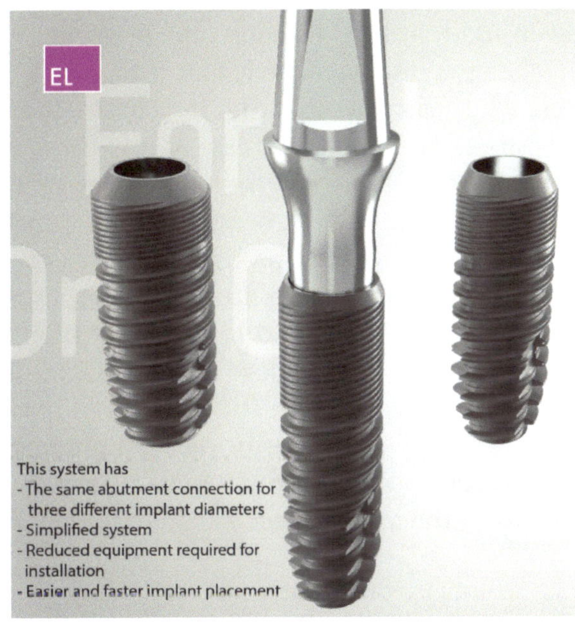

Figure 19.32. To explain to the patient the appearance of the implants used today, their characteristics and advantages.

Question: Can one of the implant systems be singled out and said to be the most perfect?

Answer: No implant system has been made, as it were; forever and ever! There are implant systems that have revolutionized oral implantology; starting with Branemark's implanted system and many after it. However the development of implant systems has progressed over time and continues today. In the large selection of implanted systems, none can be said to be the most perfect, because all systems have their advantages and disadvantages. Which system will be accepted depends on the dentist's experience and the quality of the bone. Therefore, the difference is due to the quality of the bone, which implant system will be decided by the clinician and for which design in the upper and which in the lower jaw. Many details between implant systems determine the advantage of one system over another. For example, if we compare the characteristics of two quality implant systems Nobel and El Esthetic Line. The endosellous part of both has its own characteristics; design, treatment of the implant surface, design in the neck, shape and inclination of the thread, which determines the method of implantation and the achievement of primary fixation. The screw-in abutment method for the endosseous part at Nobel is simpler, but it has disadvantages compared to the screw-in method at El Esthetic Line implants. With the Nobel, the disadvantage is that over time it can loosen, which is impossible with the construction of the El Esthetic Line implant. In case of screw breakage with this system, there is a special instrument with which to remove the abutment. Strauman belongs to the higher quality systems, but it depends on the quality of the bone whether to opt for this implant with mild threads compared to the other one that has sharp threads that achieve better primary fixation in the cancellous bone. Therefore, even though oral implantology has made the greatest progress in dental practice and science, no implant system can be said to be the most perfect.

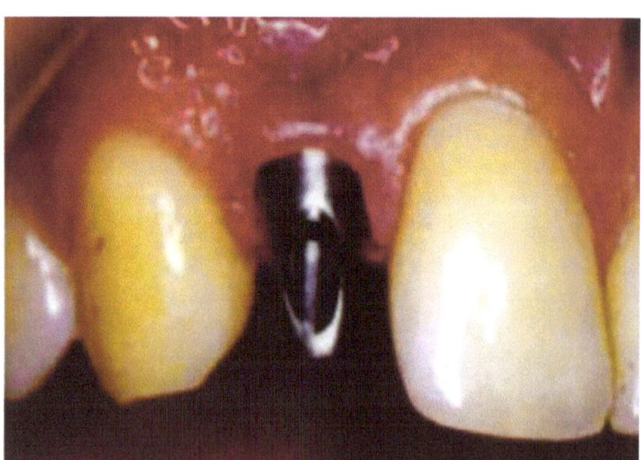

Figure 19.33. Explain to the patient what replaces the ground crown of a natural tooth and on which artificial crown should be placed.

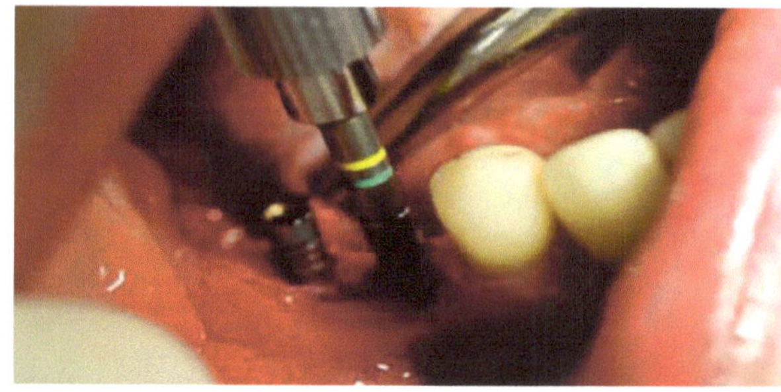

Figure 19.34. Explain to the patient that an experienced clinician, after a detailed analysis and an adopted plan, avoids a surgical incision and raising the flap, making the consequences of the procedure easier for the patient. This kind of procedure is a great relief for the patient, because after that he immediately gets teeth that he can use without any problems.

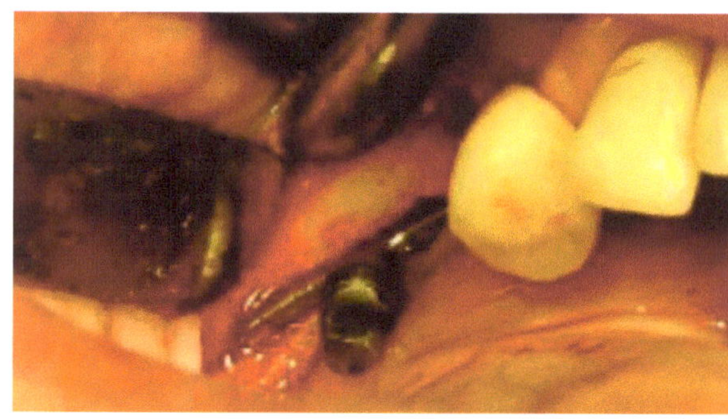

Figure 19.35. Aggressive insertion of a sheet one-piece implant. This type of implant used to be hammered into the bone with a special hammer, which is now the past and the history of the development of oral implantology.

Question: Can an implant be placed immediately after tooth extraction?

Answer: Yes! Show some of the cases you have solved. In this way, the patient gains confidence and a better understanding of what needs to be done. Often, precisely because of a lack of knowledge of what should be done, some patients visit several surgeries. If the patient expresses doubts about what is being explained to him, it must be emphasized to him that, probably, there are other opinions and, without vanity, advised to look for another opinion. Experience gives the most authoritative answers, which should also be explained to the patient. It is not desirable to promise any "guarantee periods" and, especially when dealing with a complex case, it is necessary to explain what kind of undesirable outcome can happen.

The reasoning will be based on the following points: in places where good primary stability cannot be achieved at the beginning of the surgical procedure due to poor bone quality, the possibility of predictability of success is limited. It should be explained to the patient that it takes a certain amount of time for complete healing and formation of soft tissues, as well as integration of implants and bone.

Question: What type of implant will be applied in his case?

For a clearer understanding, it is preferable to present a case that was resolved in the doctor's office using pictures. Show the patient an image illustrating the replacement of diseased teeth, particularly those with periodontal and periapical changes. Explain to them that the extraction will be painless, and that the type of implant used will depend on the conditions of the site for its installation, including the quality of the bone and the horizontal and vertical dimensions of the alveolar ridge, specifically its width and height.

If the bone is narrow, inform them that there are now advanced one-part and two-part implants available with a narrower diameter, which allow for immediate placement of teeth without a waiting period.

Additionally, explain that many American dentists often recommend removing a treated root—which could still be viable—and replacing it with an implant, which is then immediately followed by the placement of an artificial crown. This practice among American doctors, and others, is frequently influenced by commercial interests, as the installation of implants can be considerably more profitable.

However, we can also discuss the clinician's safety during the implant procedure, as it generally provides a clear predictability of a successful outcome.

While I am not in favor of doctors adopting a commercial mentality, it's important to recognize that the liability for American doctors is exceptionally high, and medical malpractice lawyers can be quite aggressive in their pursuits. Approval of such practices is more a topic for discussion among colleagues than with patients, though the reasoning applies to both contexts.

Question: When should the patient's teeth affected by periodontitis be extracted and implanted in that place?

For example, if the tooth in the frontal region is loosened, and in the apical part 4-5 mm of quality bone mass remains, such a tooth should be extracted to stop the resorption of the lamellar bone wall. Bone preparation for the implant bed would be done in a part of healthy and dense bone. In case of hesitation, whether it is more useful to keep the loosened periodontopathic teeth for a while longer, he should be informed that the loss of bone above the top of the root will be greater, which will reduce the possibility of immediate installation of the implant and its success. If a longer period of healing is waited after the extraction, without filling the alveolar wound with bone substitutes, a much smaller amount of bone will remain, both in height and in width, than if the extracted root were replaced with an implant. Why? First, in such cases, the amount of apical bone is favorable for achieving primary stability. Preservation of the alveolus, removing the granulation tissue, and filling that space with bone substitutes will speed up the osseointegration processes.

The question often depends on the patient's level of education. If the patient asks the question, what are the experiences when the lost bone is replaced, the dentist's explanation follows:

If it is necessary to perform augmentation if there are bone defects, explain to the patient and give a brief explanation. The experiences of many practitioners prove that bone regeneration is much faster and greater, and alveolar bone atrophy is slower, when substitutes for lost bone are applied. The bone substitutes surrounding the implant stimulate new bone formation. It should be explained to the patient that "artificial bone" prevents the formation of granulation tissue in the empty space between the bone and the implant, as well as around and around the neck of the implant. The penetration of the granulation tissue into the placed "artificial bone" is prevented by the collagen resorptive membrane. That is very important. By replacing a tooth with an implant, at least 2 mm of bone will be preserved and the creation of new ones around the implant will be accelerated.

The conclusion is that the formation of new bone is enhanced by bone substitutes, but the experience of practitioners shows that healing can often be successful without substitutes after implant placement. Many doctors achieve a successful result when they immediately install an implant in the post-extraction wound and recommend that immediate implant installation should be used wherever possible, which will prevent accelerated atrophy of the ridge in the vertical and horizontal direction. For primary stability, the implant threads play a crucial role (hence the longevity of even Tramonte's implants, which did not have today's technological treatment, but were embedded in the post-extraction wound, thanks to the thread design, showed exceptional primary stability and long survival in the bone).

Question: Does this mean that an artificial root is implanted in the place in the jaw, where there was a natural tooth and root, and an artificial tooth - a crown - is placed on it immediately or later? Is it complicated?

Answer: It used to be a complicated and risky surgical procedure, but today it is much less risky. That insert, which is installed in the jawbone, is called an implant. The implant should replace the natural root and tooth in all their functions that they had as a natural unit. It is a much more difficult and complicated procedure than the installation of an implant, for example, the extraction of an impacted wisdom tooth or an impacted canine tooth.

Question: Why was implant placement a complicated surgical procedure in the past, but not today?

Answer: The complexity of implant placement has always depended on the implant system. Most of the earlier implant designs were unsuitable for embedding in bone. The surgical intervention was extremely aggressive on both bone and soft tissues. In order to install an implant of the selected form, it was necessary to raise the soft tissues, i.e. uncovering the entire alveolar ridge to provide access to the bone, into which a deep groove is cut to drive the appropriate implant.

Today, it is not done that way, and the installation of modern implants is not only a much simpler surgical procedure, but also the success of the therapy is incomparably longer.

Question: How long does it take to replace lost teeth and what is the waiting period?

Answer: In the past, the wait was as long as six months. Today, the waiting time for a patient to get teeth is significantly reduced. Even today, many dentists adhere to the principle that the earliest time to load an implant, i.e. the time it takes for a patient to get teeth, is 3-4 months. However, it all depends on the case, and sometimes the optimal waiting time is 3-4 months. In some cases, that time can be much longer - 12 months, especially after augmentation (implantation of artificial bone) in the place where the implant should be placed.

Here too, it is the anatomical conveniences that determine the waiting time for new bone formation. The author of the book abandoned the principle of long waiting for the patient to get teeth.

Question: What is the success rate of implant placement and what does it depend on?

Answer: The percentage of success today is incomparably higher than thirty years ago. It is bigger than ten years ago. Thanks to the development of science, success can be predicted. The first step towards predictable success is choosing the highest quality implant from a reputable manufacturer with the appropriate certificate. Another important step for a successful outcome is the experience of the implantologist. Those two basic conditions are a guarantee of success, which today ranges up to 98%.

Of course, the patient himself contributes significantly to that percentage of success by maintaining extremely good oral hygiene, and in the case of smokers, by quitting smoking. Many experienced implantologists do not attempt implant placement in patients with poor oral hygiene and smokers. It should be explained to the patient that such patients belong to the risk group in which implant placement is not recommended.

Question: What does the implant look like?

Answer: Explain to the patient that the implant approximately imitates the root of the tooth and to a large extent takes over its role, i.e. all its functions, from reception and transmission of chewing forces to the bone to aesthetic requirements. Explain to the patient with a schematic picture. The implant is made of titanium, a material that is biocompatible with the bone, with which it integrates after a certain time.

Aesthetic metal-ceramic crowns are placed on the implant embedded in the bone, whether it is one or more, which completely functionally and aesthetically replace the natural tooth.

Question: What replaces the ground crown of a tooth on which an artificial crown is placed?

Answer: It is replaced by an extension on the implant called a support, explain with a picture.

Question: If one tooth is missing, is it necessary to grind two healthy teeth to compensate for one lost tooth?

Answer: You don't need to. Implant placement is very useful in such cases, because it saves adjacent teeth, provided there is enough bone for implant placement. From today's point of view of modern rehabilitation and high-end implantology, grinding two teeth to compensate for one tooth is an outdated procedure.

If the dentist does not deal with the installation of implants, the most useful advice for the patient is to refer to a colleague who has experience successfully doing it.

Question: What will happen if the organism does not receive that "foreign body" and why is this "artificial root" - implant not a foreign body? Can this "foreign body" harm the body?

Answer: In a certain sense, an implant is a foreign body, but it does not behave as such in the body. It has been proven that quality implants are biologically neutral and cannot cause any harmful consequences for the body, nor can they be rejected as a foreign body. The terms: "foreign body" and rejection, when it comes to the implant, i.e. the material from which it is made (titanium), we cannot consider as appropriate and valid terms. The implant can be referred to as an "artificial root", which will have the same role as a natural root, i.e. a natural tooth, in that place. And as for "rejection", it should be explained to the patient that the treatment may fail and what can influence the unsuccessful outcome, but that it is certainly not "rejection".

Question: Why can't rejection of the implant be expected, when that dead foreign body is inserted into living tissues, that is, into healthy bone? And how can there be rejection when a liver, kidney, heart or any organ in the body is transplanted? And when it comes to replacing the natural root with an artificial, dead and foreign body - an implant, why would the term "rejection" be absolutely inapplicable?

Answer: They are two completely different things. Transplantation (of organs and tissues from a donor) is a transplant, and the insertion of an implant made of dead material, titanium, into living tissues is the insertion of an implant, i.e. implantation. In contrast to transplantation, the implantation of an implant does not result in rejection of the implanted body. Adverse outcomes in organ transplantation are caused by immuno-biological conflicts, both on the part of the host (recipient) and on the part of the donor (donor). Bone transplantation also exists in oral implantology, when bone is transferred from a region where there is enough bone to a region where the bone mass is insufficient, in order to place an implant in that place. But, even then, there is no reaction of rejection of the part taken, because it is one's own tissue - autologous transplantation. When installing implants, failures arise from other reasons and several factors: operative errors, use of low-quality and inadequate implants, poor prosthetics, poor oral hygiene. But, of all the unfavorable factors, the insufficient amount of bone should be singled out in the first place, where the primary stability of the implant cannot be achieved most often. Without the primary stability of the implant, most often there is no successful outcome of implant placement.

Question: How is it scientifically explained that the implant is not a "foreign body", that it does not harm the body and that there is no rejection reaction with the implant?

Answer: It is true that the implant is made of foreign, inorganic, inanimate material of non-biological origin and that as such it is incorporated into living tissues, the organism does not reject it, as an inert material. After thorough scientific tests, it was proven that the implant does not behave like a foreign body in the biological environment, because the milieu around it is in homeostatic balance. That balance is not disturbed by the implant. The material of choice from which implants are made is titanium, which behaves neutrally in the body, i.e. biocompatible, i.e. it does not in any way disturb the homeostasis of the living tissues that surround it. Therefore, the implant is a foreign body, when it comes to the material from which it is made. The relationship of the implant with the living tissues in which it is inserted and with which it is in constant contact is such that it does not disturb the existing homeostasis of the environment and does not lead to an immune reaction. Today, joints - hip and knee - are replaced with the same material.

Question: What is homeostasis?

Answer: It is a fine physiological harmony of the organism between all its tissues and organs. Homeostasis is actually the health of the organism

Question: Which term is more correct, implanting or implanting a tooth?

Answer: Both words mean what they mean. Etymologically, the word implant comes from the Latin language, from the word implantum from the root implantare, which means to implant, to insert, to wedge in, to embed... In medicine, a huge fund of Latin words is used, and so is the word implantatio - installation of an implant or implanting, borrowed from the Latin language. As today the richest medical professional literature is in the English language, i.e. Anglo-Saxon literature, and we often use certain words from that literature as transcribed expressions in our language, avoiding a literal translation, which is often inappropriate and sloppy, the word implant adopted from Latin was introduced into German and English language, and literally translated it means implant or insert. The term most often used by patients, "tooth implantation", is therefore not wrong.

There is a defense system in the body, with which the body reacts to reject any foreign body that has entered it in any way. Often, these defensive reactions of the organism are also very violent. Inflammation is manifested by redness, pain, swelling, and suppuration around the foreign body. The question arises "Why does the organism with its defense system not react to the implant as a foreign body, which is also made of dead material and non-living inorganic origin"?

Titanium, as the material from which the implant is made, is biocompatible. The very word compatible has its roots in the Latin language - compatibilis, which means literally translated: agreeable, compatible, able to exist together with something else in the same subject, environment, means mutually tolerant and does not "cause" stimulation of immunocompetent tissue. In the biological environment, for such a material as titanium, we say that it is biocompatible. This means that in contact with living tissues it is extremely resistant to the action of tissue fluids, and the presence of surrounding tissue cells shows activity in a certain pH milieu, and this whole physiological harmony in the biological environment represents the concept of bioinertness, i.e. biological tolerance. Titanium in such a biological environment remains unchanged. For this reason, the body does not react to titanium with a defense system like a foreign body.

On the contrary, under certain conditions, following the implantological procedure, in the biological environment, the reaction of rejection is replaced by the reaction of integration, forming new bone on the surface of the implant. Such a reaction is biotolerant, and it manifests itself in the possibility of new bone formation on the entire surface of the implant lying in the bone. Over time, the connection of the newly formed bone with the surface of the implant becomes stronger and this process is called bone integration (osseointegration).

Question: Can this connection, this process of creating newly formed bone on the surface and around the implant, called bone integration, be prevented by some factors or if it has already been achieved, can this connection be weakened or completely endangered?

Answer: The very word integration (lat. root integratio) means joining, that is, the process of unification or the state of unification. Integrate (lat. integrare) means to supplement, renew, add something to the whole as its essential part. That term is used today in implantology in general, not only in oral, but also in orthopedics. The term "bone integration" was introduced by Branemark after scientific research evidence. Since that discovery, the process of integration, ie. to the process of uniting new bone that is in direct, intimate contact with the surface of the implant, many aspects of the work during the installation of the implant are subordinated: starting with the ability and experience of the oral surgeon, surgical technique, as well as the choice of a quality implant, and ending with impeccably made prosthetics. But the basic principle of all this is to assess whether or not there is enough bone. If the quantity and quality of bone is insufficient, then there is no point in embarking on an adventure that will result in failure.

Question: Are there patients who are unsuitable for implant placement?

Answer: Implantology is not immune to risks like any surgical activity. Thanks to the enormous progress of science and the development of implantology, the number of contraindications has been significantly reduced. However, there are patients who belong to risk groups for implant placement. The dentist should recognize such patients and explain in detail why it is not advisable to install implants in them. In general, most often it is about some anatomical disadvantages or a large lack of alveolar bone due to premature tooth loss. With the development of science and surgical techniques, contraindications due to anatomical limitations have been significantly reduced by implanting bone substitutes, and the term "artificial bone" is most often used.

Question: To what extent does the success of an oral implant procedure depend on the general state of health?

Answer: Some diseases of the body exclude the possibility of installing implants, which the implantologist assesses based on medical history, laboratory findings and consultations with doctors of appropriate specialties.

Question: Are there any additional restrictions, in addition to the listed disadvantages for implant installation? Is age one of the restrictions?

Answer: Age is not a limitation for implant placement. It is considered that people under the age of 18 should not get implants, but exceptions can be made in such cases. If there are all advantages, starting with anatomical, bone quantity and quality and the patient's general state of health, age is irrelevant for the success of the procedure. However, implantation is not recommended if there are some diseases, primarily metabolic bone diseases.

Question: Can pregnant women have implants installed?

Answer: That period should be avoided, and the installation of the implant can be performed later.

Question: I have receding gums on my front teeth in my upper jaw. Is it possible to have an implant?

Answer: The most common questions patients have when it comes to not installing implants are mucogingival anomalies. For the dentist to be able to give the patient a clear answer, he must know the etiology, pathogenesis, and treatment of mucogingival anomalies, he must have a good knowledge of the anatomy of the periodontium and the mucogingival complex as an integral part of the periodontium. The most common mucogingival anomalies of root co-recession of natural teeth. Explain to the patient the causes beyond his control and the patient's influence on the promotion of gingival recession by improper maintenance of oral hygiene using hard brushes.

Question: Is there receding gums around the implant?

Answer: Mucogingival anomalies and tissue diseases are related to teeth and implants, which include: gingival recession, lack of keratinized gingival zone, gingival enlargement that appears swollen with a change in the color of healthy gums and bleeding at the slightest touch with a brush or probe

Question: If the root of the tooth is too exposed and shows signs of loosening and needs to be extracted, can an implant be placed in that place?

Answer: Explain to the patient that lamellar bone loss is a large bone defect that must be compensated with artificial bone. This significantly complicates implantation procedures with the risk of achieving good aesthetics. Rehabilitation requires a longer treatment time. The success and shortening of the treatment time largely depends on the experience of the dentist.

Question: How long can an implant last?

Answer: It depends on how well everything was done right from the beginning: selection of a quality implant, suitable patient, precisely and according to the protocol performed surgical procedure, high-quality prosthetic work. Of course, for all that, the experience of the implantologist who will perform all these procedures with as little aggression as possible to the surrounding tissues is crucial.

The patient himself contributes to the success of the indicated procedures by maintaining good oral hygiene, reducing and stopping smoking, as well as mandatory regular check-ups. If the above requirements are met, such work can last for twenty or more years. This conclusion is the author's practical experience. This is also confirmed by the multi-decade duration of even some, today, outdated implant systems.

It must be emphasized that every organism, with aging, is exposed to degenerative changes, as a natural process, so a certain degree of bone loss (resorption) around the implant must be taken into account. The loss of bone around the implant is most pronounced in the marginal part, which also happens with natural teeth, especially in the interdental spaces. Natural, physiological bone resorption around the implant amounts to about 0.1 to 0.2 mm per year. Any major loss on an annual basis is an alarm to look for and remove the cause of accelerated bone loss around the implant during regular checkups. For this reason, regular six-month or annual check-ups are mandatory. The most risky are the first two years. If all the parameters of the entire procedure are respected, the most beautiful and vivid comparison of the survival of a quality implant in the bone is that of the quality of red wine: the older it is, the better it is.

Question: Can an implant "get sick" after a certain time, just like a natural tooth that the implant replaces completely can get sick?

Answer: If a natural organ in the body can get sick, it can also get sick what is forced to replace it. But that "disease" of implants is in some ways similar, but in some ways also very different from a natural tooth, primarily because of the connections in which they are tied, attached to the jawbone. For this reason, the chapter "Indications And Contraindications For Implant Placement" in this book is different from how it is written in textbooks and books in the field of oral implantology.

The most common "disease" of implants is caused by two factors: the first is inadequate loading of the implant (due to poorly executed prosthetics), and the second is the accumulation of bacterial plaque around the implant, due to insufficient or poor oral hygiene. The bacterial content of the plaque penetrates the length of the implant, which is in direct contact with the natural bone, causing inflammatory changes in the surrounding tissues (peri-implantitis). Smoking is an additional risk factor that enhances those unfavorable processes that threaten the stability of implants.

It is still debatable which of these two causes of bone decay and loss around the implant, and thus implant loss, is dominant: is it biomechanical stress-inadequate pathological load or accumulated bacterial content around the implant? If these two factors combine, the entire procedure will inevitably be compromised. The implantologist and the dental technician are responsible for the unwanted outcome. However, the responsibility of the dental technician is assumed by the doctor, because he allowed low-quality work to be placed on the implants. The consequences are multiple: the precious waiting time of several months, which was needed to achieve bone integration, was lost, and an additional and more serious consequence is a longer period of waiting to place a new implant in the same place, since the destroyed and lost bone must compensate by augmentation, i.e. by implanting a bone substitute. In order not to repeat the unfavorable outcome, the waiting time in this case must be at least 12 months.

In the conversation with the patient, attention must be paid to one phenomenon, "psychogenic pain", which is not described in any dental textbook, especially in books on oral implantology, and is very often present in everyday practice. For the reason that the phenomenon of psychogenic pain is a big unknown for dentists, and for those with a lot of experience, the author paid special attention.

Question: Can pain such as toothache occur after tooth implantation?

occurs immediately after a surgical procedure or later, without a clearly confirmed symptom and reason for the appearance of pain, it must be suspected that the pain was not caused by the dentist's mistake. When it comes to the appearance of pain in the oro-facial region and it persists without visible causes, the first suspicions of psychogenic pain arise.

It is necessary to rule out all dental causes through differential diagnosis. Painful conditions must be excluded in the differential diagnosis; from the eye (glaucoma), refraction disorder, ear pain, sinus pain, nasal disorders, cranial neuralgia, the central origin of the pain must be determined. In a conversation with the patient, find out about his wishes and expectations after the implant-prosthetic treatment.

Question: From all the answers, it can be concluded that oral implantology has progressed a lot and made the biggest step forward in that progress out of all branches of dentistry. Trust in implantology is significantly higher than in the era when the first implants were installed. If confidence has increased in line with the reach of oral implantology, can a guarantee be given for implanted implants today?

Answer: The current confidence in oral implantology compared to a few decades ago cannot be compared. Today, it is no longer a complicated oral surgical procedure thanks to its enormous progress, primarily the scientific contribution to that progress. In addition, the techniques have been completely changed, and the new ones have been greatly improved. Everything is simplified, and the patient tolerates the entire procedure very easily and painlessly. If the patient asks for a guarantee period, a clear answer must follow; that biological laws are not mechanical machines. Unforeseen events that are not the doctor's fault are always possible. The guarantee is shared by both the patient and the doctor. The best guarantee from a doctor is experience, conscience, the application of the highest quality implants and the creation of precise prosthetic works. The patient's guarantee is to follow the instructions on maintaining oral hygiene and to attend mandatory periodic check-ups.

Question: In situations where the dentist feels powerless to fulfill the patient's wishes, what answer should be given to the patient?

Answer: The dentist, without any vanity, in certain situations, must admit to the patient that he is not capable of compensating for something that has been lost for decades. Our knowledge and our professional power have a limit!

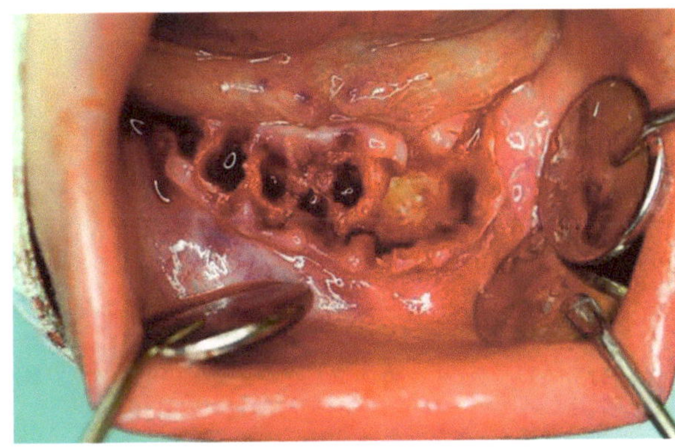

Figure 19.36. Explain to the patient that in the case of major destruction of the jawbone, the lost bone must be compensated with bone substitutes, which is termed as "artificial bone".

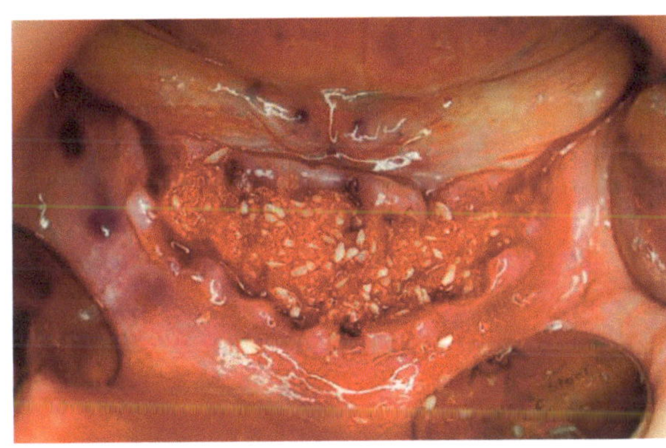

Figure 19.37. Appearance of a bone defect filled with bone substitute mixed with autologous bone chips.

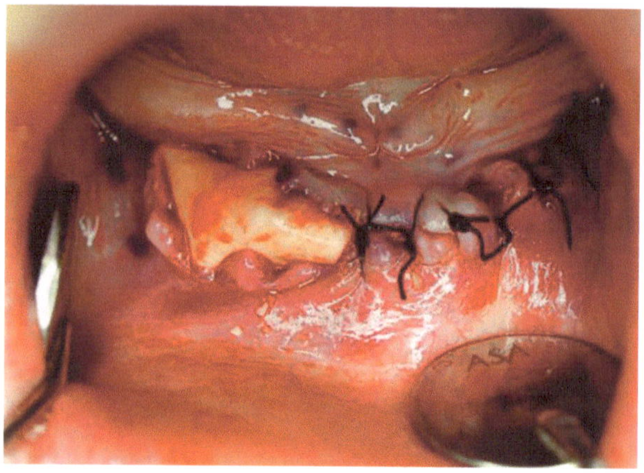

Figure 19.38. Placed substitute on the bone covered with a collagen resorptive membrane. Explain to the patient why this procedure is important.

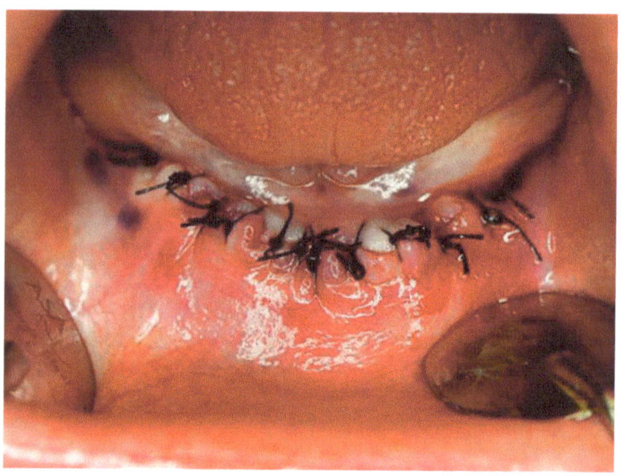

Figure 19.39. Completed the procedure of compensating the lost bone. Explain to the patient that a longer waiting time is needed for the healing of soft tissues and the formation of new bone in order to create favorable conditions for implant placement.

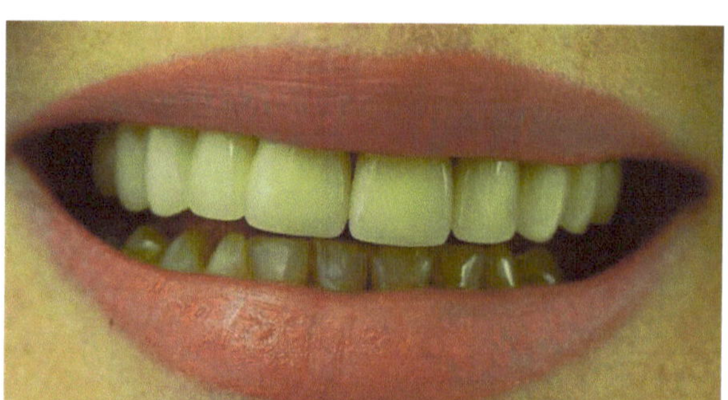

Figure 19.40. In the conversation with the patient, show the cases before the implant-prosthetic procedures and the result of the treatment.

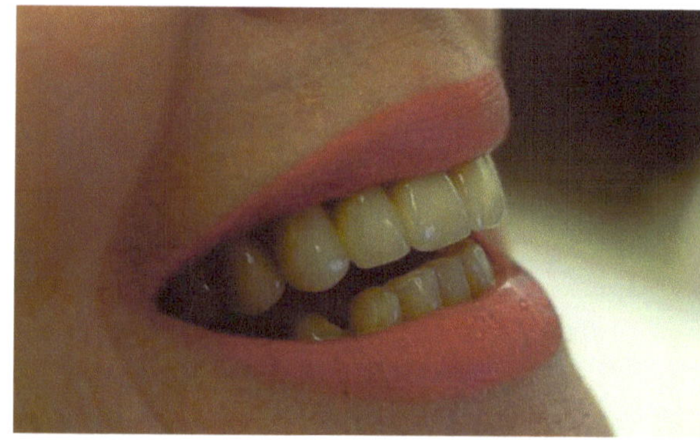

Figure 19.41. Successful aesthetic and functional result after extensive augmentation of bone defects.

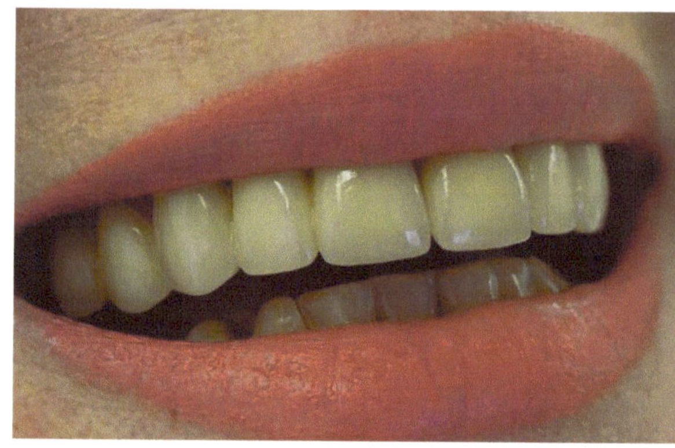

Figure 19.42. The patient's request that prosthetic work on implants be performed in zirconium should not be accepted. In the conversation with the patient, it should be explained to him that pomodorism in fashion, even in oral implatology, is not desirable. The stiffness of the materials from which the prosthetic work is made can jeopardize the achieved osseointegration.

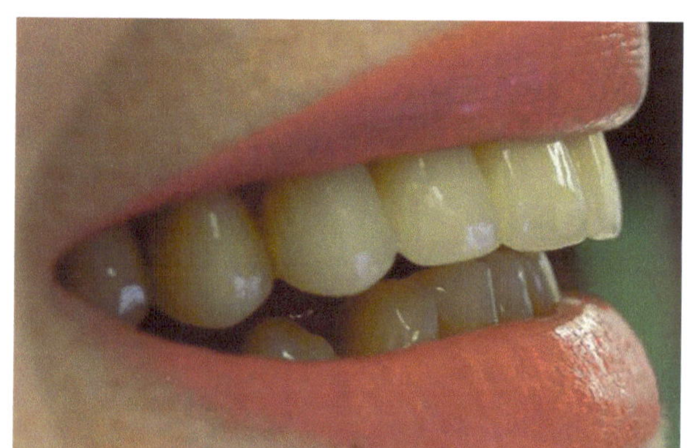

Figure 19.43. Successful aesthetic solutions are achieved by pre-esthetic work performed in metal-ceramics.

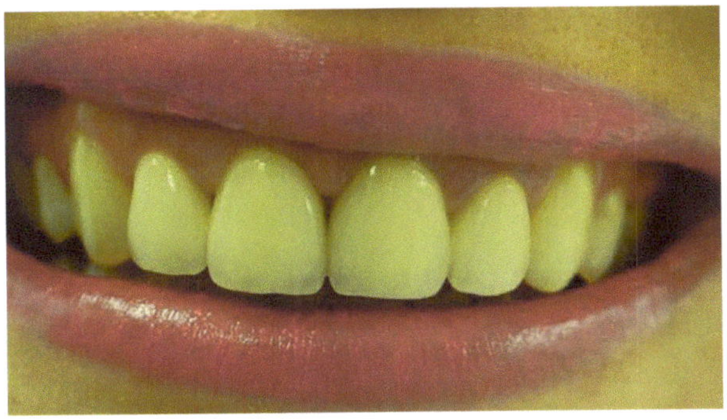

Figure 19.44. Prosthetic work on implants of lateral and central incisors performed in metal-ceramics.

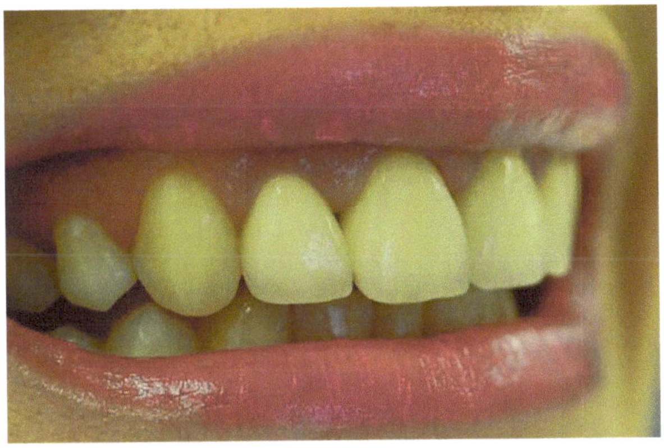

Figure 19.45. Reconstruction of the papilla is extremely important for creating a quality aesthetic solution.

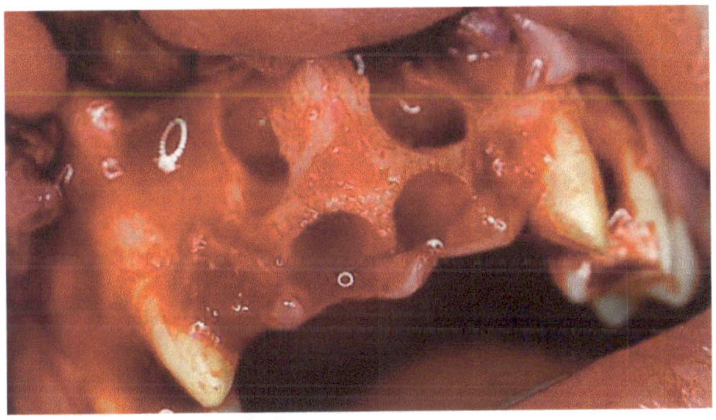

Figure 19.46. Bone defect in the apocal region of the central incisors in the upper jaw, a consequence of root resection. Required augmentation of defects with a bone substitute mixed with autologous bone (round bowl).

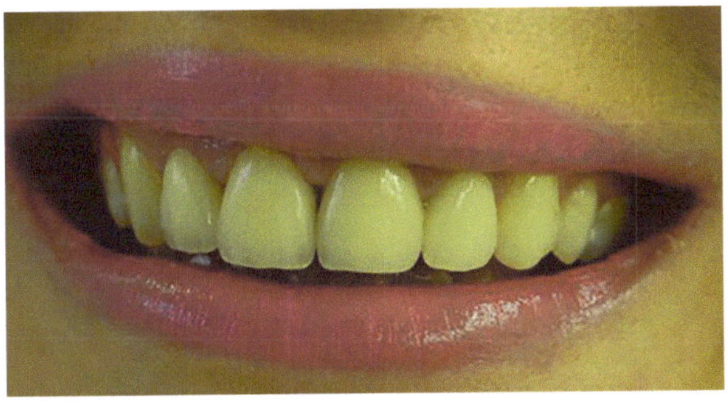

Figure 19.47. The reconstruction of the inter-implant papilla is also a successful aesthetic result. Prosthetic work on metal-ceramic implants.

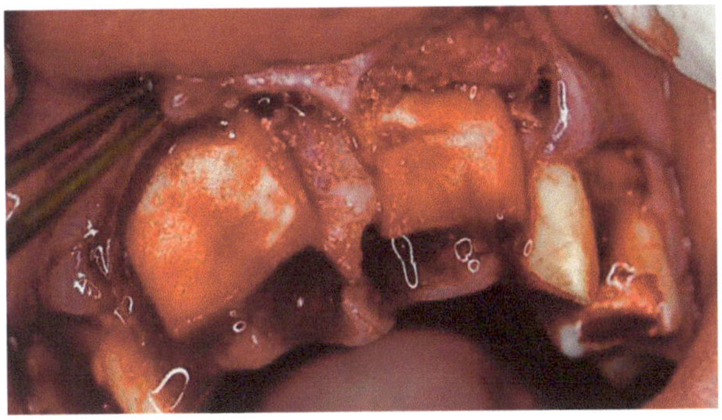

Figure 19.48. Bone defects filled with a mixture of xenogeneic bone substitute (vessel on the left) and autologous bone (vessel on the right), covered with a collagen resorbable membrane. Explain the procedure to the patient.

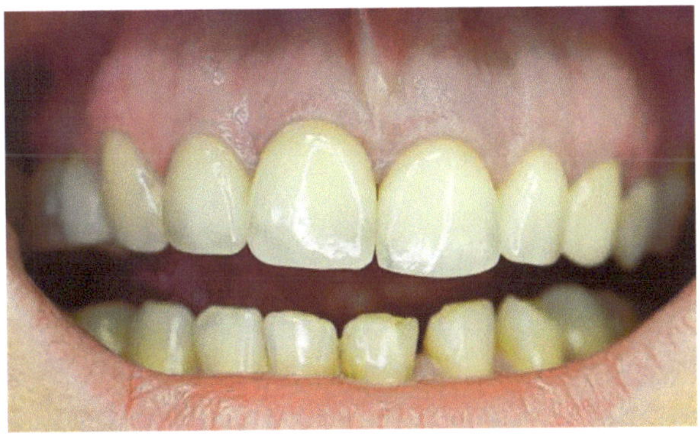

Figure 19.49. Explain to the patient the importance of successful bone defect augmentation. The appearance of completely healed bone and soft tissues.

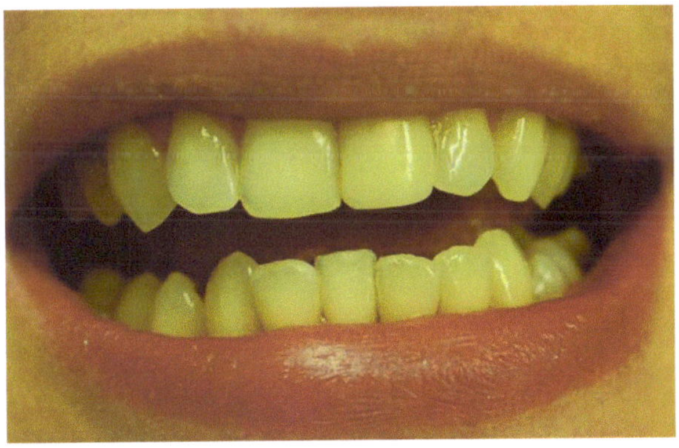

Figure 19.50. Replacement of the central incisor (21) with an implant and a metal-ceramic crown.

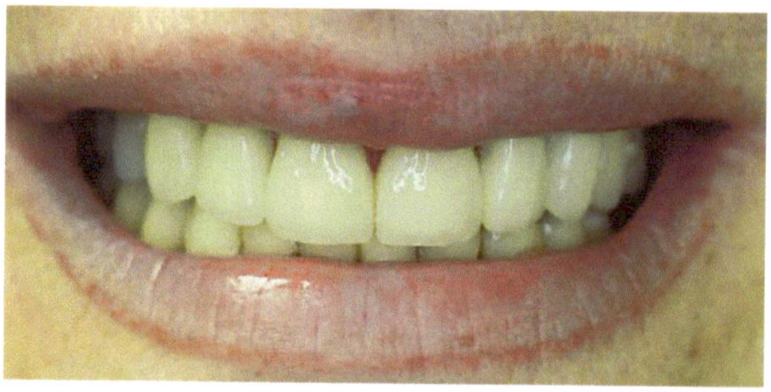

Figure 19.51. Replacement of lost teeth by implantation in both jaws. Fulfilling the patient's request for a holier color is not a failure, as it is a personal feeling.

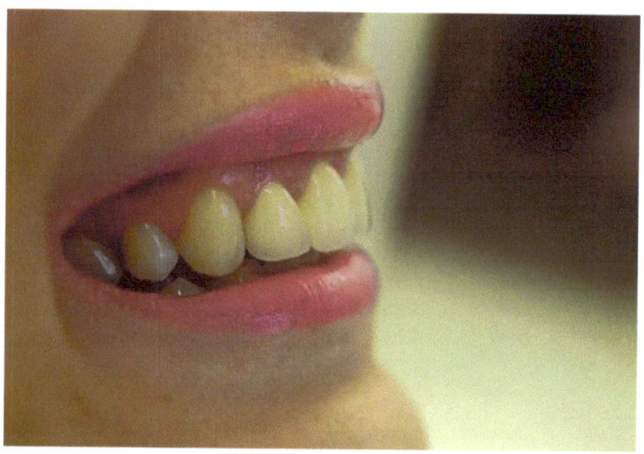

Figure 19.52. Profile view of the implant-prosthetic solution to replace the lost lateral (12) and central (11) incisor in the upper jaw.

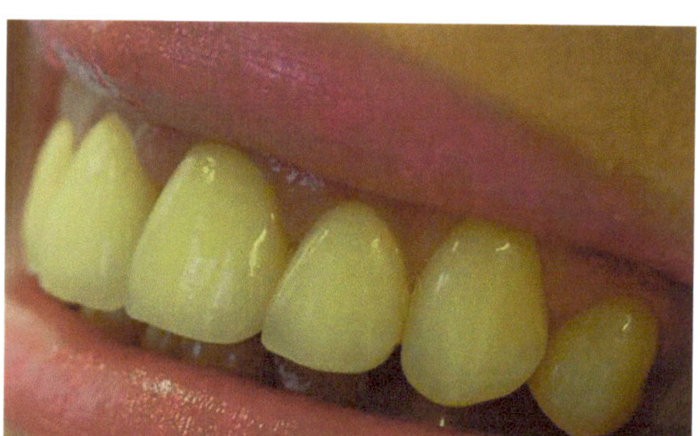

Figure 19.53. Regenerated papillae significantly contribute to achieving perfect aesthetics.

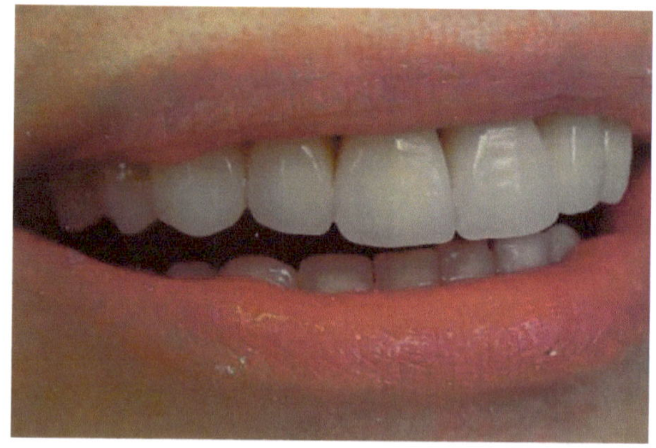

Figure 19.54. Explain to the patient the scope of oral implantology in terms of function and aesthetics. Analyze his case in detail and then give evaluations of the outcome of the entire implant-prosthetic treatment. When it comes to choosing the color of the teeth, find out the patient's request, and the trend is the lightest color, as in the case of the patient shown (prosthetic work on implants in the upper jaw).

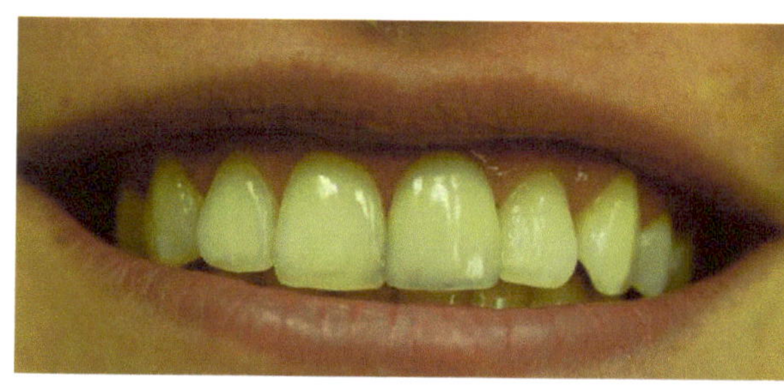

Figure 19.55. Compensation of a central incisor (21) lost in a traffic accident. Successful papilla reconstruction.

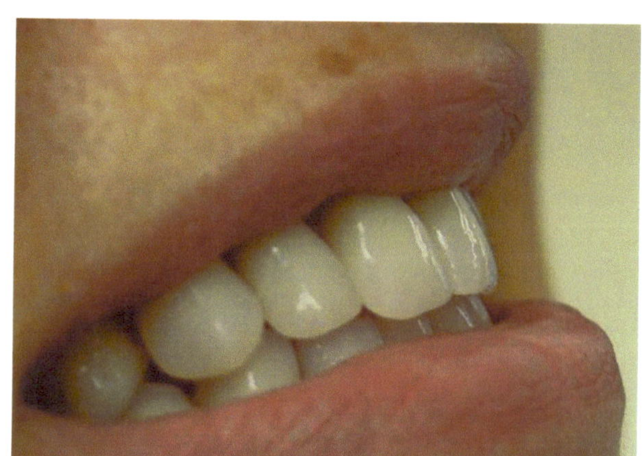

Figure 19.56. Prosthetic work on implants achieved perfect aesthetics and canine-guided occlusion.

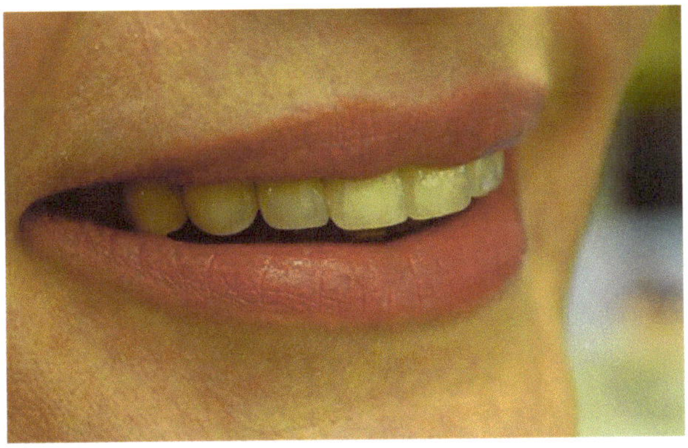

Figure 19.57. In the conversation, explain to the patient that the goal of implant prosthesis rehabilitation is to compensate for lost natural teeth in terms of function and aesthetics and to match the shape and color of prosthetic teeth with the harmony of the face.

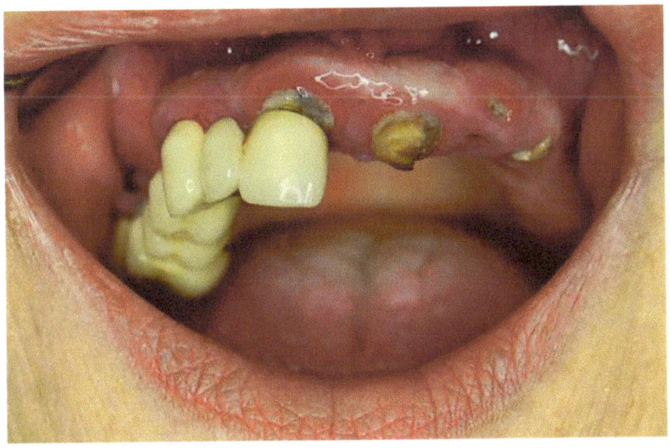

Figure 19.58. The state in the beginning. After extraction, it was necessary to shape the crestal arch by augmentation with a xenogeneic bone substitute mixed with autologous bone chips. Solution of picture 19.57.

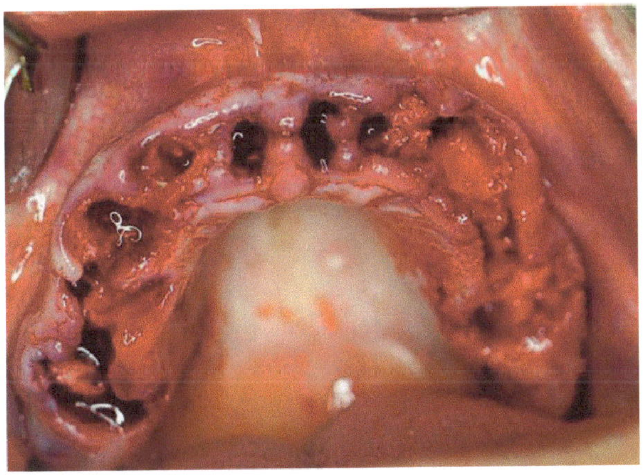

Figure 19.59. Such pictures should not be shown in a conversation with the patient. But before starting such operations, the dentist must have a well-laid plan, a planned sequence of operations and predictability of the outcome of the entire surgical and prosthetic performance.

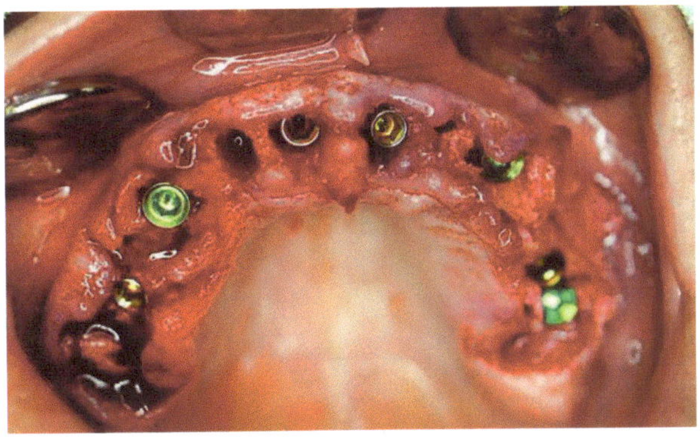

Figure 19.60. The position and number of implants must be in accordance with biomechanical laws, with a predictable outcome of function and aesthetics.

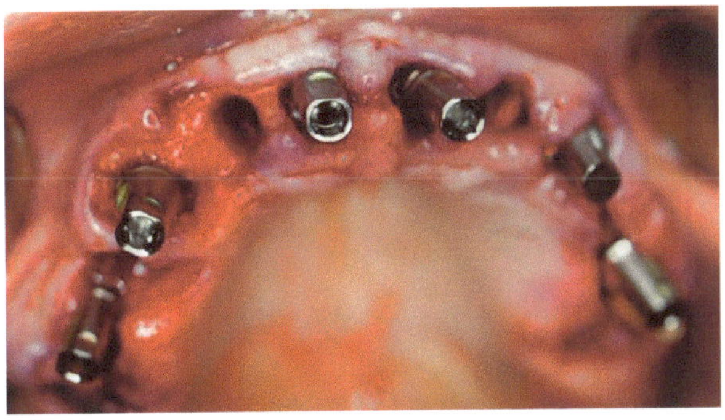

Figure 19.61. Presentation of immediately installed implants with simultaneous augmentation of bone defects, shaping of the arch of the alveolar ridge with bone substitutes. The author of the book avoids the use of caps for healing, because experience confirms faster and better healing and shaping of soft tissues around the neck of the implant and abutment.

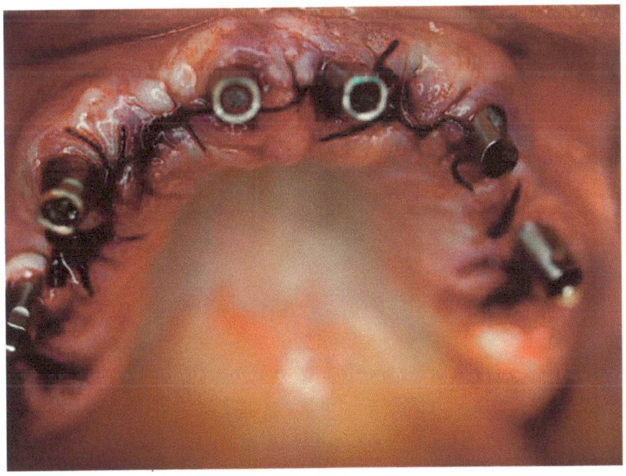

Figure 19.62. Immediately implanted with implants with definite abutments (carriers), the patient's comfort lasts for the period of healing of all tissues by making provisional prosthetic work.

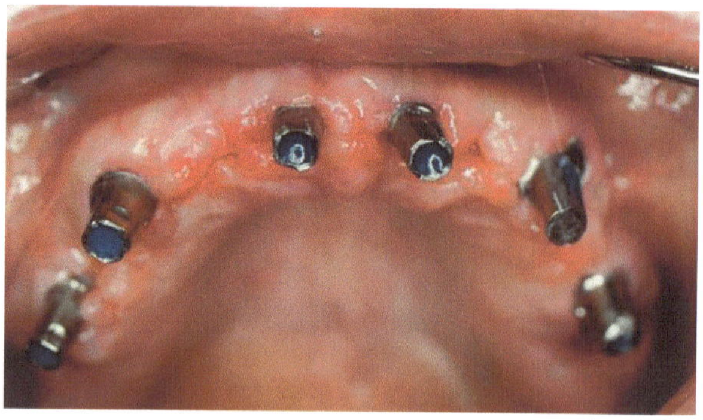

Figure 19.63. Appearance of healed tissues after 3 months. Patient comfort with temporary prosthetic work in function and aesthetics, experience advises that the healing period of soft tissues and to achieve good bone integration should be extended and that the creation of definitive prosthetic work should not be rushed.

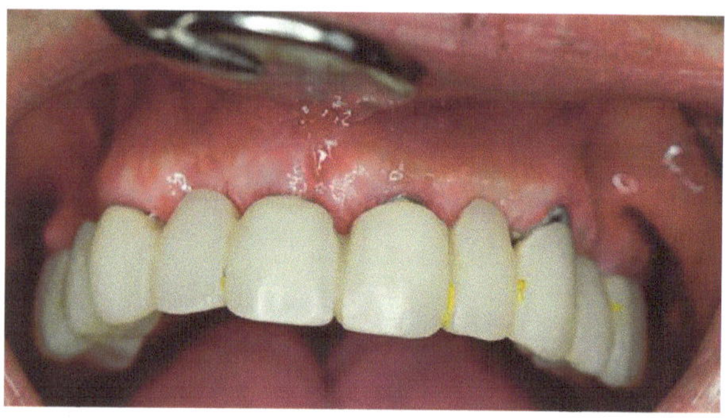

Figure 19.64. Temporary prosthetic work in composite. Healed soft tissues after 4 weeks.

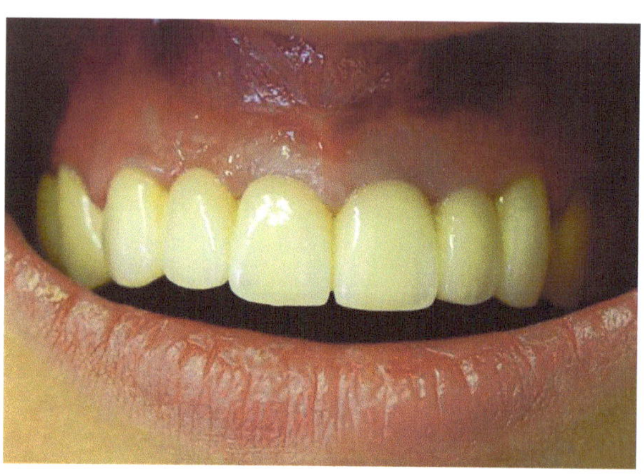

Figure 19.65. Functional and aesthetic requirements must be fully met with definitive prosthetic work in metal-ceramics. Healed bone and soft tissues after 6 months.

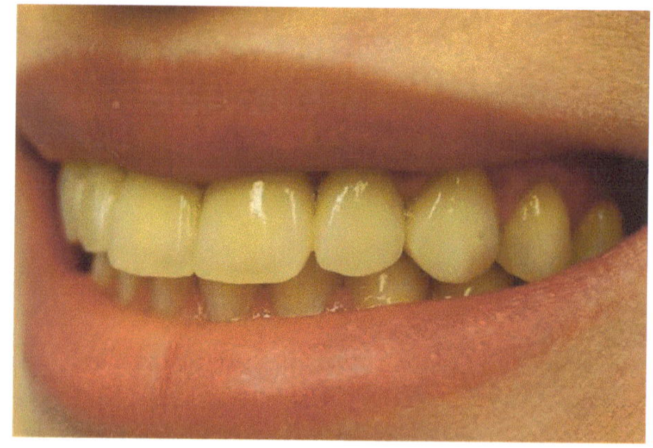

Figure 19.66. The patient's request that prosthetic work on implants be performed in zirconium should not be accepted. In the conversation with the patient, the oral implant dentistry can hinder the achieved bone integration due to the rigidity of the materials from which the prosthetic work is made. Prosthetic work in metal-ceramics.

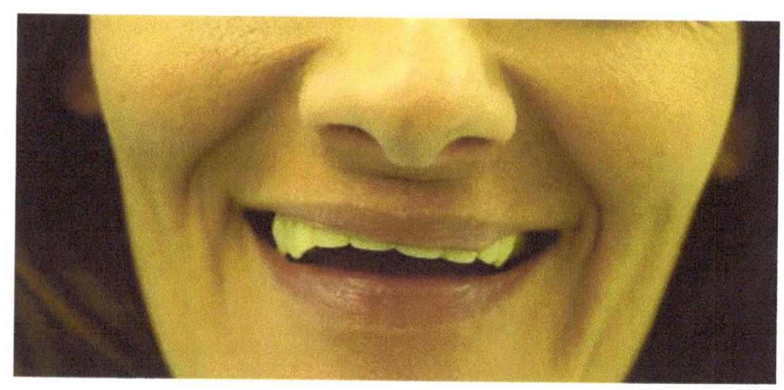

Figure 19.67. With such prosthetic works, one should not criticize a colleague, and in a conversation with the patient, say that the scope of oral implantology and prosthetics is beyond this.

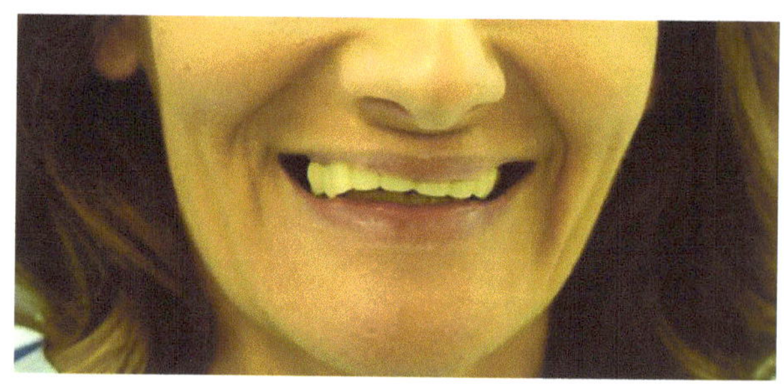

Figure 19.68. Rehabilitation in the oral cavity of four teeth (premolar and canine on the right side of the upper jaw and two premolars on the left side) should not have been solved in this way. After extraction of loosened and endodontically untreated teeth, implantation with 8 implants was performed.

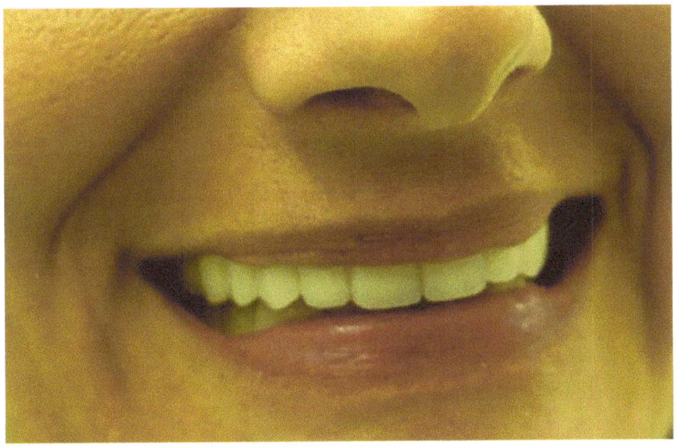

Figure 19.69. At the beginning of implant-prosthetic planning, one must have a vision of the outcome.

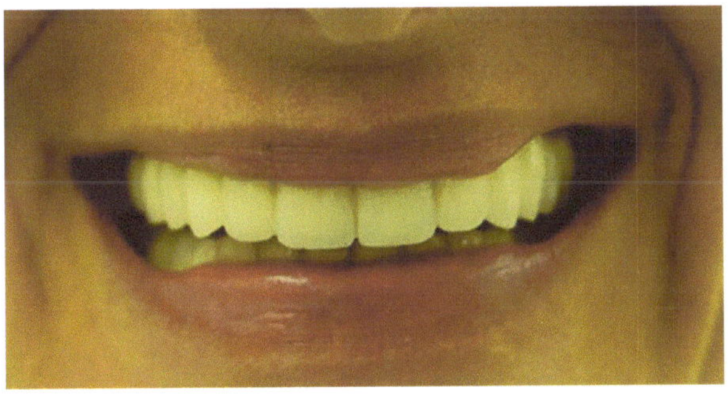

Figure 19.70. The shape of the lips and laugh line contribute to the successful realization of aesthetics.

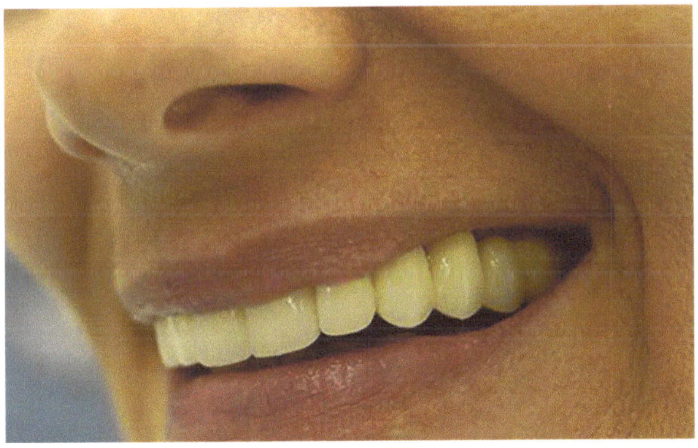

Figure 19.71. A successful aesthetic result changes facial expression with the establishment of overall harmony.

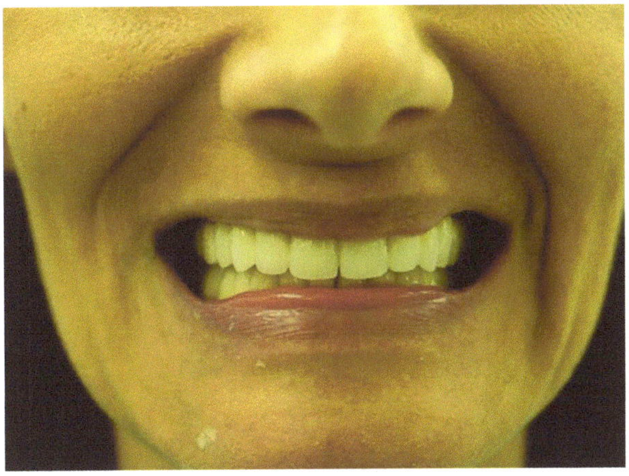

Figure 19.72. Along with successful aesthetics, good function was achieved with fixed prosthetic work in metal-ceramics

Question: How many implants can be used to avoid total acrylate prostheses covering the entire palate, when implants cannot be placed in posterior regions due to anatomical disadvantages such as low sinus floor and insufficient amount of available bone?

Answer: Successful prosthetic fixed work can be from 5 to 8 implants, and the length of distal extensions, hanging members, with one or two members, which depends on the quality and dimensions of the available bone, diameter, length of the implant and the condition of the antagonist.

Question: What solutions could be sought in this particular case?

Answer: In the presented case, prosthetic solutions could be performed in several ways: total acrylate prosthesis with and without retention clips. Possible application of Dolder's retention bar. In all variants, the palate and alveolar ridges would be covered with an acrylic plate, which would significantly reduce the comfort in the oral cavity. Without retention elements, the upper total prosthesis would not be sufficiently stable due to extreme atrophy in the posterior regions and non-existent tubercles. The patient would have to use adhesive pastes to stabilize the total acrylate prosthesis with a covered palate, which is not a pleasant feeling in the mouth.

Question: What is the most optimal solution in the presented patient?

Answer: In a conversation with the patient, you learn about his wishes and expectations.

Explain to the patient that the most comfortable is implant-prosthetic rehabilitation; by explaining the advantages, but also presenting the possible risks, due to hanging distal extensions, because when planning prosthetic works, whether it is fixed or fixed-mobile prosthetic works, biomechanical laws must be respected. Explain to the patient that in his case the advantage is the gain of 10 fixed teeth, which is an incomparably greater functional effect and a more pleasant feeling than a total mobile acrylate prosthesis.

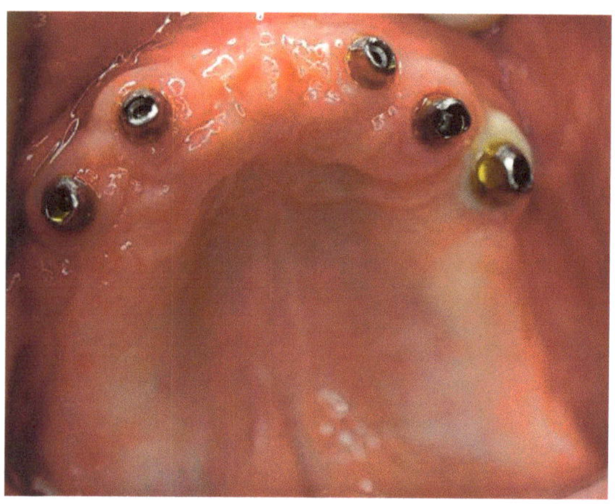

Figure 19.73. Explain to the patient why more implants could not be inserted: insufficient volume of the scrotum and low sinus floor. In order to increase the sufficient amount of bone in which the implant could be installed, an extremely complex procedure is required that requires a longer treatment time with a known increase in the price of the treatment.

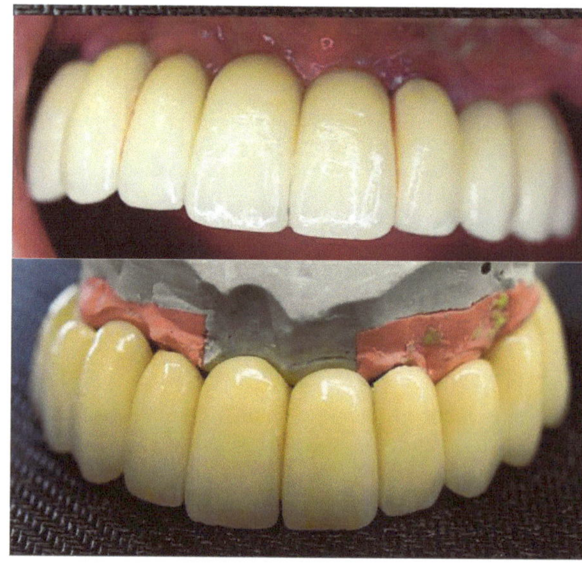

Figure 19.74. Definitive prosthetic work in metal-ceramics. Advantage of the solution; the patient received a sufficient number of teeth, which fulfilled the functional and aesthetic requirements, as well as an incomparably greater comfort in the mouth than a total unstable acrylate prosthesis.

Question: Should prosthetic work on implants be done in zirconium?

Answer: Pomodari in medicine, because of some other effects, is harmful. Likewise in oral implantology. The more we move away from natural laws, in this case in the choice of materials to replace lost natural teeth, the closer we are to failure. Porcelain, as the material of choice in prosthetics; it is two and a half times harder than natural enamel, and zirconium incomparably more. The melting point is about 18550C, and the density is 6511 kg/m3. The abrasiveness of the material, a property possessed by natural teeth, significantly affects the reception and distribution of chewing forces. If the prosthetic work is supported by the roots of the natural teeth, the reception and distribution of forces during chewing, in order to reduce the load on the periodontium of the natural tooth, depends on the stiffness of the material and compliance with gnathological principles. The performance of prosthetic works in zirconium anchored to implants has no justification for several reasons. The author's experience confirms that many patients who had prosthetic works performed in zirconium in both jaws felt much more comfortable when they were replaced with metal-ceramic prosthetic works.

Cementation of prosthetic works on implants is an extremely important stage of treatment.

Cement retention can result in serious consequences of peri-implantitis. In the rehabilitation of total edentulism, the so-called with "circular" bridges, it is necessary to periodically check the stability of the support (abutments) and the screw that connects it to the endosseous part of the implant. For this reason, for a time, fixation of prosthetic work with screws was resorted to. The author abandoned that method of prosthetic compensation for the following reason: If it is necessary to adjust the occlusion and eliminate "premature contacts", then adjusting the occlusal surfaces can destroy the screw head and the possibility of its loosening and tightening.

Then the space between the surface of the support (abutment) and the inner surface of the crown becomes a space for the deposition of plaque, bacterial content and the cause of unpleasant odor. The most convenient way of fixing prosthetic works is "Implantinekom-semi"; which fixes the definitive prosthetic work well, and is easily removed to control the condition of the soft tissues around the implant and the tightness of the abutment screwing. In prosthetic works, anchors on implants, made of zirconium, are a big disadvantage, because removing them poses a risk of zirconium breakage. If it is a question of aesthetics in implant-prosthetic rehabilitation previously shown the works are done by metal-ceramics with successful aesthetics, confirming the justification of the author's position.

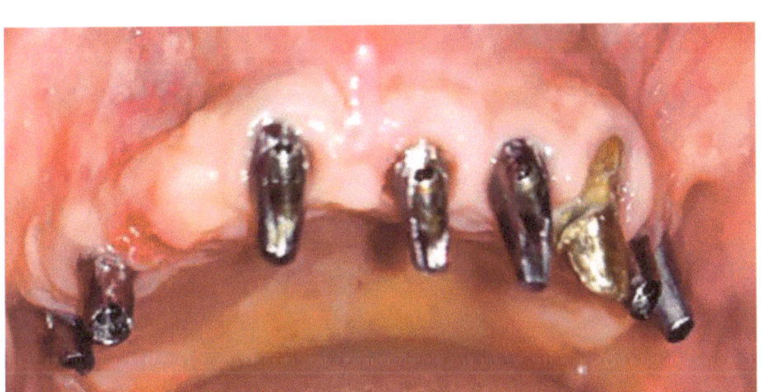

Figure 19.75. Presentation of the state of soft tissues, integrated implants and stability control of abutments (carriers) and solid screws after 15 years from implantation.

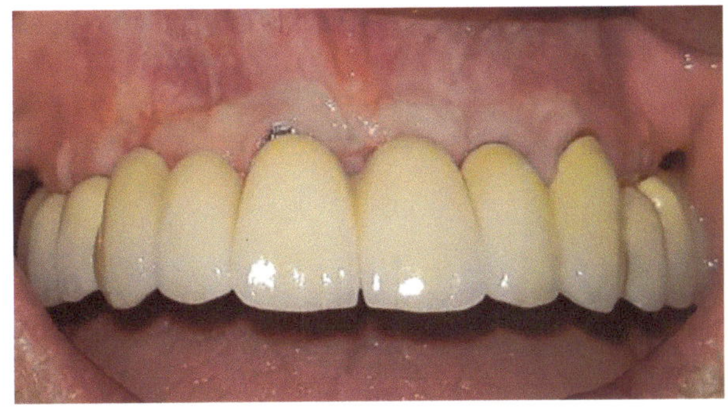

Figure 19.76. The appearance of the condition of soft tissues and fixed prosthetic work was achieved by performing for a light color of the canines. metal-ceramic placed on implants after 11 years. You can see a slight gingival recession on the central incisor (11) aggravated by the use of a stiffer brush during oral hygiene. Considering that this minimal gingival anomaly manifested itself after a long time on the titanium abutment, the possibility of complications is excluded, because all parameters are harmonized; biomechanical, gnathological, functional and aesthetic with precise prosthetic work in metal-ceramics.

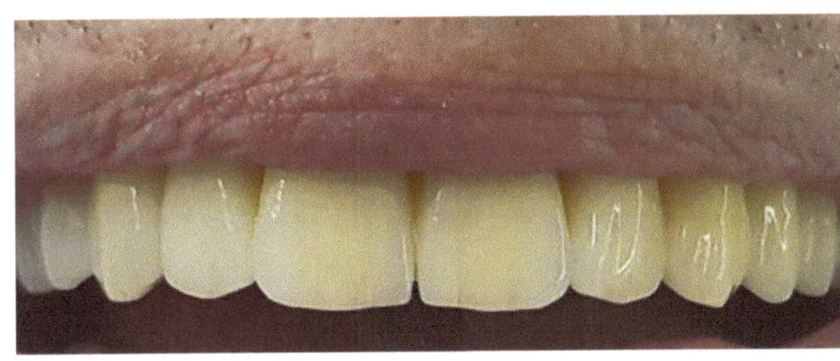

Figure 19.77. The shape of the lip increases the aesthetics achieved by implant prosthetic treatment. The color and shape of the teeth must be matched with the harmony of the face and the age of the patient. It is not a failure if the patient's desire for a lighter color Is fulfilled.

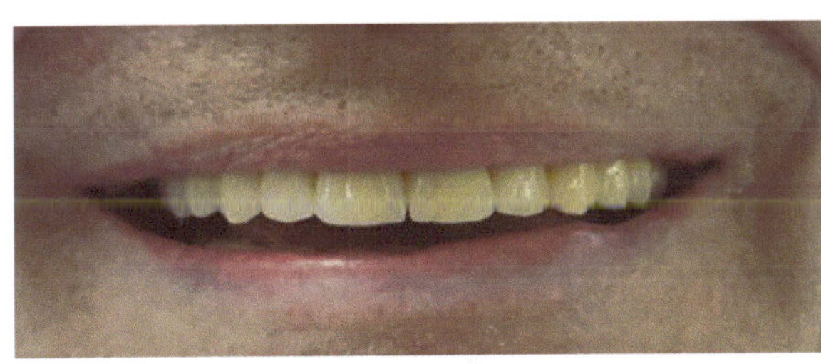

Figure 19.78. Aesthetic solution in metal ceramics. Experience confirms that a more successful solution could not have been done better in zirconium. The patient's request to harmonize the prosthetic work with the harmony of the face was fulfilled, which was achieved by implementing a light color of the canines.

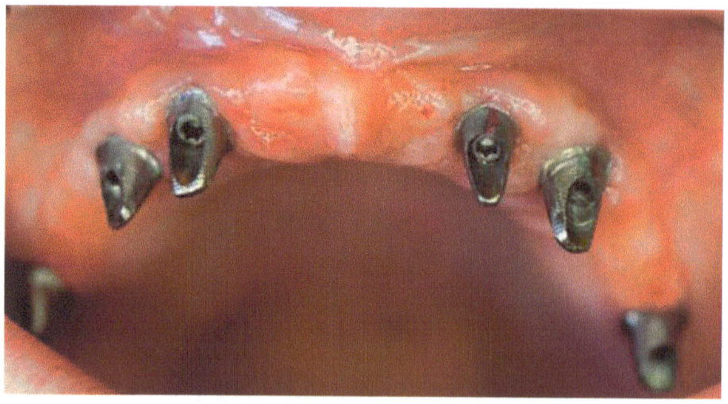

Figure 19.79. Replaced and parallelized abutments in the laboratory. Ideal fit of soft tissues around the abutments. Checked screwing with gedor up to 35Ncm.

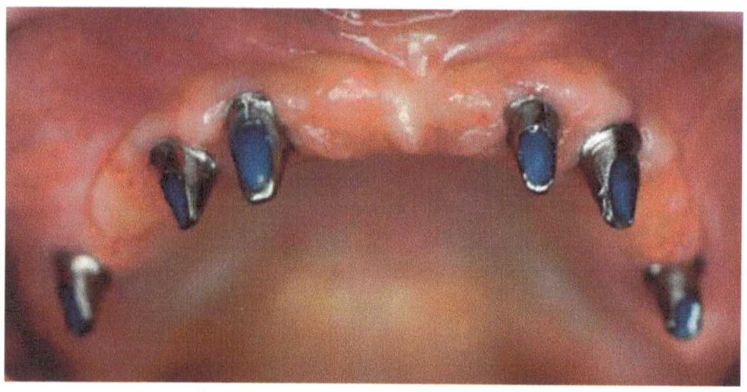

Figure 19.80. Presentation of prepared supports (abutments) for fissuring definitive prosthetic work. After checking the tension of the support with the screw for the endosseus part of the implant, ensure that in case the screw loosens and the support loosens, the tightening process can be performed again without damaging the screw head. Cover it with a thin layer of gutta-percha and fill the rest with self-polymerizing acrylate (blue color).

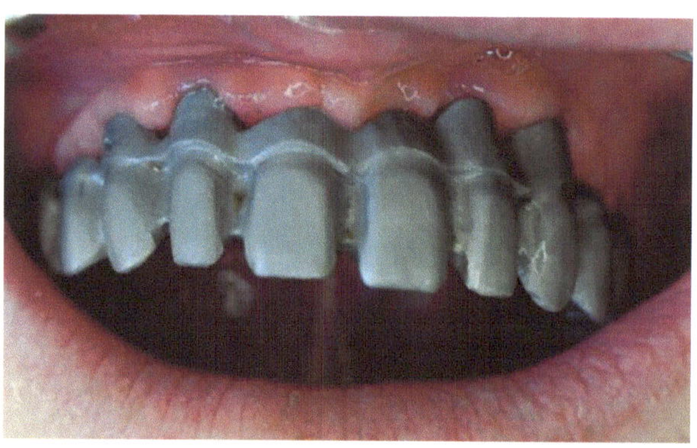

Figure 19.81. The planning and execution of the metal construction must be based on the assumption that the interjaw relations are changeable during life under the influence of several factors, which conditions the reduction and change of the interjaw relations. The first factor is abrasion and loss of individual teeth. In case of total toothlessness, unilateral or bilateral, this process is significantly accelerated, because with the aging of the organism, significant changes occur in all tissues in the oral cavity, which also manifests itself in changes in the temporomandibular joint. In the implant-prosthetic procedure, establishing ideal interjaw relationships is one of the most important stages of rehabilitation treatment.

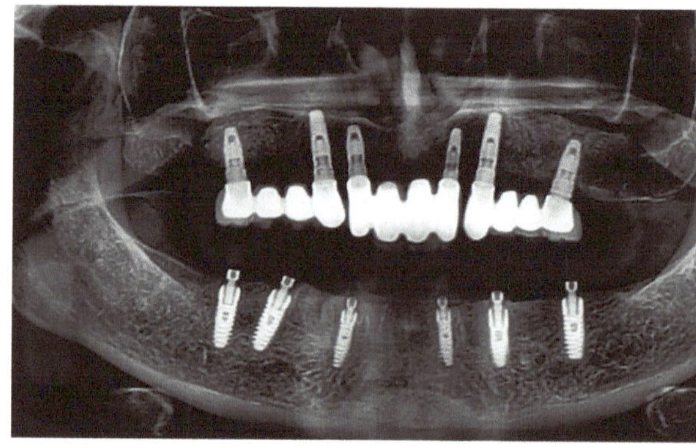

Figure 19.82. Immediately installed and immediately loaded implants in the upper jaw 12 years ago. Immediate loading performed by precise prosthetic work in the composite. The patient lives abroad, satisfied with the provisional fixed prosthetic work, decided to do the definitive prosthetic work there after some time. However, the practicing dentist made a triple mistake: from the planning of the prosthetic construction, execution and selection of the zirconium material.

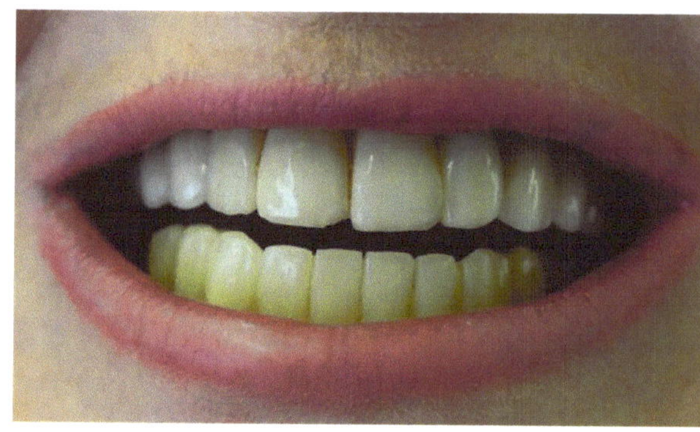

Figure 19.83. Appearance of definitive prosthetic work in zirconium, in the upper jaw, placed on the installed implants. The work was done abroad (Netherlands). In the lower jaw, the implants were inserted immediately after tooth extraction into the alveolar wounds and immediately loaded with provisional prosthetic fixed work. Appearance of precise temporary prosthetic work in composite. Fracture of zirconium on the central incisor (11).

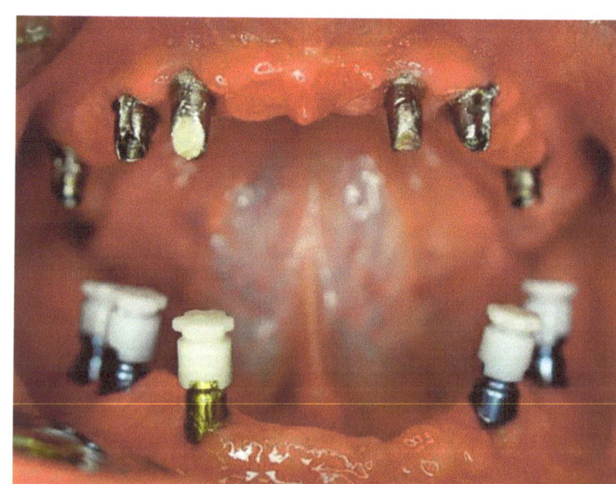

Figure 19.84. Removed prosthetic work, partially made of zirconium (frontal part of the upper jaw), and partially made of metal-ceramic. A

mistake made in the planning of the prosthetic solution; non-connection of the prosthetic support and different materials. It is necessary to replace the abutments - place the transfers, take an impression and parallelize the abutments (carriers) in the laboratory (Figure 19.85) Appearance of the placed transfers on the implants in the lower jaw. Preparation for taking an impression for making definitive prosthetic work in metal-ceramics.

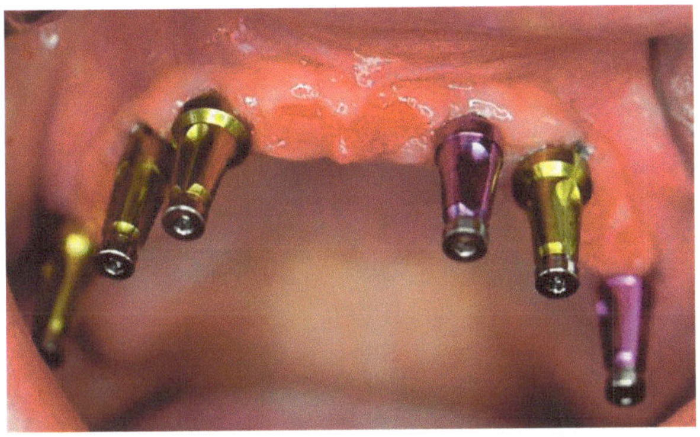

Figure 19.85. After an unforeseeable long wait (12 years) from implant placement, there was an increase in the microcrack (the connection between the implant neck and the support-abutment due to unscrewing) and the deposition of bacterial content. Due to changes in the soft tissues around the neck of implants and abutments, it is necessary to replace the existing abutments with new ones. Layout of placed transfers for the impression for parallelizing abutments (supports) in the laboratory.

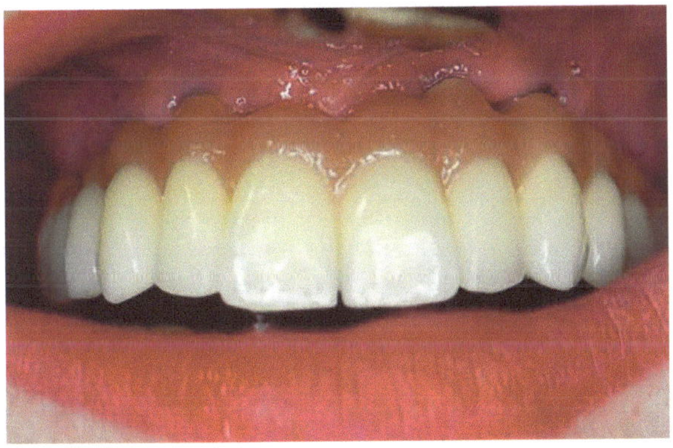

Figure 19.86. Significantly changed conception of rehabilitation planning and definitive prosthetic work.

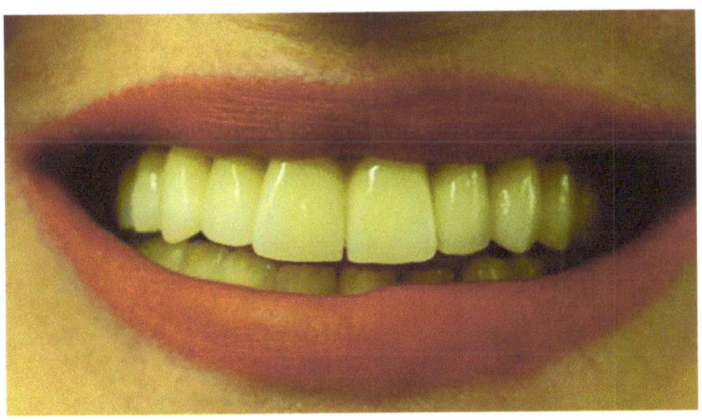

Figure 19.87. Definitive prosthetic work in metal-ceramics. Established adequate interjaw relationships, resulting in the establishment of good occlusion function and aesthetics. The shape of the lip and laugh line compensates on the prosthetic definitive work part of pink porcelain for the height of raising the bite to place the condyles in the maximum physiological distoposition.

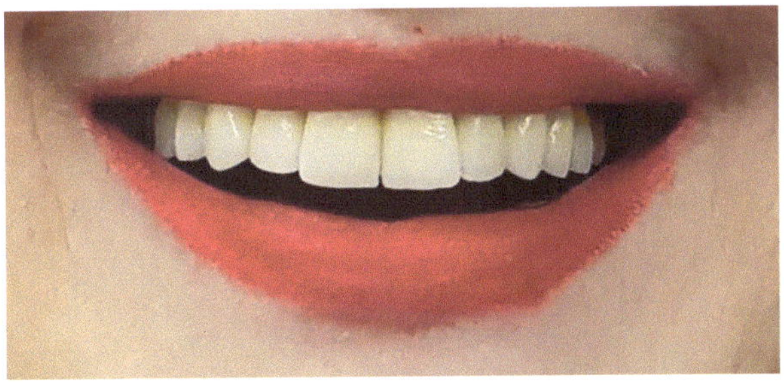

Figure 19.88. Successful outcome of complex disability in the oral cavity from immediate implantation, establishment of physiological inter-oral relations, occlusion and articulation, good function and aesthetics with prosthetic works in metal-ceramics. Works fixed "Implantlink semi" with an emphasis on mandatory periodical checks for the patient, and the material with which the prosthetic works on the implants are fixed allows for easy removal and the possibility of inspecting the stability of the implant, support and surrounding soft tissues.

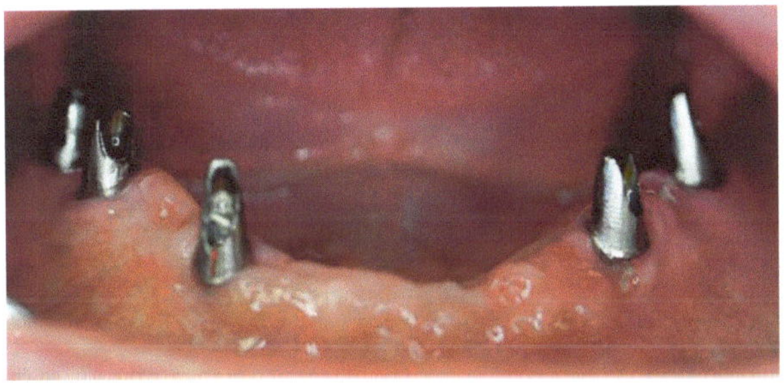

Figure 19.89. Immediately installed implants in the alveolar wound, after preservation of the alveolus, loaded with provisional fixed prosthetic work performed in the composite. Achieved good bony integration and healing of soft tissues around the support of the prosthetic work.

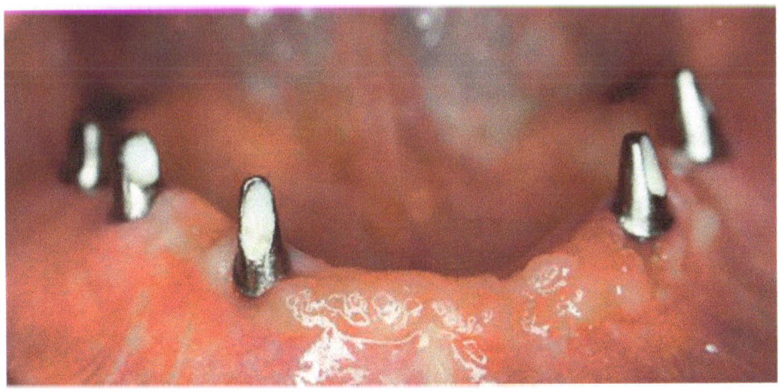

Figure 19.90. Definitive abutments placed, screw tension checked up to 35 Ncm, covered with a thin layer of gutta-percha filled with G Glasionomer, in case of loosening of the screw, re-tightening is possible without complications. Fixation of definitive prosthetic work is done with Implantlink-semi - a DETAX product. The characteristics of "Implantlink semi and forte" material for definitive fixation of prosthetic work have already been emphasized. The characteristics of this material are good fixation and work stability and easy removal for periodic checking of the

stability of the carrier and the condition of the surrounding soft tissues. In order to ensure the stability of the support and the screw, the screw head is protected by a layer of slightly heated gutta-percha supplemented with glass ionomer, which can be easily removed in order not to damage the screw head. The use of a cotton ball is not recommended.

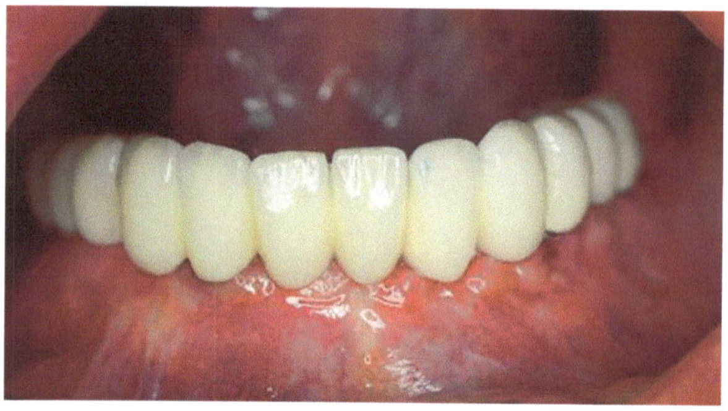

Figure 19.91. Appearance of definitive prosthetic work in metal-ceramic anchored on El Esthetic Line system implants.

Question: What are the causes of changes in interjaw relationships in relation to aging?

Answer: The process of interjaw relationship disorders begins with: abrasion, bruxism, tooth loss, degenerative changes in the masticatory muscles, i.e. weakening of their tone and elasticity, due to partial atrophy and fibrosis of muscle fibers. These changes are accompanied by degenerative changes in all structures of the temporomandibular joint (TMJ).

Establishing physiological intermaxillary relations and placing the condyle in a physiological position, i.e. in the maximum disto-position, in case of total edentulism, by surgical-implant-prosthetic procedures (see pictures 19.79. to 19.98.) is much more complex than the procedures for determining intermaxillary relations with wax templates for production of total acrylate prostheses.

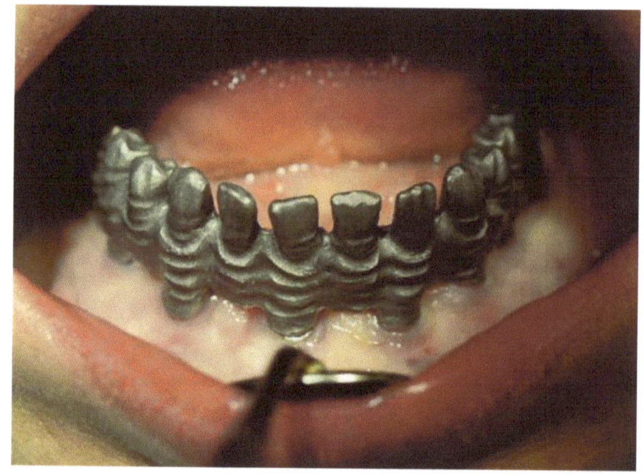

Figure 19.92. Establishing disturbed interjaw relationships due to premature tooth loss in bilaterally total edentulous jaws is an extremely complex implant-prosthetic procedure.

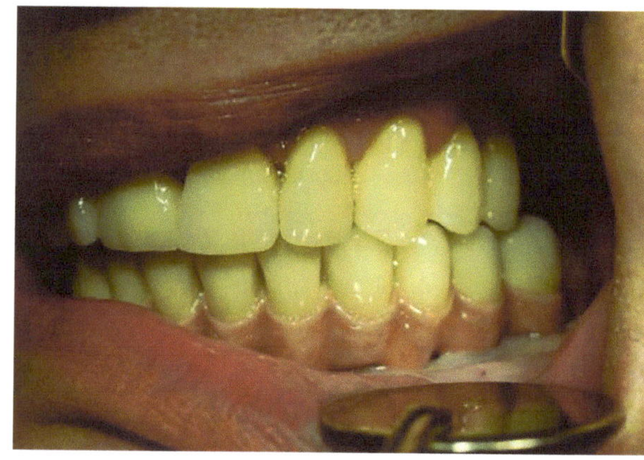

Figure 19.93. Rehabilitated impaired intervolar physiological relations (patient 60 years old), TMJ condyles placed in maximum disto-position (central occlusion) occlusion and articulation, cusps inclination, lateral movements of the lower jaw, aligned with biomechanical laws. Surgical implant-proter rehabilitation in both jaws was performed with the Branemark implant system and prosthetic works in metal-ceramics.

Question: In what way faddism is not desirable in medicine?

Answer: First of all, marketing is usually not in the desired goal of helping people, but in the profit of the producer, where ethics does not exist. Most of the advertised preparations benefit only the manufacturer, and have no effect on the person to whom the product is offered. For example, in oral surgery and oral implantology for replacement of lost bone, "Easy-graft" has been advertised as a "bone substitute". The marketing of this "substitute for bone" emphasized the "advantages"; ease of application and without the use of a collagen resorbable membrane, the cost of treatment is significantly reduced. Practice denied marketing; it turned out to be the most ordinary markentist fraud; first of all, the author of this "sensational discovery" is an engineer, not a biologist. After a short time, the implanted material was resorbed, and the new bone was not replaced

Question: When it comes to augmentation, what does it mean terminologically?

Answer: Augmentation (Augmetatio), has multiple meanings: multiplication, augmentation, enlargement, amplification, reinforcement, increase, addition, compensation, and augmentation. Therefore, this term in oral surgery and oral implantology and in aesthetic treatments of the face and lips, in contrast to implant placement, has a different meaning; method of application and results of successful treatment. The results of treatment in oral implantology are incomparably more successful and long-lasting.

Question: What is the difference between the materials used to replace lost bone in bone destruction and to increase the amount of bone in a thin bony sinus floor to create conditions for implant placement or in lip augmentation?

Answer: These two augmentation procedures are incomparable and nothing alike. First of all, increasing bone volume in oral implantology, in order to create conditions for implantation, is a biological process; the formation of new bone. The procedure of increasing bone volume by augmentation can be performed with autologous bone, i.e. sawdust or bone graft; with a bone graft taken from another region of the jaw in the patient's mouth or a xenogeneic bone substitute mixed with autologous bone chips. Increasing bone volume is not only a need for implant placement, but also as a support for soft tissues.

The conclusion is that the material used in oral implantology to increase bone volume is not a foreign body.

The materials used to enlarge lips or remove facial wrinkles is hyaluronic acid, which is a 50% ingredient in the skin of every organism. The material that is injected into the subcutaneous layer of the lips is called hyaluronic filler. Fillers are means intended as support for the skin and mucous membrane to fill facial wrinkles due to aging. The role of hyaluronic acid is to bind strongly to water. With aging, the skin becomes loose and thin, and the subcutaneous tissue loose and flabby. The volume of the skin decreases with aging, because the hyaluronic acid decreases and the skin becomes loose, dehydrated, wrinkled and inelastic. Hyaluronic fillers that are injected in the form of a gel, a synthetic substance, is unknown and foreign to the body being injected, on which the body reacts with inflammatory reactions after the injection.

Question: From the above, it can be concluded that the body reacts to materials used for lip augmentation and aesthetic treatment of facial wrinkles as a foreign body, unlike materials used in oral implantology to replace lost bone or increase bone volume in order to could an implant be safely placed in that place?

Answer: By injecting fillers, no biological material is introduced, but an artificial alloplastic material to which the body reacts with inflammatory reactions, because it is an immunobiological reaction to a foreign body. Immunobiological reactions are manifested by complications: the formation of nodules, granulomas and fibrous capsules around the foreign body. These phenomena can lead to serious deformities. The lip is thickened and stiff, not elastic. Muscle fibers are stretched and under pressure, and thus the function is weakened. This muscle condition can later lead to muscle fibrosis and atrophy. Small salivary glands are also pressed, due to which can cause a retention cyst. The enlarged soft tissues of the lips are no longer in proportion to the teeth and bony tissues. Moving the placed material from the place where it was injected, can be moved to completely different, near or far place. Cases have been described in which the substances, hyaluronic fillers injected into the lower lip, were moved even into the neck. Although this domain is much narrower than the domain of surgical-prosthetic procedures, there are more unexplained complications than in oral implantology, practically there are no such complications in oral implantology. For example, the formation of granulomas is unknown, and the dislocation of injected material and the appearance of nodules, their transformation is explained: inadequate injection technique and inadequate amount of filler. However, oral implantology is handled by competent people, and lip augmentation and facial wrinkle filling; from competent plastic surgeons to beauticians and medical technicians. Complications are also influenced by the gravity factor, under the influence of the Earth's gravity. A large amount of material wrapped in a thin capsule, which is unable to hold it, migrates downwards, from the lip to the chin. Complications are also caused by the factor of muscle movements in regions where muscle activity is strong, such as the region of the lips, during speech and chewing, the twisted "threads" of the subtance are transformed into spherical shapes by circular muscle movements, and thus nodules - balls are formed. Muscle movements can push the injected material down, like gravity, and up, against gravity. Also, muscle movements can push the placed material towards the deeper tissue layers - submucosal or towards the surface of the skin - subepidermal, so that the muscle can easily push the material out of the region where it was injected. So the entire desired goal of the patient gets the opposite outcome. There are no such complications in oral implantology.

Question: Does this mean that these lip augmentation procedures destroy the harmony of the face and that it is an unnatural process?

Answer: It is not only the facial harmony of a person who gets lip augmentation that is destroyed. The harmony of the racial peculiarity is being destroyed, the characteristic of the racial peculiarity is changing. The lips of the black population are of a different shape from the lips of white people. Lips that are filled with hyaluronic fillers will age sooner than those that are not filled. In other words, the lips will be relaxed, stretched with age-related vertical wrinkles. The procedures must be repeated after some time, because the breakdown and resorption of hyaluronic acid occurs.

The conclusion is that all this is contrary to nature. In the end, the foregoing confirms that the author's position is justified; faddism in medicine is harmful!

20

Contract With The Patient On Implant Installation And Prosthetic Work

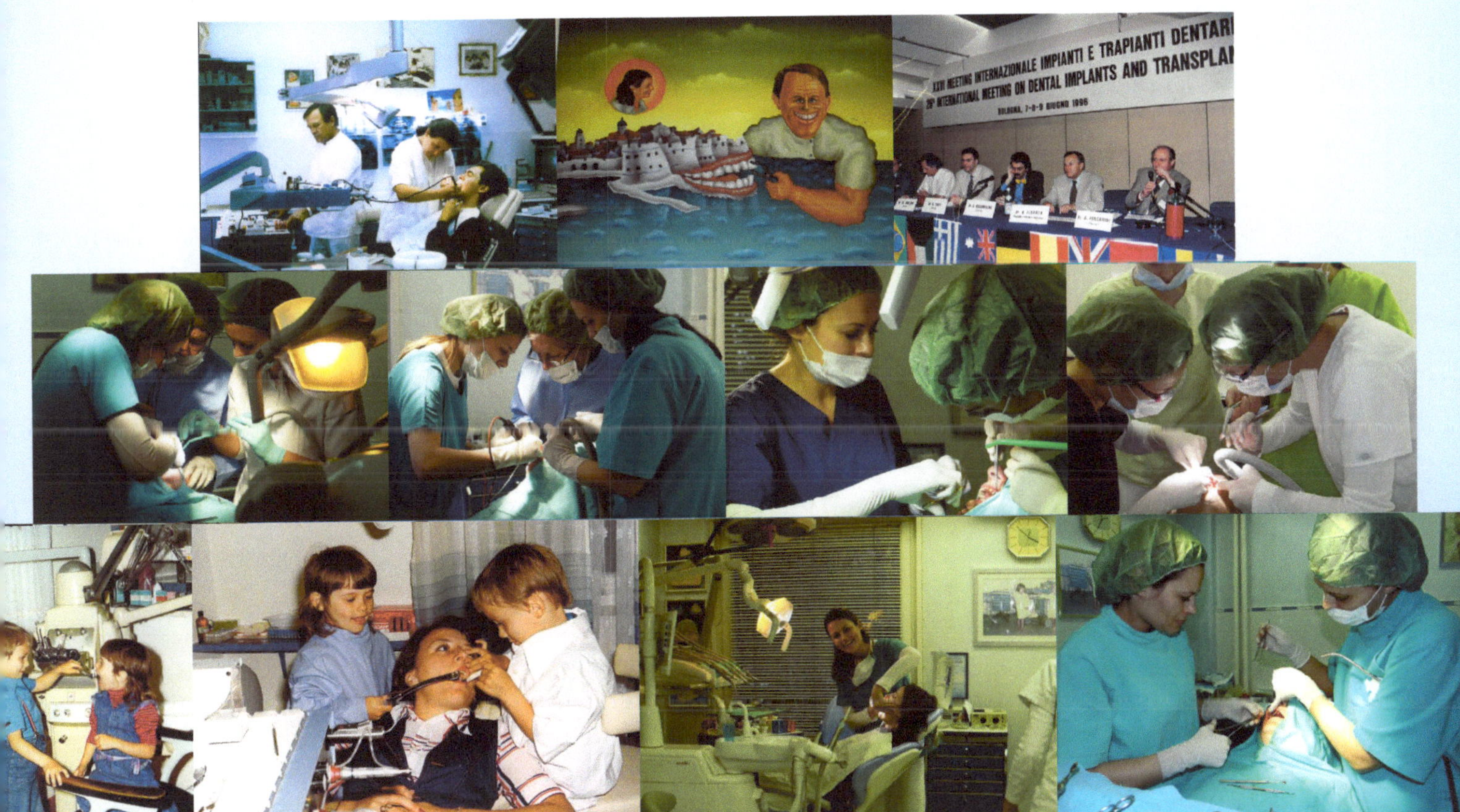

Types Of Medical Services Contracts

Despite the great progress of oral implantology, it must be remembered that risk is always possible and that an unwanted outcome can happen even to the most experienced implantologists. We can never be sure how the patient will accept it, especially if it is not explained to him well what needs to be done and what can happen outside of our expectations. Given that implant installation is a team effort in which the practicing oral surgeon and dental technician participate, all responsibility is taken by the dentist and the patient does not see another person who would be responsible in the event of an unwanted outcome.

Legal consideration

General legal considerations should be known when it comes to the contract with the patient on implant installation. Within the right to health protection, as a general human right, appropriate rules must be established so that each of the responsible parties in the patient-doctor relationship, i.e., dentist or oral surgeon, can ensure the factual and formal protection of their rights.

For a long time, there was hesitation, both in theory and in judicial practice, that the doctor-patient relationship qualifies as a contractual relationship. We assume that the reason for this is the nature of this relationship, the fact that it is to some extent susceptible to mystification and idealization, since it is related to the ethical and even to the emotional sphere, related to concepts such as trust, handover "in the hands of another", which in colloquial language excludes formalism and "dryness" which is excluded by a contractual relationship with a legally normed debt - fiduciary obligations.

However, when we get rid of such prejudices, it becomes clear from the legal point of view that the rule of thumb is to qualify the doctor-patient relationship as a contractual relationship, the best way to regulate the rights and obligations that this relationship inevitably entails. We are witnessing that more and more surgeries, not only dental ones, are subject to administrative controls. Since it is often not possible to determine at the beginning what kind of patient it is, I believe that the installation of implants can be considered one of the types of contracts for medical services. Accordingly, the installation contract implants are subject to the same legal rules and the same general characteristics that apply to contracts for medical services in general

What is the purpose of "implanting artificial teeth", would be a question for lawyers

Implantation of artificial teeth (oral implantation of implants) is the introduction (implantation) of foreign material directly into the jawbone. This procedure is performed where teeth are missing in the jaw - in legal terms. The purpose of this procedure is to strengthen prostheses or bridges for the implanted implants after the appropriate treatment, in the next phase, and after healing, and thus to improve the ability to chew, and thus the quality of life and aesthetics.

Legal nature of the dental implant contract

Since the contract on the implantation of artificial teeth (legal term) belongs to contracts for medical services, it is an obligatory synalagmatic contract. It is about an inevitable contract, about an assessment whose legal nature has differences in legal systems, although these differences are reduced more to nuances than they are of an essential character.

According to Austrian, German and Greek law, a contract for medical services, as well as a contract for dental treatment through implant placement, by its legal nature, can be considered a service or service contract. According to Swiss law, it is a contract of mandate, while French lawyers consider it a "sui generis" contract (a contract of special importance).

How is it regulated by our Law?

According to our Law on Obligations, the contract for medical services, including the contract for the installation of implants, is a work contract, where this contract has been taken into something by stretching the form, which means that in certain types of work, under the subject of the work contract, no it always implies a good result - the outcome of the treatment, even assuming that everything is made of the highest quality material and the most modern application.

The contract on the implantation of artificial teeth (insertion of implants) for the purpose of dental treatment, i.e. the legal issues related to dental treatment are the most elaborated in German legal theory and practice.

When it comes to the contract on the implantation of artificial teeth (implantation), its legal nature can be referred to either as a work contract or as a service contract. According to the provisions governing the service contract, the service provider - in this case, dentist, oral surgeon, periodontist, is only obligated to perform a certain action, while according to the norms applicable to the work contract, he is obliged to achieve success, which he must guarantee as for his work.

In the practice of the German courts, in which the contract for the provision of medical services is sometimes treated as a service contract, and sometimes as a work contract, the implant installation contract should generally be considered a service contract, and in case of a dispute, the provisions of civil law that regulate this shall apply. contract.

It should be emphasized that mobile and fixed prosthetic works (dentures and bridges) fall under a different regime.

Regarding the installation of implants, it is considered as a specific type of dental treatment. Apart from the high expertise of the dentist's skill and effort, there are factors that the dentist cannot influence or can influence to a very limited extent. It is about the physical and psychological constitution of the patient, which cannot be predicted in advance, and it is impossible to know whether the organism will accept or reject the implant as a foreign body. This is in favor of the dentist, because this legal thinking is frankly speaking, modern implantology no longer accepts the term of rejecting the implant as a foreign body, even though it is.

In the legal document "Administrative Contracts", where this topic is discussed, it is stated that the percentage of failure ranges from 20 to 30%, which absolutely does not correspond to this moment when the percentage of success ranges between 96 to 98%.

Failure is manifested by the loosening of the installed implants, so that they cannot respond to their task. Such a result, i.e. failure, can also occur in the case of implant placement performed according to all the rules of the profession, i.e. when there is no procedural error.

The dentist, therefore, cannot guarantee the success of the procedure with this specific dental treatment, which leads to the conclusion that the contract for implant placement can be considered a contract for your service. These considerations, from a legal point of view, oblige the dentist in the contract for implant installation to the following.

As previously emphasized, the dentist cannot guarantee in writing the success of the dental implant procedure undertaken, nor can he be required to do so. What can be demanded and what he is obliged to provide is making available to the patient the knowledge and experience he possesses. The dentist must perform an examination in the appropriate premises, the office, on the basis of which he makes a diagnosis. An accurate diagnosis precedes the indication for the dental procedure of installing artificial (implant) teeth.

The patient, of course, before performing the operation, i.e. installing the implant, should agree to this type of treatment. In order for the patient's consent (and in some Western countries they also have a legal representative) to be valid, it is necessary for the patient to be validly and fully informed, and also to be able to understand the information given to him. The dentist is obliged to inform the patient accurately about the method and scope of the planned procedure. This certainly includes the notification about the percentage of success or failure. In particular, it is necessary to point out in detail the possible complications of this type of procedure, about the complications that could occur, about other methods of treatment, as well as the consequences of the absence of treatment. In order for the patient's consent to be valid, it is necessary that he is able to understand the information given to him.

The dentist is obliged to inform the patient accurately about the method and scope of the planned procedure. This certainly includes notification of the percentage of success and failure, in particular, possible complications must be indicated in detail, but also that after the treatment is completed, the patient is obliged to come for regular check-ups and possible complications that could occur due to the absence of mandatory periodic checks. The question arises of the limits of informing the patient about possible risks. It is unnecessary to be informed about the risks that are possible with any surgical procedure. For example, the Federal Supreme Court of Germany considers that when informing the patient "only those risks that a reasonable person considers essential for making a decision on consent should be pointed out." Avoid confusing the patient with irrelevant questions.

In order for the patient's consent to be valid, it is certainly necessary for him to be able to do business. However, apart from this general condition, the dentist should determine whether, in a specific case, at the time of notification, reference to the necessary knowledge about the surgical procedure, the patient is capable of receiving and understanding the information given by the dentist. If for any reason it can be determined that the patient is not sober enough to understand the information given, the doctor should postpone the notification until the next, better opportunity.

In order for, from a legal point of view, specific dental treatment to be indicated by the installation of implants, it is necessary to establish an accurate diagnosis. The diagnosis should establish that the state of the masticatory system is such that, based on professional scientific knowledge and experience, it turns out to be the most effective treatment with the implant installation method. The indication for this kind of dental procedure naturally implies the consent and desire of the patient. We emphasize that for a correct indication it is necessary that there is a concurrence of both of these conditions - medical necessity and the patient's wish. The absence of one of these conditions could be a presumption for the existence of hidden, illegal physical injury.

As it was concluded earlier (see the third paragraph of the third page of this paper), when undertaking an oral surgical procedure to install an implant, the dentist cannot be required to guarantee that the procedure will succeed. But what can be demanded is the observance of certain standards, such as the conduct of doctors with appropriate medical care and in accordance with the established rules of medical science. In these cases, the question arises of the doctor's decision to strictly observe the rules of medical science, more precisely what this standard entails, strict adherence to school rules and what is the measure of its elasticity.

My legal opinion is that the dentist does not have to use the method that according to the rules of "school medicine" is the most effective, in the second case, if his expert opinion, based on medical reasons, is not in accordance with that method. They would agree with this position, say lawyers, because otherwise any progress in dental medicine and the introduction of modern procedures in treatment would not be possible. However, a certain ambivalence in judgment still arises here. If the dentist applies a tool that is not generally accepted in the profession and the procedure is successful, the problem does not arise, i.e. it is progress in the treatment. If, however, the intervention fails, the question arises from a legal point of view, how to justify the non-compliance with the prevailing rule for that type of intervention. Such legal positions made sense at a time when the pioneers of implantology were installing implants and when implantology was not accepted by any faculty at all. When installing implants, the dentist can apply, based on the appropriate diagnosis and indication, methods based on medical experience and scientific research. The duty of the dentist is to use the appropriate implant, which has a quality certificate of titanium as the material from which it is made. Also, the operative technique must be performed with the best system and finally everything must be completed with prosthetic care.

Implant failure is something that can happen regardless of knowledge, skill, experience and compliance with the rules of medical and surgical skill.

If the patient raises the question of the responsibility of the dentist, he must provide evidence that the practicing dentist did not act with the necessary care, which means that the diagnosis was not appropriate to indicate the treatment with the installation of implants or that the patient's information about the successes and risks of such treatment was not complete. or finally, that due to the incompetence or carelessness of the dentist, there were complications and failure of the surgical procedure.

Patient Obligations

The patient is obliged, since it is a mutually binding contract, to pay the dentist the compensation determined by the price list of the association or the compensation agreed between them for that type of medical service. The dentist is the one who estimates the amount of the contracted price, because often due to the specifics of the case, it is not possible to stick to the prescribed price list. According to our regulations, the price of registered services can be paid exclusively in domestic currency. Since the dinar exchange rate is variable, contracting for a specific service, the prices from the price list of the association cannot be the subject of the contract.

The obligation to pay compensation also exists in the case when the installation of the implant failed, provided, of course, that the failure was not the result of the dentist's mistake. A patient who has given his consent for specific treatment with the installation of implants, or in legal terms "treatment with the installation of artificial teeth", is obliged to undergo the entire therapy, which most often includes prosthetic rehabilitation of the jaw (placing crowns and bridges on implants). The patient should also cooperate with the dentist, i.e. to follow the dentist's instructions in maintaining oral hygiene and controlling the implanted parts of the jaw or teeth.

Conclusion

The contract on the implantation of artificial teeth (installation of implants) is, like all other contracts on medical services, an unnamed contract, which is not specifically regulated anywhere, and it seems that there is no need for a separate one regulation in this domain. This contractual relationship is largely based on mutual trust, especially the patient's trust in the chosen dentist. Therefore, in the event of a dispute, the disputed relationship must be precisely clarified and then the legal rules must be applied according to the case.

Why did I give this topic a special accent? One can never be sure what kind of patient the dentist meets and what can be born from the good intentions of the dentist and his efforts. Very often in our offices, at the end of treatment, dentists meet dissatisfied and ungrateful patients.

Such patients usually visit many surgeries. Problems arise when the patient is burdened with ill-intentioned information by a professional. Experience gives me clear and collegial guidance; such a patient should be listened to and examined in detail. If you find that the patient is right and in trouble, call the dentist and explain the patient's objections and your observations. Refer the patient to the dentist who performed the entire treatment.

In order to avoid unwanted and often very unpleasant legal disputes, the practicing dentist should invite a more experienced colleague to solve the problem and the patient's dissatisfaction together.

Afterword

The book before the reader is a "diary of work and experience." It is the result of long-term, painstaking efforts that did not tire me; rather, I approached it with the enthusiasm of a dedicated enthusiast. My curious and restless spirit drove me to leave the hilly Balkans for the even more mountainous terrain of Switzerland, a country renowned for having the best-organized dental service in the world. Its residents have the healthiest teeth, and dentists here are among the highest paid.

The journey was challenging and demanding. I began my training at the Volkszahn Klinik (People's Dental Clinic) in Basel, an institution where I gained valuable knowledge. The clinic was managed by university professors who oversaw and signed every document. Swiss doctors often referred their own children to this clinic after completing their studies, prior to allowing them to practice independently. Furthermore, private dental practices in Switzerland were highly regarded for their advanced equipment and high-quality services, with assistants selected based on the recommendations of the clinic's professors.

All private dental practices operated in competitive relationships where the primary measure of value was the quality of work and the skill of the individual dentist. Factors such as the doctor's reputation, the quality of equipment, the standard of the practice, its location, and its "fame" influenced both patient choice and pricing. Swiss doctors practiced general dentistry, and there was a wealth of knowledge to acquire that we did not have the opportunity to learn at university.

Prosthetics in Switzerland was the most advanced, not only in Europe but also in the world. This field captured my attention, as the prosthetic practices in Yugoslavia at that time were significantly below Swiss standards, lacking in both materials and execution in dental laboratories. I began writing lectures and presenting cases I had resolved. My journey started in Switzerland at professional meetings held by the Canton, and I made sure to attend every dental week and congress in Yugoslavia.

When an exceptional prosthetist, Dr. Vojin Petrović, who was a lecturer of prosthetics at the Faculty of Dentistry in Belgrade and head of prosthetics at the Academy of Medical Sciences, came to visit me, he was convinced by my claims. We became close associates, and he expressed a desire to preside over all my lectures. My curiosity drove me to gather knowledge from across Europe and around the world.

The lectures I delivered in Yugoslavia were distinctive in their presentation style and differed from the norm of the time. For instance, when discussing the restoration and compensation of lost teeth, I emphasized that achieving harmony is an essential condition. The shape of the teeth should correspond to the anatomical shape of the face, as well as to their position and color. An experienced practitioner always considers these three factors to meet aesthetic standards.

On the other hand, patients often have cosmetic preferences influenced by current trends. Many patients desire white teeth like those of a certain actor, actress, or artist. For a long time, I questioned these demands, fearing that fulfilling them might result in teeth that looked artificially created or overly prominent. However, aesthetic prosthetics and dentistry have advanced significantly, making these patient desires more valid today. Throughout my many years of practice, I have tried to avoid being a trend follower.

But, also, today I believe that modern prosthetic achievements in both materials and technology can often surpass nature itself, when it comes to aesthetic restoration in the mouth. This justifies the patient's demands that need to be fulfilled, and thus his satisfaction. I think that new techniques, materials and methods in the world were first served to dentists in Switzerland and Scandinavian countries. When I mastered the language, I accepted the "Swiss style" and grabbed innovation before others. My professional interest at the beginning was mainly related to prosthetics. Although dentistry in the field of prosthetics was the most successful medical branch of dentistry, at that time it had not yet achieved the possible perfection. True, in the field of aesthetics and cosmetics, today it is "more successful than nature". Problems remain in the field of physiology and molecular biology. Youth and an inquisitive research spirit did not allow me to be lulled into the routine work of everyday life, but I awakened my research spirit and followed, adopted and implemented innovations for the benefit of the patient. When I watched my mother holster with lower total dentures, my sphere of interest was directed towards the stabilization of total acrylic dentures, especially in the lower jaw. I tried everything, but, I must admit, it ended up with only minor improvements.

My curiosity and investigative spirit, I have followed, adopted, implemented and propagated into a work of innovation and scope of oral implatology. In the sixties of the last century, the appearance of somewhat more successful rehabilitation of disabilities in the oral cavity, with implant-prosthetic treatment, was the most revolutionary innovation in modern dentistry. Implantation is becoming an increasingly frequent therapeutic procedure in the oral cavity. From then until today, my professional interest has been directed in that direction. Through persistent work, learning and training at world clinics, contacts, following the literature and knowledge from my own practice, I "figured out" the essence of the problem of "implantation of teeth", as it is said in layman's language.

According to a Chinese wisdom, from the time of Confucius; "If we decide on a path, be it a hundred or a million steps long, the most important is the first step!" I started that first step towards oral implantology in Switzerland with one enthusiast. We presented what we tried at the professional conference in Canton. We are sometimes laughed at. From today's time distance in relation to the current scope of oral implantology, it is really funny. Lugano, one of the centers of Swiss tourism, became the place of my work and affirmation. Material possibilities allowed me to visit many famous world clinics from there, adopting new achievements in the profession. During my stay in Switzerland and later, I considered it my ethical and patriotic duty to acquaint dentists and the medical public with the achievements of the profession, and first of all with the achievements of oral implantology in the world. I regularly visited domestic congresses, symposiums and dental weeks, which were then held in the republics; showed slides, held the first lectures on prosthetics, because metal ceramics were not being made. I also held the first lectures on oral implantology. I traveled around the world, participated and presented at congresses and symposiums, persistently spreading the idea of introducing oral implantology in our dentistry as well.

When I look back, the efforts were not in vain. Progress was impossible to stop. Unfortunately, the pioneers of any progress must go through the thorny path of conservative resistance, crush ignorance and overcome the vanities so characteristic of the medical profession. But the guide and light that illuminated my planned path was biblical wisdom: "Blessed is he who knows that he does not know, and wants to know!" The book that is before the reader is, at least, a hymn of praise to the "successes" of my own practice and experience. In favor of the progress of oral implantology and the profession, I mustered the courage to present at a world scientific symposium

(Bologna, 1985) held a lecture on the topic: "My failures in oral implantology". I'm not sure if any lecture at that time caused as much interest and sincere recognition as that one. Bone integration was discussed. This world scientific meeting was led by Professor Giordano Muratori, a legend of Italian implantology, he approached me and, as a sign of recognition and gratitude, told me to lead the round table that day.

I was in a hurry to transfer the new achievements of the profession to my environment. But everything happened beyond my expectations. Since then I support enthusiasts in any business. I said that I devoted myself to oral implantology with great enthusiasm. I gathered the courage to write about it and give lectures. I overcame obstacles in an unusual way and always emerged as an enthusiastic winner. My office in Cavtat was visited by many professors of dental faculties in Yugoslavia. Among them professors from Zagreb: Ivo Miše, Vlada Amšel, Miroslav Suvin and others, and professor Čeda Ravnikar from Ljubljana with several other colleagues. The professors of the Belgrade Faculty of Dentistry, professors of the Academy of Medical Sciences, Dr. Škundrić, Dr. Škokljev, Dr. Cvetinović, Starčević and the head of the Academy of Medical Sciences, Prof. Dr. Vladimir Vojvodić, then faculty professors from Sarajevo, Skopje and Rijeka.

At the beginning of the eighties of the last century, Slovenians organized "Days of Oral Implantology" in Portorož. That group was called "Alpe-Adria". Until then, not a single implant had been installed in Slovenia. They invited two foreign lecturers; Professor Ugo Pasqualini from Milan and Professor Weinmüller from Vienna. The meeting was attended by dentists from all over Yugoslavia. VMA Belgrade was then the only institution that was known for installing implants, thanks to professors Aco Škundrić and Smiljana Matić. In many newspapers, readers asked medical questions and sought answers. There were also questions: do we "implant teeth" and where? The answers were: at the VMA and in Cavtat. "Injured by vanity", because they didn't invite us to participate as lecturers, I jokingly told Professor Aco Škundrić that we would "get revenge" on them and that I had an idea to "mine" the memorial meeting. Which came true. I told this "secret" to my friend Professor Škundrić, who always supported me, as did all my colleagues from the then famous VMA, unlike the Faculty of Dentistry. I prepared to surprise the two lecturers and everyone present with my "mischief". Especially Slovenes as organizers. When the lecturers finished their lectures, showing more schematics and much less performed implant-prosthetic works on implants, assistant professor Dr. Rode invited the attendees to ask questions to the lecturers. The packed hall came alive.

The questions came one after the other, to which the lecturers answered. I must emphasize; that the questions were truly layman's, because the essence of oral implantology was unknown to the participants. At the end, the chairman said: "If no one has any more questions, let the meeting end!" Professor Škundrić, "disappointed" thinks that I gave up on my intention, because most of those present had already stood up. However, I waited a moment, so that the surprise would be greater; raised his hand, asked the chairman to allow me a short question to the lecturers. I did not address the lecturers first, but the presiding Slovenian: "Can I ask a short question to the lecturers in their language; Italian and German?" I had prepared more than a hundred slides. Lecturer

I asked, and apologized for my "immodesty", would you allow me to briefly supplement their lectures, which I praised as exceptional and very interesting? A big surprise for the lecturers. I had the impression that the lecturers had the impression that they were the first to present the scope of oral implantology at that time in the East Block. I handed over the cassette with the slides and began my "short" supplement to the lecture, which lasted a little over an hour. In the end, when I finished "supplementing" their lectures, the situation turned into a dialogue with the lecturers, which was translated.

I forced the Slovenians to translate for me as well, because I conducted the dialogue in Italian and German. The gathering of dentists from all over Yugoslavia in Portorož started in the Slovenian language. The same thing happened again at the Congress of Dentists of Yugoslavia in Ljubljana. Both gatherings began with my "cheeky" question and proposal: "That the basic order, according to the rules of "etiquette", is for the host to adapt to the guest! Given that the majority of those present are from the Serbian-Croatian speaking area, I propose that the Congress be in a language understood by the majority, given that it is the Congress of Dentists of Yugoslavia, not Slovenia!" The proposal was accepted. How fierce the resistance to oral implantology was in our country; it is worth highlighting and recording some events that are incomprehensible today. When, at the Congress of Dentists of Yugoslavia in Budva, Dr. Zoran Atanasovski, gave a lecture on "implantation of teeth", it is impossible today to describe the ferocity and cruelty of the attacks of those present. I have never seen a sadder expression at any gathering than on the face of this enthusiast. Maltene was ridiculed! I stood up, the only one defending his views. Finally, I must point out; that I wasn't doing better myself! It is worth recording an event that was remembered by many generations. I was sad then, and today I am proud of the event that took place in the 1980s in Vrnjačka Banja, at the Congress of Dentists of Yugoslavia. They interrupted my lecture by turning off the lights in the hall. The chairman, an assistant professor at the Faculty of Zagreb, explained this: "It is illegal and frivolous to include such lectures in congress programs, where they show "foreign body" embedding in living bone, which causes cancer! I forced the Slovenians to translate for me as well, because I conducted the dialogue in Italian and German. The gathering of dentists from all over Yugoslavia in Portorož started in the Slovenian language. The same thing happened again at the Congress of Dentists of Yugoslavia in Ljubljana. Both gatherings began with my "cheeky" question and proposal: "That the basic order, according to the rules of "etiquette", is for the host to adapt to the guest! Given that the majority of those present are from the Serbian-Croatian speaking area, I propose that the Congress be in a language understood by the majority, given that it is the Congress of Dentists of Yugoslavia, not Slovenia!" The proposal was accepted. How fierce the resistance to oral implantology was in our country, it is worth highlighting and recording some events that are incomprehensible today. When, at the Congress of Dentists of Yugoslavia in Budva, Dr. Zoran Atanasovski, gave a lecture on "implantation of teeth", it is impossible today to describe the ferocity and cruelty of the attacks of those present. I have never seen a sadder expression at any gathering than on the face of this enthusiast. Maltene was ridiculed! I stood up, the only one defending his views. Finally, I must point out; that I wasn't doing better myself! It is worth recording an event that was remembered by many generations. I was sad then, and today I am proud of the event that took place in the 1980s in Vrnjačka Banja, at the Congress of Dentists of Yugoslavia. They interrupted my lecture by turning off the lights in the hall. The chairman, an assistant professor at the Faculty of Zagreb, explained this: "It is illegal and frivolous to include such lectures in congress programs, where they show "foreign body" embedding in living bone, which causes cancer!

I could not keep silent about this, because I gave that lecture in Liège (Belgium), the president of which was prof. Strel and Linkov. After my presentation, Professor Linkov stood up, satisfied with my presentations, the great speaker said excitedly: "Gentlemen, today is my happiest day. I don't have to look into the crystal ball anymore, does implantology have a future!? This man confirmed it to us, you see, the communists also successfully applied it! To tear down the communist iron curtain, no more atomic and megaton bombs are needed, my tiny implant did it! "He approached, hugged me and congratulated me. The applause lasted a long time. I was the first from the so-called Eastern Bloc.

I asked Professor Joza Perović to just allow me to give a conclusion. My conclusion was: "Dear colleagues, I came to this lectern for two reasons; the first is, I want to be remembered, and you all would like to be remembered. You will remember me for interrupting the lecture, turning off the lights. I want you to remember me more by the conclusion, and I am asking the chairman to write it down, because this event will remain in his memory and say something that he does not know today: It is very important for the coachman to see well! Even with blind oxen and horses they will reach the goal!"

It should be emphasized that the first scientific symposia in Yugoslavia, on oral implantology, were not organized by dental faculties, but by enthusiasts in Osijek and Kumanovo. They were organized by colleagues, my friends; in Osijek, the distinguished Dr. Vladimir Jokanović, maxillofacial surgeon, and in Kumanovo, Dr. Zoran Atanasovski. It should be pointed out that at that time, implantology was not available at the faculties, not only in our country. Resistance was then the majority opinion. But, in the end I have to confirm; that at that time was the majority opinion of dentists, and had the greatest support from professors of dental faculties about oral implantology. For this reason, implantology could not be learned at the university, but through visits to various seminars and trainings with eminent experts who, with their works, both practical and scientific, established themselves in this domain of oral rehabilitation in the oral cavity.

The best attitude towards oral implantology dominated in America and Sweden, but not in Switzerland. For most dentists, for a long time, implants placed in living bone were a "foreign body". If this book, which is before the reader, is a replay of Portorož and Vrnjačka Banja, it means that my efforts were not in vain. The most realistic is the judgment made by the readers. The resistance of majority opinion is stubborn and sometimes very dangerous. The truth that the earth revolves around the sun cost the great scientist his head!? Scientific and professional knowledge paves new paths, turning them into easy routines that experienced practitioners in dentistry indulge in.

AUTHOR

Gratitude

"Behind every scientific work is a team of people who stimulated and demotivated his creative work!"

While writing this book, I could not avoid the "traps" of criticism and praise. But the justification for not correcting what is written, which is well known to me, is unknown to many generations. I changed countries, places of residence, but the desire to put my "journal of professional memories" on paper and publish it never left me. I spread the accumulated professional knowledge in my immediate and distant surroundings, so that my creativity exceeded the place of creation. I confirmed this with lectures at many congresses and dental weeks throughout Yugoslavia and many foreign performances when oral implantology was a big unknown. Resistance and misunderstanding in our country made me give more lectures abroad. I feel the need to thank everyone who supported me.

I owe thanks to my friends for supporting my mission and supporting "my learning". For this reason, I first gave the written work to four eminent practitioners for verification: Dr. Veroslav Dabić and Dr. Zoran Kostić, maxillofacial surgeon, oral surgeon Dr. Marjan Marjanović and Milan Uzelac, so that their remarks would be based on what practice says. Their critical review is a valuable help, for which I am grateful. I owe special thanks to the reviewers who gave a critical review of everything presented "between the two covers". When choosing the reviewers, I tried to ensure that, in addition to top-notch professional knowledge, they were decorated with intellectual and artistic uniqueness. I am grateful to the reviewers: Dr. Vladimir Jokanović, maxillofacial surgeon, writer and eminent sculptor, Professor Dr. Asen Džolev, maxillofacial surgeon, Professor Dr. Zoran Aleksić, Professor Dr. Obrad Zelić, Professor Dr. Radmil Roncevic, maxillofacial and plastic surgeon, and Professor Dr. Zoran Lazić, Head of Dentistry. VMA in Belgrade.

I would like to express my deepest gratitude to my expert proofreaders: Dr. Smiljana Matić, a professor at the Academy of Medical Sciences, and Dr. Ljubo Todorović, a professor at the Faculty of Dentistry in Belgrade. Their dedicated effort and collaborative spirit ensured that the book was published with minimal errors.

I also wish to pay tribute to the late Professor Dr. Jovan-Joza Perović, a dear friend from my childhood and student days, whose unwavering support at every gathering meant a great deal to me.

Additionally, I extend my heartfelt thanks to the late Professor Aco Škundrić, who understood and supported me when others did not.

It is their enthusiasm and creativity that have significantly contributed to the advancement of oral implantology in our region.

Index

K

L

M

N

O

P

Q

Literature

A. Gajton, J. Hall: Translation into Serbian and editor, Prof. Dr. Vujadin Mujovič, Belgrade 2001. Medical Physiology.

Adell R. Hansson, B. O. Brenemark -Review of clinical approachs. 1970. Intra-osseous anchorage of dental prostheses.

Aghaloo TL, Moy PK. In. J. Oral Maxillofac Implants. 2007. Which hard tissue augmentation techniques are the most successful in furnishing bony support for implant placement

Aline Rivulet, Loyola University, Chicago, US, 1972. Atlas de Periodontologie

Albrektsson TO, Johansson CB, Sennebry L. Jou. Periodontol 1994. Biological aspects of implant dentistry: Osseointegration.

Alexander J. Hassel, Raed S Hahin, Alexander Kreuter, Peter Rammelsberg. Quintessence International, Berlin 2008. Rehabilitation of the edentulous lower jaw with a ceramic fixed bridge on implants

American Akademy of Periodontology. Glossary of periodontal terms. ChicagoAAP. 2001.

Anderson D, Zarb GA. Dao TT. J. Oral Maxilofac Implants. 1993. Is osteoporosis a risk faktor for ossteointegration of dental implants?

Andre Schroeder, Franz Sutter, and Gisbert Krekeler-D. Buser, B. Maeglin, S. Steinemann, H. Stich, E. van der Zypen. 1988. Georg Theime Verlag Stuttgart-New York Oral Implantology.

Anitua E, Orive G. J. Periodontal, 2919. Short implants in maxillae and mandibles: retrospective study with 1 to 8 years of follow-up.

Araujo M, Linder E, Wennstrom J, Lindhe J. socket. Int. J. Periodontics Restorative Dent. 2008. The influence of Bio-Oss Collagen on healing of extraction.

Araujo MG, et al. Clin Oral Periodontol 2005. Ridg alterations following implant placement in frech extaction sockets : an experimental study in th dog.

Araujo MG, Sukekava F, Wenrstrom JL, LindheJ. Journal Clin Periodontaol, 2005. Ridage alternations following implant placement in fresh extaction sockets: an experimental study in the dog.

Arndt Happe, Gerd Kerner. Qustessenze 2011. Implant treatment in the frontal region from an aesthetic point of view. Reasons for success and causes of risk

Arndt Happe, Gerd Korner, Daniel Rothamel. Quintesenze International. Berilin 2011. Problematici sumukoznih cementnih ostataka kod implantoloških struktura i indikacija za individualne nadogradnje.

Ashok Sethi, Thomas Kaus. Quintesence books 2005. Prakticna implatologija.

Auty C. Siddiqui. Implant Dent, 1999. Punch technique for preservation of interdental papilae at nonsubmerged implant placement.

Babbush C. A. Dent. Clin. North Amer. 1980. Endosteal blade vent implants.

Babbush, C. A. Oral Surgery 1972. Endosseous blade-vent implants.

Bahat O, Fontanessi TV. Int. Journal Periodintics RestorativeDent. 2001. Implant placement in threedimensional graft in the anterior jaw.

Bain CA. Int. J. Oral Maxillofac, 1966. Smoking and implant failure: Benefits of a smoking cessation protocol.

Barry I. Simon, Jay L. Greenfield. Quintessence Internationale, Berlin 2011. Sinus floor elevation with osteotome.

Beck, P. M, Apr. 1970. Endosseous implants.

Bergh van den JP, ten Bruggenkate CM, Disch FJ, Tuinzing DB. Clin Oral Implants Res 2000. Anatomical aspects of sinus floor elevations.

Bert, M. Quest. Odonto_Stomat, 1985. Bone Physiology and Dental Implants.

Biological complications with dental implants; Their prevention, diagnosis and treatment. Oral implants. 2000.

Biomechanical aspects of prosthetic implant-borne reconstructions. Periodontol 2000, 1998.

Block MS, Kent JN. J. Maxilofac Surg 1990. Factors associated with soft and hard-tissue compromise of endosseud implants.

Bonfante S, Bosco AF, Luize DS, de Almeida JM, Cestari TM. Int. J. Maxillofac Implants, 2008. Influenze of nikotin on healing process of autogenous bone blok grafts in the mandibule: histomophometic study in rats.

Botticelli D, J Clin Oral Periodontol, 2004. Hard-tissue alterations following immediate implant placement in extraction sites

Babbush C. A. Dent. Clin. North Amer. 1980. Endosteal blade vent implants.

Babbush, C. A. Oral Surgery 1972. Endosseous blade-vent implants.

Bahat O, Fontanessi TV. Int. Journal Periodintics RestorativeDent. 2001. Implant placement in threedimensional graft in the anterior jaw.

Bain CA. Int. J. Oral Maxillofac, 1966. Smoking and implant failure: Benefits of a smoking cessation protocol.

Barry I. Simon, Jay L. Greenfield. Quintessence Interantionale, Berlin 2011. Podizanje poda sinusa osteotomom. Beck, P. M, Apr. 1970. Endosseous implants.

Beck, P. M, Apr. 1970. Endosseous implants.

Bergh van den JP, ten Bruggenkate CM, Disch FJ, Tuinzing DB. Clin Oral Implants Res 2000 Anatomical aspects of sinus floor elevations.

Bert, M. Quest. Odonto_Stomat, 1985. Physiologie osseuse et implants dentaries.

Biological complications with dental implants; Their prevention, diagnosis and treatment. Oral implants. 2000.

Biomechanical aspects of prosthetic implant-borne reconstructions. Periodontol 2000, 1998.

Block MS, Kent JN. J. Maxilofac Surg 1990. Factors associated with soft and hard-tissue compromise of endosseud implants.

Bonfante S, Bosco AF, Luize DS, de Almeida JM, Cestari TM. Int. J. Maxillofacial Implants, 2008. Influenze of nicotine on healing process of autogenous bone block grafts in the mandibule: histomophometic study in rats. Maxillofacial D, J Clin Oral Periodontol, 2004. Hard-tissue alterations following immediate implant placement in extraction sites

Bottocelli D, Beglundh T, Lindhe J. Hard-tissue alterations flowing immediate implant placement in extraction sites. J. Clin Periodontol, 2004.

Boyne P. James, RA J. Oral Surg. 1990. Grafting of the maxillary sinus with autogenous marrow and bone

Bragger U, et al. Clin Oral Implants Res 1997 Associations between clinical parameters assessed around implants and teeth.

Brenemark, P. I. Adell, R. Albrektsson, T. Lekholm, U. Lundkvist, S. Rockler, B. Biomaterials, 1983. Osseointegrated titanium fixtures in the treatment of edentulousness

Brenemark, P. I. hesis. Brenemark, P. I. uli, 1971. Jaw reconstruction and intraosseous anchorage of dental prosthesis. Brenemark, P. I. hesis.

Brenemark, P. I. scand. J Plast. Reconstr. Surg. 1977. Osseointegrated implants in the treatment of the endontulous jaw.

Brenemark, P. I, Albreksston, T. Scand. J Plast. Reconstr. Surg. 1982. Titanium implants permanently penetrating human skin.

Brenemark, P. I, B reinen, U, AdellR, Hansson, B. O. Linnd srom, J. Olsson, A. Scand Journal Plast. Reconstr. Surg. 1969. Intraosseousnachorage of dental prostheses; experimental studies.

Brenemark, P. I, Breine, U, Scand. J. Plast. Reconstr. Surg. 1980. Reconstruction of alveolar jaw–bone. An experimental and clinical study immediate and preformed autologous bone graft in combination with osseointegrated implants.

Brgundh, T. Lindhe, J. 1996. Supportive therapy in implant dentistry. Dimensions of the peri-implant mucosa. Biological width revisited. Journal of Clinical Periodontology.

Brinkmann, E. 1976. Indicationes for endoseous implantation.

Bruno J. 1969, 1970, 1971. Trib. Odontol. Intraosseous stabilization. Result of 17 years of its application. Intraosseous stabilization. V Biological and methodological bases

Brurkhardt R, Joss A, Lang NP. Soft tissue coverage around endosseus implants; a prospective cohort study Clin Oral Implants Res 2008.

By Care, J. Drago, D. D. S, M. S. 2007. Chicago. 2000. Implant Restorations: A Step-By-Step-Guide for Dentists.

By Step Guide For Dentists. by Carl J. Drago, DDS, MS. Chicago, USA 1997 Implant Restorations Asteo.

C. Landeau, J. F. Lauret, M. Le Gall. Prosthetic synergy September 2000. Occlusal analysis of lateral movements - Comparison of clinical situations and those on articulators. Video. Analysis of lateral movements in clinical situations and those on articulators. Oral surgeons. Dentists

Cardopoli G. J. Clin Periodontol, 2003. Dynamics of bone tissue formation in tooth extraction sites. An experimental study in dogs

Catalano, L. Odontostomatol. 1967. Preliminary study on a complete itraosseous implant.

Chiapasco M, Casentini P, Zaniboni M. Bone augmentation procedures in implant dentistry. I Int J Oral Maxilo-fac Implants, 2009.

Chipasco M, Zaniboni M, Boisco M. Augmentation procedures for the rehabilitation of deficient edontulous ridges with oral implants. Clin Oral Implants Res 2006.

Clin Oral implants Res, 2008 Evans CD, Chen ST. Esthetic outcomes of immediate implant placements.

Clinical Oral Implants research, 2002. Probing around implants and teeth with healthy or inflamed peri-implant mucosa/gingiva. A histologic in cynomolgus monkeys.

Coachman C, Van Doren E, Gurel G, Calimata MA, Calgaro M, Souza Neto J. "Minimally invasive reconstruction in implant therapy: The prosthetic restoration". Quintenssence Dent Technol 2010.

Coachman C, Van Doren E, Gurel G, Calamita MA, Calgaro M, Souza Neto J. "Minimally invasive reconstruction in implant therapy: The prosthetic restoration." Quintessence Dent Technol, 2010.

Cochman C, Salama M, Garber D, CalimataM, Salama H, Gabral G. "Prosthetic gingival reconstruction in a fixed partial restoration. Part 3"

Cochman C, Salama M, Garber D, Calimata M, Salama H, Gabral G. "Prosthetic gingival reconstruction in a fixed partial restoration. Part 1: Introduction to artificial gingiva as an alternative therapy." Int J Periodontics Restorative Dent. 2009.

Cohen ES. "Atlas of cosmetic and reconstructive periodontal surgery." BC Decker, 2006.

Contempory Implant Dentisry – Carl E. Misch. MOSBY, St. Louis, Baltrimore, Boston, Chicago, London, Filadelphie, Sydney, Toronto. 1993.

Cullen, R. Dent. News, July, 1968. How do I begin endosseous implants?

Davidson's. Edited by C. R. W. Edwards, I. A. D. Bouchier, C. Haslett, E. R. Chilvers. 1995. Principles and Practice of MEDICINE.

De Santis E, Maxillofacial D, Pantani F, Periera FP, Beolochini M, Lang NP. "Bone regeneration at implants placed into extraction sockets of maxillary incisor." Clin Oral Implants Res, 2011.

Dejan Markovic, Faculty of Dentistry, University of Belgrade 2009. Dental Lexicon.

Dent. Surv. Friedman, S. 1970. 2 years clinical results with endosseous implants.

Deutsche Ausgabe von Adolf Kroncke Berlin, 1980. Mund-Krankheiten.

Deutsche Ausgabe von Heinz Spranger, Hanser I. D. Strahen, I. M. Waite. Munchen, Wien, 1980.

Deutsche Zahnarztl 1998. Diabetes mellitus-ein Risikfaktor fur enossale Implantate im zahnlosen Unterkkiefer.

Dr Jhon Mills, dr Mary T. Ho, dr Donald D. Trunkry, i 38 autora. Savremena administracija , Beograd URGENTNA MEDICINA Savremena dijagnostika i lečenje.

Dr Marfkus Schulte, Lucerne Switzerland. 2012. Immediate rehabilitation of a patient with dental phobia.

Dr Markus Schulte, Lucerne, Switzerland, EDI European Journal for dental Implantologie. 2012. Immediate rehabilitation of a patient with dental phobia

Dr. C.H. Haase, Berlin, 2008. i 2009. Godišnjak Estetska stomatologija.

E. Van Doren, Calip Crull, M. A. Calamita, M. Calopro. 2006. N. Y. USA. Minimally invasive Reconstruction in Implant Therapy: The Prosthetic Gingival Restaration. Crhristian coachman,

Eckert SE, choi YG, Sanchez AR, Koka S. Internationa J. Oral Maxillofac Implants 2005. Comparasion of dental implants systems: Quality of clinical evidence and prediction og 5-year survival.

Edited by Ralph V. McKinney, Jr, Jack E. Lemons for the American Academy of Implant Prosthodontics. Chicago, 1983. The Dental Implant-Clinical and Biological Response of Oral Tissues

Eik Scheignitz, Dr. med. Baial Al-Nawas, Prof. med. Quintessence Int. Berlin . 2014. Implantati reduciranog promera.

Ein Atlas fur die Praxis-Charles A. Babbush. Deutsche Bearbeitung: Diter Schlegel, Minchen. 1980. Implantation im Kieferbereich-Indikationen und Techniken.

Ein Symposium, Herausgegeben Von Prof. dr. dr. J. Franke, Minchen, 1980. Der heutige Stand der

Implantologi Hanser Carl Hanser Verlag Minchen Wien 1980. Herausgegeben Von Prof. Dr. Sr. J. Franke. Der heutige Stand der Implantologie-Ein Symposium-Hamburg 8. 12. 1979.

Ella B, Sedaret C, Noble Rda C. Vascular connections of the lateral wall of the sinus: surgical effect in sinus augmentation. Int J. Maxillo-fac implants, 2008.

Ellan N, Erlich B, Jalbout ZN, et al. Dent Clin North Am. 2003. Advanced concepts in implant dentistry. Creating the "aesthetic site foundation"..

Eran fermon, Ramt Hasharon. EDI Journal Evropean Juournal for Dental Implantologists. 2912. Bilatreal sinus floor elevation and simultaneous implantation. Clinical experience with a new implant in a minimally invasive procedure.

Eran Fermon. DMD, Ramat Hasharon. European Journal for Dental Implantologie, 2012. Bilateral sinus floor elevation and simultaneous implantation.

Esposit M, Hirch JM, Lekholm U. Tomsen P. Biolological factors contributing to failures of ossteointegrated oral implants. Eut. Patients at risk in implant dentistry

Esthetic Implant Dentistry-Soft and Hard TRissue Management-Patrick Placci, DDSIngvar Ericsson. Predgovor Per-Ingvar Brenemark.

Evans CD, ChenSt. Esthetic outcomes of immediate implant placements Clin Oral Implants Res 2008.

Evian Cl, CronH, Rosenberg ES Compend Contin Educ Dent. 1996. Retained interdental papilla procedure for maintaining anterior esthetics.

F. Bianchi, G. Prerrotti, L. francetti, T. Testori. Italian Oral Surgeri. Rivista di chirurgia orale parodontale implant-gare riabilitazione protesica. Masson-Milano 2002. L'esthetica in implantologia. Un caso clinico di agnesia dentale.

F. Sigmund, J. Neugebauer, F. Kistler, S. KistlerG. Bauer Quintessence Int. Bedrlin 2014.Terapijski plan, hirurški i protetski postupak i kasnije praćenje ultrakratkih implantata

Fahmer V, Saller I, Muller P, Hammerle CH. "Kriterlen fur die Auswahl reconstructiver Materiallen." Quintessence, 2011.

Ferrieri Gb, Castiglioni S, Carmagnola D, Cargnel M, Strohmenger L, Abati S. J. Oral Maxillofac Surg. 2007. Oral surgery in patients on anticoagulant treatment without therapy interruption

G. Landeau, J. F. Lauret, M. Le Gall, chirurgiens-dentistes. Synergie prothetique feb. 2001. L'analyse occlusale des mouvements lateraux. Programmation de l'articulateur Revese. Drugi deo.

Galip Gruel, Cristian Coachman. Quntessence International 2013. Postupanje s implantgatima pogrešnog smjera uzdžne osi.

Garber DA, Salama MA and Salama H. "Immediate total tooth replacement." Compend Educ Dent, 2001.

Garber DA, Salama MA and Salama H. Compend Contin Educ Dent 2001 Immediate total tooth replacement.

Gastaldo, JF. Cury, RP, Sendyk, WR. J. Periodontol 2004. Effect of the vertical and horisontal distances between adjacent implants and between a tooth and an implant on the icidence og interprximal papilla.

Gerentostomatlogija. Prvo izdanje. Urednici Dragoslav Đukanović i Vera Todorović. Autori: Hristo Anđelski, Stevan Avramov, Mihajlo Gajić, Dragoslav Đukanovič, Ankica Jakovljević, Milan Jakšić, Jovo Kolar, Zoran Lazić, Mirjana Mandić –Kolar, Jasmina Milić, Dušica Popović, Milica Popović, Vera Todorović, Asen Žolev. Pančevo 2012.

Gerseme L, Baker K. Oral Maxillfac Surgery. 1992. Use corticosteroids in oral surgery.

Giovani U, Gormelini R, Galvo JL, Tonell P, Barone A. "Bone remodeling araund Implants placed in frech extraction soocets." Int J. Periodontics Restorative Dent, 2010.

Gisbert Krekeler, Prof. dr Christian Foitzik, Quintessence international. 2006Najgori slučajevi-implantološki neuspjesi.

Gomesz- Roman G. Flap methods and implant positioning. Surcical recomandations for the single tooth gap. Z. zahanarzti Impl. 2003.

Gridler NM. J Oral Rehabilitation, 1994. Fatalsequel to dental implant surgery.

Grundlagen der neuzeitlichen Parodontalchirurgie. New.York, Tokio, Berlin 1977.

Hammerle CH, Saller I, Thoma A, Halg G, Suter A, Ramel C. "Essential aspects for clinical practice". Chikago, Quentssence, 2008.

Hartman GA, Cochran DL. J. Periodontol, 2003. Int J Periodontics Dent, 2009 Initial implant position determines the magnitude of crestal bone remodeling.

Hildebrand, Dr Susanne Nahles and MDT Juergen Mehrhof, Berlin, Germany, European Journal for Dental Imnplantologie, 2012.

Huynh/Ba-G, et al. Clin Oral Periodontol 2010. Analiyis of the socket bone wall dimensions in the upper maxilla in relation to immediate implant placement

I. D. Strahan, I. M. Waite, Paris, 1978. Farbatlas der Parodontopathien Farbatlas Parodontopathien

Ilic Aleksandar, Blagotic Milena, MalobabicSl obodan, Radonjic Vidosava, Prostran Milan i Toševski Jovo. Savremena administracija Beograd 1990. Anatomija centralnog nervnog sistema.

Immediate placement and provisionlization of maxillary anterior single implants: 1-year prospective study. Kan JY, et al. Int. J Oral Maxillofac Implant, 2003.

Implant displacment into the mandibule: an unusual complication during implant surgery. Implant dent, 2011.

Implant surgery complications: etiology and treatment. Implnt Dent. 2008.

Implants 3.3 diameter for therehibilitation of edentulous posterior regions: a retrospective clinical study with up to 11 years of follow-up. Clin Implant Dent Realt. 2011.

Inga Johanning, ZA, Tim Joda, Guido Heydecke. Zahanmedizinische Klinik Universitet Bern, SchweizQuintessenze International, Berlin 2012. Koncept rehabilitacije bezubosti u donjoj vilici. Trajnost, pacijentovo zadovoljstvo i socioekonomska analiza.

Int J. Oral Maxillofac implants 2010. On implants surfaces : a review of current knowledge and options.

Int Jou. Periodontics Dent. 1989. Immediate implant placement into extraction sites : surgical and restorative advantages.

Int. Jou. Bahat O, fontanessi RV. Periodontics Restorative Dent. 2001.Complications of grafting in the atrophic edontulous ot partially edontulous jaw.

Int. Maxillofac Impolants. 2005. Dental implant failure rates and associated risk factors.

J. Dent Educ, 2003. Davis Je. "Understanding peri-implant endosseous healing."

J. Periodontal, 2013. Academy report. Peri-implantitis mucosis and peri-implantitis: a current understanding of their diagnosis and clinical implications.

Jemt T, Lekholm U. Measurements of buccal tissue volumes at angle implant restorations after local bone grafting in maxillas: a 3 year clinical prospective study case series. Clin Implant Sent Relat Res 2003.

Jochen Tunkel. Quintessenza Internationa, Belin 2011. Vestibuloplastika prema Kazanijanun u eri implantologije.

John L . Wilson, Joseph J. McDonald. Los Altos, California. 1963. Handbook of Surgery.

Journal of Clinical Periodontology. 2008. Peri-implant diseases: diagnosis and risk indicators. Proceedings from the 6th European Workshop on Periodontology.

Journal Oral Implant Transplant-Cherche, R. Surg. 1966. The Philosophies which govened the origin, devlopment and present-day use of endosseous dental implants .

Jovanovic SA, Hunt DR, Bernard GW, Spiecermann H, Wozney UM. Bone reconstruction following implantation of rh MP 2 guided bone regeneration in canine alveolar ridge defects. Clin Oral Implants Res 2007.

Jung RE, Sienenthaler DW, Hammarle CH. J. Periodontics Restorative Dent. 2004. Postextraction tissue managament: a soft tissue punch technique.

Kammerer PW, Lehmman KM. Zahanarztl Implant 2013. Titan-Zirkon-Legirungen bei durchmesserreduzierten Implantaten.

Kan J, Rungcharassaeng K. Pract Periodontics Aestheet 2000. Immediate placement and provisionalization of maxillary anterior single implantants : A surgical and prostodontic rationale.

Kern M. Besser. Implantol 2008. Besser eines als keines? Bolje jedan implantata nego ni jedan?

Khoury F. Augmentative Fervaheren in der Implantologie. Berlin, Quintessenz, 2009.

Khouty F. The bony lid approach in periimplant and implant surgery: a prospective study 2013.

Kim Y, Oh TJ, Misch CE, Wang HL. Clin Oral Implants. 2005. Occlusal considerations in implant therapy: Clinical guidelines with biomechanical rationale

Klein M, Scheingnitz E, Al-Nawas. J Oral Maxillofac 2013. Systematic review on success of narrow diameter dental.

Klein MO, Schiegnitz E, Al Nawas B. Systematic review on success of narrow-diameter dental implants. Int J Oral Maxillofac Implants 2014.

Klein MO. Schiegntz E, Al NawasB. Syistematic rewiev on success of narrow–diameter denatal implants InzJ Oral Maxillofac Implants, 2014.

Klinicka Parodontologija. Stomatološki fakultet Univerzitet u Beogardu. Urednik Božo Dimitrijevic. Autori: Vojislav Lekovic, Obrad Zelic, Ljiljana Jankovic, Irena Ursu Magda, Saša Cakic, Dragoslav Đukanovic, Saša Jankovic, Zoran Aleksic. Zavod za udžbenike. Beograd, 2011.

Kohal RJ, Mellas P, Hurceler MB, Trejo PM, Morrision E, Caffese RG. J. Periodontol, 1998. The effects of guided bone regeneration and grafting on implants placed onto immediate extraction sockets.

Kompakt. Decembar 2002. Dentale Implantologie-Parodontologie.

Kotshovills S, Karoussis IK, Trianti M, Formuoussis I. "Therapy of peri-implantitis: a systematic review" J. Clin Periodontola, 2008.

Lames PelayoJ, Penarrocha Diego M, Marti Bowen E, Penarrocha Diego. Med oral Patol Oral Cir Bucal, 2008. Intraoperative complications during oral implantology.

Lang B, Pohl Y, Filippi A. Transplantation von Zahnen. Schweiz Monatsschr Zahanmed 2003.

Laur Wanner Nemačka, Gwendolin Manegold-Bauer Basel Švajcarska, Hans Ulrich Bauer, Nemačka, QI 2014. Neobične intraoperativne i postoperativne komplikacije kod imnplantacije endoosealnog iumplntata.

Lavori Scientifici. E. G. Bratolucci, C. Mangano, R. F. Grassi. Masson 1, 2001. Italian Oral Surgery. Chirurgia orale pardontale implantare-Riabilitazione protesica. La terapia chirurgica paradontale.

Lazzara, R. J. Rev. Int. Parodont. Dent. Rst, 1989. Immediate implant placement into extraction sites.: surgical and restorative advantages.

Lenkevikulus T, Aspew P. Quintessenze Int. Berlin 2011. Inffluenze of Abatment material on Stability of Periimplant Tissues.

Leonard I. Linkow, New York, 1983. Dental implants-Can Make your liffe wonderful again.

Lindhe J, Lijenberg B, Adielson B, Borjesson I. J. Clin Pereiodontol, 1983Use of metronidazole as a probe in the study of human periodontal disease.

Lindhe J, Meyle J. Journal of Clinical Periodontology. 2008. Periimplant diseases.

Linkow, L. Dent. Cadmos, Summer, 1966. 8 years of intraosseous implantations.

Linkow, L. Dent. Concepts. Summer, 1966. Maxillary endosseous implants.

Linkow, L. Implantologist, 1976. Development of five piece ramus frame implant.

Linkow, L. Oral Implant Transpant Surg. 1976. Clinical evaluation of the various designed endosseous implants.

Linkow, L. Promot. Dent. 1969. Assessment of the metal wire endosseous implant.

Ludlow JB, Ivanovic M. "Comparative dosimetry of dental CBCT devices and 64-slice CT for oral and maxillofacial radiology." Oral Surg. Oral Med Oral Pathol, Oral Radiol Endod 2008.

Luigi Checci, Marco Montevecchi, Vittorio Chechi, Giulio Bonetti. Quintesenze Inernational, Berlin 2010 Modificirana tewhnika ocuvanja papile.

M. Bassetti, R. Bassetti, R. R. Kaufmann, G. E Salvi, A. Sculena. Augmentacia mekog tkiva radi povećanja širine prirasle keratinizovane sluzokože oko implantata. Quintenssence, 2015.

M. Juriciuc i autori. 2008. Orealna implantologija-Stomatološki fakultet Univezitet u Beogradu

M. Sachs, M. Pohlges, D. Suwwelacg, Quintessence International, 2014. Rehabilitacija pojedinačnog zuba pomoću augmentacije kosti i krunice na implantatu uz posebno uvažaavanje estetskih aspekata.

Malmstrom HS, Fritz ME, Timmis DP, Van Dyke T. J. Periodontal 1990. Osseo-integrated implant treatment of a patient with rapidly progressive periodontitis. : a case report.

Malo P. de Argujo Nobre M. Implants(3.3 mm diameter) for the rehabilitation of endotulous posterior regions: a retrospective clinical study with up to 11 years of follow – up. Clin Implant Dent Relat Res, 2011.

Mark Bert, Patrick Missika. Edizione italiana- Giorgio Vogel, Matteo Chiapasco. MASSON, Milano-

Parigi-Barcelona 1997. Implantologia Chirurgica e Protesica

Mateo Chiapasco, Claudio Gatti, Jan Gottlow, Anna Karin Lundgren, Paulo Malo, Neil Meredith, Giovanni Polizzi, Lars Sennerby. Cordinamento scientifico di Claudio Gatti. MASSON, Milano 2002. Osteointegratione a carico imediato-Fundamenti biologici e applicazioni cliniche.

Mc Guire MK& Schezer. J. Periodontol 2010. Xenogenic Collagen Matrix eith Coronally Advanced Flap compared for the Treatment of Conenective Tissue which Coronally Avanced Flap for the Treatment of Dehiscenze-Type Recession Defects.

Meriche -Stem R- "Prosthetic considerations" Clin. Oral Dent Ossoc J 2008.

Merichke-Stern R. Zarb GA. Overdentures: an alternative implant methodology for edentolous patients. IntJ. Prosthodont, 1993.

Meyers, S. Dist. Dent-Soc. Apr, 1969. Immediate fixation using endosseous implants.

Michael Norton. London, 1995. Dental Implants- A Guide for General Practitioner.

Misch CE. Int Jou. Oral Implantol 1987 Maxillary sinus augmentation for endosteal implants: Organized alternative treatment plans.

Missika, P, Abbou, M, Actualites Odonto- Stomat. 1985. Extraction et implantations immediates.

Mithridade Davarpanah, Henry Martinez, Myriam Kebir, Jean-Francois Tecucianu, Richard J. lazzara, Renato Celletti, Daniel Etienne, Curtis Jansen, Karl Donath. Zagreb, 2006. Prirucnik dentalne implantologije.

Mombelli A, Buser D, Lang NP. Colonization of osteointegated titanium implants in edontulous patients early results. Oral Microbiol Imunol 1988.

Mombelli A, Lang NP. The diagnozis and treatment of peri-implantitis. Periodontol 2000.

Mukogingival surgical procedures. Quintessence. 1999. Muller HP Eger T. "Gingival phenotypes in young male adults." J Clin Periodontol, 2007.

Murat Yildrim, Bastian Wessing. Quintessenze Internationa, Berlin 2010.Pojedinacni implantati u frontalnoj regiji gornje vilice. Koncept zta estetskiu uzspeh

N. Y. State. Feb, 1980. Endosseous implant. A vital adjunct to rehabilitation , a four. year approach study.

Niamtu J. Oral surg Oral Med Oral Patol 2001. Near-fatal airway obstruction after routine implant placement.

Nils Weywr, Emil Endress. Quintessence International, Berlin, 2914. Kratki implantati.

Noelken R, Kunkel M, Wagner W. "Immediate implant placement and provisionalization after long-axis root fracture and complete loss of the facial bony lamela." Int J Periodontics, Restorative Dent, 2011

Oral Maxillofac Implants, 1993 The association between the failure of dental implants and cigarette smoking. Int. Jou.

PacoWeiss, AndreasFilippi, J. ThomasLambrecht. Quentessenze International. Berlin 2001. Odontogene ciste.

Periimplantitis – A New Approach for Prevention and Treatment - author is Dr. Eduardo Anitua, MD. DDS, Ph.D. Vitoria – Spain 2014. Edition 1

Posselt U. Oxfort, Blackwell. 1968. Physiology of occlusion and rehabilitation.

Praxis 1975. Cherche. Twenty years of experience with implantation. Zahnaerztl.

Prof. Dr Mihailo –Miša Vucinic, Beograd, 1999. Integralni pristup vaskularnoj medicini

Prof. dr Roko Živkovic. Medicinska knjiga Beograd-Zagreb. 1988. Interna Medicina

Prof. dr Smilja Radlović-Pantelić - Stomatološka protetika nadoknade na implantatima, Jugoslovenska knjiga 1998

Prof. dr Vladimir Lapter, Prof. dr Juraj Hraste, Globus Zagreb, 1990. Stomatološki leksikon

Prof. dr Vujadin Mujovic, Elit Medica, Beograd, 2002. Fiziološke osnove bola- Integrativna fiziologija.

Prof. dr. Vujadin Mujovic Medicinska fiziologija. Compendium

Profesor Katja Nelson, Freiburg, Dr Deflef. A treatment approach for edontulous patients. The severely resorbed alveolar ridge

Quiintessence Interenational- clinically relevant, scientifically based. Quintessenz Verlags-GmbH, Berlin, 2000-2012.

Quirynen, M. Soete, M. van SteenbergheD. Clin. Oral. Implants Res. 2002. Infectious risks for oral implants.

Radiographic bone fill of peri-implantitis defects following nonsurgical therapy : Report of three cases. Clin Oral Implants Res 2001.

Raviv E, Turcotte A, Harel-Raviv M, Quintessence International, Berlin, 2014. Short dental implants in reduced alveolar bone height.

Rene B. A. Sanderink, Urlich Peter Saxer. Quintessenze International. Berlin 2010. Terapija peri-implantitisa djelovanjem na biofilm.

Renouard F, Nisand D. Oral implantsRes 2006. Impact of implant length and diameter on survival rates.

Renvert S, Roos-Jansaker AM, Claffey N. J. Clin 2001. How do implant surface characteristics influence peri-implant disease?

Richard W. Chaikin. Quentessence Biblioteke. Berlin, Chikago, Berlin, Tokio, Rio de Janeirio. 1977. Grundlagen der neuzeitliche Parodontalchirurgie.

Robert Gauthier. Sent-Etienne, 1987. Precis D'Implantologie Dentarie.

Robert Gauthier, Paris, 1987. Precis D'Implantologie Dentarle.

Rocket Atlas of Oral Diseases. Giorg Laskaris. Universiteti of London, Second Edition, 1998.

Romeo E, Ghistolfi M, Carmagnola D. Minerva Stomatology. 2004. Peri-immplant diseases.

Rompen E, Van Dooren E, Touati B. „ Soft tissdue stability at the facial aspect of gingival converning abutments in the esthetic zone" A pilot clinical study, 2007.

Rosenquist B, Grenthe, B, Int. J. Oral Maxillofac implants, 1996. Immediate placement of implants into extraction sockets:implant survival.

Ruten L, Ruten P. "The fabrication of the full ceramic abutments in: Crown-Bridge and Implants. The Art of Harmony". Teamwork Media, 2006.

Ruten L, Ruten P. "The ovate pontic technique. In: Crown-Bridge and Implants. The Art of Harmony." Fuchstal: Teamwork Media, 2006.

Rutten L, Rutten P. The ovate pontic technique . In: Crown-Bridge and Implants. The Art of Harmony Fuchstal. Teamwork Media 2009.

S. Sivolella, E. Bressan, E. Cnocco, M. Bernego, G. Antonio Favero, Quintessence International, Berlin, 2011. Augmentacija maksilarnog sinusa bovinom kosti te stimulantna insercija dentalnog implantata u uslovima ekstremne alveolarne atrofije.

Salama H, Salama Ma, Garber D, AdarP. Pract Periodontiсts Aesthet Dent 1998. The interproximal height of bone: a guidepost to predictable aesthetic strategies and soft tissue contours in anterior tooth replcament.

Salama M, Cochman C, Garber D, Calamita D, Salama H, Gabral G. "Prosthetic gingival reconstruction in the fixed partial restoration. Part 2: Dijagnosis and tretman planing." Int Priodontics Restorative Dent, 2009.

Sanz M, et al. J. Clin Periodontol 2009. Clinical evaluation of a new collagen matrix *Mucograft prototype (to enhance the width of keratinized tissue in patients with fixed oristhetic restorations: a randomized prospective clinical trial.

Sanz M, Etienne D. 1996Identification of risk patients in oral implantology. Paradonral Implantol Orale.

Satoru Matsuda, Kenichi Norizuki . Quntessenze Int. 2008. Estetski nadomestak levog sekutica (21) nošen implantatom.

Saviodelli C, Le Page F, Santini , cortecci. Maxillar Osteonecrosis associated with bisphosphanate treatment and dental treatment.

Schou S, Berglundh T, Lang NP. "Surgical treatment of periimplantitis" Int J Oral Maxilofac Implants, 2009.

Schrott AR, et al, Clin Oral Implants Res 2009. Five-year evuluation of the influence of keratinized mucosa on periimplant softtissue health and stability around implants supporting fullarch mandibubular fixed prostheses.

Schwerpunkte in der oralen Implantologie und Rekonstruktion. J. R. Strub-B. E. Gysi-P. Scharer. Berlin 1983.

Severe osteomyelitis folowing immediate placement of a dental implant. Int J Oral Maxillofac Implants, 2008.

Short implants in paritialy edontuloolous maxillae and mandibules: a 10 to 20 yeares retrospective evoluation. Int. J. Dent, 2012.

Simon M, Jovanovic SA, TrisiP, Scarano A, Piattelli. Int. Jou. Periodontics. Resorative Dent 1998. Verticale ridge augmentaion araund dental implants using a membrane technique and autogenous bone or allografts in humans.

Simon M, et al. Biocompatibility according to ISO. J. Periodontol, 2010.

Simplified Clinical Analysis for Predictable Treatment-Second Edition- Franck Renouard, DDS- Private Practice, Paris, France Bo Rangert, PhD MeechEng,

Chief Scientist, Nobel Biocare, Gothenburg, Sweden. Quintesesnce International, 2008. Paris, Berlin, Chicago, Tokyo, London, Milan, Barcelona, Istambul, Sao Paolo, Mumbai, Moscow, Prague, and Warsaw. Risk Factors in Implant Dentistry.

Smith Ra, Berger R, Dodson TB. Int. J Oral Maxillofac Implants 1992. Risk factors associated with dental implants in healthy and medically compromised patients..

Stantfor CM. "Surface modifications of dental implants" Astr DentJ 2008.

Stefano Sivolella, Eriberto Bressan, Elissa Gnocco, Mario Berenago, Gian antonio Favero. Quintessence Internationale, Berelin 2011. Augmentacija maksilarnog sinusa bovinom kosti te simultana insercija dentalnog implantata u uslovima opsežne alveolarne atrofije.

Steigemann M, Wnag HL. J. Periodontol, 2006. Esthetic buccal flap for corection of buccal fenestration defects during flapless immediate implant surgery.

Tarnow D, Magner AW, Fietcher P. The effect of the distance from the contact point to the crest of bone on the presence or absence of the interproximal dental papillae. J. Periodontal, 1992.

Tarnow D, Elian N, Fietcher P, Mangner AV. "The effect of the distance from the contact point to the crest of bone on the presence or absence of the interproximal dental papillae. J Periodontol , 1992.

Tarnow D, Elian N, Fletcher P. "Vertical distance from the crest of bone to the height of the interproximal papillae between adjacent implants", 2003.

Tarnow DP, Cho SC, Wallance SS. J. Periodontol. 2000. The effect of inter-distace on the height of inter-implant bone cres.

Tarnow DP, Manger AW, Flether P. J. Periodontol 1992. The effect of the distance from the contact point the crest of bone on the presence or asence of the interproximal dent papilla.

Tarnow DP, Wallace SS, Froum SJ, Rohrer Md, Cho SC. Int. J Periodontics Restorative Dent 2000. Histologic and clinical comparison of bilateral sinus floor elevation with and without barrier membrane placement in 12 patients: part 3 of an ongoing prospective study.

The radiographic role in endoseous implant interventions. Chron. Omaha Dist. Dent. June, 1966.

The rationale for soft-tissue grafting and vestibuloplasty in associaton with andosseous implants: a literatur e review. J Oral Implantology. 1994.

The rationale for soft-tissue grafting and vestibuloplasty in associaton with endosseous implants. Journal Implantology 1994.

Thomas J. Nowak, A. Gordon Handfort. British Columbia Institute ofTechnology. 1994. Essentialif of Pathophysiology.

Tomasi C, et al. Clin Oral Periodontol Res 2010. Bone dimensional variations at implants placed in fresh extraction sockets: a multilevel multivariant analysis.

Tortamano P, Camargo Lo, Bello-Siva MS, kanashiro LH. Int. Journal Oral Maxillofac Implants 2010. Immediate implant placement and restoration in the esthetic zone: a prospective study with 18 months of follow up.

Ueli Grunder. Zollikon Schweiz. Quesstenze Int. Berlin 2012. Odrstranjivanje implantata.

Ugradnja jednog implantata u donjoj bezuboj vilici u centralnoj regiji sa retencionom kopcom. Mat6tias Kern. Klinik fur zahanartztliche Prothetic. Universitet zu Kiel. Quintesence International, Berlin 2012.

Uvod u naucnu studiju o smijehu ljudskom fenomenu - Francuski autori: dr Beržge. J. Berlioz, Mme Dieterlen, Mme Gratiot-Alphandry, dr Logre, A. Monnier, J. Plaquevent, M. Schweich, A. Sularac, E. Souriau, D. Victoroff, A. Villiers. Jugoslovenski autori: Boqdan Popovic, Marko Ristic, asko Popa, Bora Cosic, Vlatko Pavletic. Zagreb, 1961. Smijeh.

Van den Bergh JP, Disch Fj. Tuizing DB. Anatomical Aspectus of sinus floor elevations. Clin Oral Implant Res 2000.

Van der Weiden F, Dell'Acqua F, Solt DE. J. Clin Periodontol, 2009. Alveolar bone dimensional changes of post-extraction sockets in humans : a systematic review.

Van Steenberghe D, et al. Cli J Oral Implants Res 2000. The clinical use of deproteinized bovine bone mineral on bone regeneration in conjunction with immediate implant installation.

Vehemente VA, Chuang SK, Daher S, Muftu A, Dodson TB. J Oral Implantol 2002. Risk factors affecting dental implant survival.

V McKinney, David. E Steflik, David L. Koth. The Journal of Oral implantology. Massachusetts, 1984. Ultrastructural surface topography of the single crystal sapphire endosseous dental implant. Ralph.

Vujadin M. Mujovic. Belgrade. 2000. Integrative cardiovascular physiology.

Vujadin Mujović, Beograd, Fond solidarnosti 2012. Textbook – Medicinska fiziologija.

Warrer, K. Gotfredsen. K. Hjorting- Hansen, E, Karrring, T. Int. J. Oral Maxillo- Fac. Impl. Guided tissue regeneration ensures osseointegration of dental implants in humans.

Wide-diameter implants:surgical, loading, and prosthetic considerations. Misch CE. Dent Today, 2005.

Willian R. Tyldsley. Minchen, Wien, 1987. Mundkrankeiten. Deutsche Ausgabe fon Adolf Kroncke.

Wilson TG Jr. J Periodental 2009. The positive relationship between excess cement and peri-implant disease: a prospective clinical endoscopyc study.

Wilson TG, et al. Clin Oral implants, 1998. Implants placed in immediate extraction sites: report of histologic and histometric analyses og human biopsies

Wilson TG. Jr. The positive relationship between excess cement and periimplant disease: prospective clinical endoscopic study. J Periodontol 2009.

Wolfart S. Implantat prothetik-eine patiente norientirtes Koncept. 1. Auflage, Berlin, Quintessence, 2014.

Zitzmann, NU. Berglundh, T. Journal of Clinical Periodontology. 2008. Definition and prevalence of periimplant diseases.

ORAL IMPLANTOLOGY - PRINCIPLES AND PRACTICE

Author
Dr Blažo Zlopaša

Reviewers:
Prof. Dr Radmilo Rončević
Prof. Dr Zoran Aleksić
Prof. Dr Obrad Zelić
Academician of Medical Sciences Prof. Dr Vladimir Jokanović
Prof. Dr Smiljana Matić
Prof. Dr Zoran Lazić

Serbian language editor:
Stanka I. Marković

Expert editors:
Prof. Dr Ljubmir Todorović
Prof. Dr Smiljana Matić

Preparation for printing:
Zorica Tonjanski
Časlav Bjelica

www.ingramcontent.com/pod-product-compliance
Lightning Source LLC
LaVergne TN
LVHW071243210926
848486LV00007B/336